EARLY'S PHYSICAL DYSFUNCTION PRACTICE SKILLS

for the

OCCUPATIONAL THERAPY ASSISTANT

I would like to dedicate this book to my dear friend and mentor, Jane Clifford O'Brien, PhD, MS EdL, OTR/L, FAOTA. She believed in me enough to give me my first job in academia. She mentors me and inspires me to be the best occupational therapy educator I can be. She also gave me my first chapter to write. Without her guidance and direction, this book would not have been possible.

Fourth Edition

EARLY'S PHYSICAL DYSFUNCTION PRACTICE SKILLS

for the

OCCUPATIONAL THERAPY ASSISTANT

Mary Elizabeth Patnaude, DHSc, OTR/L
Associate Clinical Professor
Director of Admissions
Baylor University
Waco, Texas

ELSEVIER

Elsevier
3251 Riverport Lane
St. Louis, Missouri 63043

EARLY'S PHYSICAL DYSFUNCTION PRACTICE SKILLS FOR
THE OCCUPATIONAL THERAPY ASSISTANT   ISBN: 978-0-323-53084-2

Notice

Practitioners and researchers must always rely on their own experience and knowledge in evaluating and using any information, methods, compounds or experiments described herein. Because of rapid advances in the medical sciences, in particular, independent verification of diagnoses and drug dosages should be made. To the fullest extent of the law, no responsibility is assumed by Elsevier, authors, editors or contributors for any injury and/or damage to persons or property as a matter of products liability, negligence or otherwise, or from any use or operation of any methods, products, instructions, or ideas contained in the material herein.

Previous editions copyrighted 2013, 2006, and 1998.
Library of Congress Control Number: 2020945513

Senior Content Strategist: Lauren Willis
Senior Content Development Manager: Luke Held
Senior Content Development Specialist: Maria Broeker
Publishing Services Manager: Shereen Jameel
Senior Project Manager: Karthikeyan Murthy
Design Direction: Patrick Ferguson

Printed in India

Last digit is the print number: 9 8 7 6 5 4 3 2

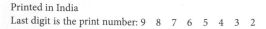

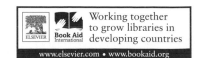

Working together
to grow libraries in
developing countries

www.elsevier.com • www.bookaid.org

CONTRIBUTORS

Denis Anson, BS, MS, OTR/L
Director of Research and Development
Assistive Technology Research Institute
Misericordia University
Dallas, Pennsylvania

Jessica Balland, MS, OTR/L
Occupational Therapy
University of New England
Portland, Maine

Caroline Beals, MS, OTR/L
Assistant Professor
Occupational Therapy
University of New England
Portland, Maine

Nichole Bell, MS, OTR/L
Occupational Therapy
University of New England
Portland, Maine

Kyle Borges, MS, OTR/L
Student Occupational Therapist
Occupational Therapy
University of New England
Seabrook, New Hampshire

Kelcey Briggs, MS, OTR/L
Occupational Therapist
North Country Kids Inc.
Plattsburgh, New York

Ann Burkhardt, BA, MA, OTD
Consultant
Higher Education/Clinical Program
    Development
Independent Consultant
Bristol, Rhode Island

Nancy Carson, PhD, OTR/L
Division of Occupational Therapy
Medical University of South Carolina
Charleston, South Carolina

Hannah Colias, MS, OTR/L
Occupational Therapy
University of New England
Portland, Maine

E. Joy Crawford, OTD, MS, OTR/L
OTA Program Coordinator
Health Sciences
Trident Technical College
Charleston, South Carolina
Contributing Faculty PPOTD Program

Health Sciences
University of Saint Augustine
Saint Augustine, Florida
Adjunct Assistant Professor
Health Professions
Medical University of South Carolina
Charleston, South Carolina

Peter Dasilva, MS, OTR/L
Occupational Therapist, OTR/L
Department of Occupational Therapy
University of New England
Portland, Maine

Christopher Delenick, OTR/L
Clinical Instructor
Health, Wellness, and Occupational
    Studies
University of New England
Biddeford, Maine

Kelly Dolyak, MS, OTR/L
Occupational Therapist
Early Childhood
South Bay Community Services
Lawrence, Massachusetts

Amanda K. Giles, OTD, OTR/L
Assistant Professor
Department of Health Professions
Medical University of South Carolina
Charleston, South Carolina

Anne Graikoski, MS, OTR/L
Clinician
Occupational Therapy
University of New England
Portland, Maine

**Deborah Greenstein Simmons, MS,
OTR/L, Advanced Practice Certificate in
Upper Quarter and Upper Extremity
Rehabilitation**
Clinical Specialist
Occupational Therapy
Spaulding Rehabilitation Cape Cod
East Sandwich, Massachusetts

Brina A. Kelly, MS, OTRL
Occupational Therapy
University of New England
Portland, Maine

Katlyn Kingsbury, MS, OTR/L
Occupational Therapist
Senior Therapy Services

Center for Physical Therapy and Exercise
Nashua, New Hampshire

Regina M. Lehman, MS
Associate Professor
Health Sciences
LaGuardia Community College
Long Island City, New York

Josh McAuliffe, MSOT, OTR/L
The Hand Center
Therapy
Glastonbury, Connecticut

Erin McGeggen, MS, OTR/L
Alumni
Occupational Therapy
University of New England
Portland, Maine

Shelby E. Hutchinson, MS, OTR/L
Occupational Therapist
Rehabilitation Services
Southern Maine Health Care
Sanford, Maine

Michele D. Mills, MA, OTR/L
Associate Professor
Occupational Therapy Assistant
    Program
LaGuardia Community College
Long Island City, New York

**Jane Clifford O'Brien, PhD, MS EdL,
OTR/L, FAOTA**
Professor
Occupational Therapy
University of New England
Portland, Maine

Mary Elizabeth Patnaude, DHSc, OTR/L
Associate Clinical Professor
Director of Admissions
Baylor University
Waco, Texas

Gina Regiacorte-Mosher, OTR/L
Outpatient Therapies Director
Rehabilitation
Southern Maine Health Care
Sanford, Maine

Regula H. Robnett, PhD, OTR/L
Professor
Department of Occupational Therapy
Associate Director

Center for Excellence in Aging and Health
University of New England
Portland, Maine

Megan Samuelson, MSOT, OTR/L
Occupational Therapist
Rehabilitation
Paxxon Healthcare Services
Chicago, Illinois

Rachael Schaier, MS, OTR/L
Occupational Therapist
Physical Medicine and Rehabilitation
STAR Program
Richmond Veteran Affairs Medical Center
Richmond, Virginia

Mary Beth Selby, MS, OTR/L, CPhT
Occupational Therapist (affiliate)
Occupational Therapy
University of New England
Portland, Maine

Dana Shah, BS, COTA/L
Inpatient Rehabilitation
Scripps Health
San Diego, California

Lori M. Shiffman, BS, MS
Owner
Private Occupational Therapy Practice
Life Balance Rehabilitation
Midlothian, Virginia

Jean W. Solomon, MHS
Occupational Therapist
Consultant
Moncks Corner, South Carolina

Erin Kelly Speeches, OTR/L
Occupational Therapist
Outpatient Neuro Rehab
Goodwill Industries of Northern New
    England
Gorham, Maine

Kristin Winston, PhD, OTR/L
Program Director and Associate
    Professor
Master of Science in Occupational
    Therapy
University of New England
Portland, Maine

Test Bank to Accompany Textbook
Mashelle K. Painter, MEd, COTA/L, CLA
OTA Program Director & Faculty
Occupational Therapy Assistant Program
Linn-Benton Community College
Healthcare Occupations Center
Lebanon, Oregon

The fourth edition of *Early's Physical Dysfunction Practice Skills for the Occupational Therapy Assistant* reorganizes and expands this text designed specifically for the occupational therapy assistant (OTA) student. The authors embrace the notion that every person has a natural and compelling desire to function and participate in activities and occupations that are meaningful, productive, and interesting. Although the practice of occupational therapy has acquired many techniques and interventions over its history, the core of practice is the restoration of ability to participate in personally selected and valued occupations. Consequently, the present text focuses quite clearly on this core of practice, as is reflected in the organization of chapters and information within chapters. Throughout, the reader will see a pervasive emphasis on occupation, participation in occupation, and engagement in functional activities.

The text presents concepts and information needed for entry-level practice in physical disabilities and has been revised to conform to the American Occupational Therapy Association's (AOTA) *Occupational Therapy Practice Framework: Domain and Process*, Third Edition (OTPF-3) and to provide major content required by the Accreditation Council for Occupational Therapy Education's (ACOTE) *Standards for an Accredited Educational Program for the Occupational Therapy Assistant*. The text may also serve as a resource for occupational therapy practitioners at all levels seeking to understand the role of the OTA in physical dysfunction practice. Strict attention has been given to AOTA guidelines for practice, supervision, and service competency.

This edition continues to provide depth of content beyond entry level so that it may continue to serve as a resource to the OTA in the clinic. This includes a new chapter on interventions for feeding and eating. We have also recognized that individual schools and practitioners in different areas of the country may need specialized material to meet the needs of their local practice environment and have tried to include this information without compromising the parameters of technical level practice or unduly enlarging the book.

Certain assumptions were made when designing this book for the technical level student. First, the student should have completed basic anatomy and physiology and foundation occupational therapy courses. Second, the student should have completed or should be taking as a corequisite a course in medical conditions or pathology. Third, the student must be willing to supplement this text with references, such as medical dictionaries and pathology texts, which will provide background information. We have made a sincere effort to write the book in such a way that it is understandable to an associate degree student, but it is not an elementary text.

The book is organized into seven sections. Part I covers theory and foundations for the role of the OTA in physical dysfunction practice. Part II explains the occupational therapy process and documentation of service. In response to user feedback, a new chapter on intervention for feeding and eating has been added. Part III provides extensive information on evaluation and includes some evaluations that are beyond entry level but in which the OTA might reasonably be expected to achieve competency, at least in certain practice environments. Part IV introduces basic principles of intervention. Performance in areas of occupation is the focus of Part V, which includes chapters on activities of daily living, mobility, work, technology, and leisure and social participation. Parts VI opens with a chapter on the special needs of the older adult, but it also includes chapters on the major intervention modalities and techniques used for physical dysfunction. Part VII provides treatment applications for a variety of clinical conditions seen in physical disabilities practice, including cerebrovascular accident, traumatic brain injury, degenerative diseases, amputations, lower and upper extremity orthopedics, spinal cord injury, burns, oncology, human immunodeficiency virus, cardiac dysfunction, and chronic obstructive pulmonary disease.

Special features include lists of key terms and objectives for each chapter, selected reading guide questions at the end of each chapter, text boxes highlighting special techniques, case studies and treatment plans, and a wealth of illustrations and photographs. A guide to selected acronyms has been included inside the front cover.

To make the best use of this text, we recommend that readers begin with the objectives, key terms, and reading guide questions for the targeted chapter. Then, making use of a medical dictionary as needed, the student should read the chapter or section completely, without taking notes and with an aim to understanding what is being read. During a separate session, the student should then do a second reading, make an outline or notes from the text, and attempt to answer the reading guide questions. This level of thoroughness and repetition is critical to mastery of the material.

Certain terms in this book have been used to describe both the occupational therapy service provider and the consumer. The consumer may be referred to as *patient, client, resident,* or *caregiver*, depending on the context of the intervention. The terms *practitioner* and *clinician* refer to providers of occupational therapy services at both levels of practice (i.e., both the occupational therapist and the OTA). The words *assistant, OTA,* and *occupational therapy assistant* are used to designate the technical-level practitioner. The terms *therapist, OT,* and *occupational therapist* indicate the professional-level practitioner. Occasionally the word *therapist* is used more generically to describe the provider of therapy but is intended to designate both levels of practitioners.

Mary Elizabeth Patnaude

ACKNOWLEDGMENTS

I would like to acknowledge my professional colleagues and students who were willing to provide the expertise and specialized information for the diverse chapters, whose professional expertise and support made this book possible. I would also like to thank my former coworkers at the University of New England who contributed: Dr. Kristin Winston, Dr. Jane Clifford O'Brien, Dr. Regula H. Robnett, Dr. Christopher Delenick, and Professor Caroline Beals. I am also thankful to Mary Beth Early and the contributors of the first three editions. I would like to make a special acknowledgment to Lorraine Williams Pedretti and her contributors whose text *Occupational Therapy: Practice Skills for Physical Dysfunction* inspired the first edition of this text.

All of the editors and staff at Elsevier have been supportive, professional, and endlessly helpful. I am grateful to Lauren Willis, Senior Content Strategist, and Maria Broeker, Senior Content Development Specialist, for their patient and reliable guidance and assistance. Thanks are also due to Karthikeyan Murthy, Senior Project Manager, for his careful scrutiny and stewardship of the production process.

I would like to acknowledge my family and friends who have supported me during this process. I would especially like to thank my husband, Jeffrey Patnaude, for his loving encouragement and support when I was in the midst of a tight deadline. I would like to thank my sons, Richard, Michael, Aaron, David, and Matthew, who light up my world. Finally, I would like to thank my cover models: Mary Lee Donovan, Ellen Mary Jahne, Luke Jahne, Aaron Patnaude, Mark Thallander, and Reverend Dennis Vincenzo. It is my hope that seeing you engaged in meaningful occupations in the midst of physical challenges will be an inspiration to both the OTAs reading this book and the clients whom they serve.

CONTENTS

Selected Abbreviations from Medicine and Rehabilitation[a]

%TBSA	percent of total body surface area (burns)	DIP	distal interphalangeal
A-P, AP	anteroposterior (also for AP, angina pectoris)	DME	durable medical equipment
		DOB	date of birth
AAROM	active assisted range of motion	DRG	diagnosis related group
ABA	American Burn Association	DTR	deep tendon reflex
ADL	activities of daily living	DVT	deep venous thrombosis
AI	aortic insufficiency	Dx	diagnosis
ALS	amyotrophic lateral sclerosis	ED	emergency department
AMA	American Medical Association; also, "against medical advice"	EEG	electroencephalogram, electroencephalograph
ARDS	acute respiratory distress syndrome	EKG	electrocardiogram
ARMD	age-related macular degeneration	EMG	electromyogram
AROM	active range of motion	EMR	electronic medical record
ASD	atrial septal defect	FAS	fetal alcohol syndrome
ASHD	arteriosclerotic heart disease	FCE	functional capacity evaluation
ASIA	American Spinal Injury Association	FBS	fasting blood sugar
AVN	avascular necrosis	FUO	fever of unknown origin
b.i.d.	twice a day (bis in die)	FWB	full weight bearing
BM	bowel movement	Fx	fracture
BMR	basal metabolic rate	GI	gastrointestinal
BP	blood pressure	GSW	gunshot wound
BSA	body surface area	GTT	glucose tolerance test
BUE	bilateral upper extremities	HCFA	Health Care Financing Administration
CAD	coronary artery disease	HOB	head of bed
CARF	Commission on Accreditation of Rehabilitation Facilities	HR	heart rate
CC	chief complaint	Hx	history
cc	cubic centimeter	IBD	inflammatory bowel disease
CHF	congestive heart failure	IBS	irritable bowel syndrome
CIMT	constraint induced movement therapy	ICD-10	*International Statistical Classification of Diseases and Related Health Problems*, 10th Edition
CLD	chronic liver disease	ICF	International Classification of Functioning, Disability and Health
CNS	central nervous system		
COPD	chronic obstructive pulmonary disease	IM	intramuscular; also, infectious mononucleosis
CORF	comprehensive outpatient rehabilitation facilities	IV	intravenous
COTA	certified occupational therapy assistant	JCAHO	Joint Commission on Accreditation of Healthcare Organizations
CPM	continuous passive motion		
CPR	cardiopulmonary resuscitation	kg	kilogram
CRPS	complex regional pain syndrome	LCVA	left cerebrovascular accident (stroke)
CPT	current procedural terminology	LOC	loss of consciousness
CSF	cerebrospinal fluid	LP	lumbar puncture
CT	computed tomography	MCP	metacarpophalangeal
CTD	cumulative trauma disorder	MD	muscular dystrophy
CTS	carpal tunnel syndrome	MDS	minimum data set (long-term care)
CVA	cerebrovascular accident (stroke)	MET	basal metabolic equivalent

[a]Some abbreviations from Brooks ML, Brooks DL: *Exploring Medical Language, A Student-Directed Approach*. 8th ed. St Louis, MO: Elsevier Mosby; 2012.

MI	myocardial infarction (heart attack)	PVC	premature ventricular complex
MP	*See* MCP	PWB	partial weight bearing
MRI	magnetic resonance imaging	q.	each, every
MRSA	methicillin-resistant *Staphylococcus aureus*	RA	rheumatoid arthritis
MS	multiple sclerosis	RAD	reactive airway disease
n	normal	RAI	resident assessment instrument (long-term care)
NDT	neurodevelopmental treatment	RAP	resident assessment protocol (long-term care)
NMES	neuromuscular electrical stimulation	RCVA	right cerebrovascular accident (stroke)
NPO, npo	nothing by mouth (*non per os*)	RHD	rheumatic heart disease
NWB	nonweight bearing	R/O	rule out (as in diagnosis)
OA	osteoarthritis	ROM	range of motion
OBS	organic brain syndrome	RPE	rate of perceived exertion
ORIF	open reduction and internal fixation (i.e., of bones)	RPP	rate pressure product
OSHA	Occupational Safety and Health Administration	RSD	reflex sympathetic dystrophy
		RSI	repetitive strain injury
OTAS	occupational therapy assistant student	RT	respiratory therapy
OTR	registered occupational therapist	RVU	relative value unit
OTS	occupational therapy student (professional level)	Rx	prescription
		SICU	surgical intensive care unit
P&A	percussion and auscultation	SCI	spinal cord injury
P-A, PA	posteroanterior; also for PA, physician assistant	SLE	systemic lupus erythematosus
		SNF	skilled nursing facility
p.c.	after meals (*post cibum*)	SOB	shortness of breath
p/o	postoperative	SROM	self range of motion
PCA	patient-controlled administration (e.g., of medication)	STSG	split-thickness (mesh of sheet) skin graft
PE	physical examination; also, pulmonary embolism	TAM	total active range of motion
		TBI	traumatic brain injury
PET	positron emission tomography	TENS	transcutaneous electrical nerve stimulation
PFM	peak flow meter		
PFT	pulmonary function test	THR	total hip replacement
PH	past history	tid	three times a day
PI	previous illness	TIA	transient ischemic attack
PIP	proximal interphalangeal	TKA	total knee arthroplasty
PLB	pursed lip breathing	TLC	tender loving care
PO, p.o.	by mouth (*per os*)	TPM	total passive range of motion
POV	power-operated vehicle	TTWB	toe-touch weight bearing
PNF	proprioceptive neuromuscular facilitation	Tx	treatment
		UE	upper extremity
PNS	peripheral nervous system	US	ultrasound
PRN, prn	as required, as needed (*pro re nata*)	VA	Veteran's Administration
PROM	passive range of motion	VF	field of vision
PT	physical therapy, physical therapist	WBAT	weight bearing as tolerated
PTA	physical therapy assistant; also, posttraumatic amnesia	WBC	white blood cell
		W/C	wheelchair
PTVS	posttraumatic vision syndrome	WHO	wrist-hand orthosis

PART I

Foundations

1

Occupational Therapy Treatment in Rehabilitation, Disability, and Participation

Mary Elizabeth Patnaude

OBJECTIVES

After reading this chapter, the student or the occupational therapy practitioner will be able to do the following:

- Review occupational therapy practice settings in the area of physical dysfunction.
- Discuss the implications of impairment in body functions and structures to occupational performance.
- Discuss the importance of skills, habits, routines, rituals, and roles in performance of occupation.
- Consider the effects of values, beliefs, and spirituality on occupational performance and on the rehabilitation process.

- Illustrate ways in which different kinds of environments and contexts affect occupational performance.
- Describe the model of human occupation and illustrate its application to a person with a physical disability.
- Describe the following approaches: biomechanical, sensorimotor/motor learning, and rehabilitation.
- Differentiate these approaches from each other and identify the practice situations in which each might be used.
- Describe the treatment continuum and its four stages: adjunctive methods, enabling activities, purposeful activity, and occupational performance and occupational roles.

KEY TERMS

Practice settings
Occupation
Areas of occupation
Performance skills
Performance patterns
Context
Activity demands
Body functions
Body structures
Client factors
Treatment continuum
Adjunctive methods
Enabling activities
Purposeful activities
Occupational roles

Models of practice
Systems model
Volition
Habituation
Performance capacity
Biomechanical approach
Kinetics
Statics
Sensorimotor approach
Neurophysiologic
Reflex
Motor learning
Rehabilitation approach
Evidence
Evidence-based practice

INTRODUCTION

Occupational therapists (OTs) and occupational therapy assistants (OTAs) provide distinct value to the individuals and populations they serve through the facilitation of engagement in occupational performance. To do this they must understand how activity demands and client performance skills enable or hinder participation in occupation (American Occupational Therapy Association, 2014b). OTs and OTAs provide services to clients with physical dysfunction in many practice settings, from the intensive care unit to the home.

Practice settings refer to the environment in which the occupational therapy occurs and includes the physical, social, and economic structures of the facility (Schultz-Krohn & Pendleton, 2018). These faculties represent the continuum of care. Regardless of setting, they should keep the focus on occupation.

Theories provide OTs and OTAs a process to understand the factors related to physical dysfunction, to apply them across practice settings with a variety of conditions (Schultz-Krohn & Pendleton, 2018). They use models of practice to apply the theory to practice. Several models of practice are commonly utilized in the area of physical dysfunction such as the model of human occupation (MOHO), biomechanical approach, sensorimotor and motor learning approach, and rehabilitation approach. Each will be discussed later in the chapter.

DISTINCT VALUE OF OCCUPATIONAL THERAPY IN REHABILITATION, DISABILITY, AND PARTICIPATION (RDP) PRACTICE

OTs and OTAs provide distinct value to the clients they serve through the facilitation of occupational performance (American Occupational Therapy Association, 2014b). This is done by utilizing the occupational therapy process, to serve clients as individuals, groups, or populations. The service provided includes analyzing the ways in which client factors interact with the environment to support healthy participation in valued occupations.

No other profession focuses on facilitating health through occupational engagement. **Occupation** includes functional life activities (e.g., grooming, working, caring for children) and is classified by performance in eight **areas of occupation** (Fig. 1.1). The main purpose of occupational therapy is to address performance issues that interfere with successful participation in occupation. For example, OTs and OTAs can help the person who has had a stroke and has weakness and impaired function of one side of the body to return to independence in dressing and self-care, working, and leisure activities.

Performance skills are the building blocks of performance in occupation. These skills (see Fig. 1.1; Table 1.1) apply flexibly and with many minute levels of precision to the entire range of human occupation, from caring for children to operating a forklift to designing webpages. The individual performing an occupation benefits from **performance patterns** such as habits, routines, rituals, and roles. Patterns help to make performance more automatic and thus less demanding of conscious attention. For example, the webpage designer who knows HTML commands thoroughly may flow through the workday without having to think much about which command applies to a given task. Conversely, the student who is learning HTML must struggle more to find the right command for the desired effect.

The performance skills and patterns of the person who is engaged in an occupation are affected by the demands of an activity and the context or environment in which it is performed. Consider, for example, opening an envelope with a letter opener in an office or negotiating a racetrack on a videogame screen. The first activity (opening a letter) may be done differently at work (a social, cultural, and physical context) than it would be at home (also a social, cultural, and physical context). The second activity (playing a videogame) is performed in a virtual context but may also have a social context if it is being played with someone else. A temporal context may also apply if racing against a clock.

The word **context** comes from the Latin *contexere*, meaning "to weave together" (Oxford University Press, 2013). A context is the background into which something is interwoven. This word is used in many ways. For example, a child who is having

TABLE 1.1 Performance Skill Categories and Examples

Category	Examples
Motor and praxis skills	Stabilizing, positioning, bending, reaching, transporting, lifting, gripping, pinching, manipulating
Sensory-perceptual skills	Positioning the body for action, locating keys by touch, timing one's movements
Emotional regulation skills	Responding to others, persisting in tasks, recovering from uncomfortable feelings without lashing out at others
Cognitive skills	Judging what is appropriate in each situation, sequencing tasks, prioritizing, organizing, multitasking

Areas of occupation	Client factors	Performance skills	Performance patterns	Context and environment	Activity demands
Activities of daily living (ADL)* Instrumental activities of daily living (IADL) Rest and sleep Education Work Play Leisure Social participation	Values, beliefs, and spirituality Body functions Body structures	Sensory perceptual skills Motor and praxis skills Emotional regulation skills Cognitive skills Communication and social skills	Habits Routines Roles Rituals	Cultural Personal Physical Social Temporal Virtual	Objects used and their properties Space demands Social demands Sequencing and timing Required actions Required body functions Required body structures
*Also referred to as *basic activities of daily living (BADL)* or *personal activities of daily living (PADL).*					

Fig. 1.1 Aspects of occupational therapy's domain. From American Occupational Therapy Association. *Occupational Therapy Practice Framework: Domain and Process.* 2nd ed. Bethesda, MD: AOTA; 2008:628.

difficulty understanding a new word encountered in reading is told to "look for context clues" such as illustrations or other words that may help the child identify the mystery word. In another common use of the word, after listening to a story or anecdote someone who knows more about the situation may remark that "you've taken that out of context," suggesting that the speaker has failed to provide enough background information to give a fair idea of what actually happened. In both examples, we can see that context gives meaning. In the case of occupation, the context supplies the background and often the meaning of the activity—how and why it is performed. Contexts provide cues about what kind of occupational performance is expected and effective; the six categories of context and environment are shown in Fig. 1.1.

Activities present their own demands (see Fig. 1.1) somewhat independent of context. **Activity demands** consider all the parameters of a specific activity. A letter opener and a videogame controller must be operated with the hands. Objects such as these and the space and timing of activities may present challenges to persons with physical disabilities affecting **body functions** and **body structures**. Someone with the use of only one hand will have problems stabilizing objects that are manipulated with the other hand (e.g., opening a can with a can opener or taking the lid off a plastic food container) or performing personal hygiene and getting dressed in a normal timeframe. Body functions and body structures are part of the client factor aspect of the occupational therapy domain (see Fig. 1.1).

Another element within client factors concerns the values, beliefs, and spiritual aspects of an individual. These elements can strongly influence the rehabilitation process. For example, a person who has a strong belief in family and obligation to family may be upset over a new disability status, fearing that she will be unable to provide for her family. This strong belief in the family may be helpful, however, if family members can be involved in caregiving and even in therapy sessions. Spiritual beliefs may also influence rehabilitation outcomes; if the person believes that the accident or injury is "God's will" or punishment for sin, then the motivation to improve in therapy may be affected.

PHYSICAL DYSFUNCTION AND ENGAGEMENT IN OCCUPATION

Physical dysfunction is associated with **client factors** (see Fig. 1.1; Table 1.2) such as changes in body functions and/or structures. Most changes that vary from the normal tend to disrupt performance of occupation. For example, a wrist fracture, with its necessary casting and period of immobilization, causes problems in dressing, bathing, handling money, driving a car, caring for a child, and so on. Some activities cannot be done independently while the cast is on (e.g., bathing an infant); others can be accomplished with modifications (e.g., donning a coat). Persons experiencing physical dysfunction cannot do the activities in the normal or customary way because of impairments in underlying abilities needed to

TABLE 1.2	**Client Factors and Examples**
Client Factor	**Examples**
Values, beliefs, and spirituality	Honesty
	Each person has responsibility to others
	Search for meaning and purpose beyond self
Body functions	Mental
	Sensory
	Neuromusculoskeletal and movement-related
	Cardiovascular, hematologic, immunologic, respiratory
	Voice and speech
	Digestive, metabolic, and endocrine
	Genitourinary and reproductive
	Skin and related structures
Body structures	Brain, central nervous system structures, spinal cord, peripheral and autonomic nervous systems
	Eye, ear
	Organs of voice and speech
	Heart, lungs, blood vessels, and immune system
	Digestive and metabolic organs
	Genitourinary and reproductive systems
	Bones, joints, muscles
	Skin and sensory receptors of skin and soft tissue

perform the activities. For example, a mother whose wrist is in a cast cannot bathe a squirming infant because she cannot hold the child with both hands; because of the cast, she lacks the necessary tactile sensitivity, strength, range of motion (ROM), and grasp.

TREATMENT CONTINUUM IN PHYSICAL DYSFUNCTION

A continuum is a "continuous series of elements passing into each other" (Oxford University Press, 2013). A **treatment continuum** begins with the onset of injury or disability and ends with the restoration of the patient to maximal independence. It is not a series of steps but a gradual movement from disease and disability toward health and ability, and a client entering it may do so at any point on the continuum (Schultz-Krohn & Pendleton, 2018). The elements of the continuum are usually provided in a variety of settings from inpatient to the community (Schultz-Krohn & Pendleton, 2018). For every patient the end point of the continuum is the maximal possible functional return. See Table 1.3 for examples of practice settings, condition applications, and occupations frequently seen in occupational therapy for physical dysfunction.

Fig. 1.2 is a model for the treatment continuum in physical disabilities practice. The stages in this treatment continuum overlap and can occur simultaneously. Although four stages are identified within it, the treatment continuum is not meant to illustrate a strict step-by-step progression. It takes the

TABLE 1.3   Practice Settings for Physical Dysfunction

Area of Practice	Setting	Conditions/Systems	Occupations	Frequency of Treatment
Acute care	Intensive care unit Step-down	Orthopedic Cardiac Neurologic (early management of CVA, TBI) Delirium Vision (basic)	ADL Rest and sleep	Daily
Rehabilitation	Acute rehabilitation Skilled nursing facility	Multitrauma Neurologic (continuing) Spinal cord injury Burns Amputations Joint arthroplasty (bariatrics or bilateral) Cardiac Congestive heart failure Chronic obstructive pulmonary disease Gastrointestinal (GI bleed) Diabetes mellitus Bowel obstruction Wounds	ADL IADL Leisure	Daily
Community based	Home health Outpatient	Dementia Chronic conditions Cognition—higher level Parkinson Multiple sclerosis Musculoskeletal (orthopedic) Outpatient neuro	ADL Medication management Community mobility Strength and conditioning ADL IADL	2–3 times per week

ADL, Activities of daily living; *CVA*, cardiovascular accident; *IADL*, instrumental activities of daily living; *TBI*, traumatic brain injury.

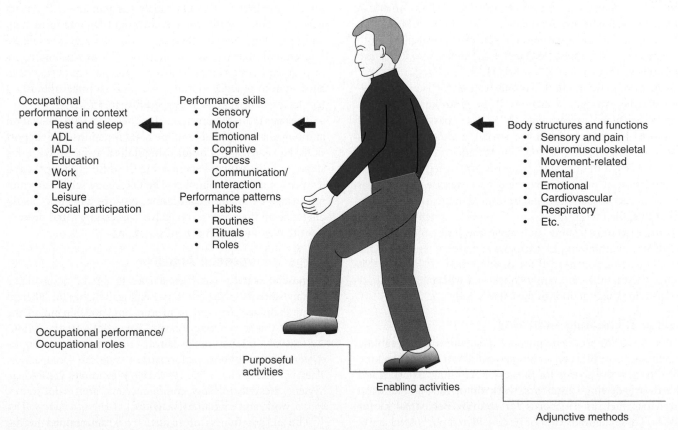

Fig. 1.2 Treatment continuum for physical disabilities practice. Courtesy Karin Boyce.

patient through a logical progression from dependence to skill development, then to purposeful activity, and finally to resumption of life roles (Reed, 1984). The treatment continuum identifies the concerns of occupational therapy practice within the context of performance of occupation and is compatible with the model of human occupation.

Stage 1: Adjunctive Methods

OTs and OTAs utilize **adjunctive methods** to prepare the patient to engage in activity (American Occupational Therapy Association, 1979). These methods may include exercise, facilitation and inhibition techniques, positioning, sensory stimulation, selected physical agent modalities, and devices such as braces and splints. Adjunctive methods are used by OTs, physical therapists, physiatrists, chiropractors, and massage therapists. OTs utilize these methods in preparation for purposeful activity, which ensures that there is no duplication of services, and provide evidenced-based, value-driven services to clients (Gillen et al., 2019).

Adjunctive methods are often used in but are not limited to the acute stages of illness or injury. During this stage the OT is likely to be most concerned with evaluating and remediating problems in body structures and functions. The OT plans the progression of treatment so that adjunctive modalities are used to prepare the patient for purposeful activity and are directed toward the achievement of maximal independence in the performance skills and areas of occupation. Some adjunctive methods, such as the application of physical agent modalities (PAMs), require the advanced education and training (and certification in some states) for both OTs and OTAs (American Occupational Therapy Association, 2004, 2008, 2014a, 2015). Others, such as the application of sensorimotor techniques to normalize muscle tone (see Chapter 20) and passive ROM, can be utilized by entry-level OTs and OTAs.

An adjunctive method that may be used for a client following a cerebrovascular accident (CVA) or stroke may be neurodevelopmental treatment (NDT) or passive range of motion (PROM). Following a stroke, a client may display hypotonia and limited strength on the affected side (hemiplegia), leaving him unable to move his arm or leg. Without the stimulation of normal movement and exercise, the muscles will contract, and motion will be limited in the future. To prevent this, the therapist may apply a quick stretch to the limb to increase muscle tone and move the limbs for the client (PROM), maintaining as normal a range as possible. PROM is a body function needed for development of skills. At this stage the therapist is mainly concerned with maintaining or remedying the functions of the client's body.

Stage 2: Enabling Activities

OTs and OTAs stimulate purposeful activities using enabling methods. Examples are sanding boards, skateboards, stacking blocks, practice boards for mastery of clothing fasteners and hardware, driving simulators, work simulators, and tabletop activities such as pegboards for training perceptual motor skills. These methods cannot be considered purposeful activity. Such activities are not likely to be as meaningful to the patient or to stimulate as much interest and motivation as purposeful activities. However, they may be necessary as a preparatory or ancillary part of the treatment program to train specific sensory, motor, perceptual, or cognitive functions necessary for performance skills and occupations.

Enabling activities require more patient involvement than do adjunctive methods. Whereas the therapy practitioner usually applies adjunctive methods to the patient who passively receives them, the patient carries out enabling activities. Enabling activities meet two of the three characteristics of purposeful activity: (1) the patient participates actively; and (2) the activity requires and elicits coordination of sensory, motor, psychosocial, and cognitive systems (Di Joseph, 1982).

However, enabling methods fail to meet the third characteristic of purposeful activity: the presence of an autonomous or inherent goal beyond the motor function required to perform the task (Ayres, 1958). In other words, getting exercise should not be the only reason for doing the activity. Although enabling methods might not be considered purposeful, they are often used as a necessary step toward the ability to perform purposeful activities.

Special equipment such as wheelchairs, ambulatory aids, assistive devices, special clothing, communication devices, and environmental control systems may also be necessary to enable independence in the performance areas and assumption of occupational roles.

Returning to our example, the patient at this stage may have some voluntary movement of his arm and leg. However, spasticity makes the movement too weak and uncoordinated for performance that would satisfy the patient's self-esteem needs. In other words, the patient might be able to pick up and place large mosaic tile pieces, but the result would be uneven and unattractive. An activity such as stacking cones or pegboard designs may be given to the patient at stage 2 to allow him to practice motions and skills (lifting, calibrating) that later will be applied to purposeful activities.

In stage 2 the therapist is still concerned with evaluation and remediation of skills and the body functions that support skills. Flexible conditions for using skills may be added at this stage, with the patient experiencing the different weights and textures of materials handled. The OTA may safely carry out most stage 2 enabling activities but must be careful to obtain guidance on the purpose, objectives, procedures, and precautions that apply to each patient situation.

Stage 3: Purposeful Activity

Purposeful activity has been a core tenant of occupational therapy since its inception. Purposeful activity has an inherent or autonomous goal and is relevant and meaningful to the patient (American Occupational Therapy Association, 1997; Ayres, 1958). It is part of the daily life routine and occurs in the context of occupational performance (American Occupational Therapy Association, 1983, 1993, 1997). Examples are feeding, hygiene, dressing, mobility, communication, arts, crafts, games, sports, work, and educational activities.

The purposefulness of an activity is determined by the individual performing it and the context in which it is performed. OTs and OTAs use purposeful activities to evaluate, facilitate, restore, or maintain a person's ability to function in life roles (American Occupational Therapy Association, 1983). Purposeful activity can be carried out in a health care facility or in the patient's home.

Following a CVA, a client at this stage may have achieved more control of the affected arm or leg. Weakness and spasticity may remain, but significant improvement has occurred. The OT or OTA at this point would teach the patient techniques for dressing, self-feeding, toileting, and transfer from the wheelchair. The patient might participate in crafts or games that have been adapted to improve performance skills in, for example, reaching and holding and pinch and release.

In stage 3 the OT or OTA is concerned with evaluating and remediating deficits in the performance of skills related to occupations. The OTA can expect to be involved prominently in the patient's treatment at this point because performance skills and engagement in occupation are the focus of the assistant's treatment skills.

Stage 4: Occupational Performance and Occupational Roles

In the final stage of the treatment continuum, the patient resumes or assumes **occupational roles** in the living environment and in the community. Appropriate tasks in activities of daily living, work, education activities, play, leisure, and social participation are performed to the patient's maximal level of independence. This level is defined by each client or patient according to personal capacities and limitations and values, interests, and goals. Residual disability may remain, but the person has learned compensatory techniques. Formal OT intervention is decreased and ultimately discontinued.

At this stage, the client who has experienced a CVA has likely achieved maximal motor return. Sensorimotor techniques have been applied to normalize abnormal tone to facilitate independence in self-care activities, such as dressing and feeding, leading to the relearning of performance skills and habits that make up daily life. The OT and the OTA work with clients to identify needs in work and home life, then select and train them in the use of appropriate adaptive devices. This allows clients to resume life in the community, shaping a new occupational life with the strategies and techniques learned in therapy. In stage 4 the OT and OTA are concerned with assisting clients to transition to community life.

THEORIES AND MODELS OF PRACTICE IN PHYSICAL DYSFUNCTION

OTs and OTAs utilize theory and **models of practice** to structure their thinking about practice situations. Some models of practice utilized in the practice of physical dysfunction include the model of human occupation, biomechanical approach, sensorimotor approach, and rehabilitation approach. Each has advantages and limitations but may help OTs and OTAs shape their thinking about each client.

Model of Human Occupation

The model of human occupation provides a clear, organized system for understanding occupational performance. The MOHO suggests how the various aspects of human occupation work together and how they are related. We can compare it to a building plan or blueprint.

Human Occupation. The core idea of MOHO (Kielhofner, 2008; Kielhofner & Burke, 1980) is that humans have an inborn drive to explore and master their surroundings. The activity generated by this drive, of exploring and attempting to control the environment, is called occupation. The drive toward occupation can be nurtured and developed, or it can be obstructed and crushed. In this model the individual and the environment are interacting with and affecting one another.

MOHO is a **systems model**. It is a holistic model (one that looks at the whole) rather than a reductionistic model (one that looks intensely at one part, such as muscular function). In this holistic model the human individual engaged in occupation is seen as a complex interaction of parts that cannot make sense viewed separately. In other words, therapists cannot look only at the right upper extremity or at the ability to sequence an activity without considering how these fit within the lives or occupation that individuals have shaped for themselves. Persons cannot be considered separately from their environments. Their families, communities, cultures, and the objects they use every day are forces that shape their nature as actors in the world.

MOHO seeks to explain complex interactions between the person, the activity or occupation, and the environment. Many reasons exist for difficulties in performing occupations. For example, a person may not be motivated; or the person may keep repeating an ineffective action or sequence of actions, perhaps out of habit. Actions may be limited or ineffective because of inability to organize information into meaningful ideas or because of lack of strength or coordination. To organize these various aspects, MOHO recognizes three interrelated components of human occupation: volition, habituation, and performance capacity (and the lived body) (Fig. 1.3).

Volition. Another word for **volition** is *motivation.* Three key elements of volition are personal causation, values, and interests. Personal causation refers to the person's beliefs about personal effectiveness: Am I in control, or am I controlled by forces outside myself? Am I good at things? Can I succeed if I try?

Values are internalized images of "what is important and meaningful to do" (Kielhofner & Burke, 1980). Values motivate behavior in many ways. For example, someone who is ill may make a special effort to get dressed and go to church. A father may neglect professional reading to spend more time helping his child with homework, because to him the child is more important.

Interests are "what one finds enjoyable or satisfying to do" (Kielhofner, 2008). Interests are the things that attract people. When people are interested, they are energized, alive, and ready to attempt new things. Together and separately, personal causation, values, and interests supply motivation or volition to engage in occupation.

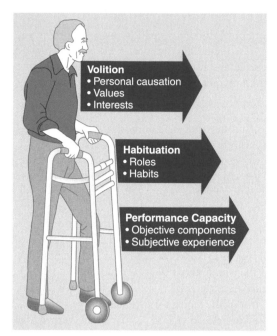

Fig. 1.3 The interrelationships within the model of human occupation. From Kielhofner G, ed. *A Model of Human Occupation: Theory and Application.* 3rd ed. Baltimore, MD: Lippincott Williams & Wilkins; 2002:22[fig. 2.6].

Habituation. **Habituation** refers to activities that have been performed enough times to become routine and customary. Two elements of habituation are habits and internalized roles. Habits are automatic routines or patterns of activity that a person seems to perform almost by reflex, with little conscious awareness. An example would be folding towels or locking a door when leaving. Habits help conserve energy; tasks are accomplished without too much effort or concentration, leaving more time and attention available for other things. Habits and habitat or environment are interdependent; the customary physical environment gives cues that are the same over time and that support regular performance of habits and role behaviors (Kielhofner, 2008).

Internalized roles are personalized occupational roles that consist of many different habits, routines, and skills. Some typical occupational roles are homemaker, student, and retiree. Although each role carries certain socially expected behaviors, these are internalized or personalized by the individual. For example, one homemaker may pay more attention to preparing food for family and guests, whereas another is more involved in keeping the house clean and organized. The internalized role of a student might reflect habits established in childhood, as when the adult student sets up to study at the kitchen table immediately on returning home, just as the person was taught to do in grade school 30 years ago. Also, it may reflect values and interests, as when the student organizes study time around a favorite television program.

Role change, or role transition, occurs as life moves forward and the person grows. Roles contract, expand, are modified, and sometimes are abandoned or replaced. Former roles are rediscovered and renewed. New ones are attempted. The grade school student becomes the high school student. The student becomes a worker. The worker becomes a student again. The worker changes to another field. Role change can be exciting or terrifying; occasionally it is both. Time for learning and adjustment is necessary before a new role becomes internalized.

Performance capacity. **Performance capacity** is "the ability for doing things" (Kielhofner, 2008). Doing things depends on the body structures and functions already discussed and on the subjective experience of them. We live our lives through our bodies, giving each of us a subjective and personal experience. For example, stiffness of the fingers from arthritis may be experienced differently by a pianist or hairdresser than by someone whose work depends less on finger flexibility.

Performance capacity and performance skills are in many cases the primary focus of occupational therapy intervention for persons with physical dysfunction. Performance skills depend on performance capacity. When the body is disabled, the sense of the lived body is different. For the person who is not disabled, there exists a seamless interaction of body and mind in which one does not notice one's body actions because these actions are effective expressions of mental intentions. Once the body is disabled, body actions become a big deal. One must notice, correct, and alter behavior because the body is not performing as previously experienced.

Complex Interactions and Interdependence. As noted, human occupation involves a complex relationship among volition, habituation, and performance capacity (as reflected in the lived body). Any of these three components will affect the others. Trends or patterns can develop. Successful completion of a goal can provide the energy and optimism to try more challenging tasks and the perseverance to keep trying despite minor setbacks. On the other hand, a perception that one has failed can reduce enthusiasm for new tasks and dampen willingness to try. The subjective experience of repeated successes, or of repeated failures, can set up and reinforce a persistent pattern. See Box 1.1 for definitions of terms used in MOHO (Kielhofner & Burke, 1980; Kielhofner, 2008).

MOHO's View of How Disability Affects Human Occupation. Now that you have a general understanding of MOHO, consider what happens when a person encounters the challenge of a physical disability. Consider the case of a young, healthy, single woman who falls and fractures both wrists while rollerblading. She will probably experience this physical disability most immediately in performance capacity of the lived body because it takes away function of the hands. She will not be able to use her hands while they are in casts and will not be able to operate many switches, doorknobs, and faucet handles.

These changes also lead quickly to changed habits and roles because the necessary performance skills are not available and thus the habits cannot be carried out. She cannot bathe herself, prepare her own food, or perform her job. Ultimately, personal causation is affected, with the normal feedback of success from participating in accustomed roles

BOX 1.1 Model of Human Occupation Definitions

Human occupation The act of doing work, play, activities of daily living, and other activities within the context of human life.

Environment Human and nonhuman object world in which human occupation is carried out.

Volition Motivation or the desire to act. Personal causation, values, and interests are aspects of volition.

Personal causation Individual's sense of own competence and effectiveness.

Values Internalized images of what is good, right, and important.

Interests Personal preferences in activities or people.

Habituation Patterns or routine behavior. Aspects of habituation include habits and internalized roles.

Habits Automatic routines. Actions carried out so regularly that they can be done without conscious effort.

Internalized roles Individual's personal interpretation and enactment of the (more general and less specific) occupational role.

Occupational roles Patterns for organizing productive activity, usually according to the product or service produced. Examples are grade-school student, homemaker, basketball player.

Role change/role transition Movement from one role to another, or movement within a role. Examples are going to work after finishing school and moving from full-time to part-time work.

Performance capacity The underlying capacities needed to do things, based on body structures and functions and on the subjective experience of them.

BOX 1.2 Model of Human Occupation Selected Concepts for Intervention

"Client change is the focus of therapy." (p. 296)

"Only clients can accomplish their own change." (p. 296)

"For doing to be therapeutic, it must involve an actual occupational form, not a contrived activity." (p. 297)

"For the client to achieve change through doing, what is done must have relevance and meaning for the client." (p. 297)

"Change in therapy involves simultaneous and interacting alterations in the person, the environment, and the relationship of the person to the environment." (p. 302)

"Change in therapy is part of a history of change in the person's life." (p. 302)

"The role of the therapist is to support and thereby enable clients to do what they need in order to change." (p. 310)

Based on information from Kielhofner G, ed. *A Model of Human Occupation: Theory and Application.* 3rd ed. Baltimore, MD: Lippincott Williams & Wilkins; 2002.

reduced or eliminated. She is confined to her home and begins to feel isolated. She no longer enjoys the company of coworkers or the feeling of satisfaction from doing her job. Discouragement, helplessness, and apathy (lack of interest) may dominate her thinking. She begins to feel worthless, depressed, and self-pitying. She is forced into a new role, that of helpless patient, in which she receives more pleasant (less demanding and less frustrating) feedback from the environment. She sees herself as less capable, more dependent on others, and more needy of support. She watches television and sleeps all day. Although such dependence may be appropriate for a time, if prolonged it might undermine the volition subsystem and reduce motivation for independent living.

Few persons who sustain a physical disability react in this way. Many respond to the challenge with inventive solutions and creative and energetic changes in behavior. Environmental supports such as family or friends can ease the adjustment so that patients feel more in control. The disability is viewed as an inconvenience but not a serious obstacle to achieving life goals. Commonly, people dealing with a physical disability experience both optimism and despair alternately and with varying intensity. Important factors are the severity of the disability and whether it is temporary or permanent. The course of adjustment is usually not just one way or the other; ups and downs are common.

General Principles of Occupational Therapy Intervention. MOHO provides guidelines for designing and carrying out occupational therapy treatment. Some of these are discussed as follows and summarized in Box 1.2 (Kielhofner & Burke, 1980; Kielhofner, 2008).

Client change is the focus of therapy (Kielhofner, 2008). Even forms of therapy in which the practitioner provides equipment or devices still require the client to incorporate the devices and ways of using them.

Only clients can accomplish their own change (Kielhofner, 2008). Engagement and participation by the individual are required. Therapy cannot be done to someone. The person must be involved and active.

For doing to be therapeutic, it must involve an actual occupational form, not a contrived activity (Kielhofner, 2008). As discussed later in the chapter, contrived or enabling activities (e.g., stacking cones) are sometimes used as part of therapy, but these do not provide the opportunity to engage in occupation in ways that are real to the person or that engage the lived body in doing in the world. By participating in activities that match their needs, interests, and abilities, individuals can improve their ability to perform in daily life activities. The OT practitioner selects and designs activities to match the patient's characteristics and goals.

For the client to achieve change through doing, what is done must be relevant and meaningful to the client (Kielhofner, 2008). Therapy practitioners must start from the client's interests and history in selecting activities for therapy. Cleverness, creativity, and careful gradation of the activity to the patient's capabilities will be necessary.

Change in therapy involves simultaneous and interacting alterations in the person, the environment, and the relationship of the person to the environment (Kielhofner, 2008). A dynamic among the person, task, and environment exists. In adjusting to a physical challenge, as well as learning new ways of doing things in the world, the person changes. The environment, too, must change to accommodate the person—and how he or she experiences the self in relation to the environment changes.

Change in therapy is part of a history of change in the person's life (Kielhofner, 2008). As noted earlier, change in roles and occupations is ongoing. The change that occurs in therapy is just another episode of change, but how the change is experienced depends greatly on how the person sees the self. People have a sense of their own occupational nature, now challenged by physical disability. Therapy provides an opportunity for the person to modify the sense of self to accommodate the disability and the solutions that work for that person.

The role of the therapist is to support and thereby enable clients to do what they need in order to change (Kielhofner, 2008). The client needs support, information, and guided experience to change because change can be difficult and results discouraging. The therapist uses many strategies to assist the client in the process of changing. The therapist may do the following:

- Validate the client's experience
- Identify ways of managing tasks
- Provide feedback on performance
- Advise clients about alternatives
- Negotiate an intermediate step when a task seems too difficult
- Structure activities to provide meaningful challenges
- Coach performance by verbal cuing
- Offer words and gestures of encouragement
- Provide physical support and adaptations as needed.

These strategies represent only a selection of the many principles in MOHO (Kielhofner, 2008) (see Box 1.2).

Other Models of Practice

The most common models of practice used with clients with physical dysfunction are the biomechanical approach, the motor learning and sensorimotor approaches, and the rehabilitation approach. As you are reading this, keep in mind the ways in which each model can be utilized and its relationship to MOHO.

Biomechanical Approach. The **biomechanical approach** to the treatment of physical dysfunction considers the human body as a living machine. Techniques in this approach derive from **kinetics**, the science of the motions of objects and the forces acting on them (Mosey, 1981). To some extent, the principles of **statics**, the study of the forces acting on objects at rest, are also used in this approach. The object here is the human body, which is studied at rest and in motion. Treatment methods use principles of physics (Schultz-Krohn & Pendleton, 2018) related to forces, levers, and torque (Box 1.3).

Typical evaluation and treatment techniques used in this approach are measurement of joint ROM and muscle strength, therapeutic exercise, and orthotics. Therapeutic activity for kinetic purposes, or the application of movement principles in the performance of activities, is also part of this approach. Sanding with a weighted sander to improve strength or weaving on an upright loom to increase shoulder

---

BOX 1.3 Biomechanical Approach Definitions

Kinetics Study of the motions of objects and the forces acting on them.
Statics Study of the forces acting on objects at rest.
Force Measurable influence acting on a body.
Lever Rigid structure fixed at a point called the fulcrum and acted on at two other points by two forces, causing movement in relation to the fulcrum; a seesaw and a crowbar are examples.
Torque Rotary or twisting force.
Joint Point where two bones meet and around which motion occurs.
Range of motion Extent, measured in degrees of a circle, to which movement can occur at a joint.
Strength Work against resistance (including the force of gravity), measured in pounds.
Endurance Exertion or work sustained over time.

ROM are examples. The goals of the biomechanical approach are to (1) evaluate specific physical limitations in ROM, strength, and endurance; (2) restore these functions; and (3) prevent or reduce deformity.

The biomechanical approach is most appropriate for patients whose central nervous system (CNS) is intact but who have lower motor neuron or orthopedic disorders. These patients can control isolated movements and specific movement patterns but may have weakness, low endurance, or joint limitation. Disabilities typically addressed with this approach include orthopedic conditions (e.g., rheumatoid arthritis, osteoarthritis, fractures, amputations, hand trauma), burns, lower motor neuron disorders (e.g., peripheral nerve injuries), Guillain-Barré syndrome, spinal cord injuries, and primary muscle diseases (e.g., muscular dystrophy). Biomechanical principles are also applied in ergonomics and work hardening, with an emphasis on proper positioning and the optimum fit between the biomechanics of the individual and the work environment.

The biomechanical approach targets the performance capacity level of MOHO and focuses on physical skills (e.g., lifting the hand) and body structures and functions that support them (e.g., ROM, strength). Its principles can also be applied directly to occupations and to contexts (e.g., when the height of a chair and a desk are lowered to fit a person of less than standard height).

Sensorimotor and Motor Learning Approaches. Methods using the **sensorimotor approach** were developed for treatment of patients who have CNS dysfunction. The normal CNS functions to produce controlled, well-modulated (regular and adjusted) movement. The damaged CNS cannot coordinate and produce such movement smoothly or with ease.

Sensorimotor approaches to treatment use **neurophysiologic** mechanisms to normalize muscle tone and elicit more normal motor responses (Rogers, 1982). They provide controlled input to the nervous system; this controlled input is meant to stimulate specific responses. Some approaches use **reflex** mechanisms, and the sequence of treatment may be

---

BOX 1.4 Sensorimotor Approach Definitions

Central nervous system (CNS) The brain and spinal cord.

Neurophysiologic Pertaining to the study of the physical and chemical nature of the nervous system.

Muscle tone Resistance of a muscle to being stretched by an external force.

Motor response Movement or muscle action evoked by sensory input; may be voluntary or involuntary.

Reflex mechanism Involuntary motor response to sensory input.

Recapitulation of ontogenetic development Theory that the organism in its development goes through the same stages as did the species in its development from lower organisms; as applied to recovery from CNS damage, also implies that recovery must go through the same stages as individual human development (i.e., from infancy).

---

based on the recapitulation of ontogenetic development (Rogers, 1982). In other words, these approaches might use primitive reflexes such as those that infants display or those that humans share with other creatures such as fish. Therapy is directed at incorporating these reflexes into purposeful activity and at integrating them so that their power is reduced, and movement becomes more controlled and voluntary. Chapter 20 describes the sensorimotor approaches. Box 1.4 lists definitions of terms related to sensorimotor approaches.

The sensorimotor approaches target the MOHO component of performance capacities. Sensorimotor approaches have been criticized when they do not include purposeful activity or the involvement of patients as creators and actors in their own occupational world. Sensorimotor approaches are used by other health practitioners, including physical therapists, speech therapists, and physiatrists. They are not exclusively used by OTs and OTAs. Although some approaches were developed by OTs, others were designed or discovered by practitioners of these other disciplines.

The principles of the sensorimotor approaches can be used when the practitioner applies them to purposeful activity. The American Occupational Therapy Association (AOTA) advises that the techniques of an approach not associated with purposeful activity may be used "to prepare the client or patient for better performance and prevention of disability through self-participation in occupation" (American Occupational Therapy Association, 1979). These techniques should be a part of occupational therapy intervention only when they are used to stimulate or condition the nervous system so that purposeful activity can be attempted, ideally during the same treatment session.

Motor learning is an approach associated with the sensorimotor approach that focuses on the acquisition of motor skills through practice and feedback (Schultz-Krohn & McLaughlin-Gray, 2018; Schmidt & Lee, 2014). Motor learning takes into account the individual's involvement in the learning process and requires active practice and reflection from the patient. It uses motor training by therapists, with opportunities for patients to create their own movement

solutions to challenges. The context or practice environment for movement activities is a major focus. Therapy practitioners attempt to design practice conditions that will challenge the person sufficiently to involve the thinking processes that guide motor behavior (Rogers, 1982). Motor control is discussed in Chapters 6 and 10.

The motor control approach addresses the volition, habituation, and performance capacity components of MOHO. The primary focus is the performance of motor functions. However, volition is involved as the person is engaged in solving movement problems. Habituation is involved through practice in a variety of situations and the generation of new movement patterns. The motor learning approach is based in learning theory.

Rehabilitation Approach. The term *rehabilitation* means a restoration to a former state or to a proper state (Phipps, 2018). In medicine it means the return to the fullest physical, mental, social, vocational, and economic usefulness that is possible for the individual. It refers to the ability to live and work with remaining capabilities. Therefore the focus in the treatment program is on abilities rather than disabilities.

Rehabilitation is concerned with the intrinsic worth and dignity of the individual and with the restoration of a satisfying and purposeful life. The **rehabilitation approach** uses measures that enable a person to live as independently as possible despite residual disability. Its goal is to help the patient learn to work around or compensate for physical limitations (Phipps, 2018).

The rehabilitation approach assumes that the patient is an active, involved, contributing member of the rehabilitation team. OTs and OTAs must identify the patient's capabilities and assets so that these can be engaged to overcome the effects of the disability on function. They must consider the best research evidence and be aware of advances in methods and equipment (rehabilitation technology). OTs and OTAs must always place primary importance on the envisioned outcome of individuals functioning as they desire in their environments of choice.

Intervention methods of the rehabilitation approach include techniques and modalities such as the following:

- Self-care evaluation and training
- Acquisition and training in assistive devices
- Acquisition and training in use of adaptive clothing
- Homemaking and child care
- Work simplification and energy conservation
- Work-related activities
- Leisure activities
- Prosthetic training
- Wheelchair management
- Home evaluation and adaptation
- Community transportation
- Architectural adaptations
- Acquisition and training in the use of communication aids and environmental control systems

In relation to occupation, the rehabilitation approach focuses on the occupations themselves and on performance skills rather than on body structures and functions. The aims of a rehabilitation program are to enable role performance and to minimize the effects of residual disability on role performance. The rehabilitation approach takes the influence of the environment into account and provides methods to adapt the environment to the individual.

The rehabilitation approach addresses most of the elements of MOHO. Including the patient as a member of the rehabilitation team engages the volition subsystem. However, the patient's values, interests, and sense of personal causation are not addressed directly. Habituation is the focus of intervention, and performance of occupation is emphasized. As mentioned, the environment and possible changes to the environment are also considered. The performance capacity level is emphasized less in this approach than in the biomechanical and sensorimotor approaches.

OTs and OTAs commonly use methods of the rehabilitation approach in combination with methods from the biomechanical or sensorimotor approach. Biomechanical or sensorimotor principles can be applied during rehabilitation activities to reinforce the functioning of sensorimotor and cognitive functions. An example is the use of cross-diagonal patterns (a sensorimotor approach) to normalize muscle tone and coordination during dressing, which complements and enhances the success of rehabilitation. At the same time it ties the sensorimotor technique to purposeful activity.

Limitations of These Practice Approaches

The three practice approaches just described have proved useful in evaluating and treating problems commonly encountered in physical disabilities practice. Used separately or together, however, they do not provide a complete view of the person. OTs and OTAs should consider not only motor control but also motor behavior—that is, "a person acting purposefully within and upon his or her environment" (Di Joseph, 1982). Ignoring the emotive and cognitive aspects of motor behavior is a reductive approach that fails to consider all factors in the production of purposeful action. Treatment goals for patients must be based on an evaluation of mind, body, and environment. These goals should be reached through activities compatible with the needs and values of the person and not necessarily with those of the therapist. Interaction between the person and the environment is essential to functional independence (Phipps, 2018). The person is mind and body, not just a motor system to be evaluated and treated (Di Joseph, 1982). This approach is essential throughout the treatment continuum.

EVIDENCE-BASED PRACTICE

Health care providers today are looking carefully at what **evidence** exists to support their practice; outcomes are usually the focus (Dirette et al., 2009; Gillen et al., 2019). Generally this takes the form of asking a question: "In a case such as this one, which approach is more likely to yield the best outcome?" To give an example, "In a 26-year-old man with C-6 spinal cord injury, what occupational therapy procedures will result in the best return to maximum functional independence?" Finding an answer to such a question is not so easy, however, because the quantity of published occupational therapy research is limited and has not yet increased to the level needed to support **evidence-based practice** (EBP) (Dirette et al., 2009; Gillen et al., 2019).

Within the field of occupational therapy much of the lore and custom of practice has been passed down from therapist to therapist but has not always been well documented or researched in a controlled way before being published in a peer-reviewed journal. Consumers and insurers are asking how we can justify our practices. Consequently, research and outcome studies have become important. The OTA of the 21st century should expect to take a role in asking and answering questions for outcomes research. This requires a thoughtful approach to practice, one that relies less on rote procedures from a textbook or classroom and more on reflective analysis of what happens in therapy. This involves considering the perspective of both the client and the OT or OTA. It requires that the OTA adopt an inquiring attitude and develop a tolerance for ambiguity and not knowing. Being able to pose clinical questions and search for information in electronic databases and print sources is also necessary. The OTA may gather data and publish outcomes studies, document and write for publication a single case study report, or work with a group of OT practitioners on a large study. All these efforts add to the knowledge base of the profession.

SUMMARY

The focus of occupational therapy in the practice of physical dysfunction is to assist or enable individuals to participate in occupations within contexts. The treatment continuum in physical disabilities practice is a process of four stages through which the patient gradually acquires the abilities to resume occupational life after disability. The OTA is most involved in the final two stages of purposeful activity and resumption of occupational roles.

The model of human occupation is a frame of reference for occupational performance. This model has three subsystems: volition, habituation, and performance capacity. People with physical dysfunction experience the most direct and visible disruption of their occupational lives at the level of performance capacity and the lived body.

Three treatment approaches commonly applied in physical disabilities practice are the biomechanical, sensorimotor/motor learning, and rehabilitation approaches. These approaches apply to specific types of disabling conditions.

The goal of occupational therapy intervention is to develop maximal functioning in occupational roles, as defined for everyone in consideration of that person's capacities and limitations. Recognizing that the client or patient is the starting point, we shape our interventions toward the individual's goals, values, and interests throughout the occupational therapy process. At the same time we must remember to research and document best practices and to consider the evidence that supports our interventions.

REVIEW QUESTIONS

1. Discuss the relationship of body structures and functions (client factors) to task demands and performance skills.
2. Differentiate holistic from reductionistic.
3. List and describe the three subsystems of MOHO.
4. Relate role change or role transition to MOHO.
5. List the typical evaluation and treatment methods used in the biomechanical approach.
6. Identify the conditions for which the biomechanical approach is most appropriate.
7. Identify the conditions for which the sensorimotor approach is most appropriate and explain why this approach is preferred for these conditions.
8. Discuss the relationship between the sensorimotor approach and purposeful activity.
9. How is the motor learning approach different from the sensorimotor approach?
10. Define rehabilitation and state the goal of the rehabilitation approach.
11. List some intervention methods of the rehabilitation approach.
12. List reasons why the three practice approaches used in physical disabilities practice have been criticized for providing an incomplete view of the patient.
13. Discuss why each of the four stages in the occupational therapy treatment continuum requires a different level of patient involvement.
14. Explain what is meant by evidence to support practice and discuss the roles of the OTA regarding gathering and documenting evidence.

REFERENCES

American Occupational Therapy Association. (1979). Resolution 532-79 (1979): occupation as the common core of occupational therapy, Representative Assembly minutes, Detroit, April 1979. *The American Journal of Occupational Therapy, 33*, 785.

American Occupational Therapy Association. (1983). Purposeful activities: a position paper. *The American Journal of Occupational Therapy, 37*, 805.

American Occupational Therapy Association. (1993). Position paper: purposeful activity. *The American Journal of Occupational Therapy, 47*, 1081–1082.

American Occupational Therapy Association. (1997). Statement: fundamental concepts of occupational therapy: occupation, purposeful activity, and function. *The American Journal of Occupational Therapy, 51*(10), 864–869, 1997.

American Occupational Therapy Association. (2004). Roles and responsibilities of the occupational therapist and the occupational therapy assistant during the delivery of occupational therapy services. *The American Journal of Occupational Therapy, 58*(6), 663–667.

American Occupational Therapy Association. (2008). Physical agent modalities, a position paper. *The American Journal of Occupational Therapy, 62*(6), 691–693.

American Occupational Therapy Association. (2014a). Guidelines for supervision, roles, and responsibilities during the delivery of occupational therapy services. *The American Journal of Occupational Therapy, 68*, S16–S22.

American Occupational Therapy Association. (2014b). Occupational therapy practice framework: domain and process, 3rd ed. *The American Journal of Occupational Therapy, 68*, S1–S51.

American Occupational Therapy Association. (2015). Standards of practice for occupational therapy. *The American Journal of Occupational Therapy, 69*, 1–6.

Ayres, A. J. (1958). Basic concepts of clinical practice in physical disabilities. *The American Journal of Occupational Therapy, 12*, 300.

Di Joseph, L. M. (1982). Independence through activity: mind, body, and environment interaction in therapy. *The American Journal of Occupational Therapy, 36*, 740.

Dirette, D., Rozich, A., & Viau, S. (2009). Is there enough evidence for evidence-based practice in occupational therapy? *The American Journal of Occupational Therapy, 63*, 782–786.

Gillen, G., Hunter, E. G., Lieberman, D., & Stutzbach, M. (2019). AOTA's top 5 Choosing Wisely® recommendations. *The American Journal of Occupational Therapy, 73*(2), 1–9.

Kielhofner, G., & Burke, J. P. (1980). A model of human occupation: 1. conceptual framework and content. *The American Journal of Occupational Therapy, 34*, 572–581.

Kielhofner, G. (Ed.). (2008). *A model of human occupation: Theory and application* (4th ed.). Baltimore, MD: Lippincott Williams & Wilkins.

Merleau-Ponty, M. (1982). *Phenomenology of perception* (C. Smith, Trans.). London, England: Routledge & Kegan Paul.

Mosby. (2008). *Mosby's medical, nursing, and allied health dictionary* (6th ed.). St. Louis, MO: Mosby.

Mosey, A. C. (1981). *Occupational therapy: Configuration of a profession*. New York, NY: Raven.

Oxford University Press. (2013). *Pocket Oxford American dictionary* (2nd ed.). New York, NY: Oxford University Press.

Phipps, S. (2018). Motor learning. In H. M. Pendleton, & W. Schultz-Krohn (Eds.), *Pedretti's occupational therapy: Practice skills for physical dysfunction* (8th ed., pp. 25–37). St. Louis, MO: Elsevier Mosby.

Reed, K. L. (1984). *Models for practice in occupational therapy*. Baltimore, MD: Williams & Wilkins.

Rogers, J. C. (1982). The spirit of independence: the evolution of a philosophy. *The American Journal of Occupational Therapy, 36*, 709.

Schmidt, R. A., & Lee, T. (2014). *Motor control and learning*. Champaign, IL: Human Kinetics.

Schultz-Krohn, W., & McLaughlin-Gray, J. (2018). Traditional sensorimotor approaches to intervention. In H. M. Pendleton, & W. Schultz-Krohn (Eds.), *Pedretti's occupational therapy: Practice skills for physical dysfunction* (8th ed., pp. 25–37). St. Louis, MO: Elsevier Mosby.

Schultz-Krohn, W., & Pendleton, H. M. (2018). Application of the occupational therapy practice framework to physical dysfunction. In H. M. Pendleton, & W. Schultz-Krohn (Eds.), *Pedretti's occupational therapy: Practice skills for physical dysfunction* (8th ed., pp. 25–37). St. Louis, MO: Elsevier Mosby.

Shumway-Cook, M., & Woollacott, M. (2001). *Motor control: Theory and practical applications*. Baltimore, MD: Lippincott Williams & Wilkins.

2

Exploring Perspectives on Illness and Disability Throughout the Continuum of Care
A Case-Based Client-Centered Approach

Michele D. Mills and Regina M. Lehman

OBJECTIVES

After reading this chapter, the student or the occupational therapy practitioner will be able to do the following:

- Realize the significance of addressing an individual's psychosocial needs and incorporate appropriate goals and intervention strategies throughout the occupational therapy process for the individual with physical disability.
- Recognize and discuss the significance of utilizing effective communication, therapeutic use of self, and clinical reasoning to collaborate with clients and their families/significant others to develop occupation-based and client-centered goals.
- Discuss the barriers to effective communication that may interfere with client-centered care for the occupational therapy practitioner.
- Describe strategies for using mindfulness and fostering connections with the client to enable client-centered care.

- Identify and discuss factors that may help or hinder individuals as they adjust within their disability experience.
- Contextualize and describe individuals' disability experience across the continuum of care. Reflect on how individuals' experience within the continuum of care may influence their adjustment to disability.
- Discuss the application of each aspect of professional reasoning/clinical reasoning to a case and the influence on a client's disability experience throughout the continuum of care.
- Discuss the importance professional/clinical reasoning as an integral component to the utilization of therapeutic use of self and mindful occupational therapy practice.
- Discuss how a client and/or the family may advocate for the client's care needs.

KEY TERMS

Disability experience
Therapeutic use of self
Effective communication
Client-centered care
Mindful practitioner
Collaboration
Continuum of care
Locus of control

Motivation
Advocate
Self-efficacy
Role competency
Clinical reasoning
Professional reasoning
Reflective practice

INTRODUCTION

The effects of physical disability extend beyond the physical body. To be truly effective, the occupational therapy practitioner must consider the psychological and social aspects of the individual's **disability experience** in unison with the presenting physical problem (Erikson, 1963). Occupational therapy practitioners must develop **therapeutic use of self** and **effective communication** along with other skills, to approach each unique situation from the client's point of view. These skills are integral to the provision of **client-centered care**. The **mindful practitioner** utilizes these skills to develop meaningful goals and occupation-based intervention in **collaboration** with the client. The practice of authentic occupational therapy (Strauss & Tinetti, 2009) includes these essential elements.

For many individuals, the disability experience includes loss and adjustment: loss of function, adjustment to a new body image, loss of social roles, adjustment to changed abilities within the performance of occupations, and adjustment to a changing personal identity. Independence and autonomy may be diminished permanently or temporarily (Dooley & Hinojosa, 2004). Individual perceptions of quality of life may change dramatically. Privacy is often surrendered, and strangers must be allowed to participate in the individual's care. Familial, social, and vocational roles are disrupted and may be seriously altered by the disability experience. The responses of the individual and significant others affect the outcome of rehabilitation (Dooley & Hinojosa, 2004). The individual must first adapt to the disability, regain essential functions (with or without assistance), and finally resume participation in meaningful life roles through engagement in occupation. These are monumental tasks that require significant adjustment (MacCormac, 2010).

This chapter considers the relationship between the psychosocial and the physical self within the context of physical disease and disability. The reader will gain an appreciation of the disability experience through a case study. The reader is prompted to examine the case in its totality and then reflect on the client's response(s), familial response(s), health care practitioner response(s), and the key factors that influence the case, throughout the **continuum of care**. The chapter concludes with attention to key variables that influence the client's disability experience and techniques for the occupational therapy practitioner to facilitate psychosocial adjustment and therapeutic use of self within the constructs of clinical reasoning and effective communication.

EXPERIENCING DISABILITY THROUGHOUT THE CONTINUUM OF CARE

The Case of Lydia: A Disability Experience

Lydia is a 79-year-old who identifies as female. She is married for over 40 years to her husband John. They live independently in a ranch-style home, in a suburban environment. Lydia is a retired public-school teacher and counselor. She began her teaching career as a math teacher and continued her education to become a school counselor. She and John have four children within a blended family. John is a retired police officer. Their four children are all college educated. Their vocations include an engineer, a lawyer, a nurse, and an occupational therapy practitioner. Their careers and success are a source of pride for Lydia and John.

Lydia is an active individual. She and John are well traveled and well read. They attend church services regularly on Sundays and volunteer in varied church-related activities throughout the week. Lydia maintains close contact with family, friends, and many of her former students. She drives herself to activities of choice and plays a large role in family decision making. She is a leader in her community and loves to participate in activities that challenge her cognitive abilities. She is well adept at playing chess and Sudoku.

Initiating the Illness and Disability Experience

While completing her morning activities of daily living (ADL) routine, John noticed that Lydia was having difficulty getting dressed, she was dropping items from her right hand, and her speech was not making sense. John contacted emergency services and notified their children. Lydia was taken to the hospital by ambulance. Medical assessment and diagnostic tests confirmed a left cerebrovascular accident (L CVA/stroke) (see Chapter 23) and a previously undiagnosed stroke. Lydia was admitted to the hospital.

Lydia's education and *strong sense of independence* prepared her to live her life to the fullest prior to the stroke. The stroke occurrence marked the beginning of change in Lydia's participation and engagement in the activities significant of her desired occupations. Immediately, change occurred within her familial role, decision-making ability, motor skills, and every aspect of her life in which she was formerly independent.

Lydia's medical history included diabetes mellitus type 2, congestive heart failure, and cardiac arrhythmia. These medical conditions were managed with medication and routine doctor visits. Two months prior to the L CVA, Lydia experienced the signs and symptoms of a stroke: numbness in her left arm and leg and a lack of sharpness in her thinking. The symptoms dissipated quickly, and Lydia's function and ability did not undergo observable change. She did not inform the medical professionals routinely managing her care nor her family about her experience of strokelike symptoms. As an avid reader, and with two children with careers in the medical field, Lydia was aware of the signs and symptoms of stroke. The experience induced fear and she did not want to alarm her family. Lydia noticed a change in her ability to solve Sudoku and crossword puzzles. Engaging in these games required more attention, concentration, and problem-solving effort. As these activities require individual performance, Lydia's family was not initially aware of her changed ability. Reflection on her activity performance and discussion with the neurologist revealed that the family noticed a reduction in text messaging. Lydia had become an avid user of text messaging to communicate and stay in touch with her family. Text messaging requires the use of the cognitive and perceptual skill set used for playing Sudoku and crossword puzzles. Lydia's initial stroke affected her virtual communication ability.

EXPERIENCES WITHIN THE CONTINUUM OF CARE

Acute Hospitalization

During her acute care hospitalization, Lydia sustained a third stroke. The third stroke occurred while she was ambulating with physical therapy staff outside of her hospital room. Diagnostic tests confirmed another L CVA. The most significant change in Lydia's motor and cognitive function occurred after the third stroke. This stroke lead to multiple decisions that needed to be made by Lydia and her family regarding the next steps in managing her care. The medical team offered Lydia and her family multiple options for managing her medical needs and the rehabilitation process:

Option 1: Return to her home with nursing and rehabilitation services and 1 to 2 days weekly of home health care. The family would have to manage the day to day care needs.

Option 2: Admission to an acute rehabilitation facility for 2 to 3 weeks with daily rehabilitation services, full medical and nursing care, and eventual return home with home health care and rehabilitation services.

Option 3: Subacute rehabilitation, with nursing and rehabilitation services and eventual return home with home health care and rehabilitation services. This option offered the potential for a longer stay than would be available within the acute rehabilitation facility.

All of these decisions were overwhelming for Lydia and her family. For Lydia, her independent lifestyle, full of self-directed decision making and ability, was slipping away from her **locus of control**. Subacute rehabilitation within a nursing home setting seemed most undesirable because a nursing home setting had a stigma, Lydia and her family were concerned that the rehabilitation would not be aggressive, and she would not be prepared for return to her home. As a previously active and independent 78-year-old woman, Lydia never thought of herself as old. The nursing home was a place for so-called old and inactive individuals. Lydia's family was fearful that she may give up if she were to be admitted to subacute rehabilitation within a nursing home facility. Ultimately, she was transferred to an acute rehabilitation facility.

Acute Rehabilitation

Lydia began to rely on her youngest daughter to assist her with day-to-day decision making while she was in the acute rehabilitation facility. Decision making was needed regarding every aspect of care. What meal options would she select? Which rehabilitation schedule was best? Which clothing choices should be made? How would she determine when toileting assistance was needed and access the toilet? These previously simple and routine decisions, among others, were difficult for Lydia.

Lydia did not like the hospital food. Her youngest daughter, a nurse, assisted her with making decisions about her meal choices. The options were not appealing. Additionally, her medical comorbidities and the new symptoms of dysphagia required both the food options and texture to change. The food consistency was infantile in its appearance. Pocketing of food, slowed swallowing ability, and coughing during meal intake placed Lydia at risk for aspirating.

During conversation with her daughter who is an occupational therapy practitioner, Lydia confided that she was most concerned about losing her independence. She shared that the members of the rehabilitation team seldom spoke to her directly about her care when family members were in the room. The members of the rehabilitation team often directed their communication to her family. Lydia felt invisible. Her participation in the planning of her care was not elicited, and discussions to assist her with understanding care plan decisions was minimal.

Lydia reported that she often felt like she was being treated in a childlike manner during the process of her rehabilitation. She noted that some of the therapists spoke to her using a tone that was more appropriate for communication with a child. The tone was high pitched. She was often referred to as "sweetie," "honey," or "dear," and the therapists would proceed with a plan of care or intervention. There was very little explanation or discussion to aid her understanding of the treatment plan or goal. No one seemed to know about her life or person prior to the stroke. Her occupational profile, history, roles, and interests were not discussed. For Lydia, the childlike communication represented a lack of concern or respect for her individuality. At times, anxiety over her slow progress, fear of failing, pain, and cognitive changes led to decreased **motivation** and intermittent refusal of therapy services.

Lydia's daughter, an occupational therapy practitioner, initiated discussion with the rehabilitation team regarding her concerns about their communication during intervention. The practitioners were not aware of their communication, Lydia's feelings, and the influence of her experience on her motivation to participate in therapy. Upon reflection, the daughter who is the occupational therapy practitioner recognized the ease in which a well-meaning clinician could easily communicate in a manner that is infantilizing and fall into the trap of planning and engaging in a client's care without the client's full participation. A therapist's mindful engagement in client-centered care is not always automatic; it is a skill set that requires development and constant attention.

Lydia's rehabilitation progression showed incremental improvement during her 3-week stay at the acute rehabilitation facility. Her family participated in the varied training sessions to facilitate her care, and all family members learned how to communicate with the team to **advocate** for her care. As the end of the 20-day stay was near, many decisions were required to determine the next phase in Lydia's care. Was Lydia ready for the next step in her care? Was Lydia's family prepared to meet her new ability challenges within the home setting? Lydia was still coughing during meals and needed moderate to maximal assistance with all aspects of her ADL and instrumental activities of daily living (IADL) upon discharge.

The acute rehabilitation staff encouraged Lydia and her family that she would continue to make slow gains at home. Return to home was recommended. The familiar surroundings of home would assist Lydia with her progression. Lydia's health insurance would cover some medical equipment but not all of the devices or equipment that would be beneficial for Lydia. The family was provided with a list and encouraged to purchase certain adaptive devices and durable medical equipment independently. Lydia's health insurance would cover rehabilitation services and nursing for a given period. Home health care services would be 1 to 2 hours weekly, for a given period. Lydia's residual deficits would require her to receive 24-hour care for their management and her safety. Eventually Lydia and her family would have to manage her day-to-day care needs independently.

Preparing for the Return Home From Acute Rehabilitation

Lydia's family prepared for her return home. The furnishings within the home were reorganized and equipment was ordered (entry ramps, rolling commode, transfer tub bench, wheelchair, walker, bathroom safety rails, and diapers). Lydia would also require a hospital bed. The hospital bed and the equipment made it necessary for a guest room to be converted into a bedroom to enable management of Lydia's care. At least temporarily she would not sleep in her bedroom and share her bed with John. Lydia's husband and children would have to take turns assisting with her care. Lydia was happy, fearful, and tearful regarding the plan for her to return home. Would her family be able to manage her care? Would she ever regain her independence?

Brief Return Home

Lydia returned home. All family members assisted with her care through the first night. Lydia did not fare well during the first night at home. The family was extremely attentive and noticed that she appeared to be weak, she continued to cough, and her responsiveness was low. Lydia was returned to the hospital by ambulance. Upon medical assessment, Lydia was diagnosed with pneumonia.

Return to the Acute Hospital

Lydia's new diagnosis of pneumonia required readmission to the hospital. Lydia received breathing treatments (from respiratory therapy) and eventual reassessment by members of the rehabilitation team. Lydia also was developing pain in her right arm and foot that were demonstrating signs of hemiparesis (see Chapter 23). The rehabilitation team's reassessment indicated regression in her functional abilities. Instead of returning to her home, the medical team recommended reconsideration of the previous options. Lydia and her family were informed that management of her care, resultant of her new diagnosis, would require another rehabilitation admission. Lydia's health insurance would cover another admission to a rehabilitation facility due to the change in her functional status.

Once again, Lydia and her family were made aware of the options for rehabilitation. They engaged in family meetings and interviews with the medical management teams at each facility option (acute rehabilitation and subacute rehabilitation). After careful decision making it was determined the potential for a longer stay and the promise for comprehensive rehabilitation and nursing care services offered by the subacute rehabilitation facility option would make it the best choice.

Subacute Rehabilitation

Lydia was transferred to the subacute rehabilitation facility, within a community-based skilled nursing facility. Initially Lydia's concerns regarding her inclusion within the care plan/goal setting were the same as they were in the acute rehabilitation setting. Based on previous experience, Lydia's family engaged in advocacy for Lydia and their involvement in

her care plan as soon as she was admitted into her new setting. Her goals and interests were shared with the rehabilitation staff. Her request to be included within care plan decisions and to be spoken to in a direct and age-appropriate manner was discussed. Lydia's family discussed dietary needs with the dietary department and the speech pathologist to advocate for early assessment and planning. Nursing and occupational therapy assessed her ADL concerns and created a care plan to address Lydia's desire for a toileting program to address toileting and hygiene with dignity, in preparation for her eventual return to home. Lydia and her family became more adept at navigating the rehabilitation and nursing care environment to optimize her participation in goal planning and engagement in meaningful activity.

Through the course of her stay in subacute rehabilitation, Lydia experienced good days and challenging days. The outcome was incremental change. Although she required time to adjust to being in a nursing home environment, Lydia began to participate in group activities led by the therapeutic recreation department to enhance her socialization and quality of life. Many of the craft activities in which she participated yielded beautiful results. She began to explore hidden talent as she continued to adjust to her new cognitive and motor abilities. Engagement in the meaningful occupation of leisure led to increasing participation in therapy goals and a greater sense of perceived **self-efficacy**. Enhanced perceived self-efficacy increased Lydia's motivation. A visit from the pastor of her church was influential in lifting her spirits and providing hope. She became willing to practice home therapy exercise activities with her family and go on brief outings.

Preparing for Return Home From Subacute Rehabilitation

Lydia and her family noticed improvement in her motor skills as she prepared for discharge. The unspoken discussion was whether Lydia would be able to return to her home. Was she medically stable? Would her family be able to manage her new care needs at home? She was participating in a toileting program. She was able to notify others when she felt the urge to urinate or required a bowel movement. She gained the ability to complete transfers with moderate assistance. She was able to walk short distances with a walker to assist with transfers and functional mobility. Toileting required maximal assistance. Dressing required moderate to maximal assistance. Selecting meal options and menu planning continued to require moderate assistance. Feeding required setup, and large food items needed to be cut into smaller pieces before intake. Lydia continued to dislike the food options that her dietary needs required. She was displeased with the requirement to chew for longer periods and drink intermittently during her meal to clear food items from her mouth. Mealtime lacked pleasure and required constant reminders to follow the steps prescribed by the speech pathologist. Additional areas of function that continued to require attention were writing, decision making, and increasing the use of the affected right upper extremity during activity performance.

Lydia experienced intermittent pain of levels 8 to 9 within the right arm and foot. When the pain occurred, these pain levels made it impossible for her to participate in therapy. She received pain medication, as needed, within the subacute rehabilitation setting. How would she manage the pain at home? Both Lydia and her family were eager for her to return home; however, they were also fearful about her return home based on their previous experience.

Adjusting to the New Home Environment and Additional Care Participants

Lydia was discharged to her home on a Friday evening. Lydia was able to make it through the initial night at home successfully, with no incidents requiring immediate medical attention. The home care nurse arrived the next day, a Saturday, and opened her case, enabling her to receive occupational therapy, physical therapy, and speech language pathology services. Lydia was also eligible for 1 to 2 hours of home health care services. All these home care services would be in place for approximately 1 month. How would Lydia and her family manage her care once her health insurance no longer covered these home health care services?

At home, Lydia realized that her **role competency** in the family had changed. She was no longer the major decision maker. Her youngest daughter, a nurse and the child living closest to her parents, now assumed that role. John was still adjusting to the changes in his wife's ability. He was active in participating in her day-to-day care and providing companionship. However, the *burden* of coping with his new role as *caregiver* for his previously very independent wife was difficult. He was reluctant to share his feelings with the family. Lydia's youngest daughter had taken a lead role in family decision making regarding her overall care. She was the communicator, the planner, the scheduler, the resource seeker, the family representative, and the one making the difficult decisions that Lydia and John could not make.

Lydia and John had to adjust to the constant flow of people coming into their home to participate in Lydia's care. Familial perceptions regarding privacy had to change to promote engagement in occupation for Lydia and each family member. In addition to the therapists and the nursing staff who came into their home daily, the family recognized the need for additional persons to assist with Lydia's care. The additional assistance was needed to enable members of the family to resume previous work, roles, habits, and routines and to develop new ones. For Lydia, striving to achieve health, well-being, and participation in life through engagement in occupation would be ongoing and require the support of her family and many individuals.

Lydia's Experience With Regaining Function at Home—3 Months Later

Lydia completed home care therapy under Medicare Part A. She participates in functional mobility within her home, for short distances, with a rolling walker and requires minimal to moderate assistance with transfers to varied surfaces. Lydia continues to require moderate assistance with toilet hygiene, bathing, and dressing. She eats independently using her nondominant left hand for utensil management. Lydia continues to desire increased use of her dominant right hand during activity performance. Motor praxis with the right hand and upper extremity continues to be a challenge. Lydia finds mealtime more pleasurable. She achieved the ability to chew and swallow her food with limited risk for aspiration. She participates in meals with her family. Although her diet continues to require special attention, she no longer requires a food texture adaptation.

Lydia is more willing to go on outings to restaurants with her family. She accepts visits from church members. She also virtually participates in live-streamed church services every Sunday. Although Lydia continues to require assistance with decision making, she demonstrates an increase in self-directing her care needs and expressing her opinion. Lydia is slowly regaining her locus of control. John and the family report seeing signs of "the old Lydia" when it comes to advocating for her needs and desires.

With all the positive changes noted, there are ongoing needs for adjustment and coping with change. Lydia's change in functional ability continues to require the support of her family and other persons. She requires 24-hour assistance with her care. She cannot remain in her home alone. During the daytime there is always a family member or a paid home health aide who assists with her care. John and his children plan their time carefully to meet their own and Lydia's personal care needs. Security measures were added to protect Lydia and their home. Lydia's health insurance will cover another brief period of rehabilitation (including occupational, physical, and speech therapy) under Medicare Part B as long as she continues to make gains in her functional abilities. The Medicare Part B level of care will be provided within Lydia's home or within an outpatient rehabilitation facility. Lydia and her family focus on her ability and recognition of the changes that she has made toward regaining function. The road ahead will continue to offer its achievements and challenges. The experience of disability has forever influenced their lives.

Authentic Engagement With the Client—Therapeutic Use of Self

Authentic engagement requires the occupational therapy practitioner to utilize mindful, effective communication strategies; use active listening; and apply sound clinical reasoning processes to gain knowledge of and collaboratively address the unique needs of the client and the disability experience as it changes through the continuum of care. While a methodical, linear approach to the occupational therapy process through the health care continuum may seem to be the most logical, this is most often not the case. The process of adjustment to loss and/or modifications in occupations, roles, and personal identity is highly personal and dependent on multiple factors both internal and external to the client. Therefore the effective practitioner can critically identify intersections in the continuum of care, where transitions with multiple possible outcomes occur, to address and meet the changing demands of the client's disability experience. Mindful engagement in client-centered care requires agility, flexibility, and multimodal reasoning skills to acknowledge and address the client's current needs while collaborating with the client and significant others to plan for the next phase of the disability experience within the continuum of care.

Ginny Stoffel, a former president of the American Occupational Therapy Association, stated: "Many of the essential elements of authentic occupational therapy are part of the foundation of our practice and involve a complex combination of factors, such as being person centered and recognizing the important occupations and environments that are part of a person's everyday life." Through the evolution of the therapeutic relationship, the occupational therapy practitioner develops an "understanding (of) the person, the occupations they want and need to engage in, the values that underlie their occupational roles, and the strengths and challenges found in their unique person—environment—occupation interface" (Strauss & Tinetti, 2009).

The concept of authentic practice lends itself well to a central tenet of occupational therapy: therapeutic use of self. Therapeutic use of self is an essential part of the occupational therapy process, whereby occupational therapy practitioners develop and manage their therapeutic relationship with clients by using principles of clinical reasoning, empathy, collaboration, and effective communication as the approach to service delivery (Taylor, 2020). Practitioners utilize themselves as therapeutic tools during the occupational therapy process to work toward developing a fundamental understanding of the client as a human being at an interpersonal level (Vargo, 1978). A "personal and subjective investment in the client" occurs "during which the therapist makes moment-to-moment decisions about how to initiate and respond to the client's reactions to therapy or the therapist" (Vargo, 1978).

The development of a collaborative relationship between the practitioner and the client fosters a better understanding of the client's experiences and desires for intervention (American Occupational Therapy Association (AOTA), 2014).

Clients bring to the occupational therapy process their knowledge about their life experiences and their hopes and dreams for the future. They identify and share their needs and priorities. Occupational therapy practitioners bring their knowledge about how engagement in occupation affects health, well-being, and participation; they use this information, coupled with theoretical perspectives and clinical reasoning, to critically observe, analyze, describe, and interpret human performance. Practitioners and clients, together with caregivers, family members, community members, and other stakeholders (as appropriate), identify and prioritize the focus of the intervention plan (p. S12) (American Occupational Therapy Association (AOTA), 2014).

Used throughout the occupational therapy process, collaboration "honors the contributions" of both the client and the practitioner (p. S12) (American Occupational Therapy Association (AOTA), 2014).

Mindful and effective interpersonal communication skills utilized by the occupational therapy practitioner facilitate a power shift in the collaborative relationship, allowing clients to reestablish their locus of control in decision making and problem solving throughout the occupational therapy process (American Occupational Therapy Association (AOTA), 2014). The development of a positive and respectful therapeutic relationship is an essential component to support effective interventions and outcomes (Cole & McLean, 2003) and provide a strong foundation for the development of flexibility and agility and the processes of clinical and professional reasoning.

Effective Communication Across the Continuum of Care

Effective communication is necessary to make meaningful connections. Our ability to communicate enables us to resolve conflict, build rapport and respect, consider new ideas, and solve problems. Lacking the ability to communicate effectively leads to conflict and misunderstanding. Effective communication requires a skill set that includes awareness of nonverbal communication, ability to listen, emotional intuitiveness, verbal communication skills (including attention to tone), and written communication skills (Davis & Rosee, 2015).

Regardless of the severity of a client's condition or level of function/ability, the occupational therapy practitioner's ability to engage the client and the family/significant others through effective communication will always be important. The client and significant others may be of a different culture (and/or ethnicity) than the occupational therapy practitioner and have strongly held values and beliefs that differ from the practitioner (Fitzgerald, 2004). Verbal communication provides directions, explains a treatment method, or expresses an idea. Nonverbal communication, such as smiles, frowns, and posture, reinforces or discourages a behavior or provides information regarding pleasure or displeasure. The occupational therapy practitioner who communicates effectively is objective, considers differing points of view, and attends to his or her (and the client's) verbal and nonverbal communication throughout the process of delivering care.

Case Application. References to ineffective communication strategies used by rehabilitation practitioners during their interactions with Lydia are significant during the early phase of her disability experience. The mindful and client-centered occupational therapy practitioner will engage in therapeutic use of self and use effective communication strategies that foster client and practitioner collaboration (Box 2.1).

BOX 2.1 Techniques for Communicating

The following is a selection of techniques that can be used to enhance the communication process between therapist and patients authored by Cheryl Joiner and Mary Hansel.

Use active listening techniques. Let people know you are interested in what they have to say and that you want to fully understand them. Free the area of distractions. Positioning yourself at their level and making eye contact tells them that you are attentive. Once patients know that you are interested in them as people and care about their needs, they are often more willing to engage in therapy.

Give choices. No matter how trivial they may seem, choices are important. If possible, offer selections among predetermined modalities. This practice helps patients have more control over what happens to them.

Problem solve to encourage involvement in the therapy process. Encourage clients to brainstorm to reinforce their worth and primary importance in the treatment effort.

Based on information from Joiner C, Hansel M: Empowering the geriatric client, OT Pract 1:2, 1996 *Joiner and Hansel (1996) Techniques for Communicating; and Practices to Foster Connection during Mindful Client-Centered Care for the Occupational Therapy Practitioner Zulman et al modified (2020).*

BOX 2.2 A Person-Centered Approach to Adaptive Equipment

- Provide education
- Identify the person in need
- Identify potential risk factors/behaviors
- Listen
- Provide education
- Promote person-environment fit
- Listen
- Provide choices
- Implement realistic solutions
- Provide education
- Follow up

Tips for Promoting Person-Environment Fit
Major points to consider when making recommendations for the modification of the home of an older adult are the following:

- Is the suggested adaptation acceptable to the person?
- Does the person understand why the adaptation is suggested?
- Is the adaptation aesthetically pleasing?
- Is the adaptation affordable, easy to obtain, and easy to apply?
- Is the person physically, emotionally, and cognitively capable of accepting the adaptation?

COMMUNICATING WITH FAMILY AND SIGNIFICANT OTHERS

The occupational therapy practitioner must develop skill in conveying information to the client's family/significant others. Health care regulations require that both the client and specified family members or significant others be informed about the type of interventions the client receives (Phillips, 2003). For many clients their family members and significant others are the most trusted people in their lives. Given the client's permission, the occupational therapy practitioner can work with the family/significant others to provide encouragement and to monitor follow-through (Taylor, 2012).

Case Application. Recognize the difference in Lydia's rehabilitation experience once her family engaged in advocacy to promote their inclusion in her care planning. The mindful occupational therapy practitioner will develop the occupational profile, perform an interest checklist, and perform a role checklist, among additional assessments and rapport-building activities, to develop occupation-based and client-centered goals and interventions in collaboration with the client and the family.

When communicating with families and significant others, explanations should be simple and provided in a respectful manner. Jargon and medical terminology should be avoided or minimized. The inclusion of effective communication strategies can promote client/practitioner collaboration and empower the client, family, and significant others to participate in the goal setting and intervention process (see Box 2.1) (*Minimum Data Set (MDS)*, 2011). The literature also shows support for collaborating with both the client and the family when making recommendations for environmental modification, equipment, and assistive devices (*Minimum Data Set (MDS)*, 2011).

Case Application. There is very little inclusion of Lydia and her family during the selection of devices and equipment that she will use when she returns to her home. Client and practitioner collaboration are not evident. Box 2.2 provides best strategies for promoting collaboration when introducing adaptive devices and equipment.

The occupational therapy practitioner who practices mindfulness during the occupational therapy process will attend to his or her ability to remain mentally present during client interactions. Zulman et al. (2020) recommend practices to foster presence and connection during the clinical encounter, including prepare with intention, listen intently and completely, agree on what matters most, connect with the client's story, and explore emotional cues. According to their study, these five practices have the potential to enhance (the practitioner's) presence and meaningful connection (with the client) during the clinical encounter (Zulman et al., 2020).

Occupational therapy practitioners must also consider the impact of a client's functional limitation on the family unit (i.e., familial role changes/role competence). Caregiver burden has been recognized as a major concern for the families/significant others of clients with significant functional limitation. Family members often feel overwhelmed when managing the care needs of their significant others who are disabled. Through effective communication and inclusion of the family and significant others in intervention and goal development, the practitioner can significantly reduce caregiver burden (Early, 2013; Humphrey & Corcoran, 2004; Livneh & Antonak, 2007). Concurrently, clients are often concerned about their changed role competence and their reliance on family and significant others to manage their care. Role competence refers to the client's "ability to effectively meet the demands of roles" (including past, current, and future roles) (American Occupational Therapy Association (AOTA), 2014, p. s8). The occupational therapy practitioner must acknowledge the client's adjustment to the change in role competence and address it within the goal-setting and intervention planning process.

Case Application. Within the case, it was noted that Lydia required 24-hour care, and John was feeling overwhelmed as he engaged in adjustment to her changed functional ability. John's feeling of being overwhelmed is a key component of caregiver burden. Often there is a sense of shame that accompanies this feeling for the caregiver. The mindful and emotionally attuned occupational therapy practitioner will recognize the signs of caregiver burden and the client's struggle with role competence. Support is needed for both the client and the caregiver(s). It is important for the occupational therapy practitioner to seek and utilize interprofessional resources to assist clients and caregivers with their needs. Within and beyond the timeframe of the case, caregiver burden and concerns regarding Lydia's role competence will surface.

An individual's religious and spiritual beliefs can be influential on his or her health and wellness outcomes. Most Americans continue to hold positive attitudes and beliefs about the efficacy of spiritual-related intervention (i.e., prayer) when coping and adjusting to disability (Crowther et al., 2002; Daaleman, 2009; Persson & Ryden, 2006). Within occupational therapy practice, spirituality is recognized as a basic human tenet (American Occupational Therapy Association (AOTA), 2014). It is suggested that prayer provides meaning, which may lessen depression/anxiety, paving a way to better long-term adjustments to a newly acquired disability (Dooley & Hinojosa, 2004). An individual may use their religious and / or spiritual beliefs as a strategy to cope, provide comfort, or motivation to achieve a task that would appear to be impossible. It is important for practitioners to consider an individual's religious beliefs and / or spirituality when designing and establishing interventions.

Case Application. A visit from her pastor was influential in lifting Lydia's spirits and increasing her motivation. Connections to her faith, both personal and virtual, proved to be important to Lydia as she copes and adjusts to her disability. A sense of hope and perceived self-efficacy enhanced by spiritual and religious beliefs and supports provided a strategy for coping and adjusting with change.

Supporting Psychosocial Adjustment to Disability

The attitude of the practitioners involved with the rehabilitation of disabled individuals is of great importance and may be highly influential in the person's response to rehabilitation. Negative reactions will result in a negative response in the client, decrease motivation, and decrease engagement. Ultimately a client's negative response to a practitioner's

---

BOX 2.3 Addressing Difficult Client Behaviors

The CALMER Approach

Catalyst for change—the patient is responsible, and we cannot change others. The question is how we can support change for the person.

Alter thoughts to change feelings—when uncomfortable feelings arise, take time to reflect on them and the thinking behind them; change the thinking and the feelings will shift.

Listen to determine what the problem is.

Make an agreement, which might be a restatement of the established plan. Make time for the client to rephrase the plan and ask questions.

Educate the client about what he or she should be doing now and before the next visit.

Reach out and discuss your feelings with your supervisor and other professional supports.

From Pomm H, Shahady E, Pomm R. The CALMER approach: teaching learners six steps to serenity when dealing with difficult patients. *Fam Med.* 2004;36:467-469.

---

negative attitude may lead to uncooperative behavior and the labeling of the client as difficult (Costa, 2008). Box 2.3 provides resources to help with communication with a client exhibiting difficult behaviors. Is the client difficult, or is his or her behavior a reaction to a negative (care-based) experience and/or adjustment to disability?

Physical illness or injury resulting in disability is a significant life stressor to which the individual brings a unique repertoire of coping mechanisms and response patterns (Patnaude, 2017). The disability experience may cause minimal or no prolonged effect on personality. However, an individual's behavior and emotions may be temporarily disordered by the crisis of physical change. Fluctuations in physical recovery and psychosocial adaptation, rather than a direct and sustained movement toward adjustment, should be expected (Chan & Spencer, 2004). There may be phase(s) within the client's disability experience in which adjustment and ability to cope may become extremely challenging. During these periods of emotional and/or physical challenge, the client may verbally or nonverbally express a lack of motivation or the client's behavior may become difficult to manage. These phases may occur at any point throughout the continuum of care. For most individuals, over time, the personality appears to be capable of drawing on its resources and integrating the crisis experience (Stoffel, 2014).

Strategies for Working With the So-Called Difficult Client

Clients who are uncooperative, who exhibit manipulative or challenging behaviors, or who appear overly dependent or unmotivated are frequently labeled difficult by staff. Although it may be difficult to work with such clients, the key to success lies in understanding the barriers to participation from the client's point of view (Early, 2013). Costa (2008) reports that the occupational therapy practitioner must attend to why the individual is engaging in the difficult behavior. Some clients have dysfunctional family histories, others are in unrelenting pain that has not been adequately addressed, and some may have had prior negative experience with health care providers. Asking questions and listening to what the client says are important first steps. The mindful and client-centered occupational therapy practitioner will use therapeutic modes such as empathizing, encouraging, and collaborating (Taylor, 2008; Taylor & Van Puymbroeck, 2013).

MacCormac (Mills & Coulanges, 2013) lists factors that may be contributing to the behavior of the client who seems unmotivated:

- Anxiety about the therapy process
- Fatigue
- Communication barriers
- Vision or hearing impairment
- Cognitive deficits
- Fear of failure
- Grief
- Worry over finances or the future
- Frustration over slow progress
- Depression (and associated problems such as poor sleep)
- Problems with social support from family and others

These factors illustrate the importance of identifying the root of the problem behavior. Each factor might call for a different response from the occupational therapy practitioner.

Case Application. During the early phase of her care, Lydia experienced many of the factors noted by MacCormac. The occupational therapy practitioner will use effective communication, therapeutic use of self, and clinical reasoning to engage the client and provide empathy.

As for managing difficult behavior and crafting a therapeutic response, several strategies have been proposed. The CALMER approach developed by Pomm et al. (2004) includes strategies that are relevant for addressing the needs of the client who presents with difficult behavior. In this approach, the occupational therapy practitioner would first recognize or remind oneself that the client is the one who is responsible for change. The second step is to alter thoughts to change feelings, which helps the practitioner identify what the client is thinking and reflect on personal responses. The third step is to listen in order to understand the problem. The fourth is to make an agreement or contract with the client, which might be a restatement of a prior agreement or plan. The fifth is to educate the client about what to do between this meeting and the next. The last is to reach out and discuss feelings with supervisors or other support systems. The CALMER approach provides systematic steps that help the clinician distance oneself from the client's behavior, avoid taking the behavior personally, and place the responsibility for change on the client, while offering the client empathy and support (see Box 2.3) (Early, 2013).

Case Application. Throughout the case there are periods in which Lydia would benefit from the inclusion of the approaches of Costa, MacCormac, Pomm et al., and Zulman et al. Utilizing the strategies discussed within the chapter, the occupational therapy practitioner must foster connection with Lydia to support her adjustment and progression within her disability experience.

Professional Reasoning and Clinical Reasoning in Occupational Therapy

Application for Mindful and Client-Centered Occupational Therapy Practice. **Clinical reasoning**, embedded in the core tenet of therapeutic use of self, is utilized by occupational therapy practitioners throughout the occupational therapy process to facilitate the client's understanding of "the information they are receiving in the intervention process, to discover meaning, and to build hope" (p. S12) (American Occupational Therapy Association (AOTA), 2014). **Professional reasoning**, the most current term adopted to describe the clinical reasoning of the occupational therapy practitioner, is a complex, multifaceted, metacognitive process utilized to "plan, direct, perform, and reflect on client care" (Boyt Schell, 2014). Professional reasoning is broader in scope than clinical reasoning as it encompasses both medical and nonmedical settings and the manner in which "outcomes of the reasoning process influence actions and outcomes of service delivery" (p. 188) (Pomm et al., 2004).

The occupational therapy practitioner considers and applies information from the client's story (narrative reasoning), the diagnosis or condition (procedural/scientific reasoning), the place on the continuum of care where services are being rendered (pragmatic reasoning), the risks and benefits of therapeutic interventions (ethical reasoning), and continuous collaborative communication (interactive reasoning) to devise an integrated, client-centered, evidence-based, flexible intervention plan that is able to respond to changes in the client and multiple, potential outcomes (conditional reasoning) (Boyt Schell, 2014; Pomm et al., 2004). Application of all levels of professional reasoning is necessary for the occupational therapy process to be effective. The occupational therapy practitioner must rapidly synthesize all the information available in any given situation and respond to address the emerging and ongoing needs of the client. Through repeated experience, application of evidence-based practice, and engagement in **reflective practice**, the practitioner moves from novice to expert, becoming adept at shifting from one type of reasoning to another throughout the occupational therapy process. Following is a brief description of the aspects of professional reasoning with an example of direct application to the case of Lydia and questions for situational query within each professional reasoning description.

Narrative Reasoning

Narrative reasoning provides the opportunity for clients to tell their story. This allows the occupational therapy practitioner to understand each client's own personal perceptions of the disability experience. The client's narrative is used to construct the occupational profile as information about the client's occupational history and experiences, patterns of daily living, interests, values, and needs is shared at the beginning of the occupational therapy process (American Occupational Therapy Association (AOTA), 2014). Central to effective narrative reasoning is the practitioner's ability to use active listening and to provide the basis for a positive therapeutic relationship. The practitioner may also tell his or her own stories when applicable to explain occupational therapy or experiences with clients in similar situations. Sharing of stories can help to create a strong bond between the client and the practitioner. Stoffel (2014) emphasized that as authentic practitioners, we offer "professional perspectives and the lived experiences we have had that might relate to the everyday life challenges they want to overcome. When our clients' occupational profiles are different from our own, we don't pretend that we know what their life is like; rather, we ask them to show us or tell us a story so we can better understand how to help them return to those meaningful desired roles, p. 631."

Case Application. Lydia shared with her daughter, the occupational therapist, that the members of the rehabilitation team seldom spoke to her directly about her care when family members were in the room. Narrative reasoning was not effectively applied to elicit the client's full participation in the therapeutic experience in the acute rehabilitation facility.

Conversely, in the subacute setting Lydia's family engaged in advocacy for Lydia and their involvement in her care plan as soon as she was admitted into her new setting. Her goals and interests were shared with the rehabilitation staff. Her request to be included within care plan decisions and to be spoken to in a direct and age-appropriate manner was discussed. Lydia and her family became more adept at navigating the rehabilitation and nursing care environment to optimize her participation in goal planning and engagement in meaningful activity. There was a significant change in her perceived self-efficacy. Lydia and her family were able to begin to realize and focus on her ability.

Questions that apply to narrative reasoning include "What is this person's life story?" "How has the health condition affected the person's life story or ability to continue his or her life story?" and "What occupational activities are the person's priorities?" (Boyt Schell, 2014).

Scientific/Procedural Reasoning

Scientific/procedural reasoning occurs when the practitioner considers the diagnosis or condition of the presenting client. Utilizing foundational knowledge from the sciences (anatomy and physiology, psychology, human development, pathophysiology, etc.), the practitioner understands the condition and formulates a hypothesis about the clinical image of the client (Pomm et al., 2004). Procedural reasoning often begins even before the occupational therapy practitioner meets the client. Information about the client, including the diagnosis or condition, is received with the referral for occupational therapy services. Based on the information in the referral, the practitioner may select theoretical models and assessments.

Case Application. How will the mindful and client-centered occupational therapy practitioner apply the following questions indicative of scientific/procedural reasoning to Lydia's case?

Questions that apply to scientific/procedural reasoning include "What is the nature of the illness, injury, or developmental problem?" "What are the common impairments that may result from the condition?" and "What theoretical models support the selection of assessments and interventions?" (Boyt Schell, 2014).

Pragmatic Reasoning

Pragmatic reasoning addresses the practical issues that impact service delivery within the context where services occur (Boyt Schell, 2014; Pomm et al., 2004). Pragmatic reasoning considers both the context of the practice setting, including the availability of resources (personnel, space, and equipment), reimbursement for services, the realities of service delivery within the setting, and the availability of family and caregiver support, and the context of the practitioners themselves related to service competence within the setting. This type of contextual reasoning allows the practitioner to identify realistic strategies for intervention to ensure the provision of appropriate care (Pomm et al., 2004).

Case Application. How will the mindful and client-centered occupational therapy practitioner apply the following questions indicative of pragmatic reasoning to Lydia's case?

Questions that apply to pragmatic reasoning include "What are the constraints of the practice setting?" "Who is paying for services and what are the guidelines for reimbursement?" "What family resources are available to support interventions?" and "What are my service competencies?" (Boyt Schell, 2014).

Ethical Reasoning

Ethical reasoning ensures that choices made during the occupational therapy process are morally justified and are in the best interest of the client (Pomm et al., 2004). The risks and benefits of interventions are considered to ensure safety. The *Occupational Therapy Code of Ethics* (American Occupational Therapy Association (AOTA), 2014) provides the foundation for ethical practice and ethical reasoning and guides the practitioner's ability to make decisions when faced with ethical dilemmas.

Case Application. How will the mindful and client-centered occupational therapy practitioner apply the following questions indicative of ethical reasoning to Lydia's case?

Questions that apply to ethical reasoning include "Are the benefits of the intervention worth the cost?" and "What should I do if I see a coworker engaging a client in an intervention that is contraindicated?" (Boyt Schell, 2014).

Interactive Reasoning

Interactive reasoning is the use of mindful, effective communication to build trust and a positive interpersonal relationship between the practitioner and the client. This is a collaborative process utilized to identify successes and solve problems during the occupational therapy process. The stories begun with narrative reasoning evolve as the continuum of care changes. The practitioner may utilize both verbal and nonverbal strategies to communicate support and to motivate the client's full participation (Boyt Schell, 2014).

Case Application. How will the mindful and client-centered occupational therapy practitioner apply the following questions indicative of interactive reasoning to Lydia's case?

Questions that apply to interactive reasoning include "How can I encourage and reassure the client?" "How can I best relate to this situation?" and "How can I put this client at ease?"

Conditional Reasoning

Conditional reasoning is a blending of all forms of professional reasoning. It allows the therapist to reason on multiple levels simultaneously to make modifications in interventions "in response to changes in conditions and to the context within which therapy is occurring" (p. 392) (Boyt Schell, 2014). The occupational therapy practitioner's ability to anticipate several possible outcomes or to envision multiple futures is based on experience and the ability to agilely interpret and apply current information. Therefore conditional reasoning ability is developed over time as the practitioner goes from novice to expert within his or her career trajectory.

Case Application. How will the mindful and client-centered occupational therapy practitioner apply the following questions indicative of conditional reasoning to Lydia's case?

Questions that apply to conditional reasoning include "How will the multiple intervention options play out given the client's health conditions, social situation, economic status, and culture?" and "Given these possible futures, what is the best action to take now?" (Boyt Schell, 2014).

Theoretical Models to Guide Practice

Utilizing effective strategies to understand the individual's occupational profile, roles, and strategy for adjusting to disability, the mindful and client-centered practitioner will apply clinical reasoning and select theoretical models to guide practice for evidence-based outcomes. The model of human occupation and Erickson's eight stages of psychosocial development are two of many potential theoretical frameworks to guide the occupational therapy process. The basic tenets of these theoretical models provide a lens through which the reader can consider the goals and hoped-for outcomes of the client, family, and practitioner within Lydia's case.

Kielhofner and Burke's 1980 model of human occupation is a useful model for considering the effects of disability on an individual. The occupational therapy practitioner who frames the occupational therapy process around this model may ask the following questions:
- What skills, habits, and roles has the individual lost or reduced resultant of this disability?

- What is the individual's sense of personal causation?
- What are the individual's values and interests?
- What is the individual's social and object environment?
- Most importantly, which interventions will assist in increasing the individual's sense of personal causation and ability to have more control within his or her environment? (Early, 2013)

Case Application. How will the mindful and client-centered occupational therapy practitioner apply Kielhofner and Burke's model of human occupation to Lydia's case? Which aspects of the case provide information for reflection and development of client-centered and occupation-based goals and intervention?

Erickson's eight stages of psychosocial development (Erickson, 1963) may be used to guide the psychosocial aspects of the occupational therapy process for a client with a physical disability. The stage in life in which an individual acquires a disability may influence his or her response and adjustment to it. Each stage of psychosocial development has its own task requirements and will influence the way an individual adjusts to the disability. With attention to the individual's age and stage within his or her psychosocial development, the occupational therapy practitioner who includes this model within the occupational therapy process may ask the following questions:
- What is this person's developmental stage?
- What developmental task(s) might be challenging for this individual?
- Based on this information, what concerns or responses might I expect from this individual?
- How can I assist this individual with identifying, stating, and achieving personal goals? (Early, 2013)

Case Application. How will the mindful and client-centered occupational therapy practitioner apply Erickson's stages of psychosocial development to Lydia's case? Which aspects of the case provide information for reflection and development of client-centered and occupation-based goals and intervention?

Developing Appropriate Occupational Therapy Goals

Goal development, although broad in nature, must reflect the client's goals and values and attend to where the client is within the process of adjusting to disability. The occupational therapy practitioner must be well versed in a variety of theoretically based interventions that are grounded in sound research and evidence (American Occupational Therapy Association (AOTA), 2014). As previously discussed, interventions are best conducted when the occupational therapy practitioner, the client, and families/significant others collaborate on the plan, and the practitioner is mindful and emotionally attuned to the client's needs (Byers-Connon & Park, 2004). The occupational therapy process is a dynamic and interactive process (American Occupational Therapy Association (AOTA), 2014). Client-practitioner interaction should be utilized throughout the process to promote client engagement in occupation. The successful intervention engages the client in meaningful activities to support participation in desired occupations (American Occupational Therapy Association (AOTA), 2014).

Case Application. Within the subacute rehabilitation phase of her care, Lydia and her family learned to advocate for her care needs with the nursing and rehabilitation practitioners involved in her care. The involvement of her family in the goal and care planning process enabled improved outcomes and increased satisfaction with the care delivery process. Further, Lydia demonstrated increased participation in leisure and social activities.

REFLECTION ON THE DISABILITY EXPERIENCE OF LYDIA AND THE COMPONENTS OF MINDFUL AND CLIENT-CENTERED PRACTICE FOR THE OCCUPATIONAL THERAPY PRACTITIONER

There are many variations of an individual's disability experience. The case study of Lydia is one representation of disability experience that spans the continuum of care. Perspectives on disability can be rigid or flexible throughout the continuum of care. The case of Lydia reveals that adjustment to disability is a dynamic process for the individual and all persons involved (including but not limited to the family/significant others and the health care professionals who participate in her care). The severity of the disability (temporary or permanent), socioeconomic status, access to health care, health care coverage, values, culture, context, and environment are all variables (among others) that influence an individual's disability experience.

SUMMARY

All aspects of the domain of occupational therapy require ongoing consideration for mindful care to be provided by the occupational therapy practitioner throughout the occupational therapy process. Aspects of the domain of occupational therapy include occupations, client factors, performance skills, performance patterns, and contexts and environments. "All aspects of the domain transact to support engagement, participation, and health" (American Occupational Therapy Association (AOTA), 2014, p. s4).

Everyone's experience of disability is unique and requires the practitioner's intentional engagement to provide mindful client-centered care while utilizing effective strategies. The case of Lydia includes situational concepts for the occupational therapy practitioner to query, consider, and address throughout the occupational therapy process and within each aspect of the continuum of care. Each concept should be explored regarding its influence on the client, the family/significant others, and the role of the occupational therapy practitioner. The psychosocial components that influence a client's physical disability experience must be realized and addressed by the occupational therapy practitioner throughout each phase of the continuum of care. It is the occupational therapy practitioner's ethical responsibility to use the comprehensive skill set indicative of reflective and authentic occupational therapy practice.

REFERENCES

American Occupational Therapy Association (AOTA). (2014). Occupational therapy practice framework: domain and process. 3rd ed. *American Journal Occupational Therapy*, 68(1), S1–S5, S12.

Boyt Schell, B. A. (2014). Professional reasoning in practice. In B. A. Boyt Schell, G. Gillen, & M. E. Scaffa (Eds.), *Willard and Spackman's occupational therapy* (12th ed.). Baltimore, MD: Lippincott Williams and Wilkins.

Byers-Connon, S, & Park, S. (2004). Opportunities for best practice in various settings. In: S. Byers-Connon, H. Lohman & R. Padilla (Eds)., *Occupational therapy with elders: Strategies for the COTA* (2nd ed.). St. Louis: Mosby.

Chan, J., & Spencer, J. (2004). Adaptation to hand injury: an evolving experience. *American Journal of Occupational Therapy*, 58, 128–139.

Cole, B., & McLean, V. (2003). Therapeutic relationships redefined. *Occupational Therapy Mental Health*, 19, 33–56. http://dx.doi.org/10.1300/J004v19n02_03.

Costa, D. M. (2008). Working with the "difficult" client. *OT Practice*, 13(13), 15–18.

Crowther, M. R., Parker, M. W., Achenbaum, W. A., et al. (2002). Rowe and Kahn's model of successful aging revisited: positive spirituality—the forgotten factor. *Gerontologist*, 42(5), 613–620.

Daaleman, T. P. (2009). Spirituality. In: J. B. Halter, J. G. Ouslander, & M. E. Tinetti (Eds.), *Hazzard's geriatric medicine and gerontology* (6th ed.). San Francisco, CA: McGraw Hill Medical.

Dooley, R. H., & Hinojosa, J. (2004). Improving quality of life for persons with Alzheimer's disease and their family caregivers: brief occupational therapy intervention. *American Journal of Occupational Therapy*, 58(5), 561–569.

Early, M. B. (2013). The disability experience and the therapeutic process. In M. B. Early (Ed.), *Physical dysfunction practice skills for the occupational therapy assistant*. St. Louis, MO: Elsevier.

Erikson, E. (1963). *Childhood and society*. New York, NY: Norton.

Fitzgerald, M. H. (2004). A dialogue on occupational therapy, culture, and families. *American Journal Occupational Therapy*, 58(5), 489–498.

Humphrey, R., & Corcoran, M. (2004). Exploring the role of family in occupation and family occupations. *American Journal Occupational Therapy*, 58(5), 487–488.

Kielhofner, G., & Burke, J. P. (1980). A model of human occupation, part 1. Conceptual framework and content. *American Journal of Occupational Therapy*, 34, 572–581.

Livneh, H., & Antonak, R. F. (2007). Psychological adaptation to chronic illness and disability. In: A. E. Dell Orto, & P. W. Power (Eds.), *The psychological and social impact of physical disability* (5th ed.). New York, NY: Springer.

MacCormac, B. A. (2010). Reaching the unmotivated client. *OT Practice*, 15(4), 15–19.

Mills, M. D., & Coulanges, K. (2013). The older adult. In M. B. Early (Ed.), *Physical dysfunction practice skills for the occupational therapy assistant*. St. Louis, MO: Elsevier.

Minimum Data Set (MDS). (2011). - *Version 3.0 resident assessment and care screening nursing home comprehensive (NC) item set*. Myers & Stauffer. Baltimore, MD: Centers for Medicare and Medicaid.

Patnaude, M. E. (2017). Clinical reasoning. In K. Jacobs, & N. MacRae (Eds.), *Occupational therapy essentials for clinical competence* (3rd ed.). Thorofare, NJ: Slack, Inc.

Persson, L., & Ryden, A. (2006). Themes of effective coping in physical disability: an interview study of 26 people who have learnt to live with their disability. *Scandinavian Journal of Caring Sciences, 20,* 355—363.

Phillips, I. (2003). Infusing spirituality into geriatric healthcare. *Top Geriatr Rehabil, 19*(4), 249—256.

Pomm, H., Shahady, E., & Pomm, R. (2004). The CALMER approach: teaching learners six steps to serenity when dealing with difficult patients. *Family Medicine, 36,* 467—469.

Stoffel, V. C. (2014). Presidential address, 2014—attitude, authenticity, and action: building capacity. *American Journal of Occupational Therapy, 68,* 628—635. http://dx.doi.org/10.5014/ajot.2014.686002.

Strauss, S. E., & Tinetti, M. E. (2009). Evaluation, management, and decision making with the older patient. In: J. B. Halter, J. G. Ouslander, & M. E. Tinetti (Eds.), *Hazzard's geriatric medicine and gerontology* (6th ed.) San Francisco, CA: McGraw Hill Medical.

Taylor, R. R. (2008). *The intentional relationship: occupational therapy and use of self.* Philadelphia, PA: FA Davis.

Taylor, R. R. (2012). Pain, fear, and avoidance: therapeutic use of self with difficult occupational therapy populations. *American Journal of Occupational Therapy, 66,* 495—496.

Taylor, R. R. (2020). *The intentional relationship: Occupational therapy and use of self (2nd ed.).* Philadelphia, PA: FA Davis.

Taylor, R. R., & Van Puymbroeck, L. (2013). Therapeutic use of self: applying the intentional relationship model in group therapy. In J. C. O'Brien, & J. W. Solomon (Eds.), *Occupational analysis and group process* (pp. 36—52). St. Louis, MO: Elsevier.

Vargo, J. W. (1978). Some psychological effects of physical disability. *American Journal Occupational Therapy, 32,* 31.

Zulman, D. M., Haversfield, M. C., Shaw, J. G., Brown-Johnson, C. G., Schwartz, R., Tierney, A. A., et al. (2020). Practices to foster physician presence and connection with patients in the clinical encounter. *Journal of the American Medical Association, 323*(1), 70—80.

3

Infection Control and Safety Issues in the Clinic

Dana Shah

OBJECTIVES

After reading this chapter, the student or the occupational therapy practitioner will be able to do the following:

- Recognize the role of occupational therapists and occupational therapy assistants in preventing accidents.
- Identify recommendations for safety in the clinic.
- Identify standard precautions and recognize the importance of following them with all clients.
- Describe proper techniques of hand washing.
- Recognize the importance of having all health care workers understand and follow isolation procedures used in patient care.

- Identify procedures for handling patient injuries.
- Describe guidelines for handling various emergency situations.
- Describe preventive positioning for clients with lower extremity amputations, rheumatoid arthritis, burns, and hemiplegia.
- Describe the purpose of special equipment.
- Identify precautions when treating clients who require special equipment.

KEY TERMS

Universal precautions
Standard precautions
Decontamination
Sterilization
Disinfectants
Isolation
Protective isolation
Shock
Seizures
Insulin reaction
Acidosis
Cardiopulmonary resuscitation
Fowler position
Intravenous lines

Turning frame
Ventilator
Endotracheal tube
Electrocardiogram
Pulmonary artery catheter
Intracranial pressure monitoring
Arterial monitoring line
Nasogastric tube
Gastric tube
Intravenous feeding
Total parenteral nutrition
Hyperalimentation
Infusion pump
Urinary catheter

INTRODUCTION

Occupational therapists (OTs) and occupational therapy assistants (OTAs) facilitate meaningful engagement in occupation. Occupational engagement requires a safe and comfortable environment (American Occupational Therapy Association (AOTA), 2014). Adherence to infection control and safety guidelines across all health care settings plays a large role in providing that safe and comfortable environment (American Occupational Therapy Association (AOTA), 2014; Centers for Disease Control and Prevention, 2017). OTs and OTAs play an important role in creating a safe environment. In the current health care delivery system, OTs and OTAs treat clients with serious and critical illnesses that require specialized equipment and knowledge of advanced safety procedures

(George, 2018). Therefore it is important for them to be aware of guidelines for handling various emergency situations and keep up to date on all recent changes.

SAFETY RECOMMENDATIONS FOR THE CLINIC

The prevention of accidents and subsequent injuries begins with consistent use of safety recommendations and infection control procedures for any health care setting, from ensuring you are working with the correct client to washing your hands before and after working with every client (Box 3.1) and by knowing where all essential safety equipment is located

---

BOX 3.1 Safety Recommendations for the Clinic

1. Wash hands for at least 40 to 60 seconds (American Occupational Therapy Association (AOTA), 2014; George, 2018) before and after treating each patient to reduce cross-contamination. Ensure that you are utilizing the proper personal protective equipment to prevent the spread of infection as well.
2. Make sure you are working with the correct patient, under the correct set of medical orders.
3. Make sure adequate space to maneuver equipment is available. Place clients where they may be protected from bumps by equipment or passing personnel. Keep the area free from clutter.
4. Do not attempt to transfer clients in congested areas or in areas where your view is blocked.
5. Routinely check equipment to be sure it is working properly.
6. Ensure that furniture and equipment in the clinic are stable. When not in use, store items out of the way of the treatment area.
7. Keep the floor free of cords, scatter rugs, litter, and spills. Avoid highly polished floors, which may be slippery.
8. Do not leave clients unattended. Use restraint belts properly to protect the clients when they are not closely observed. Follow correct protocols for restraint use (Nazarko, 2008).
9. Have the treatment area and supplies ready before the patient arrives.
10. Allow only properly trained personnel to provide patient care.
11. Follow the manufacturer's and facility's procedures for handling and storage of potentially hazardous material. Be sure such materials are marked and stored in a place in clear view. Do not store items above shoulder height.
12. Ensure that emergency exits and evacuation routes are clearly indicated.
13. Have emergency equipment such as fire extinguishers and first-aid kits readily available.

BOX 3.2 Summary of Standard Precautions

1. Wash hands immediately with soap and water before and after examining clients and after any contact with blood, body fluids, and contaminated item regardless of whether gloves were worn. Soaps containing an antimicrobial agent are recommended. Avoid wearing artificial fingernails.
2. Wear clean, ordinary thin gloves anytime there is contact with blood, body fluids, mucous membrane, and broken skin. Change gloves between tasks or procedures on the same patient. Before going to another patient, remove gloves promptly and wash hands immediately. Then don new gloves.
3. Wear a mask, protective eyewear, and gown during any patient care activity when splashes or sprays of body fluids are likely. Remove the soiled gown as soon as possible and wash hands.
4. Handle needles and other sharp instruments safely. Do not recap needles. Ensure that contaminated equipment is not reused with another patient until it has been cleaned, disinfected, and sterilized properly. Dispose of nonreusable needles, syringes, and other sharp patient care instruments in puncture-resistant containers.
5. Routinely clean and disinfect frequently touched surfaces, including beds, bed rails, patient examination tables, and bedside tables.
6. Clean and disinfect soiled linens and launder them safely. Avoid direct contact with items soiled with blood and body fluids.
7. Place a patient whose blood or body fluids are likely to contaminate surfaces or other clients in an isolation room or area.
8. To avoid injury or accidental exposure, minimize the use of invasive procedures.

(fire extinguishers, etc.). Although these recommendations seem to be common sense, it is important to make a conscious effort to use them in practice. Some questions to ask yourself include "When was the last time I washed my hands today?" "When was the last time I touched my face?" "What types of potential contamination occurred between those two events?" We know that we must maintain personal hygiene, yet it is often forgotten in the multiple tasks and demands of our lives/jobs; because of this, we suffer the consequences of exposure to germs. We must protect our clients from such careless contamination and provide the safest care we have been trained to do.

PATIENT SAFETY

The (Joint Commission's) National Patient Safety Goals (The Joint commision, 2010; Tarrac, 2008) begins with the goal of improving accuracy of patient identification before any procedure or treatment. OTs and OTAs should always use two ways to identify clients prior to any form of treatment (i.e., name and date of birth). The rest of the safety goals vary slightly across settings but include improving staff communication, using medicines safely, using alarms safely, infection prevention, identifying patient safety risks, and preventing mistakes in surgery. The complete list of goals and recommendations for performance of them is available from the referenced website (Tarrac, 2008).

INFECTION CONTROL

Infection control procedures are used to prevent the spread of diseases and infection among clients, health care workers, and others (State of Arizona, 2010). They are designed to interrupt or establish barriers to the infection cycle even when the source of infection is undetermined. The Centers for Disease Control and Prevention (CDC) first established **universal precautions** to protect the health care worker from infectious diseases such as human immunodeficiency virus (HIV), acquired immunodeficiency syndrome (AIDS), and hepatitis B virus (HBV). The CDC revised that information and now promotes **standard precautions** (Centers for Disease Control and Prevention, 2017; Tarrac, 2008) and transmission-based precautions (Box 3.2; Fig. 3.1) to apply to all body fluids, broken skin, and mucous membranes. These precautions are effective only when used with all clients, every single time, not only those identified as infected.

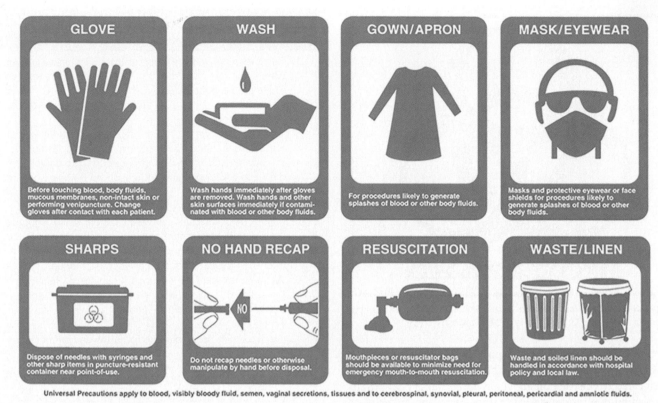

Fig. 3.1 Universal blood and body fluid precautions. (Courtesy Brevis Corp., Salt Lake City, Utah.)

The US Occupational Safety and Health Administration (OSHA) issues regulations to protect the employees of health care facilities. All treatment settings must comply with the following federal regulations (US Department of Labor, 2010):
1. Educate employees on the methods of transmission and the prevention of HBV and HIV.
2. Provide safe and adequate protective equipment and teach the employees where it is located and how to use it.
3. Teach employees about work practices used to prevent occupational transmission of disease, including but not limited to standard precautions, proper handling of patient specimens and linens, proper cleaning of body fluid spills (Fig. 3.2), and proper waste disposal.
4. Provide proper containers for the disposal of waste and sharp items; teach employees the color-coding system used to distinguish infectious waste.
5. Post warning labels and biohazard signs (Fig. 3.3).
6. Offer the hepatitis B vaccine to employees at substantial risk of occupational exposure to HBV.
7. Provide education and follow-up care to employees who are exposed to communicable disease.

OSHA has also outlined the responsibilities of health care employees, which include the following:
1. Use protective equipment and clothing provided by the facility whenever the employee comes in contact—or anticipates coming in contact—with body fluids.
2. Dispose of waste in proper containers, using knowledge and understanding of the handling of infectious waste and color-coded bags or containers.

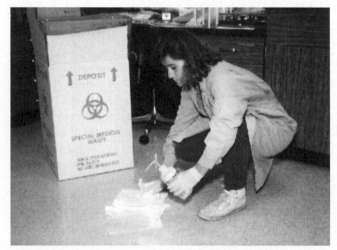

Fig. 3.2 Spills of body fluids must be cleaned up by a gloved employee, who should use paper towels and dispose of them in an infectious waste container. Then 5.25% sodium hypochlorite (household bleach) diluted 1:10 should be used to disinfect the area. (From Zakus SM. *Clinical Procedures for Medical Assistants*. 3rd ed. St. Louis, MO: Mosby; 1995.)

3. Dispose of sharp instruments and needles into proper containers without attempting to recap, bend, break, or otherwise manipulate them before disposal.
4. Keep the work and patient care areas clean.
5. Wash hands immediately after removing gloves and at all other times required by hospital or agency policy.

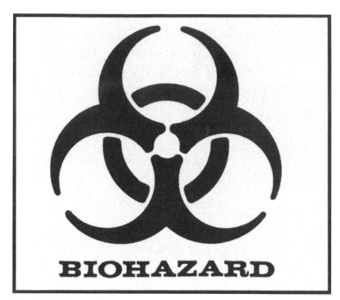

Fig. 3.3 Biohazard label. (From Zakus SM. *Clinical Procedures for Medical Assistants.* 3rd ed. St. Louis, MO: Mosby; 1995.)

6. Immediately report any exposures (e.g., needle sticks, blood splashes) or any personal illnesses to the supervisor and receive instruction about any further follow-up action.

Although eliminating all pathogens from an area or object is impossible, the risk of infection transmission can be greatly reduced. The largest source of preventable patient infection is contamination from the hands of health care workers (American Occupational Therapy Association (AOTA), 2014). Hand washing (Box 3.3) and gloves are the most effective barriers to the infection cycle. There are five opportunities for hand hygiene identified by the World Health Organization (World Health Organization, 2010). All health care workers should clean their hands (1) before touching a patient, (2) before clean/aseptic procedures, (3) after body fluid exposure/risk, (4) after touching a patient, and (5) after touching patient surroundings (Fig. 3.4). Additional personal protection measures include wearing caps, masks, and gowns and properly disposing of sharp instruments, contaminated dressings, and bed linens. Facial, or fit, masks come in various sizes; therapists should know their own size or be fitted by appropriate personnel. Be aware if you must wear long-sleeved garments so that the sleeves do not come in contact with pathogens. Hand sanitizers are being used frequently, sometimes placed in every clinic and patient room, and have their own guidelines for use (Centers for Disease Control and Prevention, 2017).

In the clinic, general cleanliness and proper control of heat, light, and air are also important for infection control. Spills should be cleaned up promptly. Work areas and equipment should be kept free from contamination.

Decontamination is a physical or chemical process of removing or inactivating pathogens on a surface or item to the point where they will not transmit infectious particles. This makes the surface or item safe for handling, use, or disposal. **Sterilization** is used to destroy all forms of microbial life, including highly resistant bacterial spores. Items to be sterilized or decontaminated should first be thoroughly cleaned to remove any residual matter. There are multiple methods used to sterilize items, including steam under pressure, ethylene oxide, dry heat, and immersion in sterilizing chemicals.

A variety of **disinfectants** may be used to clean environmental surfaces and reusable instruments. When using liquid disinfectants and cleaning agents, gloves are worn to protect the skin from repeated or prolonged contact. The CDC, local health department, or hospital infection control department can provide information regarding the best product and method to use.

A newer type of disinfection process seen in hospital settings is the use of ultraviolet (UV) lights. The UV light is placed in the room when the patient is discharged, and the combination of UVA, UVB, and UVC lights utilizes short wavelength UV radiation that kills microorganisms. The benefits of such a system are (a) it is chemical free, (b) it does not require the handling or storage of toxic chemicals, and (c) it eliminates human error. *Clostridium difficile (C. diff.)*, methicillin-resistant *Staphylococcus aureus* (MRSA), and vancomycin-resistant enterococci (VRE) are types of infections seen frequently in the hospital setting. The UV light systems are much more effective in killing these types of infections.

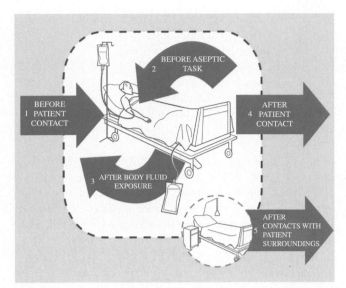

Fig. 3.4 Five opportunities for hand hygiene identified. (Sax et al., 2007)

BOX 3.4 **Summary of Transmission Risk Precautions**

Airborne Transmission
- Place the patient in an airborne infection isolation room (AIIR) where air is not circulated to the rest of the health facility. Make sure the room has a door that can be closed.
- Wear a respirator or other biosafety mask when working with the patient or in the patient's room.
- Limit patient movement from the room to other areas. If possible, place a surgical mask on the patient who must be moved.
- Wash hands thoroughly upon entering and leaving room.

Droplet Transmission
- Place the patient in an isolation room.
- Wear a respirator or other biosafety mask when working with the patient.
- Limit patient movement from the room to other areas. If patient must be moved, place a surgical mask on the patient.

Contact Transmission
- Place the patient in an isolation room and limit access.
- Wear gloves during contact with patient and with infectious body fluids or contaminated items. Reinforce hand washing throughout the health facility.
- Wear two layers of protective clothing.
- Limit patient movement from the isolation room to other areas.
- Avoid sharing equipment between clients. Designate equipment for each patient, if supplies allow. If sharing equipment is unavoidable, clean and disinfect it before use with the next patient.

Modified from Siegel JD, Rhinehart E, Jackson M, Chiarello L, Healthcare Infection Control Practices Advisory Committee. Guideline for isolation precautions: preventing transmission of infectious agents in healthcare settings. Centers for Disease Control and Prevention Web site. http://www.cdc.gov/infectioncontrol/pdf/guidelines/isolation-guidelines-H.pdf. Accessed October 28, 2010.

Instruments and equipment used to treat a patient should be cleaned or disposed of according to institutional or agency policies and procedures. Only one client at a time should use small equipment/tools such as walkers or gait belts, and the equipment should be cleansed properly. Contaminated reusable equipment should be placed carefully in a specified area or container, labeled, and returned to the appropriate department for sterilization. Contaminated disposable items should be placed carefully in a container, labeled, and disposed of properly.

Contaminated or soiled linen should be disposed of with minimal handling, sorting, and movement. It can be placed in an appropriate bag and labeled before transport to the laundry, or the bag can be color coded to indicate the type or condition of linen it contains. Other contaminated items such as toys, magazines, personal hygiene articles, dishes, and eating utensils should be disposed of or disinfected. Others should not use these items until they have been disinfected. As with all contaminated items, disposable diapers and wipes should be discarded in a secured container, and hands should be washed immediately.

Isolation Systems

Isolation systems are designed to protect a person or object from becoming contaminated or infected by transmissible pathogens. Various isolation procedures are used in different institutions. All health care workers must understand and follow the isolation approach used in their facilities to ensure protection.

Generally, clients are isolated from other clients in the hospital environment if they have a transmissible disease. Isolation involves placing the patient in a room alone or with one or more clients with the same disease to reduce the possibility of transmitting the disease to others. All who enter the patient's room must follow specific infection control techniques. These requirements are listed on a color-coded card and placed on or next to the door of the patient's room. Box 3.4 lists transmission risk precautions for the three main

forms of transmission. Protective clothing, including gown, mask, cap, and gloves, may be required. When leaving the patient, the health care professional should remove the garments in the proper sequence.

Occasionally, clients' conditions (e.g., burns, systemic infections) make them more susceptible to infection. They may be placed in **protective isolation**. With this approach, persons entering the patient's room may need to wear protective clothing to prevent transmission of pathogens to the patient. In this case, the sequence and method of donning the protective garments are more important than the sequence used to remove them.

INCIDENTS AND EMERGENCIES

OTAs should be able to respond to a variety of medical emergencies and to recognize when it is better to receive assistance from the most qualified individual available such as a physician, emergency medical technician, or nurse. Outside assistance should be easily accessible in a hospital but may require an extended time if the treatment is conducted in a patient's home or outpatient clinic. The assistant should keep emergency telephone numbers close at hand or know the correct codes to call if such a situation should arise in the acute care setting. The OTA needs to determine at the time of the incident whether to call for assistance before or after emergency care. In most cases it is advisable to call for assistance before initiating emergency care, unless the delay would be life threatening.

Many accidents can be prevented by consistently following safety measures. However, OTs and OTAs should always be alert to the possibility of an injury and should expect the unexpected. Most institutions have specific policies and procedures to follow. In general, when a patient is injured, the OTA should do the following:

1. Ask for help. Do not leave the patient alone. Prevent further injury to the patient and provide emergency care.
2. When the emergency has passed, document the incident according to the institution's policy. Do not discuss the incident with the patient or significant others. Do not admit to negligence or provide information that suggests negligence to anyone (Centers for Disease Control and Prevention, 2017).
3. Notify the supervisor of the incident and file the incident report with the appropriate person within the organization.

Falls

Staying alert and reacting quickly when clients lose their balance can prevent injuries from falls. Proper guarding techniques must be practiced. In many instances, trying to keep the patient upright is unwise. Instead, the practitioner should carefully assist the patient to the floor or onto a firm support.

If a patient begins to fall forward, the OTA should do the following:

1. Restrain the patient by firmly holding the gait belt.
2. Push forward against the pelvis and pull back on the shoulder or anterior chest.
3. Help the patient to stand erect once it is determined that the patient is not injured. The patient may briefly lean against the OTA for support.
4. If the patient is falling too far forward to be kept upright, guide the patient to reach slowly for the floor.
5. Slow the momentum by gently pulling back on the gait belt and the patient's shoulder.
6. Step forward as the patient moves toward the floor.
7. Tell the patient to bend the elbows to help cushion the fall when the hands contact the floor.
8. Ensure the patient's head is turned to the side to avoid injury to the face.

If the patient begins to fall backward, the procedure is the following:

1. Rotate your body so that one side is turned toward the patient's back, then widen your stance.
2. Push forward on the patient's pelvis and allow the patient to lean against your body.
3. Assist the patient to stand erect.

4. If the patient falls too far backward, continue to rotate your body to stay upright until it is turned toward the patient's back, then widen your stance.
5. Instruct the patient to lean briefly against your body or to sit on your thigh.
6. Consider lowering the patient into a sitting position on the floor, using the gait belt and good body mechanics.

Burns

Generally, only minor first-degree burns are likely to occur in OT practice. These can be treated with basic first-aid procedures. The OTA should contact skilled personnel for immediate care if skin is charred, missing, or blistered. For first-degree burns, where the skin is only reddened, the following steps are taken:

1. Rinse or soak the burned area in cold (not iced) water.
2. Cover with a clean or sterile dressing or bandage. A moist dressing may be more comfortable for some clients.
3. Do not apply any cream, ointment, or butter to the burn; doing so will mask the appearance and may lead to infection or a delay in healing.

Bleeding

A laceration may result in minor or serious bleeding. The objectives of treatment are to prevent contamination of the wound and to control the bleeding. To stop the bleeding, the OTA should do the following:

1. Wash hands and don protective gloves. Continue to wear protective gloves during treatment of the wound.
2. Place a clean towel or sterile dressing over the wound, then apply direct pressure to the wound. If no dressing is available, use the gloved hand.
3. Elevate the wound above the level of the heart to reduce blood flow to the area.
4. In some cases, consider cleansing the wound with an antiseptic or by rinsing it with water.
5. Encourage the patient to remain quiet and to avoid using the extremity.
6. If arterial bleeding occurs, as evidenced by spurting blood, apply intermittent, direct pressure to the artery above the level of the wound as needed. The pressure point for the brachial artery is on the inside of the upper arm, midway between the elbow and armpit. The pressure point for the femoral artery is in the crease of the hip joint, just to the side of the pubic bone.
7. Do not apply a tourniquet unless you have been trained to do so.

Shock

Excessive bleeding, changing from a supine to an upright position, or excessive heat may induce **shock**. Signs and symptoms of shock include pale, moist, and cool skin; shallow, irregular breathing; dilated pupils; a weak or rapid pulse; and dizziness or nausea. Shock should not be confused with fainting, which would result in a slower pulse, paleness, and perspiration. Clients who faint generally recover promptly if allowed to lie flat. The OT or OTA who notices a patient experiencing symptoms of shock should intervene with the following actions:

1. Determine the cause of shock, and correct it if possible. Monitor the patient's blood pressure and pulse rate.
2. Place the patient in a supine position, with head slightly lower than the legs. If head and chest injuries are present or respiration is impaired, consider keeping the head and chest slightly elevated.
3. Do not add heat, but prevent loss of body heat, if necessary, by applying a cool compress to the patient's forehead and covering the patient with a light blanket.
4. Keep the patient quiet, and ensure the patient avoids exertion.
5. After the symptoms are relieved, gradually return the patient to an upright position and monitor the patient's condition.

Seizures

Seizures may result from a specific disorder, brain injury, or medication. The OTA should be able to recognize a seizure and take appropriate action to keep the patient from being injured. A patient experiencing a seizure usually becomes rigid and statuelike for a few seconds, then begins to convulse with a whole-body jerking motion. The person will most likely turn blue and may stop breathing for up to 50 or even 70 seconds. Some clients' sphincter control may be lost during or at the end of the seizure, and they may involuntarily void urine or feces. The OTA who suspects a patient is about to have a seizure should initiate the following interventions:

1. Place the person in a safe location, away from anything that might cause injury. Do not attempt to restrain or restrict the convulsions.
2. Assist in keeping the patient's airway open, but do not attempt to open the mouth by placing any object between the teeth. Never place your finger or a wooden or metal object in the patient's mouth, and do not attempt to grasp or position the tongue.
3. If the patient's mouth is open, place a soft object between the teeth to prevent the patient from accidentally biting the tongue. A sturdy cloth object or a tongue depressor wrapped with several layers of gauze and fastened with adhesive tape may be used.
4. When the convulsions subside, turn the patient's head to one side in case of vomiting.
5. After the convulsions cease, the patient should rest. Covering the patient with a blanket or positioning a screen to provide privacy may be helpful.
6. Obtain medical assistance.

Insulin-Related Illnesses

Many clients seen in OT practice may experience insulin-related episodes. The OTA must be able to differentiate between the conditions of hypoglycemia (insulin reaction) and hyperglycemia (acidosis) (Table 3.1).

An **insulin reaction** can be caused by too much systemic insulin, the intake of too little food or sugar, or too much physical activity. If the patient is conscious, some form of sugar is provided (e.g., candy, orange juice). If the patient is

TABLE 3.1 Warning Signs and Symptoms of Insulin-Related Illnesses

Observations	Insulin Reaction	Acidosis
Onset	Sudden	Gradual
Skin	Moist, pale	Dry, flushed
Behavior	Excited, agitated	Drowsy
Breath odor	Normal	Fruity
Breathing	Normal to shallow	Deep, labored
Tongue	Moist	Dry
Vomiting	Absent	Present
Hunger	Present	Absent
Thirst	Absent	Present

Modified from Pierson FM. *Principles and Techniques of Patient Care*. 3rd ed. Philadelphia, PA: WB Saunders; 2002.

unconscious, glucose may have to be provided intravenously. The patient should rest, and all physical activity should be stopped. This condition is not as serious as acidosis, but the patient should be given the opportunity to return to a normal state as soon as possible.

Acidosis can lead to a diabetic coma and eventual death if not treated. It should be considered a medical emergency requiring prompt action, including assistance from qualified personnel. The patient should not be given any form of sugar. An insulin injection is usually necessary, and a nurse or physician should provide care as quickly as possible.

Choking and Cardiac Arrest

All health care practitioners should be trained to treat clients who are choking or experiencing cardiac arrest. Both the American Heart Association and the American Red Cross offer specific training courses. Printable posters are available online (see Resources). The following information is presented as a reminder of the basic techniques and is not meant to substitute for training.

The urgency of choking cannot be overemphasized. Immediate recognition and proper action are essential. When assisting a conscious adult or child older than 1 year, the OTA should do the following:

1. Ask the patient, "Are you choking?" If the patient can speak, or cough effectively, do not interfere with the patient's own attempts to expel the object. If the patient gives no response, call 9-1-1 or the local emergency number.
2. If the patient is unable to speak, cough, or breathe, check the mouth and remove any visible foreign object.
3. If the patient is unable to speak or cough, position yourself behind the person. Clasp your hands over the patient's abdomen, slightly above the umbilicus but below the diaphragm.
4. Use the closed fist of one hand, covered by your other hand, to give five thrusts against the person's abdomen by compressing the abdomen in and up forcefully (Heimlich maneuver). Continue to apply the thrusts until the obstruction becomes dislodged or is relieved or the person becomes unconscious.
5. Obtain medical assistance.

When assisting an unconscious adult or child older than 1 year, the OTA should take the following steps:

1. Place the patient in a supine position, then call for medical help.
2. Open the patient's mouth and use your finger to attempt to locate and remove the foreign object (finger sweep).
3. Open the airway by tilting the head back and lifting the chin forward. Attempt to ventilate using the mouth-to-mouth technique.
4. If step 3 is unsuccessful, deliver up to five abdominal thrusts (Heimlich maneuver), repeat the finger sweep, and attempt to ventilate. It may be necessary to repeat these steps.
5. Be persistent and continue these procedures until the object is removed or medical assistance arrives.
6. Consider initiating **cardiopulmonary resuscitation (CPR)** techniques to stabilize the patient's cardiopulmonary functions after the object has been removed.

The following procedures, updated in 2015, are recommended for CPR (American Heart Association, 2010). These guidelines emphasize the lifesaving value of compression and distinguish between recommendations for trained versus untrained lay rescuers. All OT practitioners should be trained lay rescuers.

1. Check quickly (within 10 seconds) for absent or abnormal breathing; if necessary, activate the emergency response system. Retrieve or send someone for automated external defibrillator (AED).
2. Unresponsive adults should be placed in a supine position on a firm surface.
3. Initiate chest compressions immediately; push hard and fast. Kneel next to the patient, place the heel of one hand on the inferior portion of the sternum just proximal to the xiphoid process, and place your other hand on top of the first hand. Position your shoulders directly over the patient's sternum; keep your elbows extended; press down firmly, depressing the sternum at least 2 to 2.4 in (5–6 cm) with each compression. Relax after each compression, but do not remove your hands from the sternum. The relaxation and compression phases should be equal in duration. This can be accomplished by mentally counting "1001," "1002," "1003," and so on, for each phase. Allow for complete chest recoil between compressions.
4. Note that the 2015 recommendations focus on the rate and depth of the compressions. In 2012 the recommended rate was at least 100 compressions per minute, whereas the new guidelines recommend 100 to 120 per minute.
5. Open the patient's airway by lifting up on the chin and pushing down on the forehead to tilt the head back.
6. Pinch the patient's nose closed, and maintain the head tilt to open the airway. Place your mouth over the patient's mouth and form a seal with your lips; perform two full breaths, then proceed to evaluate the circulation. Some persons prefer to place a clean cloth over the patient's lips before initiating mouth-to-mouth respirations. If it is available, a plastic intubation device can be used to decrease the contact between the caregiver's mouth and the patient's mouth.
7. If you are doing all CPR procedures without assistance, perform 30 chest compressions and then two breaths. Compress at the rate of at least 100 times per minute, minimizing interruptions. Continue these procedures until qualified assistance arrives or the patient is able to sustain independent respiration and circulation. If you are alone, get assistance from other persons by calling loudly for help. If a second person is present, the person should contact an advanced medical assistance unit before beginning to assist with CPR. The patient usually requires hospitalization and evaluation by a physician. (Note: Extreme care must be used to open an airway in a patient who may have a cervical spine injury. For such clients, use the chin lift, but avoid the head tilt. If the technique does not open the airway, tilt the head slowly and gently until the airway is open.)

These procedures are appropriate for adults and children 8 years of age and older. A pamphlet or booklet containing diagrams and instructions for CPR techniques can be obtained from most local offices of the American Heart Association or online (see Resources). Courses of instruction in first aid and CPR are offered through the American Heart Association, the American National Red Cross, and other organizations. OT practitioners in clinical practice should make every effort to update and maintain service competency in basic first aid, CPR, and emergency measures.

PREVENTIVE POSITIONING FOR SPECIFIC DIAGNOSES

Many clients require special positioning to prevent complications and maintain function. Staying in one position for a long time can lead to the development of contractures and skin breakdown (decubitus ulcers).

Specific patient conditions such as impaired sensation, paralysis, poor skin integrity, poor nutrition, impaired circulation, and spasticity require special attention. The patient's skin, especially bony prominences over the sacrum, ischium, trochanters, elbows, and heels, should be inspected. Reddened areas may develop from pressure within 30 minutes. Other indicators of excessive pressure are complaints of numbness or tingling and localized swelling.

Pillows, towel rolls, or similar devices may be used to provide comfort and stability but should be used cautiously to prevent secondary complications. The following examples of patient conditions demonstrate the need for specific positioning techniques. It is important to review these with both the patient and caregiver.

Clients with above-knee lower extremity amputations should avoid hip flexion and hip abduction. The time the patient may sit is limited to 30 minutes per hour. When the patient is supine, the stump is elevated on a pillow only for a few minutes. The patient should lie in a prone position to avoid contracture of the hip flexor muscles.

Clients with below-knee lower extremity amputations should avoid prolonged hip and knee flexion to prevent contractures. Again, the patient may sit only 30 minutes per hour; when supine, the patient should not keep the stump elevated for more than a few minutes. When it is elevated, the knee is maintained in extension. The patient is instructed to keep the knee extended throughout the day. Lying prone is recommended.

To avoid contractures resulting from muscle spasticity, clients with hemiplegia should avoid the following positions for prolonged periods: shoulder adduction and internal rotation, elbow flexion, forearm supination or pronation, wrist flexion, finger and thumb flexion and adduction, hip and knee flexion, hip external rotation, and ankle plantar flexion and inversion. Both the arm and the leg should be moved through the available range of motion (ROM) several times per day.

Clients with rheumatoid arthritis should avoid prolonged immobilization of the affected extremity joints. Gentle active range of motion (AROM) or passive range of motion (PROM) of the joints should be performed several times per day if the joints are not acutely inflamed.

As burns heal, scars and contractures are likely to form. Therefore avoiding prolonged static positioning of the joints affected by the burn or skin graft, especially positions of comfort, is important. The positions comfortable to the patient do not produce the stress or tension needed to maintain mobility of the wound area. When the burn is located on the flexor or adductor surface of a joint, positions of flexion and adduction should be avoided. Passive or active exercise should be done frequently to both the involved and the uninvolved joints. The patient will probably have to endure significant pain to restore normal joint function.

PRECAUTIONS WITH SPECIAL EQUIPMENT

When seeing clients at the bedside, the OTA first should contact the nurses' station to determine whether any specific positioning instructions exist. For example, a patient may need to follow a turning schedule or may be limited in time allowed to remain in one position. If the patient's current position in bed is not suitable for treatment, the treatment might be rescheduled. Other options would be to change the patient's position temporarily or to treat the patient as much as possible in the current position. If the patient's position is changed, the OTA ensures that the patient is returned to the preferred position at the end of treatment. The OTA should use common sense with any equipment. Note the position of the patient and any tubes and wires before, during, and after treatment to ensure that nothing is disconnected or disturbed to the extent that its function is impaired.

Hospital Beds

Two of the more commonly used beds in hospitals are the standard manually operated bed and the electrically operated bed. Both beds are designed to make it easier to support the patient and to change a patient's position. Other more specialized beds

are necessary for clients with more traumatic conditions. Whatever type is used, the bed should be positioned so that the patient is easily accessed and the OT practitioner can use good body mechanics (see Chapters 11 and 15).

Most standard adjustable beds are adjusted by using electrical controls attached to the head or the foot of the bed or to a special cord that allows the patient to operate them. The controls are marked according to their function and can be operated by hand or foot. The entire bed can be raised and lowered, or its upper portion can be raised while the lower portion remains unchanged. When the upper portion is raised slightly, the patient's position is called the **Fowler position**. Most beds allow the lower portion to be adjusted to provide knee flexion, which in turn causes hip flexion.

Side rails were once common on most beds as a protective measure but are now considered a form of restraint. The Resource site on Hospital Beds contains multiple website links addressing this issue and safety alternatives. Where safety rails are in use, the OTA should be aware that some rails are lifted upward to engage the locking mechanism, whereas others are moved toward the upper portion of the bed until the locking mechanism is engaged. If a side rail is used for patient security, the practitioner ensures that the rail is locked securely and has not compressed or stretched any **intravenous** (IV) **lines** or other tubing before leaving the patient.

Some beds are specifically designed to provide support and mobility for a patient, such as the **turning frame** (e.g., Stryker wedge frame), which has a front and back frame covered with canvas. The support base allows the head and foot ends, or the entire bed, to be elevated. One person can easily turn the patient horizontally from prone to supine or from supine to prone positions. This bed is used most commonly for clients with spinal cord injuries who require immobilization. The turning frame allows access to clients and permits moving them from one place to another without removing them from the frame. The skin of clients using this type of bed must be monitored frequently because the bed allows only two basic positions. Another bed for support and mobility is a posttrauma mobility bed that maintains alignment through adjustable bolsters yet can rock from side to side to reduce pressure on the patient's skin (Nazarko, 2008).

Other beds that specifically address the skin-related complications of prolonged immobility have been developed. The air-fluidized support bed (Clinitron) is a heavy, expensive bed that contains silicone-coated glass beads that simulate the properties of a fluid when heated. Pressurized air flows through the mattress to suspend a polyester cover that supports the patient. Clients feel like they are floating on a warm waterbed. The risk of developing skin breakdown is reduced because of the minimal contact pressure of the patient's body against the polyester sheet. This bed is used with clients who have several infected lesions or who require skin protection and whose position cannot be altered easily or who cannot on their own change positions easily. It helps to prevent tissue breakdown from heat, moisture, pressure, shearing, and friction. Caution should be used to prevent puncturing the polyester cover, which would cause the silicone beads to leak (Pierson & Fairchild, 2002). Another similar bed is the low air loss bed, which relies on air bladders rather than glass beads to adjust pressure; this bed was developed to reduce the incidence of pressure ulcers.

Another type of bed seen in the acute care setting is the Dolphin bed. It simulates a fluid environment, which helps prevent and treat wounds and optimizes tissue oxygenation. The pressure of the bed readjusts every 11 seconds. It helps to maintain normal blood flow and minimize soft tissue deformation. This type of bed is not recommended for clients with unstable spinal fractures. Visit https://joerns.com/product/2457/Dolphin-FIS®.aspx for more information.

Ventilators

A **ventilator** (respirator) moves gas or air into the patient's lungs and maintains adequate air exchange when normal respiration is decreased. Two frequently used types are volume-cycled ventilators and pressure-cycled ventilators. Both ventilators deliver a predetermined volume of gas (air) during inspiration and allow for passive expiration. The gas from the ventilator is usually delivered to the patient through an **endotracheal tube (ETT)**. When the tube is in place, the patient is considered to be intubated. Insertion of the ETT prevents the patient from talking. When the ETT is removed, the patient may complain of a sore throat and may have a distorted voice for a short time. It is important to avoid disturbing, bending, or kinking the tubing or accidentally disconnecting the tube of the ventilator from the ETT. A patient using a ventilator can perform various bedside activities, including sitting and ambulation, if the tubing is long enough. Because the patient has difficulty talking, the OT or the OTA should ask questions that can be answered with head nods or other nonverbal means. A patient using a ventilator may have reduced tolerance for activities and should be monitored for signs of respiratory distress such as a change in the respiration pattern, fainting, or blue lips.

Monitors

Various monitors are used to observe the physiologic state of patients who require special care. Patients who are being monitored can perform therapeutic activities if care is taken to avoid disrupting the equipment. Many of the units have an auditory and/or visual signal that is activated by a change in the patient's condition or position or by a change in the equipment's function. A nurse will need to evaluate and correct the cause of the alarm unless the OTA has received special instruction.

The **electrocardiogram (ECG)** monitors the patient's heart rate, blood pressure, and respiration rate. Acceptable or safe ranges for the three physiologic indicators can be set in the unit. An alarm is activated when the upper or lower limits of the ranges are exceeded or the unit malfunctions. A monitoring screen provides a graphic and digital display of the values for observation of the patient's responses to treatment.

Various catheters and monitors do not impede treatment as long as care is taken to leave them undisturbed by avoiding activities in muscles or joints close to the insertion point. The OTA should use common sense and due diligence with the following devices. The **pulmonary artery catheter (PAC)** is a long, plastic IV tube inserted into the internal jugular or the femoral vein and passed through to the pulmonary artery to provide accurate and continuous measurements of pulmonary artery pressures and detect subtle changes in the patient's cardiovascular system, including responses to medications, stress, and activity. The **intracranial pressure (ICP) monitor** measures the pressure exerted against the skull by brain tissue, blood, or cerebrospinal fluid (CSF). It is used to monitor ICP in clients who have experienced a closed head injury, cerebral hemorrhage, brain tumor, or an overproduction of CSF. Some of the complications associated with this device are infection, hemorrhage, and seizures. Physical activities should be limited when these monitors are in place. Avoid activities that would cause a rapid increase in ICP such as isometric exercises. Positions to avoid include neck flexion, hip flexion greater than 90 degrees, and the prone position. The patient's head should not be lowered more than 15 degrees below the horizontal plane. The **arterial monitoring line** (A line) is a catheter inserted into an artery to measure blood pressure continuously or to obtain blood samples without repeated needle punctures. Treatment can be provided with an A line in place, but care should be taken to avoid disturbing the catheter and inserted needle.

Feeding Devices

Special feeding devices may be necessary to provide nutrition for clients who are unable to chew, swallow, or ingest food. Some of the more common devices are the **nasogastric (NG) tube, gastric (G) tube**, and **intravenous (IV) feeding** tube.

The NG tube is a plastic tube inserted through a nostril and terminates in the patient's stomach. The tube may cause the patient to have a sore throat and an increased gag reflex. The patient cannot eat food or drink fluids through the mouth while the NG tube is in place. Movement of the patient's head and neck, especially forward flexion, should be avoided. If the patient needs to be placed in a supine position for any reason, the NG tube system should be placed on hold so as not to cause aspiration.

The G tube is a plastic tube inserted through an incision in the patient's abdomen directly into the stomach. During treatment the OT practitioner must avoid disturbing or removing the tube.

IV feeding, **total parenteral nutrition (TPN)**, and hyperalimentation devices are used to infuse the total calories or nutrients (**hyperalimentation**) needed to promote tissue growth without going through the digestive system. A catheter is inserted directly or indirectly into the subclavian vein. The catheter may be connected to a semipermanently fixed cannula or sutured at the point of insertion. The OTA should carefully observe the various connections to be certain they are secure before and after treatment. A disrupted or loose connection may cause an air embolus, which could be life threatening to the patient. The system usually includes an **infusion pump**, which administers fluids and nutrients at a preselected, constant flow rate. An audible alarm is activated if the system becomes imbalanced or the fluid source is empty. Treatment activities can be performed as long as the tubing is not disrupted, disconnected, or occluded and if undue stress on the infusion site is avoided. Motions of the shoulder on the side of the infusion site, especially abduction and flexion, may be restricted. Medication infusion pumps are specifically mentioned in the Joint Commission's (2010) safety goals.

Most IV lines are inserted into superficial veins. Various sizes and types of needles or catheters are used, depending on the purpose of the IV therapy, the infusion site, the need for prolonged therapy, and site availability. During treatment the OTA must be careful to avoid disrupting, disconnecting, or occluding the tubing. The infusion site should remain dry, the needle should remain secure and immobile in the vein, and no restraint should be placed above the infusion site (e.g., no blood pressure cuff applied above the site). The total system should be observed to ensure it is functioning properly when treatment begins and ends. The patient who ambulates with an IV line in place should be instructed to grasp the IV support pole so that the infusion site will be at heart level. If the infusion site is allowed to hang lower, blood flow may be affected. Similar procedures to maintain the infusion site in proper position should be followed when the patient is treated in bed or at a treatment table. The patient should avoid activities that require the infusion site to be elevated above the level of the heart for a prolonged period. Problems related to the IV system should be reported to nursing personnel. Simple procedures such as straightening the tubing may be performed by the properly trained OTA.

Urinary Catheters

A **urinary catheter** is used to remove urine from the bladder when the patient is unable to control its retention or release. The urine is then drained through plastic tubing into a collection bag, bottle, or urinal. Any form of trauma, disease, condition, or disorder affecting the neuromuscular control of the bladder sphincter may require the use of a urinary catheter. The catheter may be used temporarily or for the remainder of the patient's life.

A urinary catheter can be applied internally (indwelling catheter) or externally. Female clients require an indwelling catheter inserted through the urethra and into the bladder. Two commonly used internal catheters are the Foley and suprapubic catheters. The Foley catheter is held in place in the bladder by a small balloon that is inflated with air, water, or sterile saline solution. To remove the catheter, the balloon is deflated and the catheter withdrawn. The suprapubic catheter is inserted directly into the bladder through incisions in the lower abdomen and bladder. The catheter may be held in place by adhesive tape, but care should be taken to avoid its removal, especially during self-care activities. Males may use an external catheter. A condom is applied over the shaft of the penis and is held in place by an adhesive applied to the skin or by a padded strap or tape encircling the proximal shaft of the penis. It is connected to a drainage tube and bag.

A new device for female clients, called a PureWick™ (Fig. 3.5), is being used in some hospitals/facilities around the country. This device uses low-pressure wall suction to wick away urine from the patient and is collected in a designated collection canister. The idea behind the device is to reduce the risk of catheter-associated urinary tract infections (CAUTIs), for which females are at a higher risk. The flexible, contoured external catheter is placed between the labia and gluteus muscles. The device works by drawing urine away from the body and into the canister. The wick is replaced every 8 to 12 hours or when it is soiled with feces or blood. It is imperative that skin be assessed to see if it has been compromised in any way while the wick is in place. Proper perineal hygiene should be completed before placement of a new wick. Visit https://www.crbard.com/medical/PureWickVideo or https://www.purewickathome.com/ for more information.

When treating clients with urinary catheters, the OTA must remember the following precautions:
1. Avoid disrupting or stretching the drainage tube, and do not put tension on the tubing or the catheter.
2. Do not allow the bag to be placed above the level of the bladder for more than a few minutes.

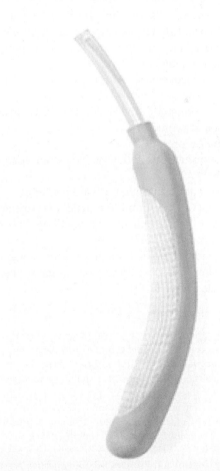

Fig. 3.5 PureWick female catheter. (From Liberator Medical Supply, Inc.)

3. Do not place the bag in the patient's lap when the patient is being transported.
4. Observe the production, color, and odor of the urine.
5. Report the following observations to a physician or nurse: foul-smelling, cloudy, dark, or bloody urine or a reduction in the flow or production of urine.
6. Be sure to empty the collection bag when it is full.

Infection is a major complication for persons using catheters, especially indwelling catheters. Everyone involved with the patient should maintain cleanliness during treatment. The OTA should not attempt to replace or reconnect the tubing unless properly trained. Health care settings that routinely treat clients with catheters have specific protocols for catheter care. (See CDC Guideline in Resources, Infection Control.)

SUMMARY

All OT personnel have a legal and professional obligation to promote safety for self, the patient, visitors, and others. The OTA should be prepared to react to emergency situations quickly, decisively, and calmly. The consistent use of safe practices helps to reduce accidents to clients and workers and decreases the time and cost of treatment.

REVIEW QUESTIONS

1. Why is it important to teach the patient and significant others guidelines for handling various emergency situations?
2. Describe at least four behaviors the OTA can adopt to improve patient safety.
3. Describe the consequences of improper positioning of clients.
4. Define the following: IV line, NG tube, TPN, hyperalimentation, and ventilator.
5. Describe standard precautions.
6. Why is it important to follow standard precautions with all clients?
7. Describe the proper technique for hand washing.
8. How should the OTA respond to a patient emergency?
9. How would you help a patient who is falling forward? A patient who is falling backward?
10. What emergency situations might require obtaining advanced medical assistance, and what situations could an OTA handle alone?

REFERENCES

American Heart Association. *Highlights of the 2010 American Heart Association guidelines for CPR and ECC*. Web site. <https://www.heart.org/idc/groups/heart-public/@wcm/@ecc/documents/downloadable/ucm_317350.pdf>.

American Occupational Therapy Association (AOTA). (2014). Occupational therapy practice framework. Domain & process. 3rd ed. *American Journal Occupational Therapy, 68*(1), S1–S51.

Centers for Disease Control and Prevention. *Core infection prevention and control practices for safe healthcare delivery in all settings—recommendations of the Healthcare Infection Control Practices Advisory Committee*. Web site. <https://www.cdc.gov/hicpac/recommendations/core-practices.html>. Accessed 15.03.2017.

George, A. H. (2018). Infection control and safety issues in the clinic. In H. M. Pendelton, & W. Schultz-Krohn (Eds.), *Pedretti's occupational therapy: Practice skills for physical dysfunction* (8th ed.). St. Louis, MO: Mosby.

Nazarko, L. (2008). Standard precautions: how to help prevent infection. *British Journal of Health Assistant, 2*(3), 119–123.

Pierson, F. M., & Fairchild, S. L. (2002). *Principles and techniques of patient care* (3rd ed.). Philadelphia, PA: WB Saunders.

Sax, H., Allegranzi, B., Ucky, I., Larson, E., Boyce, J., & Pittet, D. (2007). 'My five moments for hand hygiene': A user-centered approach to understand, train, monitor and report hand hygiene. *Journal of Hospital Infections, 67*(1), 9–21.

State of Arizona. OSHA bloodborne pathogens standard. Online publication. <http://www.blr.com/Workplace-Safety/Health/Bloodborne-Pathogens-in-Arizona>. Accessed 28.10.2010.

Tarrac, S. E. (2008). Application of the updated CDC isolation guidelines for health care facilities. *AORN Journal, 87*(3), 534–542.

The Joint Commission. *2010 national patient safety goals*. Web site. <https://www.jointcommission.org/-/media/tjc/documents/standards/national-patient-safety-goals/2020-hap-npsg-goals-final.pdf>. Accessed 21.10.2010.

US Department of Labor. Occupational Safety & Health Administration, Safety and Health Topics. Web site. <http://www.osha.gov/SLTC/healthcarefacilities/index.html> (links to all regulations). Accessed 28.10.2010.

World Health Organization. WHO guidelines on hand hygiene in health care (an evidence-based guide to everything you would want to know about handwashing). Web site. <http://whqlibdoc.who.int/publications/2009/9789241597906_eng.pdf>. Accessed 28.10.2010.

RESOURCES

Adult Basic Life Support

American Heart Association Guidelines/video: <http://www.youtube.com/americanheartassoc>.

JAMA reference article link: <http://www.emergencydispatch.org/articles/lifesupport1.htm>.

Resuscitation Council (UK) Poster of guidelines: <http://www.resus.org.uk/pages/blsalgo.pdf>.

University of Washington, Learn CPR: <http://depts.washington.edu/learncpr/>.

First Aid

American Heart Association Guidelines/CPR and First Aid links: <http://www.heart.org/HEARTORG/CPRAndECC/CPR_UCM_001118_SubHomePage.jsp>.

American Heart Association local offices, American National Red Cross: Contact for information on first aid, choking, and CPR.

Hand Washing

CDC Hand Hygiene in Healthcare Settings: <http://www.cdc.gov/handhygiene/>.

World Health Organization. WHO Guidelines on Hand Hygiene in Health Care (an evidence based guide to everything you would want to know about handwashing): <http://whqlibdoc.who.int/publications/2009/9789241597906_eng.pdf>.

Hospital Beds

US Department of Health and Human Services. US Food and Drug Administration: Medical Devices: <http://www.fda.gov/MedicalDevices/ProductsandMedicalProcedures/General HospitalDevicesandSupplies/HospitalBeds/default.htm>.

Infection Control and Universal Precautions

Centers for Disease Control and Prevention (CDC). The "An Ounce of Prevention" Campaign: <http://www.cdc.gov/ounceofprevention/>. Contains link to downloadable poster and brochure for infection control in the home.

CDC Guideline for infection control in health care settings: <http://www.cdc.gov/hai/>.

CDC Guideline for infection control in health care personnel: <http://www.cdc.gov/ncidod/dhqp/pdf/guidelines/InfectControl98.pdf>.

CDC Guideline for prevention of catheter-associated urinary tract infections: <http://www.cdc.gov/hicpac/cauti/003_cauti2009_execSum.html>.

OSHA Hazard Information Bulletins: <http://www.osha.gov/pls/oshaweb/owadisp.show_document?p_table=FEDERAL_REGISTER&p_id=16265>. Potential for occupational exposure to bloodborne pathogens from cleaning needles used in allergy testing procedures.

Restraint Use

CDC Injury Center: Falls in nursing homes: <http://www.cdc.gov/ncipc/factsheets/nursing.htm>.

PART II

Process

4

Occupational Therapy Process
Evaluation and Intervention in Physical Dysfunction

Caroline Beals

OBJECTIVES

After reading this chapter, the student or the occupational therapy practitioner will be able to do the following:

- Identify and describe the major stages in the occupational therapy process.
- Describe the flow of the occupational therapy process, and give examples to illustrate this concept.
- Identify and contrast the roles of the occupational therapist and the occupational therapy assistant in the evaluation and intervention planning stages of the occupational therapy process.
- Discuss the importance of an occupational profile client interview in the evaluation process.

- Describe the skills and behaviors of an effective interviewer.
- Differentiate standardized and nonstandardized tests.
- Discuss how to use practice models to guide planning of an occupation-centered treatment plan.
- Define treatment or intervention planning and describe the process.
- Differentiate the roles of the occupational therapist and the occupational therapy assistant in intervention planning.
- Write clear, measurable, relevant treatment goals and objectives.

KEY TERMS

Referral
Screening
Evaluation
Participation
Intervention
Targeted outcomes
Transition services
Occupational profile

Analysis of occupational performance
Occupation-centered interview
Active listening
Clinical reasoning
Treatment plan
Intervention plan
Reevaluation
Discharge planning

INTRODUCTION

Physical disabilities may impede an individual's ability to engage in daily occupational roles and routines that create meaning, purpose, and structure to their life. Occupational therapists (OTs) and occupational therapy assistants (OTAs) use a systematic process, in collaboration with clients and their support system, to create a path toward independent engagement in occupations and a restoration of function. This process begins with gathering information through an occupational profile and assessing to identify skills and abilities to develop an intervention plan. The OT completes evaluations and develops the intervention plan with input from the OTA. OTs and OTAs collaborate to provide interventions. When the process is complete, the OT develops the discharge plan with input from the OTA. This chapter provides an overview of the occupational therapy process with an emphasis on the role of the OTA and the relationship

between the client, OTA, and OT. Each step in the process requires a positive working relationship among all members of the occupational therapy team.

The occupational therapy process is a series of steps that begin with a **referral** from a physician to an OT and can occur in a hospital, nursing home, or outpatient clinic. It is client centered and collaborative in nature (American Occupational Therapy Association, 2014b). The initial referral may be oral, but a written record is also necessary. In most instances, a written referral from a physician is required for reimbursement from a third-party payer. Once a referral is received, the OT reviews pertinent data about a client to determine the need for evaluation and intervention. This initial referral and **screening** process must be performed by the OT.

Once a referral is established, the occupational therapy process includes evaluation and intervention to achieve targeted outcomes. This process occurs within the domain of the OT practitioner in collaboration with the client, is facilitated by the clinical reasoning of the practitioner, and involves analyzing the client's occupational history and performance (American Occupational Therapy Association, 2014b). The American Occupational Therapy Association (AOTA) organizes the occupational therapy process into three broad areas (American Occupational Therapy Association, 2014b):

1. **Evaluation**: The two major parts of evaluation are the occupational profile and an analysis of occupational performance. Under supervision of the OT, the OTA may carry out elements of the evaluation. The OT analyzes the evaluation data to identify the client's specific strengths and deficits.

   a. Occupational Profile: This is the initial step in the evaluation process, where the OT attempts to gather an understanding of the client's "occupational history and experiences, patterns of daily living, interests, values, and needs" (p. S10) (American Occupational Therapy Association, 2014b). During this process, the OT should also clarify the client's occupational priorities, reasons for seeking services, and concerns and perceptions about performing daily occupations. Supports and barriers to **participation** in occupations are also identified through the initial occupational profile.

   b. Analysis of Occupational Performance: Following the occupational profile, the OT performs a more in-depth analysis to determine more specific areas of deficit. Actual performance of an occupation is often observed in context to identify supports for and barriers to the client's performance. The occupation is considered as a whole, but only selected aspects of an occupation may be specifically assessed during this analysis phase. Through this analysis, the OT is able to select targeted outcomes to address during the intervention phase.

2. **Intervention**:

   a. Intervention Plan: A plan that will guide actions is developed in collaboration with the client and the client's caregivers, as appropriate (American Occupational Therapy Association, 2014b). Considering research evidence of effective treatment principles and methods, the OT develops the initial treatment plan based on selected theories and intervention approaches.

   b. Intervention Implementation: Intervention is the process of ongoing therapeutic activities that will influence and support client occupational performance. Interventions are directed toward identified outcomes or goals developed in the intervention plan. The client's response to the intervention is monitored and documented on a regular basis, as determined by the clinical facility. The OTA may have significant responsibilities for this part of the process.

   c. Intervention Review: It is important that interventions are reviewed, and progress toward targeted outcomes considered on a regular basis (American Occupational Therapy Association, 2014b). Measurement of the outcomes of treatment is critical in showing the effectiveness of the therapy intervention. The treatment plan may be modified or continue toward the set plan based on the reevaluation results.

3. **Targeted Outcomes**: Outcomes are defined by the AOTA (American Occupational Therapy Association, 2014b) as "determinants of success in reaching the desired end result of the occupational therapy process" (p. S10). Reviewing and reflecting on targeted outcomes allows the OT and OTA to determine next steps of the occupational therapy process or, in some cases, prompts discontinuation of services or progression to the next level of care if outcomes have been met.

Process and Flow

Despite the discrete stages just listed, the occupational therapy process is not a linear progression of actions and decisions related to the occupational performance of a client. Alternatively, the process is fluid, complex, and should involve a significant amount of critical thinking, clinical reasoning, and reflective practice. For the occupational therapy process to remain client centered, it is also important that this process reflects the occupational needs of the client. While a referral is often a first step in the occupational therapy process, collaboration and communication among the interprofessional team is often the key to identification of clients who may benefit from occupational therapy services. For example, a physician may consult with an OT practitioner to discuss a client's status and come to a collaborative decision around the appropriateness of an occupational therapy referral.

Similarly, evaluation and treatment are interwoven. The client is seen for a short period of time in the first evaluation, and intervention may begin that same day. As the client's skills and needs change, the OT and OTA continuously reevaluate the client's functional performance status and update the intervention plan. For example, the client's initial evaluation may include the occupation of dressing because at that time the client requires moderate assistance to complete dressing. The goal is to increase the client's independence with specific dressing tasks and decrease the level of assistance the client requires. As the client becomes more independent with dressing, the OT or OTA will assess functional status, document any improvement, and update the intervention plan. The OTA will notify the OT if a reevaluation is needed. The OTA who has achieved service competency may assume some responsibility for updating intervention plans in activities of daily living (ADL) and other areas of occupation. Communication is critical throughout each phase of this process to ensure best practice and client centered care (American Occupational Therapy Association, 2014a).

Role of the OT

According to the *Standards of Practice for Occupational Therapy* (American Occupational Therapy Association, 2015), the OT is responsible for accepting and acting on referrals and for designing and supervising individual or group screenings. The OT must be knowledgeable about the occupational dysfunction and its causes, course, and prognosis. Within the collaborative OT/OTA relationship, the OT assumes the role of manager, director, and analyst. The OT selects the areas to be evaluated, chooses appropriate evaluation instruments and procedures, and administers those evaluations or delegates their administration to another therapist or qualified OTA. The OT must be familiar with a variety of evaluation procedures, their uses, and proper administration and be able to identify evaluation procedures suitable to the client and the dysfunction. The OT documents the evaluation results, which forms the scientific foundation for the decisions in the treatment plan (Chisolm & Schell, 2019).

The OT designs, develops, and documents the treatment plan of care. The OT delegates appropriate aspects of treatment planning to the OTA but retains legal and supervisory responsibility for the plan and its implementation (American Occupational Therapy Association, 2015). The OT manages and documents treatment implementation and reevaluation even when most of the implementation is delegated to the OTA. The OT is responsible for overseeing and supervising treatment and reevaluating and documenting progress. The OT determines when service should be discontinued and develops the client's discharge plan. Parts of discharge planning may be delegated to the OTA. The OT documents all outcomes and recommendations for follow-up in the final occupational therapy report.

Role of the OTA

The OT and the OTA need to review individual state licensure laws to ensure compliance with supervision. Some state licensure laws provide more specific guidelines for the roles and responsibilities of the OTA.

The OTA can educate physicians and other potential referral sources about how to initiate occupational therapy referrals. The OTA may administer parts of the screening under OT supervision (American Occupational Therapy Association, 2015). Once the OT has selected appropriate evaluation instruments, the OTA may administer the ones that are appropriate for their experience and competency level (American Occupational Therapy Association, 2014a, 2015). They should be performed with the guidance and supervision of the occupational therapist until they have demonstrated consistent and reliable administration techniques. Effective assessment administration requires good observation skills and the ability to build rapport with a client in a short time. After administration, the OTA communicates the results, both orally and in writing. The OTA may also collaborate with the OT to educate the client and family about the purposes of the evaluation procedures.

If the OTA encounters pressure by employers to administer evaluation procedures for which they are not qualified, they should follow a course of action beginning with contacting the OT supervisor for guidance. They should then clearly explain the difference between the OT and OTA roles. If pressure continues or escalates to a level of threat, the OTA should contact the local and state practice associations and the AOTA. OTAs should never put their licensure at risk by working outside of their practice guidelines.

OTAs most commonly contribute to the intervention plan in the occupational performance areas of daily living activities (both basic and instrumental), work, education, play, and leisure (American Occupational Therapy Association, 2014a). The autonomy given to the OTA increases with experience and demonstrated service competency (American Occupational Therapy Association, 2014a). Responsibilities include implementing treatment activities, providing client and family education, and documenting the services provided.

OTAs may provide **transition services**, which help the client change from one health care facility or environment to another (American Occupational Therapy Association, 2015). For example, the client with a head injury may need to move toward independent community living. This transition might require the services of a community agency. Depending on the practice area and personal expertise, the OTA may coordinate or administer a plan, designed by the OT, for moving the client through such a transition.

Experience, Expertise, and Service Competency

OTA students or recent graduates follow the 2014 *Guidelines for Supervision, Roles, and Responsibility During the Delivery of Occupational Therapy Services* (American Occupational Therapy Association, 2014a). They also follow applicable state regulations regarding OTA services. New OTs and OTAs need and benefit from close supervision and direction in all stages of the occupational therapy process. Autonomy in service provision increases with training, experience, and continued demonstration of service competency. New graduates would benefit from securing first jobs in a setting with strong supervision; in particular, new graduates are advised to avoid working on a contract basis in settings with limited supervision.

Experienced OTAs function fairly autonomously, with only general supervision from the OT, in designated areas of evaluation and treatment planning (American Occupational Therapy Association, 2014a). In addition to years of experience, OTAs who desire more autonomy and responsibility are encouraged to seek out opportunities to increase competency through advanced training.

EVALUATION PROCEDURES

The evaluation process consists of gathering an occupational profile and an analysis of occupational performance (Fig. 4.1). The **occupational profile** describes the client's occupational history, patterns of daily living, interest, and therapy needs. The **analysis of occupational performance** looks at the client's observable performance in carrying out desired occupational tasks and ADL (American Occupational

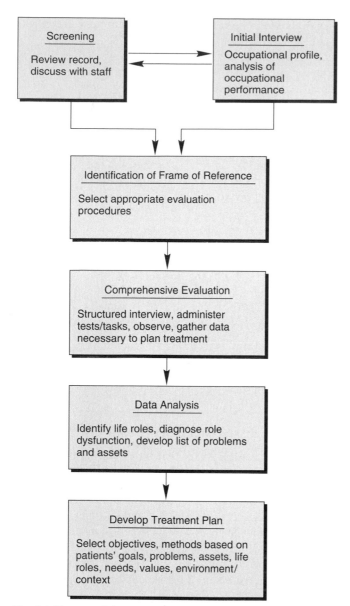

Screening		Initial Interview
Review record, discuss with staff		Occupational profile, analysis of occupational performance

Identification of Frame of Reference

Select appropriate evaluation procedures

Comprehensive Evaluation

Structured interview, administer tests/tasks, observe, gather data necessary to plan treatment

Data Analysis

Identify life roles, diagnose role dysfunction, develop list of problems and assets

Develop Treatment Plan

Select objectives, methods based on patients' goals, problems, assets, life roles, needs, values, environment/context

Fig. 4.1 Diagram of the evaluation process.

Therapy Association, 2014b). The OT observes the client's performance skills (motor skills, process skills, and/or communication and interaction skills) and evaluates client factors (such as cognitive-mental factors, physical factors, social-emotional factors) that can interfere with occupational performance. The client-centered evaluation process analyzes client factors that support or hinder occupational performance. Client goals and limitations in occupational performance become the basis for developing treatment goals or objectives and strategies to remediate or compensate for problems in occupational performance.

The OT selects an occupational therapy theory suited to determining the cause of limitations in occupational performance. The use of an occupational therapy theory helps identify the range of evaluation procedures that might be used to gather the information needed for planning treatment

(Chisolm & Schell, 2019). The OT selects and administers (or directs the OTA to administer) specific tests, clinical observations, structured interviews, standardized tests, performance checklists, and activities and tasks. The OT gathers, interprets, and analyzes the information from the evaluation procedures (American Occupational Therapy Association, 2014b). Some typical evaluation techniques that an OT will assign to the OTA, or use alone, are discussed in this chapter.

Occupation-Centered Interview

An **occupation-centered interview** consists of asking the client or family member questions relating to occupational habits and life roles, family situation, home setup, interests, values, and/or therapy goals. This is a crucial component of compiling the occupational profile. The OT gathers information on how clients perceive their life roles, physical dysfunction, health care needs, and therapy goals. This information is valuable for determining the client's values and establishing realistic possibilities for resuming former roles following occupational therapy intervention. During the initial phase of the interview, the OT explains his or her role and that of the OTA, the purpose of the interview, and how the information is to be used. As the interview progresses, the interviewer may seek the desired information by asking appropriate questions, guiding the responses, and ensuring discussion to address relevant topics. In some settings and situations (e.g., when working with occasional consultation) the OTA conducts the initial interview with a client. In general, this sort of unstructured or semistructured interview is conducted by the OT; the OTA follows a structured interview protocol with specific questions to be asked. The interview can be concluded with a summary of the major points covered, information gained, estimate of current strengths and functional problems, and plan for further occupational therapy evaluation and treatment.

The occupation-centered initial interview should take place in a quiet environment that ensures privacy. The practitioner should plan the interview in advance to know what information must be obtained and to have specific questions prepared. A specified period of time, identified by the OT or OTA and client before the interview, should be set aside. The first part of the interview may be devoted to getting acquainted and orienting the client to the occupational therapy clinic or service and to the role and goals of the OT and OTA. The rapport and trust that develop between therapist and client are important outcomes of the initial occupation-centered interview (Taylor, 2019).

The two essential characteristics of the successful interviewer are a solid knowledge base and the use of **active listening** skills. Active listening requires study, practice, and preparation. The therapist's knowledge will influence the selection of questions or topics to be covered in the interview. The interviewer who actively listens demonstrates respect for and interest in the client (Yu et al., 2018). During active listening, the receiver (interviewer) tries to understand what the sender (client) is feeling or the meaning of the message. An interviewer then rephrases the responses into his or her own words and feeds it back for verification by saying, for example, "This is what I believe you mean. Have I understood you correctly?" While listening actively, the interviewer does not send a new message such as an opinion, judgment, advice, or analysis. Rather, an interviewer relates back only what he or she thinks the client meant.

Throughout the interview the practitioner should listen to understand the client's attitude toward the physical dysfunction. A client should be encouraged to express what he or she sees as the primary problems and goals for rehabilitation. Client beliefs and preferences may differ substantially from what the therapist believes, but a client must be given careful consideration for the OT team and client to set realistic treatment goals together. As the interview progresses, the client should have an opportunity to ask questions about therapy intervention and goals.

The rapport and trust that develop between the client and the OT or OTA are based on their open and honest communication. The communication in the interview and observation phases of the evaluation are critical to all subsequent interactions and thus to the effectiveness of treatment. Clients need to sense that they have been heard and understood by someone who is caring and empathetic. Clients must be able to trust that a therapist has the skills necessary to facilitate a successful rehabilitation plan. The practitioner needs to project self-confidence in his or her own skills and in the profession. This attitude will set the tone for all future client interaction. It will enhance the development of the client's trust in the practitioner and in the potential effectiveness of occupational therapy intervention (Taylor, 2019).

The OT or OTA gathers information about the client's family and friends, community and work roles, education and work histories, leisure and social interests and activities, and living situation. Information about how the client spends and manages time is important. The OT or OTA should interview the client to obtain a detailed account of his or her activities for a typical day (or week) before the onset of physical dysfunction. Information that should be elicited in the daily schedule interview includes the following:

- Time when client wakes and gets out of bed
- Morning activities
- Typical hygiene and dressing tasks
- Breakfast routine
- Work/leisure/home management
- Child care
- Lunch
- Afternoon activities
- Work/leisure/home management
- Rest
- Dinner
- Evening activities
- Leisure and social activities
- Preparation for retiring to bed (i.e., bathing/hygiene)
- Bedtime

The amount of time spent (hours and fractions thereof) on each activity should be recorded carefully. During the interview, the OT or OTA should cue with appropriate questions so that the client will not gloss over or omit any of the daily activities. The interviewer might ask, "What time do you wake up?" "What is the first thing you do in the morning?" "When do you eat lunch?" and "Who fixed lunch for you?"

The OT or OTA reviews with the client the daily life schedule as it was before the physical disability. The client may share information freely, giving many recollections of social, community, vocational, and leisure activities. At times, allowing discussion to stray from the schedule itself is desirable to elicit a well-rounded picture of the client's roles and relationships. Although the client's needs, values, and personal goals should be revealed in a good occupation-centered interview, it is important to keep the discussion focused and to redirect the client if it becomes tangential. The interviewer should focus the client's attention on the specific daily schedule. If the client cannot remember or communicate his or her schedule, the OT or OTA should seek information from friends or family members to reconstruct the client's daily activities patterns.

The OT or OTA helps the client construct a new daily schedule of activities, focusing on the current situation in the treatment facility (or at home if the client is being seen in an outpatient clinic or at home). The interviewer must remember to ask the client who helps with each activity and how much assistance is needed and received. The therapist and client can discuss and compare the two schedules. This process will yield valuable information about the client's occupational needs, values, satisfaction/dissatisfaction with the activities pattern, primary and secondary goals for change, interests, motivation, interpersonal relationships, and fears. This information gives a basis for treatment objectives that meet the client's needs and values. Conducting an occupation-centered interview in this manner will assist the therapist in planning intervention that is meaningful to the client.

Observation

Structured and unstructured observations of the client during the interview, evaluation, and treatment provide the OT and OTA important information about the client's functioning. These interactions provide the opportunity to discover much about the client. How is the client dressed? How does he or she ambulate? What posture and gait pattern does the client demonstrate? Are musculoskeletal deformities or motor dysfunction apparent? What facial expressions, tone of voice, and manner of speech does the client exhibit? How does the client use the affected and nonaffected extremities? Does the client demonstrate any pain mannerisms such as protection of an injured part or grimaces and groans?

Structured observations are used to evaluate performance of self-care, home management, mobility, and transferring. They can be performed by either the OT or the OTA, by observing the client performing real tasks in real or simulated environments. Data from these observations yield information about the client's level of independence, speed, skill, and need for special equipment and the feasibility for further training.

Standardized Tests

Standardized tests follow a strict protocol or set of administration procedures. Standardized tests are valid and reliable. Validity is concerned with the degree to which the test measures what it is supposed to measure (construct validity). For example, a test of cognitive skills is more valid when it measures just those skills, uncontaminated by psychosocial factors or motor skill or communication/interaction factors. Validity is established by measuring the results against a sample population to demonstrate the normal ranges (norms) and abnormal ranges. This allows the score of the person being evaluated to be compared with those of a normed group (Asher, 2014). Reliability is established by measuring the consistency of results. For example, two different evaluators should be able to obtain similar results on the same client; this demonstrates interrater reliability. Also, an evaluator should be able to administer a test in the same way to each person and in the same way to the same person on two different occasions (i.e., pretest and posttest). Assuming conditions are similar, the test should yield similar results.

Standardized tests are considered superior to nonstandardized tests, and most clinicians would prefer to use standardized tests. However, relatively few standardized evaluation procedures are available in occupational therapy. Many evaluation procedures in use have unknown reliability and validity. Many are informal instruments developed by occupational therapists to suit the needs of their own practice settings. Still others are adaptations of existing evaluation instruments and are used with clients other than those for whom they were designed.

Some of the standardized tests used by OTs were designed by professionals in other disciplines. These include tests for measuring achievement, development, intelligence, manual dexterity, motor skills, personality, sensorimotor function, and vocational skills (Asher, 2014; Fleming, 1991b). Although having standardized and objective measures is desired, professional judgment and interpretation are also essential to evaluation (Schell, 2019).

OTAs can participate in the administration of standardized tests if they understand the theory that supports using the standardized tests for a specific client. They should administer those tests chosen by the OT and carefully follow the directions for the test and guidelines to score them. Typically this information can be found in the guide to administration booklet for each test. Varying from the standard testing procedure will yield unreliable results, and the results of the testing will be invalid. They should accurately communicate and document the information gathered from the assessment to the OT to interpret.

Nonstandardized Tests

Nonstandardized tests are subjective and often have no specific instructions for administration of items, no criteria for scoring, and no information on interpreting results of the test. Nonstandardized tests are valued and continue to be used because they provide subtle information that is not necessarily quantifiable but is nonetheless helpful for planning treatment. The quality of the information from such a test depends on the clinical skill, experience, judgment, and bias of the evaluator (Asher, 2014; Schell, 2019). Some nonstandardized evaluation procedures provide broad criteria for scoring and interpretation but still require considerable subjective professional judgment.

Information-Gathering Strategies

The skilled clinician combines two different approaches to gather evaluation information. Using the top-down approach, the therapist focuses on the client's report of the important occupational performance issues limiting abilities to engage successfully in ADL, IADL, work, education, leisure, and social participation. Using the bottom-up approach, the therapist focuses on evaluating the client's body structure and function deficits, as well as developing a plan to compensate for individual performance skills or client factors that interfere with occupational performance. Some OTs and OTAs use a bottom-up approach. Some OTs and OTAs emphasize the top-down approach. This often depends on their experience, the setting, and their chosen frame of reference. Most experienced OTs and OTAs will use both approaches. Taking a simultaneously top-down and bottom-up approach illuminates the client's goals (top-down) and the body functions and deficient performance skills (bottom-up) that limit participation in occupation (Weinstock-Zlotnick & Hinojosa, 2004). The OTA uses observation and active listening to gather information that will contribute to both top-down and bottom-up approaches to treatment.

Clinical Reasoning

Experienced OTs and OTAs work through a series of decisions in a process known as **clinical reasoning** to select practice model and assessment procedures they use in evaluation. Clinical reasoning is defined in the allied health literature as the many modes of thinking and decision making associated with clinical practice to understand clients and their difficulties (Fleming, 1991a; Schell & Cervero, 1993). Clinical reasoning includes but is not limited to hypothetical reasoning and problem solving; it refers to the complex processes used throughout the occupational therapy process to think about a client, the disability, the circumstances, and the meaning of the disability to the client.

Clinical reasoning has been the focus of much study in the past several decades (Coker, 2010; Henderson & Coppard, 2018; Potvin et al., 2019; Unsworth, 2005). Clinical reasoning develops professional expertise, a form of knowing that comes from doing or action. Such knowledge is difficult to articulate and in a sense exceeds the knowledge that can be expressed verbally. Clinical reasoning includes expression of theoretical reasons for clinical decisions, but it is more than that. Based on expertise gained from hands-on experience working with clients, it embodies the tacit knowledge and habitual ways of seeing and doing things and dealing with clients. Tacit knowledge is information the novice clinician learns from observing and participating in therapist-client interactions.

It develops from entry-level practice and builds with each client interaction. This knowledge determines appropriate action for the particular client at a particular time in a specific circumstance. In essence, clinical reasoning is a process of deciding how to act and what to do in a specific circumstance involving the client's well-being (Schell & Cervero, 1993).

Fleming (1991b) proposed that occupational therapists use three types of reasoning. The first is procedural reasoning, used to consider physical problems; an example is evaluating and analyzing the extent and possible causes of limited range of motion (ROM). Interactive reasoning is used to guide interactions with the client (e.g., when trying to obtain information, elicit cooperation, or develop rapport). Conditional reasoning is used to consider clients within their personal and social contexts and futures. Conditional reasoning uses a what-if approach. The therapist considers what might happen if different treatment methods, approaches, techniques, and goals were applied. Clinical reasoning is a complex, changing process for meeting the individual's unique needs for reclaiming a valued sense of self and a meaningful life (Schell & Cervero, 1993).

INTERVENTION PLANNING

Setting up the initial **treatment plan** for the client provides a design or proposal for an overall plan of care and therapeutic program. The **intervention plan** is based on the client's stated goals, the therapist's analysis of performance deficits, the unique circumstances of the individual client, and the treatment setting. Intervention planning presents a challenge because of the complexity and variety of circumstances, goals, and problems seen in clients.

The OT is responsible for the treatment plan, to which the OTA can contribute. The OTA may play a major role in intervention planning for areas of occupation included in the *Occupational Therapy Practice Framework: Domain and Process* (American Occupational Therapy Association, 2014b) such as ADL, IADL, rest and sleep, education, work, play, leisure, and social participation. Although the OTA may become more practiced, skilled, and independent with experience, the final responsibility for planning treatment rests with the OT.

An effective treatment or intervention plan should provide (1) objective and measurable goals with a specific time frame, (2) OT intervention based on theory and current evidence, and (3) a statement describing the mechanisms for service delivery (American Occupational Therapy Association, 2014b). The plan should indicate who will provide the intervention services and the types, frequency, and duration of interventions.

Specific objectives or goals must be outlined in an orderly and sequential manner so that these will be clear to the therapist, therapy assistant, client, family, and health care team. The treatment plan helps OT practitioners initiate intervention. It also provides a standard for measuring the client's progress in therapy so that the plan's effectiveness can be measured. For the OTA, a written treatment plan is essential to provide a clear structure and sequence for treatment interventions. Without a written plan, the OTA is not likely to have a clear understanding of the OT's intended direction

BOX 4.1 Questions to Be Considered in the Planning Process

- What is the most appropriate frame of reference or practice model on which to base the treatment plan?
- What are the client's goals, capabilities, and assets?
- What are the client's limitations and deficits?
- What does occupational therapy have to offer this client?
- What are the goals of treatment?
- What are specific long-term and short-term objectives or goals?
- Are the treatment objectives consistent with the client's needs and personal aspirations?
- If objectives are not compatible, how do they need to be modified?
- Which treatment methods are available to meet these objectives?
- When should the client have met the objectives?
- What standards will be used to determine when the client has reached an objective?
- How will the effectiveness of the treatment plan be evaluated?
- What is the estimated length of treatment?

and focus of treatment. This lack can lead to inconsistent client services that could jeopardize reimbursement and client outcomes. It is the OTA's responsibility to understand the treatment plan provided by the OT. Understanding the treatment plan may require asking for clarification of information about the client's intervention and directions on how to implement the plan.

In writing the treatment plan, the therapist formally documents and analyzes the proposed course of action. Some questions considered in the planning process are listed in Box 4.1.

Identifying Problems and Imagining Solutions

The occupational therapy treatment planning process (Fig. 4.2) requires identifying problems and finding their solutions. The goal is to promote health, well-being, and optimal participation in occupation in desired contexts by persons who are ill or disabled. Treatment planning is a problem-solving process that follows a logical progression. The first step is evaluation, analysis, and identification of problems. The therapist uses data gathered in evaluation to identify functions and dysfunctions in terms of areas of occupation and performance skills. A list of the client's strengths and limitations is developed. This analysis of strengths and limitations becomes the basis of the treatment plan. The therapist then explores prospective solutions and develops treatment objectives, often in close collaboration with the client. From these goals or objectives, the therapist designs and implements a plan of action—the treatment plan.

Selecting a Frame of Reference or Practice Model

The occupational therapy treatment plan derives its logic and rationale from an occupational therapy frame of reference or a specific practice model. The model or frame of reference

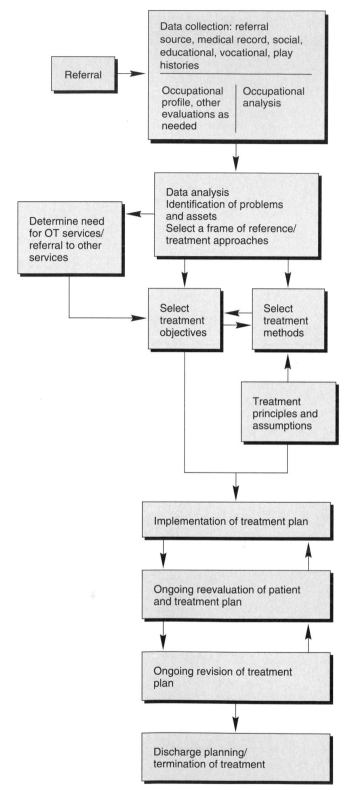

Fig. 4.2 Schematic of the treatment planning process.

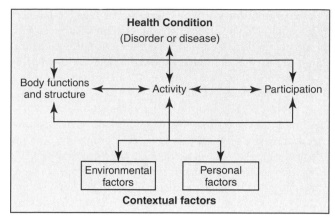

Fig. 4.3 International Classification of Functioning, Disability and Health (ICF model).

treatment, although some overlap exists. Each provides some guidelines for the clinical reasoning process in treatment planning (Gillen, 2019).

The client's motivation and goals must also be considered in planning treatment. For this reason, a frame of reference such as the model of human occupation is helpful. As noted in Chapter 1, some practice models typically used in physical dysfunction practice neglect this important element of the treatment process. (See Chapter 1 for discussions of the model of human occupation and the biomechanical, rehabilitation, sensorimotor, and motor learning practice models.) A current model used by therapists to evaluate and treat clients with physical dysfunction that highly values client interests and overall life goals is the International Classification of Functioning, Disability and Health (ICF) model (World Health Organization, 2020) (Fig. 4.3).

The ICF model emphasizes health and participation in the context of a client's disability. The first version was published by the World Health Organization for trial purposes in 1980, and the ICF has become a multipurpose classification intended for a wide range of uses in client-centered rehabilitation. The ICF is a classification of health and health-related domains—those that provide a guide to help the therapist describe changes in a client's body function and structure, determine what a client with a health condition can do in a standard environment (client level of capacity), and what a client can actually do in his or her usual environment (level of performance). These domains are classified from body, individual, and societal perspectives by means of two lists: a list of body functions and structures and a list of domains of activity and participation. In the ICF model, functioning refers to all body functions, activities, and participation, whereas disability is an umbrella term for physical impairments, activity limitations, and participation restrictions. The ICF model also considers the environmental factors that interact with all of these components. For example, a patient recovering from spinal cord injury may have several body function and structure impairments, including motor and sensory impairments below the level of the spinal cord injury. One potential activity limitation could be related to easy use of transportation in the community. This could lead to

structures the evaluation procedures, objectives, and methods that will be most appropriate for the client (Chisolm & Schell, 2019). The process of identifying problems and imagining solutions is influenced by the frame of reference or practice model being used. Each model has its particular philosophy, body of knowledge, and methods of evaluation and

participation limitations because lack of transportation limits a client's ability to resume normal roles and interests (e.g., going to church, a grocery store, or a job). A therapist using the ICF model would take a top-down approach to treatment planning to focus on the client's health and participation in important life activities. This will include treatment of the patient's physical deficits but also problem solving the client's transportation limitations to help the client resume normal daily life roles. Again, a thorough occupation-centered interview will lead the therapist to understand a client's participation deficits.

The ICF model can be used with other practice models. For example, if the therapist is treating a client with a fracture of the arm that has resulted in limited joint motion and muscle weakness from disuse, the biomechanical practice model might be selected to address specific body function and structure deficits. Evaluation procedures in this model focus on joint ROM measurement and muscle strength testing. Treatment might involve therapeutic exercise and activities. On the other hand, if the client has hemiplegia, the therapist might choose the sensorimotor practice model and the neurodevelopmental (Bobath) approach and would evaluate muscle tone and postural mechanisms. Sensorimotor treatment would be directed toward normalizing tone through positioning, handling techniques and special movement patterns, and facilitating a more normal postural mechanism through activities that demand weight shifts and weight bearing. A therapist using an ICF model would also consider how the body function and structure limitations affect the client's daily tasks and participation in community activities. Is the client able to grasp objects in the kitchen to cook meals? Can the client go back to work or resume her role as a mother with the deficits resulting from the arm fracture? A therapist incorporating the ICF model with other practice models would attach a treatment plan related to body function and structure limitations to important and valued activity and participation goals.

Selecting and Writing Treatment Goals and Objectives

The OT writes treatment goals and objectives to address the specific client problems identified in the occupational therapy evaluation. At the same time, the OT considers potential treatment interventions that could be used to improve the client's overall function in daily activities. Writing objectives and selecting treatment methods are mutually dependent elements of the treatment planning process.

Novice or entry-level OTs and OTAs need to understand that the terms *goal* and *objective* sometimes are used interchangeably; some facilities use one, while some use the other. A treatment objective or goal states what new functional activity a client will be able to perform as a result of occupational therapy intervention. A well-written goal or objective will convey clearly the change in function, performance, or behavior that the client will demonstrate when the treatment intervention or program has been completed successfully. The goal or objective will include an occupation-based

functional outcome that is clear to the reader. Whenever possible, the OT and OTA should involve the client in selecting objectives and planning. The OT, OTA, and client must consider whether objectives or goals are attainable within the time limits of the treatment program. Objectives or goals should reflect the client's life roles and interests and should be consistent with the general needs of the client as stated on the referral and determined by the occupation-centered interview and evaluation. The occupational therapy goals and/or objectives should complement those of other rehabilitation services (i.e., physical therapy, speech language pathology, nursing, and recreational therapy). When clearly defined objectives have not been stated, no sound basis for selecting appropriate treatment methods exists, and evaluating the effectiveness of the treatment program is impossible.

Writing Treatment Objectives. Writing clear treatment objectives requires time, thoughtfulness, and thoroughness. Having a method or structure to guide the process is helpful. One method for writing treatment objectives, described next, includes the concepts of the Occupational Therapy Practice Framework (American Occupational Therapy Association, 2014b).

The objective should convey the client's future functioning and performance once the objective has been achieved. It should do so in simple language and should be understandable to anyone who reads it. A comprehensive treatment objective has the following four elements (Box 4.2):

1. Occupation-based functional outcome. The functional outcome describes the occupation or occupational task in which the client will be able to engage after achieving the goal. Many goals in the areas of occupation already have implied functional outcomes that are occupational in nature (e.g., getting dressed, eating, transferring from bed to chair). However, these goals can be strengthened by

---

BOX 4.2 Elements of a Comprehensive Treatment Objective

Occupation-based functional outcome. Describes the real-life occupation or occupational task that the client will be able to engage in as a result of achieving the goal (e.g., to participate in religious services). The statement may include the context if this makes the outcome clearer (e.g., to cope with cognitive demands of a receptionist job in a medical office).

Statement of terminal behavior. Specifies the physical changes, type of behavior, or performance skill that the patient is expected to display. The terminal behavior consists of an action verb and the object receiving the action (e.g., The patient will don [action verb] a shirt [object].).

Conditions. States the circumstances required for the performance of the terminal behavior (e.g., Given verbal prompts [condition], the patient will don a shirt.).

Criterion. States the degree of competence or the performance standard by which the patient's behavior is to be measured (e.g., Given verbal prompts, the patient will don a shirt in 5 minutes with no errors [criterion].).

adding occupations that the client identifies as being of high importance (e.g., to dress for work or to participate in religious services). The statement may include the context if this makes the outcome clearer (e.g., to dress for work as a high school teacher). Including an occupation-based functional outcome is especially important for goals that focus primarily on body function and structure limitations such as ROM, muscle strength, and coordination. The emphasis should be placed on occupation—the goal within the domain of occupational therapy. A goal that emphasizes shoulder external rotation might have a functional outcome such as to brush and style hair.

2. Statement of terminal behavior. Terminal behavior specifies the observable physical change, the type of behavior, or performance skill that the patient is expected to display following treatment (Asher, 2014). The terminal behavior comprises an action verb and the object receiving the action. Consider, for example, the goal to remove the blouse. *Remove* is the action verb, and *blouse* is the object of the action.

3. Conditions. Conditions are the circumstances required for the performance of the terminal behavior. The conditions answer questions such as, "Is special equipment needed?" "Are assistive devices necessary?" "Is supervision or assistance necessary?" "Are special cues necessary?" (American Occupational Therapy Association, 2014b). An example would be, "When given verbal cues, the patient will remove the blouse." This statement indicates that the client will only be able to remove the blouse when someone is present to provide verbal cues. The phrase "when given verbal cues" represents a special circumstance or condition that enables adequate performance of the terminal behavior. Another example would be, "When using a built-up handle spoon, the patient will feed self." The patient may only be able to feed themselves if given special equipment. In this case, the adaptive equipment is an important condition needed to meet the client goal. Clients achieve many treatment objectives without any special devices, equipment, environmental modification, or human assistance. Therefore the statement of conditions is not always necessary. Conditions should be used only when some special circumstance is required to enable the performance of the terminal behavior. The treatment methodology and the treatment program's time frame are not considered conditions.

4. Criterion. The criterion is the performance standard or degree of competence the patient is expected to achieve, stated in measurable or observable terms (American Occupational Therapy Association, 2014a; Coker, 2010). The criterion answers questions such as, "How much?" "How often?" "How well?" "How accurately?" "How completely?" and "How quickly?"

The following is an objective that contains a criterion: "If given verbal cues, the patient will don the blouse within 1 minute." The criterion or performance standard indicates that the task will be completed within 1 minute. This specification might be a necessary criterion in a long-term care facility in which an aide supervises the patient's dressing; speed of performance is important so that the aide can attend to other tasks and patients.

Stating a performance standard is important to show incremental progress of a functional task over time. For example, a patient may be able to complete a transfer to the toilet with moderate assistance at the initial evaluation. The occupational performance objective may be as follows: "The patient will complete the toilet transfer with minimal assistance." Once this goal has been achieved, each new functional goal would be one step closer to the ultimate goal: "The patient will complete transfer to the toilet independently." In fact, the therapist may have set the client's long-term goals for this much desired functional outcome. Changes in muscle grades, increases in joint ROM, degree of competence in task performance, and speed of performance are possible measures for criteria.

Critiquing Sample Objectives. Studying sample objectives and analyzing their elements can help the beginner refine skills in writing clear objectives. Consider the following examples:

1. "Given assistive devices, the patient will eat independently in 30 minutes." In this objective the terminal behavior is the statement "the patient will eat," and *eat* is the action verb. No object needs to be named because the object (food) of the action is implicit. The condition is "given assistive devices." This statement indicates the special circumstances—in this case devices—that will make eating possible. The performance standards are "independently in 30 minutes." This statement reflects that the patient will be able to eat without human assistance and will complete eating a meal within 30 minutes, a reasonable amount of time for this activity. The occupation-based functional outcome is not stated separately because eating independently is an occupational task as well as a statement of behavior.

2. "The joint ROM of the left elbow will increase." As written, this objective is a good statement of terminal behavior. It indicates the type of change in physical function that is expected as a result of the treatment program. Conditions are not necessary because no special circumstances are required for the patient to demonstrate or perform the increased ROM. However, the objective does need a criterion because the amount of increase in ROM is not indicated, making it difficult to measure progress. The objective can be improved as follows: "The joint ROM of the left elbow will increase from 0-120 to 0-135 degrees." This adds the criterion of a 15-degree increase in ROM, which is measurable. More critically, the occupation-based functional outcome is missing. The objective could be further improved: "The joint ROM of the left elbow will increase from 0-120 to 0-135 degrees so that the client can prepare for return to work as a licensed practical nurse."

3. "The patient will operate the control systems of the left above-elbow prosthesis without hesitation so that he can begin practicing skills for his job as an auto-supply parts clerk." In this objective, "operate the control systems" is the terminal behavior. *Operate* is the action verb, and *control systems* is the object of the action. This outcome

is the skill (behavior) that is expected as a result of the prosthetic training program. Conditions are not necessary because the desired goal is for the patient to perform this skill under any circumstances. "Without hesitation" is the criterion. It is an observable level of skill indicative of automatic performance. The phrase "job as an auto-supply parts clerk" conveys the occupational outcome.

4. "Given assistive devices, the patient will dress herself in less than 20 minutes so that she can participate in group outings." *Dress* is the action verb that indicates the terminal behavior. The indirect object of the action (herself) is stated; the direct object (in clothes) does not need to be stated because it is implied in the action verb. The availability of assistive devices is a necessary condition for this patient to perform this task; thus the statement of conditions, "given assistive devices," is necessary. The criterion or performance standard is stated in terms of speed and indicates that dressing within 20 minutes is a reasonable expectation for this patient and for this task. Other standards could be added if formal neatness or appropriateness for a given occasion were important for the patient's life roles. The occupation-based functional outcome is "participating in group outings."

5. "Given equipment setup and assistive devices, the patient will use mobile arm supports to feed himself independently." The equipment setup and the availability of assistive devices constitute the conditions for this objective. The criterion for performance under these circumstances is "independently," which indicates that once the equipment and devices are provided, the task of eating can be performed without further human assistance. Eating is an occupational task.

Many variables and unknowns exist in the performance and functions of persons with physical dysfunction. Therefore the degree to which they can benefit from, participate in, or succeed at rehabilitation programs cannot be predicted with certainty. This fact often makes it difficult for OTs and OTAs to write comprehensive treatment objectives. However, they should attempt to write such objectives, using past experience with similar patients and knowledge gained during the evaluation process to describe desired terminal behavior, conditions, and criteria for each treatment objective. If the conditions and criteria cannot be predicted, OTs and OTAs should use a specific statement of terminal behavior until applicable conditions and criteria become apparent. The stated terminal behaviors can then be modified, as treatment progresses, to become comprehensive objectives. Unless the behavior itself is an occupational task, an occupation-based functional outcome should always be included in the occupational therapy plan of care.

Selecting Treatment Methods or Interventions

Selecting treatment methods or interventions is a challenging aspect of the treatment planning process. OTs and OTAs select a treatment method based on a principle or theory related to the problem being treated and its cause. The underlying principle may come from a frame of reference or a practice model (Gillen, 2019). For example, nerves

---

BOX 4.3 **Questions to Ask While Selecting a Treatment Method**
What is the goal for the client?
What are the precautions or contraindications that affect the occupational therapy program?
What is the prognosis for recovery?
What were the results of evaluations in occupational therapy and other services?
What other treatment is the client receiving?
What are the goals of other treatment programs, and are the occupational therapy goals compatible with these goals?
How much energy does the client expend in other therapies?
What is the state of the client's general health?
What are the client's interests, vocational skills, and psychological needs?
What is the client's physical and sociocultural environment?
What roles will the client assume in the community?
What kinds of activities or exercises will be most useful and meaningful to the client? (Chisolm & Schell, 2019)
How can treatment be graded to meet the client's changing needs as progression or regression occurs?
What special equipment or adaptations of therapeutic equipment are necessary for the client to perform maximally?
What can be provided under the terms of the reimbursement source and the facility policy?
What other means exist for providing needed interventions if the primary sources refuse to reimburse?

regenerate after peripheral nerve injury and repair. Increasing movement and strength of reinnervated muscles helps to maintain or increase the performance of the muscles in functional tasks. Improvement of function through use is a principle of the biomechanical model. This principle guides the therapist to select graded therapeutic activity or exercise as the method of choice to affect the desired goals. Box 4.3 lists other factors that influence the selection of treatment methods.

When treatment methods are selected and written, others reading the treatment plan should understand exactly how the methods will be used to reach specific objectives. Sometimes several methods may be necessary to achieve one objective, or the same methods may be used to reach several objectives.

Another aspect of treatment planning and documentation of treatment intervention concerns the requirements of the different reimbursing companies and agencies. The guidelines for writing treatment goals may need to be adjusted to suit the standards of the reimbursing entity (Box 4.4).

IMPLEMENTATION OF THE TREATMENT PLAN

The treatment plan can be implemented when at least one objective or goal and one or more treatment methods have been selected. During implementation, the OT and/or the OTA guide the client as he or she engages in the procedures that have been designed. The comprehensive treatment plan may evolve

BOX 4.4 Writing Treatment Goals to Satisfy Reimbursing Agencies

To ensure that occupational therapy services are reimbursed, practitioners must suit their documentation to the demands of insurers and Medicare and Medicaid. The following is a treatment plan that would be accepted by Medicare.

Long-Term Goals (LTGs)
1. Client will independently dress self in 3 weeks.
2. Client will demonstrate functional transfers to and from bed and toilet with equipment in 3 weeks.
3. Client will complete simple household mobility tasks with equipment in 3 weeks.

Short-Term Goals (STGs)
1. Client will require only minimal assistance for upper extremity dressing tasks in 1 week.
2. Client will demonstrate bed mobility with minimal assistance in 1 week.
3. Client will demonstrate wheelchair transfer to and from toilet with moderate assistance in 1 week.

Intervention
Client will be seen five times a week for trunk control, postural alignment, sitting balance, transfer, and dressing training.

The long-term goals are written in terms of what the OT believes the client will be able to perform after 3 weeks of occupational therapy intervention. The short-term goals are small components or steps toward meeting the long-term goals. Short-term goals are written as components of the long-term goal to show the client's gains in functional recovery. For example, the long-term goal "Client will demonstrate dressing independently in 3 weeks" may be broken down into several steps such as UE dressing with minimal assistance, lower extremity dressing with minimal assistance, and dressing independently. During the first week of treatment the short-term goal identified earlier is "Client will require only minimal assistance for UE dressing in 1 week." If the client can meet this goal within 1 week, the OT or OTA revises the plan. The long-term goal stays the same; however, the short-term goal may change to "Client will require only minimal assistance for LE dressing in 1 week." If this goal is met the following week, what might be another short-term goal that continues to lead to the long-term goal?

The next component of the treatment plan is the intervention. The purpose of the intervention is to identify clearly the OT's professional assessment of how often the client will need treatment and the focus and methods of the proposed treatment. A clear link between the goals and the intervention exists. The services provided should directly reflect what the therapists will do with the client to develop the client's abilities to meet the identified goals.

Beginning therapists frequently get confused as to the difference between an intervention and a goal. A goal is what the client will be able to do, and an intervention is what the therapist will do with the client to foster functional performance. Discussion or statement of intervention should not be included in a client's goal.

over time. For example, over the days in which a lengthy evaluation procedure (e.g., complete evaluation of basic self-care skills) is in progress, the client may begin a program of therapeutic activity to strengthen specific muscle groups. As the evaluation continues, an increasing number of problems may be identified and additional objectives or goals and methods may be added to the treatment plan. The OTA should be prepared to address continual changes in the plan.

Reevaluation/Revision of the Plan

Once the treatment plan is implemented, its effectiveness is evaluated on an ongoing basis through continuous observation and **reevaluation**. The OT and OTA must be alert observers and ask the following questions:
- Are the treatment goals and/or objectives suitable to the client's needs and capabilities?
- Are the treatment interventions most appropriate for fulfilling the treatment plan?
- Does the client engage in the treatment interventions and see them as worthwhile and meaningful?
- Are the treatment objectives realistic, and are they consistent with the client's personal goals and interests?

The OT may choose to reevaluate physical functions and performance skills with the same evaluation procedures used in the initial evaluation. Improvements and continued limitations can then be compared with baseline functions recorded at the initial evaluation. Such comparisons validate the treatment plan and provide the objective evidence of change required for reimbursement of OT services. Scrutinizing the treatment plan in this way enables the therapist to modify the plan as the need arises. The client's progress toward the stated objectives is the criterion for determining the treatment plan's effectiveness.

The therapist may recognize a need to revise or modify the initial treatment plan based on information gained from observations and reevaluation of the client, as just outlined. For example, the client's progress may be significant enough that increasing the duration, complexity, or resistance of the activity is beneficial. Conversely, the gradual decline of physical resources may necessitate a decrease in resistance, duration, and complexity of activity. This situation applies in degenerative diseases, in which a primary objective is to maintain optimal function despite declining strength and coordination.

If the client cannot see the therapeutic program as helpful or meaningful, a change in treatment approaches and methods may also be necessary. On the other hand, if the client is highly motivated and progressing well in treatment, the plan can be accelerated. The initial plan is continually revised according to the client's needs and progress. This process of reevaluation, revision, and reimplementation of the treatment plan continues throughout the course of the therapeutic program (American Occupational Therapy Association, 2014b; American Occupational Therapy Association, 2015).

DISCHARGE PLANNING AND DISCONTINUATION OF TREATMENT

Ultimately the occupational therapy treatment plan is directed to preparing the client to return to daily life roles and interests, which may include living at home or to another suitable living arrangement. **Discharge planning** is a continual process that starts at the initial evaluation and continues throughout the treatment program.

Discharge planning should be initiated as the client's treatment program in the primary health care facility is progressing. Discharge planning is a team effort that involves the client, the family, and all the rehabilitation specialists concerned with the client's care. Preparation for discharge includes discussing the client's goals for discharge, medical considerations, needs for assistive devices and mobility equipment, and considering caregiver and community support systems. This information will help the rehabilitation team recommend an appropriate discharge placement and plan a home activity or exercise program. Many times a visit to the client's home will allow a therapist to assess architectural barriers in the environment. Discharge planning should include education and training of the client and caregivers for a smooth transition. Arrangements for home care referral for continued therapies and appropriate community support agencies are also important.

The client and family must be prepared emotionally and psychologically for discharge. Therapists should not assume that clients are emotionally prepared for (or functionally capable of) managing transition to the new environment. Generalization (transfer) of learning from a health care facility to the home may be difficult for the client. The family may not know the client's capabilities or how best to give assistance. Emotional support, education, training, counseling, and information about resources are helpful measures in easing the transition. The family needs information about the client's ADL status and performance expectations; solutions to accessibility problems in the home, workplace, and community; information on home modification; how to obtain, use, and care for assistive devices or mobility equipment; and availability of community resources such as emergency care, self-help groups, respite care, and independent living centers (American Occupational Therapy Association, 2014a).

Termination of treatment requires a final reevaluation of the client. The OT should clearly indicate objectives achieved, partially achieved, or not achieved in the treatment program. The OTA may be directed to perform parts of this evaluation. The OT writes a discharge summary based on these data. The summary should indicate expected future performance of the client and potential for further rehabilitation. Termination of occupational therapy services can affirm the success of the treatment program. In reality, however, meeting all therapy goals set at the initial evaluation is not always achieved; clients may be discharged before objectives of treatment are met and treatment is concluded (Lederer, 2007). The client may be referred to another facility or to home care, with another therapist continuing the treatment program. Careful communication between therapists and agencies is necessary to ensure a smooth transition and continuity of care.

Treatment Plan Model

The model provided in Fig. 4.4 and in a more extended version in Fig. 4.5 is useful for learning what goes into treatment planning. Fig. 4.4 shows in boldface the areas that the OTA might complete. Both the model and the extended version are limited in their range; actual clinical practice will

---

Case #
Personal data
  Name
  Age
  Diagnosis
  Disability
  Occupations
  Treatment goals stated in referral
Other services
Frame of reference, practice model
OT evaluation
  Occupational profile
    Occupations of concern
    Occupational tasks of concern to client
    Performance patterns
    Contexts
Analysis of occupational performance
  ADL
  IADL
  Work
  Leisure
  Education
  Social participation
Performance skill deficit areas
  1. Motor
  2. Process
  3. Communication/interaction
Client factors, body functions and structures
  1. Mental
  2. Sensory
  3. Neuromusculoskeletal and movement-related
  4. Cardiovascular, respiratory, immunological
  5. Voice and speech
  6. Genitourinary
  7. Skin
Evaluation summary
Assets
Problem list
Outline treatment plan (OTA focuses on performance of occupational tasks)
  1. Problem
  2. Occupation-based functional outcome
  3. Objective
  4. Treatment methods
  5. Grading and adaptations

Fig. 4.4 Treatment plan model. Sections appropriate for the entry-level occupational therapy assistant are shown in boldface.

EXTENDED TREATMENT PLAN GUIDE

PERSONAL DATA
Fill in the requested information from the medical record or case study (occupational and medical history, education, occupation, work history, leisure habits, self-care habits, social relationships, cultural background).

Name	Diagnosis(es)
Age, Gender, Marital Status, Family	Disability(ies)
Occupation(s)	

OTHER SERVICES
List and describe briefly other services the client is using.

Physician	Vocational counseling
Psychology/psychiatry	Supported employment
Nursing	Educational services
Respiratory therapy	Spiritual counseling
Social service	Physical therapy
Speech pathology	Home health care
Community social groups/day care	

FRAME OF REFERENCE/TREATMENT APPROACH
State the frame of reference and treatment approach on which the treatment plan is based. More than one may be necessary.

OT EVALUATION
Occupational profile: State how this is obtained, which interviews or other assessments are or were used.
Analysis of occupational performance: State which occupations, occupational tasks are to be evaluated, including context as relevant.

Activities of daily living
  Bathing and showering
  Bowel and bladder management
  Dressing
  Eating
  Feeding
  Functional mobility
  Personal device care
  Personal hygiene and grooming
  Sexual activity
  Sleep/rest
  Toilet hygiene
Instrumental activities of daily living
  Care of others (include supervising caregivers)
  Care of pets
  Child rearing
  Communication device use
  Community mobility
  Financial management
  Health management and maintenance
  Home establishment and management

  Meal preparation and cleanup
  Safety procedures and emergency responses
  Shopping
Work
  Employment interests and pursuits
  Employment seeking and acquisition
  Job performance
  Retirement preparation and adjustment
  Volunteer exploration
  Volunteer participation
Leisure
  Leisure exploration
  Leisure participation
Education
  Formal educational preparation
  Exploration of informal personal interests
  Participation in informal personal education
Social interaction
  Community
  Family
  Peer/friend

Performance skills: For each category selected, list the specific skills, using the OTPF[4] as a guide

Motor skills
  Posture
  Mobility
  Coordination
  Strength and effort
  Energy

Process skills
  Energy
  Knowledge
  Temporal organization
  Organizing space and objects
  Adaptation

Fig. 4.5 Extended treatment plan guide. (Use of categories from American Occupation Therapy Association. Occupational therapy practice framework: domain and process. *Am J Occup Ther.* 2002;56:608–639.)

EXTENDED TREATMENT PLAN GUIDE

Communication/interaction skills
    Physicality
    Information exchange
    Relations
    Performance patterns
    Habits
    Routines
    Roles

Contexts: Discuss relationship of contexts to occupations affected by disability.

Client factors: From the list below, select the areas that are or were evaluated. For each area selected, list the specific factors, using the OTPF[4] as a guide. Indicate whether evaluation was determined by testing or by observation.

BODY FUNCTIONS
Global mental functions
    Level of arousal
    Orientation
    Motivation
Specific mental functions
    Memory
    Attention
    Perception
    Body schema
    Motor planning
    Stereognosis
    Spatial relations
    Position in space
    Figure/background
    Perceptual constancy
    Judgment
    Safety awareness
    Problem-solving ability
    Sequencing
    Abstract thinking
    Functional language skills
    Comprehension of speech/writing
    Ability to express ideas
    Reading
    Writing
    Functional mathematical skills
    Mental calculations
    Written calculations
    Self-esteem
    Self-concept
    Coping skills
    Maturity (developmental level)
    Adjustment to disability
    Reality functioning
    Rigidity
    Self-control
    Emotional expression
Sensory functions and pain
    Seeing and related functions
    Visual perception
    Visual fields
    Visual-motor coordination
    Depth perception

Fig. 4.5 (Continued).

EXTENDED TREATMENT PLAN GUIDE

Perception of vertical/horizontal elements
Eye movements
Hearing and vestibular functions
Sensations of touch, pain, temperature, proprioception, taste, smell
Pain
Neuromusculoskeletal and movement-related functions
ROM
Muscle strength
Physical endurance
Standing tolerance
Walking tolerance
Sitting balance
Involuntary movement
Movement speed
Level of motor development
Equilibrium/protective responses
Coordination/muscle control
Spasms
Spasticity
Stage of motor recovery (stroke client only)
Postural reflex mechanism
Functional movement patterns
Hand function
Swallowing/cranial nerve functions
Cardiovascular functions
Respiratory functions
Voice and speech functions
Skin integrity, wound healing, other skin functions

EVALUATION SUMMARY
Summarize findings from tests and observations.

ASSETS
List the assets of the client and his or her situation that can be used to enhance progress toward maximum independence.

PROBLEM LIST
Identify and list the problems that require occupational therapy intervention.

OBJECTIVES
Write specific treatment objectives in comprehensive form. Each should relate to a specific problem in the problem list and be identified by the corresponding number.

METHODS OF TREATMENT
Describe in detail appropriate treatment methods for the client.

GRADATION OF TREATMENT
Briefly state how treatment methods will be graded to enhance the client's progress.

Fig. 4.5 (Continued).

demand planning that is highly specific to the individual and that is focused on the main areas of need. In other words, in Fig. 4.5, every possible area for evaluation is noted; however, with an actual client or patient only a small portion of this would be relevant based on the client's specific life roles and interests. Today's health care environment demands rapid assessment and treatment, focusing on functional outcomes and improvements. The OTA student and new graduate face a great challenge in learning how to apply treatment planning principles with flexibility and focus so that objectives can be met within the time frame allowed by insurance.

A case study with an example of a treatment plan for a hypothetical client follows at the end of the chapter.

SUMMARY

The occupational therapy process begins with referral and ends with termination of therapy services. Although the process includes discrete stages that can be named and described, the process is not stepwise but rather fluid, with the stages intermingled at times. Over the course of the process, an evaluation is completed, goals and objectives are written, intervention is provided, and the discharge process is finalized. The client's motivation cannot be underestimated as a factor in treatment success.

The OT and OTA have specific responsibilities and areas of emphasis within the occupational therapy process. The OT manages and directs the process in collaboration with the OTA. Experienced OTAs are able to take on additional responsibilities and specialty roles.

The OTA is encouraged to study and practice writing clear and comprehensive treatment goals and objectives and to learn as much as possible about different intervention methods. Such study will yield great rewards: clinical clarity, effective communication, and professional self-confidence.

CASE STUDY

Sample Intervention Plan
The following plan presents a sampling of parts of a proposed intervention program; it is not a comprehensive plan. The reader is encouraged to add objectives and methods to address additional problems to make the plan more comprehensive.

Case Study
Mrs. R. is 49 years old. She has been a homemaker and mother to her two sons; one is 26 and married, and the other is 17. Mrs. R. is divorced. Before the onset of her illness, Mrs. R. lived in an apartment with her younger son. At present, she and her younger son live with her married son, his wife, and their 4-year-old boy.

Mrs. R. had Guillain-Barré syndrome. She has been left with residual weakness of all four extremities. Mrs. R. uses a standard wheelchair for mobility.

Mrs. R. appears thin and frail. She speaks in a weak voice and appears to be passive and discouraged. She says she cannot accomplish anything. The home situation is poor. Mrs. R. does not communicate with her daughter-in-law, and the couple and Mrs. R. disagree over management of the teenage son. Mrs. R. feels unable to assert her authority as his mother or to express her needs and feelings. The disability has brought about the loss of her independence and has changed her role in relation to her younger son.

Her daughter-in-law reports that Mrs. R. is dependent for self-care, never attempts to help with homemaking, and isolates herself in her room much of the time. She believes that her mother-in-law is capable of more activity "if only she would try." She says she is willing to allow Mrs. R. to do some of the household work.

Mrs. R. was referred for outpatient occupational therapy services for restoration or maintenance of motor functioning and increased independence in ADL.

Personal Data
Name: Mrs. R.
Age: 49

Diagnosis: Guillain-Barré syndrome
Disability: Residual weakness, upper and lower extremities
Treatment aims stated in physician referral: restoration or maintenance of motor functioning; increased independence in ADL

Other Services
Physician: prescription of medication, maintenance of general health, supervision of rehabilitation program
Physical therapy: muscle strengthening, ambulation and transfer training
Social service: individual and family counseling
Community social group: socialization

Frame of Reference
Model of Human Occupation

Treatment Approaches
Biomechanical
Rehabilitative
Cognitive-behavioral

OT Evaluation
Occupational profile
Occupational history (short interview)
Canadian Occupational Performance Measure
Occupational performance observation and interview
Self-care
Home management
Performance skills (to be observed in execution of occupational tasks such as dressing or housework)
Motor skills
Posture
Mobility
Coordination
Strength and effort
Energy (physical)
Process skills
Energy (mental)
Knowledge

Temporal organization
Organization of space and objects
Adaptation, adjustment, accommodation
Communication/interaction skills
Physical communication: observe gestures, eye contact, body language
Exchange of information: observe for assertiveness
Relations: observe naturally occurring interactions with family
Evaluation of client factors
Sensory and movement-related functions
Muscle strength: test
Passive ROM: test
Physical endurance: observe, interview
Walking tolerance: observe, interview
Movement speed: observe
Coordination: test, observe
Functional movement: test, observe
Sensation (touch, pain, thermal, proprioception): test
Mental functions
Energy, drive, motivation: observe, interview
Judgment: observe
Safety awareness: observe
Motor planning, sequencing movement: observe
Regulation of emotions, coping skills: observe
Adjustment to disability: observe, interview

Evaluation Summary

Before onset of illness, Mrs. R. lived independently with her 17-year-old son. Since her illness, she and her son have moved in with her 26-year-old son, his wife, and their 4-year-old son. This arrangement has proved less than ideal. Little communication occurs between Mrs. R. and her daughter-in-law. Conflicts between the couple and Mrs. R. about the management of her teenage son are a problem.

The disability has caused the loss of Mrs. R.'s independence and has changed her roles as homemaker and mother. She says she has no authority as mother of her 17-year-old; she also says she does not know how to express her needs and feelings anymore. On the Canadian Occupational Performance Measure, Mrs. R. identified the following four goals as immediately important to her. She expressed low satisfaction with her ability at present to perform in all of the following four goals:

1. To dress independently
2. To help with housework, laundry, and dishes
3. To talk with and guide her teenage son
4. To get out more to see friends as she did in the past

Mrs. R. was observed while dressing with assistance from her daughter-in-law. She needs some physical help with dressing and has difficulty with buttons and zippers. Mrs. R. reports that she manages some personal care such as washing her face, hair care, and dental care. She requires an adaptive toothbrush and needs assistance in toilet transferring and showering. Mrs. R. does not perform any home management tasks but is potentially capable of light activities such as setting the table, dusting, and folding laundry. Mrs. R.'s daughter-in-law is willing to allow her mother-in-law some household activities if an understanding about their respective roles can be established.

Throughout the interview and observation, Mrs. R. made limited eye contact, sighed deeply, and appeared passive and discouraged about her disability. She said several times that she cannot accomplish anything. She agreed with her daughter-in-law's statement that she tends to stay in her room alone.

Muscle testing revealed that all muscles are the same grades bilaterally: scapula and shoulder muscles are graded F+ to G (3+ to 4), elbow and forearm muscles are F+ to G (3+ to 4), and wrist and hand musculature is F+ (3+). Trunk muscles are G (4); all muscles of the hip are G (4) except adductors and external rotators, which are F+ (3+). Knee flexors and extensors are G (4). Ankle plantar flexors and dorsiflexors are F (3), and all foot muscles are F− (3−) to P (2).

All joint motions are within normal to functional range. Physical endurance is limited to 1 hour of light activity of the upper extremities, with some ambulation, before rest. Mrs. R. uses a wheelchair for energy conservation and propels it with both arms and legs. Slight incoordination, evident in fine hand function, is caused by muscle weakness.

Sensory modalities of touch, pain, temperature, and proprioception are intact. No cognitive deficits were observed.

Assets

Can identify own goals
Potential for good living situation
Presence of able-bodied adults who can assist
Potential for some further recovery
Some functional muscle strength
Good joint mobility
Good sensation

Problem List

1. Muscle weakness
2. Low physical endurance
3. Limited walking tolerance
4. Mild incoordination
5. Self-care dependence
6. Homemaking dependence
7. Dependent transferring
8. Isolation, apparent depression
9. Reduced social interaction
10. Lack of assertiveness

Problem 1

Muscle weakness (shoulders)

Objective

Muscle strength of shoulder flexors will increase from F+ (3+) to G (4) to allow patient more independence in self-care and resumption of a portion of homemaking tasks and role.

Method

Light progressive resistive exercise to shoulder flexion: Client is seated in a regular chair, wearing a weighted cuff one-half the weight of her maximum resistance above each elbow. Lifts arms alternately through 10 repetitions and then rests. The activity is repeated using three-quarter maximum resistance, then full resistance. Activities: reaching for glasses in overhead cupboard and placing them on the table, replacing glasses in cupboard when dry; rolling out pastry dough on a slightly inclined pastry board; wiping table, counter, and cupboard doors, using a forward push-pull motion; Turkish knotting project with weaving frame set vertically in front of her and tufts of yarn on right and left sides, at hip level.

Gradation
Increase resistance, number of repetitions, and length of time as strength improves.

Problem 1
Muscle weakness (fingers and wrists)

Objective
Strength of wrist flexors and extensors and finger flexors will increase from F+ (3+) to G (4) to allow patient more independence in self-care and resumption of a portion of homemaking tasks and role.

Method
Light progressive resistive exercises for wrist flexors and extensors: Client is seated, side to table, with pronated forearm resting on the table and hand extended over edge of table; a hand cuff, with small weights equal to one-half of her maximum resistance attached to the palmar surface, is worn on the hand; client extends the wrist through full ROM against gravity for 10 repetitions, then rests. The exercise is repeated with three-quarter maximum resistance and then full resistance. The same procedure is used to exercise wrist flexors, except that the forearm is supinated on the table, and the weights are suspended from the dorsal side of the hand cuff. Activities to improve finger flexors: tearing lettuce to make a salad; hand washing panties and hosiery. Progress to kneading soft clay or bread dough.

Gradation
Increase resistance, repetitions, and time.

Problem 5
Self-care dependence

Objective
Given assistive devices, Mrs. R. will be able to dress herself independently within 20 minutes.

Method
Putting on bra: Using a back-opening stretch bra, pass bra around waist so that opening is in front and straps are facing up; fasten bra in front at waist level; slide fastened bra around at waist level so that cups are in front; slip arms through straps and work straps up over shoulders; adjust cups and straps. Putting on shirt: Place loose-fitting blouse on lap with back facing up and neck toward knees; place arms under back of blouse and into arm holes; push sleeves up onto arms past elbows; gather back material up from neck to hem with hands and duck head forward and pass garment over the head; work blouse down by shrugging shoulders and pulling into place with hands; use button hook to fasten front opening. Putting on underpants and slacks: Sitting on bed or in wheelchair, cross legs, reach down, and place one opening over foot; cross opposite leg, place other opening over foot; uncross legs, work pants up over feet and up under thighs (a dressing stick may be used to pull pants up if leaning forward is difficult); shift hips from side to side and work pants up as far as possible over buttocks; stand, if possible, and pull pants to

waist level; then sit and pull zipper up with prefastened zipper pull; use Velcro at waist closure on slacks. Putting on socks: Using stretch socks and seated, cross one leg, place sock over toes and work sock up onto foot and over heel; cross other leg and repeat. Putting on shoes: With slip-on shoe with Velcro fasteners, use procedure for socks.

Gradation
Progress to more difficult tasks such as pantyhose, tie shoes, dresses, pullover garments.

Problem 6
Homemaking dependence

Objective
Given assistive devices, Mrs. R. will perform homemaking activities.

Method
Using a dust mitt, client dusts furniture surfaces easily reached from wheelchair such as lamp tables and coffee table; sits at sink to wash dishes; practices folding small items of clothing such as panties, nylons, and children's underwear while sitting at kitchen table; have Mrs. R.'s daughter-in-law observe activities at treatment facility; work out an acceptable list of activities and a schedule with both women. Discuss how Mrs. R. could make some contributions to home management routines; ask Mrs. R. to keep activity diary, noting any performance difficulties and successes for review at next visit.

Gradation
Increase number of household responsibilities. Increase time spent on household activities.

Problem 8
Isolation, depression

Objective
Mrs. R. will reduce time spent alone from 6 waking hours to 3 waking hours.

Method
Engage Mrs. R. in self-reflection about precursor events that discourage participation. Help Mrs. R. to restructure thinking about her own ability to participate. Establish acceptable graded activity schedule between Mrs. R. and son and daughter-in-law; include homemaking tasks and socialization with family through playing games, watching TV, preparing and eating meals, and conversing; family members encourage Mrs. R. to be with them but will be accepting if she refuses; have Mrs. R. keep activity diary for self-reflection and review; determine how time is spent and discuss how it could be more productive and enjoyable. Initiate a vocational activity such as needlework or tile mosaics to complete at home; set goals for where and how much activity will be performed.

Gradation
Increase time spent out of own room; include friends, neighbors, and family in household social activities; plan a community outing for shopping or lunch.

REVIEW QUESTIONS

1. List and describe the stages or steps in the occupational therapy process.
2. Describe and contrast the roles of the OT and the OTA with regard to each stage of the occupational therapy process.
3. Give at least one example that shows the flow of the occupational therapy process.
4. Summarize what the OTA must do to achieve greater responsibility in the occupational therapy process.
5. Discuss the purposes of occupational therapy evaluation.
6. Describe the role of the OT and the OTA in evaluation.
7. What skills must the OT and OTA possess to be an effective evaluator?
8. Define and discuss clinical reasoning.
9. Which specific areas of occupation and performance skills does the OT generally evaluate while setting up a treatment plan for patients with physical dysfunction?
10. Describe four methods of evaluation that the OT may use in the evaluation process.
11. Describe the daily schedule interview, including the information to be covered and the recommended ways of obtaining this information.
12. Discuss how the International Classification of Functioning, Disability and Health (ICF model) is used to develop client-centered OT treatment.
13. Describe the roles of the OT and the OTA in treatment planning.
14. Why should a treatment plan be based on a specific frame of reference or treatment approach?
15. List the steps in developing a treatment plan.
16. List, define, and give examples of the three elements of a comprehensive treatment objective or goal.
17. List six factors to consider while selecting treatment methods.
18. Is it necessary to develop a comprehensive treatment plan before treatment can begin? Explain.
19. Is it ever necessary to change the initial treatment plan? Why?
20. What criterion is used to evaluate the effectiveness of a treatment plan?
21. How does the therapist know when to modify or change the plan?
22. What are some of the concerns and preparations involved in termination of treatment?

REFERENCES

American Occupational Therapy Association. (2014a). Guidelines for supervision, roles, and responsibilities during the delivery of occupational therapy services. *American Journal Occupational Therapy, 68*(3), S16—S22. Available from https://doi.org/10.5014/ajot.2014.686S03.

American Occupational Therapy Association. (2014b). Occupational therapy practice framework: domain & process (3rd ed.). *American Journal Occupational Therapy, 68*(s1), S1—S48.

American Occupational Therapy Association. (2015). Standards of practice for occupational therapy. *American Journal*

Occupational Therapy, 69(3), S56—S57. Available from https://doi.org/10.5014/ajot.2015.696S06.

Asher, I. E. (2014). *Asher's occupational therapy assessment tools* (4th ed.). Bethesda, MD: AOTA Press.

Chisolm, D., & Schell, B. A. B. (2019). Overview of the occupational therapy process and outcomes. In B. A. B. Schell, & G. Gillen (Eds.), *Willard and Spackman's occupational therapy* (13th ed., pp. 352—368). Philadelphia, PA: Wolters Kluwer.

Coker, P. (2010). Effects of an experiential learning program on the clinical reasoning and critical thinking skills of occupational therapy students. *Journal of Allied Health, 39*(4), 280—286.

Fleming, M. H. (1991a). Clinical reasoning in medicine compared with clinical reasoning in occupational therapy. *American Journal Occupational Therapy, 45*(11), 988—996. Available from https://doi.org/10.5014/ajot.45.11.988.

Fleming, M. H. (1991b). The therapist with the three-track mind. *American Journal Occupational Therapy, 45*(11), 1007—1014. Available from https://doi.org/10.5014/ajot.45.11.1007.

Gillen, G. (2019). Occupational therapy interventions for individuals. In B. A. Schell, & G. Gillen (Eds.), *Willard and Spackman's occupational therapy* (13th ed., pp. 413—435). Philadelphia, PA: Wolters Kluwer.

Henderson, W., & Coppard, B. (2018). Identifying instructional methods for development of clinical reasoning in entry-level occupational therapy education. *American Journal Occupational Therapy, 72*(4), S7211505146. Available from https://doi.org/10.5014/ajot.2018.72S1-PO7010.

Lederer, J. M. (2007). Disposition toward critical thinking among occupational therapy students. *American Journal Occupational Therapy, 61*(5), 519—526. Available from https://doi.org/10.5014/ajot.61.5.519.

Potvin, M. C., Coviello, J. M., & Lockhart-Keene, L. (2019). Occupational therapy assistant students' perspectives about the development of clinical reasoning. *Open Journal Occupational Therapy, 7*(2). Available from https://doi.org/10.15453/2168-6408.1533.

Schell, B. A. (2019). Professional reasoning in practice. In B. A. Schell, & G. Gillen (Eds.), *Willard and Spackman's occupational therapy* (13th ed., pp. 482—499). Philadelphia, PA: Wolters Kluwer.

Schell, B. A., & Cervero, R. M. (1993). Clinical reasoning in occupational therapy: an integrative review. *American Journal Occupational Therapy, 47*(7), 605—610. Available from https://doi.org/10.5014/ajot.47.7.605.

Taylor, R. E. R. (2019). Therapeutic relationship and client collaboration: applying the intentional relationship model. In B. A. Schell, & G. Gillen (Eds.), *Willard and Spackman's occupational therapy* (13th ed., pp. 527—538). Philadelphia, PA: Wolters Kluwer.

Unsworth, C. A. (2005). Using a head-mounted video camera to explore current conceptualizations of clinical reasoning in occupational therapy. *American Journal Occupational Therapy, 59*, 31—40.

Weinstock-Zlotnick, G., & Hinojosa, J. (2004). Bottom-up or top-down evaluation: is one better than the other? *American Journal Occupational Therapy, 58*, 594—599.

World Health Organization. (2020). *International classification of functioning, disability and health (ICF model)*. Retrieved from http://www.who.int/classifications/icf/en/.

Yu, M. L., Brown, T., White, C., Marston, C., & Thyer, L. (2018). The impact of undergraduate occupational therapy students' interpersonal skills on their practice education performance: a pilot study. *Australian Occupational Therapy Journal, 65*(2), 115—125. Available from https://doi.org/10.1111/1440-1630.12444.

5

Effective Documentation of Occupational Therapy Services

Mary Elizabeth Patnaude

OBJECTIVES

After reading this chapter, the student or the occupational therapy practitioner will be able to do the following:

- Describe the purposes of documentation for occupational therapy services.
- List fundamental elements of documentation.
- Differentiate occupational therapy assistant and occupational therapist documentation responsibilities.
- Describe the reporting process, including initial evaluation reports, intervention plans, progress reports, and discharge summaries.

- Discuss the value of the *Occupational Therapy Practice Framework* to the documentation process.
- Describe the legal implications for complete and accurate documentation.
- Describe the opportunities and challenges of using an electronic health record.

KEY TERMS

Documentation
Referral
Screening report
Evaluation
Occupational profile
Occupational performance
Initial evaluation report
Precautions
Contraindications
Intervention plan/treatment plan

Daily notes
Progress notes
Discharge summary
HIPAA
SOAP notes
Narrative notes
Flow sheets
Functional outcomes
EHR/EMR

INTRODUCTION

Occupational therapists (OTs) and occupational therapy assistants (OTAs) provide skilled therapy services to maximize participation in meaningful occupation (American Occupational Therapy Association, 2010). To do this effectively, OTs and OTAs must choose interventions based on evidence that does not duplicate other services and promotes effective use of health care services (Gillen et al., 2019). After identifying these services, OTs and OTAs must document the services in a way that is in alignment with practice standards, settings, state laws and regulatory agencies, accreditors, and the official documents of the profession (American Occupational Therapy Association, 2018).

Documentation communicates vital information about each client, conveys the rationale for treatment, maps a chronologic record of the intervention process, and provides evidence to justify treatment (American Occupational Therapy

Association, 2018; Gillen et al., 2019). All services provided by OTs and OTAs must be supported by documentation or legally they were not done (Sames, 2015). Documentation is a continuous process that begins immediately on receipt of the initial referral. The OTA plays a valuable role in the documentation of the ongoing treatment of the client.

Referral

The occupational therapy process is initiated by a client referral. This **referral** is most often written by a physician and will specify the reason for requesting services. It is sometimes called a prescription or physician order. When a physician's referral is required, it should include the treatment diagnosis, the onset date of the treatment diagnosis, a request for evaluation and other specific treatment orders, the date, the physician's signature, and frequency and duration of occupational therapy services (American Occupational Therapy Association, 2018). Fig. 5.1 provides an

Patient Information

Name _____   Goals (functional expectations) _____

Phone: H _____ W _____   _____

Date of Onset/Exacerbation _____   Previous Therapy Results _____

Diagnosis _____

_____ Post Op: ____ Yes ____ No   Date of Surgery _____

PHYSICIAN SERVICES

☐ Consult Physical Medicine Physician   ☐ NCV _____

☐ Impairment Rating _____   ☐ EMG _____   ☐ Injections/type _____

☐ EMG/NCV _____   ☐ Other (Specify) _____

PHYSICAL THERAPY

☐ Evaluate & Treat
   ☐ Exercise
   ☐ Heat/Ice Modalities
   ☐ Massage
   ☐ Aquatics

   ☐ Electrical Stimulation
   ☐ TENS
   ☐ Ultrasound
   ☐ Phonophoresis
     __ with 10% Hydrocortisone Cream
     (Provider initials)
   ☐ Traction
   ☐ Iontophoresis
     __ Acetic Acid (MD initials)
     __ Dexa 4 mg/ml (MD initials)
   ☐ Whirlpool
   ☐ Whirlpool/Wound Care
   ☐ Gait Wt. Bearing
   _____
   ☐ Vestibular Rehabilitation

   ☐ Manual Therapy
   ☐ Other

NUMBER OF VISITS _____

BEGINNING FREQUENCY _____

NEUROPSYCHOLOGY

☐ Evaluate & Treat
☐ Neuropsych Battery (8 hour testing)
☐ Cognitive Therapy
☐ Adjustment Counseling

OCCUPATIONAL THERAPY

☐ Evaluate & Treat
☐ Splint: Type/Revision
_____
_____
_____

☐ Hand Therapy Program
_____
_____
_____

☐ Modalities _____
☐ Desensitization

☐ Upper Extremity
   Activities/Exercise
☐ Activities of Daily Living

☐ Other _____
☐ Community/Work Integration

NUMBER OF VISITS _____

BEGINNING FREQUENCY _____

WORK INJURY PROGRAM

☐ Work Hardening
☐ Work Conditioning
☐ Functional Capacity Evaluation
☐ Post Rehab Conditioning

SPEECH THERAPY

☐ Evaluate & Treat
☐ Speech/Language Therapy
☐ Dysphagia Evaluation/Therapy
☐ Modified Barium Swallow
☐ Fiberoptic Endoscopic Evaluation of
   Swallow
☐ Augmentative Device Evaluation
☐ Voice Therapy
☐ Other (Specify) _____

NUMBER OF VISITS _____

BEGINNING FREQUENCY _____

SPECIALTY PROGRAMS

☐ Adapted Driving
☐ Amputee Clinic
☐ Incontinence Program
☐ Low Vision Clinic
☐ Lymphedema Program
☐ Day Treatment – A Neurocognitive
   Development Program
☐ Orthotics Clinic
☐ Osteoporosis Clinic
☐ Spasticity Clinic
☐ Spinal Cord Follow-Up Clinic
☐ TBI Follow-Up Clinic
☐ Wheelchair Positioning Clinic
☐ Urodynamics
   ☐ Uroflow   ☐ CMG
   ☐ EMG   ☐ Erectile
            Dysfunction Study

SPECIAL PRECAUTIONS: _____

_____

Verbal/Written Order for Dr./Provider _____ Taken By _____

I hereby certify these services as medically necessary for the patient's plan of care.

Physician Signature _____ Date _____ Office Ph. _____

Other Provider Signature _____ Date _____ Office Ph. _____

Pre-Certification _____

Fig. 5.1 Physician order form. (Courtesy Baylor University Medical Center, Dallas, TX.)

Rehabilitation Clarification Orders	
Date	Primary Diagnosis: _____
	Treatment Diagnoses: _____
	_____
	Date of Onset: _____
	Treatment Frequency: _____
	Treatment Duration: _____
	Treatment Plan:
	Physician's Signature:

Fig. 5.2 Clarification order request form. (Courtesy Baylor University Medical Center—The Tom Landry Center, Dallas, TX.)

example of a physician order form that includes the entire treatment team.

When one or more of the required items for a physician's order is missing from the referral, it is important to clarify the order. Fig. 5.2 shows one type of form that can be used to clarify a physician's therapy order. The OT fills out this form after the initial evaluation is complete. The clarification order has all the required components. This order is sent to the physician along with the initial evaluation for the physician's signature.

The first entry into the client's permanent record may be to document receipt of the referral and the initial plan of action (e.g., "10/1/2011 OT referral received and client contacted by phone. OT evaluation scheduled for 10/4/2011 at 1:00 pm" or "10/1/2011 OT initial evaluation completed today with instruction in activity pacing techniques. Refer to evaluation for intervention plan"). The response time is established by each facility but is usually within 24 to 48 hours after the referral is received.

TYPES OF DOCUMENTATION (AMERICAN OCCUPATIONAL THERAPY ASSOCIATION, 2018)

Documentation provides a legal and chronologic record of the process of occupational therapy service delivery: evaluation, intervention process, intervention review, and outcomes (see Chapter 4) (American Occupational Therapy Association, 2014b, 2018). This includes the content of documentation, such as screening and evaluation reports, intervention plan, contact reports, progress reports, transition plans, and discharge/discontinuation reports (American Occupational Therapy Association, 2018).

Screening

The **screening report** provides the referral source and the reason for referral. It includes the client information, such as occupational history, medical history, diagnosis, and health status (see Fig. 5.1). It should also provide a brief occupational

profile to introduce the client's reasons for seeking services and the client's priorities and goals. Finally, it provides an overview of any assessments provided and recommendations based on those assessment results (American Occupational Therapy Association, 2018). If applicable, a full evaluation will be completed. A physician may provide a clarification of orders before a full evaluation is completed (see Fig. 5.2).

Evaluation/ Reevaluation

If the OT determines that a full **evaluation** should be completed, a client-centered process of evaluation and information gathering is instituted. The initial evaluation process begins with the OT reviewing available data obtained from the existing permanent record and interviewing referral sources, the client, and family members.

The next step of the process is the formulation of the **occupational profile**. The occupational profile "provides an understanding of the client's occupational history and experiences, patterns of daily living, interests, values, and needs" (p. S10) (American Occupational Therapy Association, 2014b). A template for completing the occupational profile can be found on the website of the American Occupational Therapy Association (AOTA), at https://www.aota.org/~/media/Corporate/Files/Practice/Manage/Documentation/AOTA-Occupational-Profile-Template.pdf. The second step is analysis of the client's occupational performance. In this step, factors that interfere with performance of functional activity are identified, and treatment goals are established (American Occupational Therapy Association, 2014b).

Occupational Profile. The occupational profile addresses the client's interests, values, and needs. The OT and OTA focus on gaining an understanding of the client to identify strengths and limitations. This information is collected not only during the initial evaluation but also during subsequent therapy visits. Outcomes are continuously modified based on information learned about the client's occupational profile. Box 5.1 outlines a list of questions that will assist in gathering data related to the occupational profile.

BOX 5.1 Data Gathering Questions for the Occupational Profile

1. Who is the client?
2. Why is the client seeking service, and what are the client's current concerns relative to engaging in occupations and in daily life activities?
3. What areas of occupation are successful, and what areas are causing problems or risks?
4. What contexts support engagement in desired occupations, and what contexts are inhibiting engagement?
5. What is the client's occupational history?
6. What are the client's priorities and desired targeted outcomes?

Modified from American Occupational Therapy Association. (2014b). Occupational therapy practice framework: domain and process. 3rd ed. *The American Journal of Occupational Therapy, 68*, S1—S51. A template is provided at https://www.aota.org/~/media/Corporate/Files/Practice/Manage/Documentation/AOTA-Occupational-Profile-Template.pdf.

Specific information that may be collected includes the client's name and address; important phone numbers; family members; third-party payers; family history; educational and work history; learning style and preferences; pertinent medical, physical, and mental status information related to specific primary and secondary diagnoses; and other information related to the client's prior level of functioning. Information regarding expected treatment outcomes and discharge plans is also pertinent.

Occupational Performance. Information related to occupational performance provides the basis for the evaluation of performance areas relevant to the client's needs. The OT identifies assessments that will allow for the observation of performance skills or client factors such as range of motion (ROM) measurements; manual muscle testing; sensory testing; perceptual/cognitive assessment results; and activities of daily living (ADL), functional mobility, home management, vocational, and leisure assessment findings.

OTs direct the evaluation process. OTAs can implement some assessments and provide verbal and written reports of observations, assessment results, and client responses to the assessment procedures (American Occupational Therapy Association, 2014a). These may include standardized and nonstandardized assessments, interviews, and checklists.

Through an analysis of occupational performance, the OT and OTA establish the client's baseline status. Accuracy in administering and recording evaluation results is critical. All future evaluation reports will compare progress to this initial baseline status, and the degree of improvement may determine the course and amount of treatment that physicians and third-party payers approve.

Outcomes are created based on the evaluative data gathered. These outcomes are developed in conjunction with the client and should address the client's areas of weakness and his or her identified priorities. While outcomes are client centered, it is also important to be aware of payer sources when establishing outcomes. For example, a client injured on the job may want to be able to play ball with his child. However, because workers' compensation is the payer source for this particular client, outcomes will need to be worded and focused on return to work. After outcomes are established, the treatment plan or intervention process is identified.

Initial Evaluation Report. The OT has primary responsibility to complete the initial evaluation (American Occupational Therapy Association, 2014a). The **initial evaluation report**, whether it is a form (Fig. 5.3) or a narrative, contains the following sections (American Occupational Therapy Association, 2018):

1. Referral information
2. Client information
3. Occupational profile
4. Assessments
5. Analysis of occupational performance

Name: _John Doe_		DOB: _12/30/27_ Date: _7/2/11_
Doctor: _Dr. J. Smith_		Diagnosis: _THA_
Therapist: _J. Gomez, OTR S. Johnson, COTA_		Precautions: _THA precautions_
Referred for: _OT THA protocol including eval + tx for ADLs_		Frequency: _3x/week_
		Duration: _1 week_
		Rehab potential: _Good_

PROBLEMS:	SHORT-TERM GOALS:	LONG-TERM GOALS:	APPROACHES:
↓ ADL: Dressing Hygiene Bathing Functional mobility	• Provided assistive devices & instructions & following THA precautions, patient will dress L/E c̄ min. assist in 3 days. • Provided raised toilet seat, patient will transfer from standing ↔ toilet c̄ min. assist following THA precautions within 3 days. • Provided tub chair and grab bars, patient will transfer from standing ↔ tub chair c̄ min. assist following THA precautions within 3 days.	• Patient will perform ADLs independently in order to return to ADL at home by D/C.	• Instruct and demo THA precautions. • Train in use of assistive devices including: reacher, dressing sticks, sock aid, long-handled shoe horn, elastic shoe laces, raised toilet seat, tub chair, grab bars. • Instruct in tub/shower, toilet and car transfers. • Provide options for work simplification, meal preparation, & item transport. • Assist in obtaining equipment as needed.

Fig. 5.3 Occupational therapy evaluation form. (Courtesy Occupational Therapy Department, Santa Clara Valley Medical Center, San Jose, CA.)

6. Summary and analysis

7. Recommendations (p. 3)

Client information includes the client's name, medical record or account number, the referring physician's name, the referral, and evaluation dates. This section should detail pertinent medical history, including the primary treatment diagnosis, related secondary diagnoses, and onset dates. **Precautions** or **contraindications** that need to be observed during treatment should also be included. The client's prior level of functioning, previous living situation, and prior vocational and leisure status are also noted. The client's priorities and desired outcomes are also identified in the section.

Analysis of the Client's Occupational Performance.

This section identifies the types of assessments used and summarizes the results of each client assessment. The OT selects specific assessments depending on the diagnosis and the individual client. For example, a brain-injured client may require a physical assessment (ROM, motor and sensory function) and perceptual and cognitive testing, while a client with a distal radius fracture may require only a physical assessment. The OTA completes certain aspects of the evaluation as identified by the OT (American Occupational Therapy Association, 2015). It is helpful to use standardized results or standardized rating scales for easy interpretation by others. Standardized scales also permit reliable replication of the evaluation process at reevaluation and discharge times.

Also included in this section is the evaluation of the client's functional performance, or how well the client performs in essential activities. A standardized scale (Table 5.1) is used so as to ensure reliable results. The focus and scope of the evaluation depend on the defined roles of the various professional departments in the facility. In the sample form (Fig. 5.4), bed mobility, transfers, wheelchair mobility, and daily living skills are assessed.

Prioritizing Areas of Occupation and Occupational Performance.

The OT, with input from the OTA, completes the evaluation summary (Fig. 5.5). This section summarizes the evaluation process and outlines priorities of the intervention plan, based on the factors most likely to impede the client's ability to achieve maximal independence in occupational performance. Previously recorded information is analyzed, and targeted outcomes are identified (American Occupational Therapy Association, 2018). The outcomes are based on procedural codes relating to the level of complexity identified in the areas of performance deficit (American Occupational Therapy Association, 2018).

The intervention process includes the intervention plan, the reports of client contact, progress reports, transition plans, and discharge reports. The OT focuses the intervention plan on areas of occupation and occupational performance needing to be addressed and expected outcomes of intervention (American Occupational Therapy Association, 2018). This includes long-term and short-term objectives and, if necessary, referrals or recommendations to other professionals (American Occupational Therapy Association, 2018). Intervention approaches and service delivery options will also be identified. Service delivery options include the frequency and duration of the occupational therapy service. This also should include a discharge plan and a section documenting discussion of goals with the client and the family. Finally, if the initial physician's order was for an evaluation only or was not specific for the treatment intervention now planned, a physician's review of the plan and verifying signature may be necessary (see Fig. 5.2).

Intervention Plan

The **intervention plan** or **treatment plan** involves organizing and interpreting the data previously gathered during the evaluation to establish a clear plan of action. This process identifies the problems impeding function and then applies clinical reasoning skills to specify predictable functional outcomes. The result is a clear set of functional outcomes and short-term objectives with an established plan of treatment to accomplish those outcomes. An intervention approach is also chosen at this time and is based on the established outcomes of therapy. The OT determines if the outcome is to create or promote a new habit or skill, to establish or restore routines, to maintain current levels of functioning, to modify

TABLE 5.1	Definitions of Levels of Assistance	
Level of Assistance	**Abbreviation**	**Definition**
Independent	Ind.	Client requires no assistance or cueing in any situation and is trusted in all situations 100% of the time to do the task safely.
Supervision	Sup.	Caregiver is not required to provide any hands-on guarding but may need to give verbal cues for safety.
Contact guard/ standby	Con. Gd./ Stby	Caregiver must provide hands-on contact guard to be within arm's length for client's safety.
Minimum assistance	Min.	Caregiver provides 25% physical and/or cueing assistance.
Moderate assistance	Mod.	Caregiver assists client with 50% of the task. Assistance can be physical and/or cueing.
Maximum assistance	Max.	Caregiver assists client with 75% of the task. Assistance can be physical and/or cueing.
Dependent	Dep.	Client is unable to assist in any part of the task. Caregiver performs 100% of the task for client physically and/or cognitively.

Critical Pathway

Physician: ___Dr. J. Smith_____
Nurse case manager: ___M. Ryan, RN_____
PT: ___R. O'Hearn, RPT; B. Crowell, PTA_____
OT: ___J. Gomez, OTR; S. Johnson, COTA_____
Speech: ___M. Swor, SLP_____
Psych: ___G. Stallig, MALP_____
Ther. rec.: ___T. Chang, TRS_____
Social worker: ___B. Kucinski, MSW_____
Dietician: ___F. Wood, RD_____

Additional team members: _____
_____
_____
_____
- -
Diagnosis: ___Right CVA Left Hemiplegia_____
Admission date: ___7/6/11_____
Discharge date: ___8/2/11_____
Length of stay: ___1 month_____

Moderate-Severe
(Right CVA Left Hemi)

Admission date: ___7/6/11_____

1	2	3	4	5	6	7
Establish bowel and bladder program Establish skin program Begin eval Oriented to unit/room Oriented to rehab program Bedside dysphagia screen Swallow risk ID band DNR/DNI status	W/C fitted Assess for positioning equipment Assess need for referral to DRS and/or CIL	Evaluations complete Assess transfers w/team Assess for dining grp Assess need for psych eval Conference	Assess need for CD referral Assess need for TR Foley out	Assess self-transport Stroke films Referral to Stroke Club		Family Day Members attended ____ ____ ____ ____ Review patient goals with patient and family

8	9	10	11	12	13	14
Assess need for adaptive equipment Reassess dysphagia Re-evaluate bowel and bladder program Re-evaluate skin program			Assess phone skills, check writing, money skills Dry run	Assess simple meal prep Assess appropriateness for self-meds	Assess need for positioning equipment/splints	Family Day Members attended ____ ____ Assess car transfer Assess light housekeeping skills W/E pass

15	16	17	18	19	20	21
Community re-entry activity Reassess dysphagia Re-evaluate bowel and bladder program Re-evaluate skin integrity		Assess anticipated equipment needs Assess home adaptation needs	Equipment ordered Wet run			Family Day Members attended ____ ____ Begin instruction in home program Assess need for DPA W/E pass

22	23	24	25	26	27	28
	D/C FIM complete Referral call to O.P. therapist					

Fig. 5.4 Occupational therapy treatment plan form.

OCCUPATIONAL THERAPY

SANTA CLARA VALLEY MEDICAL CENTER
OCCUPATIONAL THERAPY DEPARTMENT
page 1 of 2

SANTA CLARA VALLEY MEDICAL CENTER

Service _____   ☐ Inpatient   ☐ Outpatient
☐ Initial   ☐ Interim   ☐ Discharge
(Rating scale on back of form)

INFORMATION

Onset Date: _____   Referral Date: _____   Sex: M   F   Language: _____
Diagnosis

Medical History:

Precautions/Diet:

Living Situation:

A/Vocational History:

UPPER EXTREMITY

Range of Motion

☐ Refer to range of motion form

Muscle Picture

☐ Refer to muscle test form

Sensation

(Light touch, pain, kinesthesia, other)

Hand Function

Dominance: ☐ Right   ☐ Left

Splinting:

	Right			Left		
	Grip	3 point	Lateral	Grip	3 point	Lateral
Initial						
Interim/DC						
Norm						

OTHER MOTOR

(Endurance, head/trunk posture and control, sitting/standing balance, reflexes, LE picture, functional ambulation)

VISUAL PERCEPTUAL SKILLS

VISUAL	Initial	Interim/DC	PERCEPTUAL	Initial	Interim/DC	SCALE: 0 = intact; 1 = impaired; 2 = severely impaired;
Visual attention			Motor planning			3 = unable to perform
Near acuity			Graphic praxis			COMMENTS:
Distance acuity			Body scheme			
Pursuits			R/L discrimination			
Saccades			Form			
Ocular alignment			Size			
Stereopsis			Part/whole			
Visual fields			Figure ground			
Visual neglect			Position in space			Wears corrective lenses ☐ Y ☐ N Testing not indicated ☐

COGNITION AND BEHAVIOR

(Orientation, initiation, direction following, memory, judgment, organization, problem solving, impulsivity, attention span)

DISPOSITION - White - MEDICAL RECORD   Yellow - O.T. Chart   Therapist's Signature: _____

9502   SCVMC 6628-17

Fig. 5.5 Occupational therapy daily documentation and treatment record.

SANTA CLARA VALLEY MEDICAL CENTER
OCCUPATIONAL THERAPY DEPARTMENT
page 2 of 2

Service _____ ☐ Inpatient ☐ Outpatient

☐ Initial   ☐ Interim ☐ Discharge
(Rating scale on back of form)

OCCUPATIONAL THERAPY

	ACTIVITY	Initial	Interim D/C	Goal
BED MOBILITY	Rolling R			
	Rolling L			
	Bridging			
	Scooting			
	Long sit			
	Sidelying to sit			

Bed:
Positioning:

Caregiver Training:

Comments:

	ACTIVITY	Initial	Interim D/C	Goal
TRANSFERS	Bed			
	Toilet			
	Tub/shower			
	Car/van seat			
	Furniture			

Type: Equipment:
Caregiver Training:

Comments:

	ACTIVITY	Initial	Interim D/C	Goal
WHEELCHAIR	Management			
	Weight shift			
	Home			
	Community			
	In/out of car			

Type: Weight Shift Type:
Positioning/Cushion:

Caregiver Training:

Comments:

	ACTIVITY	Initial	Interim D/C	Goal
DAILY LIVING SKILLS	Eating			
	Upper body dressing			
	Lower body dressing			
	Hygiene/grooming			
	Bathing			
	Toileting			
	Kitchen			
	Homemaking			
	Community			
	Communication tasks			

Equipment:

Home Environment:

A/Vocational/Driving Skills:

Caregiver Training:

Comments:

Problems:

Goals/Recommendation: ☐ Patient/Caregiver participated in goal setting

X ___ / ___ / ___
Frequency/Session Length/Duration of Treatment

Therapist's Signature   Date   Physician's Signature

DISPOSITION - White - MEDICAL RECORD   Yellow - O.T. Chart   🌐 9502 PAGE 2 of 2   SCVMC 6628-17

Fig. 5.5 (Continued).

behaviors, or to prevent disability or injury (American Occupational Therapy Association, 2014b). Finally, the OT will determine which interventions can be provided by the OTA and which by the OT (American Occupational Therapy Association, 2018).

The client (or, when necessary, a client advocate) should be actively involved in planning treatment. The OT must consider goals that the client finds personally meaningful, valuable, and culturally relevant. Involvement in outcomes development increases client motivation and improves rehabilitation potential. Fig. 5.4 provides an example of an occupational therapy intervention plan.

Client Contact Reports

During implementation of the occupation therapy plan the OTA is responsible for documenting all interactions with the client. This documentation of client contact (daily treatment notes) takes various forms and will be determined by the facility in which the OTA works. All contact between the client and the OTA should be documented, including telephone conversations, case consultations (OTA and other professionals), and any interventions.

OTs and OTAs must complete daily records on client attendance and the treatment provided. Generally, **daily notes** are brief and reflect the treatment provided, the client's response to treatment, and progress noted. Revision of the treatment plan and outcomes or objectives are not always necessary but should be provided if applicable. These records are provided to insurance payers to verify that charges and treatment interventions are consistent. Many different formats are available to record daily documentation. Some facilities use a SOAP format, whereas others use a narrative. Figs. 5.2 and 5.3 provide some examples of daily treatment records; Box 5.2 is a sample of a brief narrative daily note.

Progress notes may be required on a weekly or biweekly basis. Weekly progress notes are more thorough and should summarize the treatment, its frequency, the client's response, and progress toward outcomes (or lack of progress, with justification). The short-term objectives should be updated, and the intervention plan revised. The new objectives and intervention plan are usually considered short-term and reflect the expected outcomes for the upcoming week's treatment regimen.

The SOAP note is one format commonly used to ensure consistency of the progress notes' content. Figs. 5.4 and 5.6 are examples of forms that can be used for either a progress or a discharge note. Boxes 5.3 and 5.4 provide some examples of progress notes.

Progress Reports (Intervention Review)

If treatment occurs over an extended period, the OT may need to complete a full reevaluation. Again, the OTA contributes to this process. The format is often the same as the initial evaluation. The primary difference is that this report reflects the differences between the initial baseline of evaluation results and the client's present clinical status. The

---

BOX 5.2   Brief Daily Note Sample

12/10/2011, 1:00-1:43 P.M. Client participated in 15 minutes of right upper extremity passive ROM and was instructed in self-mobilization techniques, followed by 28 minutes of ADL retraining to address upper body dressing. Donned pullover shirt with minimal assistance and button-front, long-sleeve shirt with moderate assistance.

BOX 5.3   Weekly Progress Note Sample

12/10/2011. Client seen 3 times this week for instruction in home exercise program, passive ROM, and ADL retraining. Upper body dressing improved from maximum assistance to moderate assistance. Continues to perform lower body dressing independently with assistive device. Short-term goal: Client will dress upper body with minimum assistance in 1 week.

BOX 5.4   SOAP Note Sample

12/10/2011

S: Client expressed frustration with her inability to fully dress herself independently.

O: Dressing lower body independent using assistive device, dressing upper body with moderate assistance for button-front shirt. Right shoulder flexion and abduction improved to 45 degrees; elbow active ROM remains at −30 degrees extension to 50 degrees of flexion.

A: Decreased active ROM of right elbow and shoulder due to tightness related to humerus fracture continues to limit upper extremity ADL independence. Short-term goal: Client will dress upper body in long-sleeve, button-front shirt with minimum assistance in 1 week.

P: Continue current plan of care, 3 times a week for 2 more weeks to address ADL deficits related to decreased active ROM.

---

reevaluation report reflects progress made toward the predicted goals and is a measure of success of the treatment intervention. Based on the new evaluation results, initial outcomes and treatment timelines can be revised. The reevaluation is an important tool for the ongoing utilization review process. It allows the OT to justify continued intervention by clearly quantifying the effectiveness and efficacy of the occupational therapy intervention.

Outcomes

Outcomes describe what the client achieved as a result of the occupational therapy process (American Occupational Therapy Association, 2014b). The outcomes are documented in a discharge/discontinuation report containing the client information, a summary of the intervention process, and recommendations (American Occupational Therapy Association, 2018). Outcomes can be directly linked to the intervention

Occupational Therapy Outpatient Treatment Record													

Demographics

Place Patient Label Here

Eval Date: _____

Dx: _____ Injury Date: _____

Order Date: _____

Freq/Duration: _____

Treatment/Supplies

Date	Start Time/ Stop Time											Additional Comments

Date	Treatment Notes

Fig. 5.6 Occupational therapy treatment record form. (Courtesy Occupational Therapy Department, Unity Hospital, Fridley, MN.)

process. Both objective and subjective terms can be used to describe outcomes (American Occupational Therapy Association, 2014b). An objective measure would be an improvement in a performance skill, such as increased independence in self-care. A subjective measure would be an improved outlook on the disease process achieved by the client, despite minimal gains in strength or endurance. Throughout the entire occupational therapy process, OTs and OTAs continually modify and adapt interventions to achieve the most meaningful outcomes for each client.

Discharge Summary Report. The **discharge summary** describes the client's final status on discharge from the facility. It provides a summary of the occupational therapy services provided to the client. It includes the dates of service, frequency and number of sessions, progress toward goals, and assessment of the effectiveness of the intervention. The OT is responsible for documenting achieved outcomes and implementing the transition or discontinuation plan. The OTA contributes to this process by documenting information related to the client's achieved goals, continuing needs, and current performance (American Occupational Therapy Association, 2010). Discharge recommendations clearly indicate the additional interventions and follow-up that may be required to ensure continued functional improvement or maintenance of the functional gains made during occupational therapy. Any home program plans or referral plans are also described.

The discharge summary reflects the client's total progress and all the accomplishments achieved. The data can be used for many purposes. Quality assurance committees may use the data to evaluate the effectiveness of treatment. The data may also be used for outcomes studies to prove overall effectiveness of treatment within certain diagnostic categories. Third party-payers may use the report to determine payment for the service. Other service agencies such as outpatient clinics will use the data to help establish continued outcomes and intervention plans in the new treatment setting. Figs. 5.7 and 5.8 provide sample forms for the discharge summary.

STANDARDS OF PRACTICE FOR DOCUMENTATION

The OT and the OTA have designated roles related to the documentation of the delivery of occupational therapy services (American Occupational Therapy Association, 2010). The OT accepts referrals and is responsible to oversee the screening, evaluation, and reevaluation process, including the evaluation results, the intervention plan, modifications to the intervention plan, outcomes, transitions, and discontinuations (American Occupational Therapy Association, 2010). The OTA administers assessments delegated by the OT, documents contacts related to intervention, and contributes to the formulation of the discharge process (American Occupational Therapy Association, 2010). Documentation of

the client's response to intervention and communications between the OTA and the client during intervention provide important contributions to the decision-making process of the OT as updates are made to the client's outcomes, transition, and discharge plans. The OTA also assists in the preparation of the intervention plan, documentation of progress, reporting of any necessary revisions in the intervention plan based on reevaluation, and completion of the discharge summary in collaboration with the OT (American Occupational Therapy Association, 2010). OTs and OTAs share the responsibility of documenting within the time frames, formats, and standards established by their practice facility, federal and state laws, payer sources, and various other regulatory programs.

Documentation and Ethics

Truth, or veracity, is a core concept of occupational therapy practice, based on the virtues of truthfulness, candor, and honesty (American Occupational Therapy Association, 2010). This means that the information OTs and OTAs provide both verbally and in writing must be true and accurate. Therefore OTs and OTAs should record and report in an accurate and timely manner to ensure that documentation is completed in accordance with applicable laws, guidelines, and regulations.

OTs and OTAs can effectively communicate a client's response to therapy and educate other health care providers and fiscal intermediaries about the value of occupational therapy by demonstrating competence in documentation. Increased health care spending in the United States continues to greatly outpace inflation (Gillen et al., 2019). This has led to a national conversation related to the utilization of health care and an initiative to reduce costs while increasing value (Gillen et al., 2019). OTs and OTAs can play a role in this initiative by providing high-quality services, supported by evidence, and by documenting about it in a clear, concise, and meaningful way (Gillen et al., 2019).

Legal Issues

OTs and OTAs must ensure that their practice meets federal and state laws (American Occupational Therapy Association, 2010). Anything done in therapy can be called into court, where the best defense is accurate, competent, and appropriate documentation. If an aspect of the intervention process is left out, it is considered not to have been done. Violations of the law can occur whether the OT or OTA knows it or not. Therefore OTs and OTAs must be familiar with all laws related to practice, including those related to documentation and privacy.

One law related to privacy is the Health Insurance Portability and Accountability Act of 1996 (**HIPAA**), which became effective in 2003. The Privacy Rule is designed to allow health care providers to share information regarding their clients yet still protect this sensitive information from the general public.

Facilities must provide clients a Notice of Privacy Practices and must gain written authorization from each client before

OCCUPATIONAL THERAPY

IP/OP Room _____

Month															
Date															
9705 OT eval/re-eval 1-15															
0959 ADL training 1-15															
0977 OT consult/care conf 1-15															
9707 Cognitive treatment 1-15															
973 Develop treatment 1-15															
9877 Environmental stim 1-15															
0970 Motor skills 1-15															
0972 Preventive skills 1-15															
0971 Sensory integration 1-15															
9785 Therapeutic adapt 1-15															
9712 Initial out/pt ADL 30															
0967 Out/Pt no show 1-15															
0968 OT eval/hand 1-15															
0969 Motor skills/hand 1-15															
0963 Preventive skills/hand 1-15															
0960 Therap adapt/hand 1-15															
0962 Splint (prefab-hand)															
0965 Splint (fabricated-H)															
97832 Splint-prefab															
609610 Splint-fabricated															
610063 2/Piece formfit TLSO															
9798 In/Pt OT adapt equip															
0964 O/P hand equip															
1008 O/P occ therapy supply															

B, Bedside; C, clinic; H, hold treatment; S, surgery; DC, discontinued; D, discharged.

Therapist's signature _____

OCCUPATIONAL THERAPY TREATMENT RECORD

Fig. 5.7 Occupational therapy progress report or discharge note. (Courtesy Baylor University Medical Center—The Tom Landry Center, Dallas, TX.)

Occupational Therapy
Hand Clinic Progress Report/Discharge Note

Patient Name: _____   Date: _____

Diagnosis: _____   Physician: _____

Treatment: _____

Number of visits: attended _____   cancelled _____   no shows _____

Treatment results/comments

_____
_____
_____
_____
_____
_____
_____

Range of Motion: Active/Passive

Wrist	Right	Left
Ext./Flex.		
RD/UD		
Sup./Pro.		

Strength:

	Right	Left
Grip		
Lateral Pinch		
Tripod Pinch		
Tip Pinch		

	Thumb	Index	Long	Ring	Small
MP ext./flex.					
PIP ext./flex.					
DIP ext./flex.					
Palmar abd.					

STG'S _____
_____
_____
_____

Established Goals

Increased range of motion	met	not met	continue
Increased strength/endurance	met	not met	continue
Decreased swelling/pain	met	not met	continue
Patient education	met	not met	continue
Improved functional activities:			
ADL self-care	met	not met	continue
ADL home management	met	not met	continue

Recommendations

I would like to request this patient:

_____ Be discharged from Occupational Therapy

_____ Continue present treatment for _____ days/week for _____ weeks.

_____ Other_____.

Thank you for your referral.

Therapist _____ phone _____

Fig. 5.8 Discharge summary form. (Courtesy Occupational Therapy Department, Unity Hospital, Fridley, MN.)

giving out health information not related to treatment or payment. Although the practice is optional under the Privacy Rule, most facilities have clients sign a consent form that allows for the release of relevant medical information related to their treatment. In addition, clients have the right to know what is in their medical record and can ask for this information. Thus the OTA must know the practices of the facility so that documentation can be disseminated in ways that protect clients' right to privacy.

Documentation is part of the legal record and may be used in court. The services that the OT practitioner documents must accurately reflect the treatment given. The legal written record is the only acceptable proof of the treatment intervention. In court, the content of the documentation within the chart will be deemed far more reliable than the memory of the OT or OTA. The standard phrase, "If it was not written, it did not happen" holds true, especially with outside reviewers looking at the documentation. Therefore completeness and accuracy of the record are essential.

The following documentation guidelines will ensure that the OT and OTA meet legal and ethical obligations:

- Accurately document date/time of all services.
- Document length of treatment/times and treatment codes/descriptions.
- Document any missed events/evaluations/intervention sessions/follow-ups and anything out of the ordinary.
- Document at the time of treatment (point of service) so that the entry will completely and accurately reflect the treatment session.
- Document using descriptive and accurate facts rather than general terms.
- Include all supportive documentation such as physicians' treatment orders or consents for release of information.
- Do not criticize the client or another health care provider in the written record.
- Do not change a legal record after the fact without clarifying the time and nature of the change. If errors occur, cross out the entry with a single line and initial over it.
- Do not leave any blank spaces. If there is space left, fill it in with lines.
- Document all instructions and evidence that the client and/or caregiver demonstrated understanding of instruction.

The AOTA "describes the purpose, types, and content of professional documentation used in occupational therapy" (p. 1) (American Occupational Therapy Association, 2018). These provide guidance based on the practice framework regardless of the method used to document the occupational therapy intervention (American Occupational Therapy Association, 2014b, 2018). Box 5.5 lists 13 elements of the documented record.

Accrediting bodies include the Joint Commission, the Commission on the Accreditation of Rehabilitation Facilities (CARF), and the Comprehensive Outpatient Rehabilitation Facilities (CORF). Medicare, Medicaid, and other third-party payers also have documentation requirements. In addition, state laws related to licensure, registration, and certification may also have specific requirements for documentation such

as cosignature of the OTA's documentation by the OT. OTAs must be familiar with the documentation requirements of the facility, third-party payers, and the state where they practice.

Quality of Documentation Content

OTs and OTAs must provide high-quality documentation. It must be well organized, contain only pertinent information, and be objective and accurate. Conciseness and brevity are critical. Considerations about who will read the documentation has an influence on what needs to be reported and how the report will be written. This includes factors such as the type of medical terminology or accepted medical abbreviations used and the amount of detail needed for accurate understanding of the report.

Many facilities undergo a quality management process for documentation. In this process, charts are audited by internal staff. The audit team will typically pull a random number of charts from each team member and will check for standard elements to ensure that these items are included in the documentation. For the OT and OTA, these chart audits can be a learning opportunity regarding one's own documentation strengths and weaknesses.

Permanent Legal Record

The documents contained in the permanent record are considered the official records related to that client. Each facility determines the official contents of this record. This may be

---

BOX 5.5 Fundamental Elements of Documentation

1. Client's full name and case number on each page of documentation
2. Date and type of occupational therapy contact
3. Identification of type of documentation and department name
4. OT practitioner's signature, with a minimum of first name or initial, last name, and professional designation
5. Signature of the recorder directly at the end of the note, without space left between the body of the note and the signature
6. Cosignature by an OT on documentation written by students and OTAs when required by law or the facility
7. Compliance with confidentiality standards
8. Facility-approved terminology
9. Facility-approved abbreviations
10. Errors corrected by drawing a single line through the mistake and the correction initialed or facility requirements followed; liquid correction fluid and erasures are not acceptable
11. Adherence to professional standards of technology when documenting
12. Disposal of records within law or agency requirements
13. Compliance with agency or legal requirements for storage of records

Modified from American Occupational Therapy Association. (2018). Guidelines for documentation of occupational therapy. *The American Journal of Occupational Therapy, 72,* 1–7.

based on requirements set by internal systems, licensing agencies, accrediting bodies, and third-party payers. The treatment team uses the record internally to understand the total client treatment plan, and reviewers use it to determine justification for continued treatment. Moreover, quality assurance teams use the record to assess overall client outcomes and services. Externally, third-party payers may use records to determine payment for services, the court system uses them for hearings and litigation, and outside agencies use the documents for continued treatment or services after discharge from the facility.

Occupational Therapy Record. The occupational therapy documents contained in the permanent legal record contain the physician's referral, initial evaluations and assessments, daily notes, ongoing weekly and monthly progress notes, reevaluation reports, and discharge summary. These records identify all tests and observations, intervention outcomes, intervention plans, and progress toward the established outcomes. The OT and/or OTA may also be required to provide entries in other sections of the permanent record such as the interdisciplinary care plan or the client care conference note.

In some facilities the occupational therapy department will maintain separate departmental files or soft charts. These files include supporting records, communication logs, notes, and worksheets, as well as copies of the reports prepared for the permanent legal record. The supporting data may include assessment results (e.g., muscle test form), treatment observations (e.g., ADL checklist), informal therapy team conference notes, or intervention plan approaches. The supporting data form the basis for the reports that become part of the permanent legal record.

Methods of Documentation

SOAP notes are often used for communicating daily or weekly information within facilities. The value of SOAP note charting is that it gives the writer a logical way to organize thoughts and the reader an easy way to review the information (Kittenbach & Shlomer, 2016; Sames, 2015). Each section of the SOAP note includes specific information, as described in the following (Kittenbach & Shlomer, 2016):

Subjective: what has been said subjectively by the client or what has been reported by significant others

Objective: observable and measurable data derived from evaluation and treatment results

Assessment: the opinion, interpretation, or assessment of the results of the client's functional performance and anticipated outcomes, including a problem list and long-term and short-term goals

Plan: the treatment plan, including the frequency and duration of treatment

Narrative notes are less structured than the SOAP format. Narrative notes can be used to document client contact that is not necessarily during treatment (Sames, 2015). Narrative notes can be used to document conversations with a client when the client cancels an occupational therapy treatment

session. They can also be used to document training with caregivers or when instructions specific to an activity or task are given outside of the treatment session. If written directly into the medical record, they should include the date and time they were written (Sames, 2015).

Flow sheets can be used to provide a large amount of information about specific client activities in a concise way (Sames, 2015). Progress flow sheets are typically in the form of a grid. They will have a slot for the dates of occupational therapy intervention and a slot for specific activities performed. Flow sheets are an efficient way to quickly document numbers of reps of an exercise or level of independence for a functional activity but have only room for objective data to be recorded and leave little room for descriptive phrases of how the client performed (Sames, 2015).

FUNCTIONAL OUTCOMES

Medicare requires that occupational therapy services be delivered under a plan of care and that will result in an improvement in the patient's level of function in a reasonable amount of time (Sames, 2015). **Functional outcomes** have four main components. First, the outcome must address performance (i.e., What is it that the client must perform?). This part of the outcome should be written using positive language. It should also be objective and observable (Sames, 2015). Second, the outcome must have measurable criteria to indicate when the outcome has been met. Third, the outcome will need to specify specific conditions under which the performance should be completed (see Table 5.1 for a list of levels of assistance that can be used to define conditions). Fourth, the outcome will need to give a time frame for completion.

Consider the following outcome: "The client will be able to independently climb three flights of stairs within 90 seconds for 4 of 5 treatment sessions while maintaining a heart rate less than 80% of max while wearing 50 pounds of protective gear so that he can return to work by 1/31/2011." This functional outcome can be broken down as follows:

- Performance: "climb three flights of stairs while wearing 50 pounds of protective gear"
- Criteria: "within 90 seconds for 4 of 5 treatment sessions while maintaining a heart rate less than 80% of max"
- Condition: "independently"
- Time frame: "by 1/31/2011"

Functional outcomes can be achieved through a series of short-term intervention goals or objectives that are designed to move the client through the intervention process, week by week. The occupational therapy evaluation will determine baseline for the client, and functional outcomes will be developed to identify the end process. The short-term objectives will then identify step-by-step progression from baseline to discharge. For example, in the previously stated functional outcome, a short-term objective may be as follows: "While carrying 25 pounds, the client will be able to climb one flight of stairs within 30 seconds with a heart rate less than 80% of max within 1 week." It is important to remember that even short-term objectives must still be measurable and must continue to describe expected performance as a result of occupational therapy treatment.

ELECTRONIC HEALTH RECORD

As part of the American Recovery and Reinvestment Act of 2009, Congress passed the Health Information Technology for Economic and Clinical Health (HITECH) Act of 2009 (Sames, 2015). One of the provisions of this act is to provide incentive payments to eligible health care professionals and hospitals who adopt **electronic health record (EHR)** technology. There are many obstacles along the path to fully implementing the EHR. However, there are also many opportunities for both the client and the OT practitioner with the use of the EHR or the **electronic medical record (EMR)**. Box 5.6 outlines both the advantages and disadvantages to using the HER (Sames, 2015).

Digital documentation can take many forms, from the simple to the complex. Using a word-processing program to type notes is the simplest form. Templates that form the basic structure of the documentation can be built; the OTA then types the required data in the appropriate section. More advanced programs will allow the OT or OTA to enter the information into a database and then merge the data into a report form. Software developed for personal data assistants and tablet-sized personal computers make the documentation process more mobile, thus allowing for documentation wherever the client may be.

With the release of the iPad by Apple and the numerous medical applications and interfaces that go along with it, the idea of the EHR is more a reality than ever before. Health care workers can have instant access to client history, including medications, x-rays, and other data. Client information can be carried by the health care provider from room to room, and information can be updated via touch screen using a writing stylus or by using a keyboard. However, this approach can distract from the human touch if practitioners become more involved in interacting with technology and spend less time focused on clients. Regardless of the type of digital documentation used, the OT or OTA who possesses basic keyboarding and word-processing skills is well prepared for the increasing use of digital documentation systems.

MEDICARE REPORTS

Medicare is the most frequent third-party payer of occupational therapy services (Sames, 2015). To get reimbursed for Medicare services, OTs and OTAs must complete reports for Medicare, Part A: Hospital Insurance Program, which pays for hospital inpatient, skilled nursing facility, home, and hospice care, and Part B: Supplemental Medical Insurance Program, which covers hospital outpatient, physician, and other professional services. Certain requirements apply to Medicare; therefore records may include prior authorizations, certification, and recertification. The OT practitioner must become familiar with Medicare regulations as they pertain to documentation. Fig. 5.9 provides an example of a Medicare B form.

SUMMARY

Documentation of occupational therapy services provides a written record about the client's status, progress, and performance. OTs and OTAs are responsible for keeping accurate records to document the client's evaluation results, the intervention plan, and the treatment outcomes.

Occupational therapy documentation includes the referral, evaluation data, initial evaluation, daily notes, progress notes, reevaluation, and discharge summary. Records and reports should reflect clear, concise, accurate, and objective information about the client. Documentation should be well organized and developed according to an agreed-upon system for internal consistency of the record.

BOX 5.6   Electronic Health Record

Advantages

- Improved patient safety (decrease in errors/alert to medication issues)
- Improved access to medical records and efficiency of time
- Improved legibility
- Decreased duplication (records/referrals)
- Streamlined billing
- Reduction of paper waste
- Decreased storage space needed
- Productivity tracking
- Identification of referral patterns

Disadvantages

- Electronic health record system cost (hardware/software/networks)
- Workforce training for use and maintenance
- Templates limit information entered may flag an audit
- Extensive time needed for design of system and implementation
- Security concerns related to privacy breach

REVIEW QUESTIONS

1. Think back to one year ago from today. At 9:30 A.M., who were you with, what were you doing, where were you, why were you there? Now do the same for six months ago, one month ago, yesterday, one hour ago. Discuss this memory exercise in relation to the requirement that occupational therapy services be documented in a timely fashion, generally the same day.
2. Write a functional outcome and a possible short-term objective for each of the following:
   a. Your client would like to be able to dress himself in a button-up shirt for church on Sunday.

DATE DISCONTINUED:	REASON:	REFERRAL OBJECTIVES:	LENGTH OF TIME PT WAS SEEN:

DIAGNOSIS:

GOALS	MET	NOT MET	REASON
STG: _____			
_____			
Pt/family will make DC plans based on level of independence at time of DC.			
LTG: _____			
_____			

PATIENT'S HOME SITUATION PRIOR TO ADMIT:	PATIENT DISCHARGED TO: ☐ Home ☐ Rehab ctr ☐ NH ☐ Other_____	LIST HELP AVAILABLE IF DC HOME:

PATIENT'S ADL STATUS AT THE TIME OF DISCHARGE

	INDEP.	ASSIST	COMMENTS
TRANSFERS			
SELF CARE			
DRESSING			
EATING			
COOKING			

ADAPTIVE EQUIPMENT (RECOMMENDED FOR) WITH PATIENT

☐ Long handled reacher   ☐ Bath sponge   ☐ Sock aide   ☐ Dressing stick   ☐ Elastic shoe laces   ☐ Walker bag

☐ Elevated toilet seat   ☐ Leg lift device   ☐ Tub grab bar   ☐ Other _____

WRITTEN MATERIAL SENT WITH PATIENT

☐ Ortho restrictions & transfer instructions   ☐ One handed ADL techniques   ☐ Adaptive dressing techniques

☐ Crutch/walker safety instructions   ☐ Back saving ADL techniques   ☐ Cognitive worksheets/instructions

☐ Dressing equipment instructions   ☐ Low vision adaptation/safety techniques   ☐ Range of motion instructions

☐ Adaptive equipment list & purchase information   ☐ Carpal tunnel prevention   ☐ Other_____

☐ Joint protection/arthritis exercises   ☐ U/E strengthening instructions

☐ Brain trauma information   ☐ U/E coordination instructions

COMMENTS: _____

_____

_____

_____

_____

_____

RECOMMENDATIONS FOR FURTHER TREATMENT OR SUPERVISION

☐ None needed   ☐ Outpatient OT is recommended   ☐ OT at new facility   ☐ Other: _____

AREAS OF CONCERN: _____

Occupational therapist signature_____ Date _____

61-00206 REV. 7/93

OCCUPATIONAL THERAPY DISCHARGE SUMMARY

OCCUPATIONAL THERAPY DISCHARGE SUMMARY

Fig. 5.9 Occupational therapy information and plan of treatment form. (Courtesy Blue Cross/Blue Shield of Minnesota, St. Paul, MN.)

b. Your client would like to be able to open the lid on a water bottle.

c. Your client would like to be able to take a shower without getting short of breath and having to stop.

3. Observe someone in your household complete a daily task such as cook a meal or get dressed.

   a. Write a narrative note about what you observed.

   b. Write a SOAP note based on your observations.

REFERENCES

American Occupational Therapy Association. (2010). Occupational therapy code of ethics and ethics standards. *The American Journal of Occupational Therapy, 64,* S17–S26.

American Occupational Therapy Association. (2014a). Guidelines for supervision, roles, and responsibilities during the delivery of occupational therapy services. *The American Journal of Occupational Therapy, 68,* S16–S22.

American Occupational Therapy Association. (2014b). Occupational therapy practice framework: domain and process. 3rd ed. *The American Journal of Occupational Therapy, 68,* S1–S51.

American Occupational Therapy Association. (2015). Standards of practice for occupational therapy. *The American Journal of Occupational Therapy, 69,* 1–6.

American Occupational Therapy Association. (2018). Guidelines for documentation of occupational therapy. *The American Journal of Occupational Therapy, 72,* 1–7.

Gillen, G., Hunter, E. G., Lieberman, D., & Stutzbach, M. (2019). AOTA's top 5 Choosing Wisely[®] recommendations. *The American Journal of Occupational Therapy, 73*(2), 1–9.

Kittenbach, G., & Shlomer, S. L. (2016). *Writing patient/client notes: ensuring accuracy in documentation* (5th ed.). Philadelphia, PA: FA Davis.

Sames, K. M. (2015). *Documenting occupational therapy practice* (3rd ed.). Boston, MA: Pearson.

RECOMMENDED READING

American Occupational Therapy Association. (2008). Occupational therapy practice framework: domain and process. 2nd ed. *The American Journal of Occupational Therapy, 62,* 625–683.

PART III

Assessment

6

Assessment of Motor Control and Functional Movement

Hannah Colias

OBJECTIVES

After reading this chapter, the student or the occupational therapy practitioner will be able to do the following:

- Delineate occupational therapy assistant/occupational therapist roles with regard to assessing motor control and functional motion.
- Describe the dynamic systems theory of motor control.
- Discuss how occupational therapy practitioners use dynamic systems theory when assessing motor control.
- Understand how postural control affects motor control and functional motion.
- Define normal and abnormal muscle tone.
- Describe specific primitive reflexes and how to assess for the presence of such reflexes.
- Describe the influence on function when primitive reflexes persist after neurologic damage in the adult client.
- Define protective extension, righting, and equilibrium responses and how to assess for the presence of these responses.

- Describe the functional significance of these responses while a client is engaged in activities.
- Describe expected motor recovery patterns in the adult with central nervous system dysfunction.
- Define levels of assistance, and give examples of functional use of an involved extremity in the adult with central nervous system dysfunction.
- List and describe simple structured tests used by the occupational therapy practitioner to evaluate coordination and dexterity.
- Define the occurrences and types of incoordination that might affect the adult with central nervous system dysfunction.
- Identify how incoordination affects one's occupational performance.

KEY TERMS

Motor control
Dynamic systems theory
Postural mechanisms
Postural tone
Muscle tone
Hypotonicity
Hypertonicity
Spasticity
Rigidity
Manual muscle testing

Primitive reflexes
Protective extension reactions
Righting reactions
Equilibrium reactions
Sensory processing
Selective movement
Brunnstrom stages of motor recovery
Neurodevelopmental treatment
Coordination
Incoordination

INTRODUCTION

Occupational therapists (OTs) and occupational therapy assistants (OTAs) facilitate engagement in desired occupations. To move through space to engage in the tasks and activities necessary for independence and life fulfillment requires motor control. Therefore OTs and OTAs must understand how clients control movement, the factors involved in skilled movement, and how to remediate motor control deficits. Knowledge of abnormal motor

patterns and how to help clients who exhibit impaired motor control is essential for helping clients engage in occupations.

This chapter will provide an introduction to the motor control frame of reference and an overview of dynamic systems theory. Motor control requires the dynamic interaction of multiple systems, including postural mechanisms and reflexes that support movement. The stages of recovery and theories for intervention will be presented.

MOTOR CONTROL

Motor control is the ability needed to regulate or direct movement to function independently during occupational performance tasks (Reuben & Siu, 1990). Information from the musculoskeletal system is relayed to and organized in the central nervous system (CNS) to create coordinated movements and skilled actions. Movement involves perception (making sense of the input), motor planning (processing input), motor execution (carrying out movement), feedback (internal and external), and biomechanics (relationship of muscles and joints to each other). Impairment or dysfunction in any of these areas may cause impairments in motor control difficulties that will interfere with function. A lesion in the brain, such as one caused by a cerebrovascular accident (CVA) (see Chapter 23), will cause difficulties in all areas of occupation and functional mobility.

Joe is a 62-year-old man who experienced a left CVA 4 weeks ago. The loss of motor control on the right side of his body means that he is unable to use his preferred right arm for self-feeding or simple oral hygiene activities. In addition, he has difficulty dressing and engaging in his leisure activity of fishing. The OT and OTA can work with Joe to help him regain motor function in his right arm so that he can return to previous activities.

Complex neurologic systems work together to make motor control possible. When an insult to the CNS occurs (e.g., stroke) or a progressive, neurologic disease develops (e.g., multiple sclerosis), motor control is affected. Functional recovery depends on the extent of the damage to the CNS and the expected neurologic recovery for a particular diagnosis (see Chapters 23 and 25 for detailed discussions of these).

DYNAMIC SYSTEMS THEORY

Dynamic systems theory proposes that movement is a function of interactions among the neuromuscular system, environment, cognition, and the task itself (McPherson et al., 1982). These systems interact with each other to influence movement. As practitioners it is important to examine the interactions of these systems with flexibility and flow, to facilitate an adaptive, creative response to occupational demands (Sinclair et al., 2018). For example, Joe may be able to complete a motor task such as preparing his fishing rod in the supportive environment at the clinic, but he may not be able to perform the same task while standing on the riverbank in the outdoors. In this example, the change in environment alters the motor demands. The goal of occupational therapy intervention is for clients to perform meaningful motor tasks in multiple environments and especially the environments of choice.

To determine how multiple systems influence the ability to engage in occupations, such as feeding, dressing, grooming, leisure, work, and social participation, requires that OTs and OTAs evaluate them. This allows them to identify areas of deficit. They can then target the intervention to remediate a deficit area or compensate for it by changing the requirements of the task to facilitate success. The practitioner may decide to target one system (motor skills) or work within multiple systems (motor skills, perceptual skills, and environment) to address motor control issues. The neuromusculoskeletal system plays an important role in motor control, so that is often the first area to be assessed when planning interventions to improve dysfunction that influences motor control.

NEUROMUSCULOSKELETAL SYSTEM

The neuromusculoskeletal system includes the nervous, muscular, and skeletal systems, which interact to influence and produce movement. Disruptions in any of these systems (such as a CVA) may result in motor control dysfunction.

When examining the neuromusculoskeletal system, practitioners evaluate the following:
- Physical appearance
- Postural mechanism
  - Postural tone
  - Muscle tone
  - Reflexes
- Coordination

Evaluation of Neuromuscular System

Physical Appearance. Symmetry of the limbs and skeleton provides the foundation for movement. The appearance of asymmetry indicates potential for a disruption in movement. When examining clients, the OTA can note deformities or injuries (e.g., contractures, burns, scarring, edema) that may mean they are unable to move in certain ways. The following questions may guide your observation of clients:
- Does the client lean to one side when sitting? Standing? Walking?
- Is the pelvis in a neutral position when seated?
- Are there any physical anomalies observed?
- Does the person have any swollen joints?
- Are both sides of the body symmetrical?
- Are the limbs of equal size?
- Are there any skeletal or muscular deficits that may interfere with movement?

Postural Mechanism

The **postural mechanisms** include postural tone, muscle tone, integration of the primitive reflexes and mass patterns of movement, righting reactions, equilibrium reactions, protective extension, and selective voluntary or intentional movement (Bobath, 1990; Charness, 1985). Adults with no movement dysfunction have developed postural support sufficient to provide stability and allow functional movement. Normal postural mechanisms are automatic, involuntary (nonintentional) movements that together provide stability and mobility during activity (Carr & Shepherd, 2003). These automatic reactions develop early in life. The postural mechanisms allow for the development of head control (stability) and mobility, trunk control and mobility, midline

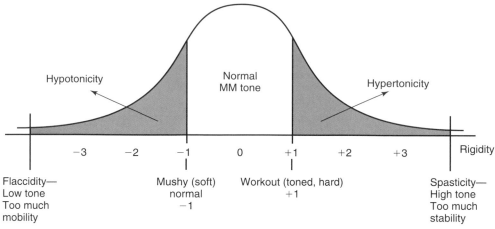

Fig. 6.1 Visual representation of the continuum of muscle tone. (Courtesy Jean W. Solomon, 1995.)

orientation of self and symmetry, weight bearing and weight shifting in all directions, balance during transitional movements, controlled voluntary limb movement, and coordination (Bobath, 1990; Charness, 1985).

> ### CLINICAL PEARL
>
> Researchers indicate that yoga can be an effective neuromuscular intervention for people at risk for falls (e.g., people who have had a traumatic brain injury [TBI], CVA, multiple sclerosis [MS]) (Green et al., 2019). Yoga can be used as an intervention in occupational therapy to strengthen postural control muscles, unify the mind and body, improve body awareness, and overcome fear of falling. Yoga promotes independence in activities of daily living (ADL) and overall quality of life. The following poses improve motor control:
> Tree Pose: Client closes eyes, brings hands together, bends one knee, and places foot on opposite leg's inner thigh.
> Mountain Pose: Client stands with base of big toes touching, heels slightly apart, squeezes inner thighs, presses shoulder blades into back (Green et al., 2019).

CNS damage, as is seen in CVA or TBI, disrupts normal postural mechanism. Abnormal muscle tone and mass patterns dominate the client's movements causing them to be slow and uncoordinated. OTs and OTAs assess the degree of damage to the postural mechanisms to understand the effect they may have on occupational performance activities.

Postural tone. **Postural tone** refers to tonus (muscle tension) in the neck, trunk, and limbs. Postural tone must be high enough to resist gravity and allow upright posture, yet low enough to allow movement (Bobath, 1990). Tone fluctuates in response to externally imposed factors, such as gravity, which allows movement. Postural tone provides the necessary proximal stability (close to the body center) to enable distal (away from the body center), voluntary, selective movements. Abnormal muscle tone may be too low, resulting in poor stability, or too high, resulting in rigidity. High or low muscle tone interferes with normal selective movement.

OTAs with service competency may help evaluate the status of the postural mechanism (and selective movement and coordination) with simple structured tests or checklists to guide in the clinical observations. Both OTs and OTAs observe how impaired motor control affects the client's functional abilities and independence during activities.

> ### CLINICAL PEARL
>
> Observe the client sitting and performing simple weight shifting from side to side as a way to determine general postural tone. This can be done during the initial interview.

Normal muscle tone. Normal **muscle tone**, a component of the normal postural mechanism, is a continuous state of mild contraction or state of readiness of a specific muscle (Ryerson, 1990). Muscle tone is the resting state of a muscle in response to gravity and emotion. It depends on the integrity of the peripheral nervous system (PNS) and the CNS mechanisms and the properties of muscles. While passively manipulating the head, trunk, or limbs, the therapist can feel the tension between the origin and insertion of the muscle. In other words, when they are passively stretched, muscles offer a small amount of involuntary resistance.

Normal muscle tone varies from one individual to another and depends on factors such as age, gender, occupation, and exercise regimen. A normal range is characterized by the following (Fig. 6.1):
1. Effective coactivation (stabilization) at axial (neck and trunk) and proximal shoulder and pelvic girdle joints
2. Ability of a limb to move against gravity and resistance
3. Ability to maintain the limb's position if it is placed passively by the therapist and then released
4. Equal amount of resistance to passive stretch between the agonist (muscle that contracts to create movement at a joint) and the antagonist (muscle that relaxes, or elongates, to allow movement at a joint) (e.g., equal

amount of resistance in the biceps and triceps muscles or in the wrist flexors and extensors)

5. Ease of ability to shift from stability to mobility, and vice versa, as needed (e.g., ability to raise arm above head and then to maintain that position while reaching for a glass in a high cabinet)
6. Ability to use muscles in groups (opening the hand to release an item) or selectively (pointing the index finger while keeping the other digits flexed) (Andric, 1984)
7. Slight resistance to passive movement (Berg et al., 1989)

Assessing muscle tone. A variety of diagnoses affecting the musculoskeletal and nervous systems require the assessment of muscle tone. Normal muscle tone is dynamic and feels different in everyone. Objective evaluation of muscle tone in the client with CNS dysfunction is difficult because of its continuous fluctuation and its relationship to the postural mechanism (Bobath, 1990; Green et al., 2019) (e.g., when muscle tone is lower when lying supported and supine than when sitting or standing unsupported upright against gravity). The level and distribution of muscle tone change as the position of the head in space changes (Bobath, 1990). When CNS damage occurs, primitive reflexes such as the asymmetric tonic neck reflex (ATNR) may reemerge. The reemergence of primitive reflexes and associated reactions alters muscle tone. Therefore muscle tone must be evaluated with regard to the postural mechanism, synergies present, the specific task, and other factors related to motor control. The OT evaluates muscle tone and its distribution. The OTA and OT observe how abnormal muscle tone interferes with occupational performance.

Sitting or standing provide the most accurate assessment of muscle tone because these positions are most often used for occupational performance tasks. During this assessment, grasp the arm proximally and distally to the joint on which the muscle acts. Move the joint slowly through the full range of motion (ROM). Note how freely and readily the limb passively moves through ROM. Record the type and distribution of muscle tone for various muscle groups or movements. This information provides a framework for formal assessment. Abnormal muscle tone is described as hypotonicity, hypertonicity, or rigidity. The therapist must be able to identify clinically the type and distribution of abnormal muscle tone to select appropriate intervention techniques.

> **CLINICAL PEARL**
>
> Practice assessing muscle tone on a variety of people to begin to feel the range of normal muscle tone.

The modified Ashworth tone scale (Bohannon & Smith, 1987) provides a uniform way to measure muscle tone in adults. This scale provides reliability in measuring muscle tone (Fig. 6.2). It is performed in the supine position and is done prior to completing goniometric testing. The scoring is as follows:

GRADE	DESCRIPTION
0	No increase in muscle tone
1	Slight increase in muscle tone, manifested by a catch and release or by minimal resistance at the end of the ROM when the affected part(s) is moved in flexion or extension
1+	Slight increase in muscle tone, manifested by a catch, followed by minimal resistance throughout the remainder (less than half) of the ROM
2	More marked increase in muscle tone through most of the ROM, but affected part(s) easily moved
3	Considerable increase in muscle tone, passive movement difficult
4	Affected part(s) rigid in flexion or extension

Fig. 6.2 Modified Ashworth scale for grading spasticity. (From Bohannon RW, Smith MB. Interrater reliability of a modified Ashworth scale of muscle spasticity. *Phys Ther.* 1987;67:206–207.)

0 = Normal tone
1 = Slight increase in muscle tone (minimal resistance at the end of range)
1+ = Slight increase in muscle tone (minimal resistance throughout less than half of the ROM following the catch)
2 = More apparent increase in muscle tone through most ROM
3 = Considerable increase in muscle tone (passive ROM is difficult)
4 = Rigid in flexion or extension (Bohannon & Smith, 1987)

> **CLINICAL PEARL**
>
> Muscle tone increases with stress or difficulty. Observe muscle tone when a client is performing an activity to better understand what types of activities are suitable for intervention.

Abnormal Muscle Tone

Hypotonicity. **Hypotonicity**, also called flaccidity, is a decrease in muscle tone. Hypotonicity is usually the result of a peripheral nerve injury, cerebellar disease, or frontal lobe damage and is found temporarily in the shock phase after a stroke or spinal cord injury. The muscles feel soft and offer no resistance to passive movement. Usually a wide or excessive passive ROM is present (Urbscheit, 1990). The flaccid limb feels heavy when moved passively. The client cannot hold a position once the limb is placed and released by the therapist. The hypotonic limb cannot resist the pull of gravity and therefore drops (Bickerstaff, 2014). Deep tendon reflexes (reflexive contractions of muscles when their tendons are tapped) are diminished or absent (Davies, 1991; Fiorentino, 1980). In clients who have CVA and spinal cord injuries, flaccidity is usually present initially but is soon replaced by hypertonicity.

Hypertonicity. **Hypertonicity**, also called **spasticity**, refers to increased muscle tone. It is commonly defined as an increased resistance to passive stretch caused by an increased or hyperactive stretch reflex (Ryerson, 1990; Snook, 1979). Any neurologic condition that alters upper motor neuron pathways may result in hypertonicity (Green et al., 2019).

Hypertonicity is characterized by hyperactive deep tendon reflexes and clonus (quick, repetitive, alternate contraction of the agonist and antagonist muscles) (*Minnesota Rate of Manipulation Test*, 1969). Hypertonic muscles offer greater than normal resistance to passive ROM. Hypertonicity usually occurs in patterns of flexion or extension (Bobath, 1990; Jewell, 1990; Okamoto, 1983). The patterns of hypertonicity typically occur in the antigravity muscles of the limbs. Flexor hypertonicity is more commonly apparent in the upper extremity and extensor hypertonicity in the lower extremity.

Hypertonicity varies with the site of the insult to the nervous system. Hypertonicity associated with cerebral damage, as occurs with stroke or head injury, is often seen in combination with other motor deficits such as rigidity or ataxia. Such hypertonicity is influenced by the client's position and the components of the postural mechanism (Green et al., 2019). Spinal cord hypertonicity is often violent, with severe episodic muscle spasms in muscle groups normally innervated below the level of the lesion (Green et al., 2019; Schneider, 1990).

Hypertonicity is often found in clients with upper motor neuron disorders such as MS, CVA, TBI, brain tumors or infections, and spinal cord injury or disease.

The postural mechanism influences the degree and patterns of hypertonicity. Therefore the positions of the body and head in space and the head in relation to the body influence the degree and distribution of abnormal muscle tone (Bobath, 1990). Many factors go into managing hypertonicity, including medical intervention (medications, surgery, injections) and physical intervention (stretching, orthotics, modalities) (Cho et al., 2013). There is no standalone treatment, so it is important to use various interventions in conjunction with each other. Extrinsic factors that influence the degree of hypertonicity include environmental temperature extremes, pain, infection, and emotional stress (Felten & Felten, 1982; Green et al., 2019). Therapeutic intervention focuses on empowering the client to reduce, eliminate, or cope with these extrinsic factors.

Hypertonicity fluctuates, making accurate measurement difficult. The degree and distribution of hypertonicity can be judged while assessing a client with CNS dysfunction. During assessment it is important to keep in mind the dynamic aspect of muscle tone and the factors that might influence a client's muscle tone. Note the influence of abnormal muscle tone while observing a client performing occupational tasks such as feeding or dressing to determine how it impairs function.

Rigidity. **Rigidity** is an increase in muscle tone in the agonist and antagonist muscles simultaneously. Both muscle groups contract continually, resulting in increased resistance to passive movement in any direction and throughout the joint ROM (DeMyer, 1974; Mayo Clinic and Mayo Clinic Foundation, 1982). Lead-pipe rigidity is identified in clients who demonstrate a constant resistance throughout the joint ROM when a limb is passively moved in any direction. With cogwheel rigidity a rhythmic give occurs in the resistance throughout the ROM, similar to the feeling of turning a cogwheel. In rigidity the deep tendon reflexes are normal or only moderately increased (DeMyer, 1974; Mayo Clinic and Mayo Clinic Foundation, 1982).

Rigidity results from lesions of the extrapyramidal system such as in Parkinson disease, certain degenerative diseases, encephalitis, tumors (deGroot, 1991), and TBI. Cogwheel rigidity occurs in some types of parkinsonism and in some cases of carbon monoxide poisoning. Rigid decerebrate posturing (full body extension) and decorticate posturing (full body flexion) may occur with diffuse brain injury or anoxia. Rigidity and hypertonicity of muscles often occur simultaneously in a client with CNS dysfunction.

Following the general guidelines for muscle tone assessment helps determine whether hypotonicity, hypertonicity, or rigidity is present. The degree of increased muscle tone, which may be mild, moderate, or severe, is determined in hypertonicity. If it is mild, resistance during passive movement of a joint through full ROM may be felt, but full ROM is attainable. Mild hypertonicity causes difficulty performing functional activities at normal speed. Moderate hypertonicity causes consistent resistance during passive movement of a joint through full ROM, but full ROM is attainable. Moderate hypertonicity causes observable deviations while performing occupational performance tasks. For example, one may be unable to incorporate forearm supination (palm up) and wrist extension (wrist in upward position) during self-feeding because of hypertonicity in the forearm pronator and wrist flexor muscles. Severe hypertonicity causes strong resistance during passive movement of a joint through full ROM. Severe

TABLE 6.1   Functional Implications With Persistence of Primitive Reflexes

Reflex[a]	Stimulus	Response	Examples of Potential Impact[b]
Suck/swallow reflex	Light touch to lips or gums	Suckling (immature protrusion and retraction of tongue as observed in neonate)	Difficulty performing oral hygiene activities Excessive tongue protrusion during eating and drinking Difficulty creating negative pressure to suck from a straw
Asymmetric tonic neck reflex (ATNR)	Head turned to one side with chin over shoulder	Extension of arm and leg on face side; flexion on arm and leg on skull side	Difficulty performing self-maintenance activities if head turned to one side
Symmetric tonic neck reflex (STNR)	Flexion of neck Extension (hyperextension of neck)	Flexion of arms and extension of legs Extension of arms and flexion of legs	Difficulty bridging (lifting buttocks off supporting surface with hips and neck flexed) Difficulty crawling reciprocally Difficulty using arms to reach over head
Tonic labyrinthine reflex (TLR)	Supine position Prone position	Extension of trunk and extremities or increased extensor postural tone Flexion of trunk and extremities or increased flexor postural tone	Difficulty performing all transitional movements that require dissociation between upper and lower body (flexion of upper body with extension of legs—e.g., moving from supine to long sitting in bed)
Positive supporting reflex (PSR)	Pressure to ball of foot	Extension in leg stimulated (hip and knee extension with plantar flexion of ankle—i.e., toe pointing downward)	Difficulty bridging Difficulty donning shoes or keeping them on Difficulty with swing-through phase of walking as it precedes toe-off phase Difficulty climbing stairs
Crossed extension reflex (CER)	Flexion of one leg	Extension of opposite leg	Difficulty bridging with both legs flexed simultaneously Difficulty walking with a reciprocal arm/leg gait pattern
Palmar grasp reflex	Pressure in palm of hand	Flexion of digits into palmar grasp	Difficulty releasing objects from a palmar grasp (e.g., drinking glass, hairbrush, mop)
Plantar grasp reflex	Pressure to ball of foot	Flexion of toes	Curling of toes in shoes Difficulty walking with foot flat Absence of equilibrium responses in foot

[a]In adults who have sustained an insult to the central nervous system (CNS), the emergence of primitive reflexes may interfere with motor control recovery. Typically these reflexes are assessed while the client is sitting or supine with the head initially in midline, with the exception of the tonic labyrinthine reflexes.

[b]In adults with CNS dysfunction while engaged in occupational performance tasks.

hypertonicity significantly limits the ability to actively control the involved extremities.

Manual muscle testing should not be completed when abnormal muscle tone is present. It can cause subluxation or dislocation of joints in clients with hypotonia. Hypertonic and rigid muscles may appear strong because of resistance during movement; however, the increased resistance to movement is involuntary, and the application of resistance utilized during manual muscle testing may tear or cause other injuries to the muscle (Bobath, 1990).

CLINICAL PEARL

Always inform the client of what is happening and the process. This will ensure the best movement and reduce anxiety that may affect muscle tone.

Reflexes. Reflexes are innate motor responses elicited by specific sensory stimuli. **Primitive reflexes** are involuntary and normally seen in young infants. They help to elongate muscle groups in preparation for voluntary control. The primitive reflexes become integrated as the infant gains voluntary motor control. Once the infant integrates them, they occur only under stress (e.g., infant is hungry or tired) and are never seen in the total complement or pattern. In cases of CNS damage, primitive reflexes should be formally assessed, typically with the client in the sitting or supine position. Table 6.1 provides the specific sensory stimulus and the expected motor response seen in reflex testing. The emergence or persistence of primitive reflexes in an adult will interfere with the recovery of the automatic protective extension, righting, and equilibrium reactions. The functional significance of the presence of specific reflexes is described next.

Suck/swallow reflex. The suck/swallow reflex causes difficulty eating and an inability to suck from a straw. The involuntary protrusion and retraction of the tongue make it difficult to keep food and liquids in the oral cavity.

ATNR. The client with a persistent ATNR may have difficulty maintaining the head in midline while moving the eyes toward or past midline (Blanchette et al., 2017). The client may be unable to extend or flex an arm without turning the head (Blanchette et al., 2017; Chusid, 1982). In addition, the client may be unable to bring the hands to midline. Thus the presence of the ATNR impedes bringing an object to the mouth, holding an object in both hands, or simultaneously looking at and grasping an object in front of the body.

Symmetric tonic neck reflex (STNR). Clients with a persistent STNR cannot support the body weight on hands and knees, maintain balance in quadruped, and creep normally (Bobath, 1985). The client struggles to move from the supine to sitting position because bending the head forward (flexed) to initiate the task increases extension in the legs. The client is unable to bend at the hips to sit upright. The client has difficulty with moving from sitting to standing. Because the arms and head are extended to initiate the movement, one or both legs may flex. Also, the client who has had a CVA may demonstrate total flexion of the affected leg, resulting in an inability to bear weight (*Crawford Small Parts Dexterity Test*, 1981).

Tonic labyrinthine reflex (TLR). The client who exhibits a poorly integrated TLR has severely limited movement. Examples of functional limitations are inability to lift the head in the supine position, to move from supine to sitting position using flexion of trunk and hips, to roll supine to prone (and vice versa), and to sit in a wheelchair for long periods (Bobath, 1985; Chusid, 1982). When the client attempts to move from supine to sitting position, extensor tone is initially dominant until halfway up, when flexor tone begins to take over. Flexor tone continues until full sitting is reached, when the head falls forward, the spine flexes, and then the client falls forward (Blanchette et al., 2017). Sitting in a wheelchair for extended periods can result in increased extensor tone as the client hyperextends the neck to view the environment. With the increased extensor tone the client slips into a semisupine position with feet off footplates (*Crawford Small Parts Dexterity Test*, 1981) (Fig. 6.3).

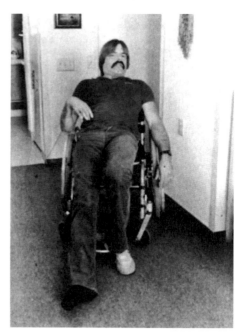

Fig. 6.3 Functional influence of tonic labyrinthine reflex (TLR) on sitting up in a wheelchair.

Positive supporting reflex (PSR). The client who exhibits a PSR has difficulty placing the heel on the ground for standing and walking. A persistent PSR interferes with foot-flat lower extremity weight bearing and weight shifting (Bobath, 1985; Chusid, 1982). The client has difficulty arising from a chair and descending steps because the leg remains stiffly in extension. The rigid leg can carry the client's body weight but cannot adjust in any balance reactions. Therefore all balance reactions are compensated with other body parts (Blanchette et al., 2017) (Fig. 6.4).

Crossed extension reflex (CER). The client who exhibits the CER has difficulty with developing a normal gait pattern because strong extension occurs in the affected leg as the unaffected leg is flexed. The client has difficulty bridging (lifting buttocks while supine with both legs flexed) in bed (Bobath, 1985; Davies, 1991).

Palmar grasp reflex. The client with a poorly integrated grasp reflex cannot release objects placed in the hand, even if active finger extension is present (deGroot, 1991).

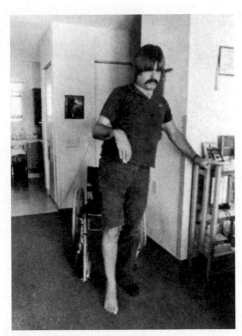

Fig. 6.4 Positive supporting reflex (PSR).

Plantar grasp reflex. The client with a poorly integrated plantar grasp reflex has difficulty keeping toes from curling in the shoes. Normal equilibrium responses in the foot do not develop if the plantar grasp reflex is present.

Functional significance. Observing a client during his or her occupational performance tasks enhances the practitioner's understanding of the functional significance of the persistence of these reflexes in clients with CNS damage. As the primitive reflexes become integrated in normal development, higher level protective extension, righting, and equilibrium reactions emerge. Automatic reactions are a part of the postural mechanism and should be evaluated as well.

Automatic Reactions

Protective extension reactions. **Protective extension reactions** (extending the arms) are used to protect the head and face when a person is off balance or falling (Farber, 1982; Fiorentino, 1980). Without these reactions, the client may fear moving or hesitate to bear weight on the affected side during bilateral or two-handed activities such as getting dressed, cutting meat with a knife and fork, or playing a game of pool.

Righting reactions. **Righting reactions** allow one to maintain or restore the normal position of the head in space (eyes parallel to the horizon) and its normal relationship with the trunk and limbs. Without effective righting responses, the client has difficulty moving from one position to another such as going from the supine position to sit or stand to arise from bed (Bobath, 1990).

Equilibrium reactions. **Equilibrium reactions** maintain and restore a person's balance in all activities (Bobath, 1990; Jewell, 1990). They ensure sufficient postural alignment when the body's supporting surface is changed, thus altering a person's center of gravity. In mature equilibrium responses,

the client's trunk elongates on the weight-bearing side. Without equilibrium responses, the client has difficulty maintaining and recovering balance in all positions and activities. The client with inadequate equilibrium reactions may be unable to sit unsupported while performing dressing activities or standing at a sink while performing oral hygiene activities.

Cognitive and physical limitations may make formal testing of protective extension, righting, and equilibrium reactions difficult. It is possible to observe the absence or presence of righting, equilibrium, and protective extension during transfers and self-maintenance activities. Equilibrium and protective extension reactions can be observed when the client shifts farther out of midline during functional activities, by noting whether the client can regain balance efficiently and effectively to complete the functional activity. If the client is unable to regain balance, note whether protective responses are used to break a fall. You should be positioned to protect the client if these responses fail. If reflexes or stereotypical patterns are not integrated and if protective extension, righting, and equilibrium reactions are impaired, the client will have difficulty using the limbs for functional self-maintenance activities.

The Berg balance test (Berg et al., 1989; 1992) and Tinetti test of balance (Smith, 1993) provide convenient protocols to measure balance in adults. These tests are easy to administer and require little equipment. They can provide practitioners with techniques to measure outcomes.

UPPER EXTREMITY MOTOR RECOVERY

OTs with input from OTAs assess upper extremity functional motion to identify where and to what extent stereotypical patterns of movement dominate the client's motor control and where and under what conditions isolated movement is present. Note the degree to which the client's abnormal postural mechanism interferes with selective volitional movement and determines in which direction of movement hypertonicity occurs and its effects on function.

The upper extremity motor recovery evaluation begins with observation of the client's overall posture. The following should be observed:

- Is the client's posture symmetrical with equal weight on both hips (if sitting) or on both feet (if standing)?
- Is the head in midline or tilted to one side?
- Is one shoulder higher than the other (elevated)?
- Is the trunk twisted or long on one side and short on the other?
- How does the client move in general?
- What is the quality of the movement?
- How does the client sequence and time movements?

Asymmetries impede the client's ability to move the limbs normally and efficiently. Clients may lean to one side and exhibit unequal muscle tone or strength. They may tilt the head to the side. Keeping one's head to the side and elevating one shoulder are signs of asymmetry and may indicate a neurologic deficit.

Asymmetrical head position may interfere with movement because the person may not accurately perceive his or her body in space. It may be that one shoulder is depressed because of hypotonicity or flaccidity. Trunk elongation on one side also indicates discrepancies in muscle tone or muscle strength.

Trunk involvement suggests that postural control is impaired. Clients with trunk involvement may experience difficulty remaining upright. Absence of sufficient stability interferes with mobility as the client is unable to position the body effectively for coordinated movement. Over time, disuse of one side of the body may lead to muscle atrophy interfering with functional movement.

Quality of movement requires stability and precision. Clients who move in smooth, coordinated patterns with ease show good quality of movement and can move as desired. A variety of factors may interfere with quality of movement: muscle tone abnormalities, neurologic processing deficits, musculoskeletal deficits, poor body awareness, and **sensory processing** difficulties. Clients who are trying to move an extremity experience changes in muscle tone that interfere with the coordinated muscle contractions of the agonist and antagonist, resulting in an uncoordinated movement. Neurologic processing deficits may cause poor timing and sequencing of muscle contractions, resulting in poor movements. These deficits may be subtle, resulting in slower reaction times (as found in clients with low cognitive abilities) or more severe as found in clients who have experienced a CVA. Many clients show poor quality of movement associated with musculoskeletal deficits such as those noted after orthopedic injuries. These quality-of-movement issues may arise as the client struggles with understanding the new sense of his or her body. Poor body awareness and sensory processing difficulties, including poor kinesthesia (awareness of movement), proprioception (awareness of muscles and joints), and tactile awareness (feeling one's body), result in poor quality of movement. All of these systems may interfere with the timing and sequencing of movements and result in poor quality of movement.

Examining how the client moves can provide insight into areas in need of remediation. Smooth, coordinated movements and an easy transition from movement to movement are the hallmarks of functional movement. Slow movements with uneasy transitions indicate processing difficulties and/or underlying motor deficits. For example, some clients who have experienced CNS damage may experience difficulty in planning movements. They may appear awkward or clumsy. They may underreach or overreach. Some clients forget how to do the movement altogether.

> **CLINICAL PEARL**
>
> Observe clients in a variety of environments and performing a variety of activities. This helps you understand the client's volition for activities and his or her reaction to different environments. Clients will perform better when doing activities that are meaningful to them or give them identity.

> **CLINICAL PEARL**
>
> Providing a mirror so a client can see his or her performance may help with adjusting movements. Provide tactile cues and simple brief verbal feedback to be effective in improving movement.

OCCUPATIONAL THERAPY INTERVENTION PROCESS

Intervention for clients with dysfunctions in motor control focuses on achieving functional motion to the extent possible to achieve maximal independence while being engaging in occupational performance. The first step in intervention involves assessing the current abilities of the client. The client usually sits during testing, but observing upper extremity control in standing may provide a better indication of the degree of impairment. This is especially true for clients who will eventually walk. In addition, many tasks (e.g., donning slacks, sweeping the floor) are performed while standing.

Following the functional motion and posture assessment, assess the amount and type of motor recovery present in the upper extremities. Assessment and intervention may occur simultaneously. For example, if asymmetry is noted, attempt to correct the asymmetry before continuing with the assessment. This process provides you with valuable information about the client's ability to respond to therapeutic touch and how the client's posture affects muscle tone and movement.

The client's goals and occupational performance desires, as well as the underlying motor control factors that need to be addressed, guide intervention planning and implementation. This includes developing activities that will challenge the motor control of the client and provide the client with practice in a supported environment. The goal of therapy is to enable independence in occupational performance in the specific contexts in which they are performed. For example, if the goal is for the client to dress at home, the practitioner analyzes the motor control movements that are required to make this happen. The goal is smoothly coordinated and effective movement patterns.

Dynamic systems theory proposes that movement is the result of many systems working collaboratively with each other. Earlier theories took a more hierarchical and linear approach toward motor recovery (Brunnstrom, 1970). Brunnstrom stages of motor recovery were developed specifically for examining clients with CVA. Brunnstrom stages do not consider multiple systems, but they provide a developmental progression that may be helpful to consider along with more current motor control concepts. OTs and OTAs may find it helpful to develop intervention using meaningful occupations while addressing the stages of motor recovery in clients after a CVA.

The *Model of Human Occupation Screening Tool* (MOHOST) (Parkinson et al., 2006) provides an occupation-based screening that allows practitioners to objectively examine a client's volition for occupations. Using this helps practitioners better understand their clients and design meaningful intervention.

Brunnstrom Stages of Motor Recovery

In the 1950s and 1960s Brunnstrom observed progressive changes in motor function and behavior during the motor recovery process after a CVA (Box 6.1) (Brunnstrom, 1970). Fig. 6.5 provides a description of the framework for assessing motor recovery developed by Brunnstrom. Brunnstrom described the following stages of motor function:

- No motion can be elicited from the involved upper extremity.
- Reflex responses are limited to generalized or localized motor responses to specific sensory stimuli (Hazboun, 1991). For example, a client with a positive palmar grasp reflex involuntarily holds an object placed in the palm of the hand (see Table 6.1 for additional examples).

- Associated reactions are abnormal increases in muscle tone in the involved extremities that occur when activity requires intensive effort of the unaffected limbs. The involved extremities often move in a synergistic, mass pattern. Associated reactions can be elicited by resisting motion at a joint in an uninvolved limb or by having the client squeeze an object with the unaffected hand. These reactions can also be observed during the client's

BOX 6.1 Brunnstrom Stages of Motor Recovery

1. No motion
2. Reflex responses
3. Associated reactions
4. Mass responses (synergistic)
5. Deviation from pattern
6. Wrist stability
7. Individual finger movement
8. Selected pattern with overlay
9. Selective movement

III. SENSORY MOTOR ASSESSMENT (continued)

F. Mass Pattern Responses: key: 0 = zero, W = weak, M = moderate, S = strong. Observe active R.O.M. and effect of heat and trunk position on motion.

	ADMISSION		DISCHARGE	
1. FLEXION PATTERN	Right	Left	Right	Left
Shoulder abduction/elevation				
Elbow flexions				

Comments: Note any motion occurring at forearm, wrist and hand.

OCCUPATIONAL THERAPY EVALUATION

	ADMISSION		DISCHARGE	
2. EXTENSION PATTERN	Right	Left	Right	Left
Shoulder Adduction/Internal Rotation				
Elbow Extension				

Comments: Note any motions occurring at forearm, wrist and hand.

Key: N = normal, WE = with ease, WD = with difficulty, U = unable, NT = not tested

G. Deviation from Patterns	ADMISSION		DISCHARGE	
	Right	Left	Right	Left
Shoulder add./Int. rot. with Elbow flexion				
Shoulder abduction with Elbow extension				
Forearm pronation with Elbow flexion				
Forearm supination with Elbow extension				

Comments:

H. Wrist and Hand Recovery: record grasp and pinch measurements	ADMISSION		DISCHARGE	
	Right	Left	Right	Left
Stable Wrist During Grasp				
Mass Grasp: Notch #				
Mass Release (3 inch cube)				
Lateral Pinch				
Palmar Pinch				
Individual Finger Motions				

Comments:

I. Selective with Pattern Overlay	ADMISSION		DISCHARGE	
	Right	Left	Right	Left
Integrate prox. to distal control (stack cones)				
Reciprocal total U.E. motion (tether ball)				
Rapid elbow flexion–extension				
Rapid wrist flexion–extension				

Comments:

HAND FUNCTION: (Functional Use Test)
Class # _____
Involved Side: _____
Describe highest function: _____

Fig. 6.5 Upper extremity motor control assessment, part of the Occupational Therapy Stroke Evaluation. (Courtesy Occupational Therapy Department, Ranchos Los Amigos, Downey, CA.)

performance of transfers and other self-maintenance activities that require effort (Fig. 6.6).

- Mass responses (synergistic) limit voluntary motion to total limb movements in flexion or extension. The client is unable to isolate individual joint motion or deviate from the stereotypical movement pattern (Bohannon & Smith, 1987; Ghez, 1991). This situation can be evaluated by asking the client to move at only one joint and observing where the motion occurs. Clients with synergistic movement responses cannot move one joint in isolation. The stereotypical patterns of movement may be seen partially or in full complement. The flexion pattern response consists of scapular adduction and elevation, humeral abduction and external rotation, elbow flexion,

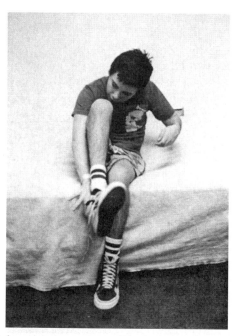

Fig. 6.6 Associated reaction elicited during lower extremity dressing.

forearm supination, wrist flexion, and digit flexion (Fig. 6.7A). The extension pattern response consists of scapular abduction and depression, humeral adduction and internal rotation, elbow extension, forearm pronation, and wrist and finger flexion or extension (see Fig. 6.7B).

- Deviation from pattern occurs when voluntary motor control deviates from the synergy through movement and is patterned predominantly when functional tasks are attempted. For example, a client may be able to actively extend the wrist when asked but unable to use wrist extension while the shoulder is flexed (e.g., reaching for an item above the head). Testing involves asking the client to perform movements that deviate from the synergies and observing the client's ability to accomplish such movements successfully. The techniques are described in the following list (Hazboun, 1991):
    1. Ask the client to touch the back of the uninvolved shoulder with the involved hand (requires scapular abduction and humeral horizontal adduction or scapular abduction with elbow flexion).
    2. Ask the client to touch, using the involved hand, the therapist's finger, which is held out to the client's involved side (requires shoulder or humeral abduction with elbow extension).
    3. Ask the client to use the involved hand to pick up an object from the therapist's hand, positioned approximately 4 in (10 cm) above the client's involved knee (requires elbow flexion with forearm pronation).
    4. Ask the client to reach out in front of the body using the involved hand to receive an object in the palm (requires elbow extension with forearm supination).

   The OT practitioner can detect whether the client is beginning to deviate from mass patterns by observing the client performing these movements. Also, observations of the client engaged in occupational performance tasks indicate when a client is beginning to deviate from these patterns.

- Wrist stability can be observed by asking the client to make a fist and observing for stability of the wrist

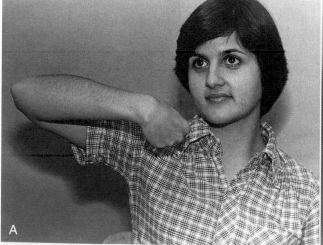
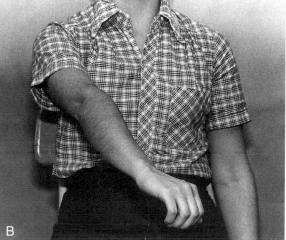

Fig. 6.7 (A) Flexion synergy in upper extremity. (B) Extension synergy in upper extremity.

joint in extension. The client must also be observed while performing tasks such as grasping a toothbrush or holding a spoon during self-feeding.

- Individual finger movements can be observed by asking the client to touch the tip of each finger with the tip of the thumb or to perform a tapping motion with the fingers against the table or the client's leg. The practitioner observes for isolated selective movements. If muscle tone is normal, grasp and pinch strength can be measured by using a dynamometer or pinch gauge.

- Selective pattern with overlay. Joint movement in the affected limb may be isolated with voluntary control, and motion may occur in a variety of planes and directions. However, when the limb is functionally stressed (e.g., client attempting to button small buttons on a shirt sleeve), synergistic patterns may be seen. Observe for compensatory movements during functional activities to see if the client is in this stage of motor recovery. The client may lean to the uninvolved side to raise the involved hand over the head. Shoulder elevation may be used to increase shoulder joint ROM on the involved side. The client in this stage has difficulty performing rapid reciprocal motions such as alternating wrist flexion and extension. During evaluation of rapid reciprocal movements, the client's uninvolved limb should be compared with the involved limb (Hazboun, 1991).

- **Selective movement** is the ability to control movements at each individual joint. The OT practitioner observes for selective movement and control while the client engages in functional activities.

In summary, Brunnstrom provided a framework for anticipated motor recovery in stroke clients. The last stage of motor recovery is selective movement. However, not all clients will reach this level of recovery. An understanding of **Brunnstrom stages of motor recovery** of the upper extremity after a CVA may help you to develop intervention strategies. This information informed by dynamic systems theory suggests that engaging in occupation-based activities will be useful to promote the use of the upper extremity. Develop activities that work for each stage and promote the progression through the stages this way. Clients will participate in activities with more intensity if they are motivated and see the activities as meaningful to them.

> ### CLINICAL PEARL
>
> Constraint-induced therapy helps clients regain motor functioning by promoting the use of the affected extremity in daily activities. Practitioners are urged to examine this intervention technique.

ASSESSMENT OF UPPER LIMB FUNCTION

An interview or occupational profile allows the OT and OTA to understand the client's occupational needs, evaluate the functional status of the involved limb, and design realistic and functional goals. This will help clients regain upper extremity functioning to return to purposeful and meaningful activities within their physical and social environments.

OTAs with service competence may assess a client's functional abilities with standardized tests. For example, the *Functional Test for the Hemiplegic/Paretic Upper Extremity* assesses the client's ability to use the involved arm for occupational performance tasks. It contains items ranging from basic stabilization to more difficult tasks requiring distal fine manipulation with proximal stability. Examples of specific tasks include holding a pouch, stabilizing a jar, wringing a wet washcloth, interlocking and zipping a zipper, folding a sheet, and installing an overhead light bulb. This test provides objective data of the client's functional abilities and is administered in 30 minutes or less (Wilson et al., 1984).

Observing a client performing self-care will help to determine functional use and potential for functional use of the involved extremities. Whether the practitioner uses a simple structured test or observations from a checklist for ADL, the level of functional assist of the involved limb must be established to set realistic goals. The following descriptors are suggested (Andric, 1984):

- Minimal stabilizing assist. The client can use the involved upper extremity to stabilize objects being manipulated by the uninvolved extremity. The involved extremity is placed, and stabilization accomplished by the limb's weight. For example, the involved upper extremity is placed on a piece of paper to stabilize it while the client writes.

- Minimal active assist. The client can use the involved upper extremity to assist actively in a single part of an activity (e.g., actively placing the hand on a piece of paper for writing, actively holding the involved arm away from the body for dressing or hygiene activities).

- Maximal active assist. The client can use the involved arm and hand in all activities that require motor control for pushing or pulling, stabilizing, and gross grasp and release. For example, while writing a letter, the client can push the paper upward with the involved arm and hand.

- Incorporation of involved upper extremity in all bilateral tasks. The client can use the involved upper extremity to assist the uninvolved extremity in most occupational performance tasks, although speed and coordination may be impaired. For example, the client can move both arms above the head to put on a pullover shirt, but movements are slow and cautious on the involved side.

The Functional Independence Measure (FIM) (Graham, 2014) is used to determine the client's ability to complete ADL. The FIM measures the type and amount of assistance required for the individual to perform activities effectively. The FIM subscales include self-care, sphincter control, transfers, locomotion, communication, and social cognition. Degrees of independence are graded on a scale of 1 (total assistance with a helper) to 7 (complete assistance with no helper).

OT practitioners also use the Physical Performance Test (Ryerson, 1990) as a measure of functioning. This test provides an overview of balance, manipulation, and basic motor skills. Although the test is not standardized, it provides a format to review performance and is readily available to clinicians. It consists of the following tasks: writing a sentence, simulated eating, lifting a book to a shelf, putting on a jacket, picking up a penny, turning 360 degrees, and walking.

Intervention

Intervention is based on the client's level of function in the areas of motor, cognition, vision, sensation, psychosocial, and occupational needs (O'Brien & Lewin, 2008) (see Chapters 10 and 20 for other approaches to motor control treatment). The following discussion offers some general guidelines for treatment.

Occupation-Based Activity. OTs and OTAs should evaluate the client's current functioning and design activities to meet his or her occupational needs. These should utilize meaningful tasks to focus on postural control and upper extremity functioning. The goal is for the client to complete activities that are closest to the actual occupations he or she will engage in on discharge from therapy. Participating in whole occupations results in the best carryover and will produce muscle coupling and better co-contraction.

OTs and OTAs should also help clients perform the actual occupation as successfully as possible, which may include adapting the activity or providing assistive technology. Success using adaptations serves as a motivator to clients and allows them to regain occupations more quickly resulting in better motor outcomes through participation. For example, instead of waiting to gain postural control before beginning a fine motor task, practitioners may decide to provide adaptive seating (external postural control) to allow the client to engage in the desired occupation. The practitioner would continue to work on postural @control, but in the meantime the client would be able to engage in the fine motor task.

Abnormal muscle tone is frequently considered an impairment to functional movement. Therefore practitioners may address muscle tone abnormalities by providing facilitation (increasing muscle tone) or inhibition (decreasing muscle tone) techniques. These techniques are supported in the **neurodevelopmental treatment** (**NDT**) frame of reference, which argues that clients must achieve typical muscle tone before moving (Bobath, 1990).

NDT proposes that practitioners first normalize muscle tone and then help clients engage in typical movement patterns by providing gentle cueing techniques at key points of control. Key points of control include the hips, pelvis, shoulders, hands, or trunk. Practitioners who understand typical movement patterns help clients move in the typical pattern. This may involve facilitating or inhibiting specific muscle groups as the client moves.

Facilitation. The increased muscle tone necessary for stability must be facilitated in clients with hypotonia and limited to no motion in the upper extremities. Weight bearing, as well as tactile and proprioceptive input, may be used to increase muscle tone. Input should be provided in a way that avoids overstimulating specific muscles or encouraging abnormal patterns of movement.

Therapeutic activities for improving strength may be used if motion is selective (i.e., not patterned) in the involved upper extremity. A primary goal of intervention should be to establish a balance of strength and tone between the agonist and antagonist muscles (Carr & Shepherd, 1987). The involved arm can be positioned as normally as possible to provide appropriate sensory feedback while the client is performing occupational tasks. Client and family education in proper positioning and joint protection is important to prevent trauma to joint structures.

Inhibition. Inhibitive techniques to decrease the abnormal muscle tone and patterns of movement should be used in clients with hypertonia. These techniques include supportive positioning, prolonged muscle stretching, splinting, motor-level stimulation, modalities, vibration, transcutaneous electrical nerve stimulation (TENS), traction, and prolonged stretching (Blanchette et al., 2017). The motor learning and sensorimotor approaches described in Chapters 10 and 20 may be appropriate, depending on the disability, severity, and distribution of the hypertonia and the associated problems. The goal of treatment is to balance the muscle tone for more normal movement. This requires inhibition of the hypertonic muscles and facilitation of the antagonist muscles, using one of the sensorimotor approaches.

Casting or Orthoses. In some clients, hypertonicity is severe enough to require progressive inhibitory casting or orthoses (Berrol, 1988; *Lincoln-Oseretsky Motor Development Scale*, 1955; O'Brien & Lewin, 2008; Schneider, 1990). Casting provides the circumferential pressure necessary to prevent soft tissue contractures and maintain the muscle's normal length for functional ROM (Keenan, 1987; Newton, 1990).

Serial casting is most successful when a soft tissue contracture has been present for less than 6 months. A series of casts is applied to obtain the maximal end range of a contracted muscle. The final cast may be bivalved (cut into two halves) and used as a night positioner (Fig. 6.8). However, many clinicians prefer bivalving all casts in the series to prevent skin breakdown (Berrol, 1988). A bivalved cast also allows the practitioner to remove the cast for therapy on a regular basis. Various types of casts can be used to decrease hypertonicity in the adult with CNS damage.

A combination of peripheral nerve blocks and casting or orthoses is often used (Berrol, 1988; Keenan, 1987; Mayo Clinic and Mayo Clinic Foundation, 1982). The physician can administer short-acting lidocaine blocks before applying an inhibitory cast to make limb positioning easier. Phenol nerve blocks, also given by a physician, can last up to 3 months.

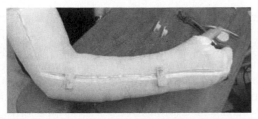

Fig. 6.8 Bi-valve cast. (From Osterman AL: Rehabilitation of the Hand and Upper Extremity, ed 6, 2011, Elsevier, Philadelphia.)

Nerve blocks allow the therapist to increase antagonist control and strength to achieve a balance of muscle control between the agonist and antagonist muscles (Keenan, 1987; Tomas et al., 1993).

Physical Agent Modalities. Physical agent modalities such as cold, heat, and neuromuscular electrical stimulation can be used in preparation for or along with purposeful activity. These modalities can help to reduce hypertonicity temporarily so as to allow for the development of antagonistic control; modalities must be provided by a practitioner with established service competency.

> ### CLINICAL PEARL
>
> In a study to assess the effectiveness of TENS on spasticity in chronic stroke clients, researchers found that the group receiving TENS showed significant reduction in spasticity compared to the control group. Using TENS prior to a treatment session may reduce hypertonicity and improve the client's functional performance (Cho et al., 2013).

Clients who experience severe pain with hypertonicity may require evaluation of the cause of pain. Drug therapy (as prescribed by the physician) and other pain management techniques may be included in the program plan. If a client has a drug therapy regimen, the OT practitioner must recognize the potential side effects. The practitioner must communicate to the medical staff any observed side effects that interfere with the client's overall function.

Although motor control may be adequate for the performance of occupational tasks, sensory and perceptual deficits may limit the client's success in performing functional activities. Perceptual deficits may alter the client's abilities, thus requiring the occupational therapist to lower expected goals (Bernspang et al., 1989) (see Chapters 9 and 22 for further discussions on perception).

Coordination

Coordination is the harmonious interaction of muscles throughout the limb that allows for the production of accurate controlled movement. Such movement is characterized by smoothness, rhythm, and appropriate speed. Voluntary control of muscle tone, postural tone, and balance among muscle groups is necessary for coordinated movement.

Coordinated movement requires that all the elements of the neuromuscular structures and functions be intact. Coordinated movement depends on the contraction of specific agonist muscles with the simultaneous relaxation of the corresponding antagonist muscles, anchored by co-contraction of the joint-stabilizing muscles. Proprioception, kinesthesia, and body schema also must be intact. The client must be able to judge space accurately and to direct body parts through space to the desired target with correct timing (Bickerstaff, 2014).

Incoordination. Coordination of muscle action is controlled by the cerebellum and influenced by the extrapyramidal tracts. Coordinated movement also requires knowledge of body schema and body-to-space relationships. Because of these multiple sources of control, many types of lesions can result in disturbances of coordination (Bickerstaff, 2014). Causes include diseases and injuries of muscles and peripheral nerves, lesions of the posterior columns of the spinal cord, and lesions of the cerebral cortex. Limb paralysis due to a PNS lesion prevents coordination testing even though CNS mechanisms are intact (Mayo Clinic and Mayo Clinic Foundation, 1982).

Common signs of **incoordination** include the following:

- Ataxia is impaired gross coordination and gait. The client with ataxia may have visible tremorlike movements. Ataxia is seen in the delayed initiation of motor responses, in errors in range and force of movement, and in errors in rate and regularity of movement. For example, an ataxic client cannot calibrate the force of grasp and might crush a Styrofoam cup. The client's gait demonstrates a wide base of support (legs far apart) with a reduced or absent arm swing. Step length may be uneven, and the client may tend to fall toward one side. Ataxia results in a lack of postural stability; clients tend to fixate or tighten specific muscle groups to compensate for the instability (Chusid, 1982; Ghez, 1991; Marsden, 1975).
- Adiadochokinesia ("not moving together") is an inability to perform rapidly alternating movements such as forearm supination and pronation or elbow flexion and extension (deGroot, 1991). For example, a client has difficulty dusting or washing windows.
- Dysmetria ("faulty distance between two points") is an inability to estimate the ROM necessary to reach the target of movement. It is evident when touching the finger to the nose or placing an object onto a table (deGroot, 1991). A client has difficulty judging distances and may knock a cup while reaching for it.
- Dyssynergia ("faulty working together") is a decomposition of movement in which voluntary movements are broken into their component parts and appear jerky. Problems in articulation (see upcoming discussion about dysarthria) and phonation may be present (deGroot, 1991).

- Tremor is an involuntary shaking or trembling motion. Tremors are classified according to their type. An intention tremor occurs during voluntary movement, is often intensified at the termination of movement, and is often seen in clients with MS. The client with an intention tremor may have difficulty performing tasks that require accuracy and precision of limb placement (e.g., drinking from a cup, inserting a key in a door). A resting tremor is present in the absence of voluntary movement (occurs while the client is not moving). A pill-rolling tremor, in which the individual appears to be rolling a pill between the thumb and index and middle fingers, is a type of resting tremor often seen in clients with Parkinson disease.
- Rebound phenomenon of Holmes ("to bounce or spring again") is a lack of the check reflex, or the inability to stop a motion quickly to avoid striking something. For example, if the client's arm is bent against the resistance of the therapist and the resistance is suddenly and unexpectedly removed, the client's hand will hit the face or body (Chusid, 1982; deGroot, 1991).
- Nystagmus is an involuntary movement of the eyeballs in an up-and-down, back-and-forth, or rotating direction. After rotation or spinning of the body and head in space, nystagmus is the normal response that helps a person regain balance and orientation. Nystagmus can interfere with head control and fine adjustments required for balance (deGroot, 1991).
- Dysarthria, or faulty speech production, is explosive or slurred speech caused by the incoordination of the speech mechanism. The client's speech may also vary in pitch, may appear nasal and tremulous, or both (Chusid, 1982; deGroot, 1991).
- Choreiform movements are uncontrolled, irregular, purposeless, quick, jerky, and dysrhythmic movements of variable distribution that may also occur during sleep (deGroot, 1991).
- Athetoid movements, or movements without stability, are slow, wormlike, arrhythmic movements that primarily affect the distal portions of the extremities. Athetosis occurs in predictable patterns in the same subject and is not present during sleep (deGroot, 1991).
- Spasms are sudden, involuntary contractions of a muscle or large groups of muscles (Chusid, 1982). In a client with a spinal cord injury, spasms often cause violent and involuntary straightening of the legs.
- Dystonia is faulty muscle tension or tone. Dystonic movements tend to involve large portions of the body and produce grotesque posturing with bizarre writhing movements (Bickerstaff, 2014; Chusid, 1982).
- Ballismus, or projectile movement, is a rare symptom produced by continuous, gross, abrupt contractions of the axial and proximal musculature of the extremity. It causes the limb to fly out suddenly and occurs on one side of the body (Chusid, 1982; deGroot, 1991).

Incoordination consists of errors in rate, rhythm, range, direction, and force of movement (Ghez, 1991). Observation is an important element of the evaluation. The neurologic examination for incoordination may include the nose-finger-nose test, the finger-nose test, the knee pat (pronation-supination) test, and the finger wiggling test (Bickerstaff, 2014; Mayo Clinic and Mayo Clinic Foundation, 1982). Such tests can reveal dysmetria, dyssynergia, adiadochokinesia, tremors, and ataxia. The neurologist usually performs these examinations.

Occupational Therapy Assessment of Coordination

Engagement in occupation is the ultimate goal of occupational therapy intervention; therefore the OTs and OTAs seek to translate the clinical evaluation to a measure of function. Selected activities and specific performance tests can reveal the effect of incoordination on function, which is the OT practitioner's primary concern. The practitioner can observe for coordination difficulties during the client's self-maintenance evaluation and training. The practitioner should observe for irregularity in the rate or force of the movement and sudden corrective movements in an attempt to compensate for incoordination. Movement during the performance of functional activities may appear irregular and jerky and may overreach the target (Mayo Clinic and Mayo Clinic Foundation, 1982).

The following general guidelines and questions can be used when assessing incoordination:

1. The OT evaluates the client's muscle tone and joint mobility.
2. The OT and OTA provide manual stability to joints proximally to distally during functional tasks and note any differences in performance with and without stabilization.
3. The OT and the OTA observe for resting or intention tremor during functional activities.
4. The OT and OTA observe for any noticeable signs of incoordination during therapy sessions.
5. The OT and OTA observe whether the client becomes more uncoordinated in distracting environments.

Smith outlines standardized tests of motor function and manual dexterity (Ryerson, 1990). These include the Purdue Pegboard (Reuben & Siu, 1990), the Minnesota Rate of Manipulation Test (Newton, 1990), the Lincoln-Oseretsky Motor Development Scale (*Lincoln-Oseretsky Motor Development Scale*, 1955), the Pennsylvania Bi-Manual Work Sample (*Pennsylvania Bi-Manual Work Sample*, 2002), the Crawford Small Parts Dexterity Test (*Crawford Small Parts Dexterity Test*, 1981), and the Jebsen-Taylor Hand Function Test (Jebsen et al., 1969). The OT and the OTA with established service competency administer one or more of these tests during the evaluation of coordination. For additional tests of upper limb function, see Table 6.2 (Carr & Shepherd, 2003).

TABLE 6.2 Tests for Upper Limb Function

Test[a]	Reference	Testing Method
Functional Tests		
Motor Assessment Scale: Upper Limb Items	Carr et al., 1985; Poole & Whitney, 1988; Malouin et al., 1994	The test consists of eight separate motor items, each measured on a 7-point scale. Three items measure upper limb function: upper arm function, hand movements, advanced hand activities. Administration is strictly standardized. For clients who achieve top scores, additional tests of dexterity such as the NHPT need to be performed.
Nine-Hole Peg Test (NHPT)	Mathiowetz et al., 1985	A measure of dexterity. Time taken to complete the test is measured as the client grasps nine pegs and places them in holes on a board.
Grip Force	Mathiowetz, 1990; Bohannon et al., 1993; Hermsdorfer & Mai, 1996	Grip-force dynamometer.
Spiral Test	Verkerk et al., 1990	A measure of coordination. Client draws a line as quickly as possible between two spirals, separated by a distance of 1 cm, without touching either spiral. Particularly useful for a client with cerebellar ataxia.
Arm Motor Mobility Test (AMAT)	Kopp et al., 1997	Measures ability to perform 13 activities of daily life composed of one to three component parts. The time taken to perform each task is measured with a stopwatch; the actions are videotaped and rated on 6-point scales.
Action Research Arm Test (ARA)	Van der Lee et al., 2001	The ability to grasp, move, and release objects of different size, weight, and shape is tested by measuring three subtests (grasp, grip, pinch) on a 4-point (0–3) scale. Points 2 and 3 are qualitative in the original scale, but subjectivity can be overcome by setting time limits for each item.
Functional Independence Measure	Uniform Data System for Medical Rehabilitation	Measures the types and amount of assistance a person requires to perform basic life activities effectively (self-care, sphincter control, transfers, locomotion, communication, social cognition): 1 (total assistance, helper) to 7 (complete independence, no helper).
Measures of Real-Life Arm Use		
Motor Activity Log: Amount of Use Scale (AOU)	Taub et al., 1993	Provides information about actual use of the limb in life situations. Client reports at semistructured interview whether and how well, on a 6-point (0–5) scale, 14 daily activities were performed during a specified period.
Actual Amount of Use Test	Taub et al., 1993	Measures actual use of the limb on 21 items using a 3-point rating scale. Clients are videotaped.
Biomechanical Tests	Trombly, 1993	Kinematic analysis of reaching.
Shoulder ROM Tests	Mngoma et al., 1990	Isokinetic dynamometry: LIDO Active System,[b] a valid and reliable measure of resistance to passive external rotation of the glenohumeral joint. Goniometer plus handheld dynamometer (to standardize force).
Tests of Isometric Strength		Handheld dynamometry, grip force[c] dynamometry, pinch force[c] dynamometry
Tests of Sensation	Lincoln et al., 1998; Carey, 1995	Nottingham Sensory Assessment Tactile Discrimination Test Proprioceptive Discrimination Test

[a]Conditions of testing must be standardized.
[b]Loredan Biomedical Inc., 3650 Industrial Boulevard, West Sacramento, CA, 95691, USA.
[c]Digital Pinch/Grip Analyser, MIE Medical Research, Leeds, England (see Sunderland A, et al. Enhanced physical therapy improves recovery of arm function after stroke: a randomised controlled trial. *J Neurol Neurosurg Psychiatr*. 1992;55:530–535).
From Carr JH, Shepherd RB. Stroke rehabilitation: guidelines for exercise and training to optimize motor skill. St Louis, MO: Butterworth Heinemann; 2003.

> **CLINICAL PEARL**
>
> Occupational therapy philosophy is based on the premise that meaningful activity helps clients reengage in meaningful occupations. Therefore meaningful occupations should be used as both a means and an end product of therapy. Research shows that clients perform movements more efficiently and with better coordination when they are engaged in a meaningful task-oriented activity. Furthermore, clients engage in more repetitions of movement. Therefore, the OT practitioner working to help clients improve motor function must first identify the activities and occupations that are meaningful to the individual client. Finding activities that are closely related to the client's occupations will help with motor recovery.

SUMMARY

Motor control is the ability to make continuous postural adjustments and to regulate body and limb movements in response to functional situations. It results from the interaction of complex neurologic systems. Evaluation of motor control includes assessment of the postural mechanism, selective movement, and coordination.

The presence of abnormal elements of motor control affects the quality of movements and the ability to perform functional tasks in all areas of occupation. The OT evaluates muscle tone and upper extremity motor recovery. The OTA assesses aspects of the postural reflex mechanism and coordination using simple structured tests. The OTA also observes for abnormal motor control while the client is engaged in functional activities. The results of the motor control evaluation along with an occupation-based interview guide the practitioner in selecting the appropriate treatment approaches, including sensorimotor approaches or rehabilitative and compensatory methods.

▍REVIEW QUESTIONS

1. What are the roles of the OT and OTA in the evaluation and treatment of an adult with CNS dysfunction who has a motor control deficit? How do these roles change with the establishment of service competency and with experience in a particular setting?
2. What are the components of the normal postural reflex mechanism?
3. Define normal muscle tone.
4. Describe the characteristics of normal muscle tone. Give an example of how normal muscle tone varies depending on the type of occupational performance task.
5. Describe the characteristics of hypotonicity.
6. Describe the characteristics of hypertonicity.
7. Diagrammatically depict the spectrum of normal and abnormal muscle tone.
8. Define specific primitive reflexes, and describe how the OT practitioner would assess for their presence.
9. Describe the functional difficulties encountered when the following primitive reflexes persist during the performance of functional activities in the adult who has sustained a CNS insult: (a) asymmetric tonic neck reflex, (b) symmetric tonic neck reflex, (c) tonic labyrinthine reflex, (d) crossed extension reflex, and (e) grasp reflex.
10. Define the expected stages of motor recovery in an adult after CNS dysfunction caused by a CVA.
11. Describe the upper extremity flexion and extension pattern responses typically observed in the client who has sustained a CVA.
12. Define fine coordination.
13. Analyze the stability and mobility necessary to perform specific occupational performance tasks such as feeding and dressing.
14. List five types of incoordination and describe the functional impact on an adult's performance of ADL (e.g., "Ataxia would interfere with self-feeding because. . .").

REFERENCES

Andric, M. (1984). Projecting the upper extremity functional level. In *Professional Staff Association of Rancho Los Amigos Medical Center: Stroke rehabilitation: State of the art*. Downey, CA: Los Amigos Research and Education Institute.

Berg, K., Wood-Dauphinee, S., Williams, J., & Gayton, D. (1989). Measuring balance in the elderly: preliminary development of an instrument. *Physiotherapy Canada, 41*, 304–311.

Berg, K. O., Maki, B. E., Williams, J. I., et al. (1992). Clinical and laboratory measures of postural balance in an elderly population. *Archives of Physical Medicine and Rehabilitation, 73*(11), 1073–1080.

Bernspang, B., Viitanen, M., & Erickson, S. (1989). Impairments of perceptual and motor functions: their influence on self-care ability 4-6 years after a stroke. *Occupational Therapy Journal Research, 9*, 27–37.

Berrol, S. (1988). The treatment of physical disorders following brain injury. In: R. Wood, & P. Eames (eds.), *Models of brain injury rehabilitation*. Baltimore, MD: Johns Hopkins University Press.

Bickerstaff, E. R. (2014). *Bickerstaff's neurological examination in clinical practice* (6th ed.). London: Blackwell.

Blanchette, A. K., Demers, M., Woo, K., Shah, A., Solomon, J. M., Mullick, A., et al. (2017). Current practices of physical and occupational therapists regarding spasticity assessment and treatment. *Physiotherapy Canada, 69*(4), 303–312.

Bobath, B. (1985). *Abnormal postural reflex activity caused by brain lesions* (3rd ed.). London: Heinemann.

Bobath, B. (1990). *Adult hemiplegia: Evaluation and treatment* (3rd ed.). London: Heinemann.

Bohannon, R. W., & Smith, M. B. (1987). Interrater reliability of a modified Ashworth scale of muscle spasticity. *Physiotherapy Canada, 67*, 206–207.

Brunnstrom, S. (1970). *Movement therapy in hemiplegia.* New York, NY: Harper & Row.

Carr, J. H., & Shepherd, R. B. (1987). *A motor relearning program for stroke* (2nd ed.). Rockville, MD: Aspen.

Carr, J. H., & Shepherd, R. B. (2003). *Stroke rehabilitation: Guidelines for exercise and training to optimize motor skill.* St Louis, MO: Butterworth Heinemann.

Charness, A. (1985). *Stroke/head injury: A guide to functional outcomes in physical therapy management.* Rockville, MD: Aspen.

Cho, H. Y., Sung In, T., Hun Cho, K., & Ho Song, C. (2013). A single trial of transcutaneous electrical nerve stimulation (TENS) improves spasticity and balance in clients with chronic stroke. *The Tohoku Journal of Experimental Medicine, 229*, 187–193.

Chusid, J. G. (1982). *Correlative neuroanatomy and functional neurology* (19th ed.). Los Altos, CA: Lange.

Crawford Small Parts Dexterity Test (1981). New York, NY: Psychological Corporation.

Davies, P. M. (1991). *Steps to follow: A guide to treatment of adult hemiplegia.* New York, NY: Springer Verlag.

deGroot, J. (1991). *Correlative neuroanatomy* (21st ed.). East Norwalk, CT: Appleton & Lange.

DeMyer, W. (1974). *Technique of the neurologic examination: a programmed text.* (2nd ed.). New York, NY: McGraw-Hill.

Farber, S. (1982). *Neurorehabilitation: A multisensory approach.* Philadelphia, PA: WB Saunders.

Felten, D. L., & Felten, S. Y. (1982). A regional and systemic overview of functional neuroanatomy. In: S. Farber (ed.), *Neurorehabilitation: A multisensory approach.* Philadelphia, PA: WB Saunders.

Fiorentino, M. (1980). *Normal and abnormal development: The influence of primitive reflexes on motor development.* Springfield, IL: Thomas.

Ghez C. (1991). The cerebellum. In: E. R. Kandel, J. H. Schwartz, & T. M. Jessel (eds.), *Principles of neural science* (3rd ed.). New York, NY: Elsevier.

Graham, J. E., et al. (2014). Reports of follow up information on patients discharged from inpatient rehabilitation programs in 2002-2010. *American Journal of Physical Medicine Rehabilitation, 93*, 231–244.

Green, E., Huynh, A., Broussard, L., Zunker, B., Matthews, J., Hilton, C. L., et al. (2019). Systematic review of yoga and balance: effect on adults with neuromuscular impairment. *The American Journal of Occupational Therapy, 73*(1), 1–11.

Hazboun, V. (1991). *Occupational therapy evaluation guide for adult hemiplegia.* Downey, CA: Los Amigos Research and Education Institute.

Jebsen, R. H., et al. (1969). An objective and standardized test of hand function. *Archives of Physical Medicine and Rehabilitation, 50*, 311–319.

Jewell, M. J. (1990). Overview of the structure and function of the central nervous system. In: D.A. Umphred (ed.), *Neurological rehabilitation* (2nd ed.). St. Louis, MO: Mosby.

Keenan, M. A. (1987). The orthopedic management of spasticity. *The Journal of Head Trauma Rehabilitation, 2*, 62.

Lincoln-Oseretsky Motor Development Scale (1955). Chicago, IL: Stoelting Co.

Marsden, C. D. (1975). The physiological basis of ataxia. *Physiotherapy, 61*, 326.

Mayo Clinic and Mayo Clinic Foundation. (1982). *Clinical examinations in neurology* (5th ed.). Philadelphia, PA: WB Saunders.

McPherson, J. J., Kreimeyer, D., Aalderks, M., & Gallagher, T. (1982). A comparison of dorsal and volar resting hand splints in the reduction of hypertonus. *The American Journal of Occupational Therapy, 36*, 664.

Minnesota Rate of Manipulation Test (1969). Circle Pines, MN: American Guidance Service.

Newton, R. A. (1990). Motor control. In: D. A. Umphred (ed.), *Neurological rehabilitation.* 2nd ed. St Louis, MO: Mosby.

O'Brien, J., & Lewin, J. (2008). Part I; translating motor control and motor learning principles into occupational therapy practice with children and youth. AOTA CEU article [invited paper].

Okamoto, G. A. (1983). *Physical medicine and rehabilitation.* Philadelphia, PA: WB Saunders.

Parkinson, S., Forsyth, K., & Kielhofner, G. (2006). Model of Human Occupation Screening Tool (MOHOST), Version 2.0. In: *Model of human occupation clearinghouse.* Chicago, IL: University of Illinois.

Pennsylvania Bi-Manual Work Sample (2002). Circle Pines, MN: Educational Test Bureau, American Guidance Service.

Reuben, D. B., & Siu, A. L. (1990). An objective measure of physical function of elderly outclients: the Physical Performance Test. *Journal of the American Geriatrics Society, 38*, 1105–1112.

Ryerson, S. (1990). Hemiplegia resulting from vascular insult or disease. In: D. A. Umphred (ed.), *Neurological rehabilitation* (2nd ed.). St Louis, MO: Mosby.

Schneider, F. (1990). Traumatic spinal cord injury. In: D. A. Umphred (ed.). *Neurological rehabilitation* (2nd ed.), St Louis, MO: Mosby.

Sinclair, C., Meredith, P., & Strong, J. (2018). Case formulation in persistent pain in children and adolescents: the application of the nonlinear dynamic systems perspective. *British Journal of Occupational Therapy, 81*(12), 727–732.

Smith, H. D. (1993). Occupational therapy assessment and treatment. In: H. L. Hopkins, & H. D. Smith (eds.), *Willard and Spackman's occupational therapy* (8th ed.). Philadelphia, PA: Lippincott.

Snook, J. H. (1979). Spasticity reduction splint. *The American Journal of Occupational Therapy, 33*, 648.

Tinetti, M. E. (1986). Performance oriented assessment of mobility problems in elderly clients. *The Journal of the American Geriatric Society, 34*, 119–126.

Tomas, E. S., et al. (1993). Nonsurgical management of upper extremity deformities after traumatic brain injury. *Physical Medicine and Rehabilitation State of the Art Reviews, 7*, 649–661.

Urbscheit, N. L. (1990). Cerebellar dysfunction. In: D. A. Umphred (ed.), *Neurological rehabilitation.* St Louis, MO: Mosby.

Wilson D. J., Baker, L. L, & Craddock, J. A. (1984). *Functional Test for the Hemiplegic/Paretic Upper Extremity.* Downey, CA: Los Amigos Research and Education Institute.

RECOMMENDED READING

Boehme, R. (1988). *Improving upper body control*. Tucson, AZ: Therapy Skills Builders.

Cech, D., & Martin, S. T. (2002). *Functional movement development across the life span* (2nd ed.). Philadelphia, PA: WB Saunders.

Pedretti, L. W., & Early, M. B. (2001). *Occupational therapy practice skills for physical dysfunction* (5th ed.). St Louis, MO: Mosby.

Shumway-Cook, M., & Woollacott, M. (2000). *Motor control: Theory and practical applications*. Baltimore, MD: Lippincott Williams & Wilkins.

Assessment of Joint Range of Motion

Kelly Dolyak and Kelcey Briggs

OBJECTIVES

After reading this chapter, the student or the occupational therapy practitioner will be able to do the following:

- Define goniometry in relation to range of motion.
- Describe functional range of motion in relation to activities of daily living.
- State 11 basic principles for joint measurement.
- Determine range-of-motion measurements of the major upper extremity joints.

- Contrast active and passive range of motion.
- Describe basic goniometry testing positions of the upper extremity.
- Recommend a therapeutic exercise program based on goniometric measurements.
- Describe the three cardinal planes of movement.

KEY TERMS

Range of motion
Joint movement
Active range of motion
Passive range of motion
Functional range of motion

Planes of movement
Goniometer
Stationary bar
Movable bar

INTRODUCTION

The study of joint **range of motion** (**ROM**) is the foundation for understanding how movement—or the lack of movement—affects how people engage in all areas of occupation (American Occupational Therapy Association, 2014). ROM is a client factor that describes the extent of movement that occurs at a joint. ROM is **joint movement**: active, passive, or a combination of both. Motion occurs in an arc; the joint acts as the axis or pivot of the arc (Fig. 7.1). **Active range of motion** (**AROM**) is the arc of motion through which the joint passes when voluntarily moved by muscles acting on the joint. **Passive range of motion** (**PROM**) is the arc of motion through which the joint passes when moved by an outside force. Normally PROM is slightly greater than AROM (Norkin & White, 2009). ROM is measured by an instrument or tool known as a goniometer.

The human body contains several types of joints, muscle tissue, tendons, and other supporting structures that allow for a high degree of joint mobility. Development and maintenance of the greatest ROM maximizes joint function. Many factors (e.g., disease processes, trauma, and periarticular changes) can decrease joint movement and thus limit an individual's participation in occupations. Normal joint movement and muscular strength are client factors that facilitate effortless movement in all areas of occupation, from simple to complex.

An occupational therapy (OT) practitioner will often measure joint ROM as part of the assessment of client factors in individuals with conditions such as cerebrovascular accident, arthritis, fractures, and general debility. The assessment of a client's baseline ROM is an important first step in evaluating client factors and creating an occupational profile. Many clients are motivated by seeing concrete improvement based on recorded ROM measures. OT practitioners should also link these measurements to an individual's participation in occupation. American Occupational Therapy Association (2014) Improvements in motion are not significant unless the person has gained in performance skills to enhance participation occupation. An example of this would be a client's improved ability to dress independently as a result of increased shoulder ROM (American Occupational Therapy Association, 1998).

ROLE OF THE OCCUPATIONAL THERAPY ASSISTANT IN JOINT MEASUREMENT

The extent of the occupational therapy assistant's (OTA's) involvement in ROM assessment is determined by the supervising OT in compliance with the practice laws and professional standards of the state in which the OTA is practicing (American Occupational Therapy Association, 2005; Asher, 2007). In many clinical practices the OTA performs basic

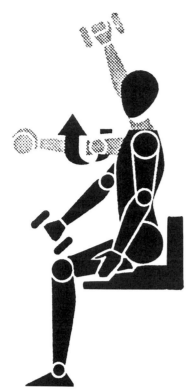

Fig. 7.1 Schematic representation of range of motion occurring around the axis of the glenohumeral joint in shoulder flexion. (Courtesy Jerry L. Pettis, VA Medical Center, Los Angeles, CA.)

goniometry of the upper extremity. The role of the OTA in this area should be based on the competency level of the practitioners. In addition, the OTA must consider legislation and restrictions governing the practice setting in which the skills are being utilized.

GENERAL PRINCIPLES OF ASSESSING JOINT RANGE OF MOTION

The OT practitioner must have complete understanding of (1) the degree and type of motion that will occur at a specific joint, (2) average or normal ROM (Greene & Heckman, 1994), and (3) how to position oneself and the client during measurement (Pendleton et al., 2012). It is important that the OT or OTA take a few minutes to establish rapport and to instruct the client about the nature and purpose of the particular ROM assessment (American Occupational Therapy Association, 1995). Before measuring, the clinician should ask the client to move the extremity through a comfortable ROM. After aligning the goniometer, the OT practitioner should note any discomfort, unusual restriction or freedom of movement, or audible noise (crepitation) from the joint.

Formal joint measurement is not necessary for all clients. The OT practitioner can measure joint movement informally by asking the client to place the affected extremity in a variety of normal positions. Comparing the movement of the affected extremity to that of the opposite, unaffected extremity allows the examiner to detect any significant limitations. The

practitioner should always check the medical record for any causes that may predispose the client to joint limitations (e.g., fused joints, previous injuries, and arthritis). Pain may limit ROM, and crepitation may be heard on movement in some conditions. Joints should not be forced when resistance is met on PROM.

Clinicians are generally concerned with **functional range of motion**. This term typically describes the minimum ROM needed to execute performance in essential areas of occupation without the use of special equipment (Killingworth, 1987). Performance in occupation is a primary goal of occupational therapy. If the client is completely independent in all areas of occupation and has adequate ROM to perform these functions, treatment to increase ROM is generally not indicated, even though the client may have less than normal ROM. ROM for any individual is affected by age, gender, and other factors, including lifestyle and occupation (Norkin & White, 2009).

ASSESSMENT OF JOINT RANGE OF MOTION

In general, most measurements are performed with the client in the anatomic position. In the anatomic position, the person stands erect with the face directed forward; the arms are at the sides, and the palms of the hands are facing forward. Motions of the body occur in three cardinal **planes of movement**: sagittal, frontal, and horizontal (Fig. 7.2). The 180-degree joint measuring system is most commonly used to measure joint ROM. In this system, 0 degrees is the starting position. To measure, the goniometer is placed on the body in the plane of movement that the joint motion will occur. The axis of the goniometer is aligned with the axis of the joint. Joint motion begins at 0 degrees and increases toward 180 degrees, for most joint measurements.

Joint ROM is assessed with a **goniometer**, derived from the Greek *gonio*, which means "angle," and *metron*, which means "a measure" (Greene & Heckman, 1994). Goniometers come in a variety of sizes and shapes, can be made from plastic or metal, and may be purchased from medical supply companies or through medical catalogs. The tool consists of a stationary (proximal) bar and a movable (distal) bar. The body of the **stationary bar** includes a small protractor (half circle) of 0 to 180 degrees or a full circle printed with a scale from 0 to 360 degrees. The **movable bar** is attached at the center or axis of the protractor and acts as a dial. As the dial rotates around the protractor, the number of degrees is indicated on the scale (Fig. 7.3).

One important feature of the goniometer is the axis, or fulcrum. The rivet that acts as the fulcrum must move freely but hold tightly enough to keep the arms at the measured position when the goniometer is removed from the body.

Two scales of figures are printed on the half circle. Each starts at 0 degrees and progresses toward 180 degrees, but in opposite directions. The key to reading the goniometer is common sense. Once the movement of the body part has exceeded 90 degrees, the larger numbers are read. A common error for beginners is to position the client and goniometer

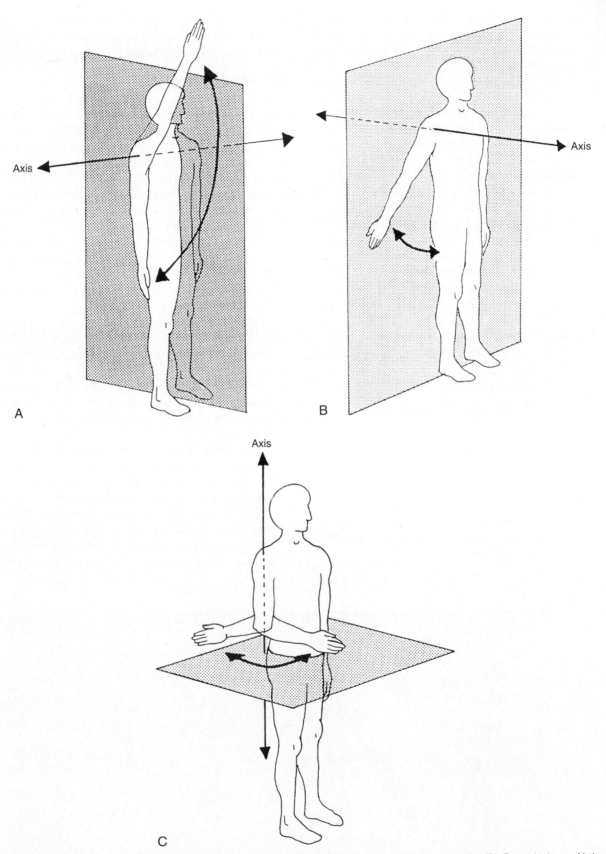

Fig. 7.2 (A) Sagittal plane. Flexion and extension occur in this anatomic plane around the coronal axis. (B) Frontal plane. Abduction and adduction occur in this anatomic plane around the anteroposterior axis. (C) Horizontal plane. Shoulder internal rotation and external rotation occur in this anatomic plane. (Courtesy Jerry L. Pettis, VA Medical Center, Los Angeles, CA.)

correctly and then misread the actual measurement. Many practitioners align the two arms first and then center the axis point over the exact anatomic landmark as an easier method to maneuver the goniometer.

Fig. 7.4 shows five styles of goniometers. The first (see Fig. 7.4A) is a full-circle goniometer. The longer arms are for use on the long bones or large joints of the body. The goniometer in Fig. 7.4B is radiopaque and can be used during x-ray examinations. The notched dial allows an accurate reading of the motion regardless of whether the convexity of the half circle is directed toward or away from the direction of motion. The finger goniometer in Fig. 7.4D has short, flattened arms designed to be used over the finger joint surfaces rather than along their sides. Small plastic goniometers are shown in Fig. 7.4C and E. These devices are inexpensive and easy to carry. The longer one can be used with both large and small joints. The dials of both goniometers are transparent and are marked and notched in two places similar to the goniometer in Fig. 7.4B. The smaller of these two goniometers is simply a larger one that has been cut to be adapted as a finger goniometer.

Other goniometers use fluid with a free-floating bubble that provides the reading after the motion is completed.

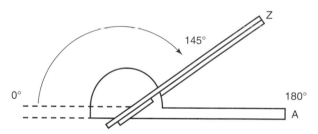

Fig. 7.3 Universal goniometer measuring 145 degrees, using the 180-degree joint measurement system. Point A represents the stationary bar and point Z the movable bar.

Digital types have a liquid crystal display (LCD) readout. Others can be attached to a body segment and have dials that register rotary motions such as pronation and supination.

Documentation of ROM

The OT practitioner most often records the ROM testing results in conjunction with the expected norms for each joint. An example of a form used to document ROM is provided in Fig. 7.5. Table 7.1 lists the norms for each joint, on a scale of 0 to 180 degrees. The practitioner must remember that these ranges are population norms, and often the client's unaffected extremity provides the closest approximation of what is normal for that client. The following points may help clarify situations that arise during measurement:

1. Alternate methods of recording ROM are possible, and the OT practitioner should adapt to the method required by the facility and to the client's ability (Asher, 1989). For example, if a client is unable to stand, measure shoulder flexion in sitting.

2. When joint measurements may be performed in more than one position (e.g., shoulder internal and external rotation), the practitioner should note the position used on the ROM form.

3. A joint measurement may not start at 0. It may start greater than 0 (−15 degrees of elbow extension) or less than 0 (15 degrees of elbow extension). If it starts at greater than 0, this is considered hyperextension. This is often seen in individuals with joint laxity. If it starts at less than 0, it is considered a limitation. This is often seen in individuals after an elbow fracture and may be exhibited as extension and flexion limitation at the elbow joint. For example, an individual may only be able to extend his elbow to 15 degrees and flex to 130 degrees. This represents a 15-degree extension and flexion limitation (60-degree total limitation) because the norm for elbow ROM is 0 to 145 degrees.

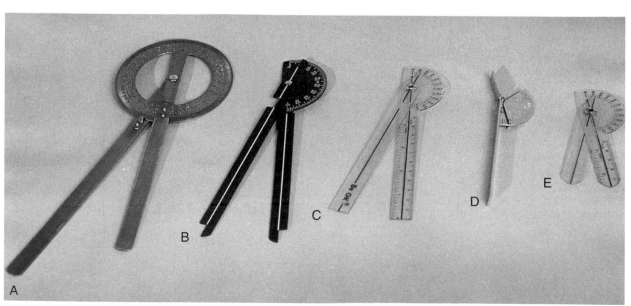

Fig. 7.4 Types of goniometers. (A) Full circle, (B) radiopaque, (C) plastic, (D) finger, (E) plastic small.

JOINT RANGE MEASUREMENTS

Patient's name _____ Chart number _____

Date of birth _____ Age _____ Sex _____

Diagnosis _____ Date of onset _____

Disability _____

LEFT				RIGHT		
3	2	1	**SPINE**	1	2	3
			Cervical spine			
			Flexion — 0 to 45			
			Extension — 0 to 45			
			Lateral flexion — 0 to 45			
			Rotation — 0 to 60			
			Thoracic and lumbar spine			
			Flexion — 0 to 80			
			Extension — 0 to 30			
			Lateral flexion — 0 to 40			
			Rotation — 0 to 45			
			SHOULDER			
			Flexion — 0 to 170			
			Extension — 0 to 60			
			Abduction — 0 to 170			
			Horizontal abduction — 0 to 40			
			Horizontal adduction — 0 to 130			
			Internal rotation — 0 to 70			
			External rotation — 0 to 90			
			ELBOW AND FOREARM			
			Flexion — 0 to 135-150			
			Supination — 0 to 80-90			
			Pronation — 0 to 80-90			
			WRIST			
			Flexion — 0 to 80			
			Extension — 0 to 70			
			Ulnar deviation — 0 to 30			
			Radial deviation — 0 to 20			
			THUMB			
			MP flexion — 0 to 50			
			IP flexion — 0 to 80-90			
			Abduction — 0 to 50			
			FINGERS			
			MP flexion — 0 to 90			
			MP hyperextension — 0 to 15-45			
			PIP flexion — 0 to 110			
			DIP flexion — 0 to 80			
			Abduction — 0 to 25			
			HIP			
			Flexion — 0 to 120			
			Extension — 0 to 30			
			Abduction — 0 to 40			
			Adduction — 0 to 35			
			Internal rotation — 0 to 45			
			External rotation — 0 to 45			
			KNEE			
			Flexion — 0 to 135			
			ANKLE AND FOOT			
			Plantar flexion — 0 to 50			
			Dorsiflexion — 0 to 15			
			Inversion — 0 to 35			
			Eversion — 0 to 20			

Fig. 7.5 Form for recording joint ROM measurements.

TABLE 7.1   Average Normal Range of Motion (180-Degree Method)

Joint	Range of Motion	Associated Girdle Motion
Cervical Spine		
Flexion	0–45 degrees	—
Extension	0–45 degrees	—
Lateral flexion	0–45 degrees	—
Rotation	0–60 degrees	—
Thoracic and Lumbar Spine		
Flexion	0–80 degrees	—
Extension	0–30 degrees	—
Lateral flexion	0–40 degrees	—
Rotation	0–45 degrees	—
Shoulder		
Flexion	0–170 degrees	Abduction, lateral tilt, slight elevation, slight upward rotation
Extension	0–60 degrees	Depression, adduction, upward tilt
Abduction	0–170 degrees	Upward rotation, elevation
Adduction	0 degrees	Depression, adduction, downward rotation
Horizontal abduction	0–40 degrees	Adduction, reduction of lateral tilt
Horizontal adduction	0–130 degrees	Abduction, lateral tilt
Internal rotation		Abduction, lateral tilt
Arm in abduction	0–70 degrees	—
Arm in adduction	0–60 degrees	—
External rotation		
Arm in abduction	0–90 degrees	—
Arm in adduction	0–80 degrees	—
Elbow		
Flexion	0 to 135–150 degrees	—
Extension	0 degrees	—
Forearm		
Pronation	0 to 80–90 degrees	—
Supination	0 to 80–90 degrees	—
Wrist		
Flexion	0–80 degrees	
Extension	0–70 degrees	
Ulnar deviation (adduction)	0–30 degrees	
Radial deviation (abduction)	0–20 degrees	
Thumb		
DIP flexion	0 to 80–90 degrees	
MP flexion	0–50 degrees	
Adduction, radial and palmar	0 degrees	
Palmar abduction	0–50 degrees	
Radial abduction	0–50 degrees	
Opposition		
Fingers		
MP flexion	0–90 degrees	
MP hyperextension	0 to 15–45 degrees	
PIP flexion	0–110 degrees	
DIP flexion	0–80 degrees	
Abduction	0–25 degrees	
Hip		
Flexion	0–120 degrees (bent knees)	
Extension	0–30 degrees	
Abduction	0–40 degrees	
Adduction	0–35 degrees	
Internal rotation	0–45 degrees	
External rotation	0–45 degrees	
Knee		
Flexion	0–135 degrees	

(Continued)

TABLE 7.1   Average Normal Range of Motion (180-Degree Method)—cont'd

Joint	Range of Motion	Associated Girdle Motion
Ankle and Foot		
Plantar flexion	0–50 degrees	
Dorsiflexion	0–15 degrees	
Inversion	0–35 degrees	
Eversion	0–20 degrees	

DIP, Distal interphalangeal; *MP*, metacarpophalangeal; *PIP*, proximal interphalangeal. Data from American Academy of Orthopedic Surgeons: *Joint Motion: Method of Measuring and Recording*, Chicago, 1965, The Academy; and Esch D, Lepley M: *Evaluation of Joint Motion: Methods of Measurement and Recording*, Minneapolis, 1974, University of Minnesota Press.

4. Glenohumeral mobility depends greatly on scapular mobility. If the scapular musculature is spastic, contracted, or orthopedically restricted, glenohumeral ROM will be affected.
5. The practitioner should observe and proceed with caution when spasticity, pain, or abnormal pathology is present.
6. ROM measurements are usually indicated in 5-degree increments. For example, if elbow flexion measures 0 to 128 degrees, the measurement would be recorded as 0 to 130 degrees. Similarly, if elbow flexion is 0 to 122 degrees, the recorded measurement should be 0 to 120 degrees.

! ALERT

The practitioner must use caution in measuring ROM when spasticity, pain, or abnormal pathology is present. Seek advice from a qualified supervisor before proceeding.

Procedure to Assess ROM

The following illustrations of and directions for measurement of included joint ROM demonstrate both goniometer placement and general orientation of the examiner in relation to the client. In most cases the examiner is squared off directly with the client so that the examiner can position the goniometer and read the result.

Factors such as degree of muscle weakness, presence or absence of joint pain, and type of ROM (passive or active) being measured determine how the examiner should hold the goniometer and support the body segment being measured. The examiner and client should be positioned for greatest degree of comfort, correct placement of the goniometer, and adequate stabilization of the joint being measured in correct anatomic plane of movement.

Box 7.1 lists principles for practitioners performing ROM testing that can be applied to the following section on measurement of upper extremity motions. The measurement section indicates the starting position and normal final position. Practitioners should record the client's final position on the form.

PROCEDURES FOR GONIOMETRIC MEASUREMENT AND TESTING OF SELECTED UPPER EXTREMITY MOTIONS

Shoulder
Shoulder Flexion: 0 to 170 Degrees (Fig. 7.6A and B).

Position of subject: Seated or supine with humerus in neutral position.

BOX 7.1   Basic Principles for Range of Motion (ROM) Testing

1. Have the client comfortable and relaxed in testing position.
2. Explain and demonstrate the what, why, and how of goniometry to the client.
3. Establish body landmarks for the measurement.
4. Stabilize joints proximal to the joint being measured.
5. Move the part passively through ROM to estimate available ROM and get a feel for joint mobility.
6. Return the part to the starting position.
7. At the starting position, place the axis of the goniometer over the axis of the joint. Place the stationary bar on the proximal or stationary bone and the movable bar on the distal or moving bone.
8. Record the number of degrees at the starting position.
9. Depending on what type of measurement is being taken (AROM or PROM), move or have the client move the part to obtain the measurement desired (e.g., shoulder flexion).
10. Reposition the movable arm of the goniometer, checking that the axis is still accurately placed, and note the number of degrees at final position.
11. Record the reading to the nearest 5 degrees, make any other appropriate notations on the form (e.g., pain, crepitation).

Position of goniometer: Axis is center of humerus just distal to acromion process on lateral aspect of humerus. Stationary bar is parallel to trunk, and movable bar is parallel to humerus.

Direction of movement: Client's arm is raised in front of body in a sagittal plane of movement.

Shoulder Extension: 0 to 60 Degrees (Fig. 7.7).

Position of subject: Seated or prone, with no obstruction behind humerus. Humerus is in neutral position.

Position of goniometer: Same as for shoulder flexion.

Direction of movement: Client's arm is to be brought in back of the body in a sagittal plane of movement. Excessive scapular motion should be avoided.

Shoulder Abduction: 0 to 170 Degrees (Fig. 7.8A).

Position of subject: Seated or prone with humerus in adduction and external rotation.

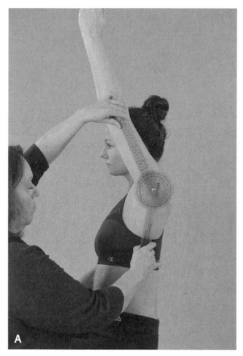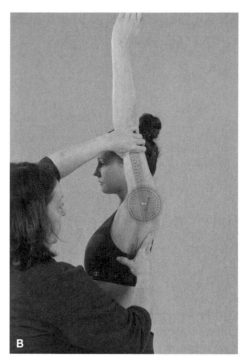

Fig. 7.6 Shoulder flexion. (A) Starting position. (B) Final position. (From Pendleton HM, Schultz-Krohn W: *Pedretti's Occupational Therapy*, ed 8, 2018, Elsevier, St. Louis.)

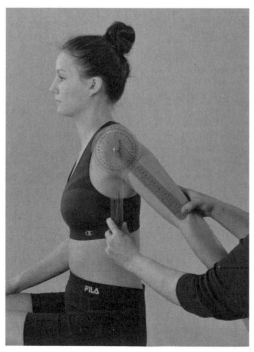

Fig. 7.7 Shoulder extension final position. (From Pendleton HM, Schultz-Krohn W: *Pedretti's Occupational Therapy*, ed 8, 2018, Elsevier, St. Louis.)

Position of goniometer: Axis is on acromion process on posterior surface of shoulder. Stationary bar is parallel to trunk, and movable bar is parallel to humerus.

Direction of movement: Client's arm is raised to side of body in a frontal plane of movement.

Shoulder Internal Rotation: 0 to 60 Degrees (see Fig. 7.8B).

Position of subject: Seated or supine with humerus abducted to 90 degrees and elbow flexed to 90 degrees.

Position of goniometer: Axis is on olecranon process of elbow, and stationary bar and movable bar are parallel to forearm.

Direction of movement: Client's forearm is swung down gently, keeping humerus parallel to floor.

(Alternate position)

Position of subject: Seated with humerus adducted against trunk, elbow at 90 degrees, and forearm in midposition and perpendicular to body.

Position of goniometer: Axis is on olecranon process of elbow, and stationary bar and movable bar are parallel to forearm.

Direction of movement: Client's forearm is swung toward body through a horizontal plane of movement. Humerus must remain adducted.

Shoulder External Rotation: 0 to 80 Degrees (Fig. 7.9A).

Position of subject: Seated or supine with humerus abducted to 90 degrees, elbow flexed to 90 degrees, and forearm pronated.

Position of goniometer: Axis is on olecranon process of elbow, and stationary bar and movable bar are parallel to forearm.

Direction of movement: Client's forearm is swung up gently, keeping humerus parallel to floor.

(Alternate position: Used in some practice settings or as preference of supervising occupational therapist.)

Position of subject: Humerus adducted, elbow at 90 degrees, and forearm in midposition, perpendicular to body.

Position of goniometer: Axis is on olecranon of elbow, and stationary bar and movable bar are parallel to forearm.

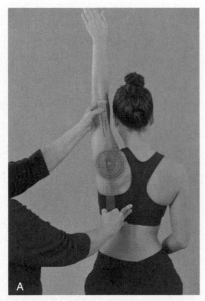
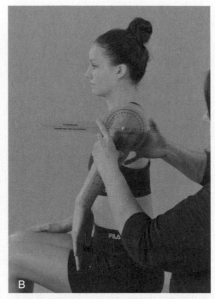

Fig. 7.8 (A) Shoulder abduction. (B) Shoulder internal rotation final position. (From Pendleton HM, Schultz-Krohn W: *Pedretti's Occupational Therapy*, ed 8, 2018, Elsevier, St. Louis.)

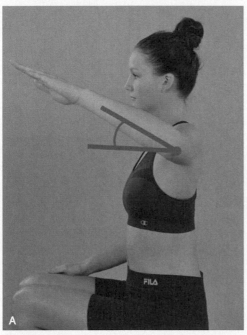
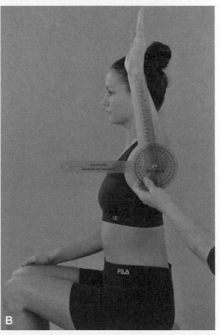

Fig. 7.9 Shoulder external rotation. (A) Starting position. (B) Final position. (From Pendleton HM, Schultz-Krohn W: *Pedretti's Occupational Therapy*, ed 8, 2018, Elsevier, St. Louis.)

Direction of movement: Client's forearm is swung out from body through a horizontal plane of movement. Humerus must remain adducted.

Elbow

Neutral Extension to Flexion: 0 to 135–150 Degrees (Fig. 7.10A and B).

Position of subject: Standing, sitting, or supine with humerus adducted and externally rotated and forearm supinated.

Position of goniometer: Axis is placed over lateral epicondyle of humerus at end of elbow crease. Stationary bar is

parallel to midline of humerus, and movable bar is parallel to radius.

Direction of movement: Client's forearm begins in extended position and is raised in a sagittal plane of movement.

Forearm

Supination: 0 to 80–90 Degrees (Fig. 7.11A and B).

Position of subject: Seated or standing with humerus adducted, elbow at 90 degrees, and forearm in midposition.

Position of goniometer: Axis is at ulnar border of volar aspect of wrist, just proximal to ulna styloid. Stationary

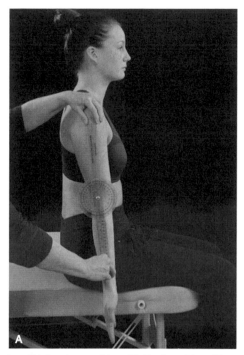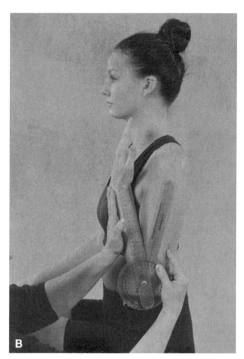

Fig. 7.10 Elbow flexion. (A) Starting position. (B) Final position. (From Pendleton HM, Schultz-Krohn W: *Pedretti's Occupational Therapy*, ed 8, 2018, Elsevier, St. Louis.)

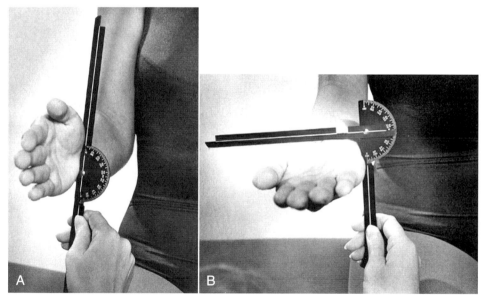

Fig. 7.11 Forearm supination. (A) Starting position. (B) Final position.

bar is perpendicular to the floor, and movable bar is resting against volar aspect of wrist.

Direction of movement: Client's forearm is rotated laterally around ulna.

Alternate Position: Used in Some Practice Settings or as Preference of Supervising OT (Fig. 7.12A and B).

Position of subject: Seated or standing with humerus adducted, elbow at 90 degrees, and forearm in midposition. A pencil is placed in subject's hand and held perpendicular to the floor.

Position of goniometer: Axis is over midshaft of third proximal phalanx. Stationary bar is perpendicular to floor, and movable bar overlays shaft of pencil.

Direction of movement: Client's forearm is rotated laterally around the ulna.

Pronation: 0 to 80–90 Degrees (Fig. 7.13A and B).

Position of subject: Seated or standing with humerus adducted, elbow at 90 degrees, and forearm in midposition.

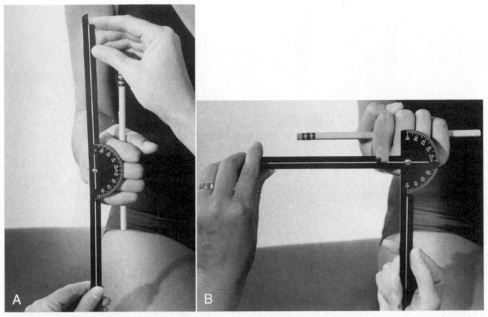

Fig. 7.12 Forearm supination, alternate position. (A) Starting position. (B) Final position.

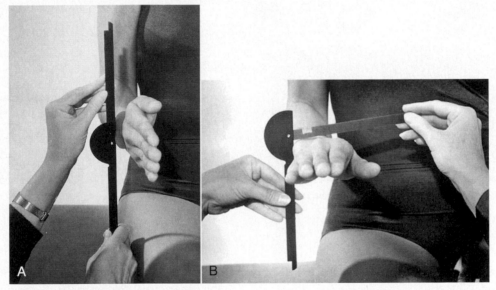

Fig. 7.13 Forearm pronation. (A) Starting position. (B) Final position.

Position of goniometer: Axis is at ulnar border of dorsal aspect of wrist, just proximal to ulna styloid. Stationary bar is perpendicular to floor, and movable bar is resting against dorsal aspect of wrist.

Direction of movement: Client's forearm is rotated medially around ulna.

Forearm Pronation: 0 to 80–90 Degrees (Fig. 7.14).

(Alternate position: Used in some practice settings or as preference of supervising occupational therapist.)

Position of subject: Seated or standing with humerus adducted, elbow at 90 degrees, and forearm in midposition. A pencil is placed in subject's hand and held perpendicular to the floor.

Position of goniometer: Axis is over third proximal phalanx. Stationary bar is perpendicular to floor, and movable bar overlays shaft of pencil.

Direction of movement: Client's forearm is rotated medially around ulna.

Wrist
Flexion: 0 to 80 Degrees (Fig. 7.15).

Position of subject: Seated with forearm in midposition and hand and forearm resting on table on ulnar border.

Position of goniometer: Axis is on lateral aspect of wrist just distal to radial styloid in anatomic snuffbox. Stationary

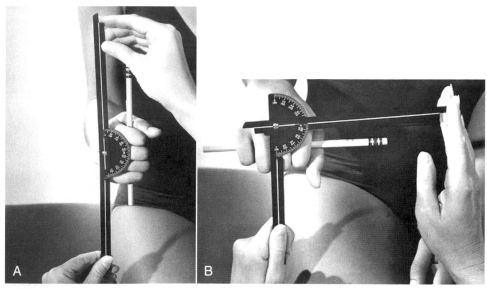

Fig. 7.14 Forearm pronation, alternate position. (A) Starting position. (B) Final position.

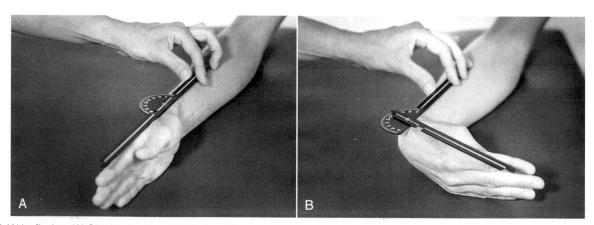

Fig. 7.15 Wrist flexion. (A) Starting position. (B) Final position.

bar is parallel to radius, and movable bar is parallel to metacarpal of index finger.

Direction of movement: Client's hand is flexed down so that palm moves closer to volar aspect of forearm.

Extension: 0 to 70 Degrees (Fig. 7.16A and B).

Position of subject: Same as for wrist flexion except fingers should be flexed.

Position of goniometer: Same as for wrist flexion.

Direction of movement: Client's hand is raised up so that back of hand moves closer to dorsal aspect of forearm.

Ulnar Deviation: 0 to 30 Degrees (Fig. 7.17A and B).

Position of subject: Seated with forearm pronated and palm of hand resting flat on table surface. Goniometer is positioned so that the third finger lines up with center of forearm.

Position of goniometer: Axis is on dorsum of wrist at base of third metacarpal. Stationary bar is positioned in center of forearm, and movable bar is parallel to third metacarpal.

Direction of movement: Client's hand is laterally extended in a horizontal plane of movement.

Radial Deviation: 0 to 20 Degrees (Fig. 7.18).

Position of subject and goniometer: Same as for ulnar deviation.

Direction of movement: Client's hand is medially extended in a horizontal plane of movement.

Fingers

Metacarpophalangeal (MP) Flexion: 0 to 90 Degrees (Fig. 7.19A and B).

Position of subject: Seated with forearm in midposition, wrist at 0 degrees neutral, and forearm and hand supported on a firm surface on ulnar border.

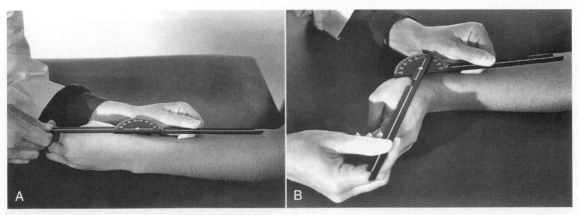

Fig. 7.16 Wrist extension. (A) Starting position. (B) Final position.

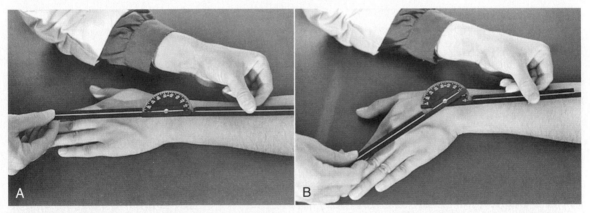

Fig. 7.17 Wrist ulnar deviation. (A) Starting position. (B) Final position.

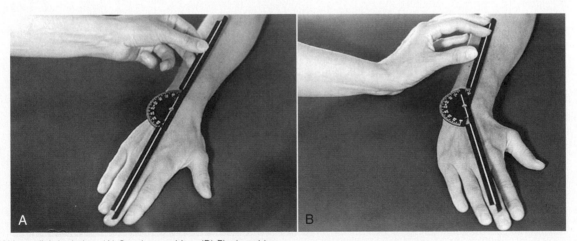

Fig. 7.18 Wrist radial deviation. (A) Starting position. (B) Final position.

Position of goniometer: Axis is centered on top of middle of MP joint. Stationary bar is on top of metacarpal, and movable bar is on top of proximal phalanx.

Direction of movement: Client's finger distal of MP joint is flexed down in a sagittal plane.

MP Hyperextension: 0 to 15–45 Degrees (Fig. 7.20A and B).

Position of subject: Seated with forearm in midposition, wrist at 0 degrees neutral, and forearm and hand supported on a firm surface on ulnar border.

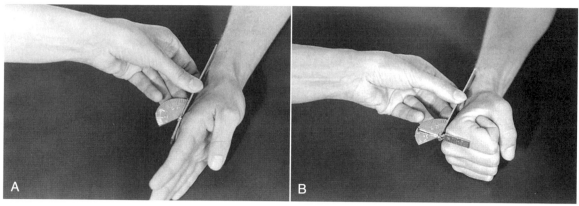

Fig. 7.19 Metacarpophalangeal flexion. (A) Starting position. (B) Final position.

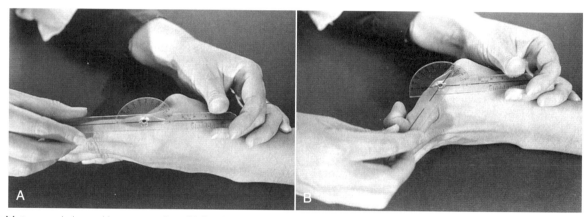

Fig. 7.20 Metacarpophalangeal hyperextension. (A) Starting position. (B) Final position.

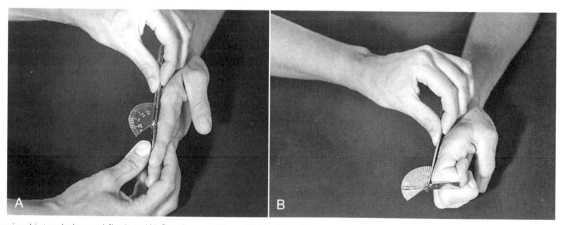

Fig. 7.21 Proximal interphalangeal flexion. (A) Starting position. (B) Final position.

Position of goniometer: Axis is over lateral aspect of MP joint of index finger. Stationary bar is parallel to metacarpal, and movable bar is parallel to proximal phalanx. MP joint of fifth finger may be measured similarly. ROM of third and fourth fingers can be estimated by comparison.

Direction of movement: Client's finger distal of MP joint is extended up in a sagittal plane of movement.

Proximal Interphalangeal (PIP) Flexion: 0 to 110 Degrees (Fig. 7.21A and B).

Position of subject: Seated with forearm in midposition, wrist at 0 degrees neutral, and forearm and hand supported on a firm surface on ulnar border.

Position of goniometer: Axis is centered on dorsal surface of PIP joint being measured. Stationary bar is placed over proximal phalanx, and movable bar is over middle phalanx.

Direction of movement: Client's finger distal of PIP joint is flexed down in a sagittal plane of movement.

Distal Interphalangeal (DIP) Flexion: 0 to 80 Degrees (Fig. 7.22).

Position of subject: Seated with forearm in midposition, wrist at 0 degrees neutral, and forearm and hand supported on a firm surface on ulnar border.

Position of goniometer: Axis is on dorsal surface of DIP joint. Stationary bar is over middle phalanx, and movable bar is over distal phalanx.

Direction of movement: Client's finger distal of DIP joint is flexed down in a sagittal plane of movement.

Thumb

MP Flexion: 0 to 50 Degrees (Fig. 7.23).

Position of subject: Seated with forearm in 45 degrees of supination, wrist at 0 degrees neutral, and forearm and hand supported on a firm surface.

Position of goniometer: Axis is on dorsal surface of MP joint. Stationary bar is over thumb metacarpal, and movable bar is over proximal phalanx.

Direction of movement: Client's thumb distal of MP joint is flexed down.

Thumb Interphalangeal (IP) Flexion: 0 to 80—90 Degrees (Fig. 7.24).

Position of subject: Same as for PIP/DIP finger flexion.

Position of goniometer: Axis is on dorsal surface of IP joint. Stationary bar is over proximal phalanx, and movable bar is over distal phalanx.

Direction of movement: Client's thumb distal of IP joint is flexed down.

Thumb Radial Abduction (Carpometacarpal [CMC] Extension): 0 to 50 Degrees (Fig. 7.25).

Position of subject: Seated with forearm pronated and hand palm down, resting flat on a firm surface.

Position of goniometer: Axis is over CMC joint at base of thumb metacarpal. Stationary bar is parallel to radius, and movable bar is parallel to thumb metacarpal.

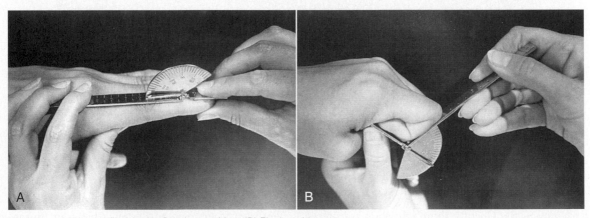

Fig. 7.22 Distal interphalangeal flexion. (A) Starting position. (B) Final position.

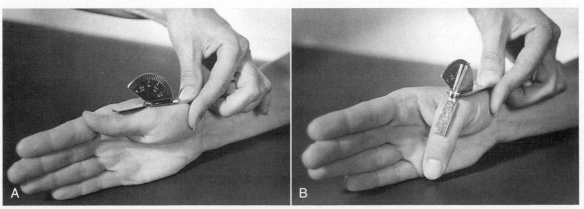

Fig. 7.23 Thumb metacarpophalangeal flexion. (A) Starting position. (B) Final position.

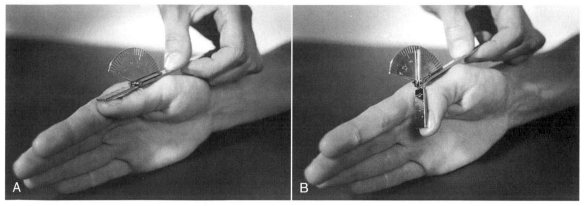

Fig. 7.24 Thumb interphalangeal flexion. (A) Starting position. (B) Final position.

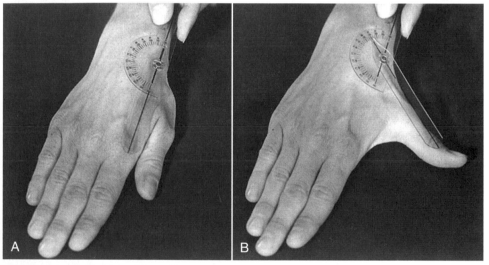

Fig. 7.25 Thumb radial abduction. (A) Starting position. (B) Final position.

Direction of movement: Client's thumb is abducted in a horizontal plane of movement.

Thumb Palmar Abduction (CMC Flexion): 0 to 50 Degrees (Fig. 7.26).

Position of subject: Seated with forearm at 0 degrees midposition, wrist at 0 degrees, and forearm and hand resting on ulnar border. Thumb is rotated and placed at right angles to palm of hand.

Position of goniometer: Axis is over CMC joint at base of thumb metacarpal. Stationary bar is over radius, and movable bar is over thumb metacarpal.

Direction of movement: Client's thumb is abducted in a horizontal plane of movement while forearm is in midposition.

Thumb Opposition (Fig. 7.27).

Position of subject: Seated with palmar aspect of hand exposed.

Position of goniometer: Distance between thumb and fifth finger pads is measured with a centimeter ruler.

Direction of movement: Client's thumb and fifth digit are opposed to one another.

SCREENING FOR FUNCTIONAL RANGE OF MOTION

Functional ROM refers to the range needed to accomplish typical and ordinary daily life activities such as self-feeding, hygiene, dressing, and grooming. This functional range is always less than the normal range given for standard measurements with a goniometer. There are many situations in which it is desirable to briefly screen a client for functional ROM. If deficits are noted in the functional range, the standard evaluation of ROM can be used to obtain more information.

The procedure for testing functional ROM is generally demonstrated by the experienced clinician to the novice or

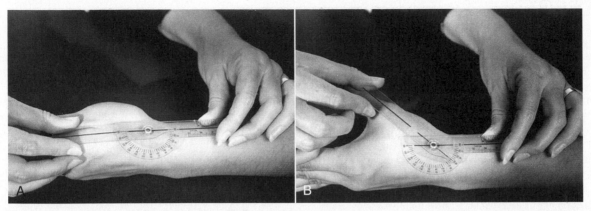

Fig. 7.26 Thumb palmar abduction. (A) Starting position. (B) Final position.

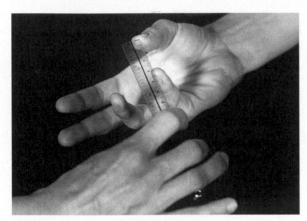

Fig. 7.27 Thumb opposition to fifth finger.

the student on fieldwork (Box 7.2). The sequence and positioning may vary. For example, testing of forearm, wrist, and finger motions of subjects who do not have the strength to maintain shoulder abduction may be done with the forearms resting on a tabletop or the arms of a chair.

SUMMARY

The medical professions have evolved to a point where positive functional outcomes are the benchmark of sound clinical practice. The assessment process is the foundation that enables the OT practitioner to target the type and scope of therapy services specific to each client's needs (American Occupational Therapy Association, 2005; American Occupational Therapy Association, 2014). The assessment of ROM cannot be based on hunches relative to the client's deficits. For an example of this process, please refer to the case study of Mr. R.

The measurement of ROM is an essential aspect of the assessment process. ROM measurement documents objectively the biomechanical changes in joint mobility that result from trauma, disease, or aging. ROM measurement lays the foundation for documenting increases in function proportional to increases in joint ROM.

BOX 7.2 Brief Screening for Functional Range of Motion

S is generally seated, preferably in a chair without arms. For each of the boldfaced motions, E gives directions (in quotes) and should also demonstrate. Alternately, E may demonstrate, saying at the same time, "Do this."

Trunk forward flexion and trunk extension: "Reach down to your toes. Come back up."

Trunk lateral flexion: "Reach down to the floor on the left with your left hand. Come back up. Reach down to the floor on the right with your right hand. Come back up."

Shoulder flexion: "Raise your arms straight up in front of you as far as you can."

Shoulder external rotation: "Place your hands behind your neck."

Shoulder internal rotation: "Reach behind your back."

Shoulder abduction: "Raise your arms out to the side."

Pronation and supination: S keeps arms in shoulder abduction position and is instructed, "Turn your palms up. Now turn your palms down."

Elbow flexion and extension: S keeps arms in shoulder abduction position and is instructed, "Bend and straighten your elbows."

Finger flexion and extension: S keeps arms in shoulder abduction position and is instructed, "Make a fist and then straighten your fingers."

Thumb opposition: S keeps arms in shoulder abduction position and is instructed, "Touch the tip of your thumb to the tips of each of the other fingers."

Wrist flexion and extension: S keeps arms in shoulder abduction position and is instructed, "Bend your wrist up. Bend your wrist down."

Wrist radial and ulnar deviation: S places hands and forearms on lap or table top and is instructed, "Turn your hands out. Turn your hands in."

REVIEW QUESTIONS

1. Describe upper extremity joint motions of the shoulder.
2. Identify major anatomic landmarks associated with joint measurements of elbow flexion and wrist flexion and extension.

CASE STUDY

Mr. R

Mr. R., a retired automobile industry executive, recently fractured his right shoulder during a fall. Mr. R. was evaluated at an urgent care center. X-ray films revealed a nondisplaced fracture of the right proximal humerus. The physician ordered immobilization of the elbow and shoulder joints for 8 weeks. Therapy was ordered after the period of immobilization. The first appointment was scheduled in the ninth week postinjury. Mr. R's chief complaint was that he was experiencing decreased independence in upper body dressing and pain around the elbow joint.

The physician provided an order for occupational therapy to evaluate and treat Mr. R. twice a week for 4 weeks.

The results of the initial assessment are as follows:
Mr. R, 62 y/o, male, SP (R) Humeral fracture. He reported generalized stiffness of the elbow and pain of 6/10 with

activity. ROM: elbow AROM 45° to 135°, PROM 30° to 150°. Strength is 4/5.

After careful assessment, the occupational therapist and OTA collaborated in developing the following course of treatment:
- PROM and AROM and progressive strength exercises for elbow extension
- Adaptive equipment (reacher and dressing stick)
- Functional activities such as bilateral reaching, balloon volleyball, and tabletop activities
- Dynamic elbow extension splint for night use and overhead pulleys for clinic and home use

After a 4-week course of therapy, Mr. R. regained normal motion of his (R) UE, became independent in dressing, and was continuing a home program of general conditioning.

---

3. Describe why the evaluation of joint ROM is an important assessment tool.
4. Describe how crepitation and discomfort can influence ROM.
5. Describe the concept of functional ROM in relation to activities of daily living.
6. Contrast AROM and PROM.
7. List the four components of a goniometer.
8. Explain the reason for the OT practitioner recording goniometric data in 5-degree increments. (HINT: Interrater reliability.)

REFERENCES

American Occupational Therapy Association. (1995). The association: clarification of the use of the terms assessment and evaluation. *Am J Occup Ther, 49,* 1072–1073.

American Occupational Therapy Association. (1998). *Effective Documentation for Occupational Therapy* (2nd ed.). Bethesda, MD: AOTA.

American Occupational Therapy Association. (2005). Standards of practice for occupational therapy. *Am J Occup Ther, 59*(6), 663–665.

American Occupational Therapy Association. (2014). Occupational therapy practice framework: domain and process. 3rd ed. *Am J Occup Ther, 68,* S1–S48.

Asher, I. E. (2007). *Occupational Therapy Assessment Tools: An Annotated Index* (3rd ed.). Bethesda, MD: American Occupational Therapy Association.

Greene, W. B., & Heckman, J. D. (1994). *Clinical Measurement of Joint Motion.* Chicago, IL: American Academy of Orthopedic Surgeons.

Killingworth, A. (1987). *Basic Physical Disability Procedures.* San Jose, CA: Maple.

Norkin, C. C., & White, D. J. (2009). *Measurement of Joint Motion: A Guide to Goniometry* (4th ed.). Philadelphia, PA: Davis.

Pendleton, H. M., & Schultz-Krohn, W. (2012). *Pedretti's Occupational Therapy: Practice Skills for Physical Dysfunction* (7th ed.). St. Louis, MO: Mosby.

RECOMMENDED READING

Cole, T., & Tobis, J. (1990). Measurement of musculoskeletal function: goniometry. In F. J. Kottke, & J. F. Lehmann (eds.), *Krusen's Handbook of Physical Medicine and Rehabilitation* (4th ed.). Philadelphia, PA: Saunders.

Everett, T., & Kell, C. (2010). *Human Movement: An Introductory Text* (6th ed.). St. Louis, MO: Elsevier.

Moore, M. L. (1978). Clinical assessment of joint motion. In J. V. Basmajian (ed.), *Therapeutic Exercise* (3rd ed.). Baltimore, MD: Williams & Wilkins.

Stedman, T. (2008). *Stedman's Medical Dictionary for the Health Professions and Nursing* (6th ed.). Baltimore, MD: Lippincott Williams & Wilkins.

8

Assessment of Muscle Strength

Kelcey Briggs and Kelly Dolyak

OBJECTIVES

After reading this chapter, the student or the occupational therapy practitioner will be able to do the following:
- Identify the six general purposes of muscle strength measurement.
- Identify the three methods of evaluating muscle strength.
- Discuss the relationship between joint range of motion and muscle strength measurement.
- Define manual muscle testing.
- Identify the four primary limitations of the manual muscle test.

- Identify and describe the two primary factors influencing muscle function.
- Identify and define the muscle grades.
- Describe the six steps of the standard procedure for manual muscle testing.
- Describe the break test.
- Demonstrate muscle testing procedures for each of the upper extremity muscle groups, including positioning, stabilization, palpation, observation, and application of resistance.

KEY TERMS

Manual muscle test
Passive range of motion
Muscle endurance
Muscle coordination
Palpation
Hypertrophy

Atrophy
Resistance
Gravity eliminated
Substitution
Muscle grades
Break test

INTRODUCTION

A variety of complex and varied movements are necessary for occupational engagement. To perform any movement requires the muscle strength to move through the environment and overcome the forces of gravity. Muscles provide the power for the human body to move. Muscles vary in size from very small (muscles surrounding the eyes) to very large (quadriceps and deltoids), but all are necessary to produce this movement.

To overcome the forces of gravity requires muscle strength, endurance, and coordination. Muscle strength is the ability of a muscle to overcome resistance in a single effort. Muscle endurance is the ability of a muscle to complete a movement repeatedly over a certain period of time. Coordination is the ability to produce smooth, rhythmic movements that are accurately controlled (Rancho Los Amigos Hospital, 1978). The **manual muscle test** (**MMT**) is a screening tool that provides resistance to a muscle to discern how strong of a contraction it can complete. Contractions can occur isotonically, isokinetically, or isometrically (Rancho Los Amigos Hospital, 1978). Occupational therapists (OTs) and occupational therapy assistants (OTAs) may use this screening procedure to identify how muscle weakness may impair occupational performance (Rancho Los Amigos Hospital, 1978). The results of this assessment may be used to

plan intervention and predict functional changes in the musculoskeletal system.

Assessment of muscle strength can be done by observing a client performing daily activities and analyzing the muscles used during specific tasks (Rancho Los Amigos Hospital, 1978). MMT is a specific assessment of muscle strength involving the active contraction of a muscle or group of muscles (Rancho Los Amigos Hospital, 1978). This screening is appropriate to utilize for many conditions, such as general debility, spinal cord injuries, Guillain-Barré syndrome, primary muscle and neurologic disease processes, traumatic conditions resulting from contractures, burns, amputation, arthritis, and fractures, among a variety of other orthopedic conditions.

Chapter 7 examined the movements of the body. This chapter discusses the muscles, especially in relation to movement, and explores how muscle function affects the ability to perform our daily occupations.

ROLE OF THE OTA IN ASSESSING MUSCLE STRENGTH

The practice standards in each state, as well as the supervising OT, determine the extent of the ability of the OTA to perform measurement for muscle testing. Each OTA must demonstrate service competency while providing services within the legislation and restrictions governing the practice setting. According to the American Occupational Therapy Association (AOTA), service competency is defined as performing the same assessments or tests in the same manner and achieving the same results.

THE EFFECTS OF MUSCLE WEAKNESS ON OCCUPATIONAL PERFORMANCE

Muscle weakness can restrict performance in all areas of occupation, including activities of daily living (ADL), instrumental activities of daily living (IADL), work, leisure, and social activities. The OT and the OTA must assess, monitor, and document the degree of limitations and improvement in strength as it relates to occupation (e.g., in performance skills required for different aspects of ADL such as the ability to carry an object and sustain an activity over time).

Given good to normal endurance, a patient with good (G) to normal (N) muscle strength can perform all ordinary ADL without undue fatigue (Kendall et al., 2005). A patient with fair plus (F+) muscle strength usually has low endurance and fatigues more easily than one with G or N strength. This patient can perform many ordinary ADL independently but may require frequent rest periods. A patient with fair (F) muscle grade can move parts against gravity and perform light tasks that present little or no resistance (Hislop & Montgomery, 2002; Kendall et al., 2005).

Low endurance is a significant problem that limits activity tolerance. As a general rule, for every 1 day of hospitalization, 3 days are necessary for a client to regain prehospitalization levels of endurance. A patient with low endurance can likely perform light ADL, such as self-feeding and face grooming, but may do so slowly and require rest periods to reach his or her goals (Kendall et al., 2005). If muscle strength in the lower extremities is only F, ambulation is not possible (Hislop & Montgomery, 2002). Poor (P) strength is considered below functional range, but the patient may be able to perform some ADL with adaptive equipment and activity modification (Hislop & Montgomery, 2002). Patients with muscle grades of trace (T) and zero (0) in a large number of muscle groups will need adaptive equipment and/or assistive technology to perform ADL without full assistance.

ASSESSMENT OF MUSCLE STRENGTH

The evaluation of muscle strength helps the examiner assess the strength of a given movement. The purposes for evaluating muscle strength are as follows (Kendall et al., 2005):

1. Determine the amount of muscle power available and thus establish a baseline for treatment.
2. Assess how muscle weakness is limiting performance of occupation.
3. Prevent deformities that can result from imbalances of strength of agonist and antagonist muscles.
4. Determine the need for assistive devices to compensate for reduced strength.
5. Aid in the selection of activities within the patient's capabilities.
6. Evaluate the effectiveness of treatment.

Muscle strength can be evaluated in several ways. As mentioned previously, this can be done through observation of the client performing functional tasks. See Chapter 13 for specifics related to the assessment of ADL. MMT provides an accurate assessment of individual muscles or muscle groups. The OT and/or OTA may perform this screening.

When the practitioner is measuring joint motion (see Chapter 7), the **passive range of motion** (**PROM**) is the measure of the range available to the patient. PROM does not, however, indicate muscle strength. One measure of muscle strength is the movement of the joint on which the muscle acts—that is, did the muscle move the joint through complete, partial, or no range of motion (ROM)? Another criterion is the amount of resistance that can be applied to the part once the muscle has moved the joint through available ROM. Available ROM is not necessarily the full average normal ROM for the given joint. Rather, available ROM is the ROM available to the individual patient.

The OT practitioner must know the patient's available PROM to assign muscle grades correctly. PROM may be limited or less than the average for a particular joint motion, but the muscle strength may be normal. For example, the patient's PROM for elbow flexion may be limited to 0 to 110 degrees because of a previous fracture. If the patient can flex the elbow joint to 110 degrees and hold against moderate resistance during the muscle test, the grade would be G. In such cases the examiner should record the limitation with the muscle grade (e.g., "0 degrees to 110 degrees/G"). If the patient's available ROM for elbow flexion is 0 to 140 degrees and the patient can flex the elbow against gravity through 110 degrees, the muscle would be graded fair minus (F−) because the part moved through only partial ROM against gravity.

MANUAL MUSCLE TESTING

The MMT is a means of measuring the maximum contraction of a muscle or muscle group. Muscle testing is used to determine the amount of muscle power and to record gains and losses in strength. The muscle test is a primary evaluation tool for patients with lower motor neuron disorders, primary muscle diseases, and orthopedic dysfunction. The criteria used to measure strength are (1) evidence of muscle contraction, (2) amount of ROM through which the joint passes, and (3) amount of resistance against which the muscle can contract, including gravity as a form of resistance (Hislop & Montgomery, 2002).

Limitations

The limitations of the MMT are the inability to measure the patient's **muscle endurance** (number of times the muscle can contract at maximum level), **muscle coordination** (smooth, rhythmic interactions of muscle function), or motor performance capabilities (use of the muscles for functional activities).

The MMT cannot be used accurately with patients who have spasticity caused by upper motor neuron disorders such as cerebrovascular accident (CVA, stroke) and cerebral palsy, for the following reasons (Brunnstrom, 1992; Davis, 1994; Killingsworth, 1976):

1. In these disorders, muscles are often hypertonic.
2. Muscle tone and ability to perform movements are influenced by primitive reflexes and the position of the head and body in space.
3. Movements tend to occur in gross synergistic patterns (several muscles and joints working together), which makes isolating muscle action and joint movement impossible for most patients, as demanded in manual muscle-testing procedures.

Examiner's Knowledge and Skill

Validity of the MMT depends on the examiner's knowledge and skill in using the correct testing procedure. Careful observation of movement, careful and accurate **palpation** (detecting muscle activity by placing the fingers over the muscle), correct positioning, consistency of procedure, and the examiner's experience are factors critical to accurate testing (Hislop & Montgomery, 2002; Kaskutas, 2019).

To be proficient in MMT, the examiner must have detailed knowledge about all aspects of muscle function. Joints and joint motions, muscle innervation, origin and insertion of muscles, action of muscles, direction of muscle fibers, angle of pull on the joints, and the role of muscles in fixation and substitution are important considerations. The examiner must be able to locate and palpate the muscles; recognize whether the contour of the muscle is normal, atrophied, or hypertrophied; and detect abnormal movements and positions. Knowledge and experience are necessary to detect substitutions and to interpret strength grades accurately (Kaskutas, 2019).

The examiner must acquire skill and experience in testing and grading muscles of normal persons of both genders and

all ages. Some muscles in normal individuals may seem to be weak, but this status may be normal for the particular person. Experience in considering the subject's age, gender, body build, and lifestyle can help the examiner differentiate normal strength from slight muscle weakness (Landen & Amizich, 1963).

General Principles of MMT

Preparation. The examiner should always perform a visual check to assess the general contour, comparative symmetry, and any apparent **hypertrophy** (overdevelopment) or **atrophy** (wasting away) of the muscle(s). When assessing the passive ROM, the examiner can estimate the muscle tone and determine resistance to that motion. During the active ROM the examiner can observe the quality of movement (speed, smoothness, rhythm, abnormal movements such as tremors).

Positioning. Correct positioning of the subject and body part is essential to effective and correct muscle evaluation. The subject should be positioned comfortably on a firm surface. Testing muscles while the subject is seated or in a wheelchair is common. Clothing should be arranged or removed so that the examiner can see the muscle or muscle groups being tested. If this accommodation is not possible, the examiner must exercise clinical judgment in approximating muscle grades (Landen & Amizich, 1963). Moreover, correct positioning, careful stabilization, and palpation of the muscle(s) and observation of movement are essential to test validity (Hislop & Montgomery, 2002).

Factors Influencing Muscle Function

Gravity. Gravity provides **resistance** to muscle power and is used as a grading criterion in tests of the neck, trunk, and extremities (Kaskutas, 2019). Therefore, when assessing muscle grade, the practitioner must consider whether a muscle has the ability to overcome the force of gravity (Kaskutas, 2019).

Movements against gravity and applied resistance are performed in a vertical plane (i.e., moving up). Graded manual resistance is used with F+ to N grades. Tests for weaker

TABLE 8.1 Muscle Grades in Manual Muscle Testing

Number Grade	Word (Letter) Grade	Definition
0	Zero (0)	No muscle contraction can be seen or felt.
1	Trace (T)	Contraction can be felt, but there is no motion.
2	Poor minus (P−)	Part moves through incomplete ROM with gravity decreased.
2	Poor (P)	Part moves through complete ROM with gravity decreased.
2+	Poor plus (P+)	Part moves through incomplete ROM (<50%) against gravity or through complete ROM with gravity decreased against slight resistance (Hislop & Montgomery, 2002).
3	Fair minus (F−)	Part moves through incomplete ROM (>50%) against gravity (Hislop & Montgomery, 2002).
3	Fair (F)	Part moves through complete ROM against gravity.
3+	Fair plus (F+)	Part moves through complete ROM against gravity and slight resistance.
4	Good (G)	Part moves through complete ROM against gravity and moderate resistance.
5	Normal (N)	Part moves through complete ROM against gravity and full resistance.

muscles (0, T, P, and P− grades) (Table 8.1) are often performed in a horizontal plane (i.e., moving sideways). The term **gravity eliminated** is often used to describe this position of testing, which reduces the resistance to muscle power by eliminating the effect of gravity.

Substitution. The brain thinks in terms of movement and not contraction of individual muscles (Hislop & Montgomery, 2002). Thus a muscle or muscle group may attempt to compensate for the function of a weaker muscle to accomplish the desired movement. This act of compensation is termed **substitution** (Kaskutas, 2019). To test the muscle or muscle group accurately, the examiner must eliminate substitutions in the testing procedure by correct positioning, stabilization, and palpation of the muscle being tested. He or she must also perform the test motion carefully, without extraneous movements. The correct body position should be maintained and movement of the part performed without shifting the body or turning the part to allow substitutions (Kaskutas, 2019). The examiner must palpate contractile tissue (muscle fibers or tendons) to detect subtle tension in the muscle group under examination. Only through correct palpation can the examiner ensure that the motion is being performed by the target muscle and not by substitution (Hislop & Montgomery, 2002). Detecting substitutions is a skill gained with experience.

Positioning for movement in the correct plane may not be possible with some patients because of confinement to bed, generalized weakness, trunk instability, immobilization devices, and medical precautions. The examiner should exercise clinician judgment to approximate muscle grades under these circumstances.

Muscle Grades. Although the definitions of **muscle grades** are standard, the assignment of muscle grades during the MMT depends on the examiner's clinical judgment, knowledge, and experience (Hislop & Montgomery, 2002). The examiner determines slight, moderate, or full resistance based on clinical expertise. The patient's age, gender, body type, occupation, and avocations all influence the amount of resistance that the examiner perceives to be appropriate.

The amount of resistance that can be given also varies from one muscle group to another (Hislop & Montgomery, 2002). For example, the flexors of the wrist take much more resistance than the abductors of the fingers. The examiner must consider the size and relative power of the muscle(s) or muscle group and accordingly adjust the leverage used when giving resistance (Kendall et al., 2005). When assessing dysfunction in a given part of the body, the examiner often uses the patient as his or her own control standard by comparing the affected side with the unaffected side when possible.

Because weak muscles fatigue easily, results of muscle testing may not be accurate if the subject is tired. Pain, swelling, or muscle spasm in the area being tested may also interfere with the testing procedure. The examiner should note such problems on the assessment form. Psychologic factors must also be considered. The examiner must assess the subject's motivation, cooperation, mood, cognitive ability, and

effort when interpreting strength (Hislop & Montgomery, 2002).

In manual muscle testing, muscles are graded according to the criteria in Table 8.1 (Hislop & Montgomery, 2002; Rancho Los Amigos Hospital, 1978).

The purpose of using plus and minus designations with muscle grades is to finetune the muscle strength grades. The experienced examiner will probably use these designations. The results attained by two examiners testing the same subject may vary up to a half grade, but they should not disagree by a whole grade (Landen & Amizich, 1963).

PROCEDURES FOR MANUAL MUSCLE TESTING

Testing should be performed according to a standard procedure to ensure accuracy and consistency. Each test is conducted following the same basic steps: (1) position, (2) stabilize, (3) palpate, (4) observe, (5) resist, and (6) grade.

First, the subject (S) should be positioned for the specific muscle test. The examiner (E) should position in relation to S. Then E stabilizes the part proximal to the part being tested to eliminate extraneous movements, isolate the muscle group, ensure the correct test motion, and eliminate the chance of substitution. E demonstrates or describes the test motion to S and asks S to perform the desired test motion. E makes a general observation of the form and quality of movement, checking for substitutions or difficulties that may require adjustments in positioning and stabilization. E then places fingers to palpate one or more of the prime movers, or the tendinous insertion(s), in the muscle group being tested and asks S to repeat the test motion. E again observes the movement for possible substitution and the amount of range completed. When S has moved the part through the available ROM, S is asked to hold the position at the end of the available ROM. E removes the palpating fingers and uses this hand to resist in the opposite direction of the test movement. E usually must maintain stabilization when resistance is given. These muscle tests use the **break test**—that is, the resistance is applied after S has reached the end of the available ROM and attempts to break the contraction.

S should be allowed to establish a maximal contraction (set the muscles) before the resistance is applied (Hislop & Montgomery, 2002; Kendall et al., 2005). E applies the resistance after preparing S by giving the command, "Hold." Resistance should be applied gradually in the direction opposite to the line of pull of the muscle or muscle group being tested.

The break test should not evoke pain, and resistance should be released immediately if pain or discomfort occurs (Hislop & Montgomery, 2002). Finally, E grades the muscle strength according to standard definitions of muscle grades (see Table 8.1). This procedure is used for the tests of strength of grades F and above. Resistance is not applied for tests of muscles from P to 0. Slight resistance is sometimes applied to a muscle that has completed the full available ROM in a gravity-decreased plane to determine if the grade is P+.

BRIEF FUNCTIONAL MUSCLE EXAMINATION OF THE UPPER EXTREMITY

Patient's name _____ Chart no. _____

Date of birth _____ Name of institution _____

Date of onset _____ Attending physician _____ MD

Diagnosis:

KEY

5	N	Normal	Complete range of motion against gravity with full resistance.
4	G	Good*	Complete range of motion against gravity with some resistance.
3	F	Fair*	Complete range of motion against gravity.
2	P	Poor*	Complete range of motion with gravity eliminated.
1	T	Trace	Evidence of slight contractility. No joint motion.
0	0	Zero	No evidence of contractility.
S or SS			Spasm or severe spasm.
C or CC			Contracture or severe contracture.

*Muscle spasm or contracture may limit range of motion. A question mark should be placed after the grading of a movement that is incomplete from this cause.

LEFT   RIGHT

					Examiner's initials					
					Date					
				SHOULDER Flexor	Anterior deltoid					
				Extensors	{ Latissimus dorsi / Teres major					
				Abductor	Middle deltoid					
				Horiz. abd.	Posterior deltoid					
				Horiz. add.	Pectoralis major					
				External rotator group						
				Internal rotator group						
				ELBOW Flexors	{ Biceps brachii / Brachioradialis					
				Extensor	Triceps					
				FOREARM Supinator group						
				Pronator group						
				WRIST Flexors	Flex. carpi rad. / Flex. carpi uln.					
				Extensors	{ Ext. carpi rad. / l. & br. / Ext. carpi uln.					
				FINGERS MP flexors	Lumbricales					
				IP flexors (first)	Flex. digit. sub.					
				IP flexors (second)	Flex. digit. prof.					
				MP extensor	Ext. digit. com.					
				Adductors	Palmar interossei					
				Abductors	Dorsal interossei					
				Abductor digiti quinti						
				Opponens digiti quinti						
				THUMB MP flexor	Flex. poll. br.					
				IP flexor	Flex. poll. l.					
				MP extensor	Ext. poll. br.					
				IP extensor	Ext. poll. l.					
				Abductors	{ Abd. poll. br. / Abd. poll. l.					
				Adductor pollicis						
				Opponens pollicis						

Additional data:

Fig. 8.1 Sample form for brief functional muscle examination of the upper extremity.

LEFT									RIGHT				
					Examiner's initials								
					Date								
					SCAPULA	Abductor	Serratus anterior						
						Elevator	Upper trapezius						
						Depressor	Lower trapezius						
						Adductors	Middle trapezius						
							Rhomboids						
					SHOULDER	Flexor	Anterior deltoid						
						Extensors	Latissimus dorsi						
							Teres major						
						Abductor	Middle deltoid						
						Horiz. abd.	Posterior deltoid						
						Horiz. add.	Pectoralis major						
						External rotator group							
						Internal rotator group							
					ELBOW	Flexors	Biceps brachii						
							Brachioradialis						
						Extensor	Triceps						
					FOREARM	Supinator group							
						Pronator group							
					WRIST	Flexors	Flex. carpi rad.						
							Flex. carpi uln.						
						Extensors	Ext. carpi rad. l. & br.						
							Ext. carpi uln.						
					FINGERS	MP flexors	Lumbricales						
						IP flexors (first)	Flex. digit. sub.						
						IP flexors (second)	Flex. digit. prof.						
						MP extensor	Ext. digit. com.						
						Adductors	Palmar interossei						
						Abductors	Dorsal interossei						
						Abductor digiti quinti							
						Opponens digiti quinti							
					THUMB	MP flexor	Flex. poll. br.						
						IP flexor	Flex. poll. l.						
						MP extensor	Ext. poll. br.						
						IP extensor	Ext. poll. l.						
						Abductors	Abd. poll. br.						
							Abd. poll. l.						
						Adductor pollicis							
						Opponens pollicis							
					FACE								

Additional data:

Fig. 8.1 (Continued).

Fig. 8.1 is a sample form for recording muscle grades. The following protocol does not include tests for the face, neck, trunk, and lower extremities and does not consider muscle grades below F.

Manual Muscle Testing of the Upper Extremity

Again, note that all the following procedures position the subject in gravity-maximized position and therefore apply to testing only muscle grades F (3) to N (5).

Motion: Shoulder Flexion (Fig. 8.2B).

Muscles (Hislop & Montgomery, 2002)	Innervation (Hislop & Montgomery, 2002)
Anterior deltoid	Axillary nerve (n.), fifth and sixth cervical n., C5, C6
Coracobrachialis	Musculocutaneous n., C6, C7

Position: S seated with arm relaxed at side of body with hand facing backward. A straight-back chair may be used to offer maximum trunk support. E stands on the side being tested and slightly behind S (Hislop & Montgomery, 2002; Rancho Los Amigos Hospital, 1978).

Stabilize: Over shoulder being tested but allowing normal abduction and upward rotation of scapula that naturally occurs with this movement (Hislop & Montgomery, 2002).

Palpate: Anterior deltoid just below clavicle on anterior aspect of humeral head.

Observe: S flexes shoulder joint by raising arm horizontally to 90 degrees of flexion (parallel to floor) (Hislop & Montgomery, 2002).

Resist: At distal end of humerus downward toward shoulder extension.

Motion: Shoulder Extension (Fig. 8.3).

Muscles (Hislop & Montgomery, 2002)	Innervation (Hislop & Montgomery, 2002)
Latissimus dorsi	Thoracodorsal n., C6, C7, or C6–C8
Teres major	Inferior subscapular n., C5, C6
Posterior deltoid	Axillary n., C5, C6

Position: S sitting or lying prone with shoulder joint adducted and internally rotated so that palm of hand is facing up. E stands on opposite side.

Stabilize: Over scapula on the side being tested.

Palpate: Teres major along axillary border of scapula. Latissimus dorsi may be palpated slightly below this point or closer to its origin parallel to thoracic and lumbar vertebrae (Hislop & Montgomery, 2002). Posterior deltoid may be found over posterior aspect of humeral head.

Observe: S lifts up arm off table, extending shoulder joint.

Resist: At distal end of humerus in a downward and outward direction, toward flexion and slight abduction (Hislop & Montgomery, 2002; Kaskutas, 2019).

Motion: Shoulder Abduction (Fig. 8.4).

Muscles (Hislop & Montgomery, 2002)	Innervation (Hislop & Montgomery, 2002)
Middle deltoid	Axillary n., C5–C8
Supraspinatus	Suprascapular n., C5

Position: S seated with arms relaxed at sides of body. Elbow on side to be tested should be slightly flexed with palms facing body. E stands behind S.

Stabilize: Over scapula on the side being tested (Hislop & Montgomery, 2002; Kaskutas, 2019).

Palpate: Middle deltoid over middle of shoulder joint from acromion to deltoid tuberosity (Hislop & Montgomery, 2002; Kaskutas, 2019; Kendall et al., 2005).

Observe: S abducts shoulder to 90 degrees. During movement, S's palm should remain down, and E should observe that no external rotation of shoulder or elevation of scapula occurs (Hislop & Montgomery, 2002; Kaskutas, 2019; Kendall et al., 2005). Supraspinatus may be difficult to palpate because the muscle lies under the trapezius muscle, but may be palpated in supraspinatus fossa (Hislop & Montgomery, 2002).

Resist: At distal end of humerus as if pushing arm down toward adduction.

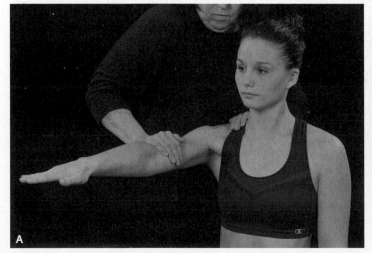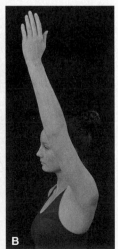

Fig. 8.2 (A) Shoulder flexion manual muscle testing. (B) Shoulder flexion. (From Pendelton HM, Schultz-Krohn W: Pedretti's Occupational Therapy, ed 8, 2018, Elsevier, St. Louis.)

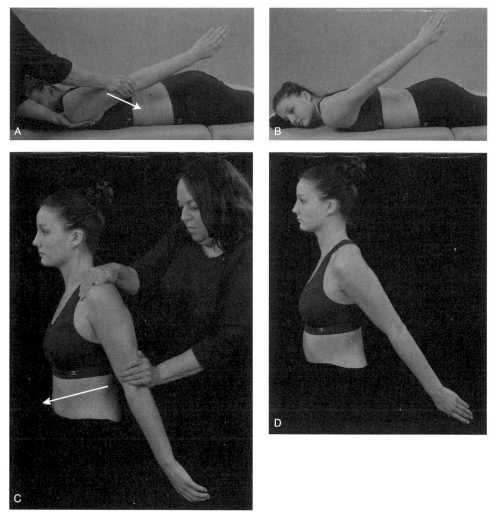

Fig. 8.3 (A) Shoulder extension manual muscle testing (prone). (B) Shoulder extension (prone). (C) Shoulder extension manual muscle testing (sitting). (D) Shoulder extension (sitting). (From Pendelton HM, Schultz-Krohn W: Pedretti's Occupational Therapy, ed 8, 2018, Elsevier, St. Louis.)

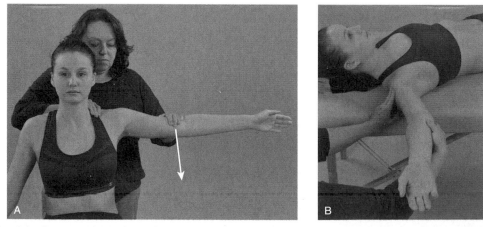

Fig. 8.4 (A) Shoulder abduction manual muscle testing (sitting). (B) Shoulder abduction manual muscle testing (supine). (From Pendelton HM, Schultz-Krohn W: Pedretti's Occupational Therapy, ed 8, 2018, Elsevier, St. Louis.)

Motion: Shoulder External Rotation (Fig. 8.5).

Muscles (Hislop & Montgomery, 2002)	Innervation (Hislop & Montgomery, 2002)
Infraspinatus	Axillary n., C5, C6
Teres minor	Axillary n., C5, C6

Position: S lying prone or seated with shoulder abducted to 90 degrees, humerus in neutral (0 degree) rotation, and elbow flexed to 90 degrees. Forearm is in neutral rotation, hanging over edge of table, perpendicular to the floor. E stands in front of supporting surface toward side being tested.

Stabilize: At distal end of humerus by placing hand under arm on supporting surface (Kaskutas, 2019).

Palpate: Infraspinatus muscle just below spine of scapula, on body of scapula, or teres minor along axillary border of scapula (Hislop & Montgomery, 2002).

Observe: Rotation of humerus so that back of hand is moving toward ceiling (Hislop & Montgomery, 2002; Kaskutas, 2019).

Resist: On distal end of forearm toward floor in direction of internal rotation (see Fig. 8.5B) (Hislop & Montgomery, 2002; Kaskutas, 2019).

Motion: Shoulder Internal Rotation (Fig. 8.6).

Muscles (Hislop & Montgomery, 2002)	Innervation (Hislop & Montgomery, 2002)
Subscapularis	Subscapular n., C5, C6
Pectoralis major	Anterior thoracic n., C5 through first thoracic nerve (T1)
Latissimus dorsi	Thoracodorsal n., C6–C8
Teres major	Subscapular n., C5, C6

Position: S lying prone with shoulder abducted to 90 degrees, humerus in neutral (0 degree) rotation, and elbow flexed to 90 degrees. Forearm is perpendicular to floor. E stands on the side being tested, just in front of S's arm.

Stabilize: At distal end of humerus by placing hand under arm and on supporting surface, as for external rotation (Hislop & Montgomery, 2002; Kaskutas, 2019).

Palpate: Teres major and latissimus dorsi along axillary border of scapula toward inferior angle.

Observe: Movement of palm of hand upward toward ceiling, internally rotating humerus (Hislop & Montgomery, 2002).

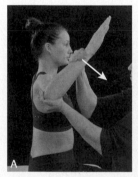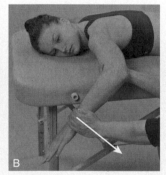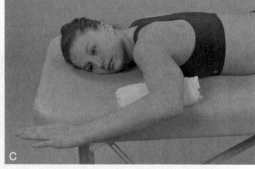

Fig. 8.5 (A) Shoulder external rotation manual muscle testing (sitting). (B) Shoulder external rotation manual muscle testing (prone). (C) Shoulder external rotation (prone). (From Pendelton HM, Schultz-Krohn W: Pedretti's Occupational Therapy, ed 8, 2018, Elsevier, St. Louis.)

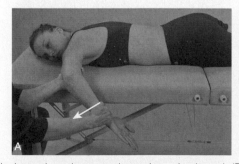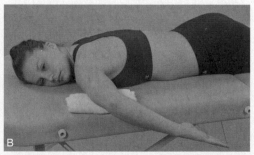

Fig. 8.6 (A) Shoulder internal rotation manual muscle testing (prone). (B) Shoulder internal rotation (prone). (From Pendelton HM, Schultz-Krohn W: Pedretti's Occupational Therapy, ed 8, 2018, Elsevier, St. Louis.)

Resist: At distal end of volar surface of forearm anteriorly toward external rotation (Hislop & Montgomery, 2002; Kaskutas, 2019).

Motion: Elbow Flexion (Fig. 8.7).

Muscles (Hislop & Montgomery, 2002)	Innervation (Hislop & Montgomery, 2002)
Biceps brachii	Musculocutaneous n., C5, C6
Brachialis	Musculocutaneous n., C5, C6
Brachioradialis	Radial n., C5, C6

Position: S sitting with arm adducted at shoulder and extended at elbow, held against side of trunk. Forearm is supinated to test primarily for biceps. E stands next to S on the side being tested or directly in front of S.

Stabilize: Humerus in adduction.

Palpate: Biceps brachii over muscle belly on middle of anterior aspect of humerus. The tendon may be palpated in middle of antecubital space (Hislop & Montgomery, 2002). Brachioradialis is palpated over upper third of radius on lateral aspect of forearm just below elbow. Brachialis may be palpated lateral to lower portion of biceps brachii, if elbow is flexed and in pronated position (Kendall et al., 2005).

Observe: Elbow flexion and movement of hand toward face. E should observe for maintenance of forearm in supination (Kendall et al., 2005).

Resist: At distal end of volar aspect of forearm, pulling downward toward elbow extension (Hislop & Montgomery, 2002; Kaskutas, 2019).

Motion: Elbow Extension (Fig. 8.8).

Muscles (Hislop & Montgomery, 2002)	Innervation (Hislop & Montgomery, 2002)
Triceps	Radial n., C7, C8
Anconeus	Radial n., C7

Position: S prone with humerus abducted to 90 degrees and in neutral rotation, elbow flexed to 90 degrees, and forearm in neutral position perpendicular to floor. E stands next to S just behind arm being tested (Kaskutas, 2019; Rancho Los Amigos Hospital, 1978).

Stabilize: Humerus by placing one hand for support under it, between S's arm and table (Kaskutas, 2019).

Palpate: Triceps over middle of posterior aspect of humerus or triceps tendon, just proximal to elbow joint on dorsal surface of arm (Hislop & Montgomery, 2002; Kendall et al., 2005).

Observe: Extension of elbow to just less than maximum range. Wrist and fingers remain relaxed.

Resist: In same plane as forearm motion at distal end of forearm, pushing toward floor or elbow flexion. Before resistance is given, E ensures elbow is not locked. Resistance to a locked elbow can cause joint injury (Hislop & Montgomery, 2002).

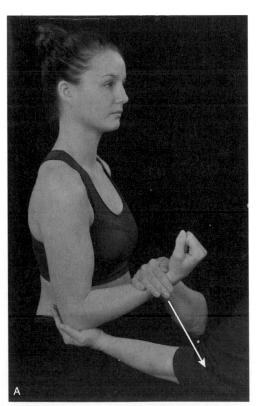 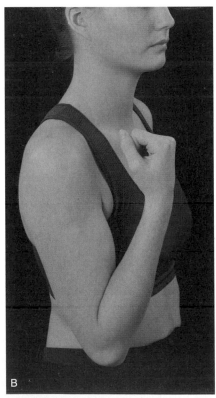

Fig. 8.7 (A) Elbow flexion manual muscle testing. (B) Elbow flexion. (From Pendelton HM, Schultz-Krohn W: Pedretti's Occupational Therapy, ed 8, 2018, Elsevier, St. Louis.)

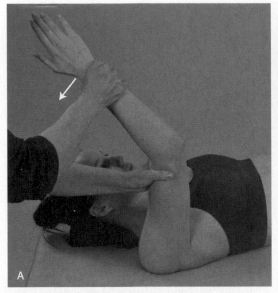
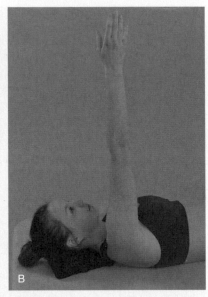

Fig. 8.8 (A) Elbow extension manual muscle testing (supine). (B) Elbow extension (supine).

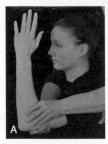
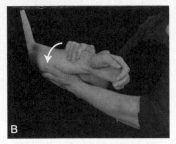
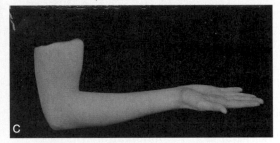

Fig. 8.9 (A) Forearm supination (Alternate position). (B) Forearm supination (Manual muscle testing). (C) Forearm supination.

Motion: Forearm Supination (Fig. 8.9).

Muscles (Hislop & Montgomery, 2002)	Innervation (Hislop & Montgomery, 2002)
Biceps brachii	Musculocutaneous n., C5, C6
Supinator	Radial n., C6

Position: S seated with humerus adducted, elbow flexed to 90 degrees, and forearm in full pronation. E stands next to S on the side being tested (Hislop & Montgomery, 2002).

Stabilize: Humerus just proximal to elbow.

Palpate: Over supinator on dorsolateral aspect of forearm, below head of radius. Muscle can be best felt when radial muscle group (extensor carpi radialis and brachioradialis) is pushed up and out of the way (Rybski, 2012). E may also palpate biceps on middle of anterior surface of humerus.

Observe: Supination, turning hand up. Gravity may assist the movement after the 0-degree neutral position is passed.

Resist: By grasping around dorsal aspect of distal forearm with fingers and heel of hand, turning arm toward pronation.

Motion: Forearm Pronation (Fig. 8.10).

Muscles (Hislop & Montgomery, 2002)	Innervation (Hislop & Montgomery, 2002)
Pronator teres	Median n., C6
Pronator quadratus	Median n., C8, T1

Position: S seated with humerus adducted, elbow flexed to 90 degrees, and forearm in full supination. E stands beside S on the side being tested (Hislop & Montgomery, 2002).

Stabilize: Humerus just proximal to elbow to prevent shoulder abduction (Hislop & Montgomery, 2002; Kaskutas, 2019).

Palpate: Pronator teres on upper part of volar surface of forearm, medial to biceps tendon and diagonally from medial condyle of humerus to lateral border of radius (Hislop & Montgomery, 2002; Kaskutas, 2019; Kendall et al., 2005).

Observe: Pronation, turning hand palm down.

Resist: By grasping around dorsal aspect of distal forearm with fingers and heel of hand, turning arm toward supination (Hislop & Montgomery, 2002).

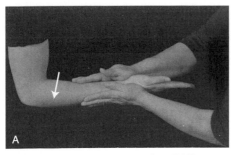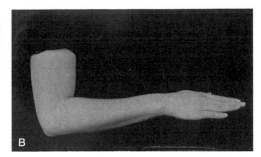

Fig. 8.10 (A) Forearm pronation manual muscle testing. (B) Forearm pronation.

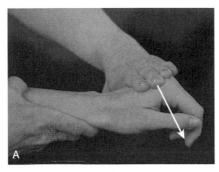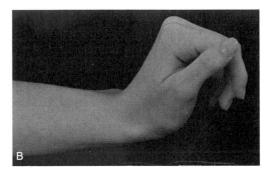

Fig. 8.11 (A) Wrist extension manual muscle testing. (B) Wrist extension.

Motion: Wrist Extension (Fig. 8.11).

Muscles (Hislop & Montgomery, 2002)	Innervation (Hislop & Montgomery, 2002)
Extensor carpi radialis longus	Radial n., C6, C7
Extensor carpi radialis brevis	Deep branch of radial n., C7, C8
Extensor carpi ulnaris	Posterior interosseous branch of radial n., C7, C8

Position: S seated or supine with forearm resting on supporting surface in pronation, wrist in neutral position, and fingers and thumb relaxed. E sits opposite S or next to S on the side being tested (Kendall et al., 2005; Killingsworth, 1976).

Stabilize: Over volar aspect of middle to distal forearm (Kendall et al., 2005; Killingsworth, 1976).

Palpate: Extensor carpi radialis longus and brevis tendons on dorsal aspect of wrist at bases of second and third metacarpals, respectively (Hislop & Montgomery, 2002; Kendall et al., 2005). Tendon of extensor carpi ulnaris may be palpated at base of fifth metacarpal, just distal to head of ulna (Hislop & Montgomery, 2002; Kendall et al., 2005; Rybski, 2012).

Observe: Wrist extension, lifting hand up from supporting surface. Movement should be performed without finger extension, which could substitute for wrist motion (Hislop & Montgomery, 2002; Kendall et al., 2005).

Resist: Over dorsum distal metacarpals toward flexion.

Motion: Wrist Flexion (Fig. 8.12).

Muscles (Kaskutas, 2019)	Innervation (Hislop & Montgomery, 2002; Kaskutas, 2019; Pact et al., 1984)
Flexor carpi radialis	Median n., C6–C8
Flexor carpi ulnaris	Ulnar n., C7–T1
Palmaris longus	Median n., C7–T1

Position: S seated or supine with forearm resting in almost full supination on supporting surface and fingers and thumb relaxed. E sits next to S on the side being tested.

Stabilize: Over volar aspect of midforearm (Hislop & Montgomery, 2002; Kaskutas, 2019).

Palpate: Muscle tendons. Flexor carpi radialis tendon can be palpated over wrist at base of second metacarpal bone. Palmaris longus tendon is at center of wrist at base of third metacarpal, and flexor carpi ulnaris tendon can be palpated at ulnar side of volar aspect of wrist at base of fifth metacarpal (Rybski, 2012).

Observe: S brings hand up from supporting surface toward face. E should observe that fingers remain relaxed during movement.

Resist: Over distal volar palm toward extension.

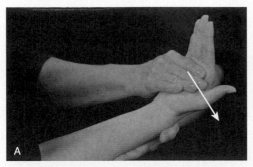
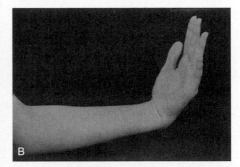

Fig. 8.12 (A) Wrist flexion manual muscle testing. (B) Wrist flexion.

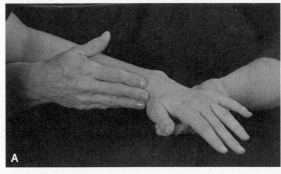
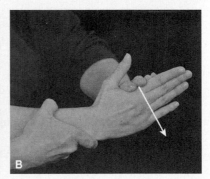

Fig. 8.13 (A) Wrist radial deviation palpation point. (B) Wrist radial deviation manual muscle testing.

Motion: Wrist Radial Deviation (Fig. 8.13).

Muscles (Kaskutas, 2019)	Innervations (Kaskutas, 2019)
Flexor carpi radialis	Median nerve, C6–C8
Extensor carpi radialis longus	Radial nerve, C6, C7
Extensor carpi radialis brevis	Deep branch of radial nerve, C7, C8

Position: S is seated with forearm in neutral rotation with wrist in slight extension and thumb pointing superiorly (Kaskutas, 2019). Fingers should be extended.
Stabilize: Radially over distal second metacarpal.
Palpate: Extensor carpi radialis brevis and longus and flexor carpi ulnaris.
Observe: S moves wrist toward the thumb (Kaskutas, 2019).
Resist: Apply pressure radially over distal second metacarpal (Kaskutas, 2019).

Motion: Wrist Ulnar Deviation (Fig. 8.14).

Muscles (Kaskutas, 2019)	Innervations (Kaskutas, 2019)
Flexor carpi ulnaris	Ulnar nerve, C7–T1
Extensor ulnaris	Posterior interosseous nerve of radial nerve, C7, C8

Position: S is seated with forearm in neutral rotation with wrist in slight extension and thumb pointing superiorly (Kaskutas, 2019). Fingers should be extended.

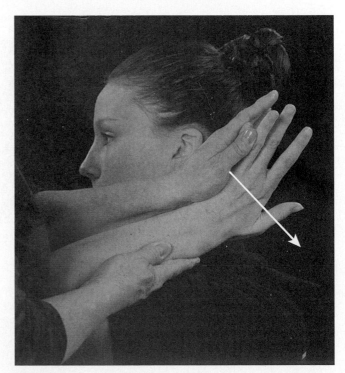

Fig. 8.14 Wrist ulnar deviation.

Stabilize: Radially over distal second metacarpal.
Palpate: Extensor carpi radialis brevis and longus and flexor carpi ulnaris.
Observe: S moves wrist toward the thumb (Kaskutas, 2019).

Resist: Apply pressure radially over distal second metacarpal (Kaskutas, 2019).

Motion: Metacarpophalangeal (MP) Flexion With Interphalangeal (IP) Extension (Fig. 8.15).

Muscles (Basmajian, 1985; Rybski, 2012)	Innervation (Hislop & Montgomery, 2002)
Lumbricales manus 1 and 2	Median n., C6, C7
Lumbricales manus 3 and 4	Ulnar n., C8, T1
Interossei dorsales manus	Ulnar n., C8, T1
Interossei palmares	Ulnar n., C8, T1

Position: S is seated with forearm in supination resting on supporting surface and wrist in neutral position (Hislop & Montgomery, 2002). MP joints are extended, and IP joints flexed (Rybski, 2012). E sits next to S on the side being tested.

Stabilize: Over palm to prevent wrist motion.

Palpate: First interosseus dorsales just medial to distal aspect of second metacarpal on dorsum of hand. The rest of these muscles are not easily palpable because of their size and deep location in hand.

Observe: S flexes MP joints and extends IP joints simultaneously (Kaskutas, 2019).

Resist: Each finger separately by grasping distal phalanx and pushing downward on finger into supporting surface toward MP extension and IP flexion, or apply pressure first against dorsal surface of middle and distal phalanges toward flexion, followed by pressure to volar surface of proximal phalanges toward extension (Kaskutas, 2019).

Motion: MP Extension (Fig. 8.16).

Muscles (Hislop & Montgomery, 2002; Kaskutas, 2019; Kendall et al., 2005)	Innervation (Hislop & Montgomery, 2002)
Extensor digitorum	Radial n., C6–C8
Extensor indicis	Radial n., C6–C8
Extensor digiti minimi	Radial n., C6–C8

Position: S seated with forearm pronated and wrist in neutral position, with MP and IP joints partially flexed (Hislop & Montgomery, 2002). E sits opposite or next to S on the side being tested.

Stabilize: Wrist and metacarpals slightly above supporting surface (Hislop & Montgomery, 2002; Kaskutas, 2019).

Palpate: Extensor digitorum tendons where they course over dorsum of hand (Hislop & Montgomery, 2002). In some people, extensor digiti minimi tendon can be palpated or visualized just lateral to extensor digitorum tendon to fifth finger. Extensor indicis tendon can be palpated or visualized just medial to extensor digitorum tendon to first finger.

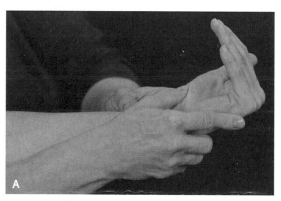 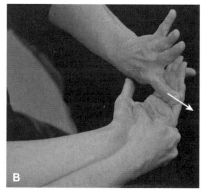

Fig. 8.15 Metacarpophalangeal (MP) flexion with interphalangeal (IP) extension. (A) Movement. (B) Manual muscle testing.

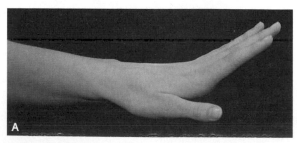 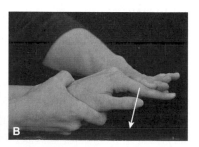

Fig. 8.16 (A) MP extension. (B) MP extension manual muscle testing.

Observe: S raises fingers away from supporting surface, extending MP joints but maintaining IP joints in some flexion.

Resist: Each finger individually over dorsal aspect of proximal phalanx toward MP flexion (Hislop & Montgomery, 2002; Kaskutas, 2019).

Motion: Proximal Interphalangeal (PIP) Flexion, Second Through Fifth Fingers (Fig. 8.17).

Muscle (Hislop & Montgomery, 2002; Kendall et al., 2005)	Innervation (Hislop & Montgomery, 2002; Kendall et al., 2005)
Flexor digitorum superficialis	Median n., C7, C8, T1

Position: S seated with forearm in supination, wrist in neutral position, fingers extended, and hand and forearm resting on dorsal surface (Hislop & Montgomery, 2002). E sits opposite or next to S on the side being tested.

Stabilize: MP joint and proximal phalanx of finger being tested (Hislop & Montgomery, 2002; Kaskutas, 2019).

Palpate: Flexor digitorum superficialis tendon on volar surface of proximal phalanx. A stabilizing finger may be used to palpate in this procedure (Kendall et al., 2005). Tendon supplying fourth finger may be palpated over volar aspect of wrist between flexor carpi ulnaris and palmaris longus tendons, if desired (Rybski, 2012).

Observe: S flexes PIP joint while maintaining distal interphalangeal (DIP) joint in extension. If isolating PIP flexion is difficult, all fingers not being tested are held in MP hyperextension and PIP extension by pulling back over IP joints. This maneuver inactivates flexor digitorum profundus (FDP) so that S cannot flex distal joint (Rancho Los Amigos Hospital, 1978; Rybski, 2012). Most individuals cannot perform isolated action of PIP joint of fifth finger even with assistance.

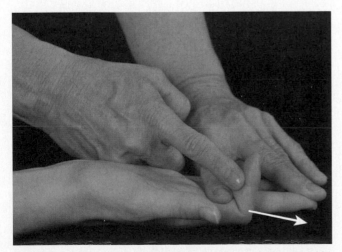

Fig. 8.17 Proximal interphalangeal (PIP) flexion, second through fifth fingers.

Resist: With one finger at volar aspect of middle phalanx toward extension (Hislop & Montgomery, 2002; Kaskutas, 2019). If index finger is used to apply resistance, middle finger may be used to move DIP joint back and forth to verify that FDP is not substituting.

Motion: DIP Flexion, Second Through Fifth Fingers (Fig. 8.18).

Muscle (Hislop & Montgomery, 2002)	Innervation (Hislop & Montgomery, 2002)
Flexor digitorum profundus	Median n., ulnar n., C8, T1

Position: S seated with forearm in supination, wrist in neutral position, and fingers extended. E sits opposite or next to S on the side being tested (Hislop & Montgomery, 2002).

Stabilize: Wrist at neutral position and PIP joint and middle phalanx of finger being tested (Rancho Los Amigos Hospital, 1978).

Palpate: Finger stabilizing middle phalanx used to simultaneously palpate FDP tendon over volar surface of middle phalanx (Hislop & Montgomery, 2002; Kendall et al., 2005).

Observe: S brings fingertip up and away from supporting surface, flexing DIP joint.

Resist: With one finger at volar aspect of distal phalanx toward extension (Hislop & Montgomery, 2002; Kaskutas, 2019).

Motion: Finger Abduction (Fig. 8.19).

Muscles (Hislop & Montgomery, 2002)	Innervation (Hislop & Montgomery, 2002)
Interossei dorsales	Ulnar n., C8, T1
Abductor digiti minimi	Ulnar n., C8, T1

Position: S seated or supine with forearm pronated, wrist in neutral position, and fingers extended and adducted. E sits opposite or next to S on the side being tested (Hislop & Montgomery, 2002).

Stabilize: Wrist and metacarpals slightly above supporting surface.

Palpate: First interosseus dorsales on lateral aspect of second metacarpal or of abductor digiti minimi manus on ulnar border of fifth metacarpal (Hislop & Montgomery, 2002). Remaining interossei are not palpable.

Observe: S spreads fingers apart, abducting them at MP joints.

Resist: First, interosseus dorsales by applying pressure on radial side of distal end of proximal phalanx of second finger in an ulnar direction; second, interosseus dorsales on radial side of proximal phalanx of middle finger in an ulnar direction; third, interosseus dorsales on ulnar side of proximal phalanx of middle finger in a radial direction; fourth, interosseus dorsales on ulnar side of proximal phalanx of ring finger in a radial direction; finally, abductor

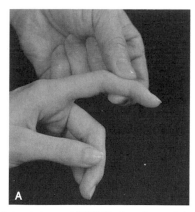
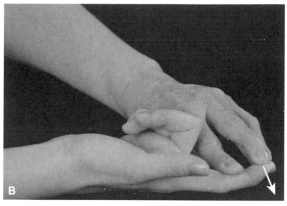

Fig. 8.18 (A) Distal Interphalangeal (DIP) Flexion, Second through Fifth Fingers. (B) DIP flexion manual muscle testing.

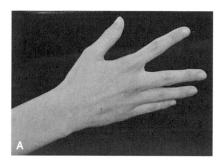
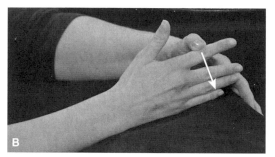

Fig. 8.19 (A) Finger abduction. (B) Finger abduction manual muscle testing.

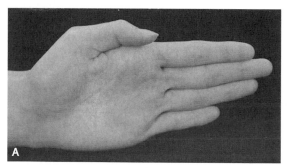
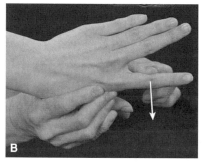

Fig. 8.20 Finger adduction A, B.

digiti minimi manus on ulnar side of proximal phalanx of little finger in a radial direction (Kaskutas, 2019).

Motion: Finger Adduction (Fig. 8.20).

Muscle (Hislop & Montgomery, 2002; Kaskutas, 2019)	Innervation (Hislop & Montgomery, 2002)
Interossei palmares	Ulnar n., C8, T1

Position: S seated with forearm pronated, wrist in neutral position, and fingers extended and abducted (Hislop & Montgomery, 2002).
Stabilize: Wrist and metacarpals slightly above supporting surface.
Palpate: Not palpable.

Observe: S adducts first, fourth, and fifth fingers toward middle finger.
Resist: Index finger at proximal phalanx by pulling in a radial direction, ring finger at proximal phalanx in an ulnar direction, and little finger likewise (Kaskutas, 2019). These muscles are small, and resistance must be modified to accommodate to their comparatively limited power.

Motion: Thumb MP Extension (Fig. 8.21).

Muscle (Hislop & Montgomery, 2002; Kaskutas, 2019)	Innervation (Hislop & Montgomery, 2002; Kaskutas, 2019)
Extensor pollicis brevis	Radial n., C6–C8

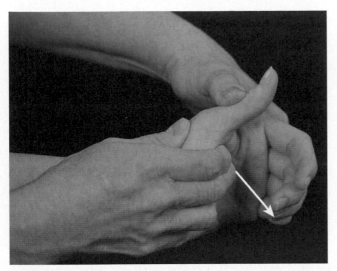

Fig. 8.21 Thumb MP extension.

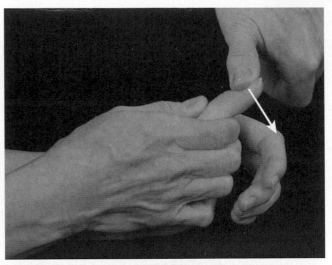

Fig. 8.22 Thumb IP extension.

Position: S seated or supine, forearm in midposition, wrist in neutral position, and hand and forearm resting on ulnar border (Hislop & Montgomery, 2002). Thumb is flexed into palm at MP joint, and IP joint is extended but relaxed. E sits opposite or next to S on the side being tested.

Stabilize: Wrist and thumb metacarpal.

Palpate: Extensor pollicis brevis (EPB) tendon at base of first metacarpal on dorsoradial aspect. The tendon lies just medial to abductor pollicis dorsoradial longus tendon on radial side of the anatomic snuffbox, which is a hollow space between extensor pollicis longus (EPL) and EPB tendons when thumb is fully extended and radially abducted (Rybski, 2012).

Observe: S extends MP joint. IP joint remains relaxed. Many people have difficulty isolating this motion.

Resist: On dorsal surface of proximal phalanx toward MP flexion (Hislop & Montgomery, 2002; Kaskutas, 2019).

Motion: Thumb IP Extension (Fig. 8.22).

Muscle (Hislop & Montgomery, 2002; Kaskutas, 2019; Kendall et al., 2005)	Innervation (Hislop & Montgomery, 2002; Kaskutas, 2019)
Extensor pollicis longus	Radial n., C6–C8

Position: S seated or supine, forearm in midposition, wrist in neutral position, and hand and forearm resting on ulnar border (Hislop & Montgomery, 2002). MP joint of thumb is extended or slightly flexed, and IP joint is flexed fully into palm. E sits opposite or next to S on the side being tested.

Stabilize: Wrist in neutral position, first metacarpal, and proximal phalanx of thumb.

Palpate: EPL tendon on dorsal surface of hand medial to EPB tendon, between head of first metacarpal and base of second metacarpal on ulnar side of anatomic snuffbox (Hislop & Montgomery, 2002; Rybski, 2012).

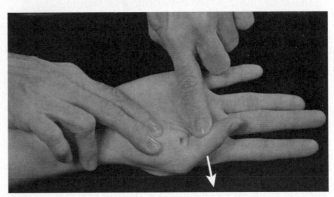

Fig. 8.23 Thumb MP flexion.

Observe: S brings tip of thumb up and out of palm, extending IP joint.

Resist: On dorsal surface of distal phalanx, down toward IP flexion (Hislop & Montgomery, 2002; Kaskutas, 2019).

Motion: Thumb MP Flexion (Fig. 8.23).

Muscle (Hislop & Montgomery, 2002; Kaskutas, 2019)	Innervation (Hislop & Montgomery, 2002; Kaskutas, 2019)
Flexor pollicis brevis	Median n., ulnar n., C6–C8, T1

Position: S seated or supine, forearm fully supinated, wrist in neutral position, and thumb in extension and adduction. E sits next or opposite to S (Hislop & Montgomery, 2002; Kaskutas, 2019).

Stabilize: First metacarpal and wrist.

Palpate: Over middle of palmar surface of thenar eminence just medial to abductor pollicis brevis (Hislop & Montgomery, 2002). Hand used to stabilize may also be used for palpation.

Observe: S flexes MP joint while maintaining extension of IP joint. Some individuals may be unable to isolate flexion to MP joint. In this case, both MP and IP flexion may be tested together as a gross test for thumb flexion strength and graded according to E's judgment.

Resist: On palmar surface of first phalanx toward MP extension (Hislop & Montgomery, 2002; Kaskutas, 2019).

Motion: Thumb IP Flexion (Fig. 8.24).

Muscle (Hislop & Montgomery, 2002; Kaskutas, 2019; Kendall et al., 2005)	Innervation (Kaskutas, 2019)
Flexor pollicis longus	Median n., C7, C8, T1

Position: S seated with forearm fully supinated, wrist in neutral position, and thumb in extension and adduction (Hislop & Montgomery, 2002). E sits next to or opposite from S.

Stabilize: First metacarpal and proximal phalanx of thumb in extension (Hislop & Montgomery, 2002; Kaskutas, 2019).

Palpate: Flexor pollicis longus tendon on palmar surface of proximal phalanx. In this case, palpating finger may be the same one used for stabilizing proximal phalanx.

Observe: S flexes IP joint in plane of palm (Hislop & Montgomery, 2002).

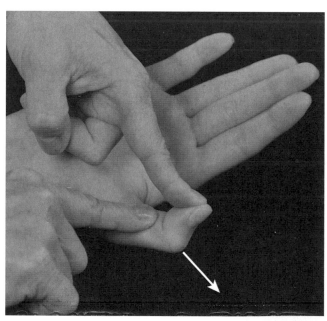

Fig. 8.24 Thumb IP flexion.

Resist: On palmar surface of distal phalanx toward IP extension (Hislop & Montgomery, 2002; Kaskutas, 2019).

Motion: Thumb Palmar Abduction (Fig. 8.25).

Muscle (Kaskutas, 2019; Kendall et al., 2005)	Innervation (Kaskutas, 2019)
Abductor pollicis brevis	Median n., C6–C8, T1

Position: S seated or supine, forearm in supination, wrist in neutral position, thumb extended and adducted, and carpometacarpal (CMC) joint rotated so that thumb is resting in a plane perpendicular to palm. E sits opposite or next to S on the side being tested (Hislop & Montgomery, 2002; Kaskutas, 2019).

Stabilize: Metacarpals and wrist.

Palpate: Abductor pollicis brevis on lateral aspect of thenar eminence, lateral to flexor pollicis brevis (Hislop & Montgomery, 2002).

Observe: S raises thumb away from palm in a plane perpendicular to palm (Kaskutas, 2019).

Resist: At lateral aspect of proximal phalanx, downward toward adduction (Kaskutas, 2019).

Motion: Thumb Radial Abduction (Fig. 8.26).

Muscle (Kaskutas, 2019)	Innervation (Kaskutas, 2019)
Abductor pollicis longus	Radial n., C6–C8

Position: S seated or supine, forearm in neutral rotation, wrist in neutral position, and thumb adducted and slightly flexed across palm. Hand and forearm are resting on ulnar border (Kaskutas, 2019). E sits opposite or next to S on the side being tested.

Stabilize: Wrist and metacarpals of fingers (Hislop & Montgomery, 2002; Kaskutas, 2019).

Palpate: Abductor pollicis longus tendon on lateral aspect of base of first metacarpal. The tendon is immediately lateral (radial) to extensor pollicis brevis tendon (Hislop & Montgomery, 2002; Rybski, 2012).

Observe: S moves thumb out of palm of hand, abducting in the plane of palm.

Resist: At lateral aspect of distal end of first metacarpal toward adduction (Hislop & Montgomery, 2002; Kaskutas, 2019).

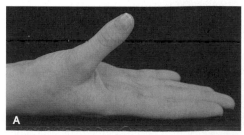
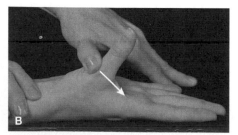

Fig. 8.25 (A) Thumb palmar abduction. (B) Manual muscle test for thumb palmar abduction.

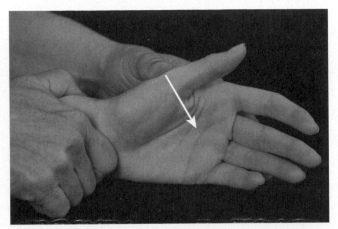

Fig. 8.26 Thumb radial abduction.

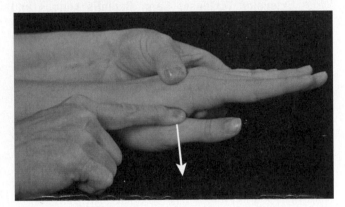

Fig. 8.27 Thumb adduction.

Motion: Thumb Adduction (Fig. 8.27).

Muscle (Hislop & Montgomery, 2002; Kaskutas, 2019)	Innervation (Hislop & Montgomery, 2002; Kaskutas, 2019)
Adductor pollicis	Ulnar n., C8, T1

Position: S seated or supine, forearm pronated, wrist in neutral position, and thumb opposed and abducted (Hislop & Montgomery, 2002; Rancho Los Amigos Hospital, 1978). E sits opposite or next to S on the side being tested.

Stabilize: Wrist and metacarpals, supporting hand slightly above resting surface (Hislop & Montgomery, 2002).

Palpate: Adductor pollicis on palmar side of thumb web space (Kendall et al., 2005).

Observe: S brings thumb up to touch palm (Hislop & Montgomery, 2002).

Resist: By grasping proximal phalanx of thumb near metacarpal head and pulling downward, toward abduction (Hislop & Montgomery, 2002).

Motion: Opposition of Thumb to Fifth Finger (Fig. 8.28).

Muscle (Hislop & Montgomery, 2002; Kaskutas, 2019)	Innervation (Hislop & Montgomery, 2002; Kaskutas, 2019)
Opponens pollicis	Median n., C6–C8, T1
Opponens digiti minimi	Ulnar n., C8, T1

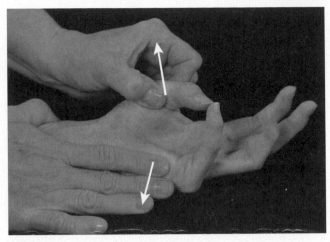

Fig. 8.28 Opposition of thumb to fifth finger.

Position: S seated or supine, forearm in full supination, wrist in neutral position, and thumb and fifth finger extended and adducted (Hislop & Montgomery, 2002; Kaskutas, 2019). E sits on the side being tested.

Stabilize: Forearm and wrist.

Palpate: Opponens pollicis along radial side of shaft of first metacarpal, lateral to abductor pollicis brevis. Opponens digiti minimi cannot be easily palpated (Hislop & Montgomery, 2002; Kendall et al., 2005).

Observe: S brings thumb out across palm to touch thumb pad to pad of fifth finger.

Resist: At distal ends of first and fifth metacarpals, exerting pressure toward, separating, and rolling away these bones and flattening palm of hand (Hislop & Montgomery, 2002).

FUNCTIONAL MUSCLE TESTING

The functional muscle test is a useful tool when screening muscles for normal strength (Hislop & Montgomery, 2002; Landen & Amizich, 1963). OTs and OTAs use functional muscle testing when specific muscle testing is the responsibility of the physical therapy service, or when the focus of the intervention plan is on functional movement only. The functional muscle test assesses the general strength and motion capabilities of the patient. The following functional muscle test should be performed while the subject is comfortably seated in a sturdy chair or wheelchair. The subject is asked to perform the test motion against gravity. The subject may perform the motion in the gravity-decreased position if the former is not feasible.

In all of the tests, the subject is allowed to complete the test motion before the examiner applies resistance. The resistance is applied at the end of the ROM while the subject maintains the position and resists the force applied by the examiner. The examiner may make modifications in positioning to suit individual needs. As in the manual muscle tests, the examiner should stabilize proximal parts and attempt to rule out substitutions. The reader should be familiar with joint motions, their prime movers, manual muscle testing, and muscle grades before performing this test. The OTA must establish service competency to ensure accurate and safe testing.

Functional Muscle Test Procedures

Shoulder Flexion (Anterior Deltoid and Coracobrachialis). With S's shoulder flexed to 90 degrees and elbow flexed or extended, E pushes down on arm proximal to elbow into extension.

Shoulder Extension (Latissimus Dorsi and Teres Major). S moves shoulder into full extension. E pushes from behind at a point proximal to elbow into flexion.

Shoulder Abduction (Middle Deltoid and Supraspinatus). S abducts shoulder to 90 degrees with elbow flexed or extended. E pushes down on arm just proximal to elbow into adduction.

Shoulder Horizontal Adduction (Pectoralis Major, Anterior Deltoid). S crosses arms in front of chest. E reaches from behind and attempts to pull arms back into horizontal abduction at a point just proximal to elbow.

Shoulder Horizontal Abduction (Posterior Deltoid, Teres Minor, Infraspinatus). S moves arms from full horizontal adduction as just described to full horizontal abduction. E pushes forward on arms just proximal to elbow into horizontal adduction.

Shoulder External Rotation (Infraspinatus and Teres Minor). S holds arm in 90 degrees of shoulder abduction and 90 degrees of elbow flexion, then externally rotates shoulder through available ROM. E supports or stabilizes upper arm proximal to elbow; at the same time, E pushes from behind at dorsal aspect of wrist into internal rotation.

Shoulder Internal Rotation (Subscapularis, Teres Major, Latissimus Dorsi, Pectoralis Major). S begins with arm as described for external rotation (90 degrees of shoulder abduction and 90 degrees of elbow flexion) but performs internal rotation. E supports or stabilizes upper arm as before and pulls up into external rotation at volar aspect of wrist.

Elbow Flexion (Biceps, Brachialis). With forearm supinated, S flexes elbow from full extension. E sits opposite subject and stabilizes upper arm against trunk while attempting to pull forearm into extension at volar aspect of wrist.

Elbow Extension (Triceps). With S's upper arm supported in 90 degrees of abduction (gravity-decreased position) or 160-degree shoulder flexion (against gravity position), elbow is extended from full flexion. E pushes forearm into flexion at dorsal aspect of wrist.

Forearm Supination (Biceps, Supinator). S or E stabilizes upper arm against trunk. Elbow is flexed to 90 degrees, and forearm is in full pronation. S supinates forearm. E grasps distal forearm and attempts to rotate into pronation.

Forearm Pronation (Pronator Teres, Pronator Quadratus). S is positioned as described for forearm supination except that forearm is in full supination. S pronates forearm. E grasps distal forearm and attempts to rotate into supination.

Wrist Flexion (Flexor Carpi Radialis, Flexor Carpi Ulnaris, Palmaris Longus). S's forearm is supported on the dorsal surface on a tabletop or armrest. Hand is moved up from tabletop, using wrist flexion. E is seated next to or opposite S and pushes on palm of hand, giving equal pressure on radial and ulnar sides into wrist extension or down toward tabletop.

Wrist Extension (Extensor Carpi Radialis Longus and Brevis, Extensor Carpi Ulnaris). S's forearm is supported on a tabletop or armrest and rests on the volar surface. Hand is lifted from tabletop by wrist extension. E sits next to or opposite S and pushes on dorsal aspect of palm, giving equal pressure at radial and ulnar sides into wrist flexion or down toward tabletop.

Finger MP Flexion and IP Extension (Lumbricales and Interossei). With forearm and hand supported on tabletop on dorsal surface, E stabilizes palm and S flexes MP joints while maintaining extension of IP joints. E pushes into extension with index finger across proximal phalanges or pushes on tip of each finger into IP flexion and MP extension.

Finger IP Flexion (Flexors Digitorum Profundus and Sublimis). S is positioned as described for MP flexion. IP joints are flexed while maintaining extension of MP joints. E attempts to pull fingers back into extension by hooking fingertips with those of S.

Finger MP Extension (IP Joints Flexed) (Extensor Digitorum Communis, Extensor Indicis Proprius, Extensor Digiti Minimi). S's forearm and hand are supported on a table surface, resting on ulnar border. Wrist is stabilized by E in 0-degree neutral position. S moves MP joints from flexion to full extension (hyperextension) while keeping IP joints flexed. E pushes fingers at PIP joints simultaneously into flexion.

Finger Abduction (Dorsal Interossei, Abductor Digiti Minimi). S's forearm is resting on volar surface on a table. E may stabilize wrist in slight extension so that the hand is raised slightly off supporting surface. S abducts fingers. E pushes two fingers at a time together at the proximal phalanges into adduction. First, index finger and middle fingers are pushed together. Then ring finger and middle fingers and finally little finger and ring fingers do the same. Resistance is modified to accommodate small muscles.

Finger Adduction (Palmar Interossei). S is positioned as described for finger abduction. Fingers are adducted tightly. E attempts to pull fingers apart one at a time at the proximal phalanges. First, index finger is pulled away from middle finger. Then ring finger is pulled away from middle finger, and finally little finger is pulled away from ring finger. In normal hand, adducted finger snaps back into adducted position when E pulls into abduction and quickly lets go. An alternate method is for E to place index finger between two of S's fingers and ask S to adduct against E's finger.

Thumb MP and IP Flexion (Flexor Pollicis Brevis and Flexor Pollicis Longus). S's forearm should be supported on a firm surface, with elbow flexed at 90 degrees and forearm in 45-degree supination. Thumb is flexed across palm. E pulls on tip of thumb into extension.

Thumb MP and IP Extension (Extensor Pollicis Brevis and Extensor Pollicis Longus). S is positioned as for thumb MP and IP flexion. Thumb is extended away from palm. E pushes on tip of thumb into flexion.

Thumb Palmar Abduction (Abductor Pollicis Longus and Abductor Pollicis Brevis). S is positioned as described for thumb flexion and extension. Thumb is abducted away from palm in a plane perpendicular to palm. S resists movement at metacarpal head into adduction.

Thumb Adduction (Adductor Pollicis). S is positioned as for all other thumb movements. Thumb is adducted to palm. E attempts to pull thumb into abduction at metacarpal head or proximal phalanx.

Opposition of Thumb to Fifth Finger (Opponens Pollicis, Opponens Digiti Minimi). S is positioned with elbow flexed to 90 degrees and dorsal surface of forearm and hand resting on a flat surface such as a tabletop or armrest. Thumb is opposed to fifth finger, making pad-to-pad contact. E attempts to pull fingers apart, applying force at metacarpal heads of both fingers.

SUMMARY

Evaluation of muscle strength contributes to the functional assessment of patients with many different physical disorders. Muscle strength is necessary to maintain body posture and to perform activities when gravity or other resistance is a factor. Evaluation of muscle strength objectively documents the physiologic and functional changes in the musculoskeletal system. Functional muscle testing is an important evaluation tool for patients with lower motor neuron dysfunction, orthopedic conditions, and muscle diseases. The role of the OTA in evaluating muscle strength must start with proven service competency and is determined by the supervising OT in accordance with practice regulations of the state and the treatment setting.

REVIEW QUESTIONS

1. List two medical conditions in which testing of muscle strength would be appropriate.
2. Define endurance; discuss the relationship of endurance to muscle testing.
3. What is the difference between spasticity and normal muscle strength?
4. Compare and contrast MMT and functional muscle testing.
5. Explain why specific positioning is used for testing of specific muscle groups.
6. How does gravity affect the tested strength of a muscle?
7. If joint range is limited, how can strength be tested, and how would this limitation be recorded?
8. Define each of these muscle grades: N (5), G (4), F (3), P (2), T (1), and zero (0).
9. Describe how muscle fatigue, pain, and muscle spasm may affect testing of muscle strength.
10. Explain the importance of knowing the patient's PROM before muscle testing.

EXERCISE

Demonstrate the muscle testing procedures for the following muscle groups: shoulder flexion, extension, abduction, external rotation, and internal rotation; elbow flexion and extension; forearm supination and pronation; and wrist flexion and extension.

REFERENCES

Basmajian, J.F. (1985). *Muscles Alive* (5th ed.). Baltimore, MD: Lippincott Williams & Wilkins.

Brunnstrom, S. (1992). *Movement Therapy in Hemiplegia*. New York, NY: Harper & Row.

Davis, P.M. (1994). *Steps to Follow: A Guide to the Treatment of Adult Hemiplegia*. Berlin: Springer-Verlag.

Hislop, H., & Montgomery J. (2002). *Daniels and Worthingham's Muscle Testing: Techniques of Manual Examination* (7th ed.). Philadelphia, PA: Saunders.

Kaskutas, V. (2019). Evaluation of muscle strength. In H. McHugh Pendleton, & W. Schultz-Krohn (eds.), *Pedretti's Occupational Therapy: Practice Skills for Physical Dysfunction* (8th ed., pp. 155–229). St. Louis, MO: Elsevier.

Kendall, F.P., McCreary, E.K., Provance, P.G., Rodgers, M., Romani, W. (2005). *Muscles: Testing and Function* (5th ed.). Baltimore, MD: Lippincott Williams & Wilkins.

Killingsworth, A. (1976). *Basic Physical Disability Procedures*. San Jose, CA: Maple.

Landen, B., & Amizich, A. (1963). Functional muscle examination and gait analysis. *Journal of the American Physical Therapy Association*, 43, 39.

Pact, V, Sirotkin-Roses, M, Beatus, J. (1984). *The Muscle Testing Handbook*. Boston: Little, Brown.

Rancho Los Amigos Hospital. (1978). Department of Occupational Therapy. *Guide for Muscle Testing of the Upper Extremity*.

Downey, CA: Professional Staff Association of Rancho Los Amigos Hospital.

Rybski, M. F. (2012). *Kinesiology for Occupational Therapy* (2nd ed.). Thorofare, NJ: Slack.

RECOMMENDED READING

American Occupational Therapy Association. (2014). *Occupational Therapy Practice Framework: Domain and Process* (3rd ed.). Bethesda, MD: AOTA.

9

Evaluation and Observation of Deficits in Sensation, Perception, and Cognition

Christopher Delenick

OBJECTIVES

After reading this chapter, the student or the occupational therapy practitioner will be able to do the following:

- Recognize the supporting role of the occupational therapy assistant in the occupational therapist's evaluation of sensation, perception, and cognition.
- Define and describe various functions and deficits in the sensory, perceptual, and cognitive systems.

- Recognize the tests and evaluation principles related to sensory, perceptual, and cognitive dysfunction.
- Describe the interrelationships among sensory, perceptual, and cognitive functions in the performance of everyday activities.

KEY TERMS

Sensation
Feedback
Thermal
Pain
Olfactory
Gustatory
Proprioception
Perception
Stereognosis
Astereognosis
Graphesthesia
Agraphesthesia
Body scheme
Asomatognosia
Praxis

Apraxia
Ideomotor apraxia
Constructional apraxia
Dressing apraxia
Cognition
Orientation
Attention
Memory
Executive functioning
Abstract thinking
Concrete thinking
Problem solving
Reasoning
Insight
Dyscalculia

INTRODUCTION

The evaluation and observation of perception, sensation, and cognition are key components of occupational therapy practice and are best evaluated and observed within the context of occupation. The official documents of the American Occupational Therapy Association (AOTA) such as Vision 2025 (American Occupational Therapy Association, 2017), AOTA's Choosing Wisely campaign (American Occupational Therapy Association, 2013), and a statement paper on cognition and occupation (American Occupational Therapy Association, 2010) strongly support this. Occupational therapists (OTs) and occupational therapy assistants (OTAs) assist clients to engage in meaningful occupation, and the use of occupation as a means to evaluate and observe the client factors of sensation, perception, and cognition is of paramount importance. Clients with physical

dysfunction may experience performance limitations in the occupations of activities of daily living (ADL), instrumental activities of daily living (IADL), rest/sleep, education, work, play, leisure, and social participation. These limitations represent the clients' inability to balance the performance skills, performance patterns, context, activity demands, and client factors to successfully participate in the desired areas of occupation (American Occupational Therapy Association, 2014).

A client with a physical dysfunction who is performing a task such as donning a shirt may have difficulty for reasons as varied as lack of sensation in the arm, neglect of body parts because of perceptual impairment, or an inability to understand the nature of the task. Each reason suggests dysfunction in a different client factor (sensation, perception, and cognition). Identification and treatment of impaired client factors are often necessary for the client to successfully engage in any occupation. A second purpose is to present a brief discussion of some of the assessments that the OT might perform. This chapter considers client factors in the areas of sensation, perception, and cognition.

The OT is primarily responsible for the evaluation of the client. The OTA may assist the OT in gathering the occupational profile and some of the assessments of client factors in areas of demonstrated competency and expertise. The complexity of the client factors related to sensation, perception, and cognition requires supervision and advanced training for both OTs and OTAs with limited experience in this area. The OTA with practice experience, advanced skills, and the opportunity to contribute to this assessment procedure should work closely with the supervising OT.

The OTA will likely observe many of the deficits discussed in this chapter when working with clients engaging in daily occupations. They are often apparent as the complexity of everyday tasks are attempted. Observations should be reported to the OT and the health care team as they are invaluable as evidence of the client's current level of function.

SENSATION

The somatosensory system provides a client the ability to perceive light touch, deep pressure, pain, temperature, taste, smell, and proprioception (Box 9.1). The somatosensory system provides essential information to allow safe and efficient task completion during daily occupations, such as brushing teeth, when the following factors come into play:

- The sense of touch allows the person to feel the toothbrush.
- Deep pressure helps the person grip the toothbrush.
- Pain alerts the person to avoid brushing a sensitive area in the mouth.
- Proprioception guides the joints of the arm and hand to complete the motion of brushing.
- Temperature sense lets the person determine if the water is at a desired temperature for rinsing the mouth.

The somatosensory system is controlled by peripheral receptors in the skin (and other sense organs). Proprioceptive receptors are located in muscles, tendons, and joint capsules. All sensory information is processed through the spinal cord

and brain. Completing the task of brushing teeth uses this entire system. Some sensations may produce a motor response before the brain even registers them. For example, the withdrawal of the hand from a hot object is driven by an automatic motor response or reflex before the object is perceived (by the brain) as being hot (Gilroy & Meyer, 1975).

Sensation and Motor Performance

Sensation is the primary means by which the body can learn about the external world and plays an important role in the control of movement. It also refers to the ability to identify the sensory modality (touch, deep pressure, pain, proprioception, and thermal sensation), its intensity, and its location. It provides **feedback** to the brain.

Sensory stimulation activates reflexive movement and plays a vital role in modulating and controlling movements (Pedretti & Early, 2001). During a motor act, a person receives sensory feedback about the effectiveness of the motion through the various sensory systems. Sensations derived from the ongoing movement are sent back to the central nervous system (CNS), where a comparison between intended action and what is actually happening is made. Consider, for example, the act of writing. If the wrong word is used or if misspelling occurs by a client without sensory impairment, visual and proprioceptive feedback signals that a motor error has occurred. The CNS processes this sensory feedback and revises the motor response, which is then carried out as the problem is corrected. See Chapter 10 for an in-depth discussion of the role of feedback and feedforward in motor control and motor learning principles.

Clients with impaired sensation have deficits in both feedback and feedforward control. Those with proprioceptive dysfunction cannot sense position and motion of joints; those with tactile dysfunction cannot sense contact with objects. Motor performance, based in part on the function of these systems, is deficient due to proprioceptive and tactile dysfunction. Vision can compensate somewhat for the loss of tactile and proprioceptive sensation. See Chapters 21 through 27 for specific deficits in sensation, perception, and motor control.

Sensory Evaluation

OTs, with input from OTAs, evaluate sensation to discern if it is adequate for the successful engagement in an occupation such as ADL (Boone & Landes, 1968; Harrell et al., 1992). They do this with the awareness the clients experiencing CNS dysfunction tend to experience sensory dysfunction over generalized areas, whereas those with peripheral nervous system (PNS) disorders tend to experience sensory dysfunction in more localized areas. These include spinal cord injury, brain injury, fractures, burns (in which sensory receptors in the skin are destroyed), arthritis (in which joint swelling may cause compression of a peripheral nerve), and traumatic hand injuries (in which skin, muscles, tendons, ligaments, and nerves may be involved). See Chapters 23 through 30. Box 9.2 lists the purposes of sensory testing.

BOX 9.1   Sensory Terms

Tactile: Referring to sensation received through the skin or hair receptors.

Deep pressure: Tactile sensation of force applied to the skin, as in the feeling of the ischial tuberosities pressing into a chair seat.

Pain: Unpleasant or noxious tactile sensation.

Thermal sensation: Tactile sensation of heat or cold.

Proprioception: Information about joint position and motion conveyed at an unconscious level from receptors in the muscles, joints, ligaments, and bone.

Sensory Supply to Specific Areas. Fig. 9.1 illustrates the sensory distribution of the major peripheral nerves of the body and limbs. The peripheral nerves (e.g., ulnar nerve) lie outside the CNS. When performing sensory tests for peripheral nerve dysfunction, the therapist focuses on the area(s) supplied by the nerve(s) affected.

Fig. 9.1 also shows the segmental or radicular distribution of nerve roots from the spinal cord. Each nerve root that exits from the spinal cord shows a specific area of sensory distribution known as a dermatome. When testing clients with spinal cord injury or disease, the therapist follows this dermatomal distribution. This procedure can help to determine the level(s) of spinal cord lesion and to detect any spared spinal cord function.

Results of the sensory evaluation indicate whether the client should be taught to protect against injury and to use compensatory techniques such as visual guidance when engaging in occupations. Results may also indicate whether a sensory retraining program is feasible.

Sensory loss may affect the use of splints or positioning equipment such as seat cushions and braces because the client may be unaware of pressure points during use and thus be at higher risk for skin breakdown. Sensory loss may also affect controlled use of a dynamic splint, which requires relatively intact sensory feedback for effective operation.

Sensory testing is subjective as the results depend heavily on the client's accurate and cooperative responses to the procedures (Gilroy & Meyer, 1975). Therefore it is important to evaluate both occupational performance and sensory functioning through task-based or occupation-based assessments, which may provide more reliable data. OTs and OTAs should observe the client for spontaneous use of the affected body part(s) during occupations, which can identify behavioral indicators of sensory deficits such as failure to protect self from injury.

Sensory Functions

Light Touch and Pressure Sensation. The ability to perceive light touch is critical to the performance of many occupations. It is needed to recognize an object in your hand and to feel if your clothes are correctly adjusted. Light touch perception is necessary for fine discriminative activities. Pressure sensation is important to occupational performance because it occurs continuously in activities such as sitting, pushing drawers and doors, crossing the knees, wearing belts and collars, and many other activities that stimulate pressure receptors. It is a protective sensation because it warns of deep or repetitive pressure that can lead to injury (Boone & Landes, 1968; Harrell et al., 1992). Pressure receptors are in subcutaneous and deeper tissue, while light touch receptors are in the superficial layers of the skin. Therefore deficits in one may not mean a deficit in both. If touch sensation is impaired, pressure sensation may assist during engagement in occupation by potentially substituting for touch feedback. Table 9.1 lists some tests for various sensory functions.

Temperature Sense. **Thermal** sensation or temperature sense is also protective and necessary to prevent injury in many ADL such as bathing, cooking, and ironing (Boone & Landes, 1968; Harrell et al., 1992). The ability to detect temperature also contributes to the enjoyment of food and the detection of uncomfortable environmental temperatures. The client can be taught temperature sense through compensatory strategies for burn prevention and precautions against injury when engaging in occupation. As in other sensory tests, the results can serve as a baseline for the client's progress. Changes in sensory status may be used to measure recovery or degeneration, depending on the diagnosis.

Superficial Pain Sensation. **Pain** allows the detection of stimuli potentially harmful to the skin and subcutaneous tissue (Boone & Landes, 1968; Harrell et al., 1992). The ability to detect painful stimuli is critical to avoidance of injury during performance of occupations and to the prevention of skin breakdown while wearing splints and braces, using a wheelchair, using crutches, and using other adaptive devices. In normal circumstances, pain sensation warns the individual, for example, to move quickly (as when withdrawing a finger from a hot surface), to adjust the position of clothing (as when an elastic leg band is binding), or to remove an offending article of apparel (e.g., a shoe that is rubbing a blister on the foot). The client who lacks the ability to detect such painful stimuli is more likely to be injured when engaging in occupation. If pain sensation is absent or impaired, the client may be taught compensatory strategies to address sensory limitations and safety awareness as part of the treatment program.

Olfactory Sensation (Smell). The sense of smell is conveyed by receptors that lie deep in the nasal cavity. Individuals with normal olfactory sensation can detect thousands of odors and at low concentrations, making smell discrimination quite extraordinary. Olfactory acuity varies greatly among normal persons and usually declines with age (Bolger, 1980). **Olfactory** sensation is associated with the pleasure of taste and is important for detection of noxious and pleasant odors. Smell is also connected to neuronal circuits that influence emotional states and evoke memories.

Hyposmia is a diminished sense of smell. It may occur in clients with cystic fibrosis, Parkinson disease, and untreated adrenal insufficiency. Loss of the sense of smell is known as anosmia. Anosmia may be specific—referring to lowered sensitivity to a specific odorant while perception of most others remains intact—or general (Bolger, 1980). Anosmia may result from local chronic or acute inflammatory nasal disease

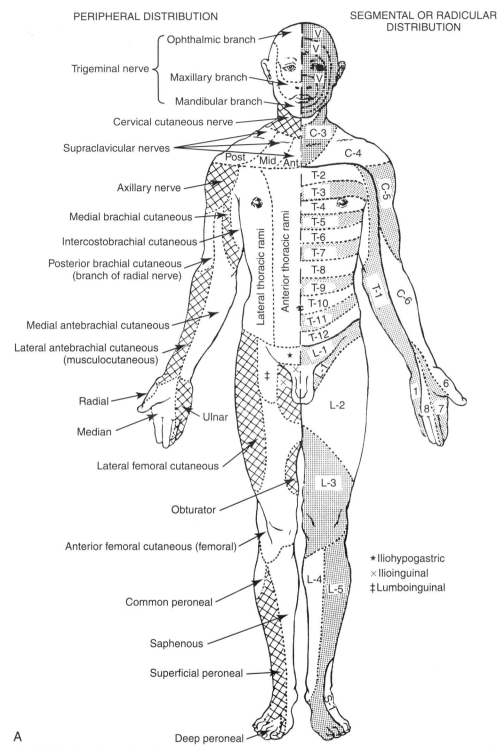

PERIPHERAL DISTRIBUTION

SEGMENTAL OR RADICULAR DISTRIBUTION

Trigeminal nerve
- Ophthalmic branch
- Maxillary branch
- Mandibular branch

Cervical cutaneous nerve

Supraclavicular nerves

Axillary nerve

Medial brachial cutaneous

Intercostobrachial cutaneous

Posterior brachial cutaneous (branch of radial nerve)

Medial antebrachial cutaneous

Lateral antebrachial cutaneous (musculocutaneous)

Radial

Median

Ulnar

Lateral femoral cutaneous

Obturator

Anterior femoral cutaneous (femoral)

Common peroneal

Saphenous

Superficial peroneal

Deep peroneal

★Iliohypogastric
×Ilioinguinal
‡Lumboinguinal

A

Fig. 9.1 (A) Sensory distribution of major peripheral nerves and dermatomes corresponding to spinal cord segments, anterior view. (B) Sensory distribution, posterior view. (From Chusid JG. *Correlative Neuroanatomy and Functional Neurology.* 19th ed. Los Altos, CA: Lange Medical Publications; 1985.)

or from intracranial lesions that may be the result of a cerebrovascular accident (CVA), head injury, tumors, and infections. In some disturbances the sense of smell is distorted. The person may perceive odors that do not exist. Pleasant odors may be distorted or perceived as noxious, a condition known as parosmia (Rustad et al., 1993).

Anosmia interferes with detection of household gas, chemicals, smoke, car exhaust, and noxious environmental odors. Anosmia is a liability for the client who has an occupation in which the sense of smell is critical to safety. The disturbance may interfere with the perception and enjoyment of food odors and taste because decreased sense of smell affects

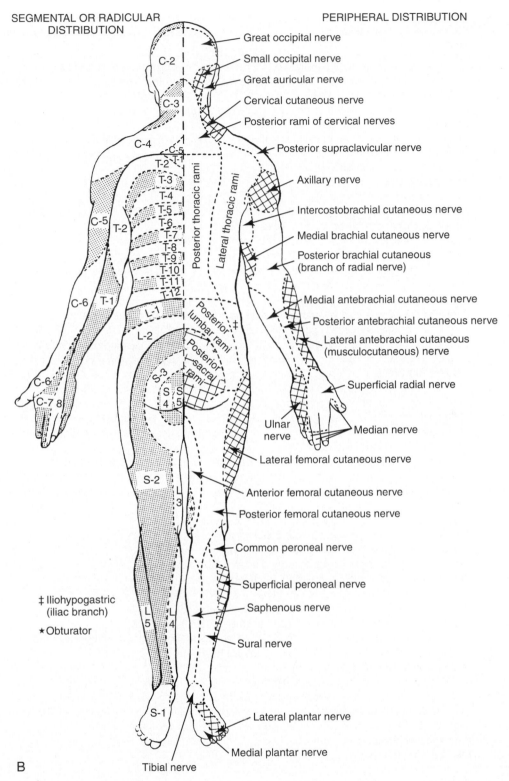

SEGMENTAL OR RADICULAR DISTRIBUTION

PERIPHERAL DISTRIBUTION

Great occipital nerve
Small occipital nerve
Great auricular nerve
Cervical cutaneous nerve
Posterior rami of cervical nerves
Posterior supraclavicular nerve
Axillary nerve
Intercostobrachial cutaneous nerve
Medial brachial cutaneous nerve
Posterior brachial cutaneous (branch of radial nerve)
Medial antebrachial cutaneous nerve
Posterior antebrachial cutaneous nerve
Lateral antebrachial cutaneous (musculocutaneous) nerve
Superficial radial nerve
Ulnar nerve
Median nerve
Lateral femoral cutaneous nerve
Anterior femoral cutaneous nerve
Posterior femoral cutaneous nerve
Common peroneal nerve
Superficial peroneal nerve
Saphenous nerve
Sural nerve
Lateral plantar nerve
Medial plantar nerve
Tibial nerve

Posterior thoracic rami
Lateral thoracic rami
Posterior lumbar rami
Posterior sacral rami

‡ Iliohypogastric (iliac branch)
★ Obturator

B

Fig. 9.1 (Continued)

Gustatory Sensation (Taste). Taste receptor cells are located in the taste buds of the tongue; in the palate; and in the pharynx, epiglottis, and esophagus. Taste sensation is conveyed to the brain by way of the facial, glossopharyngeal, and vagus nerves (cranial nerves VII, IX, and X). Generally, four basic tastes—sweet, sour, salty, and bitter—can be detected. Detection of more complex taste sensations is

the ability to taste. This may lead to secondary health complications related to nutrition and diet.

TABLE 9.1   Tests for Various Functions of Sensation, Perception, and Cognition

Function	Test
Light touch	With client's vision occluded, examiner touches client's hand lightly with cotton ball, cotton swab, etc.
	Semmes-Weinstein monofilaments—with client's vision occluded, examiner touches client's hand lightly with monofilament according to directions (Darby & Walsh, 2005; Toglia, 1993a)
Deep pressure	With client's vision occluded, examiner presses hard with cotton swab
	Semmes-Weinstein monofilaments—with client's vision occluded, examiner touches client's hand with monofilaments according to directions (Darby & Walsh, 2005; Toglia, 1993a)
Thermal sensation	Hot/cold discrimination kit—a thermometer is used to control temperatures of metal probes that contact client's skin. Client's vision is occluded
	With client's vision occluded, examiner touches the sides of test tubes filled with hot (110°F) and cool (45°F) water to client's skin
Pain	With client's vision occluded, a sterilized safety pin (new for each client) is used to touch the skin with a light prick. Examination may be contraindicated when skin atrophy (wasting of the skin) is present (Boone & Landes, 1968; Harrell et al., 1992). In this case, the end of a straightened paper clip may be used (Benton & Schultz, 1949; Kiernan et al., 1987; Montgomery, 1991; Rustad et al., 1993)
Smell (olfactory sense)	With client's vision occluded, examiner presents various scents (coffee, almond, chocolate, lemon oil, peppermint) on a cotton swab or with the cork of a bottle (Chusid, 1985; Kiernan et al., 1987; Rustad et al., 1993)
Taste (gustatory sense)	With client's vision occluded, examiner presents soft foods with various tastes
	Stimulation of the tongue may cause choking and is potentially harmful to dysphagic clients; therefore only the trained occupational therapist administers this test (McCarthy & Warrington, 1990; Miller, 1986)
Stereognosis	With client's vision occluded, examiner presents one by one various familiar objects for the client to identify. For clients with aphasia, an array of identical objects is provided so that the client can point to the same object
Graphesthesia	With client's vision occluded, examiner traces letters, forms, etc. on the client's palm
Body scheme	Examiner asks client to carry out motor actions such as pointing to body parts (Itzkovich et al., 2000; Neistadt, 1988; Webster, 1992; Werner & Omer, 1970; Wilson et al., 1985; 2008; Wilson & Moffat, 2014)
	Draw-a-person test, body and face puzzles (Ghez, 1991; Webster, 1992; Werner & Omer, 1970; Wilson et al., 1985; 2008; Wilson & Moffat, 2014).
	Examiner asks client to perform motor actions involving right and left sides of body
	Examiner asks client to name fingers or imitate finger movements (Itzkovich et al., 2000; Neistadt, 1988)
Ideomotor apraxia	The client is asked to carry out motor actions based on spoken instructions (Webster, 1992)
	The client is asked to imitate motor actions
Constructional apraxia	Test of Visual Motor Skills (TVMS) (Farber, 1985; Kent, 1965)
	Benton Visual Retention Test (Reese, 2005)
	Rey Complex Figure Test (Hécaen & Albert, 1990)
	Three-Dimensional Block Construction (Arnadottir, 1991)
	Observation of tasks such as dressing or setting the table
Dressing apraxia	Observation of client performance of dressing
Cognitive functions	Middlesex Elderly Assessment of Mental State (Gillen, 2010)
	Cognitive Assessment of Minnesota (Morrison et al., 2013)
	Mini Mental State Examination (Dodd & Castellucci, 2000; Doughtery & Radomski, 1993)
	Modified Mini Mental Examination (Sauget et al., 1971)
	Test of Orientation for Rehabilitation Patients (Cooke, 1991)
	Scales of Cognitive Ability for Traumatic Brain Injury (Adamovich & Henderson, 1992)
	Neurobehavioral Cognitive Status Screening Examination (Hécaen & Albert, 1990)
	The Arnadottir OT-ADL Neurobehavioral Evaluation (A-ONE) (American Occupational Therapy Association, 2010)
	Cognitive Skills Workbook (Deitz et al., 1990)
	The Executive Function Performance Test
	The Kettle Test
	The Multiple Errands Test
	The Complex Task Performance Assessment
Memory	Benton Visual Retention Test (Reese, 2005)
	Rey Complex Figure (Katz et al., 1989; Krotoski, 2011)
	Learning Efficiency Test (Teng & Chui, 1987)
	Rivermead Behavioral Memory Test (Toglia, 1993b); Walsh, 1987; Warren, 1981)
	Contextual Memory Test (Shumway-Cook & Woollacott, 2011)
	Subjective Memory Questionnaire (Baum et al., 2008)

thought to result from activation of combinations of the four basic taste receptors (Bolger, 1980).

Taste is basic to the enjoyment of food and helps to trigger salivation and swallowing (Pendleton & Schultz-Krohn, 2006). As with smell, taste is connected to neural circuits that control emotional states and trigger specific memories (Bolger, 1980). When the client requires a comprehensive evaluation of oral-motor mechanisms, taste sensation may be a consideration. When developing feeding-training programs, evaluation of the sensation of taste is also useful to guide intervention (Pendleton & Schultz-Krohn, 2006). Disturbances of taste may be caused by PNS or CNS lesions (Boone & Landes, 1968; Harrell et al., 1992). Smokers may demonstrate a decreased sense of taste with aging (DeJong, 2019). The test for **gustatory** sensation is usually performed by the OT. Stimulation of the tongue may cause choking or other reactions that are potentially harmful to clients with dysphagia.

Proprioception (Position and Motion Sense). Proprioception refers to unconscious information about joint position and motion that arises from receptors in the muscles, joints, ligaments, and bone. The conscious sense of motion may be referred to as kinesthesia. A partial or complete loss of position and motion senses seriously impairs movement, even if muscle function (force, tone, endurance) is within normal limits. To better understand motor dysfunction, the OT must determine whether—and to what extent—the client has a sensory loss in the area of proprioception or kinesthesia. Results of the sensory evaluation guide treatment planning with regard to developing compensatory methods or sensory retraining to address proprioceptive or kinesthetic deficits. Evaluation of position and motion sense requires specific training and the development of sensitivity in handling and positioning the client.

PERCEPTION

Perception is the mechanism by which the brain recognizes and interprets sensory information received from the environment. Perceived information is then further processed by the various cognitive functions. The end result of a client's perceptual function may be a verbal expression or motor act. For example, a woman searching for a pen to write something reaches in her purse and encounters a hard, smooth, cylindrical, oblong object (sensation). The tactile sensory data acquired through touch are then translated into a mental image of a pen (perception). The woman may then choose (cognition) to remove it (motor action) from her purse or instead to use a pen provided by someone else.

The evaluation of perception includes higher level tactile discriminative sensations, body scheme, and praxis. Evaluation of these functions is most accurate when the examiner has a thorough understanding of higher cognitive functions, their anatomic representations, and their interrelationships. The evaluation of perception is most often the responsibility of the OT with input on selected tests provided by the OTA. Some of the tests administered by the OTA include the Motor-Free

Visual Perception Test (MVPT-4) (Chusid, 1985) and the Lowenstein Occupational Therapy Cognitive Assessment (LOTCA-2) (Haines, 2012; Hartman-Maeir et al., 2009).

Evaluation of Perception

Perception may be evaluated by itself or in combination with evaluation of performance during ADL or other areas of occupation (American Occupational Therapy Association, 2010; Webster, 1992; Wilson et al., 1985; 2008). A battery of perceptual tests can be used that require verbal response, motor response, or flexible response (either mode). These variations in response mode allow the therapist to determine whether the deficit lies in the reception of information, in verbal or motor output, or exclusively in perceptual skills. This information will influence the treatment goals and approach. Analyzing the perceptual motor demands of the client's occupational engagement may provide additional and clarifying information. The OTA may observe functional performance during the client's execution of ADL and other occupations and may contribute significantly to the evaluation of perception with this information.

Perceptual Functions: Evaluation and Observation

Stereognosis and graphesthesia are tactile discriminative skills that involve discrimination of different touch sensations at a higher level of CNS synthesis than the basic tactile sensory functions of light touch and pressure already described.

Stereognosis. **Stereognosis** is the ability to identify an object through proprioception, cognition, and the sense of touch. This ability identifies common objects and geometric shapes through touch (without the aid of vision). Stereognosis is essential to daily living because it makes it possible to reach into a pocket or purse and find keys and to reach into a dark room and find the light switch. Examples are texting while watching television, sawing wood while focusing on the wood rather than the saw, and using a fork during a conversation. **Astereognosis** indicates an absence of stereognosis. Clients with astereognosis must visually monitor their hands during all activities. This may cause slow and deliberate movements, which may lead to a decrease in activity. OTAs with service competency may screen for stereognosis using specific tests (Box 9.3).

Graphesthesia. **Graphesthesia** is the ability to recognize numbers, letters, or forms written on the skin (Brand & Hollister, 1999; Ghez, 1991; Mayo Clinic and Mayo Foundation, 1998; Montgomery, 1991). The loss of this ability is called **agraphesthesia**. This is assessed by occluding vision and tracing letters, numbers, or geometric forms on the client's palm with a dull, pointed pencil or similar instrument. The client attempts to identify the symbol written (Mayo Clinic and Mayo Foundation, 1998). Pictures of the symbols may be used to indicate a response after each test stimulus in a client with aphasia.

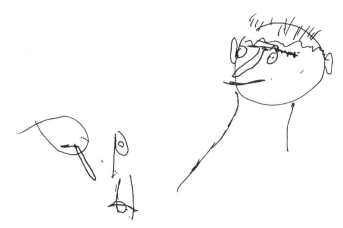

Fig. 9.2 Example of impaired body scheme. Drawing on the left is client's first attempt to draw a face. The therapist asked client to try again. Client's second effort is the drawing on the right.

BOX 9.3 Test for Stereognosis (Barco, et al., 1991; Colarusso & Hammill, 2015; Golding, 1989; Head et al., 1920; Montgomery, 1991)

Purpose
To evaluate a client's ability to identify common objects and perceive their tactile properties.

Materials
Means to occlude client's vision such as a curtain or folder. Any common objects may be used. Typical objects that could be used for identification include a pencil, fountain pen, sunglasses, key, nail, large safety pin, metal teaspoon, quarter, button, and small leather coin purse. The examiner must consider client's social and ethnic background to ensure familiarity with the objects.

Conditions
Test should be conducted in an environment with minimal distractions. The client should be seated at a table in a position that accommodates the affected hand and forearm comfortably. The test can also be completed bedside or in a wheelchair without a table. The examiner should sit opposite the client. If client cannot manipulate test objects because of motor weakness, the examiner should assist the client with manipulation of the objects.

Method
The client is provided oral instructions and a demonstration within his or her vision on an unaffected area. The client is asked to identify each item visually and verbally. The client's vision is occluded. The dorsal surface of the client's hand is in a resting position. Objects are presented in random order. The client is to use one hand only to identify the object. Manipulation of objects is allowed and encouraged. The examiner assists with manipulation of items if client's motoric hand function is impaired.

Responses
The client is asked to name object, or if unable, to describe its properties. Aphasic clients may view a duplicate set of test objects after each trial and point to a choice.

Scoring
A form may be used to score the client's responses. The examiner marks plus (+) if object is identified quickly and correctly and minus (−) if there is a long delay before identification of object or if the client can only describe its properties (e.g., size, texture, material, shape). The examiner marks zero (0) if the client cannot identify object or describe its properties.

Body Scheme. **Body scheme** awareness is the ability to identify the position of the body and its parts in relation to themselves and the environment (Farber, 1985). It includes knowledge of body construction, the anatomic elements, and their spatial relationships; ability to visualize the body in movement and its parts in different positional relationships; ability to differentiate between right and left; and ability to recognize body health and disease (Farber, 1985; Webster, 1992; Werner & Omer, 1970; Wilson et al., 2008). Body

scheme disorders include **asomatognosia**, right-left discrimination deficits, unilateral inattention or neglect, and finger agnosia.

Asomatognosia refers to a severe loss of body scheme (Folstein et al., 2010; Gardner, 2009; Gilroy & Meyer, 1975). The client with asomatognosia has a diminished awareness and recognition of a body structure or part and cannot determine the body part's relationship to the rest of his or her body. This condition is usually evaluated by having the client point to body parts on command or by imitation (Itzkovich et al., 2000; Neistadt, 1988; Webster, 1992; Werner & Omer, 1970; Wilson et al., 1985; 2008; Wilson & Moffat, 2014). Fig. 9.2 illustrates an impairment in body scheme.

Right-left discrimination deficits can occur in extrapersonal space, intrapersonal space, or both. The most basic testing of right-left discrimination abilities is intrapersonal; the client is asked to point to a body part, specifying the right or left side, on oneself. A more advanced (extrapersonal) test is to ask the client to identify right and left body parts on the examiner (Benton & Fogel, 1962).

Unilateral inattention or unilateral neglect is a failure to integrate perceptions from one side of the body or one side of body space. Fig. 9.3 illustrates evidence of left-sided neglect. The most effective evaluation of unilateral neglect as it relates to a body scheme disorder is direct observation during occupation such as ADL and IADL. Clients with unilateral inattention or unilateral neglect may exhibit occupational performance such as shaving one side of the face, applying makeup to one side of the face, or dressing one side of the body.

The client with finger agnosia has difficulty naming fingers on command or identifying which finger has been touched (Hartman-Maeir et al., 2009). The OT or OTA evaluates finger agnosia through finger localization, naming on command, or having the client imitate the therapist's finger movements (Itzkovich et al., 2000; Neistadt, 1988).

Praxis. **Praxis** is the ability to plan and perform purposeful movement. **Apraxia** is an impairment in praxis, a deficit in

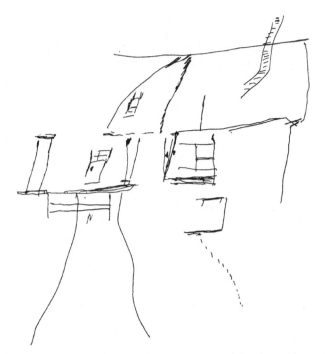

Fig. 9.3 Example of two-dimensional constructional apraxia and inattention to the left side in a client's drawing of a house. The client was a retired architect.

the ability to perform purposeful movement despite normal motor power, sensation, coordination, and general comprehension. Subtypes include ideomotor, constructional, oral, and dressing apraxias.

A client can demonstrate a single form of apraxia or a combination of subtypes. The individual with apraxia faces problems with effective planning and performance of skilled purposeful movement. Evaluation of praxis disorders is reserved for the OT.

Ideomotor apraxia. **Ideomotor apraxia** is an inability to perform a motor act on command, despite the ability to perform the act automatically. The client may be able to describe the intended motion in words but cannot execute the motor act at will. For example, the client is asked to stand up and walk across the room but instead looks at the therapist in a puzzled way and does not move. The presence of ideomotor apraxia impairs the understanding of the requested act. Later, the client gets up on his or her own and walks across the room to get a towel, indicating that the ability to perform the motor act itself is present.

Constructional apraxia. **Constructional apraxia** is a deficit in the ability to copy, draw, or construct a design, whether on command or spontaneously (Goodglass & Kaplan, 2002; Webster, 1992). It is the inability to organize or assemble parts into a whole, as in putting together block designs (three-dimensional action) or drawings (two-dimensional action). This perceptual motor impairment is often seen in persons with severe head injury or CVA and relates to a dysfunction of the parietal lobes. Constructional apraxia causes significant dysfunction in activities such as dressing,

following instructions for assembling a toy, and stacking a dishwasher. Fig. 9.3 shows evidence of left-sided neglect and demonstrates constructional apraxia. Constructional apraxia impairs dressing and other sequential ADL and can be observed by the OTA in these functional activities.

Dressing apraxia. **Dressing apraxia,** or the inability to plan and perform the motor acts necessary to dress oneself, has been linked with problems of body scheme, spatial orientation, and constructional apraxia (Lezak et al., 2004; Sivan, 1991; Webster, 1992; Wilson et al., 2008). Clinically the client may have difficulty initiating dressing or may make errors in orientation by putting the clothes on the wrong side of the body, upside down, or inside out (American Occupational Therapy Association, 2013; Webster, 1992; Wilson et al., 2008).

COGNITION

Cognitive deficits can cause difficulty with occupational performance. **Cognition** includes global mental functions (consciousness, orientation, sleep, temperament, personality, energy, and drive) and specific mental functions (attention, memory, thought, judgment, time management, problem solving, decision making, language, regulation of emotion, and experience of the self). Cognition relies on information from external sources and internally generated ideas. Cognition allows individuals to use and process sensed and perceived information and thus is intimately connected to sensation and perception. See Chapter 22 for an in-depth discussion of disturbances in and interventions for cognition.

Cognitive Evaluation

Clinical evaluation of individual cognitive deficits is challenging and complex (Box 9.4). Deficit areas are rarely seen in isolation, and interpreting a client's behavior is difficult. Therefore several important principles must be considered when evaluating cognition. When administering standardized tests adherence to the instructions is crucial to attaining valid results. Nonadherence to the instructions of a standardized assessment will negate the underlying reliability, validity, and other psychometric properties of the assessment tool.

The process of evaluating a client through observation of a task can be difficult, but it is a critical piece in the puzzle when addressing cognitive deficits. Assistance must only be provided to the client when safety is at risk. If too much assistance is given it will be difficult to gather accurate information on the client's cognitive functioning. If not enough assistance is provided, the client will become frustrated with the task and will not experience a positive sense of accomplishment.

See Table 9.1 for some of the assessments utilized. Cognitive functions are evaluated in a particular order because certain cognitive skills depend on others. For example, individuals will be unable to display effective problem-solving skills when they cannot attend to or remember a particular task. It is important to note, however, that intact function in a specific area of cognition during a client factor-focused testing does not always translate to intact function of the very same client factor during

BOX 9.4 Principles of Cognitive Evaluation

1. Cognition should always be seen in relation to other potential deficit areas. The client's sensory, language, visual, and perceptual systems affect the observable qualities of cognition. For example, the client may be unable to attend to and concentrate on a particular task because of an underlying deficit in visual scanning.
2. Cognition is best assessed by engaging a client in occupation or utilizing an occupation-based assessment tool. Engaging in occupation is complex, context dependent, and client specific. It is through the lens of occupational engagement that a client's cognitive deficits are most likely to be observed.
3. Discussions of the occupational therapy evaluation results with health professionals from other disciplines will enhance the OT practitioner's understanding of the client's capacity. The speech pathologist, physical therapist, psychologist, or neuropsychologist and the client's family can provide different perspectives.
4. The testing environment, as a function of context, also influences the results of the cognitive evaluation. A client's behavior in the foreign environment of the hospital or rehabilitation facility may differ from performance in a familiar home setting.
5. The optimal test battery involves a selection of tests—standardized and normed for the population—and a variety of occupations (e.g., homemaking). Therapists need standardized tests to provide objective, quantifiable data to measure the extent of the deficit in comparison with an established norm, to document progress, and to determine discharge planning. Occupations provide opportunities to observe the practical implications of the deficits revealed by the standardized tests and allow the therapist to better predict the person's functioning in a home environment. Observation of functional performance during occupation is the best way an OTA can contribute to the evaluation of cognitive skills.
6. When introducing a cognitive test to a client, the examiner should avoid a condescending attitude or a too cheerful, falsely positive approach. Regardless of the level of functioning, the client should be approached on an age-appropriate level. The therapist should only offer choices that he or she is willing to complete.

occupation. The following functions are discussed in the order of the recommended progression of testing.

Orientation. **Orientation** refers to an individual's ongoing awareness of the current situation, the environment, and the passage of time. Immediately after any traumatic injury, a person must develop an awareness of the events that preceded the accident and those occurring since then. After a CVA, for example, the individual is typically disoriented initially but becomes more aware as healing occurs (Webster, 1992; Wilson et al., 1992).

Orientation is related to an individual's memory capacity because a person must be able to remember past occurrences to place current events in their proper perspective. After a severe traumatic brain injury (TBI) or CVA, a person initially may be confused about personal identity, which indicates a disorientation to person (Webster, 1992). This issue is a more global deficit than an inability to speak one's name, which may occur in the case of aphasia, when a person has difficulty with the verbal expression of any message. The client may also confuse the identities of other individuals, for example, thinking that the therapist or assistant is a family member. Orientation to place refers to an individual's awareness of being in a hospital (if appropriate) or knowing the name of the immediate town, city, and state. Difficulty in monitoring the passage of time can result in time disorientation. Clients may confuse the sequence of events in time. For example, a client may report that a family member visited the previous day when that person actually came to see him a week earlier.

An unimpaired individual typically can respond to the following questions:

1. What is your name? (or be able to respond to his or her name)
2. Where are you?
3. What time is it? (i.e., what year, month, day, and time of day)

The client who can respond accurately to all three orientation questions is said to be oriented times three (the standard abbreviation is written as O × 3), or oriented to person, place, and time. If only able to answer the first two questions, the client is oriented times two, or oriented to person and place (the standard abbreviation is written as O × 2). If he or she can answer only the first question, the client is oriented times one, or oriented to person (the standard abbreviation is O × 1). Because levels of orientation can vary with time of day and other conditions, these questions must be asked several times to determine the consistency of the client's awareness.

Topographical orientation describes an individual's awareness of the position of self in relationship to the environment (e.g., the room, building, city). Functional examples of this disorder are noted when a client becomes confused or lost while attempting to leave a room and locate another therapy department or travel to the cafeteria. These clients may perform better in the familiar environment of home and community, but deficits may still be apparent. Topographical orientation is assessed by observing clients traveling from one place to another or by asking them to find their way to their room, the therapy area, or to areas within their home or community. Clients with visual field deficits may appear to have deficits in topographical orientation when in fact their difficulty in navigation is caused entirely by a deficit in vision.

Attention. **Attention** is an active process that allows the individual to focus on the environmental information and sensations relevant at a particular time. Attention involves the simultaneous engagement of alertness, selectivity, sustained effort, flexibility, and mental tracking (Shumway-Cook & Woollacott, 2011). A client must be alert and awake and able to select a relevant focus of interest. The client must be able to maintain this focus for as long as needed but be able to shift the focus if another event of interest or importance occurs. Consider, for example, attending to the task of dressing until the task is completed and shifting attention to breakfast when it arrives. The client must be able to ignore information if it is not relevant—a concept known as stimulus inhibition—and to track several types of information simultaneously. This need requires, for example, dressing without being distracted by the people in the hall while recognizing when someone brings in the breakfast tray. Because these skills underlie all aspects of cognitive functioning, the deficits can interfere with all areas of occupation, especially in clients who have experienced neurologic damage.

The two types of information processing relevant to attention are automatic and controlled processing (Webster, 1992). Automatic processing occurs at a subcortical (not deliberately conscious) level. Controlled processing is used when new information is being considered. Two disorders, focused attentional deficit and divided attentional deficit, are related to these two types of information processing. A focused attentional deficit occurs when an automatic response is replaced by a controlled response. For example, walking (an automatic response) may require focused attention and deliberate control in a client with a CVA who is concentrating on trying to walk.

A divided attentional deficit occurs when the individual cannot process all the information required for task completion. The person becomes overloaded and typically responds by reverting to focused attention. For example, if a client with a CVA is asked a question while ambulating, the client may stop movement to engage in conversation. Divided attention deficit often manifests when a client is engaged in an activity or an occupation.

Concentration requires that an individual sustain focused attention for a period of time. Clients with difficulties in this area may be distracted easily or be sensitive to events in the immediate environment that pull their focus away from the task at hand. Noting which types of stimuli (e.g., visual, auditory, tactile, gustatory) appear to distract the client easily is important. A low-stimulus environment or quiet room may be available in the hospital or rehabilitation center.

Other clients have the opposite problem: They can become deeply focused on a given stimulus or activity and have difficulty maintaining general awareness of events occurring around them. Neither extreme is desirable. Effective functioning in daily life demands the ability to focus, to remain aware of (but not distracted by) peripheral events, and to disengage and reengage concentration as needed.

Memory. **Memory** is the cognitive function that allows a person to retain and recall information. Fig. 9.4 summarizes the memory process. Consider the client who is learning one-handed dressing after experiencing a CVA. The therapist demonstrates and explains the steps in one-handed dressing. The client uses sensory input or the selective attention portion of memory. The information is moved to working memory or temporary storage as the client completes the task one or two times. Finally, after the client has repeated the task

several times, the information is stored in long-term memory for encoding and consolidation. After this phase, when the client wants to put on his or her shirt using the one-handed dressing technique, the information is retrieved (from long-term memory) and sent to the working memory. Thus the task can be completed.

A breakdown in the memory process can occur at any level. If a client cannot attend to information, it may never enter the system. Some clients can process information in short-term or working memory but never encode the information into long-term storage. Still others can store the information but have trouble retrieving it. Clients with memory deficits, who need to expend additional effort to learn new material, may also have difficulty forgetting information when it is no longer needed. For example, the client learning to use a one-handed dressing technique may repeatedly try to use the dressing technique learned before the CVA. A client whose memory is this impaired cannot learn the new technique. Memory deficits in any of these areas can result in an inability of the client to successfully implement compensatory strategies during occupational engagement.

A person's ability to recite or reproduce information is generally taken as an indication of recall and is referred to as declarative memory or explicit memory (Ghez & Krakaur, 2000; McCarthy & Warrington, 1990). Tests of declarative memory may require a client to repeat a word list or draw a set of geometric designs. Less formally, the practitioner may ask a client about events occurring earlier in the day. Declarative memory is subdivided into two categories. Episodic memory refers to an individual's personal history and lifetime of experiences. Semantic memory describes the general fund of knowledge shared by groups of people such as language and rules of social behaviour (Glogoski et al., 2006). Episodic memory and semantic memory are types of explicit memory (Ghez & Krakaur, 2000; Webster, 1992).

Some clients may have a significant deficit in declarative memory, but procedural memory (a type of nondeclarative or implicit memory) or memory for a skill or series of actions (Ghez & Krakaur, 2000; Glogoski et al., 2006; McCarthy & Warrington, 1990; Webster, 1992) may be less impaired. For example, a client who cannot tell a therapist the steps to make a sandwich and cup of coffee nonetheless may be able to perform the activity adequately.

Procedural memory may enable a client to learn new self-care techniques despite severe declarative memory deficits on standardized tests. Everyday memory refers to a person's ability to remember information pertinent to daily life

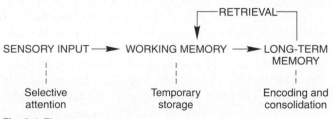

Fig. 9.4 The memory process.

(Toglia, 1993b; Walsh, 1987). In the hospital or rehabilitation facility, this term refers to learning the names and faces of the physicians, nurses, and therapy staff who work regularly with the client. Learning a schedule of appointments or the locations of various departments may be difficult and further complicated by frequent changes; therefore the hospital escort staff often assumes this responsibility for the client with impaired everyday memory. Everyday memory also includes the ability to keep track of daily events in their proper sequence. Prospective memory refers to the ability to remember events that are set to occur at some future time such as an appointment scheduled for later in the day (Toglia, 1993b; Walsh,1987).

Clients with memory deficits may confabulate, which is to fill in memory gaps with imaginary material (Callahan, 2002; Silverman & Elfant, 1979). They are unaware that they are making up stories or adding erroneous information and thus can become confused regarding past events. A client's memories are generally better for specific activities and for topics of interest or of a personal relevance. For this reason, the family may minimize a memory deficit, stating for example that "he can remember if he wants to." Staff members need to explain this inconsistent performance and educate family members to the reality of the underlying deficit. For example, a client who has difficulty with the sensory input or working memory will not remember new or recent events or activities. The same client may remember information that has been stored in long-term memory. Family members may be puzzled by the fact that a client cannot remember them visiting yesterday but can remember every detail of a birthday party last year. This memory is recalled because the birthday party is stored in the unimpaired long-term memory.

Tests (see Table 9.1) can be used to determine where the breakdown in the process occurs. For example, a client may be unable to remember information when he is asked to recall it (with no or minimal cues) but may score high on recognizing the same information. This would suggest that the information was adequately stored, but that the client has a deficit in retrieval. Treatment would then focus on the development of retrieval strategies.

Executive Functioning. **Executive functioning** includes higher order reasoning and planning functions such as goal formation, planning, plan implementation, and effective performance (Katz et al., 1989; Krotoski, 2011). Due to the complexity of executive function it is possible for a client to independently complete ADL despite an underlying impairment in executive functioning. Deficits in executive functioning are best observed by engaging a client in occupations with higher cognitive demands such as IADL. The client who cannot think of anything to fix for breakfast but who responds well to an established routine of making toast and coffee in the morning demonstrates a deficit in goal formation. Occasionally the structured schedule of a hospital or rehabilitation facility may mask goal formation deficits, which then become apparent once the client is discharged home, where externally structured goals and routines are

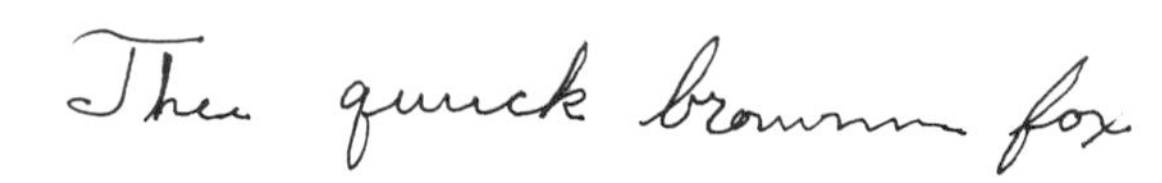

Fig. 9.5 Example of writing perseveration.

absent. Conversely, some clients may perform at a higher level during rote occupations when in the familiar contextual environment of home. Some clients may be able to verbalize an intended goal and plan a course of action but are unable to implement it. These clients often seem much more capable than their behavior actually demonstrates, which underscores the importance of engaging in occupation, particularly those with higher cognitive demands.

A client may demonstrate poor mental flexibility, resulting in perseveration or impulsivity. Perseveration refers to repeated acts or movements during functional performances as a result of difficulty in shifting from one response pattern to another (Folstein et al., 2010; Gardner, 2009). Perseveration can be seen in motor acts, verbalizations, or thought processes. Fig. 9.5 illustrates writing perseveration. Another example is seen with a client buttering toast and then moving on to eating cereal while using the motion of spreading butter with the spoon in the cereal bowl. Impulsivity, or impulsive behavior, is seen when a client begins a task or activity before formulating a plan. The impulsive client will begin a task before receiving instruction or in an unsafe manner because he or she has not generated a plan. A client in a wheelchair who tries to stand up without taking his or her feet off the foot rests or prior to locking the wheelchair brakes is one observable example of impulsivity.

Effective performance of occupations requires that clients continually monitor and adjust performance activities throughout the execution of tasks. Some clients cannot perceive their errors, and others may recognize the error but make no effort to correct the mistake.

While family members, nurses, and nursing aides can provide some information about a client's executive functioning, the true measure of executive function is best achieved through engagement in occupation. A homemaking evaluation that involves planning and simultaneously preparing a variety of dishes for a meal is useful for observing the client's executive functioning. Perseveration or impulsivity would be noted in relation to the specific environment and particular tasks. Perseveration and impulsivity may be related to other clinical deficits such as poor comprehension or apraxia or may be a sign of depression.

Reasoning and Problem-Solving Skills. **Abstract thinking** enables a person to see relationships among objects, events, or ideas; to discriminate relevant from irrelevant detail; or to recognize absurdities (Katz et al., 1989; Krotoski, 2011; Webster, 1992). Clients with frontal lobe damage often lose this ability and think only in a concrete, literal manner. This **concrete thinking** is often paired with mental inflexibility. This problem creates difficulty in problem solving and transfer of knowledge to new situations (Webster, 1992; Wilson et al., 1985; 2008; Wilson & Moffat, 2014).

The following example illustrates concrete thinking. A client is asked the interview question, "What brought you to this hospital?" The client responds, "My parents' car." The client is interpreting the question literally rather than in reference to the accident that resulted in the brain injury.

Problem solving is a complex process involving many cognitive skills. It requires attention, memory, planning and organization, and the ability to reason and make judgments. Various types of **reasoning** can be used in the problem-solving process. The client must be able to process complex information to plan strategies and to evaluate established strategies (Baum & Edwards, 1993). Formal evaluation of problem solving and reasoning is performed by the OT or the psychologist or neuropsychologist. Evaluation of a client's ability to solve problems requires observation and attention to the process the person uses to complete occupations.

The OTA may be able to apply the following questions to observations of the client's performance during occupation. He or she should decide whether the client can do the following:

1. Define the problem or recognize when a problem exists
2. Develop possible solutions to a problem
3. Choose the best solution
4. Execute the solution
5. Evaluate the outcome once the solution has been executed

INSIGHT AND AWARENESS

Consider a client with paralysis who falls out of bed trying to walk to the bathroom. This behavior may result from a denial or lack of awareness of the paralysis. Limited **insight** results in impulsive and unsafe behavior. Clients with this deficit cannot monitor, correct, and regulate the quality of their behavior (Webster, 1992; Wilson et al., 1985; 2008; Wilson & Moffat, 2014). A client's insight may increase as body scheme is modified in response to the changes imposed by the disability. This process is long and complex. Memory deficits may also complicate the client's awareness of the problem or the frequency with which it occurs. The client may remember making only a few errors, when in fact the number of errors was far greater. For example, the client may remember having difficulty recalling a nurse's name two or three times in a given day and thus judge that the memory problem is minimal. However, the incidence actually may be closer to 12 to 15 times a day. The use of a frequency check sheet, recorded by the client (with supervision), may help the client to recognize the severity of the problem. When clients with dysfunctions in insight either overestimate or underestimate their functional abilities and limitations they may be at risk for injury. This is especially important if a client lives alone or with limited support. Anosognosia refers to the total inability to recognize deficits (Folstein et al., 2010; Gardner, 2009). A team approach is necessary to distinguish between neurologic and psychologic (e.g., denial) types of awareness deficits (Archibald & Wepman, 1968).

Emotional lability is the inability to control moods and inhibit impulses that may lead to inappropriate behavior (Folstein et al., 2010; Gardner, 2009). A person experiencing this may laugh or cry or express other emotions that have no relationship to the actual emotional context of the situation. A related condition exists when the client responds with the correct category of emotion such as laughing at a humorous situation but to an exaggerated, inappropriate extent and forcefulness.

Judgment

Judgment is the ability to make realistic decisions based on environmental information (Folstein et al., 2010; Gardner, 2009). The client with poor judgment cannot use feedback to correct errors. Some typical behaviors that show impaired judgment are dressing inappropriately for the weather or driving at a rate of speed twice that of the legal limit. It can sometimes be a struggle to classify a behavior as an example of poor judgment, poor insight, or impulsivity as they can present in observably similar manners.

Sequencing

Sequencing is the ability to organize an activity in logical and timely steps (Folstein et al., 2010; Gardner, 2009). A client with poor sequencing has difficulty organizing a task in a logical sequence. For example, a client making a peanut butter sandwich may take out the peanut butter and a knife and begin to spread the peanut butter before getting the bread. Clients generally can recognize the problem as it occurs and make corrections using their problem-solving skills. The deficit is in the logical organization of the steps while completing the task. The most effective method of evaluation is to have the client engage in familiar occupations that are within physical abilities and observe the performance of sequencing the steps of the task.

Dyscalculia

A deficit in the ability to perform simple calculations, or **dyscalculia**, can have serious implications for an individual's independent functioning in the community. Various types of calculation disorders have been identified (Lezak, 1995). A client may have difficulty reading (alexia) or writing (agraphia) the numbers. The speech/language pathologist may evaluate these functions further. Spatial dyscalculia refers to a deficit in the spatial arrangement of the numbers.

SUMMARY

Sensation provides the background information to perform essential daily activities. Without intact sensation, motor performance becomes inefficient, fatiguing, and discouraging. Evaluation of sensation is important for clients with CNS disorders and peripheral nerve injuries. The OTA can assist the OT in administering some portions of the sensory assessment and provide important information regarding the functional implications of sensory deficits for the individual.

Deficits in perception and perceptual motor skills impair overall function. Deficits can vary greatly; therefore a systematic, comprehensive evaluation of perceptual motor function is crucial to facilitating achievement of the client's highest functional potential. The OTA contributes to the evaluation of perception by administering structured tests as directed, carefully observing the client's engagement during occupations, and reporting observations to the OT.

Cognition involves a complex, hierarchical, dynamic process. Many cognitive functions are necessary for optimal occupational performance. OTAs can assist in cognitive assessment through the observation of a client's occupational performance. The OT and OTA can work together to determine the best course of action in all cases.

REVIEW QUESTIONS

1. Why is sensory and perceptual evaluation necessary and important for occupational therapy?
2. Discuss the relationship between sensation and motor performance.
3. In what types of disabilities are sensory evaluations routinely given?
4. What is the functional significance of olfactory sensation?
5. Define perception and describe its role in everyday activities.
6. Define body scheme.
7. Describe how unilateral neglect can be observed.
8. List four types of apraxia and discuss how each can affect the ability to perform daily living skills.
9. What are the implications of a deficit in attention and concentration on an individual's functioning in everyday activities?
10. Differentiate between procedural and declarative memory.
11. Define confabulation and explain why patients with memory problems may confabulate.
12. What behaviors will the client with poor mental flexibility and abstraction display?

REFERENCES

Adamovich, B. B., & Henderson, J. (1992). *Scales of Cognitive Ability for Traumatic Brain Injury (SCATBI)*. Austin, TX: Pro-Ed.

American Occupational Therapy Association. (2010). Standards of practice for occupational therapy. *The American Journal of Occupational Therapy, 64*, S106–S111.

American Occupational Therapy Association. (2013). Cognition, cognitive rehabilitation, and occupational performance. *The American Journal of Occupational Therapy, 67*(6), S9–S31. http://dx.doi.org/10.5014/ajot.2013.67S9.

American Occupational Therapy Association. (2014). Occupational therapy practice framework: domain and process. 3rd ed. *The American Journal of Occupational Therapy, 68*(1), S1–S48. http://dx.doi.org/10.5014/ajot.2014.682006.

American Occupational Therapy Association. (2017). AOTA's *Centennial Vision* and executive summary. *The American Journal of Occupational Therapy, 61*, 613–614. http://dx.doi.org/10.5014/ajot.61.6.613.

Archibald, Y. M., & Wepman, J. M. (1968). Language disturbance and nonverbal cognitive performance in eight patients following injury to the right hemisphere. *Brain, 91*, 117–130.

Arnadottir, G. (1991). *The brain and behavior: Assessing cortical dysfunction through activities of daily living*. St Louis, MO: Mosby.

Barco, P. P., et al. (1991). Training awareness and compensation in postacute head injury rehabilitation. In: J. S. Kreutzer, & P. H. Wehman (eds.), *Cognitive rehabilitation for persons with traumatic brain injury*. Baltimore, MD: Brookes.

Baum, C. M., Tabor Connor, L., Morrison, T. M., Hahn, M., Dromerick, A. W., & Edwards, D. F. (2008). Reliability, validity, and clinical utility of the executive function performance test: a measure of executive function in a sample of people with stroke. *The American Journal of Occupational Therapy, 62*(4), 446–455. http://dx.doi.org/10.5014/ajot.62.4.446.

Baum, C., & Edwards, D. F. (1993). Cognitive performance in senile dementia of the Alzheimer's type: the kitchen task assessment. *The American Journal of Occupational Therapy, 47*(5), 431–436.

Benton, A. L., & Fogel, M. L. (1962). Three-dimensional constructional praxis: a clinical test. *Archives of Neurology, 7*, 347–354.

Benton, A. L., & Schultz, L. M. (1949). Observations of tactile form perception (stereognosis) in pre-school children. *Journal of Clinical Psychology, 5*, 359–364.

Bolger, J. F. (1980). Cognitive retraining: a developmental approach. *Journal of Clinical Neuropsychology, 4*, 66–70.

Boone, P., & Landes, B. (1968). Right-left discrimination in hemiplegic patients. *Archives of Physical Medicine and Rehabilitation, 49*, 533.

Brand, P. W, & Hollister, A. (1999). *Clinical mechanics of the hand* (3rd ed.). St Louis, MO: Mosby.

Brown, J. (1992). *Aphasia, apraxia, agnosia*. Springfield, IL: Thomas.

Callahan, A. D. (2002). Sensibility testing: clinical methods. In: J. M. Hunter, et al. (eds.), *Rehabilitation of the hand and upper extremity* (5th ed.). St Louis, MO: Mosby.

Chusid, J. G. (1985). *Correlative neuroanatomy and functional neurology* (19th ed.). Los Altos, CA: Lange.

Cooke, D. (1991). Sensibility evaluation battery for the peripheral nerve injured hand. *Austral Occupational Therapy Journal, 38*, 241–245.

Colarusso, R., & Hammill, P. (2015). *Motor free visual perception test* (4th ed.). Ann Arbor, MI: Academic Therapy Publications.

Darby, D., & Walsh, K. (2005). *Walsh's neuropsychology* (5th ed.). London, England: Churchill Livingstone.

Deitz, T., Beeman, C., & Thron, D. (1990). *Test of orientation for rehabilitation patients*. Tucson, AZ: Therapy Skill Builders.

DeJong, R. (2019). *The neurologic examination* (8th ed.). New York, NY: Hoeber.

Dodd, J., & Castellucci, V. F. (2000). Smell and taste: the chemical senses. In: E. R. Kandel, J. H. Schwartz, & T. M. Jessel (Eds.), *Principles of neural science*. New York, NY: Elsevier.

Doughtery, P. M., & Radomski, M. V. (1993). *The cognitive rehabilitation workbook* (2nd ed.). Rockville, MD: Aspen.

Farber, S. D. (1985). *Neurorehabilitation: A multisensory approach*. Philadelphia, PA: WB Saunders.

Folstein, M. F., Folstein, S. E, White, T., & Messer, M. A. (2010). *Mini-mental state examination* (2nd ed.). Lutz, FL: PAR.

Gardner, M. F. (2009). *The Test of Visual Motor Skills Revised (TVMS-R)*. Burlingame, CA: Psychological and Educational Publications.

Ghez, C. (1991). The control of movement. In: E. R. Kandel, J. H. Schwartz, & T. M. Jessel (eds.), *Principles of neural science*. New York, NY: Elsevier.

Ghez, C., & Krakaur, J. (2000). The organization of movement. In: E. R. Kandel, J. H. Schwartz, & T. M. Jessel (eds.), *Principles of neural science* (4th ed.). New York, NY: McGraw-Hill.

Gillen, G. (2010). *Stroke rehabilitation: A functional-based approach* (3rd ed.). St Louis, MO: Mosby.

Gilroy, J., & Meyer, J. S. (1975). *Medical neurology*. London, England: Macmillan.

Glogoski, C., Milligan, N. V., & Wheatley, C. J. (2006). Evaluation and treatment of cognitive dysfunction. In: H. Pendleton, & W. Schultz-Krohn (eds.), *Pedretti's occupational therapy: Practice skills for physical dysfunction* (6th ed.). St Louis, MO: Mosby.

Golding, E. (1989). *The Middlesex elderly assessment of mental state*. Thames, England: Thames Valley Testing.

Goodglass, H., & Kaplan, E. (2002). *Assessment of aphasia and related disorders* (2nd ed.). Philadelphia, PA: Thomas.

Haines, D. E. (2012). *Fundamental neuroscience* (4th ed.). Philadelphia, PA: Churchill Livingstone.

Harrell, M., et al. (1992). *Cognitive rehabilitation of memory: A practical guide*. Gaithersburg, MD: Aspen.

Hartman-Maeir, A., Harel, H., & Katz, N. (2009). Kettle test—a brief measure of cognitive functional performance: reliability and validity in stroke rehabilitation. *The American Journal of Occupational Therapy, 63*(5), 592—599.

Head, H., et al. (1920). *Studies in neurology*. London, England: Oxford University Press.

Hécaen, H., & Albert, M. L. (1990). *Human neuropsychology*. New York, NY: Wiley.

Itzkovich, M., Averbuch, S., Elazar, B., & Katz, N. (2000). *Lowenstein occupational therapy cognitive assessment* (2nd ed.). Wayne, NJ: Maddak Inc.

Katz, N., Itzkovich, M., Averbuch, S., & Elazar, B. (1989). Lowenstein occupational therapy cognitive assessment (LOTCA) battery for brain-injured patients: reliability and validity. *The American Journal of Occupational Therapy, 43*(3), 184—192.

Kent, B. E. (1965). Sensory-motor testing: the upper limb of adult patients with hemiplegia. *Journal of the American Physical Therapy Association, 45*, 550.

Kiernan, R. J., et al. (1987). The Neurobehavioral Cognitive Status Examination: a brief but differentiated approach to cognitive assessment. *Annals of Internal Medicine, 107*(4), 481—485.

Krotoski, J. B. (2011). Sensibility testing: history, instrumentation and clinical procedures. In: T. M. Skirven, A. L. Osterman, J. Fedorczyk, & P. C. Amadio (eds.), *Rehabilitation of the hand and upper extremity* (6th ed.). Philadelphia, PA: Elsevier.

Lezak, M. D. (1995). *Neuropsychological assessment* (3rd ed.). New York, NY: Oxford University Press.

Lezak, M. D., et al. (2004). *Neuropsychological assessment* (4th ed.). London, England: Oxford University Press.

Mayo Clinic and Mayo Foundation. (1998). *Clinical examinations in neurology* (7th ed.). Philadelphia, PA: WB Saunders.

McCarthy, R. A., & Warrington, E. K. (1990). *Cognitive neuropsychology: A clinical introduction*. San Diego, CA: Academic.

Miller, N. (1986). *Dyspraxia and its management*. Rockville, MD: Aspen.

Montgomery, P. C. (1991). *Perceptual issues in motor control. Contemporary management of motor control problems. Proceedings of the II STEP conference*. Alexandria, VA: Foundation for Physical Therapy.

Morrison, T. M., Giles, G. M., Ryan, J. D., Baum, C. M., Dromerick, A. W., Polatajko, H. J., et al. (2013). Multiple errands test—revised (MET—R): a performance-based measure of executive function in people with mild cerebrovascular accident. *The American Journal of Occupational Therapy, 67*(4), 460—468.

Neistadt, M. E. (1988). Occupational therapy for adults with perceptual deficits. *The American Journal of Occupational Therapy, 42*(7), 434—440.

Pedretti, L. W., & Early, M. B. (2001). *Occupational therapy: practice skills for physical dysfunction* (5th ed.) St Louis, MO: Mosby.

Pendleton, H., & Schultz-Krohn, W. (2006). *Pedretti's occupational therapy: Practice skills for physical dysfunction* (6th ed.). St Louis, MO: Mosby.

Reese, N. B. (2005). *Muscle and sensory testing* (2nd ed.). Philadelphia, PA: WB Saunders.

Rustad, R. A., et al. (1993). *The Cognitive Assessment of Minnesota*. San Antonio, TX: Pearson.

Sauget, J., Benton, A. L., & Hécaen, H. (1971). Disturbances of the body scheme in relation to language impairment and hemispheric locus of lesion. *Journal of Neurology, Neurosurgery, and Psychiatry, 34*, 496.

Shumway-Cook, W., & Woollacott, M. H. (2011). *Motor control theory: Translating research into clinical practice* (4th ed.). Baltimore, MD: Lippincott Williams & Wilkins.

Silverman, E. H., & Elfant, I. L. (1979). Dysphagia: an evaluation and treatment program for the adult. *The American Journal of Occupational Therapy, 33*(6), 382—392.

Sivan, A. B. (1991). *The Benton Visual Retention Test manual* (5th ed.). San Antonio, TX: Pearson.

Teng, E., & Chui, H. (1987). The modified mini-mental state (3MS) examination. *Journal of Clinical Psychology., 48*(8), 314—318.

Toglia, J. P. (1993a). Attention and memory. In: C. B. Royeen (Ed.), *AOTA self study series: Cognitive rehabilitation*. Rockville, MD: American Occupational Therapy Association.

Toglia, J. P. (1993b). *The contextual memory test manual*. San Antonio, TX: Pearson.

Walsh, K. (1987). *Neuropsychology: A clinical approach*. Edinburgh, Scotland: Churchill Livingstone.

Warren, M. (1981). Relationship of constructional apraxia and body scheme disorders to dressing performance in adult CVA. *The American Journal of Occupational Therapy, 35*(7), 431—437.

Webster, R. E. (1992). *The learning efficiency test* (2nd ed.). Novato, CA: Academic Therapy.

Werner, J. L., & Omer, G. E. (1970). Evaluating cutaneous pressure sensation of the hand. *The American Journal of Occupational Therapy, 24*(5), 347—356.

Wilson, B., Cockburn, J., & Baddeley, A. (1985). *The Rivermead Behavioural Memory Test*. Suffolk, England: Thames Valley Testing.

Wilson, B., Greenfield, E., Clare, L., Baddeley, A., Cockburn, J., Watson, P., et al. (2008). *Behavioral memory test* (3rd ed.). San Antonio, TX: Pearson.

Wilson, B. A., & Moffat, N. (2014). *Clinical management of memory problems* (2nd ed.), London, England: Chapman and Hall.

RECOMMENDED READING

Gardner, M. F. (2009). *The Test of Visual Perceptual Skills Revised (TVPS-R)*. Burlingame, CA: Psychological and Educational Publications.

Shumway-Cook, W., & Woollacott, M. H. (2011). *Motor control theory: Translating research into clinical practice*. 4th ed. Baltimore, MD: Lippincott Williams & Wilkins.

PART IV

Intervention Principles

10

Teaching and Learning
Motor Performance in Occupational Therapy

Jane Clifford O'Brien and Jean W. Solomon

INTRODUCTION

Teaching and learning are essential to the occupational therapy process. **Learning** takes place within the learner and can be defined as the acquisition of skills or information that changes a person's motor skills, behavior, attitudes, insights, or perceptions. Teaching refers to the process of instructing and helping other people acquire information and/or skills. Understanding how to best teach clients so they learn more effectively strengthens occupational therapy intervention and results in improved outcomes for clients.

Occupational therapy assistants (OTAs) teach clients motor skills by structuring the environment as well as designing and guiding the experiences that facilitate improved motor performance (e.g., gross and fine motor skills, balance, and coordination) necessary to complete one's desired occupations. OTAs instruct clients in the movement and skills that facilitate independence and occupational performance.

In this chapter, the authors explore the concepts of motor control and motor learning and the application of these concepts to occupational therapy intervention. The authors provide an overview of dynamic systems theory. They delineate the stages and types of motor learning. They outline the motor learning principles and strategies (i.e., meaningfulness, transfer of learning, feedback, distribution and variability of skill practice, and mental practice) that inform techniques to teach clients movement. The authors review the teaching-learning process to facilitate occupational performance. Case vignettes, examples, and clinical pearls are used throughout to emphasize key concepts.

Dynamic Systems Theory

Dynamic systems theorists propose that movement is the result of the interaction among multiple systems (e.g., neurologic, cardiovascular, respiratory, skeletal, muscular), which include movement expectations (e.g., activity demands, object characteristics, speed, accuracy) and environmental contexts (e.g., physical setting, social, cultural expectations). Fig. 10.1 illustrates many of the systems influencing movement. OTAs consider multiple systems and the unique interactions between systems when creating intervention plans to address occupational performance. The OTA analyzes movement using a dynamic system view by

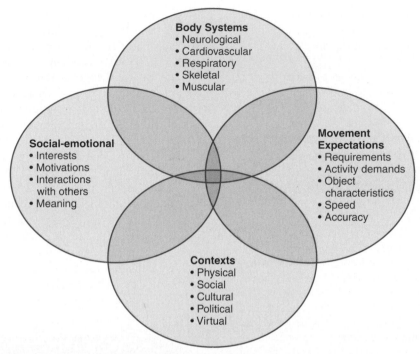

Body Systems
- Neurological
- Cardiovascular
- Respiratory
- Skeletal
- Muscular

Social-emotional
- Interests
- Motivations
- Interactions with others
- Meaning

Movement Expectations
- Requirements
- Activity demands
- Object characteristics
- Speed
- Accuracy

Contexts
- Physical
- Social
- Cultural
- Political
- Virtual

Fig. 10.1 Movement is the result of the interactions among multiple systems.

CASE 10.1

A client has difficulty reaching with her right upper extremity (R UE) after a stroke. In therapy, the OTA engages her in a variety of repetitive tasks to reach for points on the wall. She is frustrated and tearful. Her phone rings just out of reach on the table near her right side. The client stops what she is doing and reaches forward with her R UE and pushes the phone so she can pick it up with her left upper extremity (L UE). This example illustrates the role of meaning, activity demands, and environmental support on motor performance. Specifically, the client is motivated to get her phone rather than pointing to a spot on the wall. She problem-solves and adapts to get her phone. She uses her physical environment (i.e., the table) to assist her and has adequate movement to succeed by moving in a different way.

---

examining the interactions between the individual, task, and environment. This type of viewpoint requires that the OTA embrace the complexity of human occupational performance. Case 10.1 provides an example of this concept.

The OTA explores how the characteristics and limitations of each learner influence the content and speed of learning in relationship to the specific task and the **context** in which the task occurs. Importantly, OTAs view the client holistically and attend to the client's motivations, habits, routines, previous experiences, along with physical, social-emotional, and environmental factors when designing intervention to address motor performance. Targeting multiple systems and the interactions between them results in improved motor performance (Armstrong, 2012). Approaches targeting one system (e.g., reflexes, strength training) have been found to be less effective at improving motor control for occupational performance.

Occupational therapy models consistent with dynamic systems theory include Kielhofner's Model of Human Occupation (Taylor & Kielhofner, 2017); Person-Environment-Occupation-Participation (PEOP) model (Bass, et al., 2017; Baum et al., 2015); and the Canadian Model of Occupational Performance and Engagement (CMOP-E) (Canadian Association of Occupational Therapists, 1997). Each model emphasizes the complex interactions among multiple systems as affecting occupational performance. See Box 10.1 for a summary of occupational therapy models that are consistent with dynamic systems theory. The following case vignette (Maureen) exemplifies how the interactions between multiple systems as proposed in dynamic systems theory inform occupational therapy practice. Fig. 10.2 describes some of the factors within the systems influencing Maureen's occupational performance.

Case Vignette: Maureen. Maureen is a 75-year-old woman with diabetes, congestive heart failure, and difficulty walking due to arthritis in both knees. She lives at home with her husband of 50 years, who is accustomed to Maureen's care; their children live in another state. Maureen wants to prepare meals for her husband and herself.

The OTA considers the home environment, location of the kitchen, meal requirements for a diabetic client, and the meaning that Maureen ascribes to preparing meals. The context of meal preparation has significant social value for Maureen and her husband. The OTA cannot assume that all clients hold meal preparation to the same standard. For example, Maureen's daughter requires her husband make his own meal, which typically consists of a microwave dinner.

The OTA in collaboration with the occupational therapist (OT) conducts an activity analysis of meal preparation, which reveals multiple factors that influence Maureen's occupational performance. The OTA uses information from the analysis to develop an intervention plan by considering the individual, task, and environment.

Maureen must use cognitive processes to select the menu, prepare the recipe, time the cooking, and sequence the steps required to make a meal. Maureen must use motor functions to grip a knife, cut food, stir, spread, lift, and turn. She must show adequate standing balance to move around her kitchen and adequate strength and endurance to complete meal preparation. The OTA carefully considers the individual (what abilities and challenges Maureen possesses regarding physical, processing, and social interactions), the task (steps and client factors required for success), and the environment (e.g., social, cultural, personal, physical setup). Furthermore, the OT evaluates Maureen's cardiac performance for endurance and musculoskeletal functioning for strength, positioning, and coordination. The OT and OTA consider the neurologic aspects influencing performance (e.g., the influence of muscle tone, timing, sensation and perception, and movement quality on performance). The OT and OTA hypothesize how Maureen's strengths and challenges in a variety of areas influence her ability to engage in meal preparation. The OT and OTA use this information to determine if Maureen requires accommodations, adaptations, or remediation of motor skills to be successful in meal preparation and to design intervention activities.

BOX 10.1 Occupational Therapy Practice Models That Include Dynamic Systems Theory Concepts

- Model of Human Occupation (MOHO): Kielhofner's model examines the client's occupational performance in terms of volition (i.e., values, interests, personal causation), habituation (i.e., habits and roles), and performance capacity (i.e., physical, cognitive, social-emotional) within certain environmental contexts (i.e., physical, social, institutional, societal, virtual) (Taylor, 2017).
- Person-Environment-Occupation-Participation (PEOP): The PEOP examines person factors (i.e., physical, neurologic, orthopedic), environments (i.e., constraints and affordances), occupations (e.g., everyday things that people do that provide them meaning and quality of life), and participation (e.g., what a person is capable and desires to do) (Bass et al., 2017; Baum et al., 2015).
- Canadian Occupational Model of Performance and Engagement (COMP-E): The COMP-E examines the person, environment, and occupations within the context of spirituality (e.g., those things of which the person finds meaning and purpose). The model examines the interaction and influences of its components and how they influence occupational engagement (Canadian Association of Occupational Therapists, 1997).

CLINICAL PEARL

The task demands vary between washing hands at home versus washing hands in a restroom at an unfamiliar restaurant. At an unfamiliar setting, the client must problem-solve how to turn on the water and locate the towel. The client may need to complete different movements (push vs pull lever) and reach differently while standing to get the towel. The client may not have the physical support (such as grab bars) that is offered in a familiar setting. Therefore the OTA and OT consider how environment influences a client's occupational performance when creating and carrying out intervention plans.

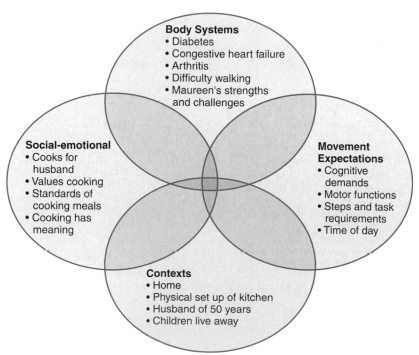

Fig. 10.2 Schematic of systems influencing Maureen's occupatioal performance.

MOTOR LEARNING

Motor learning refers to the acquisition of motor skills. It is a set of processes associated with practice or experience leading to neurologic and physical changes in the capability for responding (Schmidt & Wrisberg, 2008). In other words, motor learning is an internal neurologic process through which motor skills are acquired, refined, and become automatic while a person is engaged in daily occupations and activities. The desired outcome of motor learning is a permanent change in motor behavior or skill as a result of practice and experience. This change in behavior leads to improved neuroplasticity that is at first specific to the activity learned but in time generalizes to similar tasks in different environments. The goal of motor learning is for clients to perform meaningful activities in a variety of environments, under a variety of conditions. Motor learning addresses how one acquires motor skills and includes strategies to use in practice to teach movement required for occupational performance. The OTA considers the client's stage in the learning process when selecting the motor learning strategy.

Stages of Motor Learning

The stages of motor learning include cognitive, associative, and autonomous (Fitts & Posner, 1967). OTAs may work with clients at each stage. The OTA uses different motor learning strategies according to the stage of the client. Table 10.1 provides examples of intervention suggestions corresponding to the stage of motor learning. The following case vignette (Virgil) illustrates the stages.

Case Vignette: Virgil. Virgil is a 45-year-old male who owns a small construction company. He is married and has a 12-year-old child. Virgil's wife is a stay-at-home mom and is actively involved in community activities and her church. Recently, Virgil injured his right hand (dominant/preferred hand) while working on renovations of a neighbor's house.

TABLE 10.1   Stages of Motor Learning With Examples

Stage	Example
Cognitive	Adult learning to dance; older person who had a stroke learning to brush his teeth again; person with LE amputation learning to move around the house
Associative	Adult remembering similar movements in previous dance routine; older person picking up familiar toothbrush; person with LE amputation noticing how nice it feels to be back home
Autonomous	Adult dancing routine flawless even when the music suddenly skips; older person quickly adjusting the water temperature; person with LE amputation moving easily around the house even when the cat passes unexpectedly in front of him

Virgil receives occupational therapy intervention three times weekly at an outpatient occupational therapy clinic. As a result of his hand injury, Virgil has minimal movement of his right wrist and digits 1 through 3 (thumb, index, and middle fingers).

In the beginning stages of motor learning, individuals rely on cognition to guide movement. Frequently clients in the **cognitive stage** of learning "talk and think through" the steps. This requires more time and effort to complete the task. This stage may also be referred to as the **skill acquisition stage** as the client understands the idea of the movement but has not learned it. Errors are common, and performance is inefficient and inconsistent. Clients who are at the cognitive or skill acquisition stage respond well to simple directions of one to three words that the learner can repeat. The OTA provides the key words and allows the client to complete the task using those same words to learn the movement. During this stage, the OTA is not concerned with quality of movement but the steps and overall sequence of movement. For example, the OTA may emphasize that Virgil "bend," "straighten," or "make a fist." As Virgil bends and straightens his fingers, he repeats the verbal commands.

In the **associative stage** (also referred to as the **skill refinement stage**), the learner makes connections to previous experiences. As the client moves to this stage, he or she demonstrates improved performance, fewer and less significant errors, and increased consistency and efficiency of the movement. OTAs working with clients who are at this stage may use analogies (Bobrownicki et al., 2019; Tse et al., 2017) or familiar experiences to teach or reteach a client movement. For example, they may relate the activity to a previous pattern, such as reminding Virgil that the movement of wrist and fingers during an activity to wind up toys in the clinic (allowing him to perform the movement with little resistance) is similar to how he uses a screwdriver at work.

In the final **autonomous** or **skill retention stage**, the learner no longer thinks consciously about movements but can perform quickly and efficiently while adjusting to required changes to achieve functional goals. The objective at this stage is to retain the skill and transfer that skill to different settings. In these varied contexts, clients must modify the timing, force, sequencing, balance, postural integrity, and ongoing excitation of neurons in the brainstem and the spinal motor neurons (the motor pool) to succeed at the task. This achievement may be considered motor problem solving and is a hallmark of true motor learning. The OTA focuses on the client's quality of movement at this stage and provides opportunities to practice in a variety of situations and environments. The OTA may suggest small changes to refine movement difficulties or ask the client to identify what went well and how he/she may improve performance next time.

For example, Virgil uses a screwdriver to complete a small craft construction project in the clinic. He adjusts his motor skills to manipulate the screwdriver to handle different types of screws and positions of screws. Upon completion, he reflects on the quality of his movements and work, by stating "I think I need to retighten this screw."

Types of Motor Learning

OTAs and OTs engage clients in procedural or declarative learning. Each type demands different intervention strategies. **Procedural learning** involves mastering movements or techniques. It refers to learning how to do something. Examples include riding a bike, transferring from a wheelchair to a bed, or putting on a shirt. OTAs include demonstrative instruction followed by practice and feedback to help clients with procedural learning. Procedural learning involves practice of how to perform and is acquired through experience (Knowlton et al., 2017).

Declarative learning, on the other hand, depends more on memory of facts or events (ten Berge & van Hezewijk, 1999). Declarative learning can be verbalized or put it into words, and therefore it is more easily remembered. This type of learning identifies relationships. Learning to use a computer is an example of declarative learning as one can explain the concepts and steps. Getting dressed from start to finish is another example.

The areas of the brain involved in the storage and retrieval of motor and cognitive information as related to procedural and declarative knowledge are different (Knowlton et al., 2017; Quintero-Gallego et al., 2006). Often motor skills are first learned in a declarative way (using words and rules about movement) and later become procedural (using experiences and practice). For example, a client learns the motor steps to assemble a birdhouse (declarative) and later can perform the movements on his own (procedural) (Fig. 10.3).

Declarative learning fits within the cognitive stage of learning because learners talk through the sequence. For example, tying shoelaces or typing at a keyboard first requires intense concentration on the sequence of the steps, which may be verbalized and remembered through declarative learning. Once learned, however, speed and efficiency of movement are possible only when the person operates on a procedural level, without conscious control or attention.

Motor Learning Principles

Principles serve as guidelines for how to structure intervention. Box 10.2 lists motor learning principles. Research suggests that clients learn movements more easily if they are meaningful, practiced as a whole (vs part), and practiced in the natural context (which promotes variability and problem solving) (Hetu & Mercier, 2012; Ikudome et al., 2019; Muratori et al., 2013; Trombly, 1995). The natural context provides contextual cues that may assist the client in performing the movement. Using actual objects promotes quality of movement and enhances motor control. For example, Fig. 10.4 shows a client who loves to garden who is not able to use both sides effectively after her stroke. The client used both

---

BOX 10.2 **Principles of Motor Learning**

- Meaningful repetition (practice) promotes neuroplasticity.
- Natural contexts provide variability, which facilitates learning.
- Whole learning is preferred over part-task learning.
- Use of motor learning strategies may improve performance and learning.
- Intensity (more repetitions of movement in occupation over a short period of time promotes neuroplasticity).
- Motor performance is the result of an interaction of a variety of systems.
- People will perform movements that are intrinsically motivating and meaningful to them with more repetitions and better quality.

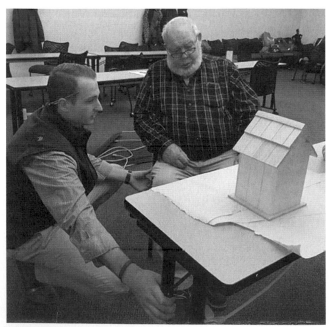

Fig. 10.3 A client learns the motor steps to assemble a birdhouse (declarative) and later is able to perform the movements on his own (procedural). (Courtesy Jane O'Brien.)

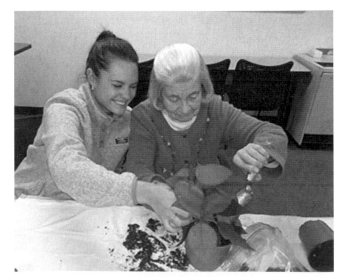

Fig. 10.4 A client who loves to garden is not able to use both sides effectively after her stroke. (Courtesy Jane O'Brien.)

upper extremities more effectively when provided with actual objects (such as soil and a plant). The client moved more quickly and was eager to complete the task although it was difficult for her. She remarked on the smell of the soil and how that reminded her of her own garden. Research suggests that intervention whereby the client is engaged in the actual occupation is superior to task-based or component-based intervention strategies (Bovend Eerdt et al., 2012; Fontana et al., 2009; Ikudome et al., 2019; Jarus & Ratzon 2005; Rapolienė et al., 2018). For example, strength training may not have the benefits of engaging the client in an occupation-based intervention. While a certain degree of strength is required to perform basic motor skills, OTAs and OTs must be mindful that engagement in meaningful, whole activities within the natural contexts (i.e., occupations) produces longer lasting results (Bovend Eerdt et al., 2012; Fontana et al., 2009; Hetu & Mercier, 2012; Ikudome et al., 2019; Jarus & Ratzon, 2005; Rapolienė et al., 2018). While some task-based interventions may be helpful during the cognitive stage of learning or as prerequisites for movement, OTAs should move to occupation-based interventions for best outcomes.

Motor Learning Strategies

Motor learning strategies are evidence-based techniques based on principles that promote motor control. Research supports the use of motor learning strategies to improve motor performance (as measured by accuracy, improved muscle co-contractions, increased repetitions of movement, and improved participation in daily activities) (Bobrownicki et al., 2019; Bovend Eerdt et al., 2012; Hung et al., 2017; Ikudome et al., 2019; Liu et al., 2004; Muratori et al., 2013; Niemeijer et al., 2006; Rapolienė et al., 2018). The *Occupational Therapy Motor Learning Strategies Worksheet* (O'Brien, 2020) (Table 10.2) was developed from the 2006 Williams (Williams et al., 2006) compilation of motor strategies. This tool may be useful in reinforcing concepts for use in practice. Occupational therapy students found the worksheet useful for implementing intervention plans (O'Brien & Patnaude, in press).

Meaningfulness. Occupational therapists have long recognized the powerful impact that meaning has upon a person's ability to perform (Fisher, 1998; Kielhofner, 2008; Trombly, 1995). It is well documented that people perform better (as measured by improved co-contractions, muscle synergies, and accuracy) when engaging in those things for which they attribute meaning or purpose (Rapolienė et al., 2018). Occupational therapists seek to understand what clients find meaningful so they can use these activities to promote motor skills. For example, a 76-year-old client, Max, was diagnosed with chronic schizophrenia in his late 20s. Max was a football player in high school and attributed purpose, memories, and feelings of competence to football. One day in group session, the OTA brought in a football instead of a beachball. Max became engaged in the session and threw the football further and with more accuracy than the beachball. He smelled the

ball, felt the ball, and ascribed meaning to it. He sat upright and told a story of how he played football in high school. This example shows the power of finding activities that are meaningful and despite months of throwing the beachball around in group, things changed when the client was reunited with a familiar pastime. Neurologically, the smell and touch of the football may have activated areas of the brain (such as the hippocampus, which is associated with previous emotionally laden memories).

> **CLINICAL PEARL**
>
> Meaningfulness refers to the value a person ascribes to an activity. Asking clients what they like to do and what activities mean to them allows OTAs to use this information to design effective intervention. Engaging clients in conversations and stories may help OTAs understand what is meaningful for each client.

Transfer of Learning

Transfer of learning or generalization refers to the ability to perform skills in the natural context. For example, a client may be able to walk to the lunchroom, buy a sandwich, and sit down at a table at the rehabilitation center. However, the same client is not able to walk to a nearby café, buy a sandwich, and sit down at a table with strangers nearby due to the additional environmental stimuli and requirements. As it turns out the flat surface and short distance at the clinic is not equivalent to the rocky path filled with people passing that the client must navigate once home. The busy café requires the client to adjust and adapt movements quickly while attending to sounds and sights.

Generalization, or transfer of learning, occurs more readily with practice in different contexts. Transfer enables an individual to perform similar tasks in a new context by drawing on experience. This ability indicates not only that the skill can be performed in a single situation, but it has been acquired and retained; this point is considered the **motor retention stage** of motor learning. For example, the client who learns to sponge-bathe the upper body in the hospital lavatory and can perform the task in the bathroom in his or her own home has transferred the learning to a new context. Although the motor skills and the practice environment are not identical in the new context, the memory of performing the required motor skills in a similar environment enables the client to perform the task.

Practice under variable conditions, with actual objects, and at the time it naturally occurs, increases generalization of learning to new situations. Dressing training, for example, can occur in the client's room some of the time and in the occupational therapy clinic's activities of daily living (ADL) area at other times. Using various types of clothing requiring similar motor patterns may reinforce generalizability. For example, the OTA may require the client put on shorts or different styles of trousers when practicing dressing. Training should occur in the environment most appropriate and most realistic for the task being performed (e.g., dressing in one's room in the morning or getting ready for bed).

TABLE 10.2 Occupational Therapy Motor Learning Strategies Worksheet

Category	Strategy	Description of Observations
Meaning	• Skill has meaning or purpose to client. • Client expresses interest in skills/chooses activities and skills. • Client acknowledges abilities and self-efficacy (belief in skills). • Client shows pleasure in activity. • Client wants to demonstrate skill.	
Transfer of Learning	• Skill experiences are presented in logical progression. • Simple, foundational skills are practiced before more complex skills. • Skill practice includes real-life and simulated settings. • Skills with similar components are more likely to show transfer effect. • Practice in natural context with actual objects is most effective.	
Feedback *Modeling or Demonstration*	• Demonstration is best if it is given to the individual before practicing the skill and in the early stages of skill acquisition. • Demonstration should be given throughout practice and as frequently as deemed helpful. • Allow client time to "figure it out."	
Feedback *Verbal Instructions*	• Verbal cues should be brief, to the point, and involve one to three words. • Verbal cues should be carefully timed to not interfere with performance. • Verbal cues should emphasize key aspects of movement. • Use of analogies may help when client is in associative stage of learning.	
Knowledge of Results (KR) and Knowledge of Performance (KP)	• Utilize a variety of both KR and KP to facilitate learning. • It is important to balance between feedback that is error-based and that which is based on "appropriate" or "correct" characteristics of the performance. • KP feedback can be descriptive or prescriptive. • KP and KR should be given close in time to but after completion of the task, but not necessarily given 100% of the time. • Learning is enhanced if KP/KR are given at least 50% of the time.	
Distribution and Variability of Skill Practice	• Shorter, more frequent practice sessions are preferable to longer, less frequent practice. • If a skill or task is complex, frequent rest periods are preferable. • It can enhance skill acquisition to practice several tasks in the same session. • Providing several different environmental contexts in which the skill is practiced facilitates learning. • Clinical judgment should be used to recognize when practice is no longer producing changes; at this time a new or different task should be introduced. • Consider intensity of training (short periods of training more frequently).	
Whole Versus Part Practice	• Whole practice may be preferable when the skill/task is simple; part practice may be preferable when the skill is more complex. • If part practice is used, be sure that the parts practiced are "natural units" that go together. • To simplify a task, reduce the nature and/or complexity of the objects to be manipulated (e.g., use a balloon for catching instead of a ball). • To simplify a task, provide assistance to the learner that helps to reduce attention demands (e.g., provide trunk support during practice of different eye-hand coordination tasks). • To simplify a task, provide auditory or rhythmic accompaniment; this may facilitate learning through assisting the learner in getting the appropriate "rhythm" of the movement.	
Mental Practice	• Mental practice helps to facilitate acquisition of new skills as well as the relearning of old skills. • Mental practice helps the person to prepare to perform a task; it should be relatively short, not prolonged. • Mental practice combined with physical practice works best.	
Intensity	• Provide challenging movements. • Allow client to repeat movements in a short time (many durations in short time). • Provide opportunity for self-reflection.	

Revised from O'Brien J. Box 16.5 Occupational therapy motor learning strategies worksheet. In: O'Brien J, Kuhaneck H, eds. *Case-Smith's Occupational Therapy for Children and Adolescents.* 8th ed. St. Louis, MO: Elsevier; 2020:405.

Feedback

Feedback and reinforcement are closely connected. Confirmation of successful responses encourages the person to continue learning. People respond best to thoughtful constructive feedback delivered in a nonthreatening and honest manner. False praise can be confusing. The person also needs feedback during the learning process to recognize mistakes and modify performance. In a motor task, however, external reinforcement may override intrinsic mechanisms and not allow for innate self-correction. When extrinsic feedback is used to assist in motor learning, feedback should be realistic, honest, and appropriate to the task (e.g., the OTA does not need to exclaim loudly in superlatives when a shoe has been tied effectively). A more appropriate reinforcer would be a low-key, positive statement that the lace is correctly tied and will effectively keep the shoe on the foot. Similarly, if the motor performance will not reach the identified goal, the OTA might suggest an alternative plan of action and repeat the instruction, possibly using a different sensory mode.

Modeling or Demonstration.
OTAs use modeling or demonstration to help clients see the desired action. Demonstration is most effective when it is given before the client practices the skill and in the early stages of skill acquisition. Demonstration should be provided as needed but should not be accompanied by verbal commentary. The OTA uses simple verbal instructions to direct the client's attention to critical cues before the skill is demonstrated.

Verbal Instructions.
Verbal instructions provide learners with cues to perform that may help them recall movement patterns for later. Verbal instructions should be brief (one to three key words), highlight the main cues, and be carefully timed. Verbal cues should be used for major aspects of the movement and repeated so that the client can use these cues. OTAs should limit verbal cues, especially when the client is performing the movement, and allow the client to experience the movement.

Intrinsic and Extrinsic Feedback.
Information about whether a movement has been successful in acting on the environment is a critical ingredient in motor learning. If learners do not receive the intrinsic feedback necessary to estimate the success of their own motor performance, learning may be poor or not occur at all.

The learner receives intrinsic feedback as a natural consequence of performing the task (Schmidt & Wrisberg, 2008). Intrinsic feedback arises from sensory stimulation to tactile receptors, proprioceptors, and visual and vestibular systems. Intrinsic feedback occurs during performance of the task (i.e., information about the movements) and after the task is completed (i.e., results of the action). This feedback may be processed at a preconscious level within the central nervous system. Preconscious processing allows the client to determine whether the motor patterns selected for task accomplishment were accurate or need refinement.

For example, a client putting on a shirt receives knowledge of performance when he or she can feel the movements of joints and muscles and the sensation of the shirt on the skin as the task progresses. The client can sense whether arms and hands are in the correct position to grasp the edge of the shirt or to push an arm through a sleeve. He or she can feel the fabric on the arms and trunk and thus knows whether a sleeve is pulled up over the shoulder. When the task is completed, the client can see the results by looking in the mirror and seeing that the shirt is properly adjusted, the buttons are buttoned, and the collar is lying flat. The client receives intrinsic feedback that the motor actions are successful. Clients with a variety of neurologic, orthopedic, or emotional conditions may have difficulty with intrinsic feedback interfering with movement.

Feedback about performance from an outside source (e.g., OTA) or a mechanical device (e.g., virtual reality program) is called extrinsic feedback. For example, the OTA may inform the client that the shirt is on backwards or not correctly buttoned. Two types of extrinsic feedback are (1) knowledge of performance and (2) knowledge of results.

Knowledge of performance. Verbal feedback about the process or performance provides the client with information about the client's progress toward the motor goal. The OTA might say, "Raise your arm a little higher" or "Hold on to the edge of the shirt tightly." Feedback on knowledge of performance (KOP) informs the performer about the quality of movement and its effectiveness in achieving the goal.

Knowledge of results. The OTA provides feedback about the outcome, product, or results of the motor actions. The OTA might say, "The shirt is put on correctly; it looks neat, and each button is lined up with its buttonhole." Knowledge of results (KOR) may point out performance errors and facilitate the revision of movement patterns. For example, the OTA could point out that the buttons are not aligned with the correct buttonhole or that the body of the shirt is twisted to one side. The client then can revise the movement plan to correct the performance.

Feedback is essential to learning and enhances the learning process. Knowledge of performance is typically given more frequently than knowledge of results during intervention sessions because knowledge of performance is directed toward the process and quality of performance. Extrinsic feedback should be decreased over time to encourage the client to rely on intrinsic feedback. To facilitate intrinsic feedback, the OTA may decrease verbal feedback about the movement and ask the client for a description of the movement (i.e., quality, accuracy, speed, effectiveness). Providing clients time to reflect on the action helps to promote intrinsic feedback and improves performance (Gredin & Williams, 2016). For example, after a dressing activity the OTA may direct the client's attention to one aspect of the movement by asking, "How did you pull on your t-shirt?"

DISTRIBUTION AND VARIABILITY OF SKILL PRACTICE

Practice involves repetition of movements, which results in brain plasticity. OTAs seek to promote practice in natural environments, which require that the client adapt and generalize movements to a variety of situations. Research suggests that neuroplasticity occurs with high-intensity, repetitive practice that stimulates multiple areas of the brain as opposed to repetitive rote exercise (Bovend Eerdt et al., 2012; Gredin & Williams, 2016; Bryck & Fisher 2012). For example, adults with a stroke who performed high-intensity training showed better retention of motor skills than adults who did not engage in 15 minutes of high-intensity exercise (Nepveu et al., 2017). This strategy suggests that OTAs engage clients in meaningful repetitive practice adapted so the client challenges his or her abilities at a high intensity.

Blocked Practice

Blocked (massed) practice involves repeated performance of the same motor skill with a short break and then repetition of the same skill. For example, the client is asked to pick up a cup from the left side of the table and place it on a saucer on the right side. The client needs to solve the motor problem only once or twice and then repeat the same motor skill. If measured during the therapy session, performance improves faster with blocked practice but does not generalize to other settings. Blocked practice provides limited learning; once he or she learns the skill, the client does not need to attend to the task because it no longer requires novel solutions. No opportunity exists for alternative activities and the reformulation of the solution to the motor problem, a process that enhances long-term learning and retention.

In early learning or with confused individuals, blocked practice may be necessary to promote learning. The person needs to practice the same movements over and over to establish the motor pattern. For example, practicing with the same open-front shirt repeatedly before introducing a jacket or housecoat that requires similar movement patterns may be helpful at the outset. The OTA should introduce novelty, problem solving, and variability for best learning and generalization, but may use blocked practice at times.

Distributed Practice

Distributed practice refers to practice that is spaced out with short breaks. Clients may practice multiple skills in each session over a longer period. Distributed practice may help clients learn complex movements better than massed practice (Kwon et al., 2015). For example, studying for short periods over a longer time is more effective for memorizing facts than trying to memorize facts the night before. Clients may benefit from rest periods when exerting themselves physically in the occupational therapy session. The OTA pays careful attention to client responses and the tasks that are required when determining the type of practice that is most beneficial.

Random Practice

Random practice occurs when several motor tasks are presented in random order and with random rest breaks. It involves the formulation of plans to solve new motor problems. This promotes motor learning because it introduces problem solving and variability. For example, the client may be asked to pick up cubes, buttons, and spheres in random order. The prehension (grasping) pattern for each is different. This variability requires that the client reformulate the solution to the motor problem each time a different object is approached. If motor skill acquisition is measured by performance during a random practice session, learning may not be as rapid as with the repetitive or blocked practice. However, the repeated regeneration of the solution to motor problems has been shown to be beneficial to retention (Schmidt & Wrisberg, 2008).

Whole Versus Part Practice

Simple and discrete tasks are learned best through **whole learning**, in which the client practices the entire task at one time. A transfer from wheelchair to bed would be considered a simple task and often can be learned as one procedure. Contrast this with learning the task in the following separate steps: (1) Lock the chair, (2) move weight forward to edge of chair, (3) shift weight over feet, (4) stand up, (5) pivot, and (6) sit down. By teaching six different steps or procedural programs as part of the transfer, the OTA increases the difficulty level unnecessarily.

Teaching tasks in steps is called **progressive-part learning**. Clients may learn intermediate skills and serial tasks more easily through progressive-part learning. For example, a dance step sequence might be considered an intermediate skill. It may require walking or stepping to a beat and various movements between and within limbs while moving on a diagonal and with a partner. If the dance has a specific sequence, learning the first few movements and then adding more steps, always starting from the beginning, is considered a progressive-part practice schedule.

Some skills can be learned through **pure-part learning**, whereby the part is learned alone. If the skill is cutting food on a plate, whether the individual cuts the meat or the vegetables first does not matter. All types of cutting are required; thus pure-part learning can be used.

Whole-to-part-to-whole learning refers to learning a part in the context of the whole and generally leads to the best retention when the client must learn a complex skill (Fontana et al., 2009). Putting on a necktie with one hand is an example of this type of skill. Knowing the whole while working on component parts helps with long-term retention. OTAs consider the client and activity demands when determining the learning approach to the task.

> **CLINICAL PEARL**
>
> Clients learn motor skills best when they are performing the actual occupation.

Occupation as Whole Learning. Motor learning research shows that the most useful motor learning occurs when the task resembles the actual task in that it is performed in a similar environment, with similar tools and requires the client adapt to a variety of situations (David & Nagaraj, 2016;

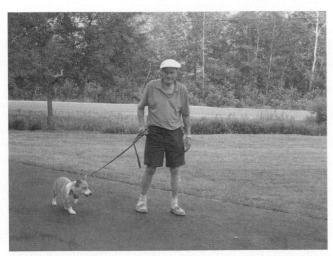

Fig. 10.5 An older man walking his dog, which he defined as a meaningful and important part of his daily routine (i.e., occupation). (Courtesy Jane O'Brien.)

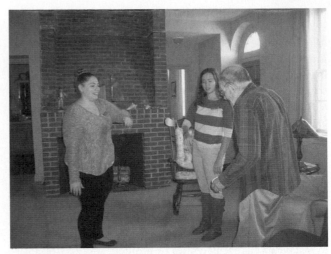

Fig. 10.6 For the older man who values walking his dog, the OTA may begin a session using stretching exercises. (Courtesy Jane O'Brien.)

Fontana et al., 2009; Hetu & Mercier, 2012; Jarus & Ratzon, 2005). Clients learn best when performing the actual **occupation** (Fisher, 1998). Occupation-based activities are those deemed meaningful to the client in terms of desired occupations in desired contexts. Occupation-based activities occur in the actual context and require the client to adapt to real situations. Fig. 10.5 shows an older man walking his dog, which he defined as a meaningful and important part of his daily routine (i.e., occupation).

In another example, caring for her children is an occupation to a young mother. Some tasks associated with this may include feeding the children, getting them ready for school, and reading to them. The OTA may visit the mother at home after school and ask that she feed the children a snack. This is considered an occupation-based activity.

Contrived activities may be used in clinical settings when replicating the exact occupation is impossible (Fisher, 1998). For example, the OTA may ask the mother to pretend she is making lunch for the children in the occupational therapy clinic. The closer the activity is to the actual experience, the more useful to learning. The OTA might make this activity more real by inviting the children to come in for lunch at the clinic.

Finally, **preparatory activities** include those activities that help the client perform the specific components of the motor tasks. These activities are the furthest from the occupation and thus should be used sparingly (Fisher, 1998). Furthermore, clients may struggle to connect these preparatory activities and their goals. For example, the OTA may decide that for the mother to begin to make her children lunch, she must show improved upper extremity control. The OTA may start therapy by performing upper extremity strengthening activities. For the older man who values walking his dog, the OTA may begin a session using stretching exercises (Fig. 10.6).

The goal of occupational therapy is for the client to perform the occupation in a variety of settings and under a variety of conditions. Thus clients benefit from practicing motor skills as they complete the desired occupation and in a variety of contexts.

Mental Practice

Mental practice involves imagery or rehearsing motor performance mentally. It is sometimes referred to as visualization, imagery, or mental rehearsal. Mental practice can help facilitate the acquisition of new skills and the relearning of old ones (Bovend Eerdt et al., 2012; Machado et al., 2019). It is most beneficial when combined with physical practice (David & Nagaraj, 2016; Malouin & Richards, 2010). Mental practice can be accomplished by requiring a client to review a videotape or watch a performance and then reflect on it before attempting it. Mental practice can involve visualizing oneself practicing the movement repeatedly. Liu et al. (2004) found that clients who experienced a stroke who used mental imagery were better able to generalize their skills to untrained tasks than the control group. OTAs are encouraged to examine this form of practice with clients as it can easily be accomplished and used as an adjunct to therapy. See Box 10.3 for strategies to promote motor learning using mental rehearsal.

TEACHING/LEARNING PROCESS

The teaching/learning process is a systematic problem-solving process designed to facilitate learning. The teaching/learning sequence, like the occupational therapy process (American Occupational Therapy Association, 2014), involves four basic elements: assessment, design of the plan, instruction, and feedback/evaluation.

Assessment

The OTA and OT assess characteristics of self, learner characteristics, learning needs, learning skills and style, and the situation during the client's evaluation. They examine client factors, including cognitive, perceptual, physical, and psychosocial, along with the client's attitudes, feelings, and emotional state in relation to occupational performance (American Occupational Therapy Association, 2014). Such information is essential for estimating the client's readiness for learning, planning appropriate intervention activities, and selecting methods of teaching.

Readiness for learning implies that the learner is prepared for the learning process and thus possesses the necessary cognitive, perceptual, and physical skills to perform and master the learning task. Assessment involves chart review, client and/or family interview, direct observation, and standardized or nonstandardized testing. The assessment information is used to understand the client's abilities, challenges, and goals. The OTA selects appropriate learning tasks and teaching methods to match the client's skills and abilities. The OTA may have to change activities to promote success, while also ensuring that the client engages in problem-solving and adapts to changes.

Design of Teaching Plan

The OT is responsible for synthesizing the assessment information and planning intervention. Specific learning or intervention objectives are written with the client and/or family's input. The OTA and OT collaborate on the intervention plan activities. Specifically, they decide on methods of instruction that suit the learner and environment (e.g., hospital, home, community).

In selecting intervention activities, the OTA considers the client's goals, interests, and sources of motivation as well as physical condition and environment. Motivation may be intrinsic or extrinsic. Intrinsic motivation is internally driven and self-initiated and occurs when the learner needs to know something and is ready to learn. Clients will perform with more intensity and practice movements more when they are intrinsically motivated (Ikudome et al., 2019; Jarus & Ratzon, 2005). Extrinsic motivation, on the other hand, comes from an external stimulus to act, such as the OTA deciding what the learner needs to learn and presenting this information. Extrinsic motivation requires more effort, concentration, and

time. Therefore OTAs and OTs create meaningful intervention that addresses those things the client finds intrinsically motivating. It is important to consider the intensity level of the intervention session designed to improve motor learning. The OTA creates intervention that challenges the client to problem-solve and perform at a slightly higher level each time.

OTAs consider the client's age, gender, interests, and cultural group when selecting relevant intervention activities. Clients are involved in the decision-making process, so the activities selected closely match the client's goals. Selecting activities that are relevant and meaningful to the client's life roles and family or social group ensures a higher level of motivation and participation than irrelevant activities (Taylor, 2017). The activities should be clearly related to the client's goals. Figs. 10.7–10.9 show some sample occupation-based

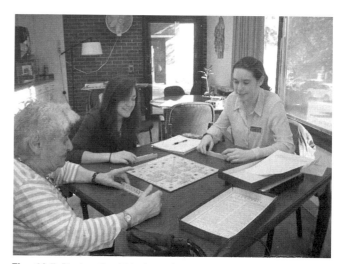

Fig. 10.7 Playing Scrabble is an important leisure activity for this client. The OTA addresses the client's motor and cognitive skills to play the game. (Courtesy Jane O'Brien.)

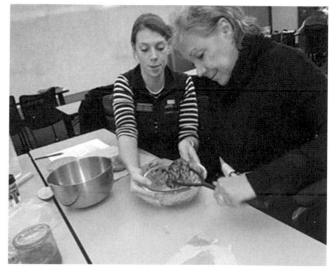

Fig. 10.8 The client makes a salad for lunch in her kitchen. The OTA addresses the client's motor and processing skills during this familiar occupation. (Courtesy Jane O'Brien.)

BOX 10.3 Suggested Strategies for Mental Rehearsal

- Demonstrate the movement in front of client. Ask client to picture completing the movement.
- Record the movement on video. Review the tape with the client, pointing out key aspects.
- Ask the client to reflect on the movement by visualizing oneself actually performing the activity.
- Work with the client to stop the visualization at key points and "correct" client's pattern.
- Ask the client to "picture" completing the movement in a variety of conditions.
- Once the client has "imagined" the movement, follow up with actually completing the movement.
- Intersperse periods of imagery with actual performance.
- Ask clients which strategies are most appealing to them.

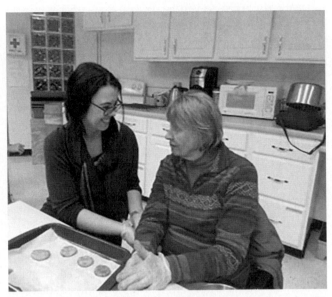

Fig. 10.9 Preparing cookies for her grandchildren is a favorite pastime. The OTA addresses the client's motor, sequencing, and memory. (Courtesy Jane O'Brien.)

BOX 10.4 **Intervention Plan**

Client's name:
Date of report:
Primary diagnosis:
Reason for referral to OT:
Occupational profile:
Interpretation (what is interfering with client's functioning in desired occupations?):
    Strengths:
    Challenges:
Intervention session:
- Expected frequency, duration, and intensity
- Location of intervention
- Anticipated discontinuation environment
- Precautions

Long-term goal
Short-term goals
    Activities to meet short-term goals:
    How can these activities be graded (easier or more challenging) for client?
Materials required:

---

intervention activities to promote daily occupations and motor performance. Otherwise, the OTA carefully describes how the activity will allow the client to resume important life activities. Box 10.4 provides an outline of an intervention plan (adapted from a lesson plan), which may help the OTA prepare for the session.

CLINICAL PEARL

Clients perform better and make more significant gains when intervention activities are meaningful to them and occupation based rather than rote and simulated activities.

Instruction

After creating meaningful goals and developing intervention activities that match the client's current performance level, the OTA selects specific activities to teach to the individual or group in an understandable and meaningful way. Repetition of instruction is important to the learning process. Clients will also learn from problem solving, asking questions, and revising performance based on feedback.

Clients are challenged to perform while still experiencing some success, which is referred to as the just-right challenge. Tasks that are too easy fail to help the client move to higher levels and those that are too difficult may frustrate the client. The OTA ensures that clients are pushing themselves at the right level through problem solving or physical activity. For example, allowing a client to reach a little further or struggle with a new movement may promote learning. Paying careful attention to the client's body position, breathing, and attention may help the OTA determine if it is necessary to assist.

Activities can be graded according to the complexity of their physical and cognitive demands and the levels of supervision and assistance provided by the therapist. Tasks are taught in a relevant environment and context. For example, practice

brushing one's hair is done as part of the normal morning hygiene activities in the client's bathroom rather than in the middle of the afternoon in the occupational therapy clinic.

The Teaching Process. The instruction phase of the teaching/learning process can be subdivided into four specific steps, which may be modified to match the client's needs.

Step 1: Preparation: Preinstruction phase. Preparation occurs before instruction. After the goals and objectives have been created based on the client's strengths and challenges and from assessment data, the OT and OTA plan the intervention session. They analyze potential intervention activities at this stage and consider the physical and cognitive demands by examining each step. Once the OT and OTA have selected the activities, the OTA prepares the environment for the therapy session (e.g., equipment, furniture, materials, space) before the client arrives.

Step 2: Demonstration: Motivation and instruction phase. The OTA puts the client at ease and introduces a meaningful and motivating activity that matches the client's needs. The OTA demonstrates the activity to the client one step at a time, using key words to emphasize important aspects of the movement. The OTA provides clear instructions and stresses key points. The OTA allows the client to ask questions and may ask the client to repeat the key points. The OTA is careful to present directions so the client can successfully master the movement. Some clients may require tactile and kinesthetic cues or gentle manual guidance along with verbal and demonstrative instruction.

Step 3: Return demonstration: Performance phase. Once the OTA has shown the activity to the client, the client performs the skill. The OTA observes the performance and corrects errors upon completion. The OTA may decide to allow some errors so that the corrections are not overwhelming to the client. The OTA may ask the client to repeat a portion of the activity after providing a few cues to allow the client to problem-solve and reflect on the performance. Asking reflective questions enables clients to use problem solving and to self-correct. For example, instead of saying to a client, "Next time, scoot up to the edge of your chair before getting up," the OTA may suggest, "Try getting up in different ways to see which way is easiest for you." Letting clients problem-solve empowers them and provides them with a sense of accomplishment.

Step 4: Follow-up: Guided independence phase. Once the client has completed the activity successfully, the OTA reinforces the movement by having the client complete the movement in a variety of situations and independently. The OTA may ask questions about aspects that need refining to see if the client can self-correct. The OTA may provide coaching to refine aspects of the movement or increase the speed or accuracy of the movement. Finally, the OTA may decide to add to the movement so the client may reach another goal.

Strategies Utilized in the Teaching Process

Pacing and grading instruction. Pacing refers to structuring the instruction and the practice so that learners progress at their own speed. Once the client is beyond the skill acquisition phase, distributing practice over time and spacing it with rests or alternative activities is more effective for retention than long periods of concentrated practice on the same task.

Tasks may be graded from simple to complex. Simple tasks are taught as a whole-movement activity (e.g., catching a ball). As movements become more complex (e.g., riding a bike), pure-part learning may be used. In pure-part learning, steps are taught singly; as each step is mastered, another step in the sequence is added to the learning process until the client masters the whole task (David & Nagaraj, 2016; Mathiowetz & Haugen, 1994).

One way to grade the client's independent performance of an activity is to use backward or forward chaining as a method of instruction. In backward chaining, the OTA assists the client through all steps of the activity and then allows the client to perform the last step independently. The activity is then graded to the last two steps, three steps, and so forth, until the client can perform the whole activity independently. The process is consistent with a whole-to-part-to-whole type of practice environment. In forward chaining, a similar process is used, except the OTA allows the client to perform the first step independently and then assists the client in performing the rest of the steps. Then the client performs the first two steps, then three steps, and so on, until the activity can be performed independently.

Active participation and repetition. Learning only occurs through active participation and repetition. Clients must be actively engaged in the movements, problem-solve how to complete the movements, and repeat them in the natural contexts. Learning is enhanced as the client experiences the visual, tactile, kinesthetic, and proprioceptive aspects of movement. The OTA designs activities to promote active engagement and problem solving in a variety of settings.

> **BOX 10.5** **Key Questions When Evaluating Effectiveness of the Teaching/Learning Process**
>
> - How did the intervention go?
> - Did the client succeed?
> - Was the client satisfied?
> - Did the client enjoy the activities?
> - Was the client interested and motivated in the session?
> - What went well?
> - What could have gone better?
> - Were treatment objectives achieved?
> - What was the extent or quality of achievement of specific objectives?

Feedback and Evaluation

Upon completion of the instruction, the OTA reflects upon the session—that is, what went well and what needs attention. The OTA considers the client's responses toward the intervention activities and progress toward the goals and adjusts for the next session. Progress can be evaluated by repeating tests that were administered on the initial evaluation or referring to the goals. The results can provide objective evidence of the effectiveness of intervention. The OTA also reflects upon his or her therapeutic use of self in relation to the intervention activities. The OTA questions how much feedback is provided, timing of feedback, clarity of instructions, choice of activities toward goals, and intensity of session. The OTA may ask for feedback from the client upon completion of the session. Box 10.5 lists questions that the OTA may use to evaluate the effectiveness of the teaching/learning process.

METHODS OF TEACHING

The OTA considers the client's cognitive level, perceptual functions, physical status, motivation, and goals of the intervention when choosing teaching methods. Occupational therapy intervention aims to allow clients to engage in their desired occupations. Teaching methods require different levels of perceptual and cognitive function and access one or more sensory systems in transmitting data to the cerebral cortex for information processing and execution of the motor plan. In therapy, the methods may be combined. The OTA finds the method that best suits the client's learning style and level of comprehension.

Teaching Through the Auditory System: Verbal Instruction

Verbal instructions are commonly used in occupational therapy intervention. The client must understand the words spoken, retain memory of the command, retrieve it from memory, and plan and execute the motor task associated with the instructions. Furthermore, the client's motivation to complete the movement may affect performance. Some clients may have difficulty following verbal instructions only (e.g., individuals with deficits in receptive language, auditory perception, auditory or visual memory, motor planning). Verbal instruction alone is generally the least effective method of teaching.

Teaching Through the Visual and Auditory Systems: Verbal Instruction and Demonstration

Demonstrating an activity while giving verbal instruction enhances learning. For example, the OTA brushes his or her own hair first and then asks the client to imitate the activity, in parallel or after the OTA finishes. This method of instruction relies less on receptive language and auditory memory skills. Instead, the client merely imitates motor acts of another person. Clients with motor-planning deficits (dyspraxia) will have difficulty imitating the OTA's demonstration. Poor visual or auditory memory may also hamper learning through this method of instruction.

Teaching Through Touch, Proprioception, and Motion

For clients who have difficulty following verbal and demonstrative instructions, the OTA may have success using tactile, proprioceptive, or movement stimuli to cue the client. The OTA may choose to provide no verbal guidance or to use short, simple commands. Some demonstration may also be appropriate. The OTA may say, "Brush your hair," then touch the client's hand and move the hand to the hairbrush. This gesture alone may be enough to cue the client to perform the task. If it is not, the OTA may lift the client's hand that is holding the hairbrush and simulate the movement pattern of hair brushing on the client's head. The feeling of the correct movements and the tactile cue to pick up the brush augment the auditory and visual input of the demonstration, which in many cases enhances learning. As learning occurs, the clinician may decrease the amount of guiding and use less intense sensory input.

Many occupational therapy intervention approaches use multisensory input in teaching motor skills. Providing tactile (touch) and proprioceptive (pressure) cues is helpful for clients with dyspraxia (difficulty with motor planning or thinking of and performing motor tasks) who cannot imitate movements or have forgotten motor patterns associated with common implements (e.g., hairbrush). Clients who have severe tactile and proprioceptive sensory losses (awareness and/or discrimination) or who resist being touched (tactile aversion or defensiveness) may not benefit from using tactile or proprioceptive approaches.

Case Application. Mary, the OTA, is working with Ken, a 35-year-old man who experienced a traumatic head injury resulting in poorly coordinated movements and balance deficits. Ken has three children and enjoys outside activity such as kayaking and hiking. He considers himself an "athlete." When planning his intervention, Mary carefully considers Ken's past occupations and what he finds meaningful. She works with him in occupational therapy on gathering the equipment for a hike with his children. Later she accompanies him outside for a short hike, and eventually she invites the children to come along. As Ken improves, Mary reduces her guidance and encourages and allows him to problem-solve solutions.

This case illustrates principles of motor learning and use of motor learning strategies. Mary has considered Ken's occupations and what he finds meaningful (children, hiking and kayaking). She guides Ken to relearn motor skills by engaging him in the tasks or actions associated with the occupations. For example, she works with him on gathering the equipment for a hike. This requires Ken to use motor skills and problem-solve, both important for motor learning and retention.

As they begin the hike, Mary provides physical guidance and verbal cues of the key points to remember. She is careful not to talk the entire way and allows Ken to receive intrinsic feedback of his performance.

Once Ken has succeeded in hiking without distractions, she invites the children to participate. This is close to the actual occupation, but she is still present to help him with his performance.

Mary skillfully used motor learning principles and strategies as she integrated Ken's occupations in her sessions.

SUMMARY

OTAs are concerned with the acquisition and retention of motor skills for occupational performance. Understanding the concepts of motor learning helps OTAs design effective intervention to help clients regain motor performance. For example, motor learning concepts may help an OTA determine whether and when to provide verbal feedback versus allowing the client to process the feedback internally. Motor learning strategies assist OTAs in remaining mindful of the type of task they present and in developing intervention plans that lead to occupation-based activity as the key to motor learning. Since teaching is an essential component of the intervention process, applying teaching and learning concepts to occupational therapy intervention allows OTAs to promote clients' learning.

SELECTED READING GUIDE QUESTIONS

1. Define motor learning.
2. What is the difference between procedural and declarative learning?
3. What is the difference between whole learning and progressive-part learning? Give examples, illustrating when it is appropriate to use each.
4. List and define the stages of motor learning.
5. Identify the different practice schedules and explain the conditions under which each is most effective.
6. How would you apply motor learning strategies in practice? Provide three examples.
7. List and define the steps in the teaching/learning process.

8. List three methods of teaching that use different sensory systems (e.g., auditory, visual, tactile, proprioceptive, and motion systems). For each method, describe how you would teach a client to use a spoon to eat mashed potatoes.

REFERENCES

American Occupational Therapy Association. (2014). Occupational therapy practice framework: domain and process. 3rd ed. *The American Journal of Occupational Therapy*, 68(1), S1–S48.

Armstrong, D. (2012). Examining the evidence for intervention with children with developmental coordination disorder. *British Journal of Occupational Therapy*, 75(12), 532–540.

Bass, J., Baum, C., & Christiansen, C. (2017). Person-environment-occupation-performance model. In J. Hinojosa, P. Kramer, & C. B. Royeen (eds.), *Perspective on human occupation theories underlying practice* (2nd ed.). Philadelphia, PA: FA Davis.

Baum, C., Christiansen, C., & Bass, J. (2015). Person-environment-occupation-performance (PEOP) model. In C. Christiansen, C. Baum, & J. Bass (eds.), *Occupational therapy: Performance, participation, well-being* (4th ed.). Thorofare, NJ: Slack.

Bobrownicki, R., MacPherson, A. C., Collins, D., & Sproule, J. (2019). The acute effects of analogy and explicit instruction on movement and performance. *Psychology of Sport and Exercise*, 44, 17–25.

Bovend Eerdt, T. J. H., Dawes, H., Sackley, C., & Wade, D. (2012). Practical research-based guidance for motor imagery practice in neurorehabilitation. *Disability and Rehabilitation*, 24(25), 2192–2200.

Bryck, R. L., & Fisher, P. A. (2012). Training the brain: practical applications of neural plasticity form the intersection of cognitive neuroscience, developmental psychology and prevention science. *The American Psychologist*, 67(2), 87–100.

Canadian Association of Occupational Therapists. (1997). *Enabling occupation: An occupational therapy perspective*. Ottawa, ON: CAOT Publications ACE.

David, N. S., & Nagaraj, A. (2016). Evaluate the effects of mental practice as compared to part/whole practice on rate of skill acquisition. *Indian Journal Physiotherapy Occupational Therapy*, 10(2), 160–164.

Fisher, A. G. (1998). Uniting practice and theory in an occupational framework: 1998 Eleanor Clarke Slagle Lecture. *The American Journal of Occupational Therapy*, 52(7), 509–521.

Fitts, P. M., & Posner, M. I. (1967). *Human performance*. Oxford, England: Brooks/Cole.

Fontana, F., Furtado, O., Mazzardo, O., & Gallagher, J. (2009). Whole and part practice: a meta-analysis. *Perceptual and Motor Skills*, 109, 517–530.

Gredin, V., & Williams, A. M. (2016). The relative effectiveness of various instructional approaches during the performance and learning of motor skills. *Journal of Motor Behavior*, 48(1), 86–97.

Helu, S., & Mercier, C. (2012). Using purposeful tasks to improve motor performance: does object affordance matter? *British Journal of Occupational Therapy*, 75(8), 367–376.

Hung, Y. C., Brandão, M. B., & Gordon, A. M. (2017). Structured skill practice during intensive bimanual training leads to better trunk and arm control than unstructured practice in children with unilateral spastic cerebral palsy. *Research in Developmental Disabilities*, 60, 65–76.

Ikudome, S., Kou, K., Ogass, K., Mori, S., & Nakamoto, H. (2019). The effect of choice on motor learning for learners with different levels of motivation. *Journal of Sport and Exercise Psychology*, 41, 159–166.

Jarus, T., & Ratzon, N. Z. (2005). The implementation of motor learning principles in designing prevention programs at work. *Work*, 24, 171–182.

Kielhofner, G. (2008). *Model of human occupation: Theory and application* (4th ed.). Philadelphia, PA: FA Davis.

Knowlton, B. J., Siegel, A. L. M., & Moody, T. D. (2017). Procedural learning in humans. In H. Eichenbaum (ed.), *Memory systems of learning and memory: A comprehensive reference* (2nd ed., pp. 295–312). Oxford, England: Elsevier Academic Press.

Kwon, Y. H., Kwon, J. W., & Lee, M. H. (2015). Effectiveness of motor sequential learning according to practice schedules in healthy adults: distributed practice versus massed practice. *Journal of Physical Therapy Science*, 27, 169–772.

Liu, K., Chan, C., Lee, T., & Hui-Chan, C. (2004). Mental imagery for promoting relearning for people after stroke: a randomized control trial. *Archives of Physical Medicine and Rehabilitation*, 85, 1403–1408.

Machado, T. C., Carrengosa, A. A., Santos, M. S., Ribeiro, N. M. D. S., & Melo, A. (2019). Efficacy of motor imagery additional to motor-based therapy in the recovery of motor function of the upper limb in post-stroke individuals: a systematic review. *Top Stroke Rehabilitation*, 26(7), 548–553.

Malouin, F., & Richards, C. (2010). Mental practice for relearning locomotor skills. *Physical Therapy*, 90(2), 240–251.

Mathiowetz, V., & Haugen, J. B. (1994). Motor behavior research: implications for therapeutic approaches to central nervous system dysfunction. *The American Journal of Occupational Therapy*, 48, 734–745.

Muratori, L. M., Lamberg, E. M., Quinn, L., & Duff, S. V. (2013). Applying principles of motor learning and control to upper extremity rehabilitation. *Journal of Hand Therapy*, 26, 94–103.

Nepveu, J. F., Thiel, A., Tang, A., Fung, J., Lundbye-Jensen, J., Boyd, L. A., et al. (2017). A single bout of high-intensity interval training improves motor skill retention in individuals with stroke. *Neurorehabilitation and Neural Repair*, 31(8), 726–735.

Niemeijer, A. S., Schoemaker, M. M., & Smits-Engelsman, B. C. M. (2006). Are teaching principles associated with improved motor performance in children with developmental coordination disorder? A pilot study. *Physical Therapy*, 86, 1221–1230.

O'Brien, J. (2020). Box 16.5 Occupational therapy motor learning strategies worksheet. In J. O'Brien, & H. Kuhaneck (eds.), *Case-Smith's occupational therapy for children and adolescents* (8th ed., p. 405). St. Louis, MO: Elsevier.

O'Brien, J., & Patnaude, M. *Validity and reliability of the occupational therapy motor learning strategies worksheet*. Portland, ME: University of New England; in press.

Quintero-Gallego, E. A., Gomez, C. M., Casares, E. V., Marquez, J., & Perez-Santamaria, E. J. (2006). Declarative and procedural learning in children and adolescents with posterior fossa tumours. *Behavioral and Brain Functions*, 2, 9.

Rapolienė, J., Endzelytė, E., Jasevičienė, I., & Savickas, R. (2018). Stroke patients motivation influence on the effectiveness of occupational therapy. *Rehabilitation Research Practice*. Available from: http://dx.doi.org/10.1155/2018/9367942.

Schmidt, R. A., & Wrisberg, C. A. (2008). *Motor learning and performance: A situation-based learning approach*. Champaign, IL: Human Kinetics.

Taylor, R. (Ed.), (2017). *Kielhofner's model of human occupation* (5th ed.). Philadelphia, PA: Wolters Kluwer.

Taylor, R., & Kielhofner, G. (2017). Introduction to the model of human occupation. In R. Taylor (ed.), *Kielhofner's model of human occupation* (5th ed., pp. 1–10). Philadelphia, PA: Wolters Kluwer.

ten Berge, T., & van Hezewijk, R. (1999). Procedural and declarative knowledge: an evolutionary perspective. *Theory and Psychology, 9*(5), 605–624.

Trombly, C. (1995). Occupation: purposefulness and meaningfulness as therapeutic mechanisms. *The American Journal of Occupational Therapy, 49*(16), 960–972.

Tse, A. C., Fong, S. S., Wong, T. W. L., & Masters, R. (2017). Analogy motor learning by young children: a study of rope skipping. *The European Journal Sport Science, 17*(2), 152–159.

Williams, H. (2006). Motor control. In J. Solomon, & J. O'Brien (eds.), *Pediatric skills for the occupational therapy assistant.* (2nd ed., pp. 474–480). St. Louis, MO: Elsevier.

11

Mealtime Occupations—Interventions for Feeding and Eating

Kristin Winston

OBJECTIVES

After reading this chapter, the student or the occupational therapy practitioner will be able to do the following:

- Discuss factors that affect the role of the occupational therapy assistant in the practice area of mealtimes.
- Identify a variety of mealtime occupations at both the ADL and IADL level.

- Name, objectively describe, and contrast differing levels of independence in the occupation of mealtime.
- Identify recommended strategies to facilitate participation in mealtimes for individuals with specific functional losses.

KEY TERMS

Activities of daily living
Instrumental activities of daily living
Task analysis
Nonskid mats
Plate guard

Scoop dish
Universal cuffs
Dominance shift
Rocker knife
Swivel spoon

INTRODUCTION

This chapter focuses on mealtime occupations, which include **activities of daily living** (ADL) such as eating and swallowing and **instrumental activities of daily living** (IADL) skills such as shopping for food, meal preparation, and cleanup (American Occupational Therapy Association, 2014). Mealtime occupations may be done in a variety of contexts and environments, alone, or with other people. Winston (Winston, 2017) states "the sharing of food and the occupations of mealtimes are frequently part of celebrations large and small; cultural events; and other social activities at home, school, in the workplace, and within the community" (p. 522). There are many skills, functions, and structures that play a role in people's varying abilities in the variety of activities/occupations that make up the broad occupation of mealtime. These abilities are often taken for granted by the average person. For persons with difficulties in this area of occupation, losing the ability to engage in mealtime ADL or IADL may affect self-esteem, create a loss of independence, and affect their overall health physically and psychologically. The loss of ability in any of the occupations and activities involved in and around mealtime may require assistance from family, friends, and other caregivers when a person cannot participate or engage independently, creating co-occupations or shared occupations, defined as those occupations where more than one person is engaged in participation (Lawlor & Mattingly, 2019).

Occupational therapists (OTs) with input from occupational therapy assistant (OTAs) assess mealtime occupations and co-occupations to determine areas of strength in occupational performance, determine areas of concern that may interfere with participation, collaborate with clients and caregivers regarding treatment objectives, and provide training or equipment to promote or facilitate participation and engagement at a level that is feasible and acceptable for each client. As a part of the occupational therapy process, OT or OTA practitioners may also help reduce or remove physical, cognitive, social, and emotional barriers that interfere with performance by addressing contextual factors that influence mealtimes (Winston, 2017). A client's need to learn new methods or to use assistive devices to participate in the various activities associated with mealtimes may be temporary or permanent, depending on a variety of factors such as diagnosis, the prognosis for recovery, or contextual or environmental factors. OTs and OTAs are frequently involved in providing ADL/IADL services in regard to mealtimes. When considering mealtime occupations, as with other occupations, an OTA functions under the supervision of an OT. OTAs with proven competency may function autonomously in areas of practice but still under supervision as per practice and licensure guidelines (American Occupational Therapy Association, 2014). The American Occupational Therapy Association (AOTA) has guidelines for both entry-level

OTAs and OTAs with advanced levels of knowledge. The AOTA (American Occupational Therapy Association, 2017) delineates roles for both knowledge levels: Entry-level OTAs may "select, administer, and adapt activities that support the intervention plan developed by the occupational therapist" (p. 3) in line with competency level; OTAs with advanced knowledge in mealtime occupations may "provide services to clients who are more medically fragile or whose problems or needs are more complex than those addressed by the occupational therapy assistant with entry level practice skills" (p. 3). All evaluation and intervention choices must be determined through OT and OTA collaboration.

EVALUATION OF OCCUPATIONAL PERFORMANCE IN ADL, SPECIFICALLY MEALTIME OCCUPATIONS

Both basic and instrumental ADL represent one of the areas of occupation that OT practitioners address with clients. A primary purpose of occupational therapy is to facilitate performance of and engagement in these essential tasks of living. The evaluation of occupational performance is conducted from a top-down approach, in which the therapy practitioner focuses on the client as a whole, including his or her occupational history and interests, what meaning various occupations hold, and what roles may be important (Trombly Latham, 2014). In the area of mealtimes, this might include eating certain foods, cooking, shopping, or eating at specific restaurants. The practitioner starts with a top-down approach to determine the client's goals and preferences and then works to determine where difficulties might exist with performance or engagement in desired occupations, in meeting goals, or in facilitating preferred participation in mealtime occupations.

The evaluation of mealtime occupations includes both standardized and nonstandardized assessment, which may include data from observation or performance analysis (American Occupational Therapy Association, 2017; Fisher & Griswold, 2019), interview, and standardized testing. An interview and observation yield important information regarding the client's engagement in mealtime occupations and his or her current performance. The role of the entry-level OTA in evaluation regarding mealtime is determined in collaboration with the supervising OT (American Occupational Therapy Association, 2017). The *Occupational Therapy Practice Framework* discusses multiple levels of analysis of an individual's occupational performance, including performance analysis where the practitioner observes the person doing an occupation, looking at the quality of motor, process, and social interaction skills related to mealtime occupations (American Occupational Therapy Association, 2014). A **task analysis** is completed to determine what factors might be influencing occupational performance, including but not limited to body functions, body structures, context, and environment (Fisher & Griswold, 2019). Task analysis as a part of an evaluation assists practitioners in determining possible causes of difficulties in occupational performance.

In summary, the OTA in collaboration with the OT would gather information from a client regarding what is important, what might be challenging, and what he or she would like to do. The next step is to observe the client perform mealtime occupations that are important, challenging, and desired; analyze the performance of the observed occupations; and determine a plan for moving forward.

INTERVENTION FOR MEALTIME OCCUPATIONS

Appropriate short-term objectives and long-term goals must be established based on evaluation findings and client priorities. The Occupational Therapy Code of Ethics (American Occupational Therapy Association, 2015) principle of autonomy states that the occupational therapy practitioner should "establish a collaborative relationship with the recipient of service and relevant stakeholders to promote shared decision making" (p. 4). The more collaborative and client driven the occupational therapy intervention is, the more likely a high level of achievement and satisfaction in desired outcomes in mealtime occupations will occur (Gagne & Hoppes, 2003).

Methods of Teaching in Intervention

The methods of teaching the client to perform ADL must be tailored to suit each client's learning style and ability. The OT or OTA, in collaboration with the client, may need to explore a variety of methods or assistive devices to reach a solution. There are a variety of ways OTs or OTAs might consider teaching and learning; a few examples to be explored with clients may include a behaviorist approach, social learning and social cognitive theories, constructivist theory, self-efficacy theory, and motivational theory (Helfrich, 2019). Many special methods used to perform specific activities also evolve through trial-and-error approaches of practitioners and their clients. Clients often have good suggestions because they live with the difficulty and are confronted regularly with the need to adapt or change the performance of daily tasks. Occasionally a solution may be presented that the client finds unacceptable as it involves excessive adaptive equipment, gadgets, or time. It is important to practice from a client-centered perspective recognizing that not all potential solutions will work for all clients.

The techniques and equipment specified in this chapter provide the reader with basic skills to approach the client with confidence but may not be appropriate for all clients in all situations.

General Decisions Regarding Grading (Remediation) and Adapting (Compensation)

The OT, in collaboration with the OTA, will determine which approach to intervention in mealtime occupations is most appropriate for a client. One primary approach is that of establish/restore (remediation/restoration), also known as grading, which aims to return a client to or as close to a prior level of function as possible (American Occupational Therapy Association, 2014). Intervention strategies will be graded as determined by current level of function and potential for improvement. The rate at which grading can occur depends on a variety of client factors, including potential for recovery, endurance, performance skills, and contextual supports.

Another approach is modifying (compensation, adaptation), also referred to as adapting, where the goal is to find ways to alter the way a client is participating in an occupation to facilitate performance and participation (American Occupational Therapy Association, 2014). As a part of this process, the practitioner and the client may explore the possibility of alternate methods of participating in desired occupations. One such method may be the use of assistive devices.

DEVELOPMENTAL STAGES

It is important to note where the client is in terms of development, as participation in mealtime occupations occurs across the lifespan and as such is different at all levels of development. The OT practitioner should consider the following: What skills does the client possess? What structures and functions are important to consider developmentally? What mealtime occupations are typically seen at a specific developmental level? What can be expected in terms of participation and engagement in mealtime occupations given developmental level?

PHASES OF EATING/DRINKING

The phases of eating/drinking include a preoral or anticipatory phase, the oral preparatory phase, the oral phase, the pharyngeal phase, and the esophageal phase.

The preoral or anticipatory phase of eating involves those activities/occupations that are precursors to the actual eating of foods and liquids (Smith, 2018). A variety of occupations occur in and around this phase of the eating process. This may include who the client will be eating with, who shops and prepares the food, whether the client experiences hunger, and how the food will be presented (Winston, 2017).

Intervention in this phase will likely focus on context and environment, habits and routines, as well as performance skills, body functions, and body structures. The OTA may be addressing concerns related to social participation in terms of mealtimes with family or friends, developing strategies for process skills needed for meal planning and meal preparation, motor skills for preparing meals, or modifications to the environment to support mealtime participation, to name a few.

Oral Versus Nonoral Eating

Most individuals are able to take in nutrition through oral means (by mouth) where they are able to bring foods and liquids to the mouth (oral preparatory phase), manage the textures and consistencies to effectively initiate a swallow (oral phase), and swallow/process those foods and liquids (pharyngeal and esophageal phases of oral eating) (Smith, 2018).

Intervention in the oral preparatory phase and oral phase may be directed at addressing performance skills, body functions, and body structures. In particular motor skills, issues of strength, tone, and range of motion (ROM) are often addressed as a part of intervention plans to improve a client's participation in eating and drinking. Intervention in the pharyngeal and esophageal phases is typically done in collaboration with physicians, nursing, speech/language pathologists, nutritionists, and other providers as indicated. Occupational therapy interventions are often aimed at safety, such as positioning for safe swallowing, assisting with transitions in diet modifications, and caregiver training to assist with mealtimes (American Occupational Therapy Association, 2017; Smith, 2018).

Individuals who experience difficulties with oral intake secondary to dysphagia, aspiration, or other medical concerns may need to receive nonoral nutritional support or parenteral nutrition via nasogastric tube, gastrostomy tube, or jejunostomy tube depending on severity of concerns (Korth & Rendell, 2015). Occupational therapy intervention will focus on working with clients and families to develop habits and routines around mealtimes with parenteral nutrition methods (Korth & Rendell, 2015).

CONCERNS THAT MAY AFFECT PARTICIPATION IN MEALTIME OCCUPATIONS AND INTERVENTION STRATEGIES TO ADDRESS AREAS OF CONCERN

Motor Skills

As noted earlier, in the oral preparatory and oral phases of eating, motor skills, including issues of strength, tone, and ROM are often addressed as part of intervention plans to improve a client's participation in eating and drinking. In collaboration with the OT, the OTA may carry out motor-based intervention strategies aimed at improving motor skills and functions. Strategies may include stretching, strengthening, modification of food textures to accommodate for performance skills related to managing a bolus of food, and use of adaptive equipment to encourage participation. Advanced training and mentoring are recommended when utilizing many motor-based strategies secondary to the complexity of many concerns related to eating, drinking, and swallowing. For more information regarding entry-level versus advanced-level practice in this area please refer to "The Practice of Occupational Therapy in Feeding, Eating, and Swallowing" (American Occupational Therapy Association, 2017).

Problems of Incoordination in Mealtime Occupations

Incoordination can result from a variety of central nervous system (CNS) disorders such as Parkinson disease, multiple sclerosis, cerebral palsy, and traumatic brain injuries (TBIs). Incoordination may take the form of tremors, ataxia, or athetoid or choreiform movements. Persons with incoordination may have difficulty maintaining safety and performance within mealtime occupations. For clients with decreased coordination, mealtime can be a challenge. Lack of control during mealtime may be frustrating and may cause embarrassment and social isolation. Thus making eating safe, pleasurable, and as independent as possible is important.

Individuals experiencing decreased coordination who have functional muscle strength can use weighted devices to help stabilize objects. For some clients, a weight attached to the arm may decrease tremors and ataxia.

Intervention Strategies for Decreased Coordination

Use plate stabilizers such as **nonskid mats**, suction bases, Dycem, or damp dishtowels to prevent slipping (Fig. 11.1).

1. Use a **plate guard** or **scoop dish** to prevent food being pushed off the plate. The plate guard can be taken from home and clipped to any ordinary dinner plate (Fig. 11.2).

2. Prevent spills during the plate-to-mouth movement by using weighted or swivel utensils to offer stability. Weighted **universal cuffs** may be placed on the forearm to decrease involuntary movements or tremors (Fig. 11.3). Choose foods that are mashed or have a texture that stays together easily versus foods that have pieces that can easily slip off a utensil.

3. To eliminate the need to bring a glass or cup to the mouth (which may cause spills), use long plastic straws with a straw clip on a glass or cup with a weighted bottom. Plastic cups or hot beverage travel containers with covers and spouts can also reduce spills.

4. Stabilize a proximal body part for better control distally. This stabilization may be accomplished by propping the elbow on a counter or tabletop and moving only the forearm, wrist, and hand in the activity. Stabilizing the arm may reduce some of the incoordination and may allow the individual to accomplish gross and fine motor movements without assistive devices. Stabilizing the trunk

using seated positioning devices may increase the fine coordination of the upper extremity (refer to Chapter 15).

5. Specific intervention strategies to assist with managing tremors during mealtime can be found at https://www.essentialtremor.org/treatments/assistive-devices/.

Note each client will likely respond differently to techniques such as adding weight or stabilization and as such should be evaluated to determine what strategies might be most effective in a variety of situations.

Hemiplegia

Hemiplegia is the most commonly seen diagnosis in which unilateral upper extremity dysfunction occurs and requires a unique approach to facilitating independence in mealtime occupations. Clients with unilateral upper extremity dysfunction resulting from amputations and temporary disorders such as fractures, burns, and peripheral neuropathy are likely to learn compensatory techniques quickly and easily if they

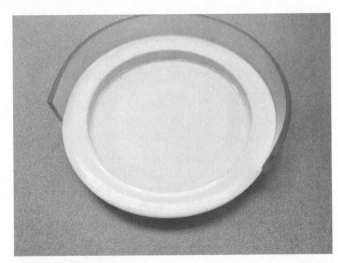

Fig. 11.2 Plate guard.

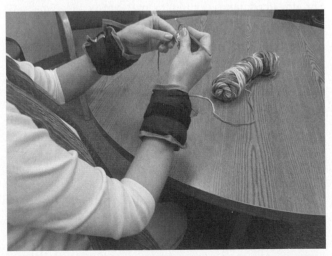

Fig. 11.3 Weighted cuffs can sometimes compensate for incoordination. (From Pendleton HM, Schultz-Krohn W: Pedretti's Occupational Therapy, ed 8, 2018, Elsevier, St. Louis.)

Fig. 11.1 Dycem.

have typical functioning of sensory, perceptual, and cognitive skills. Clients with unilateral upper extremity dysfunction may benefit from suggestions to assist with mealtimes while recovering from an injury.

Clients with hemiplegia as a result of diagnoses such as stroke or acquired brain injury may require specialized methods of teaching; many have greater difficulty learning and performing one-handed skills than do persons with orthopedic or lower motor neuron dysfunction. This is often a result of motor involvement and muscle tone changes in many areas of the body, including the head, trunk, leg, and arm. In addition, sensory, perceptual, cognitive, and speech concerns may affect the ability to regain skills or adapt to new skills in mealtime occupations. Evaluation of mealtime participation will include determining the client's needs and preferences at all levels of mealtime preoral or anticipatory phase, oral preparatory, oral, pharyngeal, and esophageal phases to establish appropriate teaching methods and intervention strategies to facilitate participation. *One-Handed in a Two-Handed World* is a good resource book for teaching ADL adaptations (Mayer, 2000).

Eating activities and other occupations related to mealtimes may require a **dominance shift**. If the patient is right-hand dominant and is experiencing right-side hemiplegia, left-hand coordination may need to be learned through practice.

As noted earlier, a variety of assistive devices can make mealtime occupations easier to perform (Koketsu, 2019). Whether the client is experiencing concerns related to the loss of function of one arm and hand (as in amputation or peripheral neuropathy) or whether both arm and leg are affected—along with possible visual, perceptual, and cognitive dysfunctions (as in hemiplegia)—makes a significant difference in planning treatment.

Strategies for Unilateral Upper Extremity Use During Mealtimes

For unilateral upper extremity use during mealtimes, the following strategies are useful (see References for further details).

1. Stabilization of items is a major problem for the individual who can use only one hand. Stabilize foods for cutting and peeling by using a board with two stainless steel or aluminum nails attached to the surface (Fig. 11.4). A raised corner on the board stabilizes bread while making sandwiches or spreading butter. Suction cups or a rubber mat under the board will keep it from slipping. Rubber stair tread, shelf liner, or Dycem may be glued to the bottom of the board (see Fig. 11.1).

2. A significant concern in mealtime when using one hand is managing a knife and fork simultaneously for meat cutting. This problem can be solved by the use of a **rocker knife** for cutting meat and other foods (Fig. 11.5). The knife cuts with a rocking motion rather than a back-and-forth slicing action. This motion holds the food in place while cutting it, therefore requiring only one hand

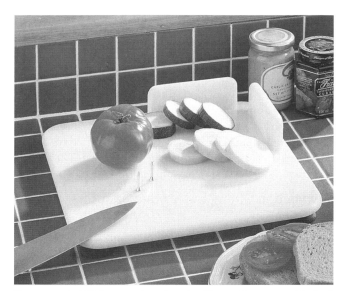

Fig. 11.4 Stabilizing cutting board. (From Patterson Medical, Warrenville, IL.)

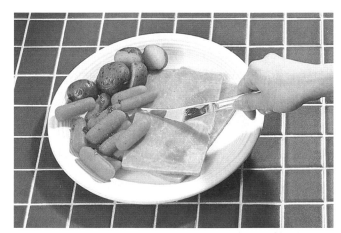

Fig. 11.5 Rocker knife. (From Patterson Medical, Warrenville, IL.)

for the task. Use of a rocking motion with a standard table knife or a sharp paring knife may be adequate to accomplish cutting tender meats and foods. If such a knife is used, the patient is taught to hold the knife handle between the thumb and the third, fourth, and fifth fingers, and the index finger is extended along the top of the knife blade. The knife point is placed in the food in a vertical position, and then the blade is brought down to cut the food. The rocking motion, using wrist flexion and extension, is continued until the food is cut.

3. Use sponge cloths, nonskid mats or pads, wet dishcloths, or suction devices to keep bowls and dishes from turning or sliding during food preparation. Use a pan holder—a steel rod frame with suction cups attached to the stove top—to keep the pot from spinning while the contents are being stirred or flipped.

4. To open a jar, stabilize it between the knees or in a partially opened drawer while leaning against it. Break

the air seal by sliding a bottle opener under the lid until the air is released; then use a wall-mounted opener (e.g., Zim Jar Opener) (Fig. 11.6). When purchasing food items in jars, ask the grocer to open and gently reseal jars before bagging them.

5. Open boxes, sealed paper bags, and plastic bags by stabilizing between the knees or in a drawer, as just described, and cutting open with a household shears. Special box and bag openers are also available from ADL equipment vendors.

6. Open an egg by holding it firmly in the palm of the hand, hitting it in the center against the edge of the bowl, and then using the thumb and index finger to push the top half of the shell up and the ring and little fingers to push the lower half down. Separate whites from yolks by using an egg separator or a funnel. Another solution is to use cholesterol-free eggs, such as Egg Beaters, from a carton.

7. Eliminate the need to stabilize the standard grater by using a grater with suction feet, or use an electric food processor.

8. Eliminate the need to use hand-cranked or electric can openers requiring two hands by using a one-handed electric can opener.

9. Use a utility cart to carry items from one place to another.

10. Use electrical appliances that can be managed with one hand to save time and energy. Some of these appliances include a lightweight electrical hand mixer, blender, and food processor. Safety factors and judgment need to be evaluated carefully for electrical appliances.

These suggestions are just a few of the possibilities to solve concerns noted in mealtime occupations for clients with the functional use of only one hand. The OT practitioner must evaluate each client to determine how the dysfunction affects performance. One-handed techniques require more time and may be difficult for some clients to master. Activities should be paced to accommodate the client's physical endurance and tolerance for one-handed performance and use of special devices.

New techniques and devices should be introduced on a graded basis as the client gains skill and comfort. Clients may also problem-solve how to participate in desired occupations by compensating for the loss of upper extremity function (whether one or both upper extremities) with other parts of the body. This exploration of alternate ways of participating should be explored as a part of the therapeutic process. Exploring compensatory techniques, low-tech adaptive equipment, and technology are all options for problem-solving how to facilitate participation.

CONTEXT

The environment and context in which a client lives or will live is an important consideration when looking to intervene in mealtime occupations. OT practitioners can provide recommendations or adaptations to many aspects of context to support participation in mealtime occupations. Consider how these questions might affect intervention choices: Will the client live alone or with family or a roommate (social context)? Will the client go to a skilled nursing facility (SNF) or to a long-term care situation? If so, will the stay be permanent or temporary? Where will the client eat meals (physical context)? How and when will the client shop for and obtain food (physical context and temporal context)?

The type and amount of assistance (social context) available in the home environment must be considered so that the caregiver can receive proper orientation and training in the appropriate supervision and assistance required. The finances available (personal context) for assisted care, special equipment, and adaptations to home environments are important considerations. Additional resources include the client's insurance and community-based or philanthropic organizations. The client's case manager or social worker can help determine eligibility for resources.

General Strategies for Mealtime Participation

1. Positioning directly affects the ability to swallow safely and efficiently across the lifespan. Positioning should be addressed as a priority with the trunk and pelvis supported with a slight anterior pelvic tilt. Smith (Smith, 2018) states "the client should be positioned symmetrically with normal alignment between the head, neck, trunk, and pelvis" (p. 685). The head and neck should be in midline with a slight chin tuck. The overall goal of positioning at meals is to promote safe swallowing, facilitate postural alignment, and prevent structural deformities (Winston, 2017) (Fig. 11.7).

2. Built-up eating utensil handles can accommodate limited grasp or prehension (Fig. 11.8). Utensils can be

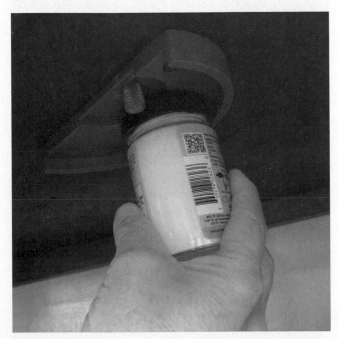

Fig. 11.6 Jar opener.

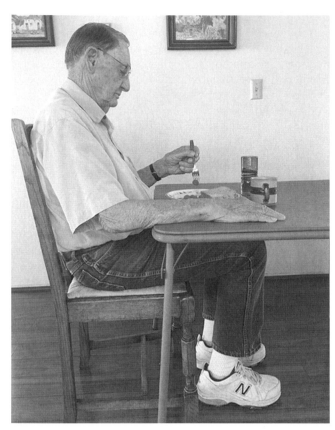

Fig. 11.7 Optimal position for sitting during eating. (From Pendleton HM, Schultz-Krohn W: Pedretti's Occupational Therapy, ed 8, 2018, Elsevier, St. Louis.)

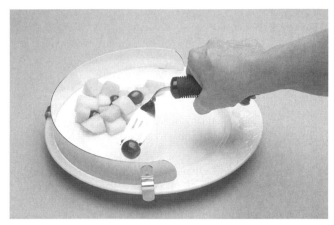

Fig. 11.9 Swivel utensil to compensate for lack of pronation and supination. (North Coast Medical, Morgan Hill, CA. www.ncmedical. com.)

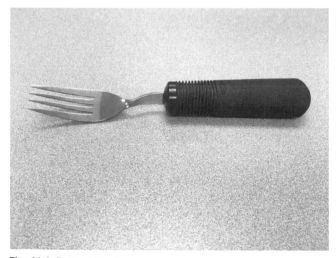

Fig. 11.8 Built up handles.

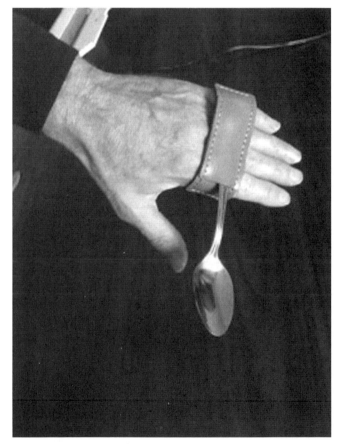

Fig. 11.10 Universal cuff.

purchased with wide handles; alternatively, cylindrical foam, which is found at hardware stores in the pipe insulation section, can be added to regular utensils.

3. Elongated or specially curved handles on spoons and forks may be necessary to reach the mouth. A **swivel spoon** or spoon-fork combination can compensate for limited supination (Fig. 11.9).

4. Long plastic straws and straw clips on glasses or cups can be used if neck, elbow, or shoulder ROM limits hand-to-mouth motion or if grasp is inadequate to hold the cup or glass.

5. Universal cuffs or utensil holders can be used if grasp is limited and built-up handles do not work (Fig. 11.10). These cuffs wrap around the palm of the hand with an opening on the first web space. A variety of items can

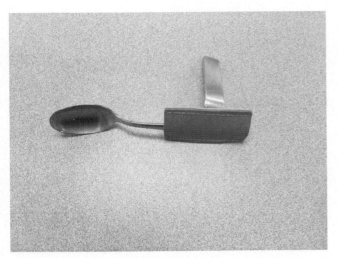

Fig. 11.11 Utensil for universal cuff.

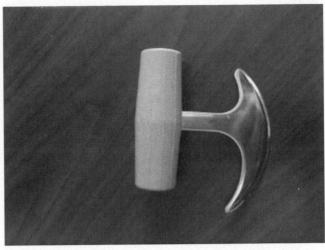

Fig. 11.13 Quad knife.

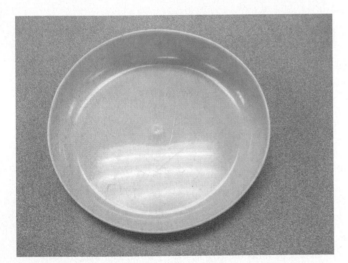

Fig. 11.12 Scoop dish.

11. Examples of these assistive devices can be found in adaptive equipment or medical equipment catalogs and websites, including:
   a. Northcoast Medical: https://www.ncmedical.com/categories/Assistive-Devices-ADL_12839533.html
   b. Rehabmart.com Skills for the Job of Living: https://www.rehabmart.com/category/daily_living_aids.htm
   c. These items can also be found online in a variety of places such as Amazon, Walmart, Walgreens, or other retail locations.
12. Many types of assistive devices exist to facilitate mealtime participation. Technology can range from low-tech items, such as a built-up handle on a spoon, to high-tech electronics. Examples of high-tech assistive devices for mealtime include:
   a. Electronic eating assist (via chin switch): https://www.assistivetechnologycenter.org/device/winsford-feeder
   b. Adaptive spoons (to address tremors): https://www.liftware.com/

be placed in the opening, including eating utensils. A utensil can then be placed in the cuff (Fig. 11.11).
6. Plate guards (see Fig. 11.2) or scoop dishes (Fig. 11.12) may be useful to prevent food from slipping off the plate if the patient lacks coordination when scooping the food with the utensil.
7. A swivel spoon-fork combination can be used when the client has minimal muscle function.
8. A long plastic straw with a straw clip to stabilize it in the cup or glass eliminates the need for picking up these drinking vessels. A bilateral or unilateral clip holder on a glass or cup allows many clients with hand and arm weakness to manage liquids without a straw.
9. Cutting food may be managed with a quad knife if arm strength is adequate to manage the device (Fig. 11.13).
10. Built-up utensils may be useful for clients with some functional grasp or tenodesis grasp.

Strategies to Increase Safety and Function in Meal Related IADLs

1. Use convenience and prepared foods to eliminate processes such as peeling, chopping, slicing, and mixing when possible.
2. Use easy-open containers or store foods in plastic containers.
3. Use heavy utensils, mixing bowls, and pots and pans to increase stability.
4. Try using various types of jar openers, including wall-mounted and portable.
5. Use nonskid mats on work surfaces. Line the kitchen sink with rubber mat cushions to prevent items from sliding or breaking.

6. Use electric appliances such as crockpots, electric fry pans, electric tea kettles, toaster ovens, and microwave ovens because they are safer to use than the range or oven.
7. Use a blender and countertop mixer because they are safer than handheld mixers and easier than mixing with a spoon or whisk.
8. Adjust work heights of counters, sink, and range to minimize leaning, bending, reaching, and lifting, whether the client is standing or using a wheelchair, when possible. Use a stool at the counter to increase balance and stability.
9. Use long oven mitts, which give greater protection than potholders.
10. Use lightweight pots, pans, casserole dishes, and appliances with bilateral handles because they may be easier to hold and manage than those with one handle.
11. Use an adaptive cutting board with stainless steel nails (see Fig. 11.4) to stabilize meats, potatoes, and vegetables while cutting or peeling. When the cutting board is not in use, the nails should be covered with a large cork. To prevent slipping, the bottom of the board should have suction cups, be covered with stair tread, or be placed on a nonskid mat.
12. Use heavy dinnerware, which offers stability and control to the distal part of the upper extremity and may be easier to handle. If dropping and breaking are problems, durable plastic dinnerware may be more practical.
13. Cover the sink, utility cart, and countertops with protective rubber mats or mesh matting to stabilize items.
14. Use a serrated knife for cutting and chopping because it is easier to control.
15. To eliminate the need to carry and drain pots of hot liquids, use a steamer basket or deep-fry basket for preparing boiled foods.
16. Use tongs to turn foods during cooking and to serve foods because tongs offer more control and stability than a fork, spatula, or serving spoon.
17. Use a bottle tipper to safely pour liquids. Velcro straps hold the bottle into a wire frame while the client controls the tipping angle by pulling down on the wire frame until liquid slowly streams out of the bottle.[37,49]
18. Use blunt-ended loop scissors to open packages.

SUMMARY

Mealtime occupations are those that allow a client to function independently, pursue meaningful participation, and assume important occupational roles. OT practitioners routinely evaluate performance in mealtime occupations to assess clients' desired engagement and participation. The OTA may choose to establish service competency and special expertise in this area of occupational therapy practice.

Evaluation and intervention are directed toward facilitating participation and engagement in desired mealtime occupations using a variety of methods and strategies to address factors such as context, performance skills, body functions, and body structures. The OTA practicing in this area should

be familiar with all aspects of mealtime participation as well as with the special equipment and methods for participation needed by the client with specific functional concerns.

REVIEW QUESTIONS

1. List at least three potential mealtime occupations at the ADL level and the IADL level.
2. List three factors that the OT practitioner must consider before beginning assessment and intervention in mealtime occupation. Describe how each could limit or affect the client's performance.
3. Describe three approaches to teaching ADL/IADL skills for a client with deficits in mealtime occupations.
4. Explain how an OTA would establish service competency and maximal independence in providing ADL services within the legal guidelines of his or her state or other local jurisdiction.

EXERCISES

1. Demonstrate the use of at least three assistive devices mentioned in the text.
2. Teach a person how to make a sandwich with only one hand.

REFERENCES

American Occupational Therapy Association. (2014). Occupational therapy practice framework. Domain and process, 3rd ed. *Am J Occup Ther*, 68(1), S2–S51.

American Occupational Therapy Association. (2014). Guidelines for supervision, roles, and responsibilities during the delivery of occupational therapy services. *Am J Occup Ther*, 68(3), S16–S22. https://doi.org/10.5014/ajot.2014.686S03.

American Occupational Therapy Association. (2015). Occupational therapy code of ethics. *Am J Occup Ther*, 69(3), S1–S8.

American Occupational Therapy Association. (2017). The practice of occupational therapy in feeding, eating, and swallowing. *Am J Occup Ther*, 71(2). S7112410015. https://doi.org/10.5014/ajot.2017.716S04.

Fisher, A., & Griswold, L. A. (2019). Performance skills: implementing performance analyses to evaluate quality of occupational performance. In B. A. B. Schell, & G. Gillen (Eds.), *Willard & Spackman's Occupational Therapy* (13th ed., pp. 335–350). Philadelphia, PA: Wolters Kluwer.

Gagne, D. E., & Hoppes, S. (2003). The effects of collaborative goal focused occupational therapy on self care skills: a pilot study. *Am J Occup Ther*, 57(2), 215–219.

Helfrich, C. A. (2019). Principles of behavior change. In B. A. B. Schell, & G. Gillen (Eds.), *Willard & Spackman's Occupational Therapy* (13th ed., pp. 693–713). Philadelphia, PA: Wolters Kluwer.

Koketsu, J. S. (2019). Activities of daily living. In H. McHugh Pendleton, & W. Schultz-Krohn (Eds.), *Pedretti's Occupational*

Therapy: Practice Skills for Physical Dysfunction (8th ed., pp. 155–229). St. Louis, MO: Elsevier.

Korth, K., & Rendell, L. (2015). Feeding intervention. In J. Case-Smith, & J. O'Brien (Eds.), *Occupational Therapy for Children and Adolescents* (7th ed.). St Louis, MO: Mosby, 389–341.

Lawlor, M., & Mattingly, C. (2019). Family perspectives on occupation, health, and disability. In B. A. B. Schell, & G. Gillen (Eds.), *Willard & Spackman's Occupational Therapy* (13th ed., pp. 196–211). Philadelphia, PA: Wolters Kluwer.

Mayer, T. K. (2000). *One-Handed in a Two-Handed World* (2nd ed.). Boston, MA: Prince-Gallison Press;.

Smith, J. (2018). Eating and swallowing. In H. McHugh Pendleton, & W. Schultz-Krohn (Eds.), *Pedretti's Occupational Therapy: Practice Skills for Physical Dysfunction* (8th ed., pp. 669–700). St. Louis, MO: Elsevier.

Trombly Latham, C. A. (2014). Conceptual foundations for practice. In M. V. Radomski, & C. A. Trombly Latham (Eds.), *Occupational Therapy for Physical Dysfunction* (7th ed., pp. 1–23). Philadelphia, PA: Wolters Kluwer.

Winston, K. (2017). Interventions to enhance feeding, eating, and swallowing. In K. Jacobs, & N. MacRae (Eds.), *Occupational Therapy Essentials for Clinical Competence* (3rd ed., pp. 521–535). Thorofare, NJ: Slack Inc.

RECOMMENDED READING

Korth, K., & Rendell, L. (2015). Feeding intervention. In J. Case-Smith, & J. O'Brien (Eds.), *Occupational Therapy for Children and Adolescents* (7th ed.). St Louis, MO: Mosby, 389–341.

Smith, J. (2018). Eating and swallowing. In H. McHugh Pendleton, & W. Schultz-Krohn (Eds.), *Pedretti's Occupational Therapy: Practice Skills for Physical Dysfunction* (8th ed., pp. 669–700). St. Louis, MO: Elsevier.

Winston, K. (2017). Interventions to enhance feeding, eating, and swallowing. In K. Jacobs, & N. MacRae (Eds.), *Occupational Therapy Essentials for Clinical Competence* (3rd ed., pp. 521–535). Thorofare, NJ: Slack Inc.

12

Occupations, Purposeful Activities, and Preparatory Activities

Brina A. Kelly

OBJECTIVES

After reading this chapter, the student or the occupational therapy practitioner will be able to do the following:

- Describe the value and use of occupations to guide therapeutic interventions.
- Describe the multidimensional interaction between the person and his or her daily occupations and the impact of this process on health and identity.
- Identify personal, contextual/environmental, and social influences on occupation.
- Discuss the role of activity analysis in the selection of therapeutic activity.
- Differentiate purposeful activity from other modalities used in occupational therapy.

- Identify the relationship between physical agent modalities and occupation in occupational therapy practice.
- Describe how grading activity can be used to heighten functional performance.
- Identify the requirements for the use of adjunctive modalities in occupational therapy practice.
- Perform an activity analysis appropriate for the treatment of physical dysfunction.
- Understand the indications, contraindications, procedures, and precautions for a variety of therapeutic protocols.

KEY TERMS

Client factors
Performance skills
Performance patterns
Purposeful activities
Preparatory tasks
Preparatory methods
Transcutaneous electrical nerve stimulation
Neuromuscular electrical stimulation

Occupational analysis
Activity analysis
Just-right challenge
Passive exercise
Active-assist exercise
Active ROM exercise
Therapeutic activity

INTRODUCTION

Occupation can be viewed as both the ends and means to the rehabilitation and habilitation of individuals (Pedretti et al., 1992). Therefore occupation can be an end product of intervention (i.e., completing the valued activity of laundry), or an agent of change (i.e., carrying a laundry basket to improve upper extremity [UE] strength), for a client who is motivated by the task of clothing care. Occupational participation empowers individuals to achieve life meaning by achieving autonomy and mastery of meaningful skills. Occupational therapists (OTs) and occupational therapy assistants (OTAs) emphasize occupation throughout the intervention process. The process of analyzing occupation and examining the way in which it can be utilized in practice will lay a strong foundation for practitioners.

OCCUPATION

OTs and OTAs utilize occupation, the activities or tasks that people need or want to do (Wilcock, 2006), to help individuals or groups meaningfully engage in daily life. Humans engage in occupation throughout the lifespan. These include activities of daily living (ADL), such as grooming, bathing, and dressing, and instrumental activities of daily living (IADL), such as meal preparation, shopping, and managing finances (see Chapter 11). The occupation of work includes employment for pay and other productive activities (volunteering). Education includes activities that fulfill one's role as a student.

Play and leisure occupations include elements of choice and creativity that are done for personal pleasure, relaxation, and amusement rather productivity (i.e., sports and recreation, time spent with animals, reading, participating in arts, listening to music, meditating, watching television, downtime on the computer or internet). Social participation includes engaging in the community and among friends, family, peers, and coworkers. Lastly, the restorative activities of sleep and rest support occupational engagement and overall health. The complexity of occupation can be masked by the fact that most daily activities seem ordinary and familiar to all members of society. However, when the interaction of the processes and tasks involved in occupation, as well as the unique purpose and value to each individual, is taken into account the complexity of them becomes more apparent.

Principles of Occupation

Occupation stimulates growth and change through the complex interaction between the individual, the task, and the environment (Box 12.1). The inherent need for mastery, self-actualization, self-identity, competence, and social acceptance direct a process of "doing, being, becoming, and belonging." (Kottke, 1971). Occupational participation improves performance skills and is useful for intervention.

These principles can be illustrated through the following example. For an individual who values and is motivated by sports, improvements to her game may change her sense of being ("I am a soccer player."). This new sense of self will lead to a motivation to increase practice time, which will likely lead to greater success ("I am a good soccer player."). The improvement in performance skills leads to her sense of becoming (hopes and aspirations) through revised future goals ("I am going to be a great soccer player."). Over time, the performance improvement alters her belonging (sense of connectedness) as a more experienced member of a team or sports community. This in turn leads to increased interaction with others and sense of control in the environment.

An injury or illness may change this process. For example, an individual who has sustained a spinal cord injury (SCI) must establish new ways of being while learning new ways of doing. OTs and OTAs, in collaboration with the individual, family, and caregivers, establish a relevant, meaningful plan to stimulate a client's growth and interaction with this process again.

Through occupational therapy intervention, the engagement in occupation provides opportunities for clients to gain or regain their health and quality of life. Therapeutic use of occupation is the way in which occupational therapy provides distinct value to clients. OTs and OTAs utilize occupation-based and client-centered practice to assist clients experiencing an abrupt change to their sense of self. This can be true of any client, but particularly those who experienced an injury or illness leading to physical dysfunction. Occupation-based treatment allows clients to rediscover a sense of doing, being, becoming, and belonging. The reestablishment of the sense of self reduces the risk for depression, improves quality of life, and increases participation in health-promoting and therapeutic activities.

BOX 12.1 Fundamental Principles of Occupational Therapy

- Occupations and activities act as a therapeutic agent to remediate or restore change because individuals have the potential to improve their performance skills, patterns (habits, routines, rituals), and body functions.
- Novel occupations, utilized as interventions, develop new performance skills and habits. This occurs because novel occupations require variations in environments and contexts. To successfully navigate these contexts, individuals performing the occupations must develop the performance skills and habits necessary to be successful.
- Valued occupations are inherently motivating because they reflect what individuals enjoy and value.
- As one experiences satisfaction through participation in occupation, he or she identifies values leading to a generation of new interests.
- Occupations provide opportunities to practice and reinforce performance skills, which carry over to other routine tasks.
- Active engagement in occupation provides corrective feedback to a client that will modify future behaviors and actions.
- Engagement in occupations facilitates mastery or competence in performing daily activities because meaningful engagement encourages ongoing practice, which leads to further change.
- Skillfully designed interventions eliminate physical and social barriers to participation and increase opportunities for social interaction between individuals and groups.
- Occupational participation facilitates self-directed change that provides individuals with tools to control their health and well-being.
- Active engagement in healthy occupations, for individuals of all ability levels, contributes to overall health and wellness.
- Self-evaluation of occupational performance influences self-perception.
- Engagement in valued occupations provides satisfaction and fulfilment by providing a means to experience personal gains that lead to goal achievement.
- Individuals decide how to spend their time based on the occupations that provide meaning.
- Active participation in occupations contributes to one's identity (Christiansen & Baum, 1999).

Data from Moyers PA, Dale L. *The Guide to Occupational Therapy Practice.* 2nd ed. Bethesda, MD: AOTA Press; 2007:45–46.

INTERPLAY OF THE PERSON, ENVIRONMENT, AND OCCUPATION

It is necessary for OTs and OTAs to evaluate and understand the "individual, system, or situation" (Hinojosa et al., 2005) as a whole to create purposeful and effective interventions. To reason and practice holistically, they must understand and consider the three components of person, environment, and occupation.

Person

Each person has specific capacities, characteristics, and beliefs that influence his or her occupational choices and performance (American Occupational Therapy Association, 2014). **Client factors** include one's value system, body functions, and body structures. Each factor can be affected by the presence or absence of illness or injury and can affect one's performance skills (American Occupational Therapy Association, 2014). **Performance skills** (motor, processing, social) demonstrate a client's abilities to perform daily occupations. For example, an injury that limits one's motor functions (i.e., lower extremity [LE] strength and voluntary control) can affect a client's functional mobility and his or her ability to transfer from one position to the next. However, a change in one performance skill can take effect on other performance skills and one's overall performance in the desired occupations. For individuals with difficulty performing transfers, an intervention may focus on increasing UE strength to improve their ability (skill) to push themselves from a chair to a standing position, compensating for LE weakness during transfers. **Performance patterns** (habits, routines, roles, rituals) can also support or hinder one's occupational performance. OT practitioners that consider a client's performance patterns will have a better understanding of how performance skills and occupations interrelate and are integrated into one's life (American Occupational Therapy Association, 2014).

Environment

A person's abilities, limitations, and overall occupations cannot be understood without the consideration of the environment. As part of a client-centered practice, OT practitioners are to evaluate aspects of the person and the occupational environment before and throughout the intervention process to understand how certain factors may support or inhibit a client's participation and ability to adapt the desired occupations. Occupations involve activities within specific settings, time, and contexts; thus there are multiple dimensions to consider.

One's physical environment is nonhuman (i.e., buildings, furniture, tools, devices, animals, terrain) and refers to the natural and built surroundings in which daily occupations take place. The physical environment may present with barriers to participation in occupation, including the size of doorways or access to entry ramps for individuals who use a wheelchair, or conversely, provide supports (i.e., grab bars, built-in shower chair). Additionally, as part of the physical environment, it is important to note sensory elements and their impact on performance: visual elements (e.g., lighting and colors), auditory (e.g., room noise level), tactile (e.g., temperature, seating structures), olfactory (e.g., presence of odors), and gustatory (e.g., presence of pleasant or offensive tastes). For example, a cold therapy gym can increase the muscle tone in the hand of a client following a cardiovascular accident (CVA), inhibiting participation. In addition, a client who demonstrates decreased attention following a traumatic brain injury may perform a multistep task better in quiet space with limited distractions rather than in a crowded gym.

One's social environment consists of the networks and relationships of family, friends, colleagues, and caregivers (Mosey, 1996). The social environment includes individual or group behavioral expectations (i.e., social roles and routines, cultural components) as well as the psychologic aspects that may have an effect on mood and stress levels. The tangible environment and the social environment guide and dictate occupational performance to the same extent that physical and mental capacities do and thus must be considered in developing an intervention plan.

Contextual domains go beyond the physical and social environment (American Occupational Therapy Association, 2014). They include cultural, personal, temporal, and virtual contexts. They strongly influence occupational performance.

The cultural context includes an awareness of and a respect for the customs, beliefs, behavioral standards, and expectations of the client's society. This context influences a person's identity and activity choices (American Occupational Therapy Association, 2014). For example, in cultures where meal preparation is a valued female role, interventions (e.g., food preparation) may be inappropriate.

The temporal context includes things such as the time of day, a client's chronologic age, and expected length of stay. It can also include anticipated duration of disability, stage of illness, or one's individual history. The virtual context refers to the environment in which communication and interactions occur by means of technology, such as computers, telephones, tablets, and video games.

OTs and OTAs should become familiar with and consider all aspects of each client's contextual environment across the lifespan and practice settings. Careful consideration allows both practitioners and clients to advocate and adapt the environment to meet individual needs (physical, sensory, psychosocial, cultural, personal, temporal, and virtual). Environmental modification and adaptation can enhance occupational participation.

Occupation. Occupation occurs within a certain environment and context, and is influenced by client factors, performance skills, and performance patterns (American Occupational Therapy Association, 2014). Occupation can be organized into many categories, such as ADL, IADL, leisure, play, social participation, education, work, rest, and sleep. Each client engages differently due to the multidimensional nature and complexity of occupation. One client may view the act of walking his or her dog as an IADL task, where another client views it as a leisure task. The steps and demands of a task will be different for each client. One reason may be that Client A lives in an apartment building and navigates six flights of stairs to reach the sidewalk, while Client B drives 10 minutes to a 1-mile wooded path to walk the dog. Prioritization of occupations varies with time. This can be demonstrated by the adaptation to each occupation during the cold winter months. Client A may continue to follow the same dog-walking routine each day, while Client B may choose not to walk the dog but let it out in the backyard each day.

To use them effectively as a therapeutic tool, OTs and OTAs analyze the unique features of each occupation, including the components of individual engagement (American Occupational Therapy Association, 2014).

METHODS USED IN OCCUPATIONAL THERAPY INTERVENTION

OTs, with input from OTAs, assess many factors to develop an intervention plan and determine the most effective methods to implement the plan (see Chapters 4 through 9). Intervention includes the actions taken, behavior demonstrated, and plans utilized to improve a client's ability to perform daily occupations. OTs and OTAs utilize therapeutic reasoning to consider how each therapeutic method may affect the targeted outcome of intervention. See the case study below, as an example of how therapeutic reasoning leads to the usage of therapeutic modalities. This reasoning leads them to use a combination of methods throughout the therapeutic process to achieve goals. The methods used in intervention include (1) therapeutic use of meaningful occupations and **purposeful activities**, (2) environmental modification, (3) activity adaptations, (4) **preparatory tasks** and **methods**, (5) education and training, (6) advocacy, and (7) group intervention (American Occupational Therapy Association, 2014) (Table 12.1).

Meaningful occupations and purposeful activities are used therapeutically to promote health and wellness, prevent disability, restore function, maintain performance capacity, and modify factors related to participation. Purposeful activities may include practicing medical management with beads and mock medication bottles or practicing shower transfers in the hospital bathroom to simulate a patient's home routine and environment. These activities are specifically designed and graded to develop, adapt, or improve performance skills (Crepeau et al., 2014). Purposeful activities can be simulated in the clinical environment or completed in a natural environment.

Environmental modifications and adaptations enhance occupational functioning, safety, and performance. OTs and OTAs analyze activities to determine what areas need to be modified. Activity analysis refers to a general consideration of how tasks are typically done under ordinary circumstances with identification of the task or activity's component parts. Once this is done, activity adaptations can be implemented to improve function and enhance skills. OTs and OTAs may use adaptive equipment, assistive technology, and orthotic devices to accomplish this (also see upcoming section on occupational and activity analysis and synthesis, as well as Table 12.2 later in the chapter).

Preparatory tasks and methods prepare for the engagement in therapeutic activities. Preparatory tasks typically include active client participation and occur in a clinical or simulated setting. Examples of preparatory tasks may include therapeutic exercise such as active stretching to restore range of motion (ROM) or an upper body ergometer (arm bike) to increase endurance for participation. Preparatory methods are passive intervention applications used to improve a specific client factor, such as "to increase participation in occupation." These include sensorimotor techniques such as the application of neutral warmth to decrease hypertonicity in a client's arm, to allow the client to use it to engage in an occupation. They also include physical agent modalities (PAMs) such as superficial thermal modalities (hot packs, paraffin wax, and fluidotherapy) and electrical modalities (**transcutaneous electrical nerve stimulation** [TENS] and **neuromuscular electrical stimulation** [NMES]). In most states, OTs and OTAs need advanced certification to utilize PAMs.

Adaptive equipment training and family education are provided to promote increased independence. Advocacy empowers clients and therapists to strive for occupational justice.

Group intervention utilizes group dynamics and social interaction across the lifespan to facilitate learning and skill acquisition (American Occupational Therapy Association, 2014).

Occupational Analysis, Activity Analysis, and Synthesis

Occupational analysis refers to systematically analyzing the aspects of an activity and how a person or group of people

TABLE 12.1	Therapeutic Methods and Intervention Application	
Therapeutic Method	**Example**	**Intervention Application**
Meaningful occupation	Care of pets	Organization, functional mobility, social participation
Activity adaptation	Long-handled sponge	Compensation for decreased range of motion or endurance
Preparatory task	Passive, active assist or active range of motion (ROM) of fingers	Increase joint ROM or decrease edema to grasp an object
Preparatory method	Application of hot pack to shoulder	Increase ROM to improve ability to brush hair
Education	Energy conservation	Improve activity participation for clients with pulmonary disease
Advocacy	Justification letter for powered mobility	Allow client with spinal cord injury to return to college
Group intervention	Social skills group	Assist clients with community reintegration following a traumatic brain injury

CASE STUDY
Olivia, Part 1

Olivia is a new patient on your caseload. She is a 55-year-old teacher and involved aunt. Her primary diagnosis is right CVA with residual shoulder/hand pain of her left upper extremity (LUE). The stroke resulted in her hospitalization and subsequent admission to an inpatient rehabilitation facility. She has a past medical history of hypertension and has exhibited reactive depression since her recent hospitalization.

Before her recent hospitalization, Olivia lived in a single-level home in a suburban neighborhood. She was widowed 7 years ago and has lived alone in her home since the loss of her husband. Her sister and nephews live close by and visit often. While gathering Olivia's occupational profile, you learned that baking is one of her favorite pastimes. Before the onset of her stroke, Olivia enjoyed researching old family recipes and sharing her baked goods with friends and family. Often her nephews would join Olivia in her baking.

The occupational profile also revealed that Olivia attended church with a community group on the weekends. She developed several friendships through this group and attends every Sunday. She pursued several other interests, including gardening, tennis, and traveling. She has been on the boards of several organizations, volunteering as secretary or treasurer of these groups. She frequently communicates with her grandchildren through social networking computer sites and text messaging. She took yearly vacations, traveling to various locations in the United States for 2 to 3 weeks a year. Olivia is also responsible for managing her personal finances.

Before her stroke, Olivia was independent in all of her basic ADL and IADL tasks. Initial evaluation revealed that Olivia currently needs moderate assistance to dress herself. She independently feeds herself. She exhibits a mild left visual field cut. She has limited active and passive ROM of the left shoulder, with pain on passive flexion of the left shoulder at end range, necessitating the use of a sling. Active ROM is limited in the LUE, but Olivia is able to grasp, pronate her forearm, flex the elbow, and internally rotate the shoulder. Her balance and mobility are impaired. Although her prospects for recovery are positive, Olivia expresses feelings of dejection about regaining her ability to resume her independence, roles, and activities.

Goals for occupational therapy intervention include the following:

- Engage in meaningful occupations to reduce depression.
- Adapt and grade activities using unilateral, bilateral, and balance activities, to enable participation in life roles.
- Reduce pain associated with movement to enable use of LUE in occupations; use sling intermittently to support LUE, apply heat to left shoulder, and provide analgesic 20 minutes before active occupation treatment.
- Increase ROM and strength of LUE.
- Improve balance and mobility through participation in activity.
- Prepare Olivia with the skills needed for her to return home.
- Prepare Olivia to resume active and social interactions with family, in person, and through the use of electronic communication devices.

Since baking is one of Olivia's favorite occupations it will provide tremendous therapeutic potential. Therefore you decide to bake chocolate chip cookies during your next intervention session. You begin this process by considering the general ingredients, equipment, demands, steps, and skills that are typically needed for this task (see Table 12.1, under "Therapeutic Method") (American Occupational Therapy Association, 2014; O'Brien, 2017).

For the next step of the intervention planning process you initiate a conversation with Olivia to better understand the meaning of baking from her perspective—being careful not to bring any assumptions to the occupational analysis process (i.e., roles, culture, values, context) (see Table 12.1, under "Example) (American Occupational Therapy Association, 2014; O'Brien, 2017). This reflects baking as one of Olivia's personal and goal-directed occupations.

After interviewing the client to identify an intervention activity that she would find meaningful, Olivia decided to pursue baking, making chocolate chip cookies for her nephews that visited her at the rehab center twice a week. Intervention was initiated in the therapy kitchen with sitting balance activities in preparation for meal preparation (baking). The client was instructed in scanning techniques to compensate for her visual field cut. Olivia learned one-handed techniques, with use of adaptive equipment, for baking (i.e., stirring, gathering supplies), gradually shifting to bilateral UE use as her strength and ROM improved. Before beginning the activity, to reduce pain in her LUE and heighten her tolerance for movement, heat was applied to her shoulder using hot packs. Over the course of therapy, to improve her balance and standing tolerance, the baking supplies were placed on a standing table.

As her performance improved, Olivia was discharged to home and returned to the clinic as an outpatient three times per week. With encouragement from her family and her therapist, Olivia completed multiple homemade recipes in therapy and expressed great satisfaction in her achievement.

Acting on suggestions from the therapist and input from the patient and family, an intervention plan was developed. The family reorganized Olivia's kitchen so her baking supplies were at counter level, enabling her to participate in this occupation at home. She navigated the kitchen with a walker, utilizing a walker basket to carry baking materials as needed. When she baked with her family, her nephews assisted by stabilizing the mixing bowl as Olivia stirred and added ingredients. Additionally, raised garden beds were added at home, she resumed her check writing, and she returned to church and volunteering for one of the boards she belonged to.

These efforts resulted in her gradual recognition that she was able to engage in an adaptive form of some of her favorite activities. As she recovered motor performance in her left arm and her balance became safer, her depression lifted. She began to use the internet to find new recipes that she and her nephews could cook and enjoy together.

Critical Thinking Questions

1. Identify occupations Olivia engaged in before her stroke, those in which she engaged during intervention, and those she assumed or resumed. Describe how her progress relied on evaluation of her occupational performance.
2. Explore the contextual and environmental factors that influenced Olivia in resuming preferred activities. Describe roles she resumed as a consequence of these influences.
3. Describe how the activities in which Olivia engaged were adapted to provide an interface between activity demands and client factors.

completes that activity (Crepeau et al., 2014). Through this process, OTs and OTAs synthesize information obtained from the **activity analysis** with assessment results to help them understand the specific situation of the client. The following questions set the stage for this analysis: What do you want or need to do? How did you do this activity before? What do you feel has changed? In what environment did this activity take place, and where might it take place in the future?

These questions provide OTs and OTAs with information that allows them to know about their clients, what their clients are interested in doing, and how to best meet their clients' needs and abilities (Creighton, 1992). A complete analysis includes all aspects of performance and reveals each activity's potential for therapeutic application. Activities should be goal directed, adaptable, gradable, meaningful, matched to individual needs, capable of eliciting participation, designed to prevent or reverse dysfunction, and capable of enhancing performance in life roles.

A careful and thorough analysis must be completed to make appropriate intervention choices. This includes looking at all the components and requirements of an activity and synthesizing it with the client and environmental factors to facilitate performance (Hersch et al., 2005). The American Occupational Therapy Association provides an occupational profile template and practice framework to assist practitioners in analyzing occupations (American Occupational Therapy Association, 2014).

Occupational Adaptation and Grading

A comprehensive analysis of occupation allows OTs and OTAs to understand how to match the task with the client's functional capabilities, strengths, and challenges to maximize participation, engagement, and performance (Thomas, 2012). It also helps them to determine **just-right challenge**, which is a careful balance between the challenge of the task and the skills of the person. If the challenge is too high and the skills of the person are low, frustration may result. If the challenge of a task is too low and the skills of the person are too high, decreased motivation and engagement may result. However, if the challenge of a task is equal or slightly above the skills of the person, then he or she will experience a state of flow, which can influence an optimal experience, occupational performance, and life satisfaction (Robeiro & Polgar, 1999). This level of challenge is ideal for learning and making therapeutic gains as it enables a client's strengths to be used optimally, independence to be maximized, and a sense of increased accomplishment. Situations that foster success improve health and satisfaction (Baum & Christiansen, 2005).

Adapting Activity (Compensation)

Activity analysis reveals which components of an occupation need to be adapted to increase participation. For example, if a client has decreased strength and endurance and needs to put on shoes, the method may need to be altered (sitting instead of standing), the environment may need to be changed (storing shoes within easy reach), or an adaptive aid may be

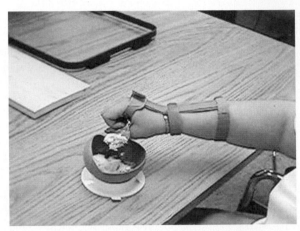

Fig. 12.1 Eating using a special splint with a utensil holder fitted to the hand.

needed (long-handled shoe horn) for the activity to be performed successfully. Another example of activity modification would be using a universal cuff utensil holder fitted to the hand (Fig. 12.1). Another environmental modification may be to use color-coded labels on dresser drawers to increase the success with dressing for a client with cognitive impairment. Compensation requires flexibility from the practitioner and the client. If a client chooses to continue to complete tasks without modification there may be a risk to his or her safety. OTs and OTAs could then find alternate activities that have the same intrinsic value that can be completed more safely.

CASE STUDY (CONTINUED)
Olivia, Part 2, Give It a Try!

Consider how the demands of baking have changed for Olivia since her diagnosis.
1. What factors affect Oliva's performance in baking?
2. What adaptations or changes can be made to the occupation process to facilitate the just-right challenge? How could the activity be made easier? More difficult?
3. What client factors could be improved via baking as a therapeutic activity?

Grading Occupations (Remediation)

To allow a client to complete a task with the just-right challenge, OTs and OTAs can grade it by increasing or decreasing activity demands (Thibodeaux & Ludwig, 1988). This facilitates skill development, increases the likelihood of success, and improves participation. As with compensation, many factors need to be considered when grading a task, especially activity demands and performance skills (American Occupational Therapy Association, 2014). There are an almost endless variety of ways to grade an activity, which makes occupational therapy both an art and a science.

Grading an activity can be done through changing the activity or the environment in which it is performed. Decreasing the challenge, sometimes referred to as grading down, means making it easier for the client. This may include

Client Factor	Increasing Challenge	Decreasing Challenge
Strength	Change plane of movement to move with gravity maximized Add wrist weights (Fig. 12.2) Utilize weighted or heavy tool	Change plane of movement to minimize gravity Use lighter utensils or adaptation (Fig. 12.3) Keep items closer to the body
Range of motion	Position materials farther away to increase joint excursion	Enlarge items with foam rubber (Fig. 12.4)
Endurance and activity tolerance	Move from light to heavy work (fold sheets and then thicker blankets) Increase time standing while completing a task (Fig. 12.5)	Sit at edge of bed while dressing Complete tasks sitting rather than standing Sponge bathe at the sink rather than taking a shower
Coordination	Increase fine motor control needed	Use larger objects requiring less coordination
Balance	Complete task on unstable surface such as plush carpet	Complete task on a stable surface such as a tile floor
Cognitive skill	Complete a task requiring multistep directions and many components	Complete tasks with fewer components in a distraction-free environment

TABLE 12.2   Specific Techniques to Grade Tasks for Targeted Client Factors

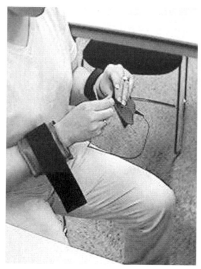

Fig. 12.2 Weight attached to the wrist increases resistance during occupation-based tasks.

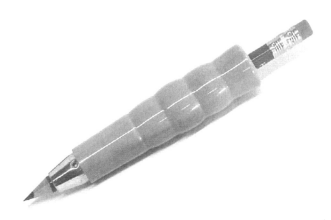

Fig. 12.3 Universal weighted grip or holder for manipulation tools (i.e., writing utensil, paint brush).

doing it at a slower pace. For a client with impaired memory, a dressing may be made easier by including visual aids to simplify the sequence of the steps to complete it.

Increasing the challenge, or grading up, means to make components of an intervention more challenging for a client. This can be done by increasing the weight of the object. For an older adult with balance deficits, dressing while standing on a foam balance pad would make the task more difficult. See Table 12.2 for examples of grading activities.

Selection of Activity

Activities for treatment of physical dysfunction are usually selected for their potential to improve functioning in sensory, movement-related, and mental factors to help sustain motivation to engage in activity. Activities selected to improve physical performance should provide desired exercise or purposeful use of affected parts. They should enable the patient to transfer the motion, strength, and coordination gained in adjunctive and enabling modalities to useful, normal daily activities.

Activities should allow for active participation. They should provide opportunities for practice, such as those

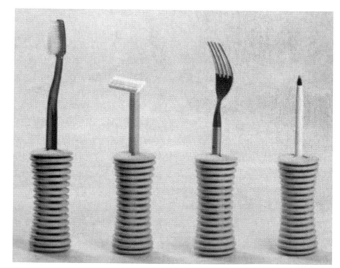

Fig. 12.4 Built-up tool handles used to assist limited digit ROM or grip strength.

involving repetition of motion to benefit the patient. Therapeutic activities allow for multiple ways of grading, such as for strength, ROM, and endurance (Hopkins et al., 1988; Spackman, 1978).

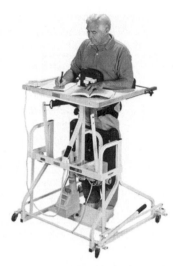

Fig. 12.5 Midland Electric Stand-In Table. Four-point support system stabilizes client at the feet, knees, buttocks, and chest. (Courtesy Performance Health, Warrenville, IL.)

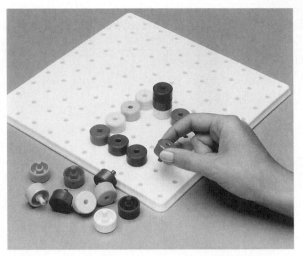

Fig. 12.6 Puzzles and other perceptual and cognitive training media are used on the tabletop. (Courtesy North Coast Medical, Morgan Hill, CA.)

Clients participate the best in motivating and interesting activities because they experience sufficient satisfaction to sustain performance of the task. It is important to guide the individual to suitable therapeutic activities at just the right level of challenge so that he or she will achieve satisfaction by engaging in the activity.

It is optimal to utilize activities in the most natural way and environment possible. However, when that is not possible, simulating appropriate active occupations to meet the patient's needs may be necessary. OTs and OTAs often devise simulated activities using equipment and found materials used in other activities. An example of this is to use a milk crate with a hand weight in it to simulate placing a turkey in the oven to bake.

Other examples are using puzzles and cognitive training media to develop visual perceptual functions, motor planning skills, memory, sequencing, and problem solving, among other skills (Fig. 12.6). Clothing fastener boards and household hardware boards may provide practice in the manipulation of everyday objects before the patient is confronted with the real task (Fig. 12.7). At a higher level of tech sophistication, commercial work simulators (see Chapter 16) and computer programs are used to train patients in physical and cognitive skills.

Enabling activities are considered nonpurposeful and generally do not meet an inherent goal, but they may engage the patient mentally and physically. The purposes of enabling activities are to practice specific motor patterns, to train in perceptual and cognitive skills, and to practice motor and process skills necessary for function in the home and community. Many enabling modalities used in occupational therapy practice facilitate perceptual, cognitive, and motor learning. Such activities may be appropriate for skill acquisition, when the patient is getting the idea of the movement and practicing problem solving. Practice should be daily or frequent, and feedback should be given often so that errors are reduced and skills refined to prepare for performance of real-life

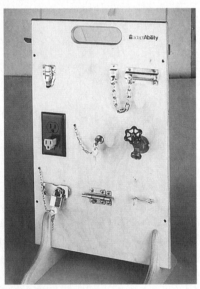

Fig. 12.7 Boards built with household fasteners are simulations used for practicing manipulation and management of common household hardware. (Reprinted with permission, S & S Worldwide, adaptAbility, 1995.)

purposeful activity. These activities should be used judiciously, and their place in the sequence of treatment and motor learning should be well planned. They can be used along with **adjunctive modalities** and purposeful activities as part of a comprehensive treatment program. Adjunctive modalities can be used as a preliminary step toward purposeful activity as they prepare the patient for occupational performance. Some examples of adjunctive modalities are therapeutic exercise, orthotics, sensory stimulation, and physical agent modalities (Thibodeaux & Ludwig, 1988).

Preparatory Tasks and Preparatory Methods. Therapeutic exercise is a preparatory task. An example involves TheraPutty

TABLE 12.3	**Physical Agent Modalities (PAMs)**		
Type of PAM	**Examples**	**Therapeutic Result**	**Contraindication for Use**
Superficial thermal (heat)	Hot packs Fluidotherapy Paraffin	Increase tissue extensibility Decrease pain	Decreased sensation Decreased vascularity Open wounds Extreme edema Malignancy
Superficial thermal (cold)	Ice packs Ice massage	Decrease swelling Decrease pain	Decreased sensation Transplanted digit
Electrical stimulation	E-Stim Neuromuscular electrical stimulation (NMES) Transcutaneous electrical nerve stimulation (TENS)	Stimulate muscle contraction Decrease pain	Cardiac patients with pacemaker Malignancy

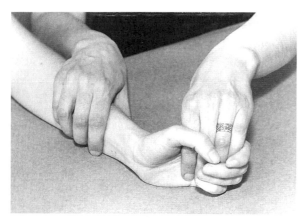

Fig. 12.8 Passive exercise of the wrist with stabilization of the joint proximal to the one being exercised.

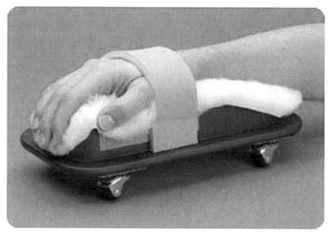

Fig. 12.9 Arm skate is equipped with ball-bearing casters for increased mobility and range of motion.

exercises to improve hand strength and dexterity. See Chapter 29 for other examples of therapeutic exercise, such as **passive** (Fig. 12.8), **active-assist** (Fig. 12.9), and **active ROM exercises**. OTs and OTAs should carefully monitor the client's response to the intervention. Physical exertion may result in muscle fatigue, pain, or muscle overload. Pain may lead to the following signs: facial grimacing, writhing, groaning or whimpering, restlessness or agitation, and withdrawal. Other troublesome signs to look for include increased perspiration, decreased respiration, distraction, decreased performance, and redness. When an OT or OTA notices signs of discomfort, the exercise or activity should be stopped and the client encourage to rest. If symptoms improve, the activity may be resumed.

Preparatory methods include physical agent modalities, such as heat, to prepare soft tissue for movement or stretch or electrical stimulation to influence soft tissue extensibility and to prepare muscles for stretch or movement (Table 12.3). Other forms of preparatory methods include manual edema mobilization or wound care, dressing changes (see Chapter 29), orthotics (see Chapter 19), and assistive technology (see Chapter 14).

Preparatory Tasks: Therapeutic Activity. Therapeutic **activities** are dynamic activities that develop or restore normal movement patterns, muscle strength, endurance,

coordination, ROM deficits, and joint contractures for improved performance in functional activities. To ensure appropriateness, the activity should always be performed in connection with the restoration of the client's desired occupations; therefore a thorough occupational analysis should always take place first. An example of a therapeutic activity is using a dressing frame fitted with laces, buckles, buttons, and zippers (Fig. 12.10) to aid manual dexterity and finger coordination; another is manipulating coins to improve manual dexterity. In both examples, the activities performed are components of occupations, such as the ADL of dressing and IADL of money management. Other activities may include walking on uneven terrain to improve community mobility, gathering beanbags from multiple heights to enhance the IADL of home management, practicing bed mobility, car transfer training, and playing a game to promote high/low reaching to improve function in various daily activities.

It is important to note that therapeutic activities are contraindicated for clients who are in a fragile medical state or are experiencing high levels of pain. Other contraindications include recent joint, tendon, and nerve surgery or repair; inflamed joints; and certain cardiopulmonary diagnoses and surgical interventions. Similarly, therapeutic activities may

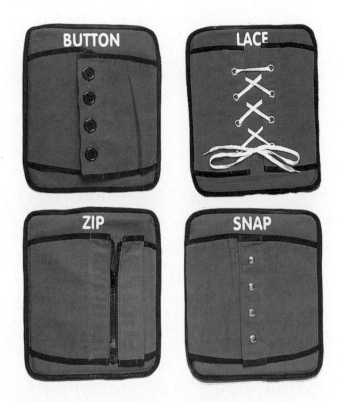

Fig. 12.10 Boards built with dressing fasteners are simulations used for practicing manipulation and management of common articles of clothing.

not be useful for a client with a permanent contracture, although most contractures can be reversed if detected before the joint is immobilized completely. Careful consideration and thorough activity analysis are required to determine the appropriate grading and use of therapeutic activities for clients who have spasticity or limited controlled movement and sensation.

SUMMARY

OTs and OTAs use occupations as the primary tools of practice. They use purposeful activity, activity analysis, adaptation, grading of activities, therapeutic exercise, simulated or enabling activities, and adjunctive modalities in the continuum of treatment, and may use these methods simultaneously toward these ends. The breadth of the OT or OTA practice skills, applied to the patient's personal and social needs, helps the patient use newly gained strength, ROM, and coordination for purposeful activity, thus preparing the patient to assume or reassume life roles. Appropriate therapeutic activity is individualized and designed to be meaningful and interesting to the patient while meeting therapeutic objectives.

Therapeutic activity may be adapted to meet special needs of the patient or the environment. It may be graded for physical, perceptual, cognitive, and social purposes to keep the patient functioning at maximal potential at any point in the treatment program. The uniqueness of occupational therapy lies in its extensive use of goal-directed purposeful activities as treatment modalities, making use of the mind-body

continuum within the tangible and social context. Purposeful activity is the core of occupational therapy practice.

In all instances, OTAs must be well trained and well qualified to deliver all aspects of practice. They should not hesitate to refer patients to supervisors and experts for treatment when appropriate.

REVIEW QUESTIONS

1. Provide two reasons why activity is valuable.
2. List at least five requirements that activities must meet to be used for therapeutic purposes.
3. What is required for an activity to be considered purposeful?
4. What is the just-right challenge in performance?
5. Grade an activity to accommodate changes in a variety of factors such as strength, ROM, endurance, coordination, and perceptual and cognitive skills.
6. How can activities be adapted to meet specific therapeutic objectives?
7. Describe the difference between preparatory tasks and preparatory methods.
8. Define and give an example of the three types of therapeutic exercise.
9. Discuss the appropriate use of enabling activities and adjunctive modalities.
10. How can the application of physical agent modalities enhance the patient's performance of activities?
11. List and describe three physical agent modalities and discuss their use as preparatory modalities for functional activity.

REFERENCES

American Occupational Therapy Association. (2008). Physical agent modalities: a position paper. *The American Journal of Occupational Therapy, 62*(6), 691–693.

American Occupational Therapy Association. (2014). Occupational therapy practice framework: domain and process. 3rd ed. *The American Journal of Occupational Therapy, 68,* S1–S48.

Baum, C., & Christiansen, C. (2005). Person-environment-performance: an occupation-based framework for practice. In C. H. Christiansen, & C. M. Baum (Eds.), *Occupational therapy: performance, participation, and well-being* (pp. 243–259). Thorofare, NJ: Slack Inc.

Christiansen, C., & Baum, C. M. (1999). Defining lives: occupation as identity: an essay on competence, coherence, and the creation of meaning. *The American Journal of Occupational Therapy, 53,* 547–558. Available from: https://doi.org/10.5014/ajot.53.6.547.

Creighton, C. (1992). The origin and evolution of activity analysis. *The American Journal of Occupational Therapy, 46*(1), 45–48. Available from: https://doi.org/10.5014/ajot.46.1.45.

Crepeau, E., Schell, B. A. B., Gillen, G., & Scaffa, M. (2014). Analyzing occupations and activity. In B. A. B. Schell, G. Gillen, & M. E. Scaffa (Eds.), *Willard and Spackman's occupational therapy* (12th ed., pp. 234–248). Philadelphia, PA: Lippincott Williams & Wilkins.

Hersch, G. I., Lamport, N. K., & Coffey, M. S. (2005). *Activity analysis: application to occupation* (5th ed.). Thorofare, NJ: Slack Inc.

Hinojosa, J., Kramer, P., & Crist, P. (Eds.), (2005). *Evaluation: obtaining and interpreting data* (2nd ed.). Bethesda, MD: AOTA Press.

Hopkins, H. L., Smith, H. D., & Tiffany, E. G. (1988). The activity process. In: H. L. Hopkins, H. D. Smith (Eds.), *Willard and Spackman's occupational therapy* (7th ed.). Philadelphia, PA: JB Lippincott.

Kottke, F. J. (1971). Therapeutic exercises to develop neuromuscular coordination. In: F. J. Kottke, G. K. Stillwell, & J. F. Lehmann (Eds.), *Krusen's handbook of physical medicine and rehabilitation* (4th ed.). Philadelphia, PA: WB Saunders.

Mosey, A. C. (1996). *Psychosocial components of occupational therapy.* New York, NY: Raven Press.

O'Brien, J. (2017). Occupational analysis worksheet [class handout]. *Occup Ther. 502.* Analysis of occupational performance. Portland, ME: Department of Occupational Therapy, University of New England.

Pedretti, L. W., Smith, R. O., Hammel, J., et al. (1992). Use of adjunctive modalities in occupational therapy. *The American Journal of Occupational Therapy, 46*(12), 1075–1081.

Robeiro, K. L., & Polgar, J. M. (1999). Enabling occupational performance: optimal experiences in therapy. *Canadian Journal of Occupational Therapy, 66*(1), 14–22.

Spackman, C. S. (1978). Occupational therapy for the restoration of physical function. In: H. S. Willard & C. S. Spackman (Eds.), *Occupational therapy* (5th ed.). Philadelphia, PA: JB Lippincott.

Thibodeaux, C. S., & Ludwig, F. M. (1988). Intrinsic motivation in product-oriented and non-product-oriented activities. *The American Journal of Occupational Therapy, 42*(3), 169–175.

Thomas, H. (2012). *Occupation-based activity analysis.* Thorofare, NJ: Slack Inc.

Wilcock, A. (2006). *An occupational perspective of health* (2nd ed.). Thorofare, NJ: Slack Inc.

Wilcock, A. (2007). Occupation and health: are they one and the same? *Journal of Occupational Science, 14*(1), 3–8.

PART V

Performance in Areas of Occupation

13

Activities of Daily Living

Nichole Bell and Erin McGeggen

OBJECTIVES

After reading this chapter, the student or the occupational therapy practitioner will be able to do the following:

1. Define the occupational therapist and occupational therapist assistant roles in promoting independence in activities of daily living (ADL) and instrumental activities of daily living (IADL).
2. Describe the ADL and IADL evaluation process, including assessments, techniques, strategies, and reporting procedures.
3. Instruct in development of individualized plans based on client factors, performance patterns, and environment.
4. Explain methods of utilization of compensatory techniques, adaptive techniques/equipment, and environmental modifications to promote client independence in ADL and IADL.
5. Identify functions and use of adaptive devices to facilitate participation in ADL and IADL for individuals with specific performance capacities.
6. Understand condition-specific strategies and treatment approaches to facilitate independence in ADL and IADL.
7. Recommend home modifications and equipment to individuals to enable maximum independence at home.
8. Describe emerging treatment approaches such as animal-assisted therapy and telehealth to further client independence at home and in the community.

KEY TERMS

Activities of daily living
Instrumental activities of daily living
Functional mobility
Adaptive equipment
Environmental modifications
Analysis of occupational performance
Occupational profile
Self-care tasks
Activity analysis
Topographic orientation
Dressing stick
Sock aid
Buttonhook

Reacher
Long-handled sponge
Tub transfer bench
Nonskid mats
Adaptive clothing
Bridging
Assistive technology
Nurturing assistance
Home assessment
Caregiver training
Bedside commode
Telehealth

INTRODUCTION

The goal of this chapter is to explain the roles of occupational therapists (OTs) and occupational therapy assistants (OTAs) in the facilitation of independence in **activities of daily living** (ADL) and **instrumental activities of daily living** (IADL). ADL include routinely performed skills related to self-care such as dressing, bathing, toileting, hygiene, grooming, sexual intercourse, **functional mobility**, and bowel/bladder management (American Occupational Therapy Association, 2014). IADL include complex living skills to support community living such as meal preparation, cleaning, financial management, transportation, shopping, child care, pet care, home management,

driving, and communication (AOTA, 2014). For a thorough discussion of interventions to improve mealtime occupations, including adaptations to facilitate feeding and eating, please refer to Chapter 11. Individuals begin to learn ADL early in life. They are practiced daily and become habits, which can be completed with little thought. Disruptions in routines and habits, which may occur with disease or injury, may challenge an individual and lead to the need for assistance with these tasks. Frequently, ADL may need to be relearned. If a client is unable to relearn how to complete them the same way as prior to illness or injury, the activities may need to be adapted or completed by another individual.

Occupational therapy practitioners provide evaluation of and training to clients needing assistance with ADL and IADL. They provide these services in a wide variety of health care settings. OTAs work with OTs to assess performance skills, determine barriers to success, select treatment objectives, and instruct in strategies to optimize independence in daily routines. This is done by developing adaptations, coaching in compensatory strategies, instructing in use of **adaptive equipment**, and facilitating **environmental modifications**. Use of these strategies may assist in removing physical, cognitive, social, and emotional barriers that interfere with a client's performance. A client may utilize adaptive methods and compensatory strategies temporarily or permanently. The timeframe for adaptation depends upon the deficits in performance skills experienced by the client, prognosis for recovery, and the environment in which the skills will be performed. Strategies to utilize adaptive equipment, environmental modifications, compensatory techniques, and other treatment methods to facilitate independence in ADL and IADL will be provided throughout this chapter.

DEFINITION OF ADL AND IADL

Daily activities can be separated into ADL (or basic ADL) and IADL. ADL require basic skills and are oriented toward the care of one's own body or person. IADL require more advanced problem-solving skills, social skills, and complex environmental interactions. IADL are oriented toward life in the community and with others. Box 13.1 provides examples and descriptions of some common ADL and IADL.

Some ADL and IADL need to be completed for an individual to participate in other ADL and IADL. For example, functional mobility involves moving from one place to another during the performance of ADL (American Occupational Therapy Association, 2014). Functional mobility includes moving one's body from surface to surface (such as wheelchair to bed), movement while on a specific surface (such as bed mobility), and moving in the environment to gather objects for a task (such as ambulation or wheelchair propulsion to gather soap and washcloths to complete bathing). Functional mobility that includes ambulation can be done with or without adaptive equipment such as canes or walkers. Communication management includes all aspects of sending and receiving information, which is necessary for the successful completion of many ADL and IADL. Communication includes not only speaking but also the ability to use tools to write, operate a personal computer, read, type, text, call with a telephone, or use special communications devices. Community mobility, another skill necessary for many IADL, refers to the ability to move around one's neighborhood or community while ambulating, using a wheelchair, operating a personal vehicle, or navigating public transportation.

CONSIDERATIONS RELATED TO ADL AND IADL

ADL and often IADL involve the personal care of one's own body, loved ones, and valued possessions. Therefore OTs and OTAs need to be aware of the client's level of comfort with exposing body parts and not be afraid to talk with the client about his or her personal preferences regarding privacy. Although in all areas of practice the client's feelings about having the body viewed and touched should be respected, this particularly sensitive area may require even more discretion. It is especially important for privacy to be maintained for toileting, grooming, and dressing tasks. If it is not possible to leave the client alone, due to safety concerns, the therapist could consider draping a towel or sheet over the patient and/or turning away while the client is on the toilet. While the OT or OTA is providing ADL training, it may be possible to discuss with the client specific feelings about personal values and culture surrounding these intimate tasks. If the client is unable to complete ADL independently or with modified independence, the clinician may include caregiver training in the sessions. Respect the client's desire for family involvement.

Other factors that influence the occupational therapy process related to ADL and IADL include level of assistance needed for completion of tasks and additional client (i.e., spirituality, values and beliefs, prior level of functioning), environmental (familial and social support), and contextual factors. The OT and OTA should be mindful of all of these

---

BOX 13.1 **Activities of Daily Living (ADL) and Instrumental Activities of Daily Living (IADL)**	
Activities of Daily Living (ADL)	**Description/ Examples**
Bathing/showering	Cleaning one's body
Toileting/toilet hygiene	Transferring to/from toileting device, clothing management, wiping self
Dressing	Donning clothing for all areas of body; often specified as upper/lower body dressing
Grooming	Hair care, makeup application, shaving
Sexual activity	Activities to satisfy sexual needs and /or reproduction
Functional mobility	Movement and transfers needed to navigate one's environment to complete ADL
Instrumental Activities of Daily Living (IADL)	**Description/ Example**
Care of others (children, pets, etc.)	Providing care for another, including feeding, etc.
Home management	Caring for and organizing one's place of residence
Driving and community mobility	Navigating around the community in a personal vehicle or utilizing public transportation
Communication	Managing interpersonal interactions in oral, written, or digital form

when formulating short-term and long-term goals and deciding the approach to treatment. For example, if a client experiences a cerebral vascular accident (CVA), there may be many performance skills and areas of occupation affected. It is therefore important to return to the occupational profile to formulate goals based on what's most important to the client. If bathing oneself independently is most important to the client, this should be the first task worked on. Many approaches to treatment could be taken. An approach to restore function may include normalizing muscle tone in a spastic upper extremity to allow the client to hold a washcloth to bath the upper body. A compensatory approach may include providing the client with an adaptive item, such as a bath mitt, to compensate for a hand with flaccidity that is unable to grip a washcloth. As the intervention process continues, the OT or OTA must continually reassess which intervention approach would be most beneficial. OTs and OTAs keep all of these factors in mind when developing individualized plans of care for each client served.

The living situation to which the client will return, as well as social and occupational roles to be performed, influences the intervention process. The following are some questions to consider when formulating the intervention plan: Will the client return home, to an assisted living facility (ALF), or to a skilled nursing facility (SNF)? What level of support will the client have? Will the client stay at the next location for a temporary period or is it a permanent placement? Will the client be returning to work or participating in other community activities?

OCCUPATIONAL THERAPY PROCESS

The occupational therapy evaluation consists of gathering an occupational history and an **analysis of occupational performance**, which can consist of standardized and nonstandardized evaluations. This is typically done by an OT with input from the OTA. The OT begins by creating an **occupational profile** about a client utilizing tools such as an interest checklist or through client interviews (American Occupational Therapy Association, 2014; Department of Veterans Affairs, 2017; Florey and Michelman, 1982; Malick & Almasy, 1998; Modlin, 2001). The interest checklist indicates degrees of interest in five categories of activities: (1) manual skills, (2) physical sports, (3) social recreation, (4) ADL, and (5) cultural and educational activities (Malick & Almasy, 1998). The Occupational Performance History Interview (OPHI-II) is an interviewing tool that can be used with a wide range of clients, is easily accessible, and consistent across cultures (Kielhofner, Mallinson, & Forsyth et al., 2001). This tool creates an occupational picture using the following areas: activity/occupational choices, critical life events, daily routine, occupational roles, and occupational behavior settings (Kielhofner et al., 2001). Occupational therapy practitioners may also conduct an unstructured interview with a client or family to gather information for the occupational profile. The assessment of occupational performance, by way of standardized and nonstandardized assessments, allows the OT to assess the client's performance skills in the areas of ADL and IADL and to

generate an intervention plan. These assessments are best when the client is observed engaging in the tasks in a natural context, such as in a bathroom. However, when the natural context is not available, a simulated version may be observed. For example, if a client typically completes bathing at the sink with a washcloth in the morning in the bathroom, the OT should observe that. If it is not possible to observe that, the OT may provide a washcloth and a basin in another context. It is important for an occupational therapy practitioner to be aware that the simulation of ADL and IADL requires the client to perform routine self-maintenance tasks at artificial times in an artificial environment. This may be difficult for clients who have difficulty generalizing or transferring learning from one situation to another.

While assessing occupational performance the occupational therapy practitioner must be aware of client factors, such as body structures and body functions, as well as environmental factors, such as the place in which the client is performing the task and any adaptations to the task that must be made.

During the performance evaluation the OT should observe the methods the client uses or attempts to use to accomplish the task. If performance deficits occur, the OT should attempt to determine their cause. Client factors and performance skills such as strength, range of motion (ROM), coordination, sensation, proprioception, and balance should be evaluated to determine potential skills and deficits in ADL performance and the possible need for special equipment. Perceptual and cognitive functions such as orientation, attention, processing skills, spatial awareness, and memory should be evaluated to determine impairments that could potentially impact performance in ADL.

Environmental and performance factors may cause performance deficits. An environmental factor may include bathroom doors that are not wide enough to get through with a walker. Performance factors include such things as decreased ROM, muscle weakness, decreased muscle of cardiovascular endurance, abnormal tone, and perceptual deficits. It is necessary to determine the cause of performance deficits to establish appropriate intervention goals.

EVALUATION OF OCCUPATIONAL PERFORMANCE IN ADL

ADL, or **self-care tasks**, involve an occupation central to one's identity and necessary for health and well-being (American Occupational Therapy Association, 2014). Occupational therapy practitioners maximize independence in ADL so that the clients they serve can achieve optimal health and well-being. The first step in this process is an occupational therapy evaluation, consisting of an occupational profile and an analysis of occupational performance. This evaluation may be conducted using a top-down or bottom-up approach. In the top-down approach, the therapist focuses on the client's occupational history and interests embedded within the home environment. The bottom-up approach focuses on identifying problems in specific client factors such as body functions and body structures. For example, the top-down approach recognizes the client's desire to dress independently. The bottom-up approach identifies a fine motor coordination impairment preventing the client from independently tying shoelaces. In practice, a blend of both approaches by the therapist is required.

ADL training may begin following the formulation of the occupational profile, the assessment of occupational performance, and the development of the intervention plan. The level and type of ADL training depends on the client's diagnosis and medical stability. All medical precautions should be followed. For example, if a client sustained a T8 spinal cord injury and needs to wear a thoracic/lumbar/spinal orthosis (TLSO) at all times while out of bed, training in bathing would need to include training in the donning and doffing of the orthosis, as well as bathing of the torso at bed level while the orthosis is off. In some cases, the client's medical fragility may mean that activities in preparation for ADL training, such as tolerance of upright posture, may need to proceed bathing. The goal of the OT or OTA in an ADL training program is for the client to achieve the maximum level of independence possible. The maximum level of independence is defined individually for each client, using clinical guidelines and clinical reasoning. A client with multiple orthopedic fractures following a motor vehicle accident is likely to achieve full independence in ADL and IADL. On the other hand, if that client also sustained a complete C7 spinal cord injury, he or she would likely return to modified independence for some ADL but need varying levels of assistance for others. A client with quadriplegia at the C7 level may achieve modified independence in self-feeding and oral hygiene utilizing assistive devices but would likely need care from a personal care attendant or family member for functional mobility.

Documentation of ADL and IADL Assessment

During the interview and performance evaluation the clinician documents the findings on an evaluation report. This evaluation report may include standardized assessments, such as the Assessment of Motor and Processing Skills (AMPS) (Koketsu, 2018) or checklists to consolidate background information gathered from the interview such as prior level of function, home environment, and prior services being used. The evaluation report also has sections to document current levels of function in categories such as self-care, mobility, and home management. OTs and OTAs may use terms to describe an individual's ability to participate in ADL (Koketsu, 2018). Terms such as *dependent, maximum assistance, moderate assistance,* and *minimal assistance* are often used, but to be useful they need to be clearly defined. The International Classification of Functioning, Disability and Health provides one way in which clinicians can document the activity limitations and participation restrictions demonstrated by a client in the area of ADL (World Health Organization, 2003). This document classifies impairments on a 0 to 4 scale (0 = no difficulty, 4 = complete difficulty). Another scale that is widely used is the Functional Independence Measure (FIM) (Department of Veterans Affairs, 2017). This assessment includes the following classifications: independent, modified independent (independent with the use of adaptive

aids such as a walker), minimal assistance ($\leq$25% help required), moderate assistance (26−50% help required), maximum assistance (51−75% help required), and dependent ($\geq$76% help required). Such terms must be defined or illustrated by supporting statements to be meaningful and useful descriptors of performance. The practitioner must specify whether the level of independence refers to a single activity, a category of activities such as dressing, or all ADL. Definitions should be modified to suit the program plan and approach of the facility at which services are delivered.

When completing the evaluation report, OTs and OTAs document body functions, mental functions, and sensory functions. These include strength, ROM, coordination, sensation, proprioception, balance, orientation, attention, processing skills, spatial awareness, and memory. For example, an evaluation report may include documentation of strength based on manual muscle testing or ROM based on goniometric measurements for upper extremity ROM. Figs. 13.1, 13.2, and 13.3 provide a sample case study, ADL and home management checklists, and summaries of an initial evaluation and progress report, respectively.

Evaluation of IADL

Home Management. Home management tasks are IADL and are evaluated as part of the assessment of occupational performance. The most accurate assessment of these skills can be achieved if done in an environment as close to the natural context as possible. This may include the treatment facility's kitchen, simulated living environment, and/or the client's home.

An **activity analysis**, which breaks the task into components that the client can perform, is important. OTs and OTAs need to understand the demands of the activity, range of skills involved in performance, and various cultural meanings ascribed to it, to perform an effective activity analysis. For example, the client may initially require assistance or cuing to retrieve items to make a sandwich. Occupational analysis can be used by the OT or OTA to grade the task, to assist the client in achieving independence in all the steps required to assemble the sandwich.

Home management roles uniquely apply to all clients depending on each person's living situation. Individuals may live independently or share home management responsibilities with their partners or families. Alteration in roles may occur following an injury resulting in physical disability. For example, if an individual sustains a traumatic brain injury, which results in decreased safety awareness managing a stove, and the person was the primary cook in the household, that role may need to be reassigned to another or modified to allow participation. A baseline level of ability to participate in IADL is required for a client to be left alone at home or at another location for an extended time. These skills include abilities to (1) prepare or retrieve a simple meal, (2) employ safety precautions and exhibit good judgment, (3) take medication, and (4) obtain emergency aid. The OT or OTA can evaluate potential for remaining at home through observation of the client while engaged in activities of home management.

Sample case study

J.V. is a 48-year-old married woman who suffered a cerebral thrombosis resulting in a CVA 6 months ago. She lives in a modest home with her husband and teenage daughter and was a full-time homemaker before the onset of her stroke. She was a cheerful and active woman who enjoyed cooking, baking, gardening, and visiting her neighbors and friends. The stroke resulted in the disturbance of cerebellar and brain stem functions. J.V. has a severe motor apraxia for speech, cannot close her mouth, drools, and walks with a broad-based ataxic gait. Since the onset of her disability J.V. has been very depressed, weeps frequently, is dependent for much of her self-care, and sits idly for long periods of time. She was referred to occupational therapy for evaluation and training in ADL, adjustment to disability, and development of drooling and swallowing control to facilitate feeding.

SAMPLE ADL PROGRESS REPORT

J.V. has attended occupational therapy 3 times weekly for 3 weeks since the initial evaluation. Further evaluation of self-care skills revealed that J.V. is capable of some hygiene skills, except a tub bath, nail care, hair care, and makeup application. However, at home she remains almost entirely dependent on Mr. V. for self-care, while crying and complaining of feeling weak.

Home management evaluation revealed considerable difficulty with most tasks except table setting, dusting, dishwashing, and sweeping, which she can perform if given cues and supervision. Performance of more complex tasks is limited by psychomotor retardation, incoordination, distractibility, inability to sequence a process, and apraxia for fine hand activities. It was necessary to supervise J.V. closely and give step-by-step instructions while she performed household tasks. A few simple homemaking tasks were performed for several training sessions, but performance did not improve.

J.V. appears to be very depressed and lacks intrinsic motivation. It was suggested to her family that they offer less assistance for self-care, and involve her with them in household tasks that she can perform, under their supervision, if possible.

The occupational therapy program will continue with greater emphasis on achieving control of mouth musculature, a primary goal of J.V. ADL training will be delayed until J.V is moving toward the achievement of this primary goal.

A

OCCUPATIONAL THERAPY DEPARTMENT

ACTIVITIES OF DAILY LIVING EVALUATION

Name ___J.V.___   Age _48_ Diagnosis ___CVA___   Dom. _Right_

Disability _Bilateral incoordination, ataxia, apraxia of mouth musculature_

Mode of ambulation ___Independent___

Grading key:
- I = Independent
- MiA = Minimal assistance
- MoA = Moderate assistance
- MaA = Maximal assistance
- D = Dependent
- NA = Not applicable
- 0 = Not evaluated

TRANSFERS AND AMBULATION

	Date	Independent	Assisted	Dependent
Tub or shower	8/1			D
Toilet	8/1		MiA	
Wheelchair	NA			
Bed and chair		I		
Ambulation			MiA	
Wheelchair management	NA			
Car			MiA	

BALANCE FOR FUNCTION

	Adequate	Inadequate
Sitting	I	
Standing	I	
Walking		MiA

B

Fig. 13.1 Activities of daily living (ADL) evaluation.

ADL SKILLS

EATING	Date	8/1	8/25			REMARKS
		Grade				
Butter bread		I				
Cut meat		I				
Eat with spoon		I				
Eat with fork		I				
Drink with straw		D				Mouth apraxia
Drink with glass		D				prevents performance
Drink with cup		D				of these activities
Pour from pitcher		D				

UNDRESS	Date	8/1	8/25			REMARKS
Pants or shorts		I				Is physically
Girdle or garter belt		MoA				capable of
Brassiere		MiA				performing the
Slip or undershirt		I				activities as
Dress		I				indicated but
Skirt		I				Mr. V. reports
Blouse or shirt		I				that J.V. is
Slacks or trousers		I				dependent on him
Bandana or necktie		NA				for much assistance,
Stockings		MoA				pleading fatigue,
Nightclothes		I				whining, and
Hair net		NA				crying for help
Housecoat/bathrobe		I				
Jacket		I				
Belt and/or suspenders		I				
Hat		I				
Coat		I				
Sweater		I				
Mittens or gloves		I				
Glasses		NA				
Brace		NA				
Shoes		MoA				
Socks		MoA				
Overshoes		MoA				

DRESS	Date	8/1	8/25			REMARKS
Pants or shorts		MiA				
Girdle or garter belt		MoA				
Brassiere		MoA				
Slip or undershirt		I				
Dress		I				
Skirt		I				
Blouse or shirt		I				
Slacks or trousers		I				
Bandana or necktie		NA				
Stockings		MoA				
Nightclothes		I				
Hair net		NA				
Housecoat/bathrobe		I				
Jacket		I				
Belt and/or suspenders		I				
Hat		I				
Coat		I				
Sweater		I				
Mittens or gloves		I				
Glasses		NA				
Brace		NA				
Shoes		MoA				
Socks		MoA				
Overshoes		MoA				

C

Fig. 13.1 (Continued).

FASTENINGS	Date	8/1	8/25			REMARKS
		Grade				
Button		I				
Snap		MoA				
Zipper		MiA				
Hook and eye		MaA				
Garters		D				
Lace		D				
Untie shoes		D				
Velcro		MiA				

HYGIENE	Date	8/1	8/25			REMARKS
Blow nose		0	I			
Wash face, hands		0	I			
Wash extremities, back		0	MaA			
Brush teeth or dentures		0	I			
Brush or comb hair		0	I			
Set hair		0	D			
Shave or put on makeup		0	MiA			
Clean fingernails		0	I, D			
Trim fingernails, toenails		0	D			
Apply deodorant		0	I			
Shampoo hair		0	D			
Use toilet paper		0	I			
Use tampon or sanitary napkin		0	NA			

COMMUNICATION	Date	8/1	8/25			REMARKS
Verbal		D				
Read		I				
Hold book		I				
Turn page		I				
Write		I				Writes name and
Use telephone		D				few words
Type		D				

HAND ACTIVITIES	Date	8/1	8/25			REMARKS
Handle money		0				
Handle mail		0				
Use scissors		0				
Open cans, bottles, jars		0				
Tie package		0				
Sew (baste)		0				
Sew button, hook and eye		0				
Polish shoes		0				
Sharpen pencil		0				
Seal and open letter		0				
Open box		0				

COMBINED PERFORMANCE

ACTIVITIES	Date	8/1	8/25			REMARKS
Open-close refrigerator		0	I			
Open-close door		0	I			
Remove and replace objects		0	I			
Carry objects during locomotion		0	D			
Pick up object from floor		0	D			
Remove, replace light bulb		0	D			
Plug in cord		0	D			

OPERATE	Date	8/1	8/25			REMARKS
Light switches		0	I			
Doorbell		0	I			
Door locks and handles		0	D			
Faucets		0	I			
Raise-lower window shades		0	D			
Raise-lower venetian blinds		0	D			
Raise-lower window		0	D			
Open-close drawer		0	I			
Hang up garment		0	I			

D

Fig. 13.1 (Continued).

SUMMARY OF EVALUATION RESULTS

Date __8/1__

Intact	Impaired	REMARKS
		SENSORY STATUS
X		Touch _____
X		Pain _____
X		Temperature _____
	X	Position sense _More marked on left_
	X	Olfaction _More marked on left_
	X	Stereognosis _____
	X	Visual fields (hemianopsia) _____
		PERCEPTUAL/ CONCEPTUAL TESTS
X		Follow directions _Verbal_
X		Visual spatial (form) _____
	X	Visual spatial (block design) _Minimal impairment_
X		Make change _____
	X	Geometric figures (copy) _Some difficulty with triangle and diamond_
		square, circle, triangle, diamond _____
	X	Praxis _Mild apraxia evident on fine hand activities_
		FUNCTIONAL RANGE OF MOTION
X		Comb hair-two hands _____
X		Feed self _____
X		Button collar button _____
X		Tie apron behind back _____
X		Button back buttons _____
X		Button cuffs _____
X		Zip side zipper _____
	X	Tie shoes _Poor balance limits_
	X	Stoop _Reach and bending for these activities_
	X	Reach shelf

E

Fig. 13.1 (Continued).

Assessment of safety awareness is often included in home management evaluations.

COMMUNITY LIVING SKILLS

Money and Financial Management

Many client factors relate to an individual's ability to use money and organize personal finances. These include cognitive and perceptual skills, as well as the ability to employ adequate judgment. The client may be capable of participating in simple transactions requiring small amounts of money, such as purchasing a candy bar, but need extensive retraining for more complex financial activities such as shopping, balancing a checkbook, paying bills, or making a budget. If the client is experiencing physical limitations, adaptive writing devices or computer software can allow the client to handle the paperwork aspects of money management. For example, online banking can help a client access financial records and complete banking transactions if going to the bank takes too much energy.

Community Mobility

Performance factors needed for community mobility include motor, process, and social interaction skills. The OT or OTA must consider client factors such as physical, perceptual, cognitive, and social skills while accurately measuring independence and safety in the area of community mobility. To train a client in community mobility OTs and OTAs must perform a multi-faceted assessment of the client's occupational performance.

Motor skills include the method of mobility (ambulation or wheelchair use). Necessary skills include managing uneven pavements, curbs, steps, ramps, and inclines and crossing streets. There are many options for the adaptation of vehicles, which are helpful for clients with limitations that do not allow them to access nonadapted vehicles. For example, an individual who utilizes a wheelchair for functional mobility may require an adaptive van (see Chapter 15). Other ways clients

OCCUPATIONAL THERAPY DEPARTMENT

ACTIVITIES OF HOME MANAGEMENT

Name ___J.V._____   Date ___8/25_____

Address ___Anytown, U.S.A._____

Age ___48___ Weight ___135___ Height ___5'5"___ Role in family ___Wife, mother_____

Diagnosis ___CVA_____ Disability ___Bilateral ataxia, apraxia of mouth___
                                                      musculature

Mode of ambulation ___Independent, no aids, mild ataxic gait_____

Limitations or contraindications for activity _____

_____

DESCRIPTION OF HOME
1.   Private house   ___✓___
      No. of rooms   ___6___ - kitchen, dining room, living room, 3 bedrooms
      No. of floors   ___2___
      Stairs   ___14___ - bedrooms on second floor
      Elevators   ___0___

2.   Apartment house   _____
      No. of rooms   _____
      No. of floors   _____
      Stairs   _____
      Elevators   _____

3.   Diagram of home layout (attach to completed form)

      Will patient be required to perform the following activities? If not, who will perform?
      Meal preparation   ___No___ Daughter_____
      Baking   ___No___ Daughter (J.V. used to bake a lot)_____
      Serving   ___Yes___ _____
      Wash dishes   ___Yes___ _____
      Marketing   ___No___ Husband_____
      Child care   ___No___ _____
         (under 4 years)   _____
      Washing   ___Yes___ _____
      Hanging clothes   ___NA___ Has dryer_____
      Ironing   ___No___ Daughter_____
      Cleaning   ___Yes___ Light cleaning_____
      Sewing   ___No___ Does not sew_____
      Hobbies or   ___Yes___ Baking and gardening would be desirable activities
         special interest   _____ _____

      Does patient really like housework? ___No___
      Sitting position: Chair ___X___ Stool ___X___ Wheelchair ___NA___
      Standing position: Braces ___NA___ Crutches ___NA___ Canes ___NA___
      Handedness: Dominant hand ___Right___ Two hands ___X___ One hand only _____ Assistive _____

A

Fig. 13.2 Activities of home management. (Modified from Activities of Home Management Form, Occupational Therapy Department, University Hospital, Ohio State University, Columbus, OH.)

navigate in the community include accessing public transportation (bus or subway), walking, or using a wheelchair. Using accessible transportation such a bus with a lift may also be included. These factors include (1) the endurance to be mobile in the community without fatigue, and (2) the ability to utilize ambulation equipment such as walkers, canes, and crutches. Community mobility skills often overlap with other areas of ADL and IADL, including managing toileting in a public restroom, handling money, and carrying objects while in a wheelchair or while using a walker.

Process skills require cognitive and perceptual processing. These skills include **topographic orientation** and problem solving. Perceptual processing is needed to read a map or recognize symbols (such as a sign for a bus stop).

Grading key: I = Independent
MiA = Minimal assistance
MoA = Moderate assistance
MaA = Maximal assistance
D = Dependent
NA = Not applicable
0 = Not evaluated

CLEANING ACTIVITIES	Date	8/25				REMARKS
		Grade				
Pick up object from floor		D				
Wipe up spills		D				
Make bed (daily)		D				
Use dust mop		I				
Shake dust mop		D				
Dust low surfaces		I				
Dust high surfaces		D				
Mop kitchen floor		D				
Sweep with broom		I				
Use dust pan and broom		MiA				
Use vacuum cleaner		D				
Use vacuum cleaner attachments		D				
Carry light cleaning tools		I				
Use carpet sweeper		I				
Clean bathtub		D				
Change sheets on bed		D				
Carry pail of water		D				

MEAL PREPARATION	Date	8/25				REMARKS
Turn off water		I				
Turn off gas or electric range		I				
Light gas with match		D				
Pour hot water from pan to cup		D				
Open packaged goods		I				
Carry pan from sink to range		D				
Use can opener		D				
Handle milk bottle		I				
Dispose of garbage		D				
Remove things from refrigerator		D				
Bend to low cupboards		D				
Peel vegetables		D				
Cut up vegetables		D				
Handle sharp tools safely		D				
Break eggs		D				
Stir against resistance		D				
Measure flour		D				
Use eggbeater		D				
Use electric mixer		D				
Remove batter to pan		D				
Open oven door		I				
Carry pan to oven and put in		D				
Remove hot pan from oven to table		0				
Roll cookie dough or piecrust		D				

B

Fig. 13.2 (Continued).

Additional processing skills needed include understanding time and schedules.

Social interaction skills are needed for community mobility. These skills include communication (to obtain directions), expression of emotion (being assertive enough to obtain an accessible table at a restaurant), and clarification (explaining to an individual that you cannot reach an item on the top shelf of a grocery store because you are unable to stand without assistance).

Health Management

Health management includes habits and routines focused on managing and maintaining good health (American Occupational Therapy Association, 2014). Skills needed

MEAL SERVICE	Date	8/25				REMARKS
		Grade				
Set table for four		I				
Carry four glasses of water to table		D				
Carry hot casserole to table		D				
Clear table		I				
Scrape and stack dishes		I				
Wash dishes (light soil)		I				
Wipe silver		I				
Wash pots and pans		MiA				
Wipe up range and work areas		MoA				
Wring out dishcloth		I				

LAUNDRY	Date	8/25				REMARKS
Wash lingerie (by hand)		D				
Wring out, squeeze dry		D				
Hang on rack to dry		I				
Sprinkle clothes		I				
Iron blouse or slip		D				
Fold blouse or slip						
Use washing machine						

SEWING	Date	8/25				REMARKS
Thread needle and make knot						
Sew on buttons						
Mend rip						
Darn socks						
Use sewing machine						
Crochet						
Knit						
Embroider						
Cut with shears						

HEAVY HOUSEHOLD ACTIVITIES. WHO WILL DO THESE?

	Date	8/25				REMARKS
Wash household laundry						
Hang clothes						
Clean range						
Clean refrigerator						
Wax floors						
Marketing						
Turn mattresses						
Wash windows						
Put up curtains						

WORK HEIGHTS SITTING/STANDING

Best height for Wheelchair _____ Chair __X__ Stool __X__

- Ironing 17½" seated
- Mixing 26" on high stool at counter
- Dish washing 26" on high stool at counter
- General work _____

Maximal depth of counter
area (normal reach) 25"

Maximal useful height
above work surface 33" if standing

Maximal useful height without
counter surface 68" if standing

Maximal reach below counter area 20" if standing

Best height for chair 17½" - can be used at adjustable ironing board

Best height for stool with
back support 24" - can be used at sink or food preparation counter

SUGGESTIONS FOR HOME MODIFICATION

- Remove scatter rugs in bedroom
- Install guard rail on both sides of toilet
- Install grab bars on wall next to bathtub
- Place nonskid strips on bottom of bathtub

C

Fig. 13.2 (Continued).

HOME EVALUATION CHECKLIST

Name _____ Date _____

Address _____

Diagnosis _____

| **Mobility status** | ☐ Ambulatory, no device | ☐ Walker |
| | ☐ Cane | ☐ Wheelchair |

Exterior

Home located on
☐ Level surface
☐ Hill

Type of house
☐ Owns house   ☐ Mobile home
☐ Apartment   ☐ Board and care

Number of floors
☐ One story   ☐ Split level
☐ Two story

Driveway surface
☐ Inclined   ☐ Smooth
☐ Level   ☐ Rough

Is the DRIVEWAY negotiable?   ☐ Yes   ☐ No
Is the GARAGE accessible?   ☐ Yes   ☐ No

Entrance

Accessible entrances
☐ Front   ☐ Side
☐ Back

Steps
Number   _____
Height of each   _____
Width   _____
Depth   _____

Are there HANDRAILS?   ☐ Yes   ☐ No
If yes, where are they located? ☐ Left   ☐ Right
HANDRAIL height from step surface?   _____
If no how much room is available for HANDRAILS? _____

Are landings negotiable?   ☐ Yes   ☐ No

Briefly describe any problems with LANDINGS: _____

Ramps   ☐ Yes   ☐ No
            ☐ Front   ☐ Back
            Height   _____
            Width   _____
            Length   _____

Are there HANDRAILS?   ☐ Yes   ☐ No
If yes, where are they located? ☐ Left   ☐ Right   Height _____
If no ramp, how much room is available for one? _____

Porch   Width   _____
            Length   _____
            Level at threshold?   ☐ Yes   ☐ No

Door   Width   _____
            Threshold height _____ Negotiable? ☐ Yes   ☐ No
            ☐ Swing in
            ☐ Swing out
            ☐ Sliding

Interior

Living room
Is furniture arranged for easy maneuverability?   ☐ Yes   ☐ No
Is frequently used furniture accessible?   ☐ Yes   ☐ No
Type of floor covering: _____
Comments _____

Hallways
Can wheelchair or walking aid be maneuvered in hallway?   ☐ Yes   ☐ No
            Hall width   _____
            Door width   _____
            Sharp turns   ☐ Yes   ☐ No
Steps?   ☐ Yes   ☐ No   Number _____
Are there HANDRAILS?   ☐ Yes   ☐ No
If yes, where are they located? ☐ Left   ☐ Right   Height _____

Bedroom ☐ Single
             ☐ Shared
Is there room for a W/C? ☐ Yes   ☐ No
Door: Width   _____
            Threshold height _____ Negotiable? ☐ Yes   ☐ No
            ☐ Swing in
            ☐ Swing out

A

Fig. 13.3 Home visit checklist. (Modified from Occupational/Physical Therapy Home Evaluation Form, San Francisco, Ralph K. Davies Medical Center, and Occupational Therapy Home Evaluation Form, Berkeley and Oakland, CA, 1993, Alta Bates Summit Medical Center.)

Bed: ☐ Twin
        ☐ Double
        ☐ Queen
        ☐ King
        ☐ Hospital bed
        Overall height _____   Accessible?   ☐ Yes   ☐ No
    Would hospital bed fit into room if needed?   ☐ Yes   ☐ No
Clothing:
    Are drawers accessible?   ☐ Yes   ☐ No
                               ☐ On right   ☐ On left
    Is closet accessible?   ☐ Yes   ☐ No
                               ☐ On right   ☐ On left
    Comments: _____

Bathroom

Door: Width   _____
         Threshold height _____   Negotiable?   ☐ Yes   ☐ No
Tub: Height, floor-rim   _____
         Height, tub bottom rim _____
         Tub width inside   _____
         Glass doors?   ☐ Yes   ☐ No
         Width of tub doors _____
         Overhead shower?   ☐ Yes   ☐ No
         Is tub accessible? ☐ Yes   ☐ No

Stall shower: ☐ Yes   ☐ No

         Door width   _____
         Height of bottom rim _____
         Accessible?   ☐ Yes   ☐ No

Sink: Height   _____
         Faucet type _____
         ☐ Open
         ☐ Closed
         Accessible?   ☐ Yes   ☐ No

Toilet: Height from floor   _____
         Location of toilet paper _____
         Distance from toilet to side wall   L   _____
                                              R   _____

Grab bars: ☐ Yes   ☐ No
         Location _____
Comments: _____

Kitchen

Door: Width   _____
         Threshold height _____   Negotiable?   ☐ Yes   ☐ No

Stove: Height   _____
         Location of controls   ☐ Front   ☐ Back
         Is stove accessible for use?   ☐ Yes   ☐ No

Oven: Height from floor to door hinge and door handle   _____
         Location of oven _____

Sink: Will w/c fit underneath?   ☐ Yes   ☐ No
         Type of faucets _____

Cupboards:
         Accessible from w/c?   ☐ Yes   ☐ No
Refrigerator:
         Hinges on   ☐ Left   ☐ Right
         Accessible from w/c?   ☐ Yes   ☐ No
Switches/outlets:
         Accessible?   ☐ Yes   ☐ No
Kitchen table:
         Height from floor   _____
         Accessible   ☐ Yes   ☐ No
Comments: _____

Laundry

Door: Width   _____
         Threshold height _____   Negotiable?   ☐ Yes   ☐ No

Steps: ☐ Yes   ☐ No

         Number   _____
         Height   _____
         Width   _____
         Are there HANDRAILS?   ☐ Yes   ☐ No
         If yes, where are they located?   ☐ Left   ☐ Right   Height _____

B

Fig. 13.3 (Continued).

Washer:
    ☐ Topload
    ☐ Front load
    Accessible?   ☐ Yes   ☐ No
Dryer:
    ☐ Topload
    ☐ Front load
    Accessible?   ☐ Yes   ☐ No

Safety

Throw rugs
    ☐ Yes   ☐ No
    Location _____
Phone
    Accessible?   ☐ Yes   ☐ No
    Location _____
Emergency phone numbers
    ☐ Yes   ☐ No
    Location _____
Mailbox
    Accessible?   ☐ Yes   ☐ No
    Location _____
Thermostat
    Accessible?   ☐ Yes   ☐ No
    Location _____
Electric outlets/switches
    Accessible?   ☐ Yes   ☐ No
Imperfect floor?
    ☐ Yes   ☐ No
    Location _____

C

Sharp edged furniture?
    ☐ Yes   ☐ No
    Location _____
Insulated hot water pipes:
    ☐ Yes   ☐ No
    Location _____
Cluttered areas?
    ☐ Yes   ☐ No
    Location _____
Fire extinguisher?
    ☐ Yes   ☐ No
    Location _____

Equipment present: _____

_____

Problem list: _____

_____

_____

_____

Recommendations for modifications: _____

_____

_____

_____

Equipment recommendations: _____

_____

_____

D

Fig. 13.3 (Continued).

for health management include medication management and initiation of contact with medical providers. This includes understanding when a physical symptom warrants a call to a physician and how to make a medical appointment.

The OT or OTA considers all performance skills necessary for a client to be proficient in the complex IADL of health management. From the information gathered in the assessment, the OT or OTA can determine which aspects of the task need to be modified to facilitate independence. For example, the occupational therapy practitioner may collaborate with a nurse to assist a client, with hemiplegia and diabetes, to independently manage insulin shots. This task requires the cognitive, perceptual, and physical abilities to decide the correct time to administer the medication, draw the measured amount out of the bottle, and properly inject it. If the client cannot safely manage the task, the occupational therapy practitioner may consider adaptations to the task. These may include using prefilled syringes, utilizing adaptive equipment to open the bottle, or changing the measuring container. Other adaptive devices to assist with medication management include pill boxes equipped with alarms and adaptive devices for application of eye drops for individuals with impaired fine motor control.

INTERVENTIONS TO IMPROVE PERFORMANCE IN ADL

The methods of teaching the client to perform ADL must be tailored to suit each client's learning style and ability. Clients who are alert and grasp instructions quickly may perform an entire process after a brief demonstration and verbal instruction. Clients who have perceptual problems, poor memory, or difficulty following instructions require a more concrete, step-by-step approach in which assistance is reduced gradually as success is achieved. First, the clinician must prepare the environment by reducing extraneous stimuli. For such individuals, it is important to break down the activity into small steps and to progress through them slowly, one at a time. The clinician's slow demonstration of the task or step in the same place and in the same manner in which the client is expected to perform is helpful. Verbal instructions to accompany the demonstration may or may not be helpful, depending on the client's receptive language skills and ability to process and integrate two modes of sensory information simultaneously.

Helpful tactile and kinesthetic modes of instruction include (1) touching body parts to be moved, dressed, bathed, or positioned; (2) passively moving the part through the desired pattern to achieve a step or task; and (3) gently guiding the part manually through the task (see Chapters 10 and 21). Such techniques can augment or replace demonstration and verbal instruction, depending on the client's best avenues of learning. Skill, speed, and retention of learning require repeated task performance. Tasks may be repeated several times during the same training session if time and the client's physical and emotional tolerance allow, or they may be repeated daily until desired retention or level of skill is achieved.

ADL training sessions allow a client to experience and practice normal movement patterns with the therapist guiding the client at key points of the body. This idea is a leading principle of neurodevelopmental technique (NDT). ADL training with NDT patterns can be a meaningful way for a client to gain strength, balance, and endurance. If the client is not expected to make physical improvements because of the nature of the physical dysfunction, the ADL training sessions should focus primarily on teaching compensatory strategies. The process of backward chaining can be used in teaching ADL skills (see Chapter 10). This method is particularly useful in training clients with cognitive impairment (Trombly, 1983).

Before beginning training in any ADL, the clinician must prepare the environment by providing adequate space and arranging equipment, materials, and furniture for maximal convenience and safety. The clinician should be familiar with the task to be performed and any special methods or assistive devices that will be used. The occupational therapy practitioner should be able to perform the adapted task in the way the client will perform it. For example, if the client is going to don pants with a dressing stick, the OT or OTA should try and master the skill first, to model it for the client.

The OT or OTA should then present the activity to the client. A multimodal approach such as one utilizing demonstration and verbal instruction would be beneficial to clients with different learning styles. The client then performs the activity—either along with the clinician or immediately after being shown, with supervision and assistance as required. Performance is modified and corrected as needed, and the process is repeated to ensure learning. Because other staff or family members often will help to reinforce the newly learned skills, family training is critical to ensure that the client carries over the skills from previous treatment sessions.

In the final phase of instruction, after mastering the task or several tasks, the client attempts to perform them independently. The OT or OTA should follow up by checking on performance in progress. Finally, the OT or OTA must check on the adequacy of performance and carryover of learning with nursing personnel, the caregiver, or the supervising family members.

Documentation of ADL Intervention

Many informal assessments, such as the ADL checklists used to record performance on the initial evaluation, have columns to record changes in abilities useful for documentation of intervention and for reevaluation. The sample checklist described earlier is designed and completed in this way (see Fig. 13.3). Progress is summarized for inclusion in the medical record. The progress record should summarize changes in the client's abilities, current level of independence, and a plan for further improvement in function. Subjective information such as the client's potential for further independence, attitudes, and motivation for ADL training may also be included. Documentation should also reflect how the client's current level of independence or assistance may affect discharge plans. For example, the client who continues to require moderate assistance with self-care may only be able to be discharged to home if care support is available. This may be provided by a family member of a personal care assistant.

ADAPTIVE TECHNIQUES UTILIZED FOR INTERVENTION IN ADL

Many situations in which clients experience a disruption in occupational performance in the area of ADL require adaptive techniques. These cases require that the OT or OTA and client explore adaptive methods or assistive devices to reach a solution. Solutions may include prefabricated or custom-fabricated devices. Many commercially available assistive devices were originally created by occupational therapy practitioners and clients. OTs and OTAs devised many adaptive methods through the skillful use of occupational analysis applied to clients of all levels of ability. These techniques often began with client suggestions and requests based on unique needs. When recommending adaptive techniques or assistive devices, the OT or OTA must respect the client's opinions throughout the entire training process. Clients have varying opinions regarding the use of adaptive techniques, and many are opposed to using assistive devices.

This chapter provides the OTA student with some techniques and equipment to provide ADL interventions for many different types of clients. It is important for OTAs to understand that they may not be appropriate for all clients. A client may resist adaptive equipment because of its aesthetic qualities, because the equipment is difficult to use, or the client may not feel ready for the change in task performance that the equipment represents. Therefore alternative strategies to the use of adaptive equipment must be also be explored. The following summary of techniques may be appropriate for clients with the following deficits in occupational performance.

Limited ROM and Strength

Range of motion may be limited by body structures and/ or precautions. Clients with severe osteoarthritis may experience decreased joint excursion. Bariatric clients may present with decreased ROM limited by girth. Some postsurgical precautions temporarily limit ROM. Clients with limited joint ROM experience a lack of reach and joint excursion. Environmental adaptation and assistive devices can compensate for decreased reach. Decreased muscle strength and endurance may also limit a client's ability to reach full joint excursion. Therefore individuals with decreased muscle strength may require some of the same devices or techniques to conserve energy and to compensate for weakness. Some adaptations and devices are outlined in the following discussion (Lift and Accessibility Solutions, 2013; Mayer, 2001; Planet Mobility, 2004; Trombly, 1983).

Dressing Activities. The following suggestions may be helpful to facilitate dressing for individuals with decreased ROM, strength, or endurance:

1. Use front-opening garments, one size larger than needed, and made of stretchable fabric.
2. Use **dressing sticks** with a garter on one end and a neoprene-covered coat hook on the other for pushing and pulling garments off and on feet and legs (Fig. 13.4) and to push a shirt or blouse over the head. Use a **sock aid** to pull on socks.
3. Use larger buttons or zippers with a loop on the pull tab.
4. Replace buttons, snaps, hooks, and eyes with Velcro or zippers (for those clients who cannot manage traditional fastenings). A cuff and collar extender installed in between the buttons of the shirt cuff widens the opening of the cuff

without the need to unfasten. A small, barely visible spring helps extend the buttons' reach.
5. Eliminate the need to bend and tie shoelaces or to use finger joints in this fine motor activity by using elastic shoelaces, shoes with Velcro closures, or slip-on shoes.
6. Facilitate donning stockings without bending to the feet by using sock aids from medical suppliers or homemade versions of garters attached to long webbing straps (Fig. 13.5). Alternatively, kitchen rubber gloves with nodules help with grasp for donning stockings or TED (thromboembolic deterrent) hose.
7. Avoid bending forward by sitting on the edge of the bed to don and doff socks and shoes without using adaptive equipment. Instruct the client to turn in bed to bring the knee up onto the bed in an externally rotated position. The foot should be hanging off the side of the bed. The client can then don/doff socks and shoes on that side and then repeat on the other side.
8. Use one of several types of commercially available **buttonhooks** if finger coordination or ROM is limited (Fig. 13.6).
9. Use **reachers** for picking up socks and shoes, arranging clothes, removing clothes from hangers, picking up objects on the floor (Fig. 13.7), and donning pants.

Interventions for Feeding and Eating. See Chapter 11.

Hygiene and Grooming. Environmental adaptations that can facilitate bathing and grooming include the following:
1. A handheld showerhead on a flexible hose for bathing and shampooing hair facilitates showering while seated

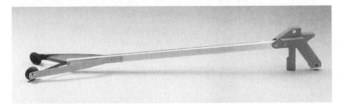

Fig. 13.4 Dressing stick or reacher.

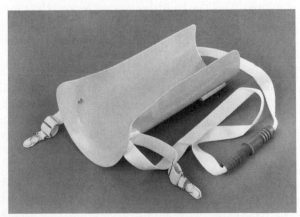

Fig. 13.5 Sock aid. (Courtesy Sammons, a BISSELL Co.)

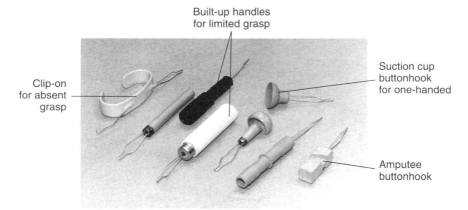

Fig. 13.6 Buttonhooks to accommodate limited grasp, special types of grasp, or amputation.

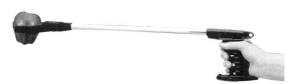

Fig. 13.7 Extended-handle reacher. (Courtesy Sorrentino SA, Remmert LN. *Mosby's Textbook for Nursing Assistants*. 10th ed. St. Louis, MO: Elsevier; 2021.)

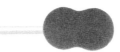

Fig. 13.8 Long-handled bath sponges. (Courtesy Sorrentino SA, Remmert LN. *Mosby's Textbook for Nursing Assistants*. 10th ed. St. Louis, MO: Elsevier; 2021.)

and allows the client to control the direction of spray. Adding cylindrical foam to the showerhead is helpful for clients with limited grasp.

2. A **long-handled sponge** with a soap holder (Fig. 13.8) or long cloth scrubber can help the user to reach the legs, feet, and back. A wash mitt and soap on a rope can aid limited grasp. Putting a bar of soap in the foot of nylon pantyhose makes it easier to grasp.

3. A position-adjustable hairdryer may be helpful for those wishing to blow-dry hair (Feldmeier & Poole, 1987). This device is useful for clients with limited ROM, upper extremity weakness, incoordination, and use of only one upper extremity. The dryer is adapted from a desk lamp with spring-balanced arms and a tension control knob at each joint. The lamp is removed, and the hairdryer is fastened to the spring-balanced arms. The device is mounted on a table or countertop and can be adjusted for various heights and direction of airflow. This frees the client's hands to style hair with brushes or combs. Specifications are available for constructing this device Feldmeier & Poole, 1987. This product is also available commer-cially under the name Hands-Free Hair Dryer Pro Stand 2000 from rehabilitation product catalogs and infomercials on television (North Coast Medical, 2004; Sammons Preston Rolyan (2004)).

4. Extended handles on a comb, brush, toothbrush, lipstick, mascara brush, and safety or electric razor may be useful for clients who have limited hand-to-head or hand-to-face movements. Extensions may be constructed from inexpensive wooden dowels or pieces of PVC pipe found in hardware stores.

5. Spray deodorant, hair spray, and spray powder or perfume can extend the reach by the distance the material sprays. Some persons may require special adaptations to operate the spray mechanism (Fig. 13.9).

6. Electric toothbrushes and the Water-Pik system may be easier to manage than a standard toothbrush. Cylindric foam to enlarge the toothbrush handle may help with grasp. Flossing aids decrease the need to directly handle and manipulate dental floss (http://sale.dentist.net/products/gripit-floss-holder).

7. A reacher can be useful to extend reach for using toilet paper. Several types of toilet tissue aids or tongs are available in catalogs of assistive devices, such as a Freedom Wand (https://www.freedomwand.com) (Active Forever, 2017).

8. Dressing sticks can be used to pull garments up after using the toilet.

9. Safety rails (Fig. 13.10) can be used for bathtub transfers, and safety mats or strips can be placed in the bathtub bottom to prevent slipping.

10. A **tub transfer bench** (Fig. 13.11), shower stool, or regular chair set in the bathtub or shower stall can eliminate the need to sit on the bathtub bottom or stand to shower, thus increasing safety.

11. Grab bars can be installed to prevent falls and to ease transfers.

Communication and Environmental Controls (See Chapter 14).

Adaptations that can facilitate communication and use of common household fixtures include the following:

1. Telephones should be placed within easy reach. A phone holder, handle or case for cellular phones, large-button

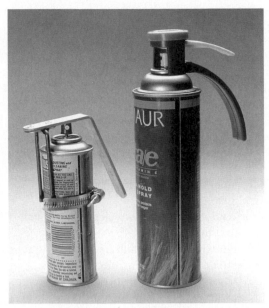

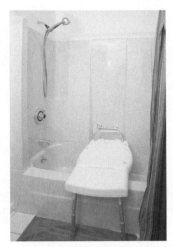

Fig. 13.11 Tub transfer bench. (From Kostelnick C. *Mosby's Textbook for Long-Term Care Nursing Assistants*. 8th ed. St. Louis, MO: Elsevier; 2020.)

Fig. 13.9 Spray can adapters. (Courtesy Sammons, a BISSELL Co.)

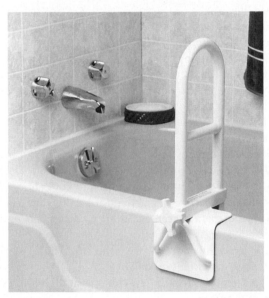

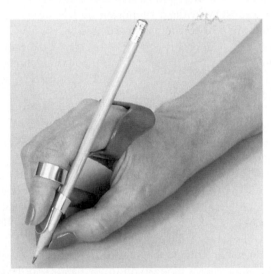

Fig. 13.12 Wanchik writing aid. (Courtesy Sammons, a BISSELL Co.)

Fig. 13.10 Bathtub safety rail. (Courtesy Sammons, a BISSELL Co.)

phone or increasing text size, speakerphone, or voice-activated features may be necessary. Dialing sticks, styluses and push-button phones, and phone cases with kickstands to support or allow for free hands are other adaptations. Teach clients how to store emergency contacts and frequently dialed telephone numbers into cellular devices. Use Bluetooth calling or a speakerphone for hands-free conversations.

2. Built-up pens and pencils with cylindric foam to accommodate limited grasp and prehension can be used. A Wanchik writer and several other commercially available or custom-fabricated writing aids are helpful (Fig. 13.12).

3. Speech-recognition software such as Dragon Naturally Speaking from ScanSoft turns speech into text and can facilitate communication for those with limited or painful joints (North Coast Medical, 2004). Many commercially available options, such as cell phones and tablets, have built-in voice recognition.

4. A slip-on typing aid attached with a Velcro strip around the palm has a pointer under the index finger and requires minimal hand strength to use.

5. Lever-type doorknob extensions (Fig. 13.13), car door openers, and adapted key holders can compensate for hand limitations.

6. Extended or built-up handles on faucets can accommodate limited grasp.

7. A wire-framed book holder or the Book Butler eliminates prolonged grasping of a book by holding the book open at a comfortable angle (Sammons Preston Rolyan, 2004).

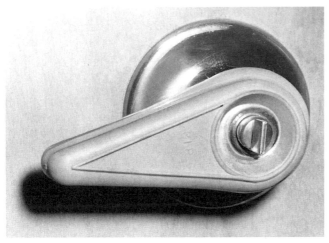

Fig. 13.13 Rubber doorknob extension. (Courtesy Sammons, a BISSELL Co.)

Functional Mobility and Transfers. The individual who has limited ROM *without* significant muscle weakness may benefit from the following assistive devices:

1. A glider chair operated by the feet can make transportation easier if hip, hand, and arm motions are limited.
2. Platform crutches can prevent stress on hand or finger joints and can accommodate limited grasp.
3. Enlarged grips on crutches, canes, and walkers can accommodate limited grasp.
4. A raised toilet seat can be used if hip and knee motion is limited.
5. A walker with padded grips and forearm troughs can be used if marked hand, forearm, or elbow joint limitations are a problem.
6. A walker or crutch bag and basket can carry objects. Some baskets include beverage holders.
7. A transfer handle at the side of the bed and a couch-cane allow clients to grasp on to the handles for leverage when transferring out of bed or the couch (North Coast Medical, 2004). Adding furniture lifters or blocks to the legs of chairs, couches, or beds increases the height of the furniture and makes it easier to stand from or transfer to another surface.

Home Management Skills. Home management activities can be made easier by a variety of environmental adaptations, assistive devices, energy conservation methods, and work simplification techniques (Klinger, Howard & Rusk Institute of Rehabilitation Medicine, 1997; Planet Mobility, 2004). Persons with rheumatoid arthritis should use the principles of joint protection (see Chapter 29). Energy conservation allows clients to perform the same task while expending less energy. Using these principles, clients with weakness due to cardiac and/or pulmonary disorders can perform daily tasks while placing less demand on the body (Branick, 2004). The demands on the body are measured by oxygen saturation levels and pulse rates. Home management for persons with

limited ROM can be eased and improved with the following energy conservation principles:

1. Plan ahead. By managing time and pacing yourself, you can limit the need for excessive motions.
2. Store frequently used items on counters when possible or on the first shelves of cabinets (just above and below counters).
3. Sit whenever possible. Use a high stool to work comfortably at counter height. Alternatively, if a wheelchair is used, attach a drop-leaf table to the wall for meal preparation.
4. Use a utility cart of comfortable height to transport several items at once.
5. Use a reacher to pull down lightweight items (e.g., a cereal box) from high shelves.
6. Stabilize mixing bowls and dishes with nonslip mats.
7. Use electric can openers and electric mixers.
8. The Black & Decker automatic jar opener opens jars of all sizes with the push of a button (Runge, 1967).
9. Eliminate bending by using extended, flexible plastic handles on dust mops, brooms, and dustpans.
10. Use pull-out shelves to organize cupboards and eliminate bending.
11. Eliminate bending by using wall ovens, countertop broilers, and microwave ovens.
12. Eliminate leaning and bending by using a top-loading automatic washer and elevated dryer and a reacher. Wheelchair users can more easily operate front-loading appliances than other types.
13. Use an adjustable ironing board to make it possible to sit while ironing.
14. For child care by the ambulatory parent or caregiver, elevate the playpen and diaper table and use a bathinette or a plastic tub on the kitchen counter for bathing. These adaptations reduce the amount of bending and reaching. The crib mattress can be in a raised position until the child is 3 or 4 months old.
15. Use large, loose-fitting garments with hook and loop (Velcro) fastenings on children.
16. Use a reacher to pick up clothing and children's toys from the floor.

Neuromuscular Coordination Deficits

Incoordination can result from a variety of central nervous system (CNS) disorders such as Parkinson disease, multiple sclerosis, cerebral palsy, and traumatic brain injuries (TBIs). Incoordination may take the form of tremors, ataxia, or athetoid or choreiform movements. Persons with incoordination may have difficulty maintaining safety and achieving adequate stability of gait, body parts, and objects to complete ADL.

Fatigue, emotional factors, and fears may increase the severity of uncoordinated movement. The client must be taught appropriate energy conservation and work simplification techniques, along with work pacing and safety methods. The client who learns to reduce fatigue and fear will perform tasks better and with increased coordination.

The uncoordinated individual with reasonable muscle strength can use weighted devices to help stabilize objects. A Velcro-fastened weight can be attached to the client's arm to decrease tremors and ataxia. Objects such as eating utensils, pens, and cups can be weighted.

Another technique that can be used throughout all ADL tasks is stabilizing the upper part of the involved upper extremity. This stabilization is accomplished by propping the elbow on a counter or tabletop, pivoting from the elbow, and moving only the forearm, wrist, and hand in the activity. Stabilizing the arm reduces some of the incoordination and may allow the individual to accomplish gross and fine motor movements without assistive devices (Australian Government, 2004; Lift and Accessibility Solutions, 2013; Parents with Disabilities, 2010). Stabilizing the trunk using seating positioning devices can greatly increase the fine coordination of the upper extremity (refer to Chapter 15).

Dressing Activities

Dressing difficulties encountered with incoordination can be reduced by using the following adaptations:

1. Front-opening garments that fit loosely can facilitate donning and removing garments.
2. Large buttons, Velcro, or zippers with loops on the tab can ease opening and closing fasteners. A buttonhook with a large, weighted handle may be helpful.
3. Elastic shoelaces, Velcro closures, other adapted shoe closures, and slip-on shoes eliminate the need for bow tying.
4. Trousers with elastic tops for women or Velcro closures for men are easier to manage than those with hooks, buttons, and zippers.
5. Brassieres with front openings or Velcro replacements for the usual hook and eye may be used with more ease. A slipover athletic-style elastic brassiere purchased one size larger may eliminate the need to manage brassiere fastenings. Regular (back-fastening) brassieres may be fastened in front at waist level and then slipped around to the back. Next the arms are put into the straps, which are worked up over the shoulders. Adaptive bras such as the Sara Bra or the Ability Bra are easy to don for women with poor coordination or limited hand and shoulder movement.
6. Men can wear clip-on ties. Alternatively, if the tie is stored loosely tied, it may be donned over the head and secured in place.
7. To compensate for balance problems and impaired fine motor control, dressing should be performed while sitting on or in the bed, in a wheelchair, or in a chair with arms.

Hygiene and Grooming. The following techniques can help a client stabilize and manipulate toilet articles:

1. If dropping is a problem, articles such as a razor, lipstick, and toothbrush can be attached to a cord. Small strips of rubber or friction tape placed around the objects help support the grasp. An electric toothbrush may be more easily managed than a regular one.

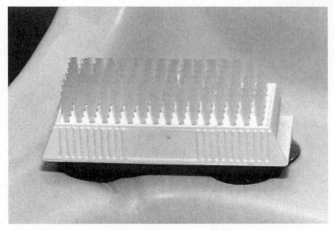

Fig. 13.14 Suction brush attached to bathroom sink for dentures or fingernails. Brush can also be used in kitchen to wash vegetables and fruit.

2. Weighted wrist cuffs may be helpful during hygiene activities requiring fine motor coordination such as applying makeup, shaving, and hair care.
3. The position-adjustable hairdryer described earlier for clients with limited ROM can be useful for those with incoordination as well (Feldmeier & Poole, 1987).
4. An electric razor rather than a blade razor offers stability and safety. A strap around the razor and the hand or neck can prevent dropping.
5. A suction nailbrush attached to the sink or counter can be used for nail or denture care (Fig. 13.14).
6. Soap should be on a rope and can be worn around the neck (if safe for the particular client) or hung over bathtub or shower fixtures during the bath or shower to keep it within easy reach. A leg from a pair of pantyhose tied over a faucet, with a bar of soap in the toe, will stretch for use and keep soap within reach. Also, liquid soap bottles with a pump dispenser can be secured near the faucet. Consider securing these dispensers to the wall or having them built into the shower or vanity of the bathroom.
7. An emery board or small piece of wood with fine sandpaper glued to it can be fastened to the tabletop for filing nails. A nail clipper can also be stabilized in the same manner.
8. Large-size roll-on or cream deodorants are controlled more easily than sprays.
9. Sanitary pads that stick to undergarments may be easier to manage than tampons.
10. A bath mitt with a pocket to hold the soap can be used for washing and eliminates the need for frequent soaping, rinsing, and wringing a washcloth.

The following recommendations can greatly increase safety during bathing. **Nonskid mats** should be used inside and outside the bathtub during bathing. Their suction bases should be fastened securely to the floor and bathtub before use. Safety grab bars should be installed on the wall next to the bathtub or fastened to the edge of the bathtub. Sitting on a bathtub seat or shower chair is safer than standing while showering or transferring to a bathtub bottom. Many uncoordinated clients require supervisory assistance during bathing. Sponge bathing while seated at a bathroom sink may substitute for bathing or showering several times a week.

Communication and General Environment.
Adaptations that can facilitate communication and the use of common household fixtures by clients with incoordination include the following:

1. Doorknobs may be managed more easily if adapted with lever-type handles or covered with rubber or friction tape (see Fig. 13.13).
2. A holder or earphones with speakers, enlarged buttons on phones or touchscreen, programmed phone numbers, or speakerphones may be helpful. Voice-activated dialing and texting is a convenient feature on cellular phones (Public Utilities Commission, 2010).
3. Writing can be managed with a weighted, enlarged pencil or pen and securing the paper with a clipboard or tape. The Wrist Hold-Down consists of a magnetized work surface and magnetized cups attached to the wrist to provide stability for writing or drawing (Runge, 1967). Computer adaptations in software and types of keyboards and mice are discussed in Chapter 14.
4. Keys can be placed on an adapted rigid key holder that extends leverage for turning the key. However, inserting the key in the keyhole may be very difficult unless the incoordination is relatively mild. Changing the lock to require a combination or remote control button eliminates the need to retrieve and manipulate the keys.
5. Extended lever-type faucets are easier to manage than push-pull spigots and knobs. To prevent burns during bathing and kitchen activities, cold water should be turned on first and hot water added gradually. External temperature controls can be added directly to the water heater to prevent water from reaching scalding hot temperatures. These controls are considered environmentally friendly and are easy to install.
6. Lamps can be wired with switches that respond to light touch or to a remote signal. Wall switches can also eliminate the need to turn a small switch manually. Environmental control units or electronic aids to daily living (EADL) provide power to specific electronic devices throughout the home in one centralized and easily accessible area. Refer to Chapter 15 for more information.

Mobility and Transfers.
Clients with problems of incoordination may use a variety of ambulation aids, depending on the type and severity of incoordination. Sometimes the OT practitioner must help the client with degenerative diseases to recognize the need for ambulation aids and accept their use. This may mean switching from a cane to crutches to a walker and finally to a wheelchair for some persons. Clients with incoordination can improve stability and mobility by using the following techniques:

1. Instead of lifting objects, slide them on counters or tabletops.
2. Use ambulation aids as appropriate. Putting weights on the sides of a walker may be beneficial for those with tremors.

3. Use a utility cart, preferably a custom-made cart that is heavy and has some friction on the wheels.
4. Remove door sills, throw rugs, and thick carpeting.
5. Install banisters on indoor and outdoor staircases with handrails on both sides if possible.
6. Substitute ramps for stairs wherever possible.

Home Management Activities.
The occupational therapy practitioner should make a careful assessment of homemaking activities performance to determine the following: (1) which activities can be done safely, (2) which activities can be done safely if modified or adapted, and (3) which activities cannot be done adequately or safely and therefore should be assigned to someone else. The major problem areas are stabilization of food and equipment to prevent spilling and accidents and the safe handling of appliances, pots, pans, and household tools to prevent cuts, burns, bruises, electric shock, and falls. Suggestions for improving safety and function in home management tasks include the following (Klinger et al., 1997; Lift and Accessibility Solutions, 2013; Trombly, 1983):

1. Use a wheelchair and wheelchair lapboard (even if ambulation is possible with devices). This saves energy and increases stability when balance and gait are unsteady.
2. If possible, use convenience and prepared foods to eliminate processes such as peeling, chopping, slicing, and mixing.
3. Use easy-open containers or store foods in plastic containers.
4. Use heavy utensils, mixing bowls, and pots and pans to increase stability.
5. Try using various types of jar openers, including wall-mounted and portable.
6. Use nonskid mats on work surfaces. Line the kitchen sink with rubber mat cushions to prevent items from sliding or breaking.
7. Use electric appliances such as crockpots, electric fry pans, electric tea kettles, toaster ovens, and microwave ovens because they are safer to use than the range or oven.
8. Use a blender and countertop mixer because they are safer than handheld mixers and easier than mixing with a spoon or whisk.
9. If possible, adjust work heights of counters, sink, and range to minimize leaning, bending, reaching, and lifting, whether the client is standing or using a wheelchair. Use a stool at the counter to increase balance and stability.
10. Use long oven mitts, which give greater protection than potholders.
11. Use lightweight pots, pans, casserole dishes, and appliances with bilateral handles because they may be easier to hold and manage than those with one handle.
12. Use a cutting board with stainless steel nails (Fig. 13.15) to stabilize meat, potatoes, and vegetables while cutting or peeling. When the cutting board is not in use, the nails should be covered with a large cork. To prevent slipping, the bottom of the board should have suction cups, be covered with stair tread, or be placed on a nonskid mat.

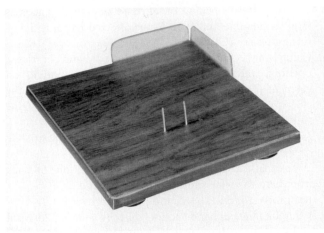

Fig. 13.15 Cutting board with stainless-steel nails, suction-cup feet, and corner for stabilizing bread is useful for patients with incoordination or lacking use of one hand. (Courtesy Sammons, a BISSELL Co.)

13. Use heavy dinnerware, which offers stability and control to the distal part of the upper extremity and may be easier to handle. If dropping and breaking are problems, durable plastic dinnerware may be more practical.

14. Cover the sink, utility cart, and countertops with protective rubber mats or mesh matting to stabilize items.

15. Use a serrated knife for cutting and chopping because it is easier to control.

16. To eliminate the need to carry and drain pots of hot liquids, use a steamer basket or deep-fry basket for preparing boiled foods.

17. Use tongs to turn foods during cooking and to serve foods because tongs offer more control and stability than a fork, spatula, or serving spoon.

18. Use a bottle tipper to safely pour liquids. Velcro straps hold the bottle into a wire frame while the client controls the tipping angle by pulling down on the wire frame until liquid slowly streams out of the bottle (North Coast Medical, 2004).

19. Use blunt-ended loop scissors to open packages (Fig. 13.16).

20. The ambulatory client may find vacuuming easier with a heavy upright cleaner. The wheelchair user may be able to manage a lightweight tank-type vacuum cleaner or electric broom.

21. Use dust mitts or old athletic socks for dusting.

22. Avoid displaying objects that are easily broken or difficult to manage such as fragile knickknacks, unstable lamps, and dainty doilies.

23. Eliminate ironing by using no-iron fabrics, timed dryer, or spray-on Downy Wrinkle Releaser. Alternatively, assign this task to other members of the household.

24. Use front-loading washers, a laundry cart on wheels, and premeasured detergents, bleaches, and fabric softeners. Purex makes three-in-one laundry "sheets" that include detergent, fabric softener, and antistatic. This product is light and reduces the need for heavy lifting, pouring, and measuring (Purex Complete 3-in-1 laundry sheet, 2019).

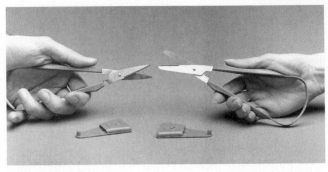

Fig. 13.16 Loop scissors.

25. Sit while working with an infant. Use foam-rubber bath aids; an infant bath seat; and a wide, padded dressing table with safety straps with Velcro fastening to offer enough stability for bathing, dressing, and diapering an infant. Child care may not be safe for individuals with significant incoordination difficulties.

26. Use disposable diapers with tape or Velcro fasteners because they are easier to manage than cloth diapers and pins.

27. Do not feed the infant with a spoon or fork unless the incoordination is mild or does not affect the upper extremities.

28. Dress the child in clothing that is large, loose, stretchy, nonslip, and fastened with Velcro.

Hemiplegia

It is tempting but misleading to classify together all conditions that may result in the dysfunction of one upper extremity. Unilateral upper extremity amputations and temporary disorders such as fractures, burns, and peripheral neuropathy may lead to unilateral upper extremity dysfunction. Clients with unilateral upper extremity dysfunction resulting from such disorders are likely to learn compensatory techniques quickly and easily if they have normal functioning of sensory, perceptual, and cognitive systems. These clients may benefit from a few suggestions to help with ADL while they recover from the injury. However, hemiplegia is the most commonly seen diagnosis in which unilateral upper extremity dysfunction occurs, and this diagnosis requires a different approach.

Clients with hemiplegia require specialized methods of teaching; many have greater difficulty learning and performing one-handed skills than do persons with orthopedic or lower motor neuron dysfunction. The reason for this is that the head, trunk, and leg, as well as the arm, are involved; consequently, ambulation and balance difficulties may be impaired. Lack of trunk control reduces coordination of the distal upper extremity for ADL tasks. In addition, sensory, perceptual, cognitive, and speech disorders may affect the ability to learn. Finally, the presence of motor and ideational apraxia sometimes seen in this group of clients can limit their potential for learning new motor skills and remembering previous ones. The client with hemiplegia needs to be evaluated for sensory, perceptual, and cognitive deficits to determine potential for ADL performance and to establish appropriate teaching methods to facilitate learning.

The major problems for the one-handed worker are reduced work speed and dexterity and poor stabilization, a function usually assumed by the nondominant arm. The major problems for the client with hemiplegia are unsteady balance and the risk of injury because of sensory and perceptual loss (Koketsu, 2018). *One-Handed in a Two-Handed World* by Tommy K. Mayer is a good resource book for teaching ADL adaptations (Matsutsuyu, 1969).

Dressing Activities. Individuals with hemiplegia may have difficulty donning and removing the clothing they wore before their disability. Suggestions for slight modifications of clothing are made throughout the following discussion on dressing. Exploring options in **adaptive clothing** can help individuals maintain independence and dignity, and the caregiver can assist with dressing without as much lifting and repositioning of the client. A number of websites (including www.easyaccessclothing.com) sell adaptive clothing and provide ideas for clients to make modifications to their own clothing. Examples of adaptive clothing include button-down shirts that open or close with Velcro tabs, pants with extended Velcro flies to allow for easy access when using a urinal or catheter, seams sewn flat to help prevent pressure sores, wrist or finger loops to help individuals lift garments when dressing, and coats with cut-out backs to eliminate sitting on excess fabric that may get caught in the wheelchair spokes or cause pressure sores. The addition of a zipper opening at the side seams from ankle to waist allows the individual to wear fitted pants without struggling to don or doff them. This concept is helpful for fitted blazers, with a zipper forming a side opening down the length of the sleeves. These solutions can be introduced to a local tailor so that discrete modifications can be added to the individual's current wardrobe to help increase safety and dressing ease.

If balance is a problem, the client should dress while seated in a locked wheelchair or sturdy armchair. Clothing should be within easy reach. Reaching tongs may be helpful for securing articles and assisting in some dressing activities. Dressing and other ADL should be approached with a minimum of assistive devices.

One-handed dressing techniques. Some dressing techniques for the client with hemiplegia employ neurodevelopmental (Bobath) treatment principles. The following one-handed dressing techniques can facilitate dressing for clients with use of one upper extremity. As a general rule, place the affected extremity in the garment first when dressing and remove last when undressing. This procedure allows more room to work with the garment when motor control is most impaired.

Shirts. Front-opening shirts may be managed by any one of three methods. The first method can be used for jackets, robes, and front-opening dresses.

Method 1: Basic Over Head—Donning (Fig. 13.17)
1. Grasp shirt collar with unaffected hand and shake out twists *(A)*.
2. Position shirt on lap with inside facing up and collar toward chest *(B)*.

3. Position sleeve opening on affected side so that it is as large as possible and close to the affected hand, which is resting on lap *(C)*.
4. Using unaffected hand, place affected hand in sleeve opening, and work sleeve over elbow by pulling on garment *(D1, D2)*. Ensuring the sleeve is placed over the elbow will prevent shoulder injuries when placing the shirt over the head.
5. Put unaffected arm into its sleeve and raise up to slide or shake sleeve into position past elbow *(E)*.
6. With unaffected hand, gather shirt up middle of back from hem to collar and raise shirt overhead *(F)*.
7. Lean forward, duck head, and pass shirt over it *(G)*.
8. With unaffected hand, adjust shirt by leaning forward and working it down past both shoulders. Reach in back and pull shirttail down *(H)*.
9. Line shirt fronts up for buttoning and begin with bottom button *(I)*. Button sleeve cuff of affected arm. The sleeve cuff of unaffected arm may be prebuttoned if cuff opening is large.

A button may be sewn on with elastic thread or sewn onto a small tab of elastic and fastened inside shirt cuff. A small button attached to a crocheted loop of elastic thread is another alternative. Also, a cuff and collar extender can be added. Slip the button on loop through buttonhole in the garment so that the elastic loop is inside. Stretch the elastic loop to fit around original cuff button. This simple device can be transferred to each garment and positioned before the shirt is put on. The loop stretches to accommodate the width of the hand as it is pushed through the end of the sleeve (Sammons Preston Rolyan, 2004). Warning: Self-buttoning is a labor-intensive and frustrating task for clients with hemiplegia. Encourage these clients to wear a larger shirt and keep most buttons fastened before donning. Clients with hemiplegia may find it easier to button before donning or to have a caregiver arrange clothing fastened ahead of time.

Method 1: Basic Over Head—Removing
1. Unbutton shirt.
2. Lean forward.
3. With unaffected hand, grasp collar or gather material up in back from collar to hem.
4. Lean forward, duck head, and pull shirt overhead.
5. Remove sleeve from unaffected arm and then from affected arm.

Method 2: Over Head On/Shrug Off—Donning. Method 2 may be used by clients who have the shirt twisted or have trouble sliding the sleeve down onto unaffected arm.
1. Position shirt as described in method 1, steps 1 to 3.
2. With unaffected hand, place involved hand into shirt sleeve opening and work sleeve onto hand, but do *not* pull up over elbow.
3. Put unaffected arm into sleeve and bring arm out to 180 degrees of abduction. Tension of fabric from unaffected arm to wrist of affected arm will bring sleeve into position.
4. Lower arm and work sleeve on affected arm up over elbow.
5. Continue as in method 1, steps 6 to 9.

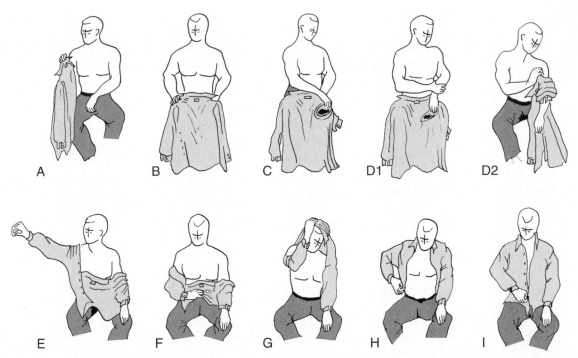

Fig. 13.17 (A–I) Steps in donning shirt: method 1 (basic over head). (Courtesy Christine Shaw, Metro Health Center for Rehabilitation, Metro Health Medical Center, Cleveland, OH.)

Method 2: Overhead/Shrug Off—Removing
1. Unbutton shirt.
2. With unaffected hand, push shirt off shoulders, first on affected side, then on unaffected side.
3. Pull on cuff of unaffected side with unaffected hand.
4. Work sleeve off by alternately shrugging shoulder and pulling down on cuff.
5. Lean forward, bring shirt around back, and pull sleeve off affected arm.

Method 3: Over Shoulder—Donning (Fig. 13.18)
1. Position shirt and work onto arm as described in method 1, steps 1 to 4.
2. Pull sleeve on affected arm up to shoulder *(A)*.
3. With unaffected hand, grasp tip of collar that is on unaffected side, lean forward, and bring arm over and behind head to carry shirt around to unaffected side *(B)*.
4. Put unaffected arm into sleeve opening, directing it up and out *(C)*.
5. Adjust and button as described in method 1, steps 8 and 9.

Method 3: Over Shoulder—Removing. The shirt may be removed using the same procedure described for method 2.

Method 4: Donning Pullover Shirt (Over Head)
1. Position shirt on lap, with bottom toward chest and label facing down.
2. With unaffected hand, roll up bottom edge of shirt back up to sleeve on affected side.
3. Position sleeve opening so that it is as large as possible, and use unaffected hand to place affected hand into sleeve opening. Pull shirt up onto arm past elbow.
4. Insert unaffected arm into sleeve.
5. Adjust shirt on affected side up and onto shoulder.

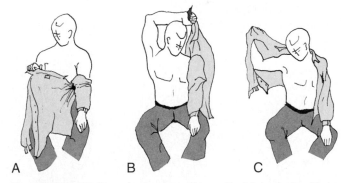

Fig. 13.18 (A–C) Steps in donning shirt: method 3 (over shoulder). (Courtesy Christine Shaw, Metro Health Center for Rehabilitation, Metro Health Medical Center, Cleveland, OH.)

6. Gather shirt back with unaffected hand, lean forward, duck head, and pass shirt over head.
7. Adjust shirt.

Method 4: Removing Pullover Shirt (Over Head)
1. Gather shirt up with unaffected hand, starting at top back.
2. Lean forward, duck head, and pull gathered fabric in back over head.
3. Remove from unaffected arm and then affected arm.

Trousers. Trousers may be managed by one of the following methods, which can be adapted for shorts and women's panties as well. Velcro or elastic may replace buttons and zippers. Trousers should be worn in a size slightly larger than worn previously and should have a wide opening at the ankles. They should be put on before the socks and shoes. Feet can slip forward when attempting to stand if the person is wearing socks; a bare foot has better traction. The client who is dressing in a wheelchair should place feet flat on the floor, not on the footrests of the wheelchair.

Method 1: Partial Standing—Donning (Fig. 13.19)

1. Sit in sturdy armchair or in locked wheelchair *(A)*.
2. Position unaffected leg in front of midline of body with knee flexed to 90 degrees. Using unaffected hand, reach forward and grasp ankle of affected leg or sock around ankle *(B1)*. Lift affected leg over unaffected leg to crossed position *(B2)*.
3. Slip trousers onto affected leg up to position where foot is completely inside of trouser leg *(C)*. Do not pull up above the knee, or it will be difficult inserting unaffected leg.
4. Uncross affected leg by grasping ankle or portion of sock around ankle *(D)*.
5. Insert unaffected leg and work trousers up onto hips as far as possible *(E1, E2)*.
6. To prevent trousers from dropping when pulling pants over hips, place affected hand in pocket or place one finger of affected hand into belt loop. If able to do so safely, stand and pull trousers over hips *(F1, F2)*.
7. If standing balance is good, remain standing to pull up zipper or button *(F3)*. Sit down to button front *(G)*.

Method 1: Partial Standing—Removing

1. Unfasten trousers and work down on hips as far as possible while seated.
2. Stand, letting trousers drop past hips or work them down past hips.
3. Sit and remove trousers from unaffected leg.

4. Cross affected leg over unaffected leg, remove trousers, and uncross leg.

Method 2: Seated Bridging—Donning. Method 2 is used for clients who are in wheelchairs (brakes locked, footrests swung away) or in sturdy, straight armchairs (back against wall) and for clients who cannot stand independently.

1. Position trousers on legs as in method 1, steps 1 to 5.
2. Elevate hips by leaning back against the chair and pushing down against the floor with unaffected leg; this is called **bridging**. As hips are raised, work trousers over hips with unaffected hand. Again, the person's feet should be able to grip the floor (do not attempt when wearing only standard socks on feet).
3. Lower hips back into chair and fasten trousers.

Method 2: Seated Bridging—Removing

1. Unfasten trousers and work down on hips as far as possible while sitting.
2. Ensure that feet are positioned securely on the floor with no-slip socks or shoes to prevent hips from slipping forward and out of the chair.
3. Lean back against the chair, push down against the floor with unaffected leg to elevate hips, and with unaffected arm, work trousers down past hips.
4. Proceed as in method 1, steps 3 and 4.

Method 3: Recumbent Bridging—Donning. Method 3 is done in a recumbent position—that is, lying down or reclining in bed. It is more difficult to perform than methods

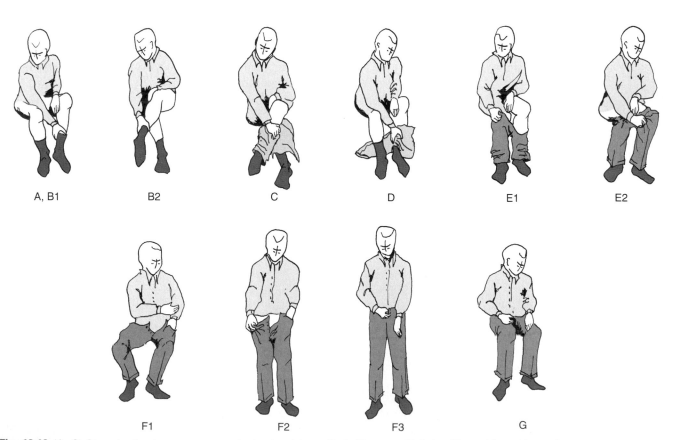

A, B1　　　　　B2　　　　　C　　　　　D　　　　　E1　　　　　E2

F1　　　　　F2　　　　　F3　　　　　G

Fig. 13.19 (A–G) Steps in donning trousers: method 1 (partial standing). (Courtesy Christine Shaw, Metro Health Center for Rehabilitation, Metro Health Medical Center, Cleveland, OH.)

done while sitting. If possible, the bed should be raised to a semireclining position for partial sitting. The firmer the mattress, the easier it is to maneuver.

1. Using unaffected hand, place affected knee in flexed position and cross over unaffected leg, which may be partially flexed to prevent affected leg from slipping.
2. Position trousers and pull onto affected leg first, up to knee. Then uncross leg.
3. Insert unaffected leg and work trousers up onto hips as far as possible.
4. With unaffected leg flexed, press down with foot and shoulder to elevate hips from bed. While in this bridged position, with unaffected arm, pull trousers over hips or work trousers up over hips by rolling from side to side.
5. Fasten trousers.

Method 3: Recumbent Bridging—Removing

1. Bridge hips as in putting trousers on in method 3, step 4.
2. Work trousers down past hips, remove unaffected leg, and then remove affected leg.

Brassiere (Back Opening)

Donning. Clothing items such as brassieres, neckties, socks, stockings, and braces may be difficult to manage with one hand. The following methods are recommended.

1. Position brassiere on lap so that shoulder strap side is toward knees and inside is facing up. Tuck one end of brassiere into pants waistband or fasten it with a clothespin, and wrap the other end around the waist (wrapping toward affected side may be easiest). Hook brassiere in front at waist level and slip fastener around to back (at waistline level).
2. Place affected arm through shoulder strap, then place unaffected arm through other strap.
3. Work straps up over shoulders. Pull strap on affected side up over shoulder with unaffected arm. Put unaffected arm through its strap and work up over shoulder by directing arm up and out and pulling with hand.
4. Use unaffected hand to adjust breasts in brassiere cups.

If the client has some function in the affected hand, a fabric loop may be sewn to the back of the brassiere near the fastener. The affected thumb may be slipped through this to stabilize the brassiere while the unaffected hand fastens it. Front-opening bras may also be adapted in this way.

In all cases, it is helpful if the brassiere has elastic straps and is made of stretch fabric. All-elastic brassieres, prefastened or without fasteners, may be put on using method 1 described previously for shirts.

Removing

1. Slip straps down off shoulders, unaffected side first.
2. Work straps down over arms and off hands.
3. Slip brassiere around to front with unaffected arm.
4. Unfasten and remove.

Necktie

Donning. Clip-on neckties are convenient. If a conventional tie is used, the following method is recommended:

1. Place collar of shirt in up position, bring necktie around neck, and adjust it so that the smaller end is at length desired when tying is completed.
2. Fasten small end to shirt front with tie clasp or spring-clip clothespin.
3. Loop long end around short end (one complete loop) and bring up between V at neck. Then bring tip down through loop at front and adjust tie, using ring and little fingers to hold tie end and thumb and forefingers to slide knot up tightly.

Removing. Pull knot at front of neck until small end slips up enough for tie to be slipped over head. Tie may be hung up in this state and replaced by slipping it over head, around upturned collar, with knot tightened as described in step 3 of donning.

Socks or Stockings

Donning

1. Sit in straight armchair or in wheelchair with brakes locked, feet on floor, and footrest swung away.
2. With unaffected leg directly in front of midline of body, cross affected leg over it.
3. Open top of stocking by inserting thumb and first two fingers near cuff and spreading fingers apart.
4. Work stocking onto foot before pulling over heel. Care should be taken to eliminate wrinkles.
5. Work stocking up over leg. Shift weight from side to side to adjust stocking around thigh.
6. Thigh-high stockings with elastic band at the top are often an acceptable substitute for pantyhose, especially for nonambulatory clients. Elastic should not be so tight as to impair circulation.
7. Pantyhose may be donned and doffed as a pair of slacks, except legs would be gathered up, one at a time, before placing feet into leg holes.

Removing

1. Work socks or stockings down as far as possible with unaffected arm.
2. With unaffected leg directly in front of midline of body, cross affected leg over it.
3. Remove sock or stocking from affected leg. Some clients may require dressing stick to push sock or stocking off heel and foot.
4. Lift unaffected leg to comfortable height or seat level and remove sock or stocking from foot.

Shoes. If possible, select slip-on shoes to eliminate lacing and tying. The client who uses an ankle-foot orthosis (AFO) or short leg brace usually needs shoes with fasteners.

1. Use elastic laces and leave shoes tied.
2. Use one-handed shoe-tying techniques (Fig. 13.20).
3. Client can learn to tie a standard bow with one hand, but this requires excellent visual perceptual and motor planning skills along with much repetition.

Ankle-Foot Orthosis. A client with hemiplegia who lacks adequate ankle dorsiflexion to walk safely and efficiently often uses an AFO. The custom AFO is often issued after the client is discharged, so it may be necessary to practice this skill before the client receives it.

Donning (Fig. 13.21)

1. Sit in straight armchair or wheelchair with brakes locked and feet on floor (A). Fasteners are loosened,

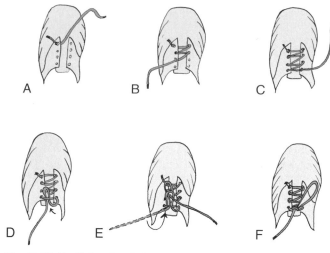

Fig. 13.20 (A–F) One-handed shoe-tying method. (Courtesy Christine Shaw, Metro Health Center for Rehabilitation, Metro Health Medical Center, Cleveland, OH.)

and tongue of shoe is pulled back to allow AFO to fit into shoe *(B)*.

2. AFO and shoe are placed on the floor between legs but closer to affected leg, facing up *(C)*.
3. With unaffected hand, lift affected leg behind knee and place toes into shoe *(D)*. It is important to keep or reposition affected leg, shoe, and AFO directly under affected knee, as much as possible.
4. Reach down with unaffected hand and lift AFO by the upright. Simultaneously, use unaffected foot against affected heel to keep shoe and AFO together *(E)*.
5. Heel is not pushed into shoe at this point. With unaffected hand, apply pressure directly downward on affected knee to force heel into shoe, if leg strength is not sufficient *(F)*.
6. Fasten Velcro calf strap and fasten shoes *(G)*. Affected leg may be placed on footstool to assist with reaching shoe fasteners.
7. To fasten shoes, one-handed bow tying may be used. Elastic shoelaces, Velcro-fastened shoes, or other commercially available shoe fasteners may be required if the client cannot tie own shoes.

Removing: Variation 1.
1. While seated, cross affected leg over unaffected leg.
2. Unfasten straps and laces with unaffected hand.
3. Using unaffected hand, push down on AFO upright until shoe is off foot.

Removing: Variation 2
1. Unfasten straps and laces.
2. Straighten affected leg by putting unaffected foot behind heel of shoe and pushing affected leg forward.
3. Push down on AFO upright with unaffected hand and at same time push forward on heel of AFO shoe with unaffected foot.

Hygiene and Grooming. With the use of alternate methods and some assistive devices, hygiene and grooming activities can be accomplished using only one hand or one side of the body. Suggestions for achieving hygiene and grooming with one hand include the following:

1. Use an electric razor rather than a safety or disposable razor.
2. Use a bathtub seat or chair in the shower stall or bathtub. Use a suction-based bathmat, wash mitt, long-handled bath sponge, safety rails on the bathtub or wall, soap on a rope or suction soap holder, and suction brush for fingernail care.
3. Sponge-bathe while sitting at the toilet, using the wash mitt, suction brush, and suction soap holder.

The uninvolved forearm and hand can be washed by placing a soaped washcloth on the thigh and rubbing the hand and forearm on the cloth.

1. Use the position-adjustable hairdryer previously described. Such a device frees the unaffected upper extremity to hold a brush or comb to style the hair during blow-drying (Feldmeier & Poole, 1987).
2. Care for fingernails as described previously for clients with incoordination.
3. Use Dycem on the sink to secure the toothbrush in place while applying toothpaste. Alternatively, squeeze the toothpaste directly into the mouth before brushing teeth.
4. Use a suction denture brush for care of dentures. The suction fingernail brush may also serve this purpose (see Fig. 13.14). Use a flossing aid with one hand for oral hygiene, such as a Gripit floss holder (http://sale.dentist.net/products/gripit-floss-holder).

Communication and General Environment. Suggestions to facilitate writing, reading, and using the telephone include the following:

1. The primary problem in writing is stabilization of the paper or tablet. Stability can be achieved by using a clipboard or paperweight, or by taping the paper to the writing surface. In some instances, the affected arm may be positioned on the tabletop to stabilize the paper passively.
2. The individual who must shift dominance to the non-dominant extremity may need to practice to improve speed and coordination in writing. One-handed writing and keyboarding instruction manuals are available.
3. Book holders may be used to stabilize a book while reading or holding copy for typing and writing practice. For reading while seated in an easy chair, the client can position a soft pillow on the lap to stabilize a book.
4. To write while using the telephone, a speaker phone or an earpiece can be used.

Mobility and Transfers. Chapter 15 describes principles of transfer techniques for clients with hemiplegia.

Home Management Activities. A variety of assistive devices make home management activities easier to perform. The nature and severity of the disability determine how many home management activities realistically can be performed, which methods can be used, and how many assistive devices can be managed. Whether the client is disabled solely by the loss of function of one arm and hand (as in amputation or peripheral neuropathy) or whether both arm and

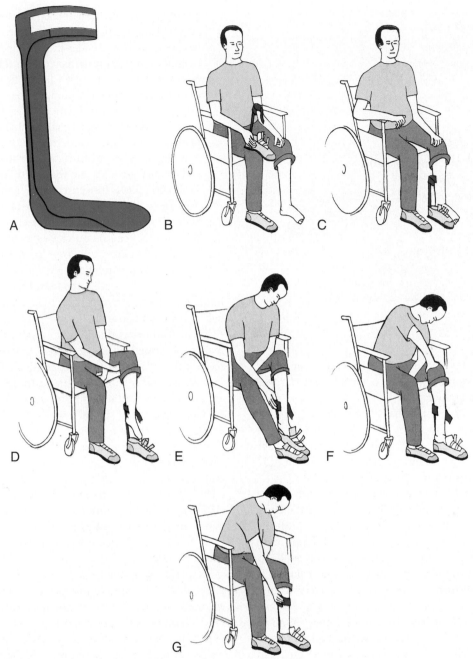

Fig. 13.21 (A–G) Seven steps in donning ankle-foot orthosis (AFO).

leg are affected—along with possible visual, perceptual, and cognitive dysfunctions (as in hemiplegia)—makes a significant difference in planning treatment. Suggestions regarding home management for the client with use of one hand include the following (see References for further details) (Klinger et al., 1997):

1. Stabilization of items is a major problem for the homemaker who can use only one hand. Stabilize foods for cutting and peeling by using a board with two stainless steel or aluminum nails in it. A raised corner on the board stabilizes bread while making sandwiches or spreading butter. Suction cups or a rubber mat under the board will keep it from slipping. Rubber stair tread, shelf liner, or Dycem may be glued to the bottom of the board.

2. Use sponge cloths, nonskid mats or pads, wet dishcloths, or suction devices to keep bowls and dishes from turning or sliding during food preparation. Use a pan holder—a steel rod frame with suction cups attached to the stove top—to keep the pot from spinning while the contents are being stirred or flipped (Runge, 1967).

3. To open a jar, stabilize it between the knees or in a partially opened drawer while leaning against it. Break the air seal by sliding a bottle opener under the lid until the air is released; then use a wall-mounted opener like

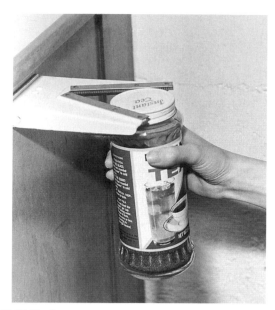

Fig. 13.22 Zim jar opener.

the Zim jar opener (Fig. 13.22). When purchasing food items in jars, ask the grocer to open and gently reseal jars before bagging them.

4. Open boxes, sealed paper bags, and plastic bags by stabilizing between the knees or in a drawer, as just described, and cutting open with a household shears. Special box and bag openers are also available from ADL equipment vendors (North Coast Medical, 2004).

5. Open an egg by holding it firmly in the palm of the hand, hitting it in the center against the edge of the bowl, and then using the thumb and index finger to push the top half of the shell up and the ring and little fingers to push the lower half down. Separate whites from yolks by using an egg separator or a funnel. Another solution is to use cholesterol-free eggs, such as Egg Beaters, from a carton.

6. Eliminate the need to stabilize the standard grater by using a grater with suction feet, or use an electric food processor.

7. Eliminate the need to use hand-cranked or electric can openers requiring two hands by using a one-handed electric can opener.

8. Use a utility cart to carry items from one place to another. A cart that is weighted or constructed of wood may be used as a minimal support during ambulation for some clients with mild balance or coordination impairments.

9. Transfer clothes to and from the washer or dryer by using a clothes carrier on wheels.

10. Use electrical appliances that can be managed with one hand to save time and energy. Some of these appliances include a lightweight electrical hand mixer, blender, and food processor. Safety factors and judgment need to be evaluated carefully for electrical appliances.

11. Floor care becomes a problem if ambulation and balance are affected in addition to the upper extremity. For clients with involvement of one arm only, a standard dust mop, carpet sweeper, or upright vacuum cleaner should present no problem. A self-wringing mop may be used if the mop handle is stabilized under the arm and the wringing lever operated with the unaffected arm. Floor cleaning systems such as Swiffer or Clorox Ready Mop dispense the cleanser through a pump, wipe up the floor with a disposable cleaning pad, and are easy to manage with one hand. Clients with balance and ambulation problems may manage some floor care from a sitting position. Dust mopping or using a carpet sweeper may be possible if gait and balance are adequate without the aid of a cane.

12. To easily push furniture aside and avoid scratching flooring while cleaning or rearranging, attach Magic Sliders to the bottoms of the feet or base of furniture. This product can be purchased at hardware stores.

13. Use a gas lighter with one hand (instead of a match requiring two hands) to light candles.

These suggestions are just a few of the possibilities to solve home management problems for clients with use of only one hand. The occupational therapy practitioner must evaluate each client to determine how the dysfunction affects performance of homemaking activities. One-handed techniques require more time and may be difficult for some clients to master. Activities should be paced to accommodate the client's physical endurance and tolerance for one-handed performance and use of special devices. Work simplification and energy conservation techniques should be employed.

New techniques and devices should be introduced on a graded basis as the client masters one technique and device and then another. Family members must be oriented to the client's skills, special methods, and work schedule. The clinician may help plan homemaking responsibilities with the family and client, focusing on which tasks will be shared with other family members and the procedures for supervising the client, if needed.

If special equipment and assistive devices are needed for ADL, obtaining them, if possible, while the person is receiving occupational therapy treatment is advisable. The OT or OTA can then train the client in their use and demonstrate to a family member before the items are used at home. After training, the clinician should provide the client with sources to replace items independently such as a consumer catalog or websites of adaptive equipment (North Coast Medical, 2004).

Paraplegia

Clients who are confined to a wheelchair need to find ways to perform ADL from a seated position, to transport objects, and to adapt to an environment that is intended for standing and walking. Given normal upper extremity function, the wheelchair-dependent client can most likely perform seated level activities independently. To do so, the client should have a stable spine, and mobility precautions should be clearly identified. Energy conservation techniques should be utilized during the ADL routine. For example, it is important to minimize transfers during self-care tasks because they require a lot of energy and can be a safety risk when fatigued. Planning out the order of the self-care routine can reduce the number of transfers required and save energy for other meaningful activities throughout the day.

Dressing Activities. Wheelchair-dependent clients should put clothing on in this order: stockings, undergarments, braces (if worn), trousers or slacks, shoes, shirt, or dress (Koketsu, 2018).

Socks or stockings
Donning
1. Put on socks or stockings while seated on bed or in wheelchair.
2. Pull one leg into flexion with one hand and cross over other leg.
3. Use other hand to slip sock or stocking over foot and pull it on.

Soft stretch socks or stockings are recommended. Pantyhose that are slightly large may be useful. Elastic garters or stockings with elastic tops may lead to skin breakdown and should be avoided. Dressing sticks or a sock aid may be helpful to some clients.

Removing. Remove socks or stockings by flexing leg as described for donning, then pushing sock or stocking down over heel. Dressing sticks may be needed to push sock or stocking off heel and toe and to retrieve it.

Trousers. Trousers and slacks are easier to fasten if they button or zip in front. If braces are worn, zippers in the side seams may be helpful. Wide-bottom slacks of stretch fabric are recommended. The following procedure is for putting on trousers, shorts, slacks, and underwear.

Donning
1. Long sit (thighs and calves on bed, knees extended) on bed with feet hanging off the foot of the bed and reach forward toward feet, or sit on bed and pull knees into flexed position.
2. While holding top of trousers, flip pants down to feet.
3. Work pant legs over feet and pull up to hips. Crossing ankles may help work pants on over heels.
4. In semireclining position, roll from hip to hip and pull up garment. When lying on the left hip, pull the trousers up over the right hip and vice versa.
5. Reaching tongs or fabric loops on the waistband may be helpful to pull garment up or position garment on feet if the client has impaired balance or limited ROM in the lower extremities or trunk.

Removing. Remove pants or underwear by reversing procedure for putting on. Dressing sticks may be helpful to push pants off feet.

Slips and skirts
Donning
1. Sit on bed, slip garment overhead, and let it drop to waist.
2. In semireclining position, roll from hip to hip and pull garment down over hips and thighs.

Slips and skirts slightly larger than usually worn are recommended. A-line, wraparound, and full skirts are easier

to manage and lie more smoothly while the client is seated in a wheelchair than do narrow skirts. Long skirts and jackets may get caught in the wheel of the wheelchair during mobility and should be avoided for safety reasons.

Removing
1. In sitting or semireclining position, unfasten garment.
2. Roll from hip to hip, pulling garment up to waist level.
3. Pull garment off over head.

Shoes. Because of sensory loss and paralysis, shoes should be donned before any transfers to prevent the foot from slipping forward and to protect the foot from bruises.

Donning
1. Sit on edge of bed or in wheelchair.
2. Cross one leg over other and slip shoe on.
3. Put foot on footrest and push down on knee to push foot into shoe.

Removing
1. Cross leg as described earlier.
2. Remove shoe from crossed leg with one hand while maintaining balance with other hand, if necessary.

Shirts. Shirts, pajama jackets, robes, and dresses that open completely down the front may be put on while the client is seated in a wheelchair. If it is necessary to dress in bed, the following procedure can be used.

Donning
1. Balance body by putting palms of hands on mattress on either side of the body. If balance is poor, assistance may be needed. Propping two pillows to support the back can leave both hands free.
2. If difficulty is encountered in customary methods of applying garment, open garment on lap with collar toward chest. Put arms into sleeves and pull up over elbows. Then hold on to shirttail or back of dress, pull garment overhead, adjust, and button.

Fabrics should be wrinkle resistant, smooth, and durable.

Roomy sleeves, backs, and full skirts are more suitable styles than fitted garments.

Removing
1. While sitting in a wheelchair or bed, open fastener.
2. Remove garment in usual manner.
3. If step 2 is not feasible, grasp collar with one hand while balancing with other hand. Gather material up from collar to hem.
4. Lean forward, duck head, and pull shirt over head.
5. Remove sleeve from supporting arm and then from the working arm.

Hygiene and Grooming. Face and oral hygiene and arm and upper body care should present no problem. Reachers may be helpful to retrieve towels, washcloths, makeup, deodorant, and shaving supplies from storage areas, if necessary.

Adjusting the sink height and removing the cabinetry below the sink may be necessary to allow the wheelchair to fit directly under the sink. A wall-mounted swivel-adjustable-arm mirror may be useful for makeup and face care. Tub baths or showers require some special equipment. Chapter 15 discusses transfer techniques for the toilet and bathtub. Suggestions to make bathing activities easier for the wheelchair-dependent client include the following:

1. Use a handheld showerhead, and keep a finger over the spray to determine sudden temperature changes in water. This method will help prevent burning the skin in areas with sensory loss.
2. Use long-handled bath brushes with soap insert for ease in reaching all parts of the body.
3. Use soap bars attached to a cord around the neck.
4. For sponge bath in a wheelchair, cover the chair with a sheet of plastic.
5. Use padded shower chairs or bathtub seats with cut-out bottom to allow for full body cleansing from a seated position.
6. Increase safety during transfers by installing grab bars on wall near the bathtub or shower and on the bathtub.
7. Fit bottom of the bathtub or shower with nonskid mat or adhesive material.
8. Remove doors on the bathtub and replace with a shower curtain to increase transfer space.

Communication and General Environment. With the exception of difficulty with reaching in some situations, wheelchair-dependent clients should have no problem using the phone. Numbers can be entered with a short, rubber-tipped stylus. These clients should be able to use writing implements, computers, and tape recorders with no difficulty, if the devices are placed on an easily accessible tabletop.

Managing doors may present some problems. If the door opens toward the client, opening it can be managed by the following procedure:

1. If doorknob is on the right, approach door from right and turn doorknob with left hand.
2. Open the door as far as possible and move wheelchair close enough so that it helps keep door open.
3. Holding door open with left hand, turn wheelchair with right hand and wheel through door.
4. Start closing door when halfway through.

If the door is heavy and opens out or away from the client, the following procedure is recommended (California Department of Aging, 2020):

1. For a doorknob on the right, back up to door so that knob can be turned with right hand.
2. Open door and back through so that back wheels keep it open.
3. Also use left elbow to keep door open.
4. Wheel backward with right hand.

Mobility and Transfers. Chapter 15 discusses transfer techniques.

Home Management Activities. For a wheelchair-dependent person, the major home management problems are work heights; adequate space for maneuverability; access to storage areas; and transfer of supplies, equipment, and materials from place to place. If funds are available for kitchen remodeling, lowering counters and range to a comfortable height is recommended. However, such extensive adaptation is often not feasible. Suggestions for home management include the following (Klinger et al., 1997):

1. Remove lower cabinet doors to eliminate the need to maneuver around them for opening and closing. Commonly used items should be stored on counters or toward the front of easy-to-reach cabinets above and below the counter surfaces.
2. If entrance and inside doors are not wide enough, use a narrower wheelchair or make doors slightly wider by removing strips along the doorjambs. Offset hinges can replace standard door hinges and increase the doorjamb width by 2 inches (5 cm) (Fig. 13.23).
3. Increase the client's height with a wheelchair cushion so that standard countertops can be used.
4. Use detachable desk arms and swing-away detachable footrests to allow the client to roll close to counters and tables and also to stand at counters, if possible.
5. Transport items safely and easily by using a wheelchair lapboard. The lapboard can also serve as a work surface for preparing food and drying dishes. It also protects the lap from injury from hot pans and prevents utensils from falling into the lap (Fig. 13.24).
6. Fasten a drop-leaf board to a bare wall or a slide-out board under a counter to provide the wheelchair-dependent cook with a work surface at a comfortable height in an otherwise standard kitchen.
7. Fit cabinets with custom-made or ready-made lazy Susans or pull-out shelves to eliminate the need to reach to the rear of the space (Fig. 13.25).
8. Ideally, ranges should be at a lower level than standard height. If this is not possible, place controls at the front of the range and hang a mirror over the range, angled at such a degree that the client can see contents of pots. Oven-stove mirrors are commercially available from rehabilitation catalogs (North Coast Medical, 2004).
9. Substitute small electric cooking units such as a portable electric range, toaster oven, and microwave ovens for the range if the client cannot use the range safely.
10. Use front-loading washers and dryers.
11. Vacuum carpets with a carpet sweeper or tank-type cleaner that rolls easily and is lightweight or self propelled. A retractable cord may be helpful to prevent tangling the cord in the wheels.

Quadriplegia

In general, clients with muscle function from spinal cord levels C7 and C8 can follow the methods just described for paraplegia. Clients with muscle function from C6 can be relatively independent with adaptations and assistive devices.

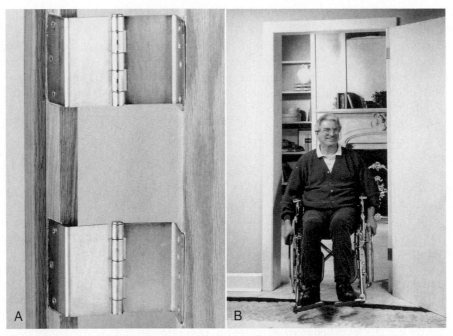

Fig. 13.23 (A) Offset hinges. (B) Offset hinges widen doorway for wheelchair-dependent patient.

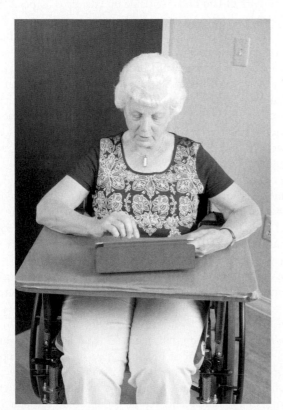

Fig. 13.24 Wheelchair lapboard is used to transport items. (Courtesy Sorrentino SA, Remmert LN. *Mosby's Textbook for Nursing Assistants.* 10th ed. St. Louis, MO: Elsevier; 2021.)

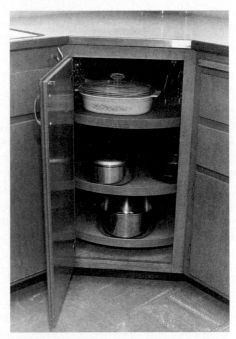

Fig. 13.25 Lazy Susan in kitchen storage cabinet.

However, those with muscle function from C4 and C5 require considerable special equipment and assistance. Clients with muscle function from C6 may benefit from the use of a wrist-driven flexor hinge splint or tenodesis splint. Externally powered splints and arm braces or mobile arm supports are recommended for C3, C4, and C5 levels of muscle function.

Dressing Activities. Determining whether a client meets the criteria for beginning dressing activities is a professional-level responsibility. However, the OTA can assist in the determination and should always closely observe client appropriateness for this or any other activity.

Criteria. Training in dressing can begin once the spine is stable (Buchwald, 1952; Renda & Lape, 2018). Before spinal stability is achieved, the client may require assistance donning a cervical or cervical thoracic orthosis as specified by doctor's orders. Minimal criteria for upper extremity dressing are the following: (1) fair to good muscle strength in deltoids, upper and middle trapezii, shoulder rotators, rhomboids, biceps, supinators, and radial wrist extensors; (2) ROM of 0 to 90 degrees in shoulder flexion and abduction, 0 to 80 degrees in shoulder internal rotation, 0 to 30 degrees in external rotation, and 15 to 140 degrees in elbow flexion; (3) sitting balance in bed or wheelchair, which may be achieved with the assistance of bed rails, an electric hospital bed, or a wheelchair safety belt; and (4) finger prehension, achieved with adequate tenodesis grasp or a wrist-hand orthosis.

Additional criteria for dressing the lower extremities are the following: (1) fair to good muscle strength in pectoralis major and minor, serratus anterior, and rhomboid major and minor; (2) ROM of 0 to 120 degrees in knee flexion, 0 to 110 degrees in hip flexion, and 0 to 80 degrees in hip external rotation; (3) body control for transfer from bed to wheelchair with minimal assistance; (4) ability to roll from side to side, balance in side lying, or turning from supine to prone position and back; and (5) vital capacity of 50% or greater (Renda & Lape, 2018).

Contraindications. Dressing is contraindicated if any of the following factors are present: (1) unstable spine at site of injury; (2) unhealed pressure sores or tendency for skin breakdown during rolling, scooting, and transferring; (3) uncontrollable muscle spasms in legs; and (4) less than 50% vital capacity (Buchwald, 1952; Renda & Lape, 2018).

Sequence of dressing. The recommended sequence for training to dress is to put on underwear and trousers while still in bed, then transfer to a wheelchair to put on shirts, socks, and shoes (Renda & Lape, 2018). Some clients may choose to put the socks on before the trousers because socks may help the feet slip through the trouser legs more easily.

Expected proficiency. Clients with total spinal cord lesions at C7 and below can achieve total dressing, which includes both upper and lower extremity dressing skills. Although people with lesions at C6 can achieve total dressing, lower extremity dressing may be difficult in terms of time and energy.

Clients with lesions at C5 to C6, with some exceptions, can independently achieve upper extremity dressing. However, these clients find it extremely difficult to put on a brassiere, tuck a shirt or blouse into a waistband, or fasten buttons on shirt fronts and cuffs. Factors such as age, physical proportions, coordination, coexistent medical problems, and motivation affect the client's degree of proficiency in dressing skills (Buchwald, 1952).

Types of clothing. Clothing should be loose and have front openings. Trousers need to be a size larger than usually worn to accommodate the urine collection device or leg braces, if worn. Avoid jeans or pants with thick seams during the first few months after onset of injury to avoid potential skin breakdown. The easiest fasteners to manage are zippers and Velcro closures. Because the quadriplegic client may use the thumb as a hook to manage clothing, loops attached to

zipper pulls, underwear, and even the back of the shoes can be helpful. Belt loops on trousers are used for pulling and should be reinforced. Brassieres should have stretch straps and no underwires. Front-opening brassieres can be adapted by fastening loops and adding Velcro closures; back-opening styles can have loops added at each side of the fastening.

Shoes should be one-half to one size larger than normally worn to accommodate edema and spasticity and to avoid pressure sores. Shoe fasteners can be adapted with Velcro, elastic shoelaces, large buckles, or flip-back tongue closures. Loose woolen or cotton socks without elastic cuffs should be used initially. Ridgeless socks, available from ADL catalogs, can help protect the skin from breakdown and are easier to don. As skill is gained, nylon socks, which tend to stick to the skin, may be introduced. If neckties are used, the clip-on type or a regular tie that has been preknotted and can be slipped over the head may be manageable for some clients (Buchwald, 1952; Runge, 1967).

The following techniques can make dressing easier for clients with upper extremity weakness.

Trousers and Undershorts

Donning

1. Sit on bed with bed rails up (long-sitting position). Trousers are positioned at foot of bed with trouser legs over end of bed and front side up (Renda & Lape, 2018).

2. Sit up and lift one knee at a time by hooking right hand under right knee to pull leg into flexion; then put trousers over right foot. Return right leg to extended or semi-extended position and repeat procedure with left hand and left knee (Buchwald, 1952). It is important to maintain one leg at a time in flexion by holding it with one arm or by taking advantage of spasticity. If neither of these strategies works, a dressing band may be used to secure the leg. This is a piece of elasticized webbing sewn into a figure-8 pattern, with one small loop and one large loop. Small loop is hooked around foot and large hoop anchored over knee. Band is measured for each client so that its length is appropriate to maintain desired amount of knee flexion. Once trousers are in place, knee loop is pushed off knee and dressing band removed from foot with dressing stick (Easton & Horan, 1979).

3. Work trousers up legs, using patting and sliding motions with palms of hands. Secure a piece of nonslip material such as Dycem to the palms of hands or wear push gloves to help grip and pull the material into place.

4. While still sitting with pants at midcalf height, insert dressing stick in front belt loop. Dressing stick is gripped by slipping its loop over the wrist. Pull on dressing stick while extending trunk, returning to supine position. Return to sitting position and repeat this procedure, pulling on dressing sticks and maneuvering trousers up to thigh level (Renda & Lape, 2018). If balance and flexibility are adequate, an alternative is for client to remain seated and lean on left elbow and pull trousers over right buttock, then reverse process for other side. Another alternative is for the client to remain in supine position and roll to one side; throw opposite arm behind back; hook thumb in waistband, belt loop, or pocket; and pull trousers up over

hips. These maneuvers can be repeated as needed to pull trousers over buttocks (Buchwald, 1952).

5. Using palms of hands in pushing and smoothing motions, straighten trouser legs.
6. In supine position, fasten trouser placket by hooking thumb in loop on zipper pull, patting Velcro closed, or using hand splints and buttonhooks if buttons are present (Buchwald, 1952; Renda & Lape, 2018).

Donning: Variation. For step 2, substitute the following: Sit up and lift one knee at a time by hooking right hand under right knee to pull leg into flexion, then cross foot over opposite leg above knee. This position frees up foot to place trousers more easily and requires less trunk balance. Continue with all other steps.

Removing

1. Lying supine in bed with bed rails up, unfasten belt and placket fasteners.
2. Placing thumbs in belt loops, waistband, or pockets, work trousers past hips by stabilizing arms in shoulder extension and scooting body toward head of bed.
3. Use arms as described in step 2, and roll from side to side to slide trousers past buttocks.
4. Coming to sitting position and alternately pulling legs into flexion, push trousers down legs (Renda & Lape, 2018).
5. Trousers can be pushed off over feet with dressing stick or by hooking thumbs in waistband.

Cardigans or Pullover Garments. Cardigan and pullover garments include blouses, vests, sweaters, skirts, and front-opening dresses (Buchwald, 1952; Renda & Lape, 2018). Upper extremity dressing is often performed in the wheelchair for greater trunk stability.

Donning

1. Position garment across thighs with back facing up and neck toward knees.
2. Place both arms under back of garment and in armholes.
3. Push sleeves up onto arms past elbows.
4. Using a wrist extension grip, hook thumbs under garment back and gather material up from neck to hem.
5. To pass garment over head, adduct and externally rotate shoulders and flex elbows while flexing head forward.
6. When garment is over head, relax shoulders and wrists and remove hands from back of garment. Most material will be gathered up at neck, across shoulders, and under arms.
7. To work garment down over body, shrug shoulders, lean forward, and use elbow flexion and wrist extension. Use wheelchair arms for balance if necessary. Additional maneuvers to accomplish task are to hook wrists into sleeves and pull material free from underarms or lean forward, reach back, and slide hand against material to aid in pulling garment down.
8. Garment can be buttoned from bottom to top with aid of buttonhook and wrist-hand orthosis if hand function is inadequate.

Removing

1. Sit in wheelchair and wear wrist-hand orthosis. Unfasten buttons (if any) while wearing splints and using buttonhook. Remove splints for remaining steps.

2. For pullover garments, hook thumb in back of neckline, extend wrist, and pull garment over head while turning head toward side of raised arm. Maintain balance by resting against opposite wheelchair armrest or pushing on thigh with extended arm.
3. For cardigan garments, hook thumb in opposite armhole and push sleeve down arm. Elevation and depression of shoulders with trunk rotation can be used to have garment slip down arms as far as possible.
4. Hold one cuff with opposite thumb while elbow is flexed to pull arm out of sleeve.

Brassiere (Back Opening)

Donning

1. Place brassiere across lap with straps toward knees and inside facing up.
2. Using a right-to-left procedure, hold end of brassiere closest to right side with hand or reacher and pass brassiere around back from right to left. Lean against brassiere at back to hold it in place while hooking thumb of left hand in a loop that has been attached near brassiere fastener. Hook right thumb in a similar loop on right side, and fasten brassiere in front at waist level.
3. Hook right thumb in edge of brassiere. Using wrist extension, elbow flexion, shoulder adduction, and internal rotation, rotate brassiere around body so that front of brassiere is in front of body.
4. While leaning on one forearm, hook opposite thumb in front end of strap and pull strap over shoulder, then repeat procedure on other side (Buchwald, 1952; Renda & Lape, 2018).

Removing

1. Hook thumb under opposite brassiere strap and push down over shoulder while elevating shoulder.
2. Pull arm out of strap and repeat procedure for other arm.
3. Push brassiere down to waist level and turn around as described previously to bring fasteners to front.
4. Unfasten brassiere.

Alternatives to a back-opening bra are (1) a front-opening bra with loops to use a wrist extension grip, or (2) a fully elastic bra, one size larger, with no fasteners. The larger bra can be donned like a pullover sweater.

Socks

Donning

1. Sit in wheelchair (or on bed if balance is adequate) in cross-legged position with one ankle crossed over opposite knee.
2. Pull sock over foot with wrist extension grip and patting movements with palm of hand (Buchwald, 1952; Renda & Lape, 2018).
3. If trunk balance is inadequate and cross-legged position cannot be maintained, prop foot on stool, chair, open drawer, or edge of bed, keeping opposite arm around upright of wheelchair for balance.
4. Fastening wheelchair safety belt or leaning against wheelchair armrest on one side are alternatives to maintain balance.

5. Use sock aids (see Fig. 13.5) or soft sock aid to assist in putting on socks while in this position. Apply sock-to-sock aid by using thumbs and palms of hands to smooth sock out on cone.
6. Place cord loops of sock cone around wrist or thumb and throw cone beyond foot.
7. Maneuver sock aid over toes by pulling cords using elbow flexion. Insert foot as far as possible into cone.
8. To remove aid from sock after foot has been inserted, move heel forward off wheelchair footrest. Use wrist extension of one hand behind knee, and with other hand continue pulling cords of cone until it is removed and sock is in place on foot. Use palms to smooth sock with patting and stroking motion (Renda & Lape, 2018).
9. Two loops can also be sewn on either side of sock top so that thumbs can be hooked into loops and socks pulled on.
   Removing
1. While sitting in wheelchair or lying in bed, use dressing stick or long-handled shoehorn to push sock down over heel. Cross legs if possible.
2. Use dressing stick with cup-hook on end to pull sock off toes (California Department of Aging, 2020).
   Shoes
   Donning
1. For putting on shoes, use same position as for donning socks.
2. Use extended-handle dressing aid and insert it into tongue of shoe; then place shoe opening over toes. Remove dressing aid from shoe and dangle shoe on toes.
3. Using palm of hand on sole of shoe, pull shoe toward heel of foot. Use one hand to stabilize leg while pushing other against sole of shoe to work shoe onto foot. Use thenar eminence and sides of hand for pushing motion.
4. With feet flat on floor or on wheelchair footrest and knees flexed 90 degrees, place long-handled shoehorn in heel of shoe and press down on flexed knee.
5. Fasten shoes (Renda & Lape, 2018).
   Removing
1. Sitting in wheelchair as described for donning socks, unfasten shoes.
2. Use shoehorn or dressing stick to push on heel counter of shoe, dislodging it from heel; then shoe will drop or can be pushed to floor with dressing stick.

Hygiene and Grooming. General suggestions to facilitate hygiene and grooming are the following (Koketsu, 2018):
1. Use a shower or bathtub seat and transfer board for transfers.
2. Extend reach by using long handled bath sponges with loop handle or built-up handle.
3. Eliminate need to grasp washcloth by using terry cloth or sponge bath mitts.
4. Hold comb and toothbrush with a universal cuff (Koketsu, 2018).
5. Use the position-adjustable hairdryer described previously (Feldmeier & Poole, 1987). Use a universal cuff to hold brush or comb for hair styling while using this mounted hairdryer.
6. Use a clip holder for electric razor.
7. Use a suppository inserter for bowel program.
8. Use skin inspection mirror with long stem and looped handle for independent skin inspection (Fig. 13.26). The degree of weakness must be considered for each client when selecting devices and when selecting and adapting methods.
9. Adapted leg-bag clamps to empty catheter leg bags are also available for clients with limited hand function. Velcro straps may substitute for elastic leg-bag straps. Use a clothespin with a bungee cord to help manage clothing during self-catheterization.

Communication and General Environment. Suggestions for facilitating communication include the following:
1. Turn pages with an electric page turner, mouthstick, or head wand if hand and arm function is inadequate (Fig. 13.27).
2. For keyboarding, writing, and painting, insert a pen, pencil, typing stick, or paintbrush in a universal cuff that has been positioned with the opening on the ulnar side of the palm.
3. Enter telephone numbers with the universal cuff and a pencil positioned with the eraser down. The phone may need to be stabilized on lap or on table with rubber grip case and positioned for listening on speakerphone or adapted to use holder to place to ear (Fig. 13.28). Set up and use programmed number options on the phone. For

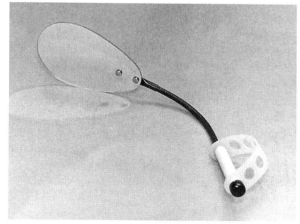

Fig. 13.26 Skin inspection mirror.

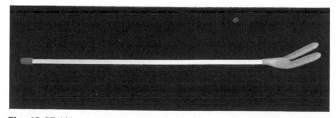

Fig. 13.27 Wand mouthstick. (Courtesy Sammons, a BISSELL Co.)

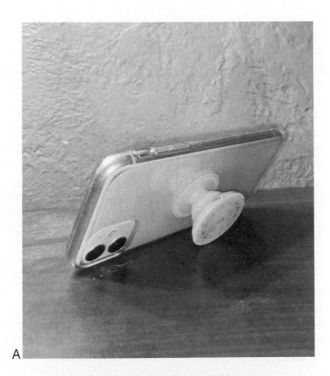

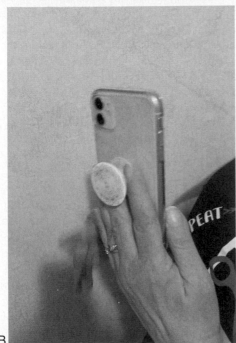

Fig. 13.28 Smartphone holder popsocket. (A) Kickstand; (B) phone holder.

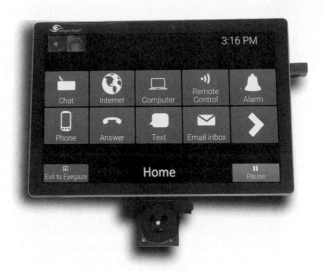

Fig. 13.29 Eye gaze technology. (Courtesy Eye Gaze Edge.)

clients with no arm function, a voice-to-text or voice recognition programs can be used to initiate a call, text, surf the internet, or use social media.

4. Use personal computers with voice activation software, head pointers, or adaptive switches. With higher level spinal cord injuries, eye gaze technology is available wherein a person may use a tablet programmed to complete commands based on the direction of gaze (Fig. 13.29).

5. Built-up pencils and pens or special pencil holders are necessary for clients with hand weakness. The Wanchik writer is an effective adaptive writing device (see Fig. 13.12). The slip-on writing aid holds the pen at an adjustable angle in the first web space and with a heat gun can be custom-fit to contour to the hand.

6. Sophisticated augmented communication devices operated by mouth, pneumatic controls, and head control are available for clients with no upper extremity function (Nuance-Dragon, 2010) (see Chapter 14).

7. Audiocassettes may still be used by some clients. Kelly (1983) described two mouthsticks and a cassette tape holder that allow persons with C3, C4, or C5 quadriplegia to operate a tape recorder or radio independently. The first mouthstick, a rod about 20 inches (50 cm) long with a friction tip, is used to depress the operating buttons and adjust the radio's volume and selector dials. The second mouthstick is a metal rod that separates into two prongs at its end. These prongs are 4 inches (10 cm) apart, and the mouthstick is used to insert cassettes from the cassette holder into the tape recorder and to remove cassettes from the recorder. The vertical cassette tape stand is made of metal, tilted backward at a 70-degree angle, and designed to hold eight tapes at its eight levels. Kelly (1983) offers specifications on construction of these devices.

8. For managing knobs or controls that require a strong lateral pinch, the person can use a potato masher to interlace around the knob and use the entire hand to twist the knob.

9. Place a terry cloth wristband around a glass or mug to protect the hand from excessive hot or cold and to provide friction to require less force to hold.

Assistive Technology. For clients with severe physical impairments, options in **assistive technology** can help improve independence with ADL. According to the Human Activity Assistance Technology (HAAT) model, a person choosing the best system for a client must consider the person using the technology, the activity the technology will be used to perform, and the environment in which the technology will be used, to set up the best system for the client (Purex complete 3-in-1 laundry sheets, 2019). The client's tolerance of technology and adaptive devices and his or her ability to learn complex commands should be considered. A complete discussion of assistive technology is provided in Chapter 14. Technology rapidly introduces new products to the general public. The OT and OTA should always stay up to date with the newest opportunities to enhance a client's independence. Subscribing to product catalogs such as the *Disabled Dealer* (www.disableddealer.com) or attending yearly expositions such as the Abilities Expo (www.abilitiesexpo.com), the American Occupational Therapy Association (AOTA) national conference, or state occupational therapy association conferences are some ways to remain knowledgeable about current products. The *Computer Resource for People with Disabilities*, a book presented by the Alliance for Technology Access, provides product information on making a personal computer more accessible.

All individuals in modern society rely on EADL, products that use electricity to perform an activity. Some basic examples of EADL are radios and lamps. Some EADL require mobility and physical abilities to control (Planet Mobility, 2004). By setting up a central unit, the therapist enables the client to control a number of appliances around the home from a centralized area.

Quartet Technology's Simplicity line is an example of a unit that can control a vast number of EADL in the environment (Purex complete 3-in-1 laundry sheets, 2019). This device can perform tasks such as operating a personal computer, activating the controls normally performed by a remote control on a television or stereo, dialing and receiving options on a phone, controlling the lighting and temperature in the room or house, and adjusting the exact position of a hospital bed. The therapist can work with the client to find the easiest way to operate the system. This product responds to voice, sip and puff, switches, and radio remote.

A control device can be linked to all adaptive devices in the house, thus allowing a client to independently perform detailed tasks such as turning a page in a book, dialing or texting a friend on the phone, opening a door, listening to favorite music, and checking email (Planet Mobility, 2004).

A unique product for increasing independence for clients with significant physical impairments is the Assistant Robot Manipulator (ARM) (Exact Dynamics BV, 2004). This robotic arm is attached to the power wheelchair and can be controlled with a joystick or switch to perform a wide variety of ADL. It can be used to assist with self-feeding, brushing teeth, picking up objects from the floor or overhead, and opening the door to a microwave or toaster. If a client is cognitively capable of performing tasks but cannot physically participate, the ARM helps bridge this gap. With precise training, the client can learn to perform enough tasks to rely less on caregiver assistance (Exact Dynamics BV, 2004).

An important factor to consider when recommending assistive technology is cost. Many new products are not covered by insurance. The therapist should consider whether the cost of the product can be justified if it will cut back on personal assistant or home modification needs. The OT and OTA should be realistic about the client's training abilities. If the client will be unable to use the full capabilities of the product, a more basic option should be considered.

Mobility and Transfers. Chapter 15 discusses principles of wheelchair transfer techniques for the quadriplegic client. Mobility depends on degree of weakness. Power wheelchairs operated by hand, chin, or pneumatic (sip and puff) controls have greatly increased the mobility of clients with severe upper and lower extremity weakness. Vans and public buses fitted with wheelchair lifts and stabilizing devices have provided such clients with transport to pursue community, vocational, educational, and avocational activities with an assistant. In addition, adaptations for hand controls have allowed many clients with at least C6-level function to drive independently.

Home Management Activities. Many wheelchair-dependent clients with upper extremity weakness are dependent or partly dependent for homemaking activities. Clients with muscle function of C6 or better may be independent for light homemaking with appropriate devices, adaptations, and safety awareness. Many of the suggestions for wheelchair maneuverability and environmental adaptation outlined for the paraplegic client apply to these clients as well. In addition, the client with upper extremity weakness needs to use lightweight equipment and special devices. The *Mealtime Manual for People with Disability and the Aging* contains many excellent and specific suggestions that apply to the cook with weak upper extremities (Klinger et al., 1997).

SEXUAL ACTIVITY

Sexual activity and sexual intercourse are ADL that often go underaddressed in occupational therapy practice. As a sensitive and sometimes uncomfortable subject to address, the OT and OTA must understand appropriate guidelines for practice. One model to guide practice is the PLISSIT model (Hattjar, 2017). This involves four key areas including permission, limited information, specific suggestions, and intensive therapy (Hattjar, 2017). It is within the OT's scope of practice to address sexual intimacy with clients, and thus it is important for practitioners to understand their own comfort levels and knowledge when addressing this area (Hattjar, 2017). Once the OT and OTA have addressed their strengths and limitations in this area and have gotten to know the client, they may then offer information regarding occupational therapy intervention. This may include a private sexuality questionnaire, one-on-one conversation at the comfort of the client, or noninvasive open-ended questions. Once the client provides permission to therapists to address these areas, the OT and OTA may build trust and offer specific suggestions based upon client conditions as aforementioned (Hattjar, 2017). This may include positioning techniques for clients with decreased strength and ROM, offering alternative means of intimacy, collaboration with spouse or significant other as permitted, or techniques for self-pleasure. The OT and OTA should always consider sexual activity when treating and assessing their adult clients, even if the area is not outwardly addressed or the topic of focus.

PARENTING FOR INDIVIDUALS WITH A DISABILITY

The need for OTs and OTAs to address the ADL of parenting or caregiving is growing. An increasing number of people with disabilities are choosing to raise their own families. Some clients may already be parents at the time of injury or illness leading to a disability. Familiarizing such clients with helpful child care products available for the general public (universal design) may be especially advantageous for a parent with a disability (Pardessus, Puisieux, & Di Pompeo et al., 2002). The practitioner may need to assist the client in customizing products to meet more specific needs.

Funding for services and products may be available in the form of direct government financial assistance. Federal agencies provide funds to assist parents with disabilities. Rehabilitative engineering departments at local hospitals often offer assistance in fabrication of custom products. The Rehabilitation Institute of Chicago and the National Rehabilitation Hospital in Washington, DC, have renowned rehabilitation engineering departments and are worth consulting. Volunteers for Medical Engineering is a philanthropic organization that helps create custom products.

Through the Looking Glass is a research, training, and service center devoted to families in which a parent or child has a disability (Parent Empowerment Network, 2010). This center, located in Berkeley, California, publishes a number of resources to help parents with disabilities perform child care tasks independently. These resources discuss caregiving techniques, adaptive aids, and current research. The website, www.lookingglass.org, shows inspiring photos, information on obtaining publications, and updates on nationwide conferences, workshops, and support groups. Parents can also be referred to the Parent Empowerment Network to connect with other parents and find commercially available child care products and tips (Pardessus et al., 2002).

Adapting the environment and introducing the client to a variety of parenting assistive devices can increase the client's independence with child care activities. A client may have a physical disability too severe to allow him or her to care for the child safely. **Nurturing assistance** involves a hired aide who provides physical assistance to parents with young children (Parents with disabilities, 2010). The parent directs the nurturing assistant through the tasks. This process facilitates parental involvement to fulfill the emotional need for the parent and can help strengthen the parent-child bond (Parents with disabilities, 2010).

The following discussion lists ready-made or custom-made products to help assist with child care activities for parents with a variety of disabilities. A full evaluation of the parent's abilities to physically and cognitively perform all

child care tasks is necessary to determine the safety of the parent and child.

The Babee Tenda Safety Convertible Crib is a crib with a toddler gate that allows a parent to retrieve the baby from the crib at wheelchair level. It reduces risks that may occur when parents with upper extremity weakness or pain attempt to reach over a standard, drop-down crib.

Velcro disposable diapers allow the parent to position and reposition closures without ripping the diaper. This product helps those with dexterity impairments change diapers with ease.

Childproofing the home can be a difficult feat when the parent has impairments in strength or dexterity. Standard safety locks and gates block access to the parent with a disability, as well as the child. Tot-loks is a safety lock for cabinets that is released when a strong magnet is held up to the exact location of the latch.

Holding the child when the parent uses a wheelchair poses a safety problem. The Baby B'Air Airline Safety Harness was created for babies seated in the parent's lap during an airplane flight. It is threaded through the airline safety belt; however, it can also be used to secure the baby onto a parent in a wheelchair by threading it through the wheelchair safety belt.

A variety of baby holders that may be helpful for a parent who requires use of an assistive device when ambulating are commercially available. Some examples include the Baby Bjorn, the Over the Shoulder Baby Holder, and the Sling Rider. Depending on the temperament of the baby and the physical needs of the parent, one product might work better than others.

Positioning for breast-feeding may be problematic for clients with upper extremity weakness. "Meals on Wheels" was created specifically for a mother with cerebral palsy who was struggling with positioning her baby for breastfeeding while seated in her wheelchair. A rehabilitation engineer modified a wheelchair lap tray that was secured on the armrests of the chair to hold a baby positioning device on top.

Helping the parent with a disability maintain independence for child care tasks is a dynamic activity. The OT and OTA must consider the ever-changing needs of a growing child and potential changes in the physical or cognitive status of the parent. Continual reassessment of child care tasks is necessary to ensure the safest and easiest solutions.

TRAVELING WITH A DISABILITY

The prospect of traveling can bring up numerous issues and concerns for individuals with disabilities. The practitioner should encourage clients to plan ahead for trips and provide them with the resources needed to help with planning. Travelers with a disability need to be educated about their rights and the resources available to them.

During airline travel, clients may encounter a variety of obstacles. The Air Carrier Access Act, passed in 1986, ensures that people with disabilities receive consistent and nondiscriminatory treatment when traveling by air (Pendleton and Schultz-Krohn, 2013). The client is required to provide the airline with at least a 48-hour notice to allow accommodations to be made. Most wheelchairs do not fit in the aisle of the plane, so the client needs to transfer to an aisle chair to get to a seat (see www.casa.gov.au/airsafe/disable/wheeltips.htm) (Traveling With a Disability, 2004). If the flight is long, the client should request that the aisle chair be available during the flight to allow access to the bathroom.

All power wheelchairs must be stowed as checked luggage. Removing seat cushions or any other loose parts that could get lost during the flight is helpful. Attaching instructions on how to assemble or disassemble the chair for storage can help the flight crew properly handle the chair. For international travel, including illustrations or pictures on the instruction sheet, may be wise (The Humane Society of the United States, 2019). If the client is traveling with a manual wheelchair that can be folded, he or she can request that it be stowed in the onboard coat closet. Traveling with basic wheelchair maintenance tools is helpful if problems occur during the flight. Clients should be advised to research ahead to have a list of wheelchair vendors at the destination in case repairs are needed.

Transferring while on the airplane can be difficult. The person with a disability should be proactive in finding out about the plane's specifications while making reservations. If requested, the airline may provide a free upgrade to first class to clients traveling with wheelchairs to allow for a safer and more efficient boarding process. Some of the larger and newer aircraft have an accessible restroom with outward swinging doors and handrails; they are large enough to fit the aisle chair inside. Alternatively, it may be possible to swing and clip the doors to increase the space. If no accessible restrooms are available, there may be an area of the plane with a privacy curtain to allow a companion to assist with toileting activities or changing clothing.

It is important to know about the environment where the disabled person will be staying. If booking a hotel room, the disabled person should request an accessible room and specify particular needs. The person should ensure that the room and restroom have ample space for a wheelchair, if necessary, and should learn what bathroom equipment such as a shower chair or commode can be requested. If the person calling is not specific about needs, the hotel representative may claim that a room is accessible simply because grab bars are installed in the restroom.

The travel industry has recently become involved in making traveling easier for individuals with varying degrees of disabilities. Accessible bus tours, trains, and cruises are available (Pendleton & Schultz-Krohn, 2013). One can rent an accessible van or arrange for basic hand controls to be installed into a rental car if needed. Providing clients with information on all the available resources may encourage them to travel.

DISCHARGE PLANNING

As a person nears the end of the occupational therapy stay, the OT and OTA will begin to prepare for discharge from services. Discharge or discontinuation of services occurs when a client has reached his or her maximum potential in performance of ADL and IADL. Discharge planning is essential to ensure that the client is able to function at his or her highest practical level of performance and promote quality of life. This planning and preparation process may include **home assessment**, **caregiver training**, reassessment of skill performance, referral to community resources, equipment training and recommendations, and development of home programs.

HOME ASSESSMENT

As a client nears the end of the in-patient stay, a home assessment is often performed to more readily prepare the client for return to the community and optimize independence in his or her living environment. Home evaluations help bridge the gap between inpatient care and life at home after discharge. Ideally, physical therapists (PTs) and OTs should perform the evaluation together on a visit to the client's home. This allows for an interdisciplinary approach to optimize performance in all aspects of reintegration into the home. The client, family members, roommates, or caregivers are typically present. Time, budget, necessity, willingness, and topographic limitations may not allow two clinicians to go to the client's home or may inhibit ability to perform the assessment in person. Therefore one discipline may perform the evaluation, or a virtual home assessment may be completed. A virtual home assessment may be performed if a client lives a great distance from the treating facility, is cognitively intact, or functions at a higher level requiring minimal adaptations within the facility. This assessment may include family or caregiver interviews, photographs of the client's home, measurements, and existing equipment or adaptations. The client, family member, friend, roommate, or caregiver may provide this information. If unable to gather dimensions and photos, a detailed interview may be conducted with the client.

The evaluator should begin by explaining the process and procedures to the client and family, friend, or caregiver. After the client has demonstrated understanding, the therapist should then gather information about expectations for discharge home, including supports available, financial aid, willingness for adaptations, and client routines to focus the home assessment based on individual client needs. For instance, if a client plans to go home with caregiver or family assistance for cooking and cleaning, the therapist will not focus on areas such as kitchen safety adaptations and use of appliances. After gathering this information, the therapist should assess client performance in completing necessary ADL and IADL tasks within the natural environment. Sufficient time to allow the client to demonstrate these necessary skills should be scheduled for the home visit. During the evaluation the client should demonstrate the use of any ambulation aids and assistive devices. The clinician should bring a tape measure to measure the width of doorways, height of stairs, height of the bed, and other key dimensions.

It may be helpful to sketch the size and arrangement of rooms for later reference and to attach the sketch to the home visit checklist (see Fig. 13.3). For more information on a variety of checklists, see the Letts et al. research (Letts, Law & Rigby et al., 1994).

During the performance evaluation the clinician should observe safety factors, ease of mobility and performance, and limitations imposed by the environment. If relevant, the client's ability to use the entrance to the home and transfer to and from an automobile should be included in the home evaluation. If the client requires assistance for transfers and other activities, the caregiver should be instructed in appropriate methods. The client may also be instructed in methods to improve maneuverability and simplify performance of tasks in a small space.

Before mentioning possible home modifications, educating the client on legal rights of a tenant or renter with a disability is important (Willard, Spackman, & Neistadt et al., 1998). Federal and state fair housing laws require the property owner to make reasonable modifications to the housing unit at their expense. Examples of these modifications include the installation of an access ramp and grab bars and widening the interior doorways. The person with a disability can also request a handicapped parking space be placed in a convenient location. If the client is planning to move to a new rental unit, the law grants disabled applicants the right to be judged on the same basis as all other tenants. Additionally, even if the building does not allow pets, the law requires a property owner to allow service animals for residents with a disability (Willard, Spackman, & Neistadt, 1998). Basic education on these rights can help ease the transition from hospital to home.

At the end of the home evaluation the clinician can list problems and recommend modifications, additional safety equipment, and assistive devices. The most commonly needed changes are the following (Trombly, 1983):
- Addition of a ramp or railings at the entrance to the home
- Addition of safety grab bars around the toilet and bathtub (Caution: It is not safe to rely on a towel rack for balance.)

- Removal of scatter rugs, door sills, and extra furniture
- Securing of electrical cords away from walkways
- Rearrangement of kitchen storage and of furniture to accommodate a wheelchair
- Lowering of the clothes rod in the closet
- Additional transfer equipment and fall reduction items such as tub bench, shower chair, or bed rail

For clients with balance impairments, an area for small children's toys, pet care items, or other low-lying furniture or objects must be designated so that walkways are free of obstacles. A bell on the collar of a cat or small dog is also recommended. Fold-away hinges increase the doorway capacity by 2 inches and allow wheelchair access to the room without reframing the opening.

The client may have trouble accessing and maneuvering in the bathroom with a wheelchair or walker. The clinician may recommend a **bedside commode** until a bathroom can be made accessible or modified to allow for independence with toileting (Fig. 13.30). Shower seats can be used in the tub (if the client can transfer safely over the edge of the tub) and can also be used in a shower. A tub transfer bench (see Fig. 13.11) is recommended for individuals who cannot step over the edge of the tub safely or independently. A handheld shower increases access to the water and also eliminates the need for standing or risky turns while bathing. Consider installing a clamp to secure the shower head in a location within reach when seated. Clamps can secure the shower head to the shower chair arm or the grab bar for convenience. A removable rubber threshold ramp allows a wheelchair to glide over high thresholds for exterior doors or sliding glass doorways (Lift and Accessibility Solutions, 2013).

For clients with severe physical impairments or who have progressive diseases, major home modifications may be necessary. For example, an automatic door opener allows the client to open locked interior or exterior doors from a remote

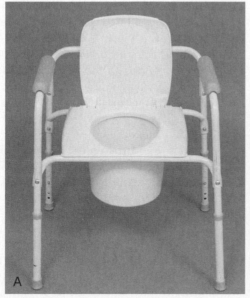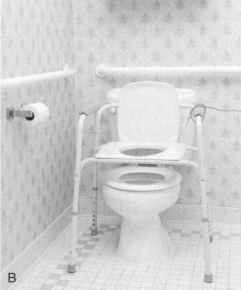

Fig. 13.30 All-purpose commode. (A) Bedside; (B) over toilet. (From Kostelnick C. *Mosby's Textbook for Long-Term Care Nursing Assistants.* 8th ed. St. Louis, MO: Elsevier; 2020.)

location. Electronic stair lifts allow the client to ascend or descend stairs while seated, thus providing access to another floor of the home. A platform lift may be more economical and aesthetic than a large ramp extending into the street for front entry. Overhead lift tracking systems lift and transfer a person from a wheelchair to various locations in the home while seated in a sling. If a client spends most of the time in a wheelchair, the walls and door jambs will most likely be scuffed and scratched. Installation of scratch-resistant plastic surfaces on the walls and door jambs can prevent such structural and cosmetic damage (Lift and Accessibility Solutions, 2013).

Some additional safety measures should be considered. It is helpful to notify the local fire and police department that an individual with a disability resides in the home. An emergency exit plan should be established with two accessible exits, if possible. The evaluator should check whether smoke detectors work properly and that a fire extinguisher is within reach. The client should keep important phone numbers on display near the phone or on the phone itself. The list should include family, neighbors, doctors, police and fire department, and the poison control center (Cason, 2012). The therapist may consider recommending a lifeline or life alert programmed with an emergency contact and will dial 911 in emergencies.

When the home evaluation is completed, the evaluator should write a report summarizing the information on the form and describing the client's performance in the home. The report should conclude with a summary of the environmental barriers and the client's functional limitations. Recommendations should include equipment or alterations, with specifics in terms of size, building specifications, costs, sources, and specialized training required. Recommendations may also include further functional goals to improve independence at home.

Home evaluation recommendations must be reviewed carefully with the client and family. The OT and OTA must use tact and diplomacy to present options and involve the client in a frank discussion of the recommendations. The client is free to refuse or consider alternative possibilities, and the OT and OTA should facilitate client choice. Cultural values, aesthetic preferences, and family finances may be limiting factors in implementing needed changes. A social worker may help with handling funding for equipment and modifications, and the client should be made aware of this service when cost is discussed (Trombly, 1983).

The evaluator should include recommendations regarding the feasibility of the client remaining in or managing the home alone or being discharged to the home environment, as applicable. Other considerations include the finances available for assisted care, special equipment, and home modifications. Additional resources include the client's insurance and community-based or philanthropic organizations. The client's case manager or social worker can help determine eligibility for resources. For example, a client with the resources, who uses a wheelchair, may be able to make major modifications in the home such as installing an elevator or lift, lowering kitchen counters, widening doorways, and replacing deep pile carpeting to accommodate a wheelchair lifestyle. Less costly modifications, which can be made for those with fewer financial resources, include things such as removing scatter rugs and door sills, installing a plywood ramp at the entrance, or attaching a handheld shower head to the bathtub faucet.

If any question regarding the client's ability to return home safely and independently exists, the home evaluation summary should include the functional skills the client needs to return home. The OT must remember to focus on preservation of autonomy and safety. Clients who do not receive home evaluations as a treatment intervention are more likely to lose autonomy after discharge than similar clients who received the evaluations (Nygard et al., 2004).

After the home assessment is complete, the treating clinician may additionally supply clients with home exercise routines or schedule of activities to continue with certain technique to reduce the risk for decline after discharge from the treatment facility. If the client will be returning home with family or caregivers, these individuals should participate in treatment sessions for education in safe caregiving strategies as well as techniques to reduce caregiver burden and prevent injury. Collaboration with social services or a case manager should be completed to guarantee that appropriate services and modifications are prepared for the client prior to return home.

INNOVATIONS FOR ADL AND IADL

Telehealth is an emerging area of practice for OTs and OTAs, which allows therapists to provide services to clients who are in different physical locations than themselves. The definition of telehealth from AOTA is "the application of evaluative, consultative, preventative, and therapeutic services delivered through telecommunication and information technologies" (American Occupational Therapy Association, 2013). Occupational therapy practitioners are using telehealth to develop skills, incorporate assistive technology and adaptive techniques, modify work/home/school environments, and create health-promoting habits and routines (Cason, 2014). Potential benefits of telehealth include increased accessibility to clients who live in remote areas or underserved communities and increased access to practitioners and specialists who may not be available otherwise. Other benefits include clients receiving care without prolonged delays and the opportunity for practitioners to practice their skills without being isolated (Christiansen & Baum, 1991).

There is potential for telehealth to be applied to many populations and areas of occupational therapy, including children and youth, productive aging, health and wellness, mental health, rehabilitation, disability and participation, and work and industry (Cason, 2014). A study conducted by Renda and Lape (2018) sought to determine the feasibility and effectiveness of using a smartphone, tablet, or computer in providing occupational therapy services to increase home safety and to measure client perception of performance of daily activities (Quartet Technology, 2019). The findings demonstrated increased home safety and an improved perception of performance and satisfaction in daily activities. These findings support the conclusions made from similar studies suggesting that telehealth can be an effective method in providing services to clients (AOTA, 2013). Overall, telehealth has the potential to improve access to high-quality care and reduce barriers such as travel, social stigma, socioeconomic issues, and cultural issues (Cason, 2014; AOTA, 2013).

Service Animals

Service animals can help to enhance independence in occupational performance for individuals with physical disabilities. Service animals can do much more than guide individuals with vision impairments. They can reduce the reliance on other people to perform tasks disabled individuals have difficulty performing on their own. Service animals are also known to help increase community participation, social contact, personal skill development, adjustment to challenges, and sense of responsibility (Canine Companion Service, 2020). Service animals often evoke feelings of "always having someone to watch over" and being "like an able-bodied person again" (https://www.cci.org/assistance-dogs/our-dogs/service-dogs).

Some OTs work with these animals during rehabilitation treatment sessions. These animals can provide the added mental, physical, and emotional support when clients are trying to learn or relearn living skills. These sessions can also screen clients for the need and appropriateness of a skilled companion or service animal of their own. Rehabilitation professionals can become advocates for their clients in obtaining, training, and adjusting to living with a service dog (https://www.cci.org/assistance-dogs/our-dogs/service-dogs).

Numerous organizations throughout the United States train animals to become assistance dogs. Canine Companions for Independence pairs the participant and dog together and establishes a training team (https://www.cci.org/assistance-dogs/our-dogs/service-dogs). The team consists of the student, the service dog or skilled companion, and a facilitator to teach the handling process and help extend the abilities of the dog. The goal is to help develop the maximum amount of independence that a team can achieve with an assistance dog. This organization also trains animals to work directly with the health care professional as facility-based service animals and prepares dogs to work with individuals with hearing impairments (https://www.cci.org/assistance-dogs/our-dogs/service-dogs).

Helping hands—monkey helpers (http://www.helpinghandsmonkeys.org) is an organization that trains Capuchin monkeys to assist individuals with quadriplegia with daily activities (https://www.cci.org/assistance-dogs/our-dogs/service-dogs). Their intelligence and fine motor dexterity allow these monkeys to perform a wide variety of tasks such as assisting with feeding or retrieving and placing a tissue on the nose after a sneeze. These monkeys have small hands, but they can be trained to don splints to allow them to expand their reach and allow them to open a large jar lid or respiration equipment valve. The affectionate and responsive nature of these animals allows them to become companions and improve mental and emotional quality of life (Unknown, 2010b).

During the evaluation of occupational performance, the OT can screen clients for the appropriateness of introducing an assistance dog or skilled companion. Providing clients with knowledge and resources about service animals early after onset of a disability can inspire them to readjust their expectations for independence.

SUMMARY

ADL and IADL are tasks of self-maintenance, mobility, communication, home management, and community living skills that allow a client to function independently and assume important occupational roles.

ADL and IADL are major life activities that consume significant time even for persons without disabilities. OTs and OTAs routinely evaluate performance in ADL to assess a client's level of functional independence. The OTA may establish service competency and special expertise in this practice area. Evaluation is performed through the interview and observation of performance. Evaluation results and ongoing progress are recorded on one of many available ADL checklists, and the content is summarized for the permanent medical record.

Treatment is directed toward training in independent living skills using methods in such activity areas as eating, dressing, mobility, home management, communication, and community living. The OTA practicing in this area should be familiar with the special equipment and methods for performing ADL needed by the client with specific functional problems.

REVIEW QUESTIONS

1. Define and differentiate between ADL and IADL. List three subcategories in both ADL and IADL.
2. Describe the role of occupational therapy in restoring ADL and IADL independence.
3. List at least three activities for each of the following subcategories of skills: self-care, mobility, communication, home management, and community living.
4. List three factors that the OT or OTA must consider before commencing ADL performance evaluation and training. Describe how each could limit or affect the client's ADL performance.
5. Discuss the concept of maximal independence, as defined in the text.
6. List the general steps in the procedure for ADL evaluation.
7. What is the purpose of the home evaluation?
8. List the steps in the home evaluation.
9. Who should be involved in a comprehensive home evaluation?
10. What other areas or factors are assessed in a home evaluation?
11. How does the OT or OTA record and report results of the home evaluation and make the necessary recommendations?

12. How does the OT or OTA, with the client, select ADL and IADL training objectives after an evaluation?
13. Describe three approaches to teaching ADL skills to a client with perception or memory deficits.
14. List the important factors to include in an ADL progress report.
15. Give an example of a health and safety management issue.
16. Explain how an OTA would establish service competency and maximal independence in providing ADL services within the legal guidelines of a state or other local jurisdiction.

EXERCISES

1. Demonstrate the use of at least three assistive devices mentioned in the text.
2. Teach a person to don a shirt, using one hand.
3. Teach another person how to don and remove trousers, as if the person had hemiplegia.
4. Teach a person how to make a sandwich with only one hand.
5. Teach a different person how to don and remove trousers, as if the person's legs were paralyzed.

REFERENCES

Active Forever. Bottom Buddy Toilet Aid. (2017). <https://www.active-forever.com/bottom-buddy-toilet-tissue-aid-model-92008>.

American Occupational Therapy Association. (2013). Telehealth [Position paper]. *The American Journal of Occupational Therapy, 67,* S69–S90. Available from: https://doi.org/10.5014/ajot.2013.67S69.

American Occupational Therapy Association. (2014). The occupational therapy practice framework: domain and process (3rd ed.). *The American Journal of Occupational Therapy, 68,* S1–S51.

Australian Government. (2004). Travel tips for wheelchair users. <http://www.casa.gov.au/airsafe/disable/wheeltips.htm>.

Branick, L. (2004). Integrating principles of energy conservation during everyday activities. *Caring, 22*(1), 30–31.

Buchwald, E. (1952). *Physical rehabilitation for daily living.* New York, NY: McGraw Hill.

California Department of Aging. (2020). Home safety checklist. California Department of Aging, Senior Housing Information and Support Center.

Canine companion service. (2020). <https://www.cci.org/assistance-dogs/our-dogs/service-dogs>.

Cason, J. (2012). Telehealth opportunities in occupational therapy through the affordable care act. *The American Journal of Occupational Therapy, 66*(2), 131–136.

Cason, J. (2014). Telehealth: a rapidly developing service delivery model for occupational therapy. *International Journal Telerehab, 6*(1), 29–35. Available from: https://doi.org/10.5195/ijt.2014.6148.

Christiansen, C., & Baum, C. M. (1991). *Occupational therapy: Overcoming human performance deficits.* Thorofare, NJ: Slack.

Department of Veterans Affairs. (2017). Functional independence measure user's manual (FIM). <https://www.va.gov/vdl/documents/Clinical/Func_Indep_Meas/fim_user_manual.pdf>.

Easton, L. W., & Horan, A. L. (1979). Dressing band. *The American Journal of Occupational Therapy, 33,* 656.

Exact Dynamics BV. Edisonstraat 96, NL-6942 PZ, Didam, the Netherlands Assistive Robotic Manipulator Product Information. 2004. <http://www.exactdynamics.nl/>.

Feldmeier, D. M., & Poole, J. L. (1987). The position-adjustable hair dryer. *The American Journal of Occupational Therapy, 41,* 246.

Florey, L. L., & Michelman, S. M. (1982). Occupational role history: a screening tool for psychiatric occupational therapy. *The American Journal of Occupational Therapy, 36*(5), 301–308. Available from: https://doi.org/10.5014/ajot.36.5.301.

Freedom Wand toilet aid self-wipe, sanitary, wiping aid. <https://www.freedomwand.com>.

Gripit floss holder. <http://sale.dentist.net/products/gripit-floss-holder>.

Hattjar, B. (2017). Addressing sexual activity: a structured method for assisting clients with intimacy. *OT Pract, 22*(19), 8–10, 12.

Helping hands—monkey helpers for the disabled. <http://www.helpinghandsmonkeys.org>.

Kelly, S. N. (1983). Adaptations for independent use of cassette tape recorder/radio by high-level quadriplegic patients. *The American Journal of Occupational Therapy, 37*(11), 766–767. Available from: https://doi.org/10.5014/ajot.37.11.766.

Kielhofner, G., Mallinson, T., Forsyth, K., et al. (2001). Psychometric properties of the second version of the occupational performance history interview (OPHI-II). *The American Journal of Occupational Therapy, 55*(3), 260–267.

Klinger, J. L., Howard, A., & Rusk Institute of Rehabilitation Medicine. (1997). *Mealtime manual for people with disabilities and the aging.* West Deptford Township, NJ: Slack.

Koketsu, J. S. (2018). Activities of daily living. In H. M. Pendleton, & W. Schultz-Krohn (Eds.), *Pedretti's occupational therapy: Practice skills for physical dysfunction* (8th ed.). St. Louis, MO: Mosby.

Letts, L., Law, M., Rigby, P., et al. (1994). Person-environment assessments in occupational therapy. *The American Journal of Occupational Therapy, 48*(7), 608–618. Available from: https://doi.org/10.5014/ajot.48.7.608.

Lift and Accessibility Solutions. (2013). San Francisco Bay Area stairlifts | Lift & accessibility solutions. <https://liftandaccessibilitysolutions.com>.

Malick, M. H., & Almasy, B. S. (1998). Assessment and evaluation: life work tasks. In H. L. Hopkins, & H. D. Smith (Eds.), *Willard and Spackman's occupational therapy* (6th ed.). Philadelphia, PA: Lippincott Williams & Wilkins.

Matsutsuyu, J. (1969). The interest checklist. *The American Journal of Occupational Therapy, 23,* 323–328.

Mayer, T. K. (2001). *One-handed in a two-handed world* (2nd ed.). Boston, MA: Prince-Gallison Press.

Melvin, J. L. (1982). *Rheumatic disease: Occupational therapy and rehabilitation.* Philadelphia, PA: Davis Publications.

Modlin, S. (2001). From puppy to service dog: raising service dogs for the rehabilitation team. *Rehabilitation Nursing., 26*(1) 12–17. Available from: https://doi.org/10.1002/j.2048-7940.2001.tb02202.x.

North Coast Medical. (2004). Rehabilitation products, equipment & supplies. <http://www.ncmedical.com>.

Nuance-Dragon. (2010). Naturally speaking. <http://www.nuance.com>.

Nygard, L., Grahn, U., Rudenhammar, A., et al. (2004). Reflecting on practice: are home visits prior to discharge worthwhile in geriatric inpatient care? Clients' and occupational therapists' perceptions. *Scandinavian Journal of Caring Sciences, 18*(2), 193–203. Available from: https://doi.org/10.1111/j.1471-6712.2004.00270.x.

Pardessus, V., Puisieux, F., Di Pompeo, C., et al. (2002). Benefits of home visits for falls and autonomy in the elderly: a randomized trial study. *American Journal of Physical Medicine & Rehabilitation, 81*(4), 247–252. Available from: https://doi.org/10.1097/00002060-200204000-00002.

Parent Empowerment Network. (2010). Website. <http://www.disabledparents.net>.

Parents with Disabilities. (2010). Through the looking glass visits Japan. <http://lookingglass.org/index.php>.

Pendleton, H. M., & Schultz-Krohn, W. (2013). *Pedretti's occupational therapy: Practice skills for physical dysfunction* (7th ed.). St. Louis, MO: Elsevier Mosby.

Planet Mobility. (2004). Accessible air travel & airline. <www.planetmobility.com/go/travel/air>.

Public Utilities Commission. (2010). Deaf & disabled telecommunications program. <http://www.ddtp.org>.

Purex complete 3-in-1 laundry sheets. (2019). Amazon. <https://www.amazon.com/Complete-Tropical-Detergent-Softener-Anti-static/dp/B0028OP0QK/ref = sr_1_3?crid = 1CD21T6QEY4IK&keywords = purex + 3 + in + one + sheet + laundry&qid = 1568506842&s = hpc&sprefix = purex + 3 + in%2Chpc%2C140&sr = 1-3>.

Quartet Technology. (2019). Website. <https://qtiusa.com/>.

Renda, M., & Lape, J. E. (2018). Feasibility and effectiveness of telehealth home modification interventions to improve safety and perception of performance. *The American Journal of Occupational Therapy, 72*(1), 3–14. Available from: https://doi.org/10.5014/ajot.2018.72s1-po8030.

Runge, M. (1967). Self-dressing techniques for patients with spinal cord injury. *The American Journal of Occupational Therapy, 21*(6), 367–375.

Sammons Preston Rolyan. (2004). *Professional Rehabilitation Catalog*. Bolingbrook, IL: SPR.

The Humane Society of the United States. (2019). The Fair Housing Act and assistance animals. <https://www.humanesociety.org/resources/fair-housing-act-and-assistance-animals>.

Traveling With a Disability. (2004). Ebility.com. <http://ebility.com/articles/accessible_travels.shtml>.

Trombly, C. A. (1983). Activities of daily living. In C. A. Trombly (Ed.), *Occupational therapy for physical dysfunction*. Baltimore, MD: Williams & Wilkins.

Trombly, C. A. (1995). Retraining basic and instrumental activities of daily living. In C. A. Trombly (Ed.), *Occupational therapy for physical dysfunction*. Baltimore, MD: Williams & Wilkins.

Willard, H. S., Spackman, C. S., Neistadt, M. E., et al. (1998). *Willard and Spackman's occupational therapy* (6th ed.). Philadelphia, PA: Lippincott Williams & Wilkins.

World Health Organization. (2003). *International classification of functioning, disability, and health*. Geneva, Switzerland.

14

Assistive Technology

Denis Anson

OBJECTIVES

After reading this chapter, the student or the occupational therapy practitioner will be able to do the following:

- Define assistive technology and contrast it with rehabilitative technologies.
- Explain why universal design is not considered assistive technology.
- Describe the human interface assessment model.
- Discuss the pros and cons of electronic aids to daily living for different populations.
- Consider augmentative and alternative communications used both for augmentative and for alternative communication and explain considerations for each use.
- Discuss the pros and cons of different technologies for keyboarding for persons with disabilities.
- Discuss the advantages and disadvantages of current speech input and voice output technologies.
- Explain why Braille is mandated by the Individuals With Disabilities Education Act of 1997.

KEY TERMS

Rehabilitation technology
Assistive technologies
Universal design
Human interface assessment (HIA) model
Electronic aids to daily living (EADL)
Power switching
X-10 system
Feature control
Subsumed devices
Augmentative and alternative communication
Message composition
Message transmission
Physical keyboard

Virtual keyboard
Pointing systems
Eye tracking
Switch encoding
Speech input
Scanning input
Rate enhancement
Semantic compaction
Compression/expansion
Visual output
Speech output
Tactile output

CASE STUDY
Mary, Part 1

Mary is a 26-year-old aspiring lawyer. Her path to the legal profession is complicated by her C4-level complete spinal cord injury, which she sustained 12 years ago in an automobile accident that killed her parents. Mary is bright, articulate, and exceptionally popular in her rural community. She recently received a new wheelchair with sip-and-puff controls, which allows her mobility in her home and community, and now she would like to attend law school. Ultimately, Mary would like to specialize in disability rights, to support the civil rights of others with profound disabilities. She believes her inside perspective on the issues might make her arguments more compelling when workers with disabilities are seeking reasonable accommodations.

The admissions office at the nearby university—which includes a law program—suggests that Mary may have a difficult time completing the required work. As a law student, Mary will have to research legal precedence in case law and write briefs. She can get into the library, which meets many of the requirements of the Americans With Disabilities Act, but she will need to be able to navigate the legal record, take notes of her findings, and write formal responses to legal challenges. The counselor believes that Mary, who has no movement below her neck, may find the challenges of the legal profession to exceed her capabilities.

Mary does have full-time attendant care, and the attendant would be allowed to sit with Mary in the classroom and take notes for her. (The school also provides lecture notes to disabled students within 3 days of a class session, if requested.) However, because Mary's attendant must constantly monitor Mary, her ability to focus on the lecture may be impaired. Also, because the attendant does not have the interest or background to study law, her ability to tell what is important is limited. Finally, because Mary generally changes attendants every 6 months or so, the attendant will not have a complete background to help with interpretation of the material Mary is studying. In her home life, Mary would very much like to be able to adjust the lights, the room temperature, and radio station (she prefers to study with music in the background) that is playing without interrupting her attendant. She knows that she will always be dependent on others for bathing, dressing, meal preparation, and many other aspects of her activities of daily living. However, she feels that her attendants might be able to remain in her employ longer if she were able to do more for herself and make fewer demands on them.

Mary has had an assistive technology consult and has obtained some of the recommended adaptations to allow her to attend law school.

1. What training strategies might help Mary learn to use her assistive technologies?
2. How would a clinician know that the assistive technology is performing as intended?
3. Now that Mary has assistive technology, would it be reasonable to expect her to perform like her able-bodied peers?
4. Now that Mary has assistive technology, is it reasonable to expect her to succeed in her goal of becoming a lawyer?

INTRODUCTION

A discussion of assistive technology (AT) should begin with a description of the general limits of the topic. This is made difficult because the legal definitions of AT are not uniform. Assistive technologies are sometimes included in the category of rehabilitation technology (Neighborhood Legal Services, 2004). In other cases, rehabilitation technology is considered an aspect of AT (Assistive Technology Act of 1998, 1998; Assistive Technology Act of 2004, 2004). A third category, universal designed technologies, does not seem to fit into either category (Center for Universal Design, 2004). For purposes of this discussion, the author presents a set of definitions that is within current practice but not necessarily congruent with any particular statute.

REHABILITATIVE/ASSISTIVE/UNIVERSAL TECHNOLOGIES

The category into which an enabling technology falls depends largely on its application, not on the nature of the device. What is for some people a convenience may for another be an AT.

Rehabilitation Technology

To rehabilitate is to restore to a prior level of function. To be consistent with general usage, therefore, the term **rehabilitation technology** should be used to describe those technologies that are intended to restore an individual to a previous level of function following the onset of pathology. (For clients with developmental delays, who have not yet reached a certain level of function, these can be called habilitative technologies, but generally they are grouped as rehabilitative.) When an occupational therapist (OT) uses a technologic device to establish, restore, or modify functioning in the client, the OT is using a rehabilitative technology. Note that occupational therapy is, by definition, using meaningful activity to affect health and function; the rehabilitation technologies used in occupational therapy may look exactly like assistive technologies.

Rehabilitative technologies are generally intended to be used within a therapy setting, by trained professionals, and over a (relatively) short period of time. The expectation is that the professional may have significant training before applying the technology. The professional guiding the use of such technologies is expected to ensure the correct application of the technology and to protect the safety of the individual using the device. Physical agent modalities such as ultrasound, diathermy, paraffin, and functional electric stimulation, which may be used in occupational therapy as preparation for participation in meaningful activity, are examples of rehabilitative technologies. When these technologies have done their job, the client will have improved intrinsic function, and the technology will be removed.

For some clinicians, augmentative and alternative communication (AAC) is another type of rehabilitative technology, in that it can be used to improve a client's native communication abilities. Many computer applications have been developed to teach basic life skills, money management, and other activities of daily living (ADL). All of these would be considered rehabilitative technologies because once the skill has been learned, the client will no longer require the technology.

Assistive Technology

Central to occupational therapy is the belief that active engagement in meaningful activity supports the health and well-being of the individual. An individual who has functional limitations secondary to some pathology may not have the cognitive, motor, or psychologic skills demanded by a desired meaningful activity and may require assistance to participate.

To assist is to help, aid, or support. There is no implication of restoration in assistance. **Assistive technologies** therefore are those technologies that assist a person with a disability in performing tasks. More specifically, ATs are those technologies, whether designed for a person with a disability or designed for mass market and used by a person with a disability, that allow a person to perform tasks that an able-bodied person can do without technologic assistance. It may be that an able-bodied person would prefer to use a technology to perform a task (e.g., using a television remote control), but it does not rise to the level of AT so long as it is possible for the able-bodied person to perform the task without the technology.

ATs replace or support an impaired function of the user without being expected to change the client factors that relate to the functioning of the individual. A wheelchair, for example, replaces the function of walking but is not expected to teach the user to walk. Similarly, forearm crutches support independent standing but do not, of themselves, improve strength or bony integrity, so they will not change the ability of the user to stand without them.

Because they are not expected to change the native ability of the user, ATs have different design considerations. They are expected to be used over prolonged periods of time, by individuals with limited training, and possibly with limited cognitive skills. The controls of the device must be readily understood so that constant retraining will not be required, although some training may be required to use the device. The device should not require deep understanding of its principles and functions to be useful.

One significant difference between rehabilitation technology and AT occurs at the end of the rehabilitation process. At this point, the client no longer uses rehabilitation technologies but may have just completed training in the use of AT. The AT goes home with the client; the rehabilitation technologies generally remain in a clinic. Some technologies do not fit neatly into these categories because they may be used differently with different clients. The distinction is not with the technology but with the application. Some clinicians use assisted communication as a tool to train unassisted speech for their clients. For other clients, assisted communication may be used to support or replace speech. In the first case, the technology is rehabilitative. In the second, the same technology may be assistive.

Universal Design

Universal design is a relatively new category of technology. The principles of universal design were published by the Center for Universal Design at North Carolina State University in 1997, and their application is still limited. The concept of **universal design** is simple: If devices are designed to meet the needs of people with a wide range of abilities, they will be more usable for all users, with and without disabilities.

This design philosophy could, in some cases, make AT unnecessary. A can opener that has been designed for one-handed use by a busy housewife will also be usable by the cook who has had a cerebrovascular accident (CVA) and now has use of only one hand. Because both individuals are using the same product for the same purpose, it is just technology, not AT. Some eBook readers include a feature to allow them to be used as talking books. In an interesting reversal of the typical relationship, the Apple iPad includes this ability to allow blind users to access onscreen content, but the same feature can be used by commuters while driving. No adaptation is necessary because accommodations for the special needs of the person with a disability have already been designed into the product.

ROLE OF ASSISTIVE TECHNOLOGY IN OCCUPATIONAL PARTICIPATION

The *Occupational Therapy Practice Framework* (American Occupational Therapy Association Inc, 2014) defines the appropriate domain of occupational therapy as including the analysis of the performance skills and patterns of the individual and the activity demands of the occupation the individual is attempting to perform.

Human Interface Assessment

Anson's **human interface assessment (HIA) model** provides a detailed look at the skills and abilities of a person in the skill areas of motor, process, and communication/interaction, as well as the demands of an activity (Fig. 14.1A). The HIA model suggests that when the demands of a task do not exceed the skills and abilities of an individual, no AT is required even when a functional limitation exists (see Fig. 14.1B). On the other hand, when a task makes demands that exceed the native abilities of the individual, the individual will not be able to perform the task in the socially accepted manner (see Fig. 14.1C). In these cases, an AT device may be used to bridge the gap between the demands and abilities (see Fig. 14.1D).

Although an AT must be able to assist in performing the desired task, it also presents an interface that must match the needs of the client. A careful match among the sensory, cognitive, and motor abilities of the human and the input and output capabilities of ATs is necessary.

When assisting a client to learn to use an AT, the attention of the occupational therapy assistant (OTA) should first focus on whether the individual can control the technology. (Does the AT make demands beyond the ability of the client?) Once it is determined that the client can control the device, the focus should shift to the ability of the client to perform the tasks for which the AT was recommended. Unless the client's ability to perform the task has improved, the AT is not effective. A great risk in providing AT is the tendency to focus on the ability of the person to use the technology, while overlooking the tasks for which it should be used. If a man with a spinal cord injury is provided with an electronic aid to daily living (EADL), for example, is he able to independently control the temperature of the environment to avoid overheating?

TYPES OF ELECTRONIC ENABLING TECHNOLOGIES

Although modern technology can blur some of the distinctions presented as follows, it is useful to consider assistive technologies in categories for which they are applied. This chapter deals only with electronic assistive technologies, which, in terms of their primary application, may be considered to fall into three categories: EADL, AACs, and general computer applications.

Electronic Aids to Daily Living

Electronic aids to daily living are devices that can be used to control electrical devices in the client's environment. Before 1998 (MacNeil, 1998), this category of device was generally known as an environmental control unit (ECU), although technically this terminology should be reserved for furnace thermostats and similar controls. The more generic EADL applies to control of lighting and temperature but may also extend to control of radios, televisions, telephones, and other electrical and electronic devices in a client's environment (Fig. 14.2) (Anson, 2006; Barnes, 1994; Center for Assistive

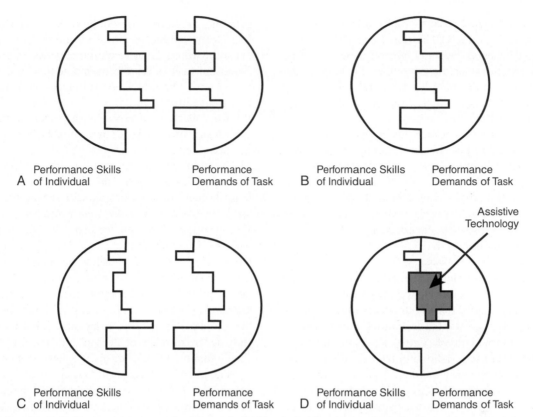

A Performance Skills of Individual — Performance Demands of Task

B Performance Skills of Individual — Performance Demands of Task

C Performance Skills of Individual — Performance Demands of Task

D Performance Skills of Individual — Performance Demands of Task

Fig. 14.1 (A) Skills of the individual and the demands of the task. (B) Match of skills of the individual with the demands of the task. (C) Skills of the individual and demands of the task mismatch. (D) Assistive technology used to bridge gap between the skills of the individual and the demands of the task.

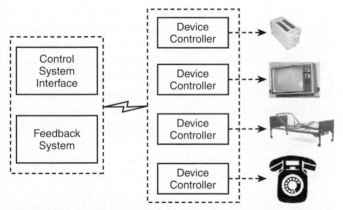

Fig. 14.2 Components of an electronic aids to daily living system.

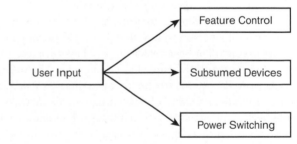

Fig. 14.3 Electronic aids to daily living control components.

Technology, 2004; Cook & Hussey, 2001; Efthimiou et al., 1981; McDonald et al., 1989).

EADL systems may be characterized by the degree and types of control that they provide to the user. These levels of control are simple power switching, control of device features, and subsumed devices (Fig. 14.3).

Power Switching. The simplest EADL provide simple **power switching** of the electrical supply for devices in a

room. Although not typically classified as EADL, the switch adaptations for switch-adapted toys provided to children with severe disabilities would formally be included in this category of device. Primitive EADL systems consisted of little more than a set of electrical switches and outlets in a box that is connected to devices within a room via extension cords. Second-generation EADL systems use various remote control technologies to switch power to electrical devices in the environment.

Regardless of the means used to communicate between the device and the controller, the user must know which control operates which device. Some systems, such as the TASH Ultra-4 (Tash Inc.), use colored markers on the control device and switch box to make this connection. Other systems, such as the **X10 system** (Smarthome, Inc.), use encoding switches so that any control module can be controlled by any input of the controller. So long as the client is able to turn on the intended device reliably, the coding is not relevant. However, systems like X10 can offer more options than Ultra-4.

When working with a client on a power-switching EADL, it is important to ensure that the client can operate the controls of the device, recognize which control operates which light or appliance, and be able to turn devices on and off at will. Ability to control devices should be evaluated when the client is relaxed and rested, as well as when fatigued. Unless the client can control his or her environment all through the day, the EADL will not be effective.

Feature Control. As electronic systems became more common in the home, devices that simply switched lights and coffee pots on and off failed to meet the needs of the individual with a disability who wanted to control the immediate environment. With wall current control, a person with a disability might be able to turn radios and televisions on and off but would have no control beyond that. A person with a disability might want to be able to surf cable channels as much as an able-bodied person with a television remote control. When advertisements are blaring from the speakers, a person with a disability might want to be able to turn down the sound or tune to another radio station. Nearly all home electronic devices are now delivered with a remote control, generally using infrared signals. Most of these remote controls are not usable by a person with a disability, due to demands for fine motor control and good sensory discrimination.

EADL systems designed to provide access to the home environment of a person with a disability must provide more than on/off control of home electronics. They must also provide **feature control** of home electronic devices. Because of this need, EADL systems frequently have hybrid capabilities and incorporate a means of switching power directly to remote devices, often using X10 technology. This allows operation of devices such as lights, fans, and coffee pots, as well as electrical door openers and other specialty devices (Quartet Technology, 2004, 2005). These EADL systems typically also incorporate some form of infrared remote control, allowing them to mimic the signals of standard remote control devices. This control is provided either by programming in the standard sequences for all commercially available VCRs, televisions, and satellite decoders or through teaching systems, in which the EADL learns the codes beamed at it by the conventional remote. The advantage of the latter approach is that the EADL can learn any codes, even those that have not yet been invented. The disadvantage is that the controls must be taught, requiring more setup and configuration time for the user and caregivers.

Infrared remote control, as adopted by most entertainment system controllers, is limited to approximate line-of-sight control. Unless the controller is aimed in the general direction of the device to be controlled (most have wide dispersion patterns), the signals will not be received. This means that an EADL cannot directly control, via infrared, any device located in another room. However, infrared repeaters, such as the X10 Powermid (asiHome), can overcome this limitation by using radio signals to send the control signals received in one room to a transmitter in the room of the device to be controlled. With a collection of repeaters, a person would be able to control any infrared device in the home from anywhere else in the home.

The proliferation of remote control devices is a problem shared by EADL users and able-bodied consumers alike. Many homes now are cluttered with separate remote controls for the television, the cable/satellite receiver, the DVD player/ VHS recorder (either one or two devices), the home stereo/ multimedia center, and other devices, all in the same room. Universal remote controls allow switching control from one device to another but are often cumbersome to operate and do not provide the full features of the controlled devices. As the number of devices to be controlled by an EADL increases, the complexity of the device does also. It is important to make sure, as the number of devices and options grow, that the client remains able to control the environment easily.

With the rise of electronic assistants and the Internet of Things (IoT), many aspects of the EADL have moved from assistive technologies to general technologies. Agents such as Alexa, Siri, and Google can be called upon by voice (for those who can speak) to turn lights on and off, adjust thermostats, tune the television, and much, much more. Because these abilities are embedded in mainstream telephones and smart speakers, they are aspects of universal design rather than assistive technology.

Subsumed Devices. The concept of a **subsumed device** is that what were, in the past or in mainstream technology, independent devices have been rolled into a single multipurpose device. The modern smartphone is no longer only or even primarily a telephone. It is often a method to control the environment ("There's an app for that!"), a messaging system, and an entertainment system incorporated into a device that fits into a pocket. The capacity for voice-dialing has been expanded to dictate messages or letters, switch power through smart-home interfaces, and monitor the home.

Controlling Electronic Aids to Daily Living. EADL systems are designed to allow the individual with limited physical capability to control devices in the immediate environment. As such, the method used to control the EADL must be within the capability of the client. Because these controls for EADL have features in common with other forms of electronic devices, the control strategies are discussed next.

Augmentative and Alternative Communication

The term **augmentative and alternative communication** is used to describe systems that supplement (augment) or replace (alternative) communication by voice or gestures between people (Lloyd et al., 1996). As used in AT, AAC may be defined as the use of technology to allow communication in ways that an able-bodied individual would be able to accomplish without assistance. Thus using a pencil to write a letter to Aunt May would not be an example of AAC for a person who is unable to speak because an able-bodied correspondent would be using the same technology (pencil and paper) for the same purpose (social communication). However, when a woman who is nonvocal uses the same pencil to explain to the doctor that she has sharp pains in her right leg, it becomes an AAC device because an able-bodied person would communicate this by voice.

There are two different reasons an individual might have a communication disorder. In a language disorder, the individual has difficulty in understanding and/or formulating messages, regardless of means of production. A person with a language disorder, in most cases, will not benefit from AAC. On the other hand, an individual with difficulty in motor control or muscle tone may be perfectly able to understand and formulate messages but not be able to speak intelligibly because of difficulty in controlling the oral musculature. Such a person has no difficulty with language composition, only with language transmission. This person may well benefit from an AAC device.

AAC devices range from extremely low technology to extremely high technology in design. In hospital intensive care units, low-tech communication boards can allow a person on a respirator to communicate basic needs (Fig. 14.4). A low-tech communication board can allow a client to deliver basic messages or spell out more involved messages in a fashion that can be learned quickly. For a person capable only of yes/no responses, the communication partner can indicate the rows of the aid one at a time, asking if the desired letter is in the row. When the correct row is selected, the partner can move across a row until the communicator indicates the correct letter. This type of communication is inexpensive, quick to teach, and slow to use. In settings where there are limited communication needs, this type of AAC is adequate but will not serve for long-term or fluent communication needs.

To meet the communication needs of a person who will be nonvocal over a longer period of time, clinicians frequently recommend electronic AAC devices (Fig. 14.5).

An AAC system used solely for expression of needs and wants can be fairly basic. The vocabulary used in this type of communication is limited, and because the expressions tend to be fairly short the communication rate is not of paramount importance. In some cases the communication system may consist only of an alerting buzzer, indicating that the individual is in need, to summon a caregiver. Low-tech communication systems such as that described earlier can meet basic communication needs for individuals whose physical skills are limited to eye blinks or directed eye movement.

Most development in AAC seems to be focused around communicating basic needs and information transfer. Information transfer presents some of the most difficult technologic problems because the content of information to be communicated cannot be predicted. Making these unpredictable bits of information available for fluent communication is the ongoing challenge of AAC development.

Social communication and social etiquette present significant challenges for users of AAC devices. Although the information content of these messages tends to be low, because the communication is based on convention, the dialogue should be both varied and spontaneous. AAC systems such as the Dynavox (DynaVox Systems LLC) have provisions for preprogrammed messages that can be retrieved for social conversation, but providing both fluency and variability of social discourse through AAC remains a challenge.

The Fat Cat Chat series of communication apps for iOS or Android devices provide up to 20 ways to communicate phatic messages, which indicate that the listener is involved in the conversation. These quirky applications help keep a conversation going but do not allow generation of novel ideas.

Devices currently available allow moderately effective communication of wants. They are not nearly so effective in discussing dreams.

Message Composition. Most of the time, able-bodied people and individuals with disabilities plan their messages before speaking. (Many of us can remember the taste of foot when we have neglected this process.) An AAC device should

A	B	C	D	E	F	I Hurt
G	H	I	J	K	L	I'm thirsty
M	N	O	P	Q	R	Head/Neck
S	T	U	V	W	X	Trunk
Y	Z	1	2	3	4	Arms
5	6	7	8	9	0	Legs

Fig. 14.4 Low-technology alternative and augmentative communications system.

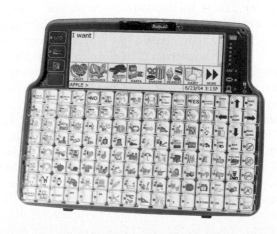

Fig. 14.5 High-technology alternative and augmentative communications system Pathfinder.

allow the user to construct, preview, and edit communication utterances before they become apparent to the communication partner. This gives the user of an AAC device the ability to think before speaking. It also allows compensation for the rate difference between **message composition** via AAC and communication between able-bodied individuals.

Able-bodied individuals typically speak between 150 and 175 words per minute (wpm) (Miller, 1981). Augmentative communication rates are more typically on the order of 10 to 15 wpm, resulting in a severe disparity between the rate of communication construction and expected rate of reception. Although input techniques (discussed later) offer some improvement in message construction rates, the rate of message assembly using AAC is such that many listeners will lose interest before an utterance can be delivered. If words are spaced too far apart, an able-bodied listener may not even be able to assemble them into a coherent message!

Perhaps the most difficult challenge when working with a new AAC user is convincing the client to use the device. Initially the process of message composition and **message transmission** is so slow and difficult that the client may wish to continue to use his or her poorly understood natural voice. Indeed, in the early stages, such communication may be faster and allow easier communication. (To understand a person with a severely distorted voice, the communication partner must pay close attention. This close attention may also be sought by the communicator because this ensures continued attention.) To teach an individual to use an AAC device, it may be important for the clinician to be unable to understand the communicator's voice and to encourage him or her to use the AAC device to continue the conversation. Over time, using the AAC device will become more automatic for the client, both with the clinician and with others.

General Computer Access

The third category of electronic enabler is general computer access. Although computer use is ubiquitous among able-bodied individuals, it is an AT for individuals with a wide range of disabilities because the computer allows them to perform tasks for which they have no alternative method. Computers can be used to write messages or to research school subjects. For the person with a print impairment, the computer can provide access to printed information either through electronic documents or through optical character recognition of printed documents, which can convert the printed page into an electronic document. Once a document is stored electronically it can be presented as large text for the person with a visual acuity limitation or read aloud for the person who is blind or profoundly learning disabled. Computers can allow the manipulation of virtual objects to teach mathematical concepts, form constancy, and develop spatial relations skills that are commonly learned by manipulation of physical objects (Intellitools, 2004). Smartphones and small personal electronics may be useful for the busy executive but may be the only means available for a person with attention deficit hyperactivity disorder (ADHD) to get to meetings on time. For the executive they are conveniences, but for the person with ADHD they can be assistive technologies.

Individuals using computers can locate, organize, and present information at levels of complexity that are not possible without electronic aids. Through the emerging area of cognitive prosthetics, computers can be used to augment attention and thinking skills in people with cognitive limitations. Computer-based biofeedback can monitor and enhance attention to task. Research in temporal processing deficits has led to the development of computer-modified speech programs that can be used to enhance language learning and temporal processing skills (Merzenich et al., 1996; Tallal et al., 1996).

Beyond such rehabilitative applications, the performance-enhancing characteristics of the conventional computer can allow a person with physical or performance limitations to participate in activities that would be too demanding without the assistance of the computer. An able-bodied person would be able to write a note by hand. A person with a disability may lack the physical capacities to hand write a note and would thus rely on the abilities of the computer. For the able-bodied person, the computer is a convenience. For the person with a disability, it is an AT because the task cannot be accomplished without it. The computer applications appropriate for a person with a disability include all the computer applications available to an able-bodied person.

For the person with cognitive or learning disabilities, the computer can provide support for acceptable learning and life experiences. Most nondisabled people use spelling checkers for their written communication to identify typographic errors. Some people with learning disabilities of various types cannot learn to spell fluently. Rather than force these students to struggle with a skill that they will never acquire, it is better to accommodate the functional limitation with a tool that supports or replaces that skill. Similarly, grammar checkers can assist those who lack the ability to assemble sentences in the socially approved structure. For students with language processing disorders, computers can read text aloud, while highlighting each word or phrase as it is being spoken. This can have extraordinary effects on learning and retention.

CONTROL TECHNOLOGIES

All electronic enabling technologies depend on the ability of the individual to control them. Although the functions of the various devices differ, the control strategies share common characteristics. Because the majority of electronic devices were designed for use by able-bodied persons, the controls of ATs may be categorized in the ways that they are adapted from the standard controls. Electronic control may be divided into three broad categories: input adaptations, output adaptations, and performance enhancements.

Input to Assistive Technologies

A wide range of input strategies are available to control electronic enablers; these can be more easily considered in subcategories. Different authors have created different taxonomies for the categorization of input strategies, and some techniques are classified differently in these taxonomies. The categorization presented here should not be considered as uniquely correct but merely as a convenience. Input strategies may be classified as those using physical keyboards, those using virtual keyboards, and those using scanning techniques.

Physical Keyboards. **Physical keyboards** generally supply an array of switches, with each switch having a unique function. On more complex keyboards, modifier keys may change the function of a key, usually to a related function (Anson, date; 2001). Physical keyboards appear on a wide range of electronic technologies, including computers, calculators, telephones, and microwave ovens. In these applications, sequences of keys are used to generate meaningful units such as words, checkbook balances, telephone numbers, and the cooking time for a baked potato. Other keyboards may have immediate action when a key is pressed. The television remote control has keys that switch power or raise volume when pressed, for example.

Physical keyboards can be adapted to the needs of the individual with a disability in a number of ways (Fig. 14.6). Most alphanumeric keyboards, for example, are arranged in the pattern of the conventional typewriter. This pattern was intentionally designed, for reasons relating to mechanical limitations, to slow down the user. Modern computers can accommodate higher speeds of keyboarding, and the QWERTY (Anson et al., 2005) layout of the standard keyboard is no longer required for anyone but is what most people have learned.

The QWERTY pattern of keys is seldom optimum for ATs. Alternative keyboard patterns include the Dvorak Two Handed, Dvorak One Handed, and Chubon (Fig. 14.7) (Anson, 1997). These patterns offer improvements in efficiency of typing that may allow a person with a disability to perform for functional periods of time (Anson et al., 2001, 2005; Fong Lee, 1995; Interactive MaM, 2003; Kincaid, 1999; Struck, 1999a, b; Trumbull, 1995; Zecevic et al., 2000).

Initially the process of using an alternative keyboard layout will be frustrating to users of standard keyboards because the keys are considered to be in the wrong places. In assisting a client to learn to use the new keyboard layout, the clinician may need to use highly engaging activities where speed is relatively unimportant. Email would be more effective than chat rooms, for example, because chat occurs quickly so a slow typist can be left behind, whereas an email exchange can be conducted at the speed of the typist. Word games depend more on the quality of typing than the speed of typing. Careful documentation of typing speed and accuracy can also be helpful because it allows the client to see progress from day to day.

The scale of the standard keyboard is designed to fit the fine motor control and range of motion (ROM) of an able-bodied adult. The client with limitations in either ROM or motor control may find the conventional keyboard difficult to use. If the client has limitations in motor control, a keyboard with larger keys and/or additional space between keys may allow independent control of the device. This adaptation may also assist the person with a vision limitation, as larger keys provide area for larger labels. However, providing an equivalent number of options on larger keys increases the size of the keyboard, which may make it unusable for the person with limitations in ROM.

To accommodate limitations in ROM, the keyboard controls can be reduced in size. Smaller controls, placed closer together, will allow the selection of the full range of options with less demand for joint movement. However, the smaller controls will be more difficult to target for the person with limited motor control. A mini-keyboard is usable only by a person with good fine motor control and may be the only scale of keyboard usable by a person with limited ROM.

To accommodate both limited ROM and limited fine motor control, a keyboard can be designed with fewer options. Many augmentative communication devices can be configured with 4, 8, 32, or 64 keys on a keyboard of a single size. Modifier or paging keys can allow access to the full range of options for the keyboard but with reduced efficiency. In this approach, the person uses one or more keys of the keyboard to shift the meanings of all other keys on the keyboard. Unless this approach is combined with a dynamic display, the user must remember the meanings of the keys.

When the client is using either an expanded or a mini-keyboard, the clinician must monitor whether task performance is actually better. Does typing speed measurably improve? Can the client complete a homework assignment in a reasonable amount of time? What kinds of errors are being made with the keyboard? Does the client strike elsewhere than the intended key? Does he or she drag across keys in the middle of the keyboard? The type of mistake can indicate what modifications are necessary.

Virtual Input Techniques. When an individual lacks the motor control to use an array of physical switches, a virtual keyboard may be used in its place. **Virtual keyboards** provide the functionality of a physical keyboard system, allowing the user to select directly from the array of options by performing a specified action. Instead of using physical switches for the

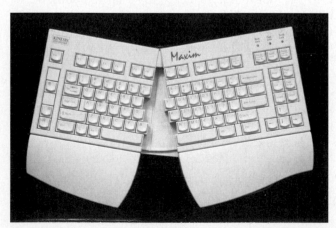

Fig. 14.6 Physical keyboard with adaptive features—the myKey keyboard.

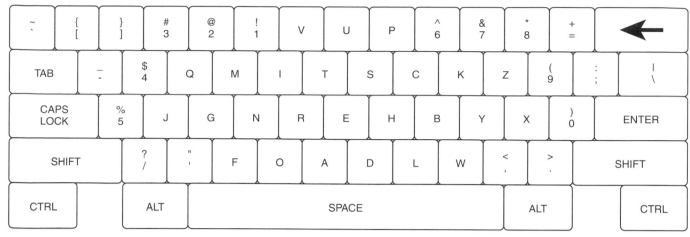

The Chubon Keyboard Layout

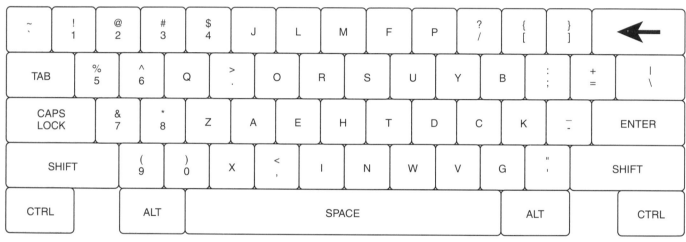

The Right-Handed Dvorak Layout

Fig. 14.7 Alternative keyboard patterns.

actions to be performed, the meaning of the selection action may be encoded spatially (via pointing) or temporally (via sequenced actions).

Pointing Systems. Pointing systems are analogous to using a physical keyboard with a physical pointer such as a head or mouthstick (DeVries et al., 1998). In these systems a graphical representation of a keyboard is presented to the user, and the user makes selections from it by pointing to a region of the virtual keyboard and performing a selection action. The selection action is typically either the operation of a single switch (e.g., clicking the mouse) or the act of holding the pointer steady for a period of time.

The use of pointing systems decreases the demands of using a keyboard but increases demands on the ability to control the mouse pointer. The conventional mouse can be easily changed for a trackpad or trackball, using off-the-shelf replacements from the local office supply store. For people with more involved motor limitations, various mouse emulators might be needed.

A roller mouse is available that looks like a wrist rest for the keyboard. This rest has a cylinder, which can either roll on a rod or slide from side to side on a rod. Rolling the cylinder causes the mouse pointer to move up and down on the screen, while sliding it moves the pointer from side to side. Pressing down on the cylinder can produce a mouse click. Such devices remove the need to grasp a mouse to provide control.

Other mouse emulators can track the movement of body parts in space and move the mouse pointer to match the movements. For example, head-tracking systems move the mouse pointer side to side as the user turns his or her head. Similarly, looking toward the top or bottom of the screen moves the pointer up and down. **Eye-tracking** systems work in a similar fashion but generally require the user to hold the head still and move only the eyes. Clicks can be produced with either an adaptive switch positioned to operate by another action (e.g., sip-and-puff or finger twitching) or by simply holding the mouse pointer in the same location for a period of time.

Most augmentative communication systems now use a dynamic display, on which the graphical keyboard can change as the user makes selections so that the meaning of each location of the keyboard changes as a message is composed. Dynamic displays free the user from having to remember the current meaning of a key or having to decode a key with multiple images on it.

Pointing systems behave much like physical keyboard systems, and many of the considerations of physical keyboards apply. The key size must balance the demands for fine motor control with the ROM available to the client. The keyboard pattern should be selected to enhance function. The selection technique should facilitate intentional selections while minimizing accidental actions.

Switch Encoding Inputs. The individual who lacks the ROM or fine motor control necessary to use a physical or graphical keyboard may be able to use a switch encoding input method. In **switch encoding**, a small set of switches (from one to nine) is used to directly access the functionality of the device. The meaning of the switch may depend on the length of time it is held closed, as in Morse code (Anson et al., 2004a, b; Jarus, 1994; King, 1999; McDonald et al., 1982), or on the immediate history of the switch set, as in the Tongue Touch Keypad (TTK; see later for more extended discussion of this device).

In Morse code, a small set of switches is used to type. In single-switch Morse, a short switch closure produces an element called a dit, which is typically written as "*." A long switch closure produces the dah element, which is transcribed as " − ." Patterns of switch closures produce the letters of the alphabet, numbers, and punctuation. Pauses longer than five times the short switch closure indicate the end of a character. Two-switch Morse is similar, except two switches are used— one to produce the dit element and a second to produce the dah. Because the meaning of the switches is unambiguous, it

is possible for the input time of the dit and dah to be the same length, potentially doubling typing speed. Three-switch Morse breaks the time dependence of Morse by using a third switch to indicate that the generated set of dits and dahs constitute a single letter.

Morse code is a highly efficient method of typing for a person with severe motor control limitations and, unlike other virtual keyboard techniques, can eventually become completely automatic (Anson et al., 2004b; McDonald et al., 1982). Many Morse code users indicate that they do not know Morse code. They think in words, and the words appear on the screen, just as happens in touch-typing. Many Morse code users type at speeds approaching 25 wpm, making this a means of functional writing.

Many therapists shy away from Morse because they do not know it themselves, and they are unwilling to ask a client to perform a task that they cannot. However, it is clear from clinical experience that Morse code is like touch-typing. When it is first being learned, it is difficult and frustrating; once learned, it becomes automatic and users are reluctant to go back to slower methods. The role of the therapist therefore is to provide the encouragement necessary for the client to get beyond the difficult and frustrating stage.

Another type of switch encoding uses immediate history (recent use) for selection. The Tongue Touch Keypad from New Abilities uses a set of nine switches on a keypad built into a mouthpiece resembling a dental orthotic.

Early versions of the product used an onscreen keyboard called Miracle Typer (Fig. 14.8). When using this input method, the first switch selection chose a group of nine possible characters, and the second switch action selected a specific character. This approach to typing was somewhat more efficient than Morse physically but required the user to observe the screen to monitor the current switch meaning. Later

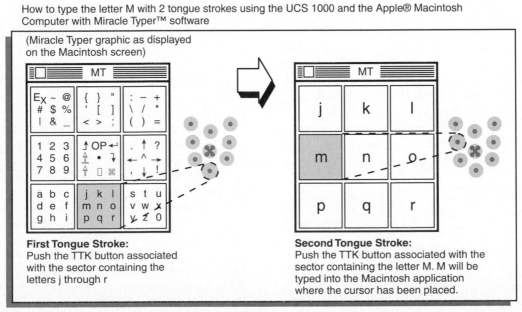

Fig. 14.8 MiracleTyper enabling character selection by selection history.

versions of the TTK used the keypad only as a mouse emulator, allowing the user to select any onscreen keyboard desired for text entry.

A different approach to switch encoding is provided by the T9 keyboard (Fig. 14.9) (Tegic Communications, 2001). In this novel interface, each key of the keyboard has several letters on it but the user types as if only the desired character were present. The keyboard software determines from the user's input what word might have been intended. The disambiguation process used in the T9 keyboard allows a high degree of accuracy in determining which character the user intended and allows rapid learning of the keyboard. The T9 keyboard is provided as an input method for text messaging in many flip-style cell phones. For those with physical disabilities, this input technology is potentially compatible with pointing systems, described earlier, providing an excellent balance of target size and available options. However, because it depends on the user striking all the correct keys, it does not work accurately for a person who cannot spell.

The developers of the T9 keyboard have also developed an input method that looks like a traditional onscreen keyboard but adds the disambiguation of the T9. The Swype input method, as this new technique is called, does not require the user to tap each key of a word. Instead, the user touches the first letter, then moves over each letter of the desired word, releasing at the last letter. Because of the disambiguation, the system does not require a high degree of precision in dragging over the letters. The Swype method has been so successful that it is now common in cell phone onscreen keyboards from most manufacturers.

Speech Input. For many, **speech input** has a magical allure. What could be more natural than to speak to an EADL or computer and have one's wishes carried out? When first introduced by Dragon Systems (Dragon Systems, Inc.) in 1990, large vocabulary speech input systems were enormously expensive and, for most, of limited utility. Although highly dedicated users were able to type using voice in 1990, almost no one with the option of the keyboard would choose to use voice for their daily work. These early systems required the user to pause between each word so that the input system could recognize the units of speech. Today (2019), the technology has evolved to allow continuous speech, with recognition accuracy greater than 90% (Koester, 2003). (The companies producing speech products claim accuracy of >95%.) Although this advance in speech technology is remarkable, it does not mean that speech input is the input method of choice for people with disabilities, for a number of reasons.

Speech recognition requires consistent speech. Although it is not necessary that the speech be absolutely clear, the user must say words the same way each time for an input system to recognize them. Because of this, the majority of people with speech impairments cannot use a speech input system effectively. Slurring and variability of pronunciation will result in a low recognition rate.

Speech input requires a high degree of vigilance during training and use. To provide the highest initial accuracy, many current speech technologies must be trained to understand the voice of the intended user. To do this, the system presents onscreen text, which the potential user must read into the microphone of the recognition system. If the user lacks the cognitive skills to respond appropriately to the presented cues, the training process will be difficult. A few clinicians have reported success in training students with learning disabilities or other cognitive limitations to use speech input systems, but in general the success rate is poor. Even after training, the user must watch carefully for misrecognized words and correct them at the time the error is made. Modern speech recognition systems depend on context for their recognition. Each uncorrected error slightly changes the context, until the system can no longer recognize the words being spoken. Spell-checking a document will not find misrecognized words because each word on the screen is a correctly spelled word. It just may not be the word the user intended.

On some devices, such as cell phones, no training is required for recognition. However, such systems do not perform the recognition on the device being used. The speech is recorded on the device and transmitted to cloud-based recognition engines. The speech is translated to text, which is sent back to the application in use. Because the speech and text are not encrypted while being transmitted, this recognition should not be used for private information.

Speech input is intrusive. One person in a shared office space talking to a computer will reduce the productivity of every other person in the office. If everyone in the office were talking to their computers, the resulting noise would be intolerable to many. Speech input may be acceptable for a person who works or lives alone but is not a good input method for most office or classroom settings (Koester, 2003).

The type of speech system used depends on the device being controlled. For EADL systems, discrete speech ("lights—on") provides an acceptable level of control. The number of options is relatively small, and there is seldom a need for split-second control. Misrecognized words are unlikely to cause difficulty. Text generation for narrative description, however, places higher demands for input speed and transparency, and it may call for a continuous input method. Other computer applications, however, may work better with discrete rather than continuous input methods. Databases and spreadsheets typically have many small input areas, with limited information in each. These applications are much better suited to discrete speech than continuous.

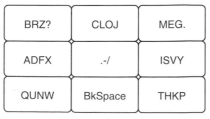

Fig. 14.9 T9 keyboard on a Palm V.

Current research suggests that the most limiting and frustrating aspect of speech recognition is error correction. When teaching a client to use speech recognition, the methods used to correct errors should be a major focus of training. Where a speech system may offer a large number of correction methods, the clinician should focus on teaching the client to use one method consistently and accurately. Only after one method of error correction is mastered should other options be introduced.

Scanning Input Methods. For the individual with limited cognition and/or motor control, some variation in row-column scanning is sometimes used (Anson, 1997; Cook & Hussey, 2001; Glennen & DeCoste, 1996). In **scanning input**, the system to be controlled sequentially offers choices to the user, and the user indicates assent when the correct choice is offered. Typically such systems first offer groups of choices and, when a group is selected, offer the items of the group sequentially. Because the items were, in early systems, presented as a grid being offered a row at a time, such systems are commonly referred to as row-column scanning, even when no rows or columns are present.

Scanning input allows selection of specific choices with limited physical effort. Generally the majority of the user's time is spent waiting for the desired choice to be offered, so the energy expenditure is relatively small. Unfortunately, the overall time expenditure is generally relatively large. When the system has only a few choices from which to select, as in most EADL systems, scanning is a viable input method. The time spent waiting while the system scans may be a minor annoyance, but the difference between turning on a light now, versus a few moments later, is relatively small. EADL systems are used intermittently throughout the day, rather than continuously, so the delays over the course of the day are acceptable in most cases.

For AAC or computer systems, however, the situation is different. In either application, the process of composing thoughts may require making hundreds or thousands of selections in sequence. The cumulative effect of the pauses in row-column scanning will slow productivity to the point that functional communication is tedious and may be impossible. Certainly when productivity levels are mandated, the communication rate available via scanning input will not be adequate.

Rate Enhancement Options. For EADL systems, rate of control input is relatively unimportant. As noted earlier, the number of control options is relatively limited, and selections are rarely severely time constrained. However, for AAC and computer control systems, the number of selections to be made in sequence is high and rate can be critical. **Rate enhancement** technologies may increase the information transmitted by each selection when a person with a disability is unable to make selections as quickly as an able-bodied person.

To understand how rate enhancement works, one must appreciate how language production works. In general, language can be expressed in one of three ways: letter-by-letter

spelling, prediction, and compaction/expansion. The latter two options allow enhancement of language generation rates.

Letter-by-letter spelling.* Typical typing is an example of letter-by-letter representation and is relatively inefficient. In all languages and alphabets there is a balance between the number of characters used to represent a language and the number of elements in a message. English, using the conventional alphabet, averages about 6 letters (selections) per word (including the spaces between words). When represented in Morse code, the same text will require roughly 18 selections per word. By comparison, the basic vocabulary of a person speaking Chinese can be produced by selecting a single ideogram per word. However, each ideogram must be selected from an array of thousands of choices. In general, having a larger number of characters in an alphabet allows each character to convey more meaning but may make the selection of each specific character more difficult.

Many AAC systems use an expanded set of characters in the form of pictograms or icons to represent entire words that may be selected by the user. Such **semantic compaction** allows a large vocabulary to be used within a device but requires a system of selection that may add complexity to the device (Conti, 2004). For example, a device may require the user to select a word group (e.g., *food*) before selecting a specific word (e.g., *hamburger*) from the group. Using subcategories, it is theoretically possible to represent a vocabulary of more than 2 million words on a 128-key keypad with just three selections.

Prediction.* Because messages in a language tend to follow similar patterns, it is possible to produce significant savings of effort using prediction technology. There are two types of prediction used in language production: word completion and word/phrase prediction.

In word completion, a communication system (AAC or computer based) will, after each keystroke, present a number of options to the user representing possible words that begin with these keystrokes. When the appropriate word is presented by the prediction system, the user may select that word directly rather than continuing to spell out the word. Overall, this strategy may reduce the number of selections required to complete a message (Anson et al., 2005; Hunnicutt & Carlberger, 2001; Koester, 2002; Koester & Levine, 1996; MacArthur, 1998; Newell et al., 1992; Tam et al., 2002). However, it may not improve typing speed (Anson, 1993; Anson et al., 2005; Koester, 2002; Koester & Levine, 1996; Williams, 2002; Zordell, 1990). Anson (1993) demonstrated that when typing from copy using the keyboard, typing speed was slowed in direct proportion to the frequency of using the prediction list. The burden of constantly scanning the prediction list overwhelms the potential speed savings of word completion systems under these conditions. However, when typing using an onscreen keyboard or scanning system, in which the user must scan the input array in any case, word completion does appear to increase typing speed and reduce the number of selections made.

Because most language is similar in structure, it is also possible, in some cases, to predict the word that will be used following a specific word. For example, after a person's first name is typed, the surname is often the next item typed. When this prediction is possible, the next word may be generated with a single selection. When combined with word completion, next-word prediction has the potential to decrease the effort of typing substantially. However, in many cases, this potential is unrealized. Many users, even when provided with next-word prediction, become so involved in spelling words that they ignore the predictions even when they are accurate. The cognitive effort of switching between typing mode and list scanning mode may be greater than the cognitive benefit of not having to spell a word out (Gibler & Childress, 1982).

Compression/expansion. **Compression/expansion** strategies allow limited sets of commonly used words to be stored in unambiguous abbreviations. When these abbreviations are selected, either letter by letter or through word completion, the abbreviation is replaced by the expanded form of the word or phrase (Anson, 2001; Cook & Hussey, 2001).

Because the expansion can be many selections long, this technology offers an enormous potential for saving energy and time. However, the potential savings are available only when the user remembers to use the abbreviation rather than the expanded form of a word. Because of this limitation, abbreviations must be carefully selected. Many abbreviations are already in common use and can be stored conveniently. Most people will refer to the television by the abbreviation TV, which requires just 20% of the selections to represent. With an expansion system, each use of TV can automatically be converted to *television* with no additional effort of the user. Similarly, TTFN might be used to store the social message *Ta-ta for now*.

Effective abbreviations will be unique to the user rather than general to all. An example of an effective form of abbreviation is found in the language shortcuts commonly used in note taking. These abbreviations form a shorthand generally unique to the individual that allows complex thoughts to be represented on the page quickly in the course of a lecture. A clinician should work carefully with the client to develop abbreviations that will be useful and easily remembered.

Another form of abbreviations that is less demanding to create is common spelling errors. For persons, either students or adult writers, who have cognitive deficits that influence spelling skills, expansions can be created to automatically correct misspelled words. In these cases the abbreviation is the way that the client generally misspells the word, and the expansion is the correct spelling of the word. Once a library of misspelled words is created, the individual is relieved of the need to worry about the correct spelling. There are those who will maintain that this form of adaptation will prevent the individual from ever learning the correct spelling. In cases where the client is still developing spelling skills, this is probably a valid concern, and the adaptation should not be used. For the individual with a cognitive deficit, however, normal spelling skills may not be a priority. In cases where remediation is not possible, accommodation through compression/expansion technology is a desirable choice.

The implementation of abbreviation-expansion in mainstream cell phones, in the form of autocorrect, has been of limited success and frequent dismay or humor. "Damn you, autocorrect" is a frequent internet meme and has at least three websites devoted to documenting the funniest or worst autocorrections. This failure appears to be caused by the increased autonomy of the corrections, such that the user is not involved in producing the expansions and has little control to repair them. This should not be taken to mean that the more controlled abbreviation/expansion of disability-related applications should be avoided.

None of these technologies will allow a person with a disability to produce messages at the same rate as an able-bodied person. However, individually and collectively, these technologies can make message generation significantly more efficient than it would be without them. The techniques are not mutually exclusive. Icons can be predicted using next-word techniques. Abbreviations can be used in conjunction with word completion and word prediction technologies.

Output Options

The control of assistive technologies involves a cycle of both human output and human input, matched to technology input and technology output. Individuals who have sensory limitations may have difficulty controlling assistive technologies (or common technologies) because they are unable to perceive the messages that are being sent to them by the technology. For these individuals, adaptations of the output of the technology may be required. These adaptations generally depend on one of three sensory modalities: vision, hearing, or tactile sensation.

Visual Output. The default output of many types of electronic technology is visual. Computer screens are designed to resemble the printed page. AAC systems have input that looks like a keyboard and, generally, a graphic message composition area. EADL use display panels and lighted icons to show the current status of controlled devices. The perception of all these controls depends on the user having visual acuity at nearly normal levels. When the client has some vision, but that vision is limited, adaptations may be required.

Colors and contrast. Many types of visual impairment affect the ability to separate foreground and background colors. In addition, bright background colors can produce a visual glare that makes the foreground difficult to perceive. In accommodating visual deficits, the clinician should explore the colors that are easily perceived by the individual and those that are difficult. Background colors, for most people, should be muted soft colors that do not produce a strong visual response. Icons and letters, on the other hand, may be represented in colors that provide visual contrast with the background. Very bright or strident colors should be avoided in both cases, and the specific colors and contrast levels required by the user must be selected on an individual basis.

Image size. Visual acuity and display size present difficulties in output displays that closely mirror the issues that ROM and fine motor skills present in keyboard design. In most cases, a person with 20/20 vision can easily read text that is presented in letters about 1/6 inch high (equivalent to a page printed in a 12-point font). On a typical display, this allows the presentation of between 100 and 150 words of text at a time or a similar number of icons for selection. If the user has lower visual acuity or limited ability to process visual stimuli, the letter/icon size must be increased to accommodate that loss of acuity. Larger icons, however, require either fewer letters shown at a time or increased display size. For people with severe vision limitations, as with individuals with severe fine motor limitations, it would be impractical to display all choices at once.

Screen enlargement programs (Anson, 2001) typically overcome this limitation by enlarging only part of the screen at a time and moving the portion that is expanded to the area most likely of interest to the user. The visual effect is similar to viewing the screen through a magnifying glass that the user moves over the display. Most programs can be configured to follow the text insertion point, the mouse pointer, or other changes on the display. With all such programs, a serious weakness is navigation. When the user can see only a small portion of the screen at a time, the landmarks that are normally available to indicate the layout of the text on a page may be invisible because they are not in the field of view. To be usable by the client, a screen enlargement program must provide a means of orienting to the location on the screen.

AAC systems can accommodate the needs of a user with low visual acuity using precisely the same techniques used for the person with limited fine motor control. The keyboard of the device can be configured with fewer, larger keys, each of which has a larger symbol to represent its meaning. However, as with keyboards for those with physical limitations, the result is either fewer communication options or a more complex interface for the user. Also, these accommodations frequently do not adapt the size of the message composition display, which may be inaccessible to the user with vision limitations.

Speech Output. **Speech output** is a useful tool in two cases: (1) when it replaces voice for a person with a disability and (2) when the user is not able to use vision to access the technology. AAC devices using voice provide the most normal face-to-face communication available. Able-bodied people, in most conditions, communicate by voice.

People with disabilities generally want to communicate in similar fashion. In voice output, the device communicates with the user using an auditory stimulus, converting printed words or commands into voice. Voice output technology has been in existence for much longer than voice input and is a more mature technology—not perfect, but more mature. The demands of voice output are different depending on the application and the intended listener. It is helpful to consider separately the systems where a second person is the listener and the systems where the user is the listener.

Second person as listener. Second person as listener systems substitute for speech when the user cannot be understood using normal speech. When used in AAC applications, voice output is almost always intended to be understood by a second person who may have little experience with synthetic voices. For example, if an AAC user is at the corner market

buying 2 lb of hamburger for dinner, the butcher is unlikely to have had much experience with a synthetic voice. When the AAC user is asking for directions on the street corner, the listener will face the additional challenge of hearing the AAC's voice over the sounds of trucks and buses.

To be understandable by novice listeners in real-world environments, a synthetic voice should be clear and as humanlike as possible. The voice will be easily understood to the extent that it sounds like what the listener expects to hear. Ideally the voice should provide appropriate inflection in the spoken material and should be able to convey emotional content. Current AAC systems do not convey emotional content well, but high-end voices sound much like a human speaker. Under adverse conditions they will remain less understandable than a human speaker because facial and lip movements (which provide additional cues as to the sounds being produced) do not accompany synthetic voices.

User as listener. When used for computer access or EADL, voice quality need not be as humanlike. In either case, the user has the opportunity to learn to understand the voice in training. In EADL applications, there will be relatively few utterances that must be produced, and they can be designed to sound as different from each other as possible so that there is little chance of confusion. General voice output for an entire language is somewhat more difficult, however, because many words sound similar and are easily confused.

For general text reading, however, the primary issue is voicing speed. As noted earlier, humans generally produce between 150 and 175 wpm. However, most humans also read between 300 and 400 wpm. A person who depends on a human-sounding voice for reading printed material will be limited to reading at less than half the speed of able-bodied readers. To be an effective text access method, synthetic voice must be understandable at speeds in excess of 400 wpm. This will obviously require significant training because untrained people without disabilities cannot understand speech at such speeds. However, with training, speech output is a useful way for a person with a vision limitation to access printed material.

Another application of voice output is eyes-free control. In the mass market for able-bodied consumers, these applications include presenting information over the telephone while driving or in other settings where a visual display might be difficult to use. These situations are important for people with disabilities as well. In addition, ATs using voice output may be intended for use by people with print impairments. The category of print impairment includes conditions that result in low vision and/or blindness, as well as conditions that result in the inability to translate visual stimuli to language and those that make manipulation of printed materials difficult.

Voice output technologies are problematic for people who are developing language skills. Because English is an irregular language, with many letter combinations making similar sounds, it is almost impossible to learn spelling by listening to the sound of words. Children who are blind from birth may not be good candidates for speech output as the primary language access method because the structure of words is lost when converted to speech. For these children, and for many

CASE STUDY
Mary, Part 2

Now that Mary, from the chapter-opening case study, has her AT, she must be trained to use it. As with all aspects of occupational therapy, her training should focus on meaningful activities. When Mary is using aids that are intended to allow her to write, she should use them to write. Initially, sending email to friends is a good activity because it is highly engaging, is not rate dependent, and friends are likely to be forgiving of misspellings. When Mary is using her EADL device, she should use it to control lights as it gets dark, to turn the television to her preferred channel, and to adjust the volume as needed. The hardest task for the clinician training Mary is to refrain from helping when Mary is able to perform the task, although with difficulty.

1. Success in an AT intervention is determined by Mary's ability to perform tasks independently. Can she write a paper for her professor within the allotted time? Can she control the lights, furnace, and entertainment devices in her home? Can she communicate with friends? One of the best indicators of success is when Mary expands her ambitions. This tells the clinician that, for Mary, the range of what is possible has expanded.

2. The AT will not make tasks as easy as they are for her able-bodied peers. Tasks will still be more difficult but not impossible. AT does not guarantee success. It can, and does, give Mary the chance to succeed. Whether or not she does succeed depends on her drive, her innate capabilities, and her belief in herself. Once AT has made it possible for Mary to succeed, it is the job of the therapist to help her believe that she can.

others, tactile access is a better tool and is in fact mandated under the Individuals With Disabilities Education Act (IDEA) (Tegic Communications, 2001).

Tactile Output. The oldest method for individuals with vision deficits to access printed material is Braille. In 1829, Louis Braille developed the idea of adapting a military system that allowed writing secret messages and aiming artillery in darkness to provide a method of reading for students at the National Institute for the Young Blind in Paris (Canadian National Institute for the Blind, 2004). Over time, this original system has been extended to allow communication of music, mathematics, and computer code to readers without vision (**tactile output**). Basic Braille uses an array of six dots to represent letters and numbers. Traditional Braille, however, is usable only for static text such as printed books. Dynamic information cannot be represented by raised dots on a sheet of paper.

Technology access requires the use of refreshable Braille. Refreshable Braille displays use a set of piezoelectric pins to represent Braille letters. Changing electrical signals to the display moves the pins up and down, allowing a single display to represent different portions of a longer document.

Braille is not widely used among individuals who are blind (Canadian National Institute for the Blind, 2004). By some estimates, only 10% of the blind population know and use Braille. It is not usable by those who have limited tactile sensation in addition to blindness. However, Braille is a skill that probably should be taught to a person who is blind and has good tactile discrimination. Most Braille readers are employed. Most people who are blind but do not read Braille are not employed. Although Braille may not be an essential skill for employment, the ability to learn Braille certainly correlates with the ability to hold a job (Canadian National Institute for the Blind, 2004).

SUMMARY

The OT practitioner must remember that although disability makes few things impossible, it does make many things harder, and some sufficiently hard that they are not worth the effort. ATs can make many things easier for the person with a disability. Because ATs make them easier, many activities that were previously not worth the effort can become reasonable for a person with a disability. ATs will never, in the terminology of the model of disability, remove the functional limitation. They can, however, allow engagement in occupation despite the functional limitation.

The key issue in all ATs is whether the individual is more able to perform desired tasks using the AT than without it. In many cases, an AT device that is provided for a specific task will have little utility in other tasks. This is not a new concept for OTs. A built-up handle toothbrush makes brushing teeth easier, but a different device is necessary for brushing hair. In the same manner, an AT that is intended to allow a student to keep up on homework assignments may not be appropriate or adequate for chatting with friends online. The technology must match the task and must allow the individual to perform the task at a higher level with it than without it. At the current state of the art, however, ATs cannot fully compensate for disability. Most tasks will still be hard, and some small number may not be worth the effort. The OT practitioner who uses an interactive, collaborative, client-centered approach to consider AT solutions is likely to achieve the optimum result in terms of engagement in occupation.

REVIEW QUESTIONS

1. Compare and contrast rehabilitative and assistive technologies.
2. In what way do devices using universal design assist individuals with disabilities? Why are they not considered to be ATs?
3. According to the human interface assessment model, why might a person with a disability not require any ATs in the completion of some tasks?
4. In pediatric applications, complex EADL devices might not be considered appropriate. What sort of EADL might be used with a very young child?

5. Some EADL devices allow control of the features of devices in the environment. Discuss the benefit of providing such control. What additional load does this place on the user?

6. AAC devices can be used to provide alternative or augmentative communication. Discuss the difference between these two strategies. Might an AAC device be a rehabilitation technology in some applications?

7. What is the value of having a message composition area that is independent from the message transmission feature of an AAC device? Discuss the value for the communicator and for the communication partner.

8. How does a language disorder differ from a communication disorder? What sort of AAC device would help a person with a language disorder?

9. Consider the keypad providing control to a microwave oven. How might the keypad present difficulty to an individual who is blind? How might it be modified by an OT to improve its usability?

10. Word prediction and word completion are often touted as means to improve typing speed, yet the research suggests that they do not. What advantage might these technologies offer to improve productivity for a person with a disability?

11. Abbreviation expansion is generally considered as a means to type long words and phrases with only a few keystrokes, though this requires the user to remember the abbreviation. How else can this technology be used for individuals with learning disabilities, in ways that do not require memorization of keystroke sequences?

12. Refreshable Braille is expensive, whereas text to speech is inexpensive. Yet Braille training is mandated by IDEA. What factors support the learning of this old technology for individuals who are blind?

REFERENCES

American Occupational Therapy Association Inc. (2014). *Occupational Therapy Practice Framework: Domain and Process* (3rd ed.). Bethesda, MD: AOTA Press.

Anson, D. (1988). Environmental control. In: J. G. Webster (Ed.), *Encyclopedia of Medical Devices and Instrumentation.* (Vol. 3). Hoboken, NJ: John Wiley & Sons (pp. 211–215).

Anson, D. (1993). The effect of word prediction on typing speed. *American Journal of Occupational Therapy, 47*(11), 1039–1042.

Anson, D. (1997). *Alternative Computer Access: A Guide to Selection.* Philadelphia, PA: FA Davis.

Anson, D. (2001). The future of computer access. *American Journal of Occupational Therapy, 55,* 106–108.

Anson, D. (2006). Environmental Control. In J. G. Webster's (Ed.). *Encyclopedia of Medical Devices and Instrumentation* (3rd ed.). Hoboken, NJ: John Willey & Sons.

Anson, D., Ames, C., Fulton, L., Margolis, M., Miller, M. (2004). Patterns for life: a study of young children's ability to use patterned switch closures for environmental control. <http://atri.misericordia.edu/Papers/Patterns.php>.

Anson, D., Eck, C., King, J., Mooney, R., Sansom, C., Wilkerson, B., Cychulis D. (2001). Efficacy of alternate keyboard configurations: Dvorak vs. reverse-QWERTY. <http://atri.misericordia.edu/Papers/Dvorak.php>.

Anson, D., George, S., Galup, R., Shea, B., & Vetter, R. (2001). Efficiency of the Chubon versus the QWERTY keyboard. *Assist Technology, 13*(1), 40–45.

Anson, D., Glodek, M., Peiffer, R. M., Rubino, C. G., Schwartz, P. T. Long-term speed and accuracy of Morse code vs. head-pointer interface for text generation. Paper presented at the RESNA 2004 Annual Conference, Orlando, Florida.

Anson, D., Moist, P., Przywara, M., Wells, H., Saylor, H., Maxime, H. The effects of word completion and word prediction on typing rates using on-screen keyboards assistive technology. In Press.

asiHome, 36 Gumbletown Rd CS1, Paupack PA 18451, phone: 800-263-8608, http://www.asihome.com/cgi-bin/ASIstore.pl?user_action=detail&catalogno=X10PEX01.

Assistive Technology Act of 1998. Pub. L. No. S. 2432 (1998).

Assistive Technology Act of 2004. Pub. L. No. HR 4278 (October 25, 2004).

Barnes, M. P. (1994). Environmental control systems—an audit and review. *Clinical Rehabilitation, 8,* 326–366.

Canadian National Institute for the Blind. Braille Information Center. Website. <https://cnib.ca/en/search/node?keys=braille%20information&region=gta>.

Center for Assistive Technology. Environmental control units. Website. <http://cat.buffalo.edu/newsletters/ecu.php>.

Center for Universal Design. What is universal design? Principles of UD. <https://projects.ncsu.edu/ncsu/design/cud/about_ud/about_ud.htm>.

Conti, B. Semantic compaction systems—the home of Minspeak. <https://minspeak.com/about/>.

Cook, A. M., & Hussey, S. M. (2001). *Assistive Technologies: Principles and Practice* (2nd ed.). Philadelphia, PA: Mosby International.

DeVries, R. C., Deitz, J., Anson, D., et al. (1998). A comparison of two computer access systems for functional text entry. *American Journal of Occupational Therapy, 52*(8), 656–665.

Dragon Systems, Inc., 320 Nevada Street, Newton, MA 02460, phone: +1-617-965-5200, fax: +1-617-965-2374.

DynaVox Systems LLC., 2100 Wharton Street, Suite 400, Pittsburgh, PA 15203, phone: 1-800-344-1778. http://www.dynavoxsys.com.

Efthimiou, J., Gordon, W. A., Sell, G. H., & Stratford, C. (1981). Electronic assistive devices: their impact on the quality of life of high-level quadriplegic persons. *Archives of Physical Medicine and Rehabilitation, 62,* 131–134.

Fong Lee, D. (1995). Alternative keyboards. *Canadian Journal of Occupational Therapists, 62,* 175.

Gibler, C. D., & Childress, D. S. (1982). Language anticipation with a computer-based scanning communication aid. Paper presented at the IEEE Computer Society Workshop on Computing to the Handicapped, Charlottesville, Virginia.

Glennen, S. L., & DeCoste, D. C. (1996). *The Handbook of Augmentative and Alternative Communication.* San Diego, CA: Singular Publishing Group.

Hunnicutt, S., & Carlberger, J. (2001). Improving word prediction using Markov models and heuristic methods. *Augmentative and Alternative Communication, 17,* 255–264.

Intellitools. Number concepts 2. <https://abledata.acl.gov/product/intellitools-classroom-suite>.

Interactive MaM. The Dvorak keyboard. <http://www.maxmon.com/1936ad.htm>.

Jarus, T. (1994). Learning Morse code in rehabilitation: visual, auditory, or combined method? *British Journal of Occupational Therapy, 57,* 127—130.

Kincaid, C. (1999). Alternative keyboards. *Except Parent, 2,* 34—35.

King, T. W. (1999). *Modern Morse Code in Rehabilitation and Education: New Applications in Assistive Technology.* Boston, MA: Allyn and Bacon.

Koester, H. H. Word prediction—when does it enhance text entry rate? Paper presented at the RESNA 2002, Minneapolis, Minnesota.

Koester, H. H. Abandonment of speech recognition by new users. Paper presented at the RESNA 26th International Annual Conference 2003, Atlanta Georgia.

Koester, H. H., & Levine, S. P. (1996). Effect of a word prediction feature on user performance. *Augmentative and Alternative Communication, 12,* 155—168.

Lloyd, L. L., Fuller, D. R., et al. (1996). *Augmentative and Alternative Communication: A Handbook of Principles and Practices.* Boston, MA: Allyn and Bacon.

MacArthur, C. A. (1998). Word processing with speech synthesis and word prediction: effects on the dialogue journal writing of students with learning disabilities. *Learning Disability Quarterly, 21,* 1—16.

MacNeil, V. (1998). Electronic aids to daily living. *Team Rehab Rep, 9*(3), 53—56.

McDonald, D. W., Boyle, M. A., & Schumann, T. L. (1989). Environmental control unit utilization by high-level spinal cord injured patients. *Archives of Physical Medicine and Rehabilitation, 70,* 621—623.

McDonald JB, Schwejda P, Marriner NA, Wilson WR, Ross AM. (1982). *Advantages of Morse Code as a Computer Input for School Aged Children with Physical Disabilities. Computers and the Handicapped.* Ottawa, Canada: National Research Council of Canada.

Merzenich, M., Jenkins, W., Johnston, P., Schreiner, C., Miller, S., & Tallal, P. (1996). Temporal processing deficits of language-learning impaired children ameliorated by training. *Science, 271,* 77—81.

Miller, G. A. (1981). *Language and Speech.* San Francisco, CA: Freeman.

Neighborhood Legal Services. Commission for the Blind and Visually Handicapped. CBVH manual, rehabilitation technology 8.20. <https://ocfs.ny.gov/main/cb/>.

Newell, A. F., Arnott, J., Booth, L., Beattie, W., Brophy, B., & Ricketts, I. W. (1992). Effect of "PAL" word prediction system on the quality and quantity of text generation. *Augmentative and Alternative Communication, 8,* 304—311.

Quartet Technology, Inc., 87 Progress Avenue, Tyngsboro, MA 01879, phone: 1.978.649.4328.

Quartet Technology. Frequently asked questions. <https://qtiusa.com/contact-form7/faq/>.

Quartet Technology. News. <https://qtiusa.com/products/>.

Smarthome, Inc. 16542 Millikan Avenue, Irvine, CA 92606-5027, phone: (949) 221-9200 x109.

Struck, M. (1999). Focus on. One handed keyboarding options. *OT Practice, 4,* 55—56.

Tallal, P., Miller, S., Bedi, G., Byma, G., Wang, X., Nagarajan, S., et al. (1996). Language comprehension in language-learning impaired children improved with acoustically modified speech. *Science, 271,* 81—84.

Tam, C., Reid, D., Naumann, S., & O'Keefe, B. (2002). Effects of word prediction and location of word prediction lists on text entry with children with spina bifida and hydrocephalus. *Augmentative and Alternative Communication, 18,* 147—162.

Tash Inc., 3512 Mayland Ct., Richmond, VA 23233, phone: 1-800-463-5685 or (905)686-4129, <http://www.tashinc.com>.

Tegic Communications, 2001 Western Avenue, Suite 250, Seattle, WA 98121, <https://www.nuance.com/index.html>.

Trumbull, M. (1995). Dvorak keyboard layout makes comeback 60 years later. *Christian Science Monitor, 87,* 9.

Williams, S. C. (2002). How speech feedback and word prediction software can help students write. *Teach Except Child, 34*(3), 72—78.

Zecevic, A., Miller, D., & Harburn, K. (2000). An evaluation of the ergonomics of three computer keyboards. *Ergonomics, 43,* 18—22.

Zordell, J. (1990). The use of word prediction and spelling correction software with mildly handicapped students. *Closing Gap, 9*(1), 10—11.

15

Moving in the Environment

Amanda K. Giles

OBJECTIVES

After reading this chapter, the student or the occupational therapy practitioner will be able to do the following:

1. Define functional ambulation.
2. Discuss the roles of the occupational therapist and occupational therapy assistant in functional ambulation.
3. Identify appropriate interventions to promote functional ambulation within occupational therapy treatment.
4. Identify safety issues in functional ambulation.
5. Recognize basic lower extremity orthotics, prosthetics, and ambulatory assistive devices.
6. List the advantages and disadvantages of power chairs and their options for wheelbase, seating system, control options, and access device.
7. Understand the factors considered during wheelchair evaluation, wheelchair measurement, and prescription completion.
8. Identify wheelchair safety considerations.
9. Follow guidelines for proper body mechanics.
10. Apply principles of proper body positioning.
11. Identify the steps necessary in performing various transfer techniques.
12. Identify considerations necessary to determine the appropriate transfer method based on the patient's clinical presentation.
13. List the elements of a driving evaluation.
14. Describe the contribution of occupational therapy to the assessment of the disabled individual's driving.

KEY TERMS

Section I. Functional Ambulation
Functional ambulation
Pathologic gait
Gait training
Ankle-foot orthosis (AFO)
Foot drop
Knee-ankle-foot orthosis (KAFO)
Ambulatory assistive device
Prosthesis
Section II. Wheelchair Selection and Evaluation
Skin breakdown
Rehabilitation technology supplier (RTS)
Assistive Technology Professional (ATP)
Seating and Mobility Specialist (SMS)
Complex rehabilitation technology supplier (CRTS)
Medical necessity
Manual chair frame
Push handle
Armrest
Leg rest
Foot plate
Mag wheel
Spoke wheel
Handrim

Recline
Tilt-in-space
Manual power assist
Power chair
Front-wheel drive
Mid-wheel drive
Rear-wheel drive
Proportional control
Nonproportional control
Joystick
Section III. Bed Mobility and Transfers
Body mechanics
Stand pivot transfer
Squat pivot transfer
One-person dependent transfer
Two-person dependent transfer
Transfer board
Mechanical lift
Section IV. Importance of Driving and Community Mobility
Driving evaluation
Clinical evaluation
Pre-driving tasks
Driving cessation
Community mobility

INTRODUCTION

The basic capacities to move within the environment, to reach objects of interest, to explore one's surroundings, and to come and go at will are considered universal and customary abilities for most people. For persons with disabilities, however, mobility is rarely taken for granted or considered automatic. A disability may prevent one from being able to walk to the bathroom, ascend the stairs to a bedroom, or operate the controls on a motor vehicle.

Safe and successful movement requires the integration of multiple sensorimotor, cognitive, perceptual, and psychosocial abilities; therefore breakdown in just one area can affect function. Cardiopulmonary conditions may limit aerobic capacity and endurance, requiring frequent rest breaks and prioritization of activities. Deficits in motor coordination may limit activities that require a combination of mobility (e.g., walking or moving in the environment) and stability (e.g., holding the hands steady as one must when carrying a cup of coffee or a watering can). Lack of depth perception and visual acuity impairments can slow mobility, even in individuals with conscious awareness of deficits. Visual field and visual processing deficits can impose safety risks when moving in congested, uneven, or unfamiliar environments. Safe sequencing of transfers requires the cognitive ability to learn and retain new information. Generally speaking, the more complex the environment, the greater the demand is on all performance components.

Occupational therapists (OTs) and occupational therapy assistants (OTAs) help individuals with mobility restrictions to achieve maximum access to environments and objects of interest to them. Clinicians at both levels must analyze the activities and environments most difficult for their clients and select the appropriate remedial or compensatory treatment approach. They must effectively communicate and collaborate with the client, caregivers, and the medical team, including the physical therapist (PT) and physical therapy assistant (PTA). Further, they must use clinical reasoning and expertise to anticipate any future changes that may arise given an individual's medical history, prognosis, and developmental status. The OTA should always discuss any change in status, progression or lack of progression, the need for goal revisions, and plans for continuation or discharge with the OT. With additional hours of specialty training and experience, the OT, OTA, PT, and PTA have the option to gain additional specialty certification through demonstrated competence in selecting, measuring, and instructing in the use of mobility devices.

The rest of this chapter will speak directly to the role of the OTA in functional mobility with the understanding that the OT and OTA are working in collaboration. Four main topics will be explored:

1. The first section addresses functional ambulation, the act of walking for a purposeful and meaningful outcome, which may necessitate the use of orthotics, prosthetics, and/or ambulatory assistive devices such as canes, crutches, and walkers.
2. The second section concerns wheelchair selection and measurement, including the key features of manual and power chairs.
3. The third section focuses on how to facilitate safe and efficient transfers to and from the wheelchair using proper body mechanics and equipment when necessary.
4. The fourth section covers community mobility, the act of getting from one place to another via private or public transportation (e.g., bike, car, bus, train).

Improving and maintaining the functional mobility of persons with disabilities can be one of the most gratifying practice areas in the profession. Consumers experience tremendous energy and empowerment when they can access and explore broader and more interesting environments.

SECTION I. FUNCTIONAL AMBULATION

FUNCTIONAL AMBULATION

Functional ambulation, a subcomponent of functional mobility, is "the ability to walk, with or without the aid of appropriate assistive devices (such as canes or walkers), safely and sufficiently to carry out mobility-related activities of daily living (ADLs)" (Heart and Stroke Foundation of Canada, date). Functional ambulation is a self-identified goal for many clients because it supports the achievement of functional outcomes such as carrying a plate to the table or carrying groceries from the car to the house. If the individual is using an ambulatory assistive device and simultaneously has a need to carry an object, goal completion becomes significantly more complex, if not impossible. Functional ambulation may be difficult for individuals after lower extremity (LE) amputation, cerebrovascular accident, acquired brain injury, total hip replacement, etc. The OTA works in collaboration with the PT to increase functional ambulation, including assessing, adapting, and modifying the home or other environments to facilitate participation in everyday activities, community mobility, and return to work.

BASICS OF AMBULATION

"Walking not only involves the ability to move the legs, but also requires the intricate coordination of neural commands to regulate upright balance and posture and the ability to adapt gait to environmental constraints" (Lam, Noonan, & Eng, 2008). The gait cycle is the repetitive pattern used when walking and consists of a stance phase (the period in which weight is shifted onto one leg while the opposite leg swings) and a swing phase (the period in which the leg bearing weight lifts off the ground and swings forward to contact the ground in front). Individuals may exhibit **pathologic gait** because of biomechanical or neurophysiologic deficits. Problems noted may include decreased walking velocity, decreased weight bearing, increased swing time of the affected LE, or an abnormal base of support. Functional deficits may include unsafe ambulation and insufficient energy to achieve a desired outcome. Depending on the cause of the gait problem, orthotics and/or ambulation aids may be recommended. It is important that the OTA communicates with the PT to reinforce consistent **gait training** recommendations during treatment.

DEVICES USED DURING AMBULATION

Lower Extremity Orthotics

For individuals with abnormal posture of the ankle, an **ankle-foot orthosis (AFO)** may be recommended. An AFO is an external device commonly made of lightweight thermoplastic splinting material and applied to the ankle area to protect or compensate for joint instability and/or weakness (Anderson, Anderson, & Glanze, 2002). The traditional AFO is rigid and supports a fixed dorsiflexed position as a means to prevent **foot drop**, the inability to lift the toes and clear the ground during stepping. The downside of the rigid AFO is that it also locks the ankle in plantar flexion, which prevents the user from shifting weight forward and unlocking the knee at the appropriate time. New dynamic AFOs are now available that allow the user to push off, or plantar flex, and consequently improve the quality of the gait pattern. Common diagnoses that may result in the use of an AFO include cerebral palsy, acquired brain injury, stroke, and multiple sclerosis.

For individuals with knee collapse or hyperextension, an external means of knee control such as a **knee-ankle-foot orthosis (KAFO)** may be recommended. A KAFO includes offset knee joints combined with a rigid AFO (Esquenazi & Hirai, 1995). Similar to the AFO, KAFOs are traditionally rigid and lock the knee in a fixed position; however, newer models allow the user to lock and unlock the knee at the appropriate phase in the gait cycle. Common diagnoses that may result in the use of a KAFO include muscular dystrophy and spinal cord injury.

The LE orthotic is typically recommended by the PT in collaboration with the orthotist and then custom fabricated, if necessary, by the orthotist. The OTA's role is to promote the client's independence in everyday activities while using and managing the orthotic. For example, the occupational therapy treatment goals may state, "Client will don and doff the RLE (right lower extremity) AFO independently" or "Client will ambulate from sink to BSC (bedside commode) with mod A (moderate assistance) using KAFO and walker." Of note, the orthotic should be worn over a cotton sock, donned in a seated position, snugly fastened, and worn with a shoe. If balance is impaired, the use of a LE orthotic may be combined with the use of an **ambulatory assistive device**, such as a cane, crutch, or a walker.

Lower Extremity Prosthetics

For individuals with LE amputation, a prosthetic limb may be recommended to improve function and/or cosmetic appearance. A LE **prosthesis** provides an artificial joint(s) above or below the knee, depending on the length of the available residual limb. A variety of suspension systems are available to

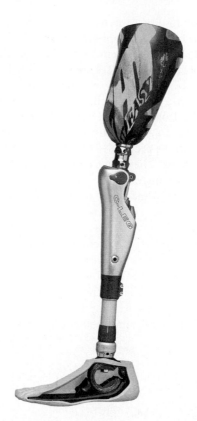

Fig. 15.1 Components of a lower extremity prosthesis. (From Black JM, et al. *Black's Medical-Surgical Nursing: Clinical Management for Positive Outcomes.* 1st ed. India: Elsevier; 2009.)

connect the residual limb, including a gel liner with locking mechanism, a harness system with a strap or belt, or more commonly, a suction apparatus that creates an airtight seal (Fig. 15.1). Advances in technology have allowed modern prostheses to be equipped with more realistic, lighter weight, and stronger materials as well as updated sensor technology and microprocessors that allow the prosthesis to adapt automatically to specific tasks and environmental conditions.

The LE prosthetic is typically recommended by the PT in collaboration with the prosthetist and then custom fabricated by the prosthetist. Similar to orthotics, the OTA's role is to promote the client's independence in everyday activities while using and managing the prosthesis. For example, the occupational therapy treatment goals may state, "Client will doff LE (lower extremity) prosthesis independently while seated in preparation for bathing" or "Client will transfer into the passenger side of car with supervision while wearing prosthesis." Of note, a liner or sleeve may be worn under the prosthesis as a protective cover and flexible cushioning to reduce the risk of skin breakdown. If balance is impaired, the use of a LE prosthesis may be combined with the use of an ambulatory assistive device(s).

Ambulatory Assistive Devices

Ambulatory assistive devices, such as crutches, canes, and walkers, may be recommended for use during ambulation to compensate for impaired balance, decreased strength, non-weightbearing status on one LE, pain during weight bearing on one or both LEs, and/or absence of a LE. Common diagnoses that result in the use of an ambulatory assistive device include LE fracture, amputation, stroke, acquired brain injury, knee or hip replacement, and Parkinson disease.

Ambulatory assistive devices are numerous. Basic devices, from those providing the most support to the least, are a walker, crutches, a single crutch, bilateral canes, and a single cane (Pezenik, Itoh, & Lee, 1984). The client may begin ambulation with a device that provides maximal support or stability and then be progressed to a device that provides less support or stability. The OTA's communication with the PT is essential to keeping abreast of any changes in the client's ambulation device(s) and/or the use of the device(s).

Walkers. The walker is the most common device used during the early stages of gait training because it provides the most stability. A walker can be used to restrict weight bearing after LE fracture. A walker can be folded for storage, but it is still large and bulky and can make navigating small spaces difficult.

A variety of options exist for walkers (Fig. 15.2): (1) The standard walker offers the most stability in standing (Figs. 15.3),

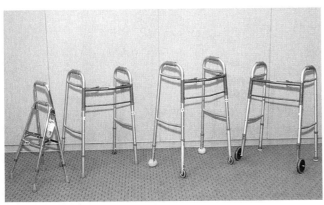

Fig. 15.2 A variety of walkers. (From Fairchild SL. *Pierson and Fairchild's Principles & Techniques of Patient Care.* 5th ed. St Louis, MO: Saunders; 2013.)

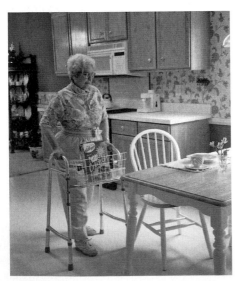

Fig. 15.3 Functional ambulation with a walker and walker basket.

(2) the rolling or front wheeled walker is the most common and allows for a more normal gait pattern, (3) the rollator provides a seat for those who fatigue easily, and (4) the platform walker can be used for clients who cannot bear weight through the wrist or hands (Giles & Kraft, 2020).

Crutches. Crutches offer an advantage over the walker because they allow increased variability of gait patterns and can be used on stairs. Crutches can also be used to restrict weight bearing but require more advanced motor planning than the walker. Crutches limit the use of hands for functional activities and pose a risk to axillary nerves and vessels with improper use. Two crutches or one crutch may be used depending on the client's needs.

Axillary crutches are the most common type of crutch in the United States and are typically lightweight aluminum (Fig. 15.4). Forearm or Lofstrand crutches allow more dynamic movement and control in small spaces but require more trunk stability than axillary crutches (see Fig. 15.4) (Giles & Kraft, 2020).

Canes. The cane typically fits easily in tight spaces and allows the most environmental freedom (Fig. 15.5). However, it is the least stable, requires weight bearing, and promotes asymmetry with improper use. Two canes or one cane may be used depending on the client's needs.

A standard cane allows the most freedom of movement (Fig. 15.6). A quad cane offers additional stability with four points of contact with the ground but results in a slower gait pattern (see Fig. 15.6) (Giles & Kraft, 2020).

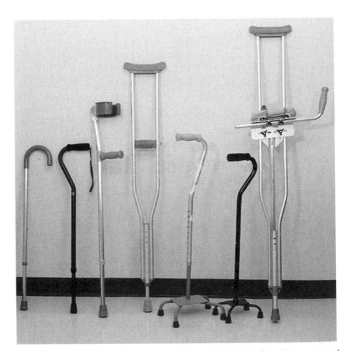

Fig. 15.4 A variety of crutches. (From Fairchild SL. *Pierson and Fairchild's Principles & Techniques of Patient Care.* 5th ed. St Louis, MO: Saunders; 2013.)

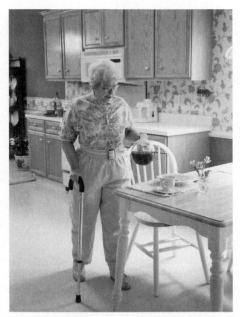

Fig. 15.5 Functional ambulation with a straight cane.

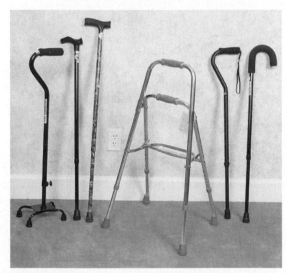

Fig. 15.6 A variety of canes. (From Fairchild SL. *Pierson and Fairchild's Principles & Techniques of Patient Care.* 5th ed. St Louis, MO: Saunders; 2013.)

TECHNIQUES FOR INSTRUCTION AND SAFETY

Preparation for Ambulation

Before beginning functional ambulation training, the OTA should review the medical record for the client's current status and precautions. As part of this review, the OTA should confer with the PT regarding the client's current ambulatory status, endurance level, gait techniques, and potential equipment needs (ambulation aids, orthosis, or prosthesis) (Table 15.1). With this information in mind, the OTA can plan ahead and prepare for the unexpected. If the client fatigues easily, it may be helpful to have a wheelchair, chair, or stool readily available for use as needed. Additional layers of prosthetic socks may be added to achieve proper fit. If the

client's abilities are unknown or unpredictable, the OTA may need to bring a wheelchair or assistive device in case the activity proves to be too difficult.

To prepare for functional ambulation, the client should wear safe and appropriate footwear, such as well-fitting nonskid shoes. Socks and slippers should be avoided. Nonslip hospital socks should be worn in the absence of shoes. A gait belt should be utilized in anticipation of possible fall risk (Fig. 15.7). To decrease anxiety, the client should be given clear instructions and expectations prior to starting ambulation.

Safety During Ambulation

During functional ambulation on a level surface, the OTA should be positioned slightly behind and to one side of the client. In most cases, it is preferable to guard on the client's involved or weaker side; however, when maneuvering in a small space (e.g., a bathroom), the OTA should stand on the side that causes the least obstacles. The OTA should grasp the gait belt with the inside arm (closest to the client), leaving the outermost hand free to assist with the functional activity and/or to give physical cues for standing upright. In some cases, the OTA may need to facilitate ambulation with both hands on the client's hips to cue weight shifts and directional movements. During ambulation, the OTA should move with (in the same direction as) the client. The OTA's outermost lower extremity should move forward with the ambulation device.

When guiding the client up the stairs, the OTA should stand slightly behind the client on the side opposite the railing. When guiding the client down the stairs, the OTA should stand slightly in front of the patient on the side opposite the railing. If using a cane or crutches, the client should step up with the unaffected leg first, leaving the opposite leg and assistive device to follow. When descending, the client should step down with the affected leg and assistive device together followed by the unaffected leg (Giles & Kraft, 2020).

The OTA should be aware of diagnosis-specific precautions and respond appropriately. Physiologic responses should be monitored and documented, including a change in breathing patterns, perspiration, reddened skin, a change in mental status, and decreased responsiveness. The OTA must not leave the client unattended during functional ambulation. The OTA should be certain that the environment is free of any potential risks or safety hazards such as obstacles and wet floors. Box 15.1 summarizes these important points.

THE ROLE OF OCCUPATIONAL THERAPY IN AMBULATION TRAINING

Functional ambulation may be incorporated during activities of daily living (ADL), work and productive activities, and play or leisure activities. Using an occupation-based treatment approach, the OTA should consider the client's abilities within the context of a meaningful activity. Further, the OT must analyze the relationship of the environment to the client's abilities and preferred task(s). During activity

TABLE 15.1   Functional Mobility Analysis

SITUATION: 53-YEAR-OLD HOMEMAKER WITH ANKLE AMPUTATION AMBULATING WITH A CANE

Task Analysis Approach	Example
1. Identify the task(s) and specify the long-term (LTG) and short-term (STG) goals.	Task: Meal preparation; LTG: To prepare meal for family; STG: To prepare muffins from a mix
2. Gather necessary information concerning the following:	Necessary information specific to this client includes the following:
a. The action, including classification of the action and the movement	What motor skills are needed for this activity? What is the client's endurance level?
b. The environment, including the influence of both direct and indirect conditions	What are the environmental conditions for conducting this task? What supplies, people, and setting are required?
c. The client, including his or her interests and abilities and whether the minimal prerequisite skills for success are present	What information is known about the client? Interests and activities? What are the strengths and weaknesses from the occupational therapy assessment?
d. The prerequisite skills or performance components required of the client	What performance components are needed for functional ambulation to successfully bake muffins?
e. The expectations of outcome and movement	*Client successfully will bake muffins while ambulating with cane.*
3. Develop a strategy to make up for any deficits identified in step 2.	Strategy: What adaptations will be necessary to accommodate availability of unilateral upper extremity to carry supplies because of use of an ambulation aid?
4. Plan the intervention strategy based on the preceding information concerning the individual-activity-environment interaction.	*Arrange supplies on countertop near oven to limit need for long distances of ambulation while carrying objects; use countertop or wheeled cart to transport bowls, pans, and other items.*
5. Effect the strategy.	Implement the task with the client.
a. Observe task and performance of the patients.	Observe and record outcomes.
b. Record what happened: What was the outcome and what was the approach and effect of the movement solution?	
6. Evaluate the observation.	*Evaluate whether the client was successful in baking muffins.*
a. Compare expectations and what happened.	Provide feedback to the client.
b. Provide feedback based on the comparison above and assist the patient in making decisions about the next attempt.	Plan next activity with client.
c. With the client, plan the next activity.	

Data from Higgins JR, Higgins S. The acquisition of locomotor skill. In Craik RL, Oatis CA, eds. *Gait Analysis: Theory and Application.* St Louis, MO: Mosby; 1995.

analysis, the OTA asks the following questions: (1) What role(s) does the client desire to perform? (2) What tasks does this role require of the client? (3) What client factors and/or performance skills are necessary for successful task completion? (4) Which one or more of those factors/skills are difficult for the client? (5) Is remediation of skills possible or are equipment and/or compensatory methods necessary? (6) How is the environment impacting function? (7) How might a change in the task or environmental demands alter performance? These questions are asked during the initial occupational therapy evaluation, but they should be revisited during treatment as the client progresses. The OTA is ultimately focused on achievement of confident, efficient, and safe functional ambulation during valued occupational roles and tasks.

FUNCTIONAL AMBULATION APPLICATION

Functional ambulation impairments invite creative problem solving from the OTA and the client. The following three

CASE 15.1

Betty: Kitchen Ambulation
Betty enjoys cooking meals for her family but struggles with maneuvering in the kitchen due to left hemiplegia from her recent stroke. For increased safety during ambulation, the PT recommended a quad cane to be held in Betty's right hand. The OTA teaches Betty to approach cabinet doors, drawers, the stove, and the refrigerator from the left to open them with her unaffected right extremity.

With assistance from the OTA, Betty ambulates with her quad cane to the left of the refrigerator and then assumes a wide base of support as she rests her cane on the ground and retrieves a tomato, lettuce, and turkey from the refrigerator. The OTA instructs Betty to transport food items to the sink by moving them along the countertop in progression. Betty stands as close as possible to the sink to wash the tomato and lettuce, then she sits on a tall stool at the counter to make her grandson a sandwich.

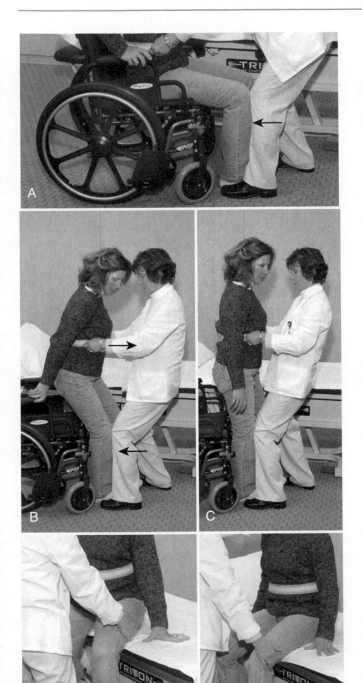

Fig. 15.7 Safe transfer with gait belt. (From Fairchild SL. *Pierson and Fairchild's Principles & Techniques of Patient Care.* 5th ed. St Louis, MO: Saunders; 2013.)

case studies provide examples of OTA intervention with specific functional ambulation activities in the kitchen, bathroom, and during home management. The OTA must use clinical judgment when applying these interventions to other cases.

CASE 15.2

John: Bathroom Ambulation

The most important goal for John is to manage his personal hygiene without having to hire a caregiver or rely on his wife. Due to his Parkinson disease, John has difficulty in safely ambulating to the sink, toilet, and bathtub. Due to the many risks associated with water and hard surfaces, the OTA educates John about dangerous tripping hazards, such as spills on the floor and loose bathmats.

During the treatment session, John uses his rolling walker to approach as close to the sink as possible to perform grooming and hygiene activities. The OTA stands to the side and slightly behind John while holding his gait belt. Since John's walker has a walker basket that prohibits him from positioning close to the sink, the OTA instructs him to cautiously maneuver the walker to one side and then carefully move forward toward the sink.

After brushing his teeth safely at the sink, John reassumes the walker and begins to ambulate toward the toilet with guidance. Since it is hard for John to perform more than one task at a time, the OTA intentionally stays quiet and allows John to focus on walking. When John gets stuck, the OTA cues him to stop, take a deep breath, stand tall, and start again. The OTA knows that it is safer to pivot the least distance possible to prevent John from losing his balance. Since John's toilet is to the left, the OTA cues him to pivot clockwise approximately 90 degrees upon approaching the toilet. (Note: If the toilet was on the right, he would have been cued to pivot counterclockwise.) The OTA stands on John's right side to stay out of his way. John has a bedside commode positioned over his toilet to raise the height of the seat and provide arm rests as support when sitting and standing.

Because John has a tub/shower combination, he must step over the tub to get into the shower, which is more difficult than a walk-in shower. While using his walker and cues from the OTA, John positions himself in a spot next to the tub that requires the least distance or extraneous movement for the tub transfer. (Note: This is the same technique when using any ambulatory assistive device.) The use of a grab bar and shower chair is recommended for John. If John was nonweightbearing on one or more limbs or unable to step into the shower safely, the OTA would recommend a tub transfer bench, which stretches over the tub so that the client can sit before transferring into the tub (Fig. 15.8).

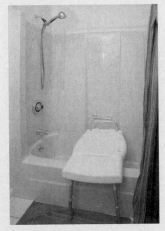

Fig. 15.8 Tub transfer bench. (From Kostelick C. *Mosby's Textbook for Long-Term Care Nursing Assistants.* 8th ed. St Louis, MO: Elsevier; 2019.)

1. Know the client (e.g., status, orthotics and aids, precautions).
2. Use appropriate footwear.
3. Clear potential hazards.
4. Monitor physiologic responses.
5. Guard by standing slightly behind and out to the side.
6. Use a gait belt in case of loss of balance.
7. Think ahead for the unexpected.
8. Do not leave the client unattended.

CASE 15.3

Sophia: Home Management Ambulation

Sophia is a stay-at-home mom whose primary need is to manage her home, including clothing care, cleaning, and household maintenance. Clothing care includes sorting, laundering, folding, and storing of clothing. Cleaning includes tidying up, vacuuming, sweeping and mopping floors, dusting, and making beds. Household maintenance includes maintaining the home, yard, garden, appliances, and vehicles. For all of these activities, Sophia needs assistance with functional ambulation due to her lower extremity amputation, even with her new prosthesis. As with any occupational therapy intervention, the OTA consults with Sophia first to determine the home management activity (or activities) that she most values.

Sophia's first goal is to make the bed. Since Sophia uses a cane during ambulation, the OTA encourages her to use one arm on the cane for stabilization while using the other arm to pull up sheets and bedcovers. The OTA takes extra caution to guard Sophia when she bends down and stands back up because her dynamic balance is more susceptible to falls.

Because Sophia is a gardener, her second goal is to maintain the yard. However, the uneven surface and obstacles with the yard make this especially difficult for Sophia. She requires more assistance from the OTA to carefully ambulate with her cane to her rose bushes on the other side of the yard. The OTA instructs Sophia to carry small yard tools (e.g., pruning shears and gloves) in a bag hung over her arm. While pruning her roses, Sophia sits on a gardening stool and moves it to the next location as the yard work progresses.

SUMMARY

Functional ambulation is the purposeful movement from one position or place to another. Gait training may be necessary for persons at any age with biomechanical and neurologic impairment. The OTA can incorporate functional ambulation during interventions related to ADL, work, and leisure activities as a means of maximizing independence. Successful outcomes depend on effective communication between all members of the health care team.

SECTION II. WHEELCHAIR SELECTION AND EVALUATION

When ambulation is impossible or impractical, a wheelchair can provide individuals with increased access to environments and occupations. A wheelchair can be the primary means of mobility for someone with a permanent or progressive disability such as cerebral palsy, brain injury, spinal cord injury, multiple sclerosis, or muscular dystrophy. A wheelchair may also be necessary as a temporary means of mobility for someone with a short-term illness or orthopedic problem. In addition to mobility, the wheelchair can substantially influence the total body positioning, skin integrity, overall function, and general well-being of the client.

Whether the client requires a temporary, noncustom rental wheelchair or a custom wheelchair for use over many years, an individualized prescription clearly outlining the specific features of the chair is necessary to ensure optimal performance, mobility, and function. A wheelchair that has been prescribed by an inexperienced or untrained person is potentially hazardous and costly to the client. An ill-fitting wheelchair can, in fact, contribute to unnecessary fatigue, **skin breakdown**, and trunk or extremity deformity and can inhibit function (Pezenik et al., 1984). A wheelchair is an extension of the patient's body and should act to facilitate rather than inhibit good alignment, mobility, and function (Box 15.2).

BOX 15.2 **Considerations in Recommendations for a Wheelchair**

Who will pay for the wheelchair?
Who will determine the preferred durable medical equipment provider—the insurance company, the patient, or the therapist?
What is the specific disability?
What is the prognosis?
Is range of motion limited?
Is strength or endurance limited?
How will the patient propel the chair?
How old is the patient?
How long is the patient expected to use the wheelchair?
What was the patient's lifestyle, and how has it changed?
Is the patient active or sedentary?
How will the dimensions of the chair affect the patient's ability to transfer to various surfaces?
What is the maneuverability of the wheelchair in the patient's home or in the community (e.g., entrances and egress, door width, turning radius in bathroom and hallways, floor surfaces)?
What is the ratio of indoor to outdoor activities?
Where will the wheelchair be primarily used—in the home, at school, at work, or in the community?
Which mode of transportation will be used? Will the patient be driving a van from the wheelchair? How will it be loaded and unloaded from the car?
Which special needs (e.g., work heights, available assistance, accessibility of toilet facilities, and parking facilities) are recognized in the work or school environment?
Does the patient participate in indoor or outdoor sports activities?
How will the wheelchair affect the patient psychologically?
Can accessories and custom modifications be medically justified, or are they luxury items?
What resources does the patient have for equipment maintenance (e.g., self, family, caregivers)?

WHEELCHAIR EVALUATION AND ORDERING PROCESS

The constant evolution of technology and variety of manufacturers' products make it helpful to have an experienced, knowledgeable, and certified specialist on the ordering team, particularly when the client's needs are complex. The OT or PT, depending on the respective role at a treatment facility, is usually responsible for evaluating, measuring, and selecting a wheelchair and seating system for the client. The OTA may be responsible for gathering information for the evaluation, communicating with suppliers and specialists, and teaching wheelchair safety and mobility skills to clients and their caregivers. OTAs with clinical experience and advanced training may assume some of the evaluation and measurement responsibilities in some settings, under local guidelines. The OTA may work closely with any of the following experts during the wheelchair selection and training process:

- **Rehabilitation technology supplier (RTS):** The RTS is a durable medical equipment (DME) supplier who is proficient in ordering custom items and can offer an objective and broad mechanical perspective on the availability and appropriateness of the options being considered. The RTS is the client's resource for insurance billing, repairs, and reordering when returning to the community (National Registry of Rehabilitation Technology Suppliers, 2020).
- **Assistive Technology Professional (ATP):** The ATP is a certified expert in selecting and instructing clients with disabilities in the use of all types of assistive technology, including wheelchair positioning devices, computer accessibility, vehicle and home modifications, and environmental control units. The ATP is an interprofessional certification that is open to OTs, OTAs, PTs, PTAs, RTSs, and others, but the amount of training and work experience required for achievement varies depending on one's education background (Rehabilitation Engineering and Assistive Technology Society of North America, 2020).
- **Seating and Mobility Specialist (SMS):** The SMS is a specialty certification for ATPs who work primarily on seating assessment and intervention (Rehabilitation Engineering and Assistive Technology Society of North America, 2020).
- **Complex rehabilitation technology supplier (CRTS):** The CRTS is an experienced ATP (minimum 3 years) who configures wheelchairs and seating systems for individuals with specific and unique needs (National Registry of Rehabilitation Technology Suppliers, 2020).

After specific measurements, modifications, and accessory needs have been determined, the wheelchair prescription is formally written as a letter of medical necessity (LMN). The LMN should be concise and specific so that everything requested can be accurately interpreted by the DME supplier, who will submit a sales contract for payment authorization. Payment may be denied if clear reasons are not given to substantiate the need for every item and modification requested. Before-and-after pictures can be helpful in illustrating **medical necessity**. Before the wheelchair is delivered to the patient, the chair should be checked against the specific prescription to ensure that all specifications and accessories are correct. When a custom chair has been ordered, it is strongly recommended that the client be fitted by the ordering therapist to ensure that the chair fits and that it provides all the elements that were expected when the prescription was generated.

THERAPEUTIC GOALS OF THE WHEELCHAIR SEATING SYSTEM

The primary goals of the wheelchair seating system may include one or more of the following: (1) postural control and deformity management, (2) pressure management, (3) comfort, and (4) increased function.

Postural Control and Deformity Management

Good posture promotes optimal respiratory function and interaction with the environment. Posture may be affected by abnormal tone and reflexes as well as asymmetric skeletal alignment and muscle contractures. These deformities may be flexible (able to be corrected with support) or fixed (stuck in a position despite support). Flexible deformities are often due to weakness or hypotonia in which passive range of motion (ROM) is possible. In this case, the seating system can be designed with external supports to facilitate a symmetric posture and prevent contractures. Fixed deformities are often due to contractures or hypertonia, which can limit ROM. In this case, the seating system can be designed to accommodate for the problem rather than trying to change the physical status of the wheelchair user. The type of cushion, height of backrest, and angle of the seat can also contribute to improved posture.

Pressure Management

Individuals with impaired sensation and movement are at high risk for pressure sores, particularly if they are sitting upright in a wheelchair for extended periods. In this case, the goal of the seating system is to prevent tissue breakdown via appropriate cushions, backrests, and lateral supports. Wheelchair cushion selection depends on the needs, abilities, and funds of the wheelchair user. For example, basic foam cushions are the least expensive and can provide comfort but are not as good at relieving pressure. Some foam cushions have a layer of liquid (gel or water) on top that provides better pressure relief but can make the cushion hot and heavy. Cushions with air pockets are lightweight with excellent pressure distribution but require maintenance and offer poor postural stability. Specialized foam cushions are custom cut based on a computerized pressure distribution map to offload bony prominences and support posture, making them the most desirable and most expensive. Even with the most supportive cushion, pressure relief training is still a necessary requirement.

Comfort

Individuals are healthier when they are out of bed and active, and they are more likely to stay up and active in their wheelchair when it is comfortable. Thus comfort is one of the most important considerations. Wheelchair cushions, lateral supports, and back rests can contribute to a comfortable (or uncomfortable) wheelchair. Importance should also be given to the proper width of the chair and the type and angle of the rear wheels (e.g., air-filled wheels provide better cushioning). Further, if the rear wheels are not placed at the appropriate height, the user's arms may fatigue earlier than necessary, which can not only be uncomfortable but also lead to secondary shoulder complications.

Increased Function

The overarching goal for most clients and their caregivers is to have a seating system that provides all the necessary ingredients to maximize function. Increased independence can be accomplished through attention to postural support, pressure management, and comfort, as discussed. For example, postural supports can make it possible for users to reach beyond their base of support to engage in activities such as putting on a shirt, opening a door, and playing a board game. Specialized cushions can maximize active time in the chair through improved sitting tolerance. In addition, adapting the chair with meaningful accessories can increase the ability to engage in functional activities.

WHEELCHAIR SELECTION PROCESS

The OTA should be familiar with the following features of manual and power chairs to facilitate the wheelchair selection, ordering, and training processes.

Manual Chairs

A **manual chair** requires the client or caregiver to propel the chair with his or her own strength (Fig. 15.9A). Individuals

benefiting from a manual wheelchair should have sufficient strength and endurance to propel the chair at home and in the community over varied terrain. The effects of manual propulsion on upper extremity (UE) joint health should be considered when recommending a manual chair. Specific features of a manual chair are discussed in this section.

Weight: Standard, Lightweight, and Heavy Duty. Standard manual wheelchairs exceed 35 pounds; they can be difficult to maneuver and transport due to weight (Fig. 15.10). A lighter-weight manual wheelchair is recommended for longer-term use (Anderson et al., 2002). A lighter-weight wheelchair requires less force to propel, is usually made with more durable components (e.g., aluminum or titanium), and offers more adjustability. Heavy-duty wheelchairs are available for clients in excess of 250 pounds, and extra-heavy-duty wheelchairs can support clients weighing more than 300 pounds. A heavy individual must be able to propel the chair or be pushed by others and may require a power chair as a result.

Frame: Folding Versus Rigid. A folding frame allows for the wheelchair to be folded for storage. Folding frames typically have swing-away and/or removable leg rests and arm rests, which make transfers easier (Fig. 15.11A). Individuals who propel with the unaffected arm and leg after stroke may use a folding hemiheight frame, which is lower to the ground and has one leg rest removed. Rigid frames do not fold but are lighter weight because they have fewer moving parts (see Fig. 15.11B). Rigid frames can also be disassembled by popping off the rear wheels, making it lighter for transporting into and out of a car. Further, rigid frames require less maintenance and less energy to navigate.

Push Handles. All manual chairs can have a **push handle** (or push bar) on the rear, which can be used for dependent propulsion when needed. Some fully independent clients opt

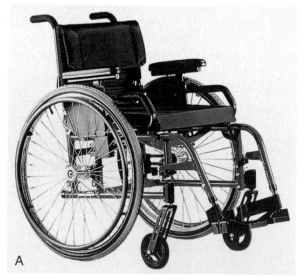
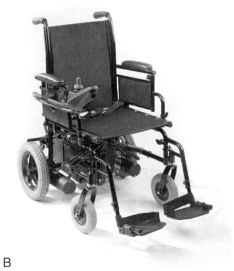

A   B

Fig. 15.9 Manual versus electric wheelchair. (A) Rigid frame chair with swing-away footrests. (B) Power-driven wheelchair with hand control. (A, Courtesy Quickie Designs; B, Courtesy Invacare Corporation.)

to go without the push handle because they do not want to invite others to push them unnecessarily. Folding push handles allow the handles to be discreetly folded when help is unwanted, but quickly unfolded when needed.

Armrests: Flip-Away, Detachable, or Fixed. Armrests come in different shapes and features. The fixed armrest is a continuous part of the frame and is not detachable. The flip-away armrest is the most common on a folding chair, which allows the arm rest to be positioned out of the way during a side approach (pivot) transfer. Some armrests are completely detachable, which increases the risk of misplacing it but allows the option to go with or without it. Tubular arms are available on lightweight frames. If the client has good trunk control, the armrest may be removed for greater freedom of

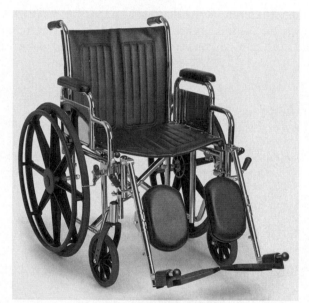

Fig. 15.10 Standard folding frame (more than 35 pounds) with swing-away footrests. (Courtesy Quickie Designs.)

movement. Reclining arms are attached to the back post and recline with the back of the chair. Armrests often block the user from positioning close to a table for a functional activity. Adjustable-height armrests or armrests that are lower on the front end (desk length) can increase accessibility.

Leg Rests: Swinging, Detachable, Elevating, or Fixed. Folding frames often have swinging **leg rests** that are detachable. Swinging leg rests make it easier to approach the bed, bathtub, or car during a transfer. A rigid frame has a fixed (immobile) leg rest, or cradle, which can make transfers more difficult. Elevating leg rests have an adjustable angle between 70 and 180 degrees with supporting calf pads, which may provide comfort for clients with a LE cast or recent operation. Articulating leg rests can be lengthened when elevated to allow more room for the extended leg.

Foot Plates. The **foot plate**, or footrest, allows the user to rest the feet at the base of the leg rest. Foot plates have a heel loop to keep the foot from sliding off. A toe strap or calf strap can also provide stability for spastic muscles when riding over bumpy terrain.

Wheels. Composite **mag wheels** are the most common rear wheels because they are inexpensive and maintenance free; however, for the long-term wheelchair user, lighter-weight **spoke wheels** are preferred. Spoke wheels are like bike wheels in that they are made of metal and require frequent maintenance.

The front wheels, or casters, are available in small and large sizes. Small casters are lighter weight and more responsive for maneuvering. Large casters move better over uneven terrain but may interfere with the footplate and/or rear wheels.

Tires. Tires can be solid or pneumatic. Solid tires require no maintenance but are not as comfortable of a ride as pneumatic tires. Pneumatic tires are lighter weight, more readily

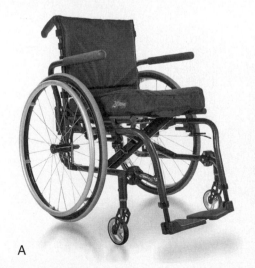

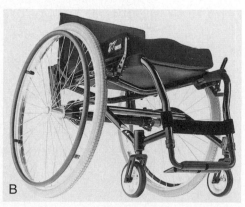

Fig. 15.11 Folding versus rigid wheelchair. (A) Lightweight folding frame with swing-away footrests. (B) Rigid aluminum frame with tapered front end and solid foot cradle. (A, Courtesy Quickie Designs; B, Courtesy Invacare Corporation.)

absorb shock, and grab better onto uneven surfaces. Tire treads should be chosen according to the client's needs (e.g., knobby for frequent outdoor use and smooth for least resistance indoors). During propulsion, the client places the hands on the **handrims** around the wheel rather than directly on the tires. Various wheel locks are available, including lock extension bars that make it easier to lock the wheels using leverage. Side guards can also be added to the sides of the seat to prevent water and debris from flipping off the tires onto the client's clothing.

Recline. A reclining feature can be medically justified for individuals with a fixed hip angle, quadriplegia, trunk casts or braces that limit upright positioning, or excessive trunk extensor tone (Fig. 15.12A). Reclining is also beneficial for self-catheterization of the bladder, relieving orthostatic hypotension, and reducing edema. Although reclining redistributes pressure, it does not count as a full pressure relief and can still lead to a pressure sore.

Tilt-in-Space. If a client is dependent for pressure reliefs, a **tilt-in-space** feature may be medically justified (see Fig. 15.12B, C). A tilt-in-space allows the client's posture and pelvic position to remain in a fixed position while the entire body rotates back. During the tilt, weight is shifted from the ischial tuberosities and thighs onto the sacrum and back. A tilt-in-space on a manual chair must be operated by a caregiver.

Manual Power Assist. **Manual power assist** propulsion technology provides supplemental power to a manual wheelchair, which can be turned on and off as needed. By adding on to the manual frame, a battery-powered system assists the client in propelling the chair, thus minimizing the energy and endurance required, especially on hills or uneven terrain. Of note, the power assist chair can be more difficult for the caregiver to propel.

Safety Features. Seat belts can be added for security. As long as the client is able to unbuckle the belt, it is not considered a restraint. Antitip devices are typically added to the rear

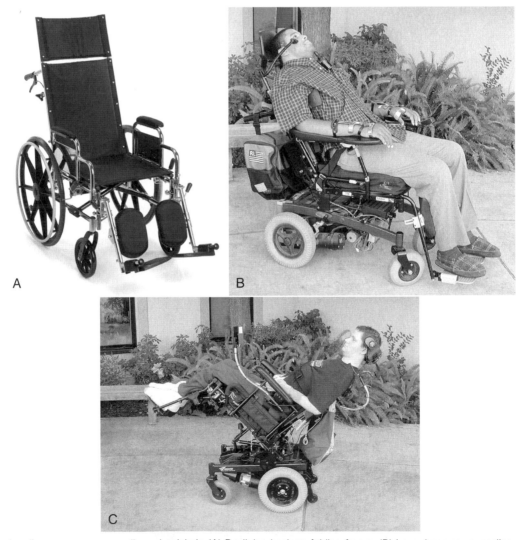

Fig. 15.12 Manual recline versus power recline wheelchair. (A) Reclining back on folding frame. (B) Low-shear power recline with collar mount chin control on electric wheelchair. (C) Tilt system with head control on electric wheelchair. (A, Courtesy Quickie Designs; B, C, Courtesy Luis Gonzalez, SCVMC.)

of the chair and can be flipped down to prevent the client from tipping backward. Antitip devices can be flipped up when they block the ability to ascend a high curb. Head supports and lateral supports keep the body in proper alignment.

Power Chairs

A **power chair** is considered for those who have minimal or no use of the UEs, limited endurance, or shoulder dysfunction due to aging, medical condition, or pain (see Fig. 15.9B). Power chairs are also preferred for inaccessible outdoor terrain (Bailey, 2007). Power wheelchairs have a wide variety of features and can be programmed to be driven by foot, arm, head, or neck or pneumatically controlled. Given today's sophisticated technology, assuming intact cognition and perception, even a person with the most severe physical limitations is capable of independently driving a power wheelchair.

However, the benefits of power chairs must be stacked next to the limitations. First, power chairs are bulky, making navigation difficult, especially in small spaces. Second, power chairs are heavy, requiring significant accommodations to travel by car. Third, power chairs are expensive and require a substantial LMN to obtain even partial coverage. Finally, power chairs demand routine maintenance, such as keeping up battery power, which may necessitate considerable forethought before a trip. Nevertheless, the benefits far exceed the limitations for many clients who would not otherwise experience access to their home and community.

The anatomy of a power chair consists of four components: (1) base, (2) seating system, (3) control options, and (4) access devices. The base can be powered by **front-wheel drive**, **mid-wheel drive**, or **rear-wheel drive**; each type offers its own advantages and disadvantages. For turning in small spaces, for example, the mid-wheel drive offers more maneuverability. However, the front-wheel drive facilitates curb climbing more readily with its anterior pulling power. When it comes to directional stability (or ability to move in a straight line), the rear-wheel drive is preferred over the front-wheel power chair's fishtailing tendency.

The seating system can be outfitted with add-on features that must be justified in a LMN, such as tilt, recline, tilt/recline combination, and standing features. The control options, **proportional** or **nonproportional**, must also be individually selected based on the client's needs and abilities. A proportional control works much like a gas pedal in that the harder one pushes, the faster the chair goes. A nonproportional control turns on and off at a preselected fixed speed (e.g., slow, medium, or fast). Fortunately a large number of options exist for access devices. A **joystick** requires some degree of coordination but can be adapted to require less fine motor ability (including being placed under the chin). If UE motor control is severely limited, a head array allows the power chair to be controlled by moving one's head on switches located near the head. The head array can be combined with a sip-n-puff mechanism that uses breath control (e.g., sips or puffs) to start or stop the power chair. Alternatively, a tongue-touch keypad allows the user to touch key points in the mouth to control the chair. New technologies using eye gaze to steer the power chair are currently being researched (Anderson et al., 2002).

CONSIDERATIONS FOR WHEELCHAIR SELECTION

When determining an appropriate wheelchair, the evaluator must be familiar with the client's roles, interests, and responsibilities and have a broad perspective of the client's clinical, functional, and environmental needs. The client's age, specific diagnosis, prognosis, and current abilities and disabilities (e.g., tone, ROM, strength, endurance) may affect wheelchair use. For insurance reimbursement, a detailed LMN must clearly explain why certain features of a wheelchair are necessary, particularly when upgraded features are recommended (e.g., reclining backrest, power tilt, or air cushion). The following questions should be considered when designing an appropriate wheelchair:

- Is the chair required for part-time or full-time use?
- Is the user active both indoors and outdoors? Will the chair be primarily for indoor or sedentary use?
- Will this frame style improve potential for independent mobility?
- Is the user a growing adolescent, or does he or she have a progressive disorder requiring later modification of the chair? Does the client have a limited life expectancy?
- Are custom features, specifications, or positioning devices required?
- Will this be the primary wheelchair?
- Is substantial durability unimportant? Does the user need the stability of a standard-weight chair?
- Does the client demonstrate sufficient endurance and functional ability to propel a manual wheelchair independently at home and in the community? Does the user have the ability to propel a standard-weight chair?
- Will the client's ability to propel the chair or handle parts be enhanced by a lighter-weight frame?
- Are custom features (e.g., adjustable height back, seat angle, axle mount) necessary?
- Does manual mobility enhance functional independence and cardiovascular conditioning of the wheelchair user?
- Does the client demonstrate progressive functional loss that makes powered mobility an energy-conserving option?
- Is lightweight or powered mobility needed to increase independence at school, at work, and in the community?
- Do the client and/or caregiver demonstrate ability to responsibly care and maintain equipment?
- Can the client or caregiver load and fit the chair into necessary vehicles?
- Is the client's home accessible for use of the manual or power chair?
- Will the caregiver be propelling the chair at any time?
- Is the client able to perform weight shifts and position changes or can the caregiver assist?

- Will the client benefit from the improved energy efficiency, decrease in weight, and performance of a rigid frame?
- Does the client have significant spasticity that is facilitated by hip and knee extension during the recline phase?
- Is the client unable to sit upright because of hip contractures, poor balance, or fatigue?
- Does the client have hip or knee contractures that prohibit his or her ability to recline fully?
- Will the client require quick position changes in the event of hypotension and/or autonomic dysreflexia?
- Does the client prefer a traditional-looking chair?
- Is the folding frame needed for transport, storage, or home accessibility?
- Which footrest style is necessary for transfers, desk clearance, and other daily living skills?
- Is cost a consideration? Has a reimbursement source been identified for a given add-on feature?
- What will be the long-term effects of the propulsion choice?
- Has the user been educated regarding the benefits and disadvantages of power assist versus straight power and been guided objectively in making the appropriate selection?
  Considerations Specific to Power Chairs:
- Does the client demonstrate physical, cognitive, and perceptual ability to operate a power-driven system safely?
- What is the optimal driving control and seated posture for the client in a power chair?
- Has the client in a power chair been educated regarding the rear-wheel, mid-wheel, and front-wheel drive systems and been guided objectively in making the appropriate selection?
- Will a power recline or tilt decrease or make more efficient use of caregiver time?
- Will a power recline or tilt reduce the need for transfers to the bed for catheterizations and rest periods throughout the day?

PEDIATRIC WHEELCHAIR CONSIDERATIONS

Rarely does a standard wheelchair meet the fitting requirements of a child. Custom seating systems specific to the pediatric population are often necessary and should consider a chair that will accommodate the child's growth. The child's ability to propel the chair relative to his or her developmental level will also affect the selection process. For children younger than 5 years of age, using a stroller base instead of a standard wheelchair base is an option. In fact, using a stroller in lieu of a wheelchair is an option for young children who are not able to participate in propulsion and do not need special supports or cushions.

WHEELCHAIR MEASUREMENT PROCEDURES

Ideally, the client should be measured in the style of chair and seat cushion that most closely resembles those being ordered. If the patient will use a brace, body jacket, or any additional device(s) in the chair, these should be in place during the measurement. Observation skills are important during this process. Measurements alone should not be used. The entire body position is eyeballed every step of the way (Adler, 1987; Everest & Jennings booklet 1, 1979). The procedures listed in this section are provided as an aid for the OTA in understanding the process while working with service-competent practitioners who complete the wheelchair measurement and prescription.

Seat Width
Objectives
- To distribute weight over the widest possible surface
- To keep the overall width of the chair as narrow as possible

Measurement
- Measure across the widest part of either the hips or thighs while the patient is seated (Fig. 15.13A).
- Add 0.5 to 1 inch on each side of the seat width measurement to prevent hips or thighs from rubbing on the edge of seat.
- Place the flat palm of the hand between the client's hip or thigh and the wheelchair skirt and armrest to check for pressure points.

Considerations
- Potential weight gain or loss
- Accessibility of varied environments
- Overall width of wheelchair (affected by camber and axle mounting position, rim style, and wheel style)

Seat Depth
Objective
- To distribute body weight along the entire length of the thigh to just behind the knee to (a) minimize risk of pressure sores on the buttocks and lower back and (b) gain optimal muscle tone normalization

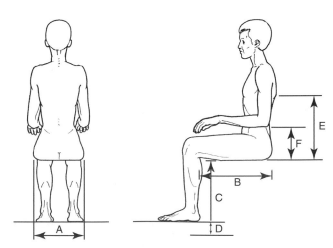

Fig. 15.13 What and where to measure. (A) Seat width. (B) Seat depth. (C) Seat height from floor. (D) Footrest clearance. (E) Back height. (F) Armrest height.

Measurement

- Measure from the base of the back post to the inside of the bent knee (see Fig. 15.13B).
- Decrease 1 to 2 inches from the seat depth measurement to prevent the back of the knee from rubbing the seat edge.
- Check clearance behind the knees to prevent contact of the front edge of the seat upholstery with the popliteal space.

Considerations

- Braces or back inserts that may be pushing the patient forward
- Postural changes throughout the day from fatigue or spasticity
- Thigh length discrepancy; the depth of the seat may be different for each leg
- If considering a power recliner, one should assume the client will slide forward slightly throughout the day and should make depth adjustments accordingly.
- Seat depth may need to be shortened to allow independent propulsion with the lower extremities.

Seat Height From Floor and Foot Adjustment
Objectives

- Supporting the body while maintaining the thighs parallel to the floor
- Elevating the foot plates to provide ground clearance over varied surfaces and curb cuts

Measurements

- The client's thighs are kept parallel to the floor so that the body weight is distributed evenly along the entire depth of the seat. The lowest point of the footplates must clear the floor by at least 2 inches (see Fig. 15.13C, D).
- Measure the top of the seat post to the floor or the popliteal fossa to the bottom of the heel (see Fig. 15.13C, D).
- Slip fingers under the client's thighs at the front edge of the seat upholstery.

Considerations

- A custom seat height may be necessary to obtain footrest clearance. An inch of increased seat height raises the footplate 1 inch.
- If the knees are too high, increased pressure at the ischial tuberosities puts the patient at risk for skin breakdown and pelvic deformity.
- Sitting too high off the ground raises the patient's center of gravity, potentially a safety and stability problem.
- Sitting too high may interfere with visibility and seat height for transfers if the patient is driving a van from the wheelchair.

Back Height
Objective

- To provide back support consistent with physical and functional needs

Measurements

- For full trunk support, measure from the top of the seat post to the top of the shoulders.
- For minimum trunk support, the top of the back upholstery should permit free arm movement, not irritate the skin or scapulae, and provide good total body alignment (see Fig. 15.13E).
- The chair back should be low enough for maximal function and high enough for maximal support.

Considerations

- Adjustable-height backs (usually offer a 4-inch range)
- Adjustable upholstery
- Lumbar support or another commercially available or custom back insert to prevent kyphosis, scoliosis, or other long-term trunk deformity

Arm Height
Objectives

- To maintain posture and balance
- To provide support and alignment for UEs
- To allow change in position by pushing down on armrests

Measurements

- Measure from the seat post to the bottom of a bent elbow (see Fig. 15.13F).
- The height of the top of the armrest should be 1 inch higher than the above measurement.
- Check that the client's posture looks correct. If possible, the shoulders should not be slouched forward, subluxated, or forced into elevation when the patient is in a normal sitting posture with flexed elbows slightly forward on armrests.

Considerations

- Other uses of armrests such as increasing functional reach or holding a cushion in place
- Certain styles of armrests can increase the overall width of the chair.
- Necessity of armrests
- The patient's ability to remove and replace the armrest from the chair independently
- Review all measurements against standards for a particular model of chair. Manufacturers have lists of the standard dimensions available and the cost for custom modifications.

SUMMARY

The client's physical and cognitive abilities, lifestyle and environment, available resources, transportation options, and reimbursement sources are major factors when determining the most effective seating system. A wheelchair evaluation is not complete until the seat cushion, back support, and other positioning devices are carefully thought out and integrated into daily life. Optimal body alignment has a profound effect on sitting tolerance, skin integrity, tone normalization, overall

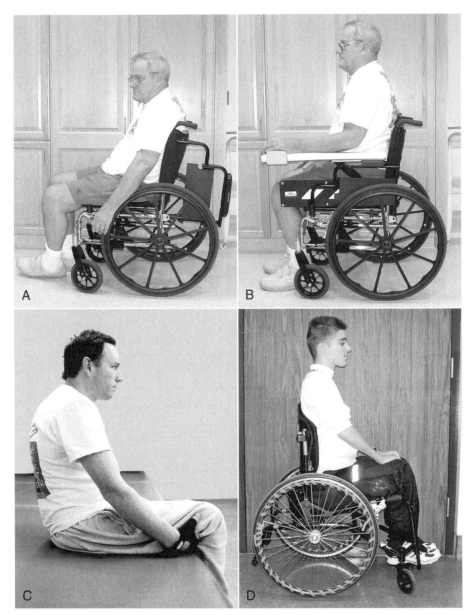

Fig. 15.14 (A) Stroke patient seated in wheelchair. Poor positioning results in kyphotic thoracic spine, posterior pelvic tilt, and unsupported affected side. (B) Stroke patient seated in wheelchair with appropriate positioning devices. Seat and back insert support upright midline position with neutral pelvic tilt and equal weight bearing throughout. (C) Spinal cord–injured patient sitting with back poorly supported results in posterior pelvic tilt, kyphotic thoracic spine, and absence of lumbar curve. (D) Spinal cord–injured patient with rigid back support and pressure-relief seat cushion, resulting in erect thoracic spine, lumbar curve, and anterior tilted pelvis.

functional ability, and general well-being (Fig. 15.14) (Adler, 1987). The OTA plays a role during and after the wheelchair selection process by communicating the client's needs and training the client in the use of his or her new chair.

SECTION III. BED MOBILITY AND TRANSFERS

Transferring is the process of moving a client's body from one surface to another. Transfer may be done by the client unaided, by the client with the aid of caregivers, or by

caregivers. Transfer includes the sequence of events that must occur both before and after the move, such as the pretransfer sequence of bed mobility and the posttransfer phase of wheelchair positioning.

The OTA should be familiar with as many types of transfers as possible so that new challenges can be resolved as they arise. Many classifications of transfers exist and are based on the amount of assistance provided. Classifications range from dependent, in which the client cannot participate in the transfer and relies entirely upon the OTA, to independent, in which the client moves on his or her own. To facilitate independence, the OTA should only provide as much assistance as necessary. In many cases, the client needs a simple verbal and/or tactile cue to initiate the direction of movement. Begin with minimal cueing and provide additional assistance as needed. Allow the client time to process what steps are needed, particularly when new motor learning or cognitive deficits are involved.

Many clinicians are unsure of the transfer type and technique to employ or feel perplexed when a particular technique does not succeed with a given client. It is important to remember that each client, clinician, and situation is different. This chapter does not include an outline of all possibilities but presents transfer techniques that are most commonly employed in practice: (1) stand pivot, (2) squat pivot, (3) one-person dependent, and (4) two-person dependent. In addition, the use of transfer boards and mechanical lifts are discussed, followed by tips for functional transfers in the home environment. Each transfer must be adapted for the particular client's needs and environment. Trial and error of technique is advised to allow for optimal facilitation of independence, safety, and the clinician's proper **body mechanics**.

BED MOBILITY

Bed mobility includes rolling and moving from supine to sit on the edge of the bed. These tasks are a necessary part of toileting in the bed, dressing in the bed, performing a pressure relief, and/or getting out of the bed in preparation for a transfer.

Rolling

- Cue the client to bend the knees.
- Cue the client to reach toward the direction of intent.
- Guide the client through the roll with one hand around the client's scapula and the other at the client's bent knee.

Side-Lying to Sitting

- Position one hand under the client's head and around the scapula as far as possible.
- Cue the client to push up from the surface.
- Bring the client's feet off the edge of the bed.
- At the same time, cue the client to sit up by shifting your arm from the scapula to the upper body.
- Facilitate the client to shift weight down onto the bed and assume an upright sitting position.
- Cue the client to place hands on the bed to help maintain balance.

PREPARING FOR THE TRANSFER

The transfer process begins with setting up the environment, positioning the wheelchair, helping the client into a pretransfer position, and checking one's own body position. The OTA must also understand and utilize the biomechanics of movement to prevent personal or client injury.

Preparing the Equipment and Environment

1. Place the manual wheelchair at approximately a 30-degree angle to the surface to which the client is transferring. If using a power chair, position parallel to the transfer surface.
2. Lock the wheels on the wheelchair and the bed when applicable. Check that all locks are in good working condition.
3. Flip back or remove the armrest on the side closer to the bed.
4. Swing away or remove the leg rest on the side closer to the bed.
5. If applicable, remove the pelvic seat belt, chest belt, and trunk or lateral supports.
6. If necessary, ensure that the transfer board or assistive device(s) are within reach.
7. Check the height of the bed (or surface) in relation to the wheelchair. Can the heights be adjusted?
8. Ensure that all unnecessary bedding and equipment have been moved out of the way.

Preparing the Client

1. Consider the client's medical condition and any special precautions.
2. Ensure that the client is dressed properly, including nonskid socks or shoes.
3. Secure a transfer (gait) belt around the waist to offer a place to grasp if needed during transfer. The belt should not be allowed to slide up the client's trunk.
4. Explain what is going to happen to minimize fear or confusion.
5. Cue the client to scoot forward in the chair. If needed, guide the client to shift weight to one side, then cue the client to bring the unweighted side forward. Repeat on the opposite side.
6. Cue the client to position both feet firmly on the floor with at least 90 degrees of knee flexion. This position allows the weight to be shifted easily onto and over the feet.
7. Cue the client to position the client's heels toward the surface to which the client is transferring. The feet can easily pivot in this position, and the risk of twisting or injuring an ankle or knee is minimized.
8. Cue the client to position the arms in a safe position in which he or she can assist in the transfer. If one or both of the upper extremities is nonfunctional, the arms should be placed in a safe position that will not be in the way during the transfer (e.g., in the client's lap). If the client has partial or full movement, motor control, or strength, he or she can assist in the transfer either by reaching toward the surface to be reached or by pushing off from the starting surface. The OTA's decision is based on prior knowledge of the client's motor function.
9. Cue the client into a neutral or slightly anterior pelvic tilt position to move the center of mass forward over

the center of the client's body (Santa Clara Valley Medical Center, Physical Therapy Department, 1985).

10. Cue the client to assume and maintain a midline trunk position before and during the transfer.

Preparing the Clinician

1. Get close to the client or move the client closer to you.
2. Square off with the client (face head on).
3. Bend knees; use the legs, not the back.
4. Keep a neutral spine (not bent or arched back).
5. Keep a wide base of support.
6. Acknowledge your own physical abilities and limitations. Do not tackle more than you can handle; ask for help or use equipment when needed.
7. Do not combine movements (i.e., avoid rotating at the same time as bending forward or backward).
8. Allot enough time for safe execution of a transfer. Do not be in a hurry.
9. Anticipate the unexpected.

STAND PIVOT TRANSFERS

The **stand pivot transfer** requires the client to be able to come to a standing position and pivot on one or both feet.

Method

The following method assumes that the necessary preparatory activities (preparing the wheelchair, environment, client, and clinician) are completed, as outlined earlier.

1. Stand on the client's affected side with hands either on the client's scapulae or around the client's waist or hips.

2. Stabilize the client's foot and knee with your own foot and knee.
3. Provide assistance by guiding the client forward as the buttocks are lifted up and toward the transfer surface (Fig. 15.15A).
4. Cue the client to reach toward the destination surface and/or push off the surface from which he or she is transferring (see Fig. 15.15B).
5. Guide the client toward the transfer surface and gently help him or her down to a sitting position (see Fig. 15.15C).

SQUAT PIVOT TRANSFER

The **squat pivot transfer** is used when the client cannot initiate or maintain a standing position. Keeping a client in the bent knee position allows the OTA to perform a safer and easier assisted transfer by providing optimal trunk and LE support. A transfer board may also be utilized.

Method

The following method assumes that the necessary preparatory activities (preparing the wheelchair, environment, client, and clinician) are completed, as outlined earlier.

1. Shift the client's weight forward from the buttocks toward and over the client's feet by positioning the arms on the client's waist, trunk, or under the buttocks (Fig. 15.16A). Do not grasp under a client's weak arm or pull a weak arm.
2. Cue the client to either reach toward the surface he or she is transferring to or push from the surface from which he or she is transferring (see Fig. 15.16B).

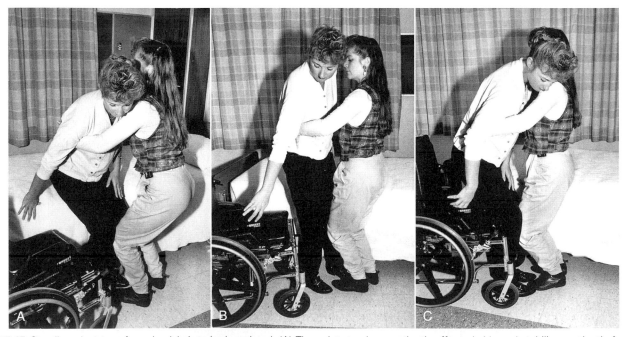

Fig. 15.15 Standing pivot transfer; wheelchair to bed, assisted. (A) Therapist stands on patient's affected side and stabilizes patient's foot and knee. She assists by guiding patient forward and initiates lifting buttocks up. (B) Patient reaches toward transfer surface. (C) Therapist guides the patient toward transfer surface. (Courtesy Luis Gonzalez, SCVMC.)

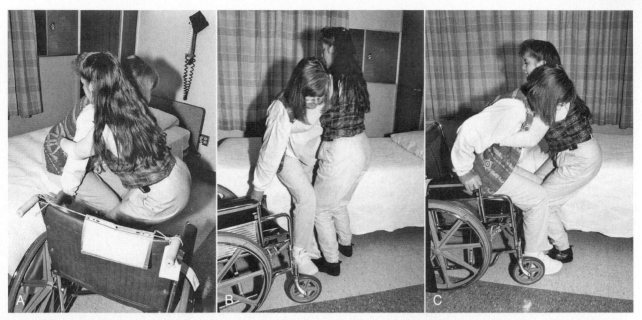

Fig. 15.16 Bent pivot transfer; bed to wheelchair. (A) Therapist grasps patient around trunk and assists in shifting patient's weight forward over feet. (B) Patient reaches toward wheelchair. (C) Therapist assists patient down toward sitting position. (Courtesy Luis Gonzalez, SCVMC.)

3. Assist the client by guiding and pivoting him or her around toward the transfer surface (see Fig. 15.16C). Do not allow the client to pivot to the destination surface until after leaning far enough forward to reach his or her center of mass (balance point).

ONE-PERSON DEPENDENT TRANSFER

The **one-person dependent transfer** is designed for use with the client who has minimal to no functional ability. If this transfer is performed incorrectly, it is potentially hazardous for both clinician and client. The clinician should be keenly aware of correct body mechanics, as well as his or her own physical limitations. This transfer should be practiced with able-bodied persons and initially used with the client only when another person is available to assist (Adler, Musik, & Tipton-Burton, 1994). With more dependent clients, it is always best to use the two-person transfer or at least have a second person available to spot the transfer. A transfer board is also recommended. If the client has no ability to participate, a mechanical lift may be an appropriate alternative. Even though the client is dependent, it is still important that he or she is cooperative and willing to follow instructions.

Method

The following method assumes that the necessary preparatory activities (preparing the wheelchair, environment, client, and clinician) are completed, as outlined earlier (Fig. 15.17A).

1. Place a transfer board under the client's inside thigh, midway between the buttocks and the knee, to form a bridge from the bed to the wheelchair. The transfer board is angled toward the client's opposite hip.

2. Stabilize the client's feet by placing your own feet laterally around the client's feet.

3. Stabilize the client's knees by placing your own knees firmly against the anterolateral aspect of the client's knees (see Fig. 15.17B).

4. Help the client lean over the knees by pulling him or her forward from behind the shoulders (do not pull on the humerus). The client's head and trunk should lean opposite the direction of the transfer. The client's hands can rest on the lap.

5. Reach under the client's outside arm and grasp under the buttock or as far as possible. On the other side, reach over the client's back under the buttock or as far as possible (see Fig. 15.17C).

6. After your arms are positioned correctly, lock them to stabilize the client's trunk. Keep your knees slightly bent and brace them firmly against the client's knees.

7. Communicate with the client to "lean forward" while holding your knees tightly against the client's knees and transfer the client's weight over his or her feet. Keep your back straight to maintain good body mechanics (see Fig. 15.17D).

8. Communicate with the client to "turn and sit" while pivoting with the client and moving onto the destination surface (see Fig. 15.17E).

9. Secure the client on the bed by easing him or her against the back of an elevated bed or on the mattress in a side-lying position, then by lifting the legs onto the bed (see Fig. 15.17F).

10. The transfer on this one-person dependent transfer board can be adapted to move the client to other surfaces. It

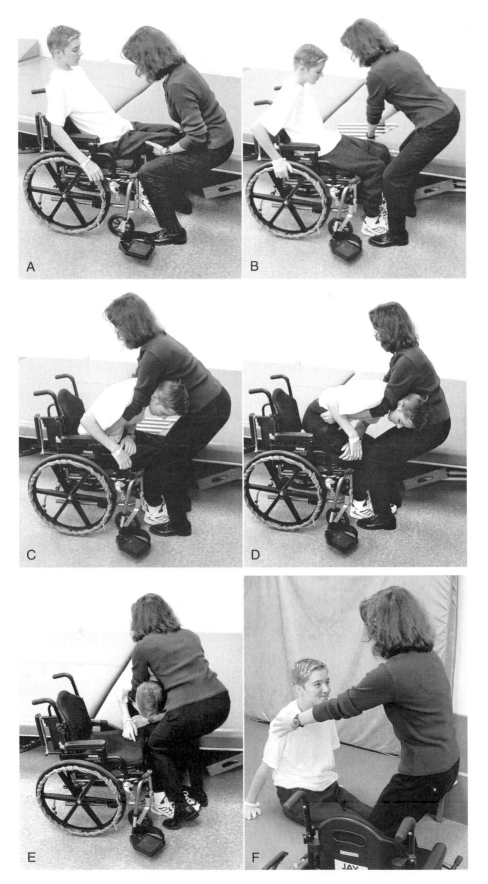

Fig. 15.17 One-person dependent sliding board transfer. (A) Therapist positions wheelchair and patient and pulls patient forward in chair. (B) Therapist stabilizes patient's knees and feet after placing sliding board. (C) Therapist grasps patient's pants at lowest point of buttocks. (D) Therapist rocks with patient and shifts patient's weight over patient's feet, making sure patient's back remains straight. (E) Therapist pivots with patient and moves patient onto sliding board. (F) Patient is stabilized on bed. (Courtesy Luis Gonzales, SCVMC.)

should be attempted only when the clinician and client feel secure with the wheelchair-to-bed transfer.

TWO-PERSON DEPENDENT TRANSFERS

The **two-person dependent transfer** essentially follows the same procedure as a squat pivot transfer or one-person dependent transfer except there is one clinician positioned in front of the client facilitating the client's trunk and legs while a second clinician is positioned in back facilitating the client's hips and buttocks. The two-person dependent transfer allows increased clinician interaction and support as well as greater control of the client's trunk and buttocks during the transfer. It is often used with neurologically involved clients because trunk flexion and equal weight bearing are often desirable with this diagnosis. A transfer board may also be utilized for the two-person dependent transfer.

Method

The following method assumes that the necessary preparatory activities (preparing the wheelchair, environment, client, and clinician) are completed, as outlined earlier.

1. One clinician assumes a position in front of the client and the other in back.
2. The clinician in front stabilizes the client's knees and feet by placing his or her knees and feet lateral to each of the client's knees.
3. The clinician in back is positioned squarely behind the client's buttocks, placing his or her hands under the buttocks (Fig. 15.18A).
4. The client's head and trunk should lean in the direction opposite the transfer.
5. The clinician in front reaches over the shoulders to grasp below the ribs or as far as possible and guides the client to lean forward and shift weight off the buttocks. The client's hands can rest on the lap (see Fig. 15.18B).
6. The clinician in back pivots the client's buttocks in the direction of the transfer.
7. This process can be repeated two or three times, making sure the client's buttocks land on a safe, solid surface. The clinicians should reposition themselves and the client to maintain safe and proper body mechanics (see Fig. 15.18C).
8. The clinicians should be sure they coordinate the time of the transfer with the client and one another by counting to three aloud and instructing the team to initiate the transfer on three. Typically, the clinician in front is the leader.

TRANSFER BOARDS

Transfer boards provide a bridge between surfaces so that the client does not have to transfer all the way from one surface to another in one move; rather, the client can break down the transfer into a series of smaller transfers across the transfer board. Transfer boards are often employed with individuals who have lower extremity amputations or spinal cord injuries but can be used for any individual struggling with effective transfers, regardless of diagnosis. In fact, transfer boards can be used as a temporary device to increase confidence in clients who are fearful or anxious. Transfer boards can be used during a sit pivot transfer, one-person dependent transfer, two-person dependent transfer, or modified independent transfer.

Method

The following method assumes that the necessary preparatory activities (preparing the wheelchair, environment, client, and clinician) are completed, as outlined earlier.

1. Cue the client to lean away and lift the leg closer to the transfer surface.
2. Place the board under the midthigh angled toward the opposite hip. The board must be firmly under the thigh and firmly on the surface to which the client is transferring (Fig. 15.19).
3. Stabilize the client's knees by placing your own knees firmly against the anterolateral aspect of the client's knees.
4. Instruct the client to place one hand on the edge of the board and the other hand on the wheelchair seat. Be careful that the client does not wrap fingers under the board where they might be pinched.
5. Cue the client to lean forward and push up with arms to lift weight off buttocks.
6. The client should pivot his or her buttocks across the board while moving his or her head and upper body weight in the direction opposite direction.
7. Assist the client where needed to shift weight and support the trunk.

MECHANICAL LIFTS

Some clients, because of body size, extent of disability, or the health and well-being of the caregiver, require the use of a **mechanical lift**. A variety of manual and electric lifting devices can be used to transfer clients of any weight (Fig. 15.20). A properly trained caregiver, even one who is considerably smaller than the client, can learn to use the mechanical lift safely and independently (Everest & Jennings. booklet 2, 1979). The client's physical size, the environment in which the lift will be used, and the instances to which the lift will be used must be considered to select the appropriate mechanical lift. The client and caregiver should demonstrate safe use of the lift before the OT prescribes it.

FUNCTIONAL TRANSFERS

Transfer to Sofa or Chair

Wheelchair-to-sofa and wheelchair-to-chair transfers are similar to wheelchair-to-bed transfers (Fig. 15.21); however, a few unique concerns should be assessed.

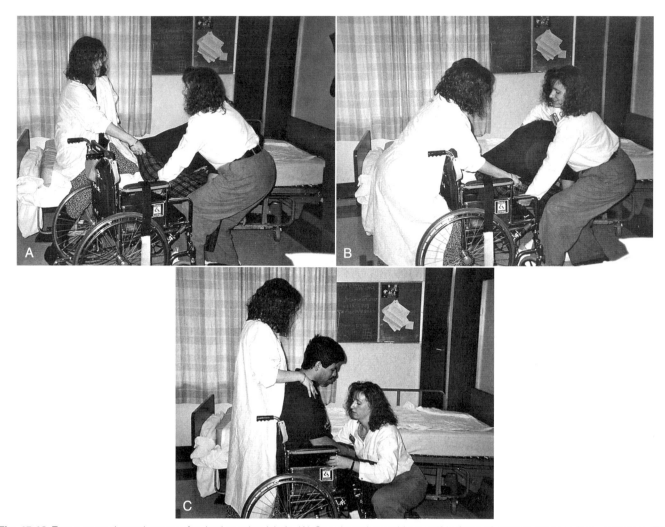

Fig. 15.18 Two-person dependent transfer, bed to wheelchair. (A) One therapist positions self in front of patient, blocking feet and knees. The therapist in back positions self behind patient's buttocks and assists by lifting. (B) Person in front rocks patient forward and unweights buttocks as the back therapist shifts buttocks toward wheelchair. (C) Both therapists position patient in upright, midline position in wheelchair. Seat belt is secured and positioning devices are added. (Courtesy Luis Gonzales, SCVMC.)

The chair may be light and not as stable as a bed or wheelchair. When transferring to the chair, the client must be instructed to reach for the seat of the chair. The client should not reach for the armrest or back of the chair because this action may cause the chair to tip over. When moving from a chair to the wheelchair, the client should use a hand to push off from the seat of the chair as he or she comes to standing.

Standing from a chair is often more difficult if the chair is low or the seat cushions are soft. Dense cushions or layers of blankets may be added to increase height and provide a firm surface to which to transfer.

Transfer to Toilet

In general, wheelchair-to-toilet transfers are difficult because of the confined space in most bathrooms and the inability and lack of support of a toilet seat. The OTA and client should attempt to position the wheelchair next to or at an appropriate angle to the toilet. The OTA should analyze the space around the toilet and wheelchair to ensure no obstacles are present.

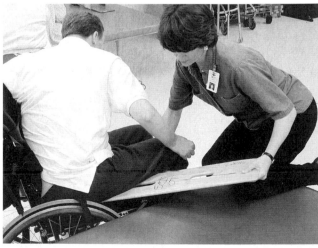

Fig. 15.19 Positioning sliding board. Lift leg closest to transfer surface. Place board midthigh between buttocks and knee, angled toward opposite hip. (Courtesy Luis Gonzalez, SCVMC.)

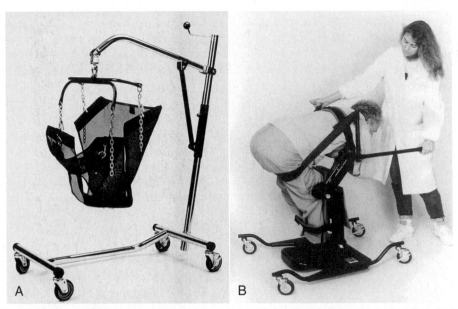

Fig. 15.20 (A) Traditional boom-style mechanical lift. (B) Patient lift useful in transferring individuals with spinal cord injury. (A, Courtesy Trans-Aid Lifts, Sunrise Medical; B, Courtesy EZ-Pivot, Rand-Scott.)

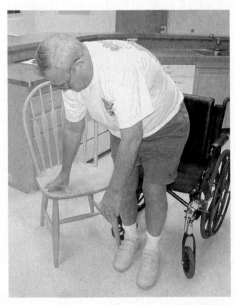

Fig. 15.21 Stroke patient in midtransfer reaches for seat of chair, pivots, and lowers body to sitting. (Courtesy Luis Gonzales, SCVMC.)

Adaptive devices such as grab bars and raised toilet seats can be installed for additional stability and independence. However, raised toilet seats can be poorly secured to toilets and may be unsafe for some clients. Alternatively, a bedside commode can be placed over the toilet, which raises the seat height and offers arm rests for support.

Bathtub

The OTA should be cautious when teaching bathtub transfers because the bathtub is one of the most hazardous areas of the home. Transfers from the wheelchair to the bottom of the bathtub are extremely difficult and used only with clients who have good bilateral UE strength and motor control. A commercially produced shower chair or tub transfer bench is often used for seated bathing (see Fig. 15.8); however, most are not covered by insurance.

If the client is unable to step into the tub, the tub transfer bench is a safer option. A tub transfer bench extends from the inside to the outside of the tub, allowing the client to transfer to the bench using his or her preferred wheelchair-to-chair transfer before placing the lower extremities into the bathtub. The confined space may complicate wheelchair placement.

If the client requires assistance, a transfer sling is an additional option during a bare bottom transfer. The cloth sling is placed under the client's trochanters, and the sling handles are used in the same manner as if grabbing the sides of the client's pants. The sling can either be removed or remain in place during bathing.

Car Transfers

A car transfer can be the most challenging because it involves trial-and-error methods to develop a technique that is not only safe but also easy for the client and caregiver to carry out. The OTA often uses the client's existing transfer technique. The client's size, degree of disability, and vehicle style (two-door vs. four-door model) must be considered. These factors will affect level of independence and may necessitate a change in the usual technique to allow a safe, easy transfer.

The following are some additional considerations when making wheelchair-to-car transfers:

1. In general, it is difficult to get a wheelchair close enough to the car seat, especially with four-door vehicles.
2. For most ambulatory clients, it may be easier to back up to the car seat using an appropriate assistive device, then bend forward and sit down before bringing the legs into the vehicle.

3. Car seats are often much lower than the standard wheelchair seat height, which makes the uneven transfer much more difficult, especially from the car seat to the wheelchair.

4. For clients wearing a brace, such as a halo body jacket or lower extremity cast or splint, the clinician may need additional time and cueing to accommodate these devices.

5. The clinician may suggest use of an extra-long transfer board to compensate for the large gap between transfer surfaces.

6. Because uphill transfers are difficult and the level of assistance may increase for this transfer, the clinician may choose a two-person assist instead of a one-person assist transfer to ensure a safe and smooth technique.

SUMMARY

A wheelchair that fits well and can be managed safely and easily by its user and caregiver is one of the most important factors in the client's ability to perform ADL with maximal independence (Andrew, 2019). Wheelchair users must learn the capabilities and limitations of the wheelchair as well as safe methods to perform self-care and mobility skills. If present, the caregiver needs to be thoroughly familiar with safe and correct techniques of handling the wheelchair, positioning equipment, and assisting the client while maximizing as much independence as possible.

Transfer skills are among the most important activities that the wheelchair user must master. The ability to transfer increases the possibility of participation in activities. However, transfers can be hazardous if safe methods are not learned and followed (Everest & Jennings. booklet 2, 1979). Many wheelchair users with exceptional abilities have developed unique methods of wheelchair management through innovative problem solving. The basic procedures outlined here provide the most recommended starting point for safe mobility training.

SECTION IV. IMPORTANCE OF DRIVING AND COMMUNITY MOBILITY

Driving and community mobility are key instrumental activities of daily living (IADL) that play a pivotal role in community independence and social interactions. A driver's license symbolizes a rite of passage to adulthood for the teenager. Driving is the primary means of transportation in any area that lacks or has only limited mass transit options. Most adults rely on driving to access employment, medical care, and leisure activities; maintain relationships with friends and family; and carry out responsibilities such as shopping and transporting others. The ability to drive is instrumental in obtaining and maintaining an independent lifestyle.

For some people, public transportation and walking may be just as critical to accessing the community as driving, depending on the environmental culture. Community mobility can include walking, biking, using a scooter or wheelchair in the community, and riding as a passenger in a motor vehicle or mass transit system. The OTA addresses driving and other aspects of community mobility with clients of all ages. Interventions may include addressing the client's ability to be safe as a pedestrian or cyclist, to safely access mass transportation, and/or to ride as a passenger in a motor vehicle. Interventions may also include addressing the needs of clients who are first-time drivers with special needs or experienced drivers after an injury or illness (American Occupational Therapy Association, 2005).

OCCUPATIONAL THERAPY AND DRIVING

Driving requires continuous integration of visual, perceptual, cognitive, and motor skills. For example, every action a driver takes begins with searching the environment for critical information while ignoring unnecessary information, processing what is seen, making a decision, making a plan to respond, and then physically reacting to the situation, all in a timely manner. Driving is a complex task that holds more risk than other IADL or ADL. Consequently, evaluation of the ability to drive is critical for individuals whose medical condition or disability may impair skills needed for driving safely and successfully. The OTA can identify clients who may be at risk if they are learning to drive, resuming driving, or continuing to drive.

Where concern exists, the primary OTA can refer the client to an OT or OTA who specializes in driver rehabilitation. These practitioners typically work within a driver rehabilitation program. They often have additional training as a driving school instructor or working with a driving school instructor. For example, the OT may provide low-vision driver training techniques, prescribe adaptive equipment, teach a driver to use adaptive driving equipment, and identify strategies to compensate for cognitive limitations in the driving task. The driver rehabilitation program can be a resource to help identify driving competency at any stage of the driving process. The OT is responsible for the overall **driving evaluation** but may delegate specific assessments and aspects of the treatment plan to the OTA.

Driving assessment and intervention are relevant across all practice areas in occupational therapy. The OTA should decide whether the client's need can be managed within the OTA's expertise or whether the need requires the intervention of driving specialist. The OTA working in the school systems can begin addressing predriving skills with students who have learning disabilities. Predriving skills include community independence, such as crossing streets, financial management, and appropriate social interactions. Children who use wheelchairs may require occupational therapy services to address safe transfers in and out of vehicles as well as vehicle transportation options. As students with disability approach driving age, there may be a need for additional resources within a driver rehabilitation program.

PURPOSE OF THE DRIVING EVALUATION

A client entering a driving rehabilitation program for the first time is initially seen for an evaluation to help establish a baseline of skills, areas needing improvement, and appropriate goals. The outcome of the evaluation could be one of the following:

- The client is safe to drive without further intervention.
- The client needs further driver rehabilitation services to be safe when driving.
- The client is unsafe to continue driving and would not benefit from further driver rehabilitation.

The OTA must address alternative transportation holistically when driving cessation is recommended, as discussed later in the chapter. If the client requires further driver rehabilitation services to be safe to drive, driving skills may be relearned in the car or in the clinic. Interventions may address areas of cognition, vision, perception, and/or motor skills. Driver evaluations may form the basis for a plan of care to address driver training with adaptive equipment and may serve as a template for identifying vehicle modifications when appropriate.

CANDIDATES FOR DRIVING ASSESSMENT

Health care professionals, including physicians, therapists, and case managers, play an important role in identifying individuals who require a driver evaluation. According to the American Medical Association, "physicians have an ethical responsibility to assess client's physical or mental impairments that might adversely affect driving abilities. A physician may suggest that the individual seek further assessments and evaluation in occupational therapy" (American Medical Association and the National Highway Traffic Safety Administration, 2003). By thoroughly screening referrals for appropriateness, occupational therapists can conserve client resources and provide cost-effective treatment. For example, a client with a cognitive impairment who is unsafe in the kitchen or in managing his or her medications would not be a good candidate to return to driving until assessed as independent in these skill areas.

To drive, a person must have the cognitive skills to be safe at home and in the community. Further, vision skills must meet the state's licensing requirements before the client can be referred to a driver rehabilitation program. A referral to a qualified driver evaluation program should be considered if any of the following conditions arise and the OT or OTA feels the person's cognitive skills are appropriate for driving:

1. The client, family, or health care professional expresses concerns about the driver's safety or competence behind the wheel.
2. The client has limitations that preclude use of the standard driving pattern of two-handed steering and right foot on the gas and brake.
3. The client has a neurologic condition (e.g., traumatic brain injury, cerebrovascular accident, peripheral neuropathy,

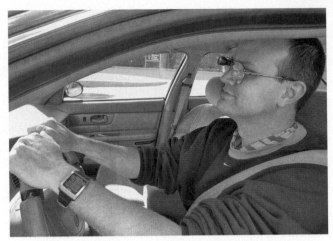

Fig. 15.22 Driver with low vision driving with bioptic lenses.

Parkinson disease, dementia, multiple sclerosis, muscular dystrophy, polio).
4. The client has impaired or low vision but meets the vision requirements for licensing in the state of residence. A variety of lenses that enable driving for persons with low vision (Fig. 15.22) are available.
5. The client is a student with learning impairments or physical disabilities (e.g., cerebral palsy, spina bifida, attention deficit disorder, autism spectrum disorder).

DRIVING EVALUATION

Driver rehabilitation programs vary greatly in the types of services offered. Some programs offer clinical evaluations or road test simulations. Simulation programs are valuable in general problem identification, but research shows that performance during simulation tests does not predict road performance. A comprehensive driver evaluation program includes both a clinical component and a driving component in an evaluation vehicle (Kostyniuk & Shope, 2003a, 2003b; Lam et al., 2008).

One of the important elements of a driving evaluation is direct observation of driving behavior. A driver who tailgates and speeds will be at a much greater risk than the individual who keeps a large following distance and stays at or below the speed limit. With a mild delay in cognitive processing speed, the risk to be tailgater or a speeder increases. What may seem insignificant in the clinic may take on large significance on the road. Conversely, what may seem to be a significant deficit in the clinic may be a minimal factor behind the wheel. In general, people are not good critics of their own driving behaviors, and therefore self-report is not always reliable.

Clinical Evaluation

The **clinical evaluation**, also referred to as a prescreening evaluation or predriving evaluation, aims to identify strengths and weaknesses related to driving. This evaluation is conducted by the OT, who may delegate assessments to the OTA. The clinical evaluation begins with a review of medical information such as medical history, vision history, medication and side effects, episodes of seizure, or loss of consciousness. An interview concerning ADL and IADL is conducted to determine routines, supports, and independence levels at home and in the community. The interview should include driving history, driving goals, and routine driving environments. The driving environment section includes questions such as: (1) Does the driver plan to drive in city traffic or in a small local community? and (2) Does the driver restrict driving to daytime hours and familiar routes?

Vision Screening. A comprehensive vision assessment includes acuity, ocular-motor skills, peripheral fields, and depth perception. Standards for distance acuity and peripheral field vary by state jurisdiction. Comprehensive vision screening is important because vision is the primary sense used to gather information required for driving-related decision making (see Chapter 21).

Motor and Sensory. Muscle strength, active ROM, grip, and right foot reaction time are often cited as the basic required measurements (Carp, 1972; Kostyniuk & Shope, 2003a; Sabo & Shipp, 1989; Easterseals, 2020; Toglia, 2001). In addition, muscle tone, dynamic sitting and standing balance, transfer status, ambulation status, type of ambulation device, and endurance are also important components to the evaluation (Stav Beth, 2004). Awareness of light touch, deep pressure, kinesthesia, and proprioception are critical for the right LE to locate the pedals and apply appropriate pressure. UE sensory awareness is also important to locate and operate the turn signals, air controls, and wiper controls while keeping eyes on the road. Coordination is necessary to control the steering wheel, move the foot accurately between the pedals, and manipulate levers, dials, gear selectors, and the seat belt (Stav Beth, 2004). During the assessment of physical and sensory measurements, the potential need for equipment or modifications, if any, should be identified and used during the road evaluation. Sensory and physical deficits may indicate the need for adaptive equipment. However, given intact cognitive skills, many persons with motor impairments can drive successfully with adaptive equipment (Fig. 15.23).

Cognitive and Visual-Perceptual Skills. Driving requires adequate reliable perception of a rapidly changing environment, blending both cognitive and visual-perceptual skills. Specific mental functions that require assessment include processing speed, selective and divided attention, attention shift, problem solving, judgment, auditory and visual memory (Stav Beth, 2004), and, most importantly, self-awareness of how the disability affects one's driving skills. Visual perception determines how the driver interprets what he or she sees in the driving environment. Components of visual perception include visual organization, visual search and scanning, spatial relations, and visual processing speed (Kostyniuk & Shope, 2003a; Lillie, 1993; Sabo & Shipp, 1989; Easterseals, 2020; Toglia, 2001). Standardized tests that assess these skills in relation to driving performance should be used to identify the driver's abilities and areas for potential intervention.

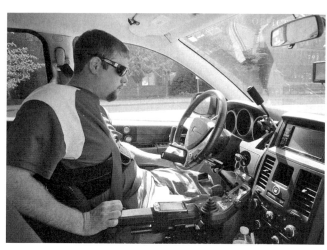

Fig. 15.23 Driver with spinal cord injury driving while seated in a wheelchair in a modified van.

Road Evaluation

Most driver rehabilitation programs use an evaluation vehicle owned by the rehabilitation facility. The vehicle may be a car or a specialized van. The vehicle should be equipped with an instructor's brake and rearview mirror for the evaluator, similar to a driver education vehicle. Any adaptive equipment recommended in the clinical evaluation should be available in the evaluation vehicle during the assessment.

Predriving tasks should be evaluated, including mobility to the vehicle, entering and exiting the vehicle, inserting and turning a key (or keyless entry operation), opening and closing the door, loading and unloading mobility devices (cane, walker, wheelchair), adjusting the driver seat and mirrors, and fastening the seat belt.

The route for the driving evaluation is critical for assessing specific skills. A new driver should be evaluated in an appropriate environment, such as an empty parking lot or low-traffic residential setting. Emphasis should be placed on maneuvering the vehicle for braking, accelerating, and turning. A driver education background or the assistance of a driver educator is helpful during the road evaluation.

The environment for an experienced driver learning adaptive equipment should be similar to that for a new driver and should address the same skills. An individual with paraplegia driving with hand controls to operate the accelerator and brake will need to master the controls in a controlled or low-traffic driving environment before progressing to more complex traffic. Clients who have overcome strokes or other paralyzing injuries might have to learn to use different foot accelerators than before their injury.

The road evaluation should always begin in low-traffic environments. Eventually, such clients must be evaluated in a traffic environment that will test any cognitive and visual-perceptual deficits; this testing should include complex environments that require cognitive skills such as rapid visual scanning, quick decisions, visual perception, and divided attention.

BOX 15.3 Skills Assessed in Road Evaluations

1. Maneuvering the vehicle
   Acceleration and braking
   Turning
   Speed control
   Lane changes
   Parking and backing
2. Skills at varying types of intersections and driving environments
   Rural roads
   Parking lots
   Residential
   Business traffic
   Interstate
3. Executive functions
   Route planning
   Decision and problem solving
   Judgment and insight

An individual with memory deficits should be evaluated in familiar geographic areas where they can be challenged with trip planning. For example, the evaluator may ask the driver to travel to three routine destinations such as the client's grocery store, post office, and church. Recall of the driving route and destinations can distract an individual with memory deficits from the driving task, causing him or her to make a driving error. If the evaluator compensates by providing directions (such as "turn right at the next block"), the accuracy of the assessment is compromised. For individuals with memory deficits, the role of driver rehabilitation is often to identify if the individual is safe to drive.

Drivers who limit themselves to a few local destinations may be able to be evaluated from home. This concept of modifying the driving environment for the road assessment is similar to that used in a cooking activity. If an individual prepares only microwave meals, the therapist would not ask him or her to cook a Thanksgiving dinner as part of the evaluation. However, making certain the driver has the ability to manage detours and other unexpected driving situations is necessary even in a limited driving environment. Skills assessed in the road evaluation are shown in Box 15.3.

Interpretation of the Evaluation

The clinical evaluation helps to identify which deficits are affecting the driving performance. For example, missing a red light may result from decreased speed of the right foot moving between the gas and brake or from problems in visual scanning or cognitive processing speed.

Careful evaluation of the benefit of recommended adaptive equipment used during the evaluation is critical for individuals who require modifications. The equipment can be costly and is often paid for out of pocket. Further evaluation and training may be necessary before any final recommendations are made.

DRIVER REHABILITATION

Rehabilitation of driving skills can take many forms and may occur in the clinic or while driving. The OT may delegate the rehabilitation to the OTA, a driving school instructor, or family members. Toglia identifies three areas that rehabilitation can address: the person, the environment, and the task (Gourley, 2000; Toglia, 2001).

A person may be able to learn strategies to compensate for deficits or to improve visual skills, specific mental functions, or physical abilities. For example, the individual with disorganized visual scanning may be instructed on new search patterns while driving, riding as a passenger, or using tools such as a visual scanning board in the clinic. Driving simulators or computerized programs can be appropriate in some cases to develop cognitive and visual skills for driving.

The driving environment may need to be adjusted. For example, a client with decreased cognitive processing speed may benefit from limitations on driving conditions such as confining driving to daytime hours, avoiding rush hours, or revising driving routes to avoid complex intersections.

The driving task can be altered to make it easier by adding a spinner knob for an individual with an UE deficit or installing blind spot and rearview convex mirrors for an individual with limited neck rotation. Adaptive equipment such as hand controls, reduced effort steering, and electronic gas/brake systems may be recommended to reduce the physical demands of driving. The person should be trained with the adaptive equipment in a variety of traffic conditions.

DRIVING CESSATION

The OTA practicing in the area of driver rehabilitation may have to recommend **driving cessation** when appropriate. It is critical to attend to the emotional impact on the individual who is unable to drive. Having medical supports and community resources in place prior to the conversation is critical. Working closely with the client's physicians, other medical professionals, and family members can aid in transition. The OTA should address plans for alternative transportation so that the client can maintain and participate in as many community roles as possible. If a transition plan is not provided and implemented, isolation and depression could follow.

Studies have shown that many older Americans who do not drive stay home because transportation options are lacking. As a group, they are less likely to use alternatives to the automobile (Kostyniuk & Shope, 2003a; Strano, 1987). Most rely on family and friends for transportation (Kostyniuk & Shope, 2003a; Taira, 1989) and in doing so experience feelings of indebtedness that become burdensome and demeaning (Carp, 1972; Latson, 1987). Resources such as the Area Agency on Aging (AAA) can provide information on transportation alternatives.

MODES OF COMMUNITY MOBILITY

Community mobility is defined by the Occupational Therapy Practice Framework as "moving [oneself] in the community and using private or public transportation" (American Occupational Therapy Association, 2008; Gourley, 2000). Community mobility may be achieved by driving or using the bus, train, subway, taxi, volunteer drivers, friends, family, and special paratransit services. A holistic approach is crucial for addressing community mobility. This includes assessment of the individual's goals, purposes for community access, and performance skills. Educating individuals on transportation options and their cost is important for making the driving cessation process run smoothly.

TASK DEMANDS

Environments

Urban areas often offer public transit systems by bus, rail, or both. However, many people live outside these areas. In rural areas of the country, nondrivers have limited options for transportation and oftentimes rely on family and friends. Those who are capable may ride a bicycle or walk. Walking can be an option but is not an appropriate mode of community transportation for everyone. One in 3 older nondrivers walks on a given day in denser areas, as compared with 1 in 14 in more spread-out areas (American Medical Association and the National Highway Traffic Safety Administration, 2003; Andrew, 2019). Inclement weather affects conditions for walking.

Motor

Motor demands in the community may challenge endurance, functional balance, and use of a mobility device in public settings. For example, the individual may need to be assessed for the ability to climb the stairs of a bus and for transfers in and out of the vehicle. For the individual who requires physical assistance, the caregiver and the client need training together with the vehicle. Loading and unloading of the walker or wheelchair will also need to be addressed.

Poor sidewalk conditions or hills or wet or icy conditions may challenge an individual's balance for walking or may prevent inefficient propelling of a manual wheelchair.

Mental Function

The mental function needed for community mobility is varied. Examples may include navigation, safety in public settings, and use of public transit systems. For example, an individual may have difficulty interpreting a bus system schedule. People with limited social skills may not know how to address strangers on the bus route, and individuals with cognitive limitations may need to develop the skills for arranging rides from volunteer drivers and taxi services. Other relevant tasks may be limited because of cognitive impairments; these include time management, financial management, and trip planning.

Visual Functions

Vision limitations can affect individuals in a number of different ways. The individual with low acuity may find reading a bus schedule or a bus route sign challenging. The client with visual field cuts walking in a parking lot may not be aware of cars backing up. People with visual-motor deficits may find it challenging to scan the environment accurately and efficiently to cross the street.

INTERVENTION

Mass Transit

In urban areas, the OTA can provide bus (or subway) training to assist the individual to develop the cognitive skills for using the transit system. The following progression could be used for a client with a learning disability, brain injury, or stroke who may otherwise have the capabilities to use mass transit:

- Stage 1 focuses on comprehension of the task. This involves working with the individual to read and understand the system schedule. To build skills gradually, the OTA would ask the individual to plan a route to get to a destination that does not involve transfers to another bus or subway line.
- Stage 2 consists of close supervision while the person performs the task. For example, this may mean riding with the individual in the same seat to acquaint him or her to the idea of paying the fare, talking to the bus driver, or reading the schedule to ensure that the right train or bus is taken.
- Stage 3 provides distant supervision to ensure independence in the task. The OTA would ride with the individual but not next to him or her. This allows the OTA to observe whether the individual can carry out the steps in stage 1 and 2 without support.
- Stage 4 provides supervision at a further remove. For example, the OTA might follow in a car behind a bus or in the next train car if the individual is traveling by train. The goal in stage 4 is to be out of sight but available to rescue the client, if need be. If the individual can plan the route, manage the time responsibilities, and address the financial aspects, he or she may have reached independence in a simple route.

When the task is completed successfully to stage 4, increased complexity (i.e., bus or train transfers) can be added. Depending on the individual's skills and deficits, training for increased complexity may start at stage 1; for the more capable client, stage 3 may be an appropriate place to begin.

Transportation as a Passenger

The OTA can educate the caregiver who is providing transportation. Proper body mechanics, communication techniques to prevent agitation, and assistive devices are a few of the areas that can be taught (Sabo & Shipp, 1989). Another role for the OTA is to identify appropriate candidates for paratransit services (State of California Department of Rehabilitation Mobility, 1990). Typically, these services provide wheelchair-accessible vehicles for those who cannot ride regular public transportation.

PEDESTRIAN SAFETY

A pedestrian must exercise a wide range of skills. In addition to the motor and visual components, the pedestrian uses topographic orientation, abstract thinking, problem solving, and reasoning skills to move in various environments. Once an OT has completed the evaluation of pedestrian safety, an OTA can train an individual with cognitive deficits to cross the street and ambulate safely in the community. If the person has visual or motor limitations, additional training techniques would be necessary. For example, the individual may require skills to move a mobility device such as a walker or wheelchair safely in the community. For a client with a vision impairment, proficiencies in visual scanning may be necessary.

SUMMARY

Driving and community mobility is essential for fulfilling many areas of human occupation: education, work, leisure, and social participation. The OTA must consider the client's community mobility needs in the context of desired occupations and participation. Interventions for driving and community mobility can be provided across all practice areas. The OTA may recognize deficits in performance skills necessary for driving and should discuss recommendations with the OT to make a referral to a specialized driver rehabilitation program or recommend driving cessation when appropriate.

In the United States, the automobile has become the primary mode of community mobility. Driving is the IADL most likely to affect the safety of other people. All health care professionals need to anticipate which clients may impose a safety risk to themselves or to others. The medical community views occupational therapy as a key resource for information and evaluation of driving skills. The American Occupational Therapy Association (AOTA) has helpful information regarding community mobility and driving safety for the generalist therapist and the therapist specializing in driving and community mobility. Additional resources are offered through a number of organizations (Box 15.4).

Community mobility can be achieved by a variety of means, by walking or using public or private transportation. The client's performance skills, goals for accessing the community, and community resources are important considerations when addressing community mobility. The OTA can help identify the appropriate means for community mobility and provide a rehabilitation approach to help individuals reach a level of independence for routine and novel transportation situations.

REFERENCES

Adler, C. (1987). *Wheelchairs and seat cushions: A comprehensive guide for evaluation and ordering*. San Jose, CA: Santa Clara Valley Medical Center, Occupational Therapy Department.

Adler, C., Musik, D., & Tipton-Burton, M. (1994). *Body mechanics and transfers: Multidisciplinary cross-training manual*. San Jose, CA: Santa Clara Valley Medical Center.

American Medical Association and the National Highway Traffic Safety Administration. (2003). *Physician's guide to assessing and counseling older drivers*. Chicago, IL: American Medical Association.

American Occupational Therapy Association. (2008). *Occupational therapy practice framework: Domain and process* (2nd ed.). Bethesda, MD: American Occupational Therapy Association.

American Occupational Therapy Association. (2005). Statements driving and community mobility. *The American Journal of Occupational Therapy*, 59(6), 666–669.

Anderson, K. N., Anderson, L. E., & Glanze, W. D. (2002). *Mosby's medical, nursing and allied health dictionary* (6th ed.). St Louis, MO: Mosby.

Andrew, M. (2019). Geronimo, taking the eye road: a new access method for powered mobility in amyotrophic lateral sclerosis. *Muscle & Nerve*, 60(5), 493–495.

Bailey, L. O. (2007). *Aging Americans: stranded without options, executive summary*. Washington, DC: Surface Transportation Policy Project. <www.transact.org>. http://www.transact.org/category/equity-livability/.

Carp, F. M. (1972). Retired people as automobile passengers. *Gerontologist*, 12, 73–78 [Cited in Kostyniuk, L. P., & Shope, J. T. (2003). Driving and alternatives: older drivers in Michigan. *Journal of Safety Research*, 34(4), 407–414.].

Easterseals. (2020). *Transportation solutions for caregivers: a starting point*. <www.easterseals.com/transportation>.

Esquenazi, A., & Hirai, B. (1995). Gait analysis in stroke and head injury. In R. L. Craik, & C. A. Oatis (Eds.), *Gait analysis: Theory and application*. St Louis, MO: Mosby.

Giles, A. K., & Kraft, S. (2020). MOBI—mobility aids. <https://itunes.apple.com/us/app/mobi-mobility-aids/id1205309397?mt = 8 and https://play.google.com/store/apps/details?id = com.goodbarber.testgiles>.

Gourley, M. (2000). OT assessments save thousands for paratransit service. *OT Practice*, 5(23), 11.

Heart and Stroke Foundation of Canada. *Stroke engine*. <https://www.strokengine.ca/en/glossary/functional-ambulation/>.

Kostyniuk, L. P., & Shope, J. T. (2003a). *Reduction and cessation of driving among older drivers: Focus groups*. Ann Arbor, MI: The

---

BOX 15.4 Additional Resources

Websites for Pertinent Associations

AAA Foundation for Traffic Safety
  Publishers of consumer pamphlets and products
  http://www.aaafts.org

ADED, the Association for Driver Rehabilitation Specialists
  CDRS information, disability fact sheets, bulletin board for driver evaluators
  http://www.driver-ed.org

American Association of Retired Persons
  Information and publication on older driver issues
  http://www.aarp.org

National Mobility Equipment Dealers Association
  Product manufacturers and equipment installers
  http://www.nmeda.org

National Highway Traffic Safety Administration
  Airbag on-off switch and consumer information
  http://www.nhtsa.gov

University of Michigan Transportation Research Institute; [Rep. No. UMTRI-98-26].

Kostyniuk, L. P., & Shope, J. T. (2003b). Driving and alternatives: older drivers in Michigan. *Journal of Safety Research, 34*(4), 407—414.

Lam, T., Noonan, V., & Eng, J. J. (2008). A systematic review of functional ambulation outcome measures in spinal cord injury. *Spinal Cord, 46*(4), 246—254.

Latson, L. F. (1987). Overview of disabled drivers' evaluation process. *Physical Disability (Special Interest Section Newsletter), 10*(4).

Lillie, S. M. (1993). Evaluation for driving. In: T. T. Yoshikawa, E. L. Cobbs, K. Brummel-Smith (Eds.), *Ambulatory geriatric care.* St Louis, MO: Mosby.

National Registry of Rehabilitation Technology Suppliers. (2020). About. <https://nrrts.org/about/>.

Pezenik, D., Itoh, M., & Lee, M. (1984). Wheelchair prescription. In: A. P. Ruskin (Ed.), *Current therapy in physiatry.* Philadelphia, PA: WB Saunders.

Rehabilitation Engineering and Assistive Technology Society of North America. (2020). *ATP General Info.* <https://www.resna.org/atp-general-info>.

Sabo, S., & Shipp, M. (1989). *Disabilities and their implications for driving.* Ruston, LA: Center for Rehabilitation Sciences and Biomedical Engineering, Louisiana Tech University.

Santa Clara Valley Medical Center, Physical Therapy Department. (1985). *Lifting and moving techniques.* San Jose, CA: Santa Clara Valley Medical Center.

State of California Department of Rehabilitation Mobility. (1990). *Statement of assurances for providers of driver evaluation services.* Downey, CA: State of California Department of Rehabilitation Mobility Evaluation Program.

Stav Beth, W. (2004). *Driving rehabilitation: A guide for assessment and intervention.* San Antonio, TX: PsychCorp.

Strano, C. M. (1987). Driver evaluation and training of the physically disabled driver: additional comments. *Physical Disability (Special Interest Section Newsletter), 10*(4).

Taira, E. D. (1989). *Assessing the driving ability of the elderly.* Binghamton, NY: Hayworth.

Toglia, J. (2001). *The Multicontextual Approach to Rehabilitation of Awareness, Memory and Executive Function Impairments.* Workshop presented at the Rehabilitation Institute of Chicago, Chicago, IL.

(1979). *Wheelchair prescription: Measuring the patient.* Camarillo, CA: Everest & Jennings [booklet 1].

(1979). *Wheelchair prescription: Wheelchair selection.* Camarillo, CA: Everest & Jennings [booklet 2].

16

Work

Gina Regiacorte-Mosher

OBJECTIVES

After reading this chapter, the student or the occupational therapy practitioner will be able to do the following:

1. Describe the history of occupational therapy's involvement with work rehabilitation and development.
2. Recognize names of assessments and evaluations used in general work evaluations.
3. Describe the purpose of a functional capacity evaluation.
4. Describe the services provided in work hardening programs.
5. Discuss the purpose of transitional work and modified duty programs.
6. Explain why and how preemployment testing is conducted.
7. Describe the process and requirements of a school-to-work transition program.
8. Explain how a work readiness program differs from other work programs.

KEY TERMS

Vocational rehabilitation
Occupational rehabilitation
Ergonomics
Engineering controls
Work practice controls

Administrative controls
Job demand analysis
Prework screening tool
Functional capacity evaluation
Worksite evaluation

INTRODUCTION

The role of work is critical in the development of identity, social relations, and a sense of mastery. It also provides a means of economic independence regardless of a person's ability or disability status (American Occupational Therapy Association, 2012). According to the employment population ratio data in the 2018 Bureau of Labor Statistics (BLS), 65% of those without a disability were employed and 19% identified as having a disability were employed (US Department of Labor, 2020). The data released for this report in 2019 indicated that there was a marked decrease in unemployment for both. The increased overall employment rate supports the continued need for the unique and holistic skill set of occupational therapists (OTs) and occupational therapy assistants (OTAs) to support individuals in the workforce.

HISTORY OF OCCUPATIONAL THERAPY INVOLVEMENT IN WORK PROGRAMS

The psychosocial importance of the role in our overall quality of life as humans is one of the cornerstones of the profession of occupational therapy. In Europe, in the late 18th and early 19th centuries, the first providers of occupationally based therapy acknowledged the importance of work related to the profession's purpose and future focus (Harvey-Krefting, 1985).

The concept of using work tasks as a means of achieving rehabilitation goals also surfaced at Massachusetts General Hospital in Boston when Dr. Herbert Hall collaborated on a program called "The Work Cure" (Harvey-Krefting, 1985). In both cases the treatment centered on restoring the impaired body to its maximum level of function and on return to the highest quality of life. "Work Cure" program participants produced goods that were then sold for profit, which they subsequently shared in.

The end of World War I brought with it a pressing need to rehabilitate large numbers of wounded soldiers so that they could return either to military service or home to resume their role as the bread winner of their families (Jacobs & Baker, 1995). With the new demand for rehabilitation of military personnel, the federal government created the US Board of Vocational Education. The program produced the first reconstructive aides. These aides provided the foundation for the professions of occupational and physical therapy.

Vocational rehabilitation continued to evolve with the Vocational Rehabilitation Act of 1943 (Public Law 78–113) to include both physical and mental limitations. Later in the 1960s occupational therapy experienced a rise in participation with prevocational testing and training activities. This time period was marked by the development of the Testing, Orientation, and Work Evaluation in Rehabilitation (TOWER) system, which utilized job simulation to develop prevocational and vocational skills. Professionals such as Florence S. Cromwell worked to establish norms for prevocational testing for adults with cerebral palsy. Also, in the 1960s and early 1970s Mary Reilly was instrumental in the development of occupational behavior theory and its premise that people achieve healthy living with a balance of work, rest, and play.

Since the 1970s occupational therapy practitioners have actively engaged in work and industrial rehabilitation programs and have been recognized for their skill set and expertise. This includes understanding the value of the work role to the individual.

The Americans with Disabilities Act (ADA) (Public Law 101–336) was passed in the 1990s. During this time, the American Occupational Therapy Association (AOTA) established the Work and Industry Special Interest Section (WISIS) to support OTs and OTAs who were providing services to this population (American Occupational Therapy Association, 2014).

Last, the ongoing efforts of the Occupational Safety & Health Administration (OSHA) to reduce the incidents of musculoskeletal disease (MSD) and work-related injuries supports the work of the valuable and unique skill set of occupational therapy in working to achieve its goal.

OCCUPATIONAL REHABILITATION

Society continues to focus on increasing the numbers of individuals in the workforce and decreasing the incidents of injury. OTs and OTAs can use their expertise in activity analysis and the wholistic view of the individual to provide many services related to **occupational rehabilitation**. These include:
1. Ergonomic oversite, injury prevention
2. Job demand analysis (JDA)
3. Prework screen development (PWS)
4. Vocational evaluations
5. Functional capacity evaluations (FCE)
6. Workstation evaluations and associated modified-duty activity
7. Work hardening and work conditioning
8. Transition services from school to work

ERGONOMICS

Ergonomics is the applied science concerned with designing and arranging things people use so that the people and things (e.g., tools) interact most efficiently and safely (Merriam-Webster's Dictionary, 2020). This concept is also recognized as biotechnology and human engineering. Ultimately the focus is on maximum production with minimum or no injury.

The skills of OTs and OTAs are a natural fit to provide all levels of ergonomic services. Their training in understanding client factors, the functional understanding of the biopsychosocial aspects of the whole person, and the effects of illness and injury on both make them an asset to any ergonomic program.

There are several factors within the role of work that can detract from the ergonomic synergy between the worker and the job. This imbalance and may increase the risk of injury. Fig. 16.1 provides a checklist of ergonomic risks. These factors include:
1. Repetition: Performing the same motion continually/frequently or for an extended period (e.g., data entry tasks)
2. Force: Including pushing, pulling, lifting heavy objects, maintaining control of heavy equipment (e.g., grip force required to operate a forklift)
3. Awkward/malaligned positioning: Twisting, kneeling, crawling (increases stress to the body structures)
4. Static positions: Maintaining a posture for an extended amount of time (e.g., standing on a production line)
5. Prolonged direct pressure to soft tissue: Leaning against a sharp edge, such as a counter edge, or the edge of a desk while typing
6. Vibration: To whole body or hands/arms, increases forces required to maintain control (e.g., using a pneumatic staple gun)
7. Extreme heat or cold exposure: Hot conditions, for example, that require the body to cool itself off and may dehydrate muscles resulting in them fatiguing more quickly and may contribute to strains
8. Light: Too light or dark can result in eye strain
9. Ill-fitting tools: Tool handles, for example, that are too large and thus require increased forces to manipulate them accurately

The presence of more than one risk factor can substantially increase the risk for injury. The goal of ergonomics or biotechnology is to decrease or eliminate risk factors that can contribute to injury while at the same time supporting efficient work practices. Ergonomic interventions to address the presence of risk factors fall under three areas of control: engineering controls, work practice controls, and administrative controls.

Engineering controls involve the design and/or modification of a workspace and/or tools. The goal of engineering control is to reduce or eliminate the presence of any combination of the risk factors. An example of an engineering control may be to install adjustable work tables on a production line so that the height of the workspace can be adjusted to the worker, on his or her shift, and subsequently adjusted at the beginning of the next shift for the next worker.

Work practice controls include the policies and procedures the employer can implement to support safe work practices. These may include a comprehensive orientation program that ensures that newly hired employees understand how to operate equipment safely and develop good ergonomic work habits.

Administrative controls address the duration frequency and severity of exposure to particular risk factors. They are more often implemented when factors are not adequately reduced by other areas of control (engineering or work practice). Administrative action addresses processes, including tasks/job rotation and use of PPE. A grocery distribution center whose workers move product in and out of a walk-in freezer may be required to wear specially insulated uniforms to reduce the risk factor of extremely low temperatures.

The understanding of ergonomics and the related integral ergonomic interventions is an integral part of any work-related activity pertaining to worker performance and safety. The concepts are a cornerstone to any area of vocational rehabilitation. They are also key to ergonomic and injury prevention activities.

General Ergonomic Risk Analysis Checklist

Check the box if your answer is "yes" to the question. A "yes" response indicates that an ergonomic risk factor that requires further analysis may be present.

Manual Material Handling
- ❏ Is there lifting of loads, tools, or parts?
- ❏ Is there lowering of loads, tools, or parts?
- ❏ Is there overhead reaching for loads, tools, or parts?
- ❏ Is there bending at the waist to handle loads, tools, or parts?
- ❏ Is there twisting at the waist to handle loads, tools, or parts?

Physical Energy Demands
- ❏ Do tools and parts weigh more than 10 lbs?
- ❏ Is reaching greater than 20 inches?
- ❏ Is bending, stooping, or squatting a primary task activity?
- ❏ Is lifting or lowering loads a primary task activity?
- ❏ Is walking or carrying loads a primary task activity?
- ❏ Is stair or ladder climbing with loads a primary task activity?
- ❏ Is pushing or pulling loads a primary task activity?
- ❏ Is reaching overhead a primary task activity?
- ❏ Do any of the above tasks require five or more complete work cycles to be done within a minute?
- ❏ Do workers complain that rest breaks and fatigue allowances are insufficient?

Other Musculoskeletal Demands
- ❏ Do manual jobs require frequent, repetitive motions?
- ❏ Do work postures require frequent bending of the neck, shoulder, elbow, wrist, or finger joints?
- ❏ For seated work, do reaches for tools and materials exceed 15 inches from the worker's position?
- ❏ Is the worker unable to change his or her position often?
- ❏ Does the work involve forceful, quick, or sudden motions?
- ❏ Does the work involve shock or rapid buildup of forces?
- ❏ Is finger-pinch gripping used?
- ❏ Do job postures involve sustained muscle contraction of any limb?

Computer Workstation
- ❏ Do operators use computer workstations for more than 4 hours a day?
- ❏ Are there complaints of discomfort from those working at these stations?
- ❏ Is the chair or desk nonadjustable?
- ❏ Is the display monitor, keyboard, or document holder nonadjustable?
- ❏ Does lighting cause glare or make the monitor screen hard to read?
- ❏ Is the room temperature too hot or too cold?
- ❏ Is there irritating vibration or noise?

Environment
- ❏ Is the temperature too hot or too cold?
- ❏ Are the worker's hands exposed to temperatures less than 70° F?
- ❏ Is the workplace poorly lit?
- ❏ Is there glare?
- ❏ Is there excessive noise that is annoying, distracting, or producing hearing loss?
- ❏ Is there upper extremity or whole body vibration?
- ❏ Is air circulation too high or too low?

General Workplace
- ❏ Are walkways uneven, slippery, or obstructed?
- ❏ Is housekeeping poor?
- ❏ Is there inadequate clearance or accessibility for performing tasks?
- ❏ Are stairs cluttered or lacking railings?
- ❏ Is proper footwear worn?

Fig. 16.1 Ergonomic risk assessment checklist. (From Cohen AL, Gjessing CC, Fine LJ, et al. *Elements of Ergonomics Programs: A Primer Based on Workplace Evaluation of Musculoskeletal Disorders*. Washington, DC: US Government Printing Office; 1997.)

Tools

- ❏   Is the handle too small or too large?
- ❏   Does the handle shape cause the operator to bend the wrist in order to use the tool?
- ❏   Is the tool hard to access?
- ❏   Does the tool weigh more than 9 pounds?
- ❏   Does the tool vibrate excessively?
- ❏   Does the tool cause excessive kickback to the operator?
- ❏   Does the tool become too hot or too cold?

Gloves

- ❏   Do the gloves require the worker to use more force when performing job tasks?
- ❏   Do the gloves provide inadequate protection?
- ❏   Do the gloves present a hazard of catch points on the tool or in the workplace?

Administration

- ❏   Is there little worker control over the work process?
- ❏   Is the task highly repetitive and monotonous?
- ❏   Does the job involve critical tasks with high accountability and little or no tolerance for error?
- ❏   Are work hours and breaks poorly organized?

Fig. 16.1 (Continued).

JOB DEMAND ANALYSIS

The **job demand analysis** (JDA) quantifies the physical and environmental demands/components of a job and subsequently provides a comprehensive description of its physical, psychosocial, and environmental requirements (Tables 16.1, 16.2, and 16.3). OTs and OTAs are highly qualified to perform the analysis with their understanding of task analysis and the wholistic workings of human beings. The quantified data from JDA are instrumental in the development of legally compliant job descriptions that clearly define the physical, psychological, and environmental demands of a job. Once the demands of a job are clearly defined, the employer can also use supporting JDA data to design a meaningful prework screen. This tool can provide analysis information and be helpful in determining appropriate return-to-work plans for injured employees.

The JDA process requires gathering information and data from several sources. These include interviews with supervisors and workers, observations of job task performance, and formal measurements (heights, weights, cycle times, etc.).

Although subjective, the interview sheds light on the practical knowledge of the work experience by the individuals performing the job. This can aid in identifying risk factors that may have otherwise been overlooked in the objective data gathering.

The object data are best gathered using standardized process. Standardized tools will objectively quantify the data and support consistency in its analysis. This information can then be used to determine the objective physical demands of the job. Subsequently it can be integrated into a job description and then into the related prework screen for that job. The *Dictionary of Occupational Titles* is a useful resource in defining the physical demands by occupation (see Table 16.1). It can assist in identifying specific criteria or work demands to be measured at the job site, including weights of tools, forces required to move items and reach distances/frequency, as well as sitting or standing times. Once the data are gathered,

each work demand is weighted in relation to the common standard to attain the essential functional requirement of the job analyzed. These calculations can be done manually or with software products.

Prework Screening

As previously mentioned, one of the products that benefits from the data gathered in the JDA is a **prework screening tool** (PWS). The PWS typically includes a host of testing components used to assess a perspective employee's abilities to perform the essential requirements of the job prior to hire.

Employers who use the PWS process are encouraged to have policies and procedures in place to support its use. This becomes particularly pertinent if a potential candidate fails the screen. Typically, the employer is notified of a candidate's passing or failing. Based on the established policies and procedures, the employer may choose to rescind the offer. In other cases, however, an employer may choose to adopt reasonable accommodations and continue with the hiring process (Snodgrass, 2004).

Vocational Evaluation

Occupational therapy evaluations tell us information about a person's functional status at the time of the evaluation relative to a diagnosis. The information is typically used as a baseline for future patient goals and plans. An OTA can participate in gathering objective data during the process. This will be used to collaborate with the OT on interpreting assessment results, setting goals, and developing an intervention plan.

The vocational or work evaluation can be customized to test the individual's potential to perform a type of work relative to returning to a job. It can also be adapted to a generalized format to assist in identifying an individual's abilities relative to overall employment options. A specific vocational evaluation may be administered to a person who is seeking to return to work at a lumberyard after suffering a stroke. After a review of the person's medical history, the valuation may

TABLE 16.1 Definitions for Overall Level of Work

Level of Work	Definition
Sedentary	Exerting up to 10 pounds of force occasionally or a negligible amount of force frequently to lift, carry, push, pull, or otherwise move objects, including the human body. Sedentary work involves sitting most of the time but may involve walking or standing for brief periods of time. Jobs are sedentary if walking and standing are required only occasionally, but all other sedentary criteria are met.
Light	Exerting up to 20 pounds of force occasionally, or up to 10 pounds of force frequently, or a negligible amount of force constantly to move objects. Physical demand requirements are in excess of those for sedentary work. Although the weight lifted may be only a negligible amount, a job should be rated light work when it requires walking or standing to a significant degree, when it requires sitting most of the time but entails pushing or pulling of arm or leg controls, or when the job requires working at a production rate pace entailing the constant pushing or pulling of materials even though the weight of those materials is negligible. NOTE: The constant stress and strain of maintaining a production rate pace, especially in an industrial setting, can be physically demanding of a worker even if the amount of force exerted is negligible.
Medium	Exerting 20 to 50 pounds of force occasionally, 10 to 25 pounds of force frequently, or greater than negligible up to 10 pounds of force constantly to move objects. Physical demand requirements are in excess of those for light work.
Heavy	Exerting 50 to 100 pounds of force occasionally, 25 to 50 pounds of force frequently, or 10 to 20 pounds of force constantly to move objects. Physical demand requirements are in excess of those for medium work.
Very Heavy	Exerting force in excess of 100 pounds of force occasionally, more than 50 pounds of force frequently, or more than 20 pounds of force constantly to move objects. Physical demand requirements are in excess of those for heavy work.

Data compiled from US Department of Labor, Employment and Training Administration. *Revised Dictionary of Occupational Titles.* 4th ed. Washington, DC: US Government Printing Office; 1991: vol. I/II; US Department of Labor, Employment and Training Administration. *The Revised Handbook for Analyzing Jobs.* Indianapolis, IN: JIST Works; 1991.

TABLE 16.2 Definitions for Physical Demand Frequencies

Physical Demand Frequency	Definition
Never	Activity or condition does not exist
Occasionally	Up to 1/3 of the day
Frequently	1/3 to 2/3 of the day
Constantly	2/3 to full day

Data compiled from US Department of Labor, Employment and Training Administration. *Revised Dictionary of Occupational Titles.* 4th ed. Washington, DC: US Government Printing Office; 1991: vol. I/II; US Department of Labor, Employment and Training Administration. *The Revised Handbook for Analyzing Jobs.* Indianapolis, IN: JIST Works; 1991.

TABLE 16.3 Strength Demands of Work

	FREQUENCY OF FORCE EXERTION OR WEIGHT CARRIED		
Strength Rating	Occasional (up to 1/3 of the day)	Frequent (1/3 to 2/3 of the day)	Constant (over 2/3 of the day)
Sedentary	10 lb	Negligible	Negligible
Light	20 lb	10 lb	Negligible
Medium	20–50 lb	10–25 lb	10 lb
Heavy	50–100 lb	25–50 lb	10–20 lb
Very Heavy	Over 100 lb	50–100 lb	20–50 lb

Data compiled from US Department of Labor, Employment and Training Administration. *Revised Dictionary of Occupational Titles.* 4th ed. Washington, DC: US Government Printing Office; 1991: vol. I/II.

the individual. The information from the evaluation may also be useful for the employer who is interested in providing accommodations.

A generalized vocational evaluation is an overall assessment of an individual's vocational potential. These evaluations are appropriate for someone who has never worked before or cannot return to a previous job for any reason. The general vocational evaluation identifies abilities and interests. The data can then help to determine appropriate and suitable employment options. A doctor may request this type of evaluation for a patient who suffered permanent injury following a car accident and is unable to return to the job as a welder but wants to work. Neither the doctor nor the patient knows what the patient's vocational potential is, and the evaluation can help determine the individual's physical abilities, cognitive abilities, and tolerance, which can aid with future employment opportunities.

In the evaluation process the OT completes the initial intake. An OTA who has completed additional training in standardized work testing and vocational assessments can assist in gathering data for portions of the evaluation. The OT will then complete the final analysis and summary, offering recommendations for the individual's vocational goals.

include testing to assess his/her ability to attend to tasks safely considering distractions in the work environment (e.g., noise, temperature, movement). Manual skills, balance, and agility may also be appropriate testing components depending on

Functional Capacity Evaluation

The **functional capacity evaluation** (FCE) is an extensive vocational evaluation that takes anywhere from 4 to 8 hours and sometimes may occur over 2 days (Fig. 16.2; Box 16.1). The data and their interpretation identify an individual's abilities to perform work. Requesters of the evaluation vary. Employers may request an FCE to determine if an employee can safely return to a job. Workers' compensation insurance companies may request the evaluation to determine if the individual is employable. Last, an evaluation may be required to decide on disability status.

There are several data points crucial to the overall evaluation. They include:

1. Review of the past medical history and current health status.
2. Preevaluation interview with the individual: although subjective, the information is helpful in appropriately planning the evaluation process.
3. Evaluation of cardiopulmonary function and musculoskeletal status (e.g., blood pressure [BP], range of motion, balance, flexibility, heart rate). The data will aid in determining if the individual can safely participate in the battery of FCE tests.
4. Standardized tests of functional work performance are preferable. They offer a higher rate of reliability and validity to published values. Informal evaluations that are developed by individuals exist, but data are not supported by standard testing methods and therefore are less reliable. The Matteson and Workwell systems are examples of FCE products with extensive research and data that support their reliability. They also provide clear testing definitions, equipment required, standard instructions, and scoring procedures. These components reduce variations in the testing process, which subsequently increases the reliability of the data. Another important aspect to the standardized products is a component built in to validate the sincerity of effort by the individual. Those individuals that give less than full effort will decrease its validity and utility in providing accurate and helpful results.

With added training, OTAs can participate in gathering the objective data for portions of the evaluation that do not require interpretation. All information collected from past medical history through the standardized testing is used in the interpretation process.

OTs have expertise in the biopsychosocial components of human performance and skill in task analysis to produce the final FCE report. Depending on the requester's expectations, the final FCE product can:

1. Set realistic goals for rehabilitation
2. Identify residual work capacity of an injured worker
3. Determine disability status
4. Identify abilities toward new employment opportunities
5. Identify the individual's functional status for closing a workers' compensation case

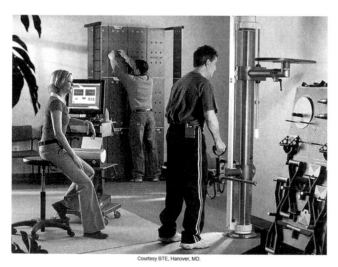

Fig. 16.2 The Eval Tech Functional Testing System, an example of a functional capacity evaluation system. (Courtesy BTE, Hanover, MD.)

WORKSITE EVALUATION

A **worksite evaluation** (WSE) takes place at the individual's place of employment. It compares the essential functional requirements of the job with the identified worker's abilities to perform them safely (Box 16.2).[39] The evaluation report will include ergonomic recommendation and potential accommodations that support safe work performance for the employee.

The request for a WSE can originate from a medical provider overseeing the care of an injured worker or from the employer. Gathering information prior to the evaluation will aid in preparing the OT and OTA for the onsite data gathering and areas of focus. The employee injury record will provide the demographic information to consider, date of injury, reported injury event, and course of medical care to date (Spencer, 2000). These data points will aid the OT in determining areas to focus attention. The job description will describe the essential functions of the job and provide insight into the actual job tasks that should be evaluated.

Worksite evaluations require various tools to gather data, which are dependent on the components of the job tasks.

BOX 16.1 VARIOUS FUNCTIONAL CAPACITY EVALUATION SYSTEMS

Blankenship	Medigraph
BTE Technologies	Occucare
DSI	Procomp
Ergoscience	Valpar-Joule
Evaluwriter	West/Epic
J-Tech	Workhab
Key	Worksteps
Matheson	Workwell

BOX 16.2 Twenty Physical Demands of Work

Lifting	Kneeling
Standing	Crouching
Walking	Crawling
Sitting	Reaching
Carrying	Handling
Pushing	Fingering
Pulling	Feeling
Climbing	Talking
Balancing	Hearing
Stooping	Seeing

Data compiled from US Department of Labor, Employment and Training Administration. *Revised Dictionary of Occupational Titles.* 4th ed. Washington, DC: US Government Printing Office; 1991: vol. I/II.

Pictures and videos are often very helpful. They capture actual work performance. Their data are used for both performance interpretation and future education opportunities for the individual and employer.

Additional tools that are often needed include measuring tape, force gauge, and supplies to record work layout and production of work process.

The most accurate data are typically gathered when the individual's supervisor and the employee are present. In some instances, the employee may invite safety representatives, process engineers, and/or a fellow employee to attend the evaluation.

The supervisor's input is critical in providing information about the company's expectation of the work process relative to safety measures in place and production expectations. At the same time, it provides an opportunity for the OT and OTA to engage management in understanding and supporting future recommendations and/or accommodations.

The employee may be asked to perform the job tasks during the evaluation if he or she is able and it is safe to do so. If the individual is unable, there are two ways to gather the needed data. The employee may describe how the job tasks are performed or another employee may be asked to demonstrate. Optimally the evaluator wants to observe the job tasks being performed. This allows the OT and OTA to determine actual disconnects between the essential job functions and how the employee is executing them.

The report generated from the worksite evaluation should include:
- Name of the requestor of the evaluation
- Name of the employee
- Injury or reason for request
- Names of all attendees and their titles
- Identified challenges to safe work performance and the associated recommendations/accommodations
- Recommended resources to help the recommendations be implemented (when possible)

The onsite portion of the evaluation allows the attendees the opportunity to share practical information related to tasks and the nuances of the processes they feel may be of concern relative to safety. It also allows for immediate insight and education to the attendees on potentially safer ergonomic work practices.

Occupational therapy's foundations in human performance, activity analysis and adaptation skill set, and understanding of ergonomics aid in the production of meaningful recommendations. The recommendations fall into the three areas described earlier in the chapter. They may include modification recommendations to movement patterns (e.g., body mechanics), workflow, job duties (e.g., modified duties, equipment or adaptive equipment), and/or schedule changes.

The Job Accommodation Network (JAN) is a tool that may be useful in identifying appropriate accommodation options. This tool was originally developed by the President's Committee for the Employment of People with Disabilities. It continues to be a relevant resource and is available at http://askjan.org.

There are numerous evaluation templates available for use in data gathering and recommendation generation. Figs. 16.3, 16.4, and 16.5 provide examples of ergonomic assessment and risk factors for computer and hand tool users.

WORK HARDENING AND WORK CONDITIONING

Work hardening and work conditioning are two levels of programming tasked with returning individuals to work. In either program meaningful work activities are incorporated into the plan as a means of rehabilitation. This concept is not only relevant to the return-to-work process but is at the very core of the profession of occupational therapy.

A correlation has been identified between individuals who were out of work for an extended amount of time and the rate of return to work. Early intervention was discovered to be critical in reducing the development of symptoms magnification and/or assuming a "sick roll"—both of which significantly delay return to work. The programming initiating 6 to 12 weeks postacute injury or symptoms identification tended to elicit the best result in returning individuals to work.

Work hardening is a highly structured and individualized program first developed in the 1970s to improve the return-to-work rates. In 1977 Leonard Matheson was one of the first to formalize and illustrate the extensive process. By the 1980s the Commission on Accreditation of Rehabilitation Facilities (CARF) developed specific guidelines for work hardening programs and an associated certification (Jacobs, 1995). The formal process involves close collaboration by an interdisciplinary team, which can include a psychiatrist, physical therapist, OT, psychologist, vocational counselor, among others.

Components of the work hardening program include physical conditioning, work simulation activities, education related to good ergonomic movement patterns, and psychosocial interventions that address topics such as stress. The time commitment is extensive and typically requires several hours per day 5 days per week for 4 to 8 weeks.

In the 1980s, to meet the need for a less intensive program, the American Physical Therapy Association (APTA) developed the Work Conditioning Program. One discipline oversees the plan, which requires much less time commitment in

Symptoms Survey: *Ergonomics Program*

Date _____/_____/_____/

_____   _____   Job Name _____
Plant   Dept #

_____   _____   _____ years _____ months
Shift   Hours worked/week   Time on THIS Job

Other jobs you have done in the last year (for more than 2 weeks)

_____   _____   _____   _____ months _____ weeks
Plant   Dept #   Job Name   Time on THIS Job

_____   _____   _____   _____ months _____ weeks
Plant   Dept #   Job Name   Time on THIS Job

(If more than 2 jobs, include those you worked on the most)

Have you had any pain or discomfort during the last year?

☐ Yes   ☐ No (If NO, stop here)

If YES, carefully shade in area of the drawing which bothers you the MOST.

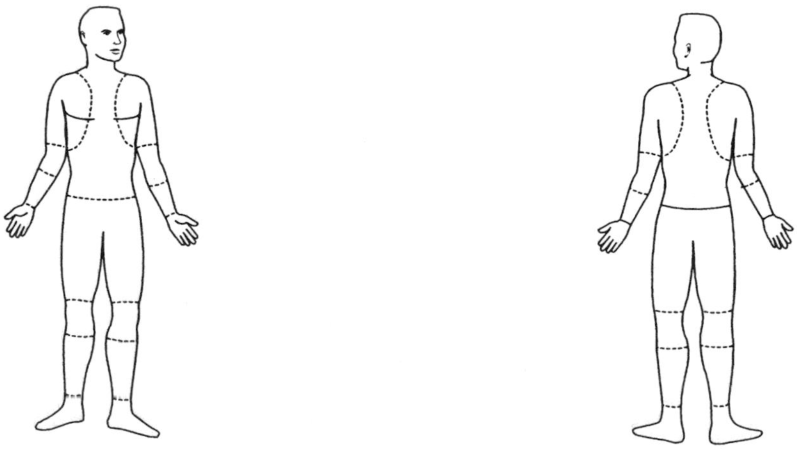

Front   Back

(Continued)

Fig. 16.3 Ergonomic assessments, pages 1 and 2. (From Cohen AL, Gjessing CC, Fine LJ, et al. *Elements of Ergonomics Programs: A Primer Based on Workplace Evaluation of Musculoskeletal Disorders.* Washington, DC: US Government Printing Office; 1997.)

(Complete a separate page for each area that bothers you)

Check Area: ☐ Neck ☐ Shoulder ☐ Elbow/Forearm ☐ Hand/Wrist ☐ Fingers
☐ Upper Back ☐ Low Back ☐ Thigh/Knee ☐ Low Leg ☐ Ankle/Foot

1. Please put a check by the words(s) that best describe your problem

☐ Aching   ☐ Numbness (asleep)   ☐ Tingling
☐ Burning   ☐ Pain   ☐ Weakness
☐ Cramping   ☐ Swelling   ☐ Other
☐ Loss of Color ☐ Stiffness

2. When did you first notice the problem?_____ (month)_____ (year)

3. How long does each episode last? (Mark an X along the line)

_____/_____/_____/_____/_____/
1 hour   1 day   1 week   1 month   6 months

4. How many separate episodes have you had in the last year?_____

5. What do you think caused the problem?_____
_____

6. Have you had this problem in the last 7 days? ☐ Yes ☐ No

7. How would you rate this problem? (mark an X on the line)
   NOW

   _____
   None   Unbearable
   When it is the WORST

   _____
   None   Unbearable

8. Have you had medical treatment for this problem?   ☐ Yes ☐ No

   8a. If NO, why not?_____

   8b. If YES, where did you receive treatment?

   ☐ 1. Company Medical   Times in past year _____
   ☐ 2. Personal doctor   Times in past year _____
   ☐ 3. Other   Times in past year _____
        Did treatment help? ☐ Yes ☐ No _____

9. How much time have you lost in the last year because of this problem?_____days

10. How many days in the last year were you on restricted or light duty because of this problem?
    _____ days

11. Please comment on what you think would improve your symptoms
_____
_____
_____
_____

Fig. 16.3 (Continued)

Risk Analysis Checklist for Computer-User Workstations

"No" responses indicate potential problem areas which should receive further investigation.

1. Does the workstation ensure proper worker posture, such as

- horizontal thighs? ☐ Yes ☐ No
- vertical lower legs? ☐ Yes ☐ No
- feet flat on floor or footrest? ☐ Yes ☐ No
- neutral wrists? ☐ Yes ☐ No

2. Does the chair

- adjust easily? ☐ Yes ☐ No
- have a padded seat with a rounded front? ☐ Yes ☐ No
- have an adjustable backrest? ☐ Yes ☐ No
- provide lumbar support? ☐ Yes ☐ No
- have casters? ☐ Yes ☐ No

3. Are the height and tilt of the work surface on which the keyboard is located adjustable? ☐ Yes ☐ No

4. Is the keyboard detachable? ☐ Yes ☐ No

5. Do keying actions require minimal force? ☐ Yes ☐ No

6. Is there an adjustable document holder? ☐ Yes ☐ No

7. Are arm rests provided where needed? ☐ Yes ☐ No

8. Are glare and reflections avoided? ☐ Yes ☐ No

9. Does the monitor have brightness and contrast controls? ☐ Yes ☐ No

10. Do the operators judge the distance between eyes and work to be satisfactory for their viewing needs? ☐ Yes ☐ No

11. Is there sufficient space for knees and feet? ☐ Yes ☐ No

12. Can the workstation be used for either right- or left-handed activity? ☐ Yes ☐ No

13. Are adequate rest breaks provided for task demands? ☐ Yes ☐ No

14. Are high stroke rates avoided by

- job rotation? ☐ Yes ☐ No
- self-pacing? ☐ Yes ☐ No
- adjusting the job to the skill of the worker? ☐ Yes ☐ No

15. Are employees trained in

- proper postures? ☐ Yes ☐ No
- proper work methods? ☐ Yes ☐ No
- when and how to adjust their workstations? ☐ Yes ☐ No
- how to seek assistance for their concerns? ☐ Yes ☐ No

Fig. 16.4 Checklist of risks for computer user workstation. (From Cohen AL, Gjessing CC, Fine LJ, et al. *Elements of Ergonomics Programs: A Primer Based on Workplace Evaluation of Musculoskeletal Disorders.* Washington, DC: US Government Printing Office; 1997.)

both frequency and duration. The work conditioning program limits its focus on work-related physical conditioning interventions and does not include the psychosocial components.

In either the work hardening or work conditioning programs, return to full-duty work is the primary goal; however, if the individual is unable to accomplish the goal then the focus may evolve to maximizing work capacity. Transitional work and modified duty may become viable options. These may support the individual returning to employment in some capacity other than full duty.

Handtool Risk Factor Checklist

"No" responses indicate potential problem areas which should receive further investigation.

1. Are tools selected to limit or minimize

   - exposure to excessive vibration?   ☐ Yes   ☐ No
   - use of excessive force?   ☐ Yes   ☐ No
   - bending or twisting the wrist?   ☐ Yes   ☐ No
   - finger pinch grip?   ☐ Yes   ☐ No
   - problems associated with trigger finger?   ☐ Yes   ☐ No

2. Are tools powered where necessary and feasible?   ☐ Yes   ☐ No

3. Are tools evenly balanced?   ☐ Yes   ☐ No

4. Are heavy tools suspended or counterbalanced in ways to facilitate use?   ☐ Yes   ☐ No

5. Does the tool allow adequate visibility of the work?   ☐ Yes   ☐ No

6. Does the tool grip/handle prevent slipping during use?   ☐ Yes   ☐ No

7. Are tools equipped with handles of textured, non-conductive material?   ☐ Yes   ☐ No

8. Are different handle sizes available to fit a wide range of hand sizes?   ☐ Yes   ☐ No

9. Is the tool handle designed not to dig in the palm of the hand?   ☐ Yes   ☐ No

10. Can the tool be used safely with gloves?   ☐ Yes   ☐ No

11. Can the tool be used by either hand?   ☐ Yes   ☐ No

12. Is there a preventive maintenance program to keep tools operating as designed?   ☐ Yes   ☐ No

13. Have employees been trained

    - in the proper use of tools?   ☐ Yes   ☐ No
    - when and how to report problems with tools? ☐ Yes   ☐ No
    - in proper tool maintenance?   ☐ Yes   ☐ No

Fig. 16.5 Checklist for hand tool user. (From Cohen AL, Gjessing CC, Fine LJ, et al. *Elements of Ergonomics Programs: A Primer Based on Workplace Evaluation of Musculoskeletal Disorders.* Washington, DC: US Government Printing Office; 1997.)

TRANSITION SERVICES FROM SCHOOL TO WORK

The 1997 amendments to the 1990 Individuals with Disabilities Education Act (IDEA) stated that transitional planning should be a part of the student's Individualized Education Plan (IEP). The OT is a formal participant in the transition plan for the student who requires these services. OTAs offer valuable contributions when working with such students in the transition activities themselves. IDEA defined transition services as "a coordinated set of activities for a student designed within an outcome-oriented process, which promotes movement from school to post-school activities, includes post-secondary education, vocational training, integrated employment (included supported employment), continuing and adult education, adult services, independent living, or community participation." The

OT's unique focus on occupational performance is a strong asset to the overall intention of the plan.

There are three functions in which OTs participate in the transition plan: (1) transition-related evaluation, (2) service planning, and (3) service implementation. OTAs can be an integral part of the service implementation activities. The OT is typically responsible for evaluation and plan development. Both the OT and the OTA contribute vital functional information about the student's performance and needs in the transition domains of domestic, vocational, school, recreation, and community.

In the transition process, the evaluator uses nonstandardized interviews, situational observation, and activity analysis. In addition, it is very important that all service providers consider what the student wants or needs. Subsequently they identify the occupational performance issues related to the challenges to the student achieving their goal. A transition team will help the student identify a positive and shared vision of the future. The vision may include goals such as living alone or with others in the community, attending postsecondary school or training programs, working as a volunteer or for pay, using community services, and participating in activities of interest. The OT, OTA, and other members of the team collaborate to identify the student's current interests and abilities as they relate to the transition goals. Areas of ongoing support and resources to achieve the vision will also be identified.

The team works together collaboratively with the student to write their goals of the individual's transition plan. For example, a student with limited arm and hand function may have a goal to complete written assignments independently. The OT may assist the student by evaluating alternative writing methods such as assistive technology and make recommendations. If the team supports the recommendations, the team may also assign equipment acquisition and training to the OT, OTA, and student.

The OT and OTA collaborate with the student and their team throughout the transition plan as appropriate. They may assist the student in goal achievement in the areas of domestic activities, vocational activities, school, recreation, and community. Typically, services are provided to the student in the natural environment. This can entail the OT or OTA working with the student at the school, workplace, home, or other community setting. Collaborative problem solving is essential in assisting the student to develop adapted methods to achieve goals and/or successfully complete activities. For example, an OTA may train a teacher to use assistive technology to help the student access it to complete homework assignments. The OTA can provide direct or consultative services to maximize success for the student with their goals. Evaluating goal achievement should be an outcome measure completed by the OT.

Work readiness programs are another avenue to support vocational goals. The program is designed for individuals who desire to work but cannot return to their employment due to an illness or major injury. The person has a desire to participate in some type of meaningful work but needs guidance and support to identify his or her vocational goals. Work readiness programs help the individual identify practical vocational options that match specific interests, skills, and abilities. Work readiness activities may take place in a group venue or individual session as needed and can be led by an OTA. Subject matter addressed in the sessions may include work values, habits, goals, work skills, vocational interests, job hunting, skill development, and exploration of community resources.

SUMMARY

This chapter provides an overview of the numerous opportunities OTs and OTAs have to support individuals in integrating or reintegrating the role of work into their daily lives through data collection, program facilitation, and treatment with the ongoing community. The focus is on increasing employment for both able and disabled individuals, and the increasing opportunities for OTAs to continue to be an integral part of the initiative. Boxes 16.3 and 16.4 provide additional resources for advanced training opportunities and regulatory agencies related to work rehabilitation, respectively.

BOX 16.3 Education and Training Opportunities in Ergonomics

Education and training beyond occupational therapy entry-level practice is necessary for achieving advanced competence in ergonomics.

- University-sponsored graduate certificate programs in ergonomics are available through Texas Women's University, Cleveland State University, University of Central Florida, and the University of Massachusetts. These graduate-level courses typically require four to five courses for a total of 12 to 16 credit hours.
- Continuing education providers offer several-day courses that earn the occupational therapist eligibility for certifications such as the Ergonomics Evaluation Specialist available through Roy Matheson and Associates, Inc. (www.roymatheson.com) and the Certified Ergonomics Assessment Specialist available through the Back School of Atlanta (www.thebackschool.net).
- The Oxford Research Institute (www.oxfordresearch.org) offers the following advanced-level certifications: Certified Industrial Ergonomist, Certified Associate Ergonomist, and Certified Human Factors Engineering Professional.
- The Board of Certification in Professional Ergonomics (BCPE) (www.bcpe.org) offers the highest level of certification in the field of ergonomics: the Certified Professional Ergonomist. Other advanced-level certifications available through the BCPE include Associate Ergonomics Professional, Certified Ergonomics Associate, Certified Human Factors Professional, and Associate Human Factors Professional.

From Snodgrass J. Getting comfortable: developing a clinical specialty in ergonomics has its own challenges and rewards. *Rehab Management* 2004(July):24—27.

BOX 16.4 OSHA AND NIOSH

The Occupational Safety and Health Act of 1970 created both the National Institute for Occupational Safety and Health (NIOSH) and the Occupational Safety and Health Administration (OSHA). Although NIOSH and OSHA were created by the same act of Congress, they are two distinct agencies with separate responsibilities.

OSHA is under the US Department of Labor and, as a regulatory agency, is responsible for developing and enforcing workplace safety and health regulations. OSHA developed the following publication guidelines to assist industries in developing in-house ergonomic programs:

- Ergonomic Program Management Guidelines for Meatpacking Plants (1993) (OSHA Publication 3123)
- Guidelines for Nursing Homes: Ergonomics for the Prevention of Musculoskeletal Disorders (Revised 2009) (OSHA Publication 3182)
- Guidelines for Retail Grocery Stores: Ergonomics for the Prevention of Musculoskeletal Disorders (2004) (OSHA Publication 3192-05 N)
- Guidelines for Poultry Processing: Ergonomics for the Prevention of Musculoskeletal Disorders (2004) (OSHA Publication 3213-09 N)
- Guidelines for Shipyards: Ergonomics for the Prevention of Musculoskeletal Disorders (2008) (OSHA Publication 3341-03 N)

These publications can be ordered at www.osha.gov or by calling 1-800-321-OSHA.

NIOSH is part of the Centers for Disease Control and Prevention (CDC) within the US Department of Health and Human Services. NIOSH is an agency established to conduct research and make recommendations for preventing work-related injury and illness. NIOSH and OSHA often work together toward the common goal of protecting worker safety and health.

NIOSH currently offers several publications to assist with ergonomic intervention efforts. The following may be of interest to OTAs wanting to get involved with ergonomics:

- Elements of Ergonomic Programs: A Primer Based on Workplace Evaluations of Musculoskeletal Disorders (1997) (NIOSH Publication 97-117)
- Simple Solutions: Ergonomics for Construction Workers (2007) (NIOSH Publication 2007-122)
- Ergonomic Guidelines for Manual Material Handling (2007) (NIOSH Publication 2007-131)
- Safe Lifting and Movement of Nursing Home Residents (2006) (NIOSH Publication 2006-117)
- Conference Proceedings: Prevention of Musculoskeletal Disorders for Children and Adolescents Working in Agriculture (2004) (NIOSH Publication 2004-119)
- Easy Ergonomics: A Guide to Selecting Non-Powered Hand Tools (2004) (NIOSH Publication 2004-164)
- Simple Solutions: Ergonomics for Farm Workers (2001) (NIOSH Publication 2001-111)
- Ergonomic Interventions for the Soft Drink Beverage Delivery Industry (1996) (NIOSH Publication 96-109)

These publications (and others) can be ordered from the CDC-NIOSH website: http://www.cdc.gov/niosh/ or by calling NIOSH at 1-800-CDC-INFO (1-800-232-4636); outside the United States, 513-533-8328.

REVIEW QUESTIONS

1. How has the occupational therapy process in work programs evolved over the years?
2. What is the role of the OTA in work programs?
3. Describe the difference between a functional capacity evaluation and a vocational evaluation.
4. Name the common applications of the results of a job demands analysis.
5. What are the possible outcomes of postoffer testing?
6. Describe the optimal sequence for postoffer screening.
7. Describe the difference between work hardening and work conditioning.
8. Why is having actual work equipment for use during simulation beneficial?
9. What is ergonomics?
10. What are work-related musculoskeletal disorders, and why would an ergonomic consultant be concerned with these disorders?
11. Name two excellent government resources for the OTA who is interested in practicing in the area of ergonomics and injury prevention.
12. What is the OTA's role in school-to-work transition programs?
13. What kind of client can benefit from participation in a work readiness program?

REFERENCES

American Occupational Therapy Association. (2012). *Occupational therapy services at the workplace: transitional return-to-work programs.* <https://www.aota.org/~/media/Corporate/Files/AboutOT/Professionals/WhatIsOT/WI/Facts/Transitional.pdf>.

American Occupational Therapy Association. (2014). Occupational therapy practice framework: domain and process (3rd edition). *The American Journal of Occupational Therapy, 68*(1), S2–S51.

Harvey-Krefting, L. (1985). The concept of work in occupational therapy: a historical review. *The American Journal of Occupational Therapy, 39,* 301–307.

Jacobs, K. (1995). Preparing for return to work. In C. A. Trombly (Ed.), *Occupational therapy for physical dysfunction* (4th ed.). Baltimore, MD: Williams & Wilkins.

Jacobs, K., & Baker, N. A. (1995). The history of work-related therapy in occupational therapy. In B. L. Kornblau, & K. Jacobs (Eds.), *Work: Principles and practice.* Bethesda, MD: AOTA.

Merriam-Webster's Dictionary. Definition of ergonomics.

Snodgrass, J. E. (2004). Getting comfortable: developing a clinical specialty in ergonomics has its own challenges and rewards. *Rehab Management, July,* 24–27.

Spencer, K. (2000). Transition from school to adult life. In B. Kornblau, & K. Jacobs (Eds.), *Work: principles and practice.* Bethesda, MD: AOTA.

US Department of Labor. Office of Disability Employment Policy (ODEP). Website. <www.dol.gov/agencies/odep>.

17

Promoting Engagement in Leisure and Social Participation

Nancy Carson

OBJECTIVES

After reading this chapter, the student or the occupational therapy practitioner will be able to do the following:

1. Identify the characteristics that distinguish leisure and social participation from other areas of occupation.
2. Apply the Occupational Therapy Practice Framework to leisure and social participation with clients.
3. Explain the contribution of leisure and social participation to life satisfaction, quality of life, well-being, and health for all persons.
4. Appreciate the leisure and social challenges faced by some persons with physical disabilities.
5. Apply different client-centered methods to gather information about the importance and meaning of leisure and social participation.
6. Implement occupational therapy intervention that promotes the benefit of engaging in leisure and social activities.

KEY TERMS

Leisure
Social participation
Life satisfaction
Well-being

Quality of life
Health
Client-centered

 QUOTES

Because we freely choose them, our play and leisure activities may be some of the purest expressions of who we are as persons. Anita C. Bundy (Bundy, 1993)

CASE STUDY

Winnie, Part 1: Engaging in Valued Daily Life Activities[a]
Maintaining a healthy balance between work and leisure can be a challenge, as many people struggle to make time for activities they enjoy. Winnie, a 74-year-old woman, has never had this problem. Throughout her life, Winnie maintained a beneficial balance between work and leisure activities, enjoying the best of both. As a young woman, she enjoyed dance lessons, traveling, and attending the theater while also working various jobs as a model, bookkeeper, and secretary. She raised five children and volunteered at her children's school.

After her children left home, she worked full time as an administrative secretary in the allied health division at a community college. Since her retirement, Winnie continues to maintain an active life. Her leisure pursuits are many; she

particularly enjoys gardening, embroidery, cooking, and swimming. Winnie and her husband Bill often go out to dance, and she is a member of a tap-dancing group that performs at various fundraising activities in association with the local Elks Club. Winnie is also an active volunteer at her church and is responsible each Sunday for the altar flower arrangements.

Family and friends are the center of Winnie's life. At regular family gatherings with children and grandchildren, everyone enjoys a good meal (particularly Winnie's cheesecake) and the friendly competition of a board game. Winnie attends her grandchildren's sporting events, rarely missing a game. Winnie hand-embroidered a unique Christmas stocking for each of her children and grandchildren. Her sense of humor, ready smiles, and bountiful laugh are familiar to many. She and several friends who were born in May are known as the "May Babies." Every year they celebrate their birthdays by going to the beach, where they enjoy playing cards, cooking their favorite seafood stew, and visiting the local casino.

Two and a half months before her 75th birthday, Winnie had a stroke.

[a]People generally use first names in leisure and social situations, so we refer to clients (including elders) in this chapter by their first names.

LEISURE AND SOCIAL PARTICIPATION

QUOTES

There are many ... rhythms ... the big four—work and play and rest and sleep, which our organism must be able to balance even under difficulty. Adolf Meyer (Meyer, 1922)

Over 100 years ago, the founders of occupational therapy emphasized the importance of a healthy balance in daily activities, including a focus on leisure activities (Cromwell, 1977; Meyer, 1922; Peloquin, 1991; Schwartz, 2009). This remains a core focus of occupational therapy today as occupational therapists (OTs) and occupational therapy assistants (OTAs) address well-being through the broad array of activities in which individuals and populations engage. Participation in life through engagement in a variety of daily activities (occupation) is the primary focus and outcome for clients receiving occupational therapy services. **Leisure** and **social participation** (also called leisure and social activities) are two of the areas of occupation, the others being activities of daily living (ADL), instrumental ADL (IADL), rest and sleep, education, work, and play (Box 17.1) (American Occupational Therapy Association, 2014).

Although the American Occupational Therapy Association (AOTA) defines each area of occupation, what specifically identifies a daily activity as leisure, social participation, or another area such as play? One occupational therapy perspective (Primeau, 2014) considers *play* and *leisure* as synonymous terms. Varying definitions of play and leisure are consolidated into four categories: "(1) plan and leisure as discretionary time, (2) play and leisure as context, (3) play and leisure as observable behavior or activity, and (4) play and leisure as disposition or experience" (Primeau, 2014, p. 698).

When considering leisure as discretionary time it can be conceptualized as time away from obligatory activities (Primeau, 2014). For example, Robin travels for work, meeting with clients during the day and often during mealtimes. These engagements take up much of her time on the road; she spends her free time in the hotel reading novels, relaxing in the bath, and phoning friends. The activities associated with work are considered obligatory; her free-time activities are considered discretionary. Thus, from this perspective, if an activity is not identified as obligatory, by default it is designated as leisure.

Leisure as context identifies leisure activities according to beliefs of the individual's culture, including the conditions or context in which the leisure activity occurs (Primeau, 2014).

BOX 17.1 Occupational Therapy Practice Framework Leisure and Social Participation

Leisure

Leisure is "nonobligatory activity that is intrinsically motivated and engaged in during discretionary time, that is, time not committed to obligatory occupations such as work, self-care, or sleep" (Parham & Fazio, 1997, p. 250).

- Exploration: Identifying interests, skills, opportunities, and appropriate leisure activities.
- Participation: Planning and participating in appropriate leisure activities; maintaining a balance of leisure activities with other occupations; and obtaining, using, and maintaining equipment and supplies as appropriate.

Social Participation

Social participation is "the interweaving of occupations to support desired engagement in community and family activities as well as those involving peers and friends" (Gillen & Boyt Schell, 2014, p. 607); involvement in a subset of activities that can involve social situations with others (Bedell, 2012) and that support social interdependence (Magasi & Hammel, 2004). Social participation can occur in person or through remote technologies such as telephone calls, computer interaction, and video conferencing.

- Community: Engaging in activities that result in successful interaction at the community level (i.e., neighborhood, organization, workplace, school, religious or spiritual group).
- Family: Engaging in activities that result in "successful interaction in specific required and/or desired familial roles" (Mosey, 1992, p. 340).
- Peer, Friend: Engaging in activities at different levels of interaction and intimacy, including engaging in desired sexual activity.

Modified from American Occupational Therapy Association. Occupational therapy practice framework: domain and process. 3rd ed. *Am J Occup Ther.* 2014;68(1):S1—S48.

Common features among Western societies include pleasurable, creative, stimulating, physically or mentally challenging, relaxing, artistic, energetic, competitive, and social. If an activity typically embodies one these features, it is customarily identified as leisure. These features can be used to differentiate leisure activities such as active versus sedentary, relaxing versus energetic, or social versus solitary. For example, Brad likes to pursue more solitary and physically challenging activities such as running through the park and swimming laps. Geneva enjoys more social and mentally challenging activities such as playing chess and participating in a book club. Thus many activities are considered leisure by society, although they can take different forms, and different societies may value different characteristics (Suto, 2004). Categorizing leisure activities by their common features acknowledges the social nature commonly associated with leisure; however, not all social activities involve leisure and not all leisure activities are social activities. A potential problem exists when conceptualizing leisure as free-time, discretionary activities or as activities identified by society as leisure. For any one person, not all free time may be experienced as leisure (at times, free time can be boring) and activities identified by society as leisure may not be experienced by a person as leisure.

Leisure as an observable behavior or activity allows for leisure activities to be categorized and thereby quantified and measurable; however, it does not consider the client's experience of activity engagement (Price et al., 2011). Leisure as disposition or experience considers the subjective experience and the personal meaning of leisure activities that arise from activity engagement. Leisure as experience is essential to understanding the client perspective. While understanding leisure from the perspectives of time, context, and as an observable, quantifiable activity yields useful information about the client, understanding leisure as experience is essential for incorporating leisure into practice and in addressing the leisure needs of the individual (Primeau, 2014).

The same leisure activity can be conceptualized and experienced differently by the individuals participating in the leisure activity. Each person has a unique perspective of and meaning associated with his or her engagement in the activity. For example, Tyrell attends a going-away party for a coworker and experiences the party as leisure. Scott attends the same party, considering it obligatory, and experiences it more as work. To confuse matters even more, it is a social activity for both. To account for each person's unique perspective and the fact that most activities could be experienced as leisure, professionals need to understand leisure as an experience—a state of mind unique to each person (Bundy, 1993; Suto, 1998).

Although different activities may be experienced as leisure, research highlights qualities that characterize an activity as more leisurely than work (Box 17.2) (Ball et al., 2007; Chen & Chippendale, 2018; Sellar & Boshoff, 2006; Suto, 1998). To consider an activity as leisure, a person does not need to experience each and every quality. Rather, if the person experiences many of these qualities, the activity will more likely be experienced as leisure. More importantly, the greater the intensity of each characteristic experienced, the more the activity will be experienced as leisure (Bier et al., 2009; Bonder et al., 2004). Given the qualities associated with experiencing leisure, how are these related to **life satisfaction**, **well-being**, **quality of life**, and **health**?

IMPORTANCE OF LEISURE AND SOCIAL ACTIVITIES IN EVERYDAY LIFE

Leisure engagement and leisure satisfaction is strongly associated with subjective well-being (Kuykendall et al., 2015).

BOX 17.2 Characteristics of Leisure Activities

Freedom of choice: The person freely chooses the activity (nonobligatory).

Sense of control: The person feels in charge during the activity.

Sense of enjoyment: The activity evokes pleasurable feelings.

Timelessness: Time seems to fly by while engaged in the activity.

Sense of competence: The person feels a sense of proficiency and accomplishment.

Spontaneity: The person could participate in the activity on the spur of the moment.

Intrinsic satisfaction: The person feels a sense of doing something worthwhile.

Companionship: The person experiences a sense of camaraderie and friendship.

Lack of external judgment: The person's performance is not evaluated by others.

Relaxation: The person feels a sense of relief from physical effort and emotional tension.

Novelty: The person engages in something new and different.

Freedom: The activity provides an escape from the daily necessities of life.

Considerable evidence suggests that participation in meaningful leisure and social activities positively influences a person's well-being, life satisfaction, quality of life, and health, particularly for older adults (Akbaraly et al., 2009; Caldwell, 2005; Clark et al., 1997; Dahan-Oliel et al., 2008; Gabriel & Bowling, 2004; Herzog et al., 2002; Horowitz & Vanner, 2010; Law, 2002; Pereira & Stagnitti, 2008). Older adults who are more active tend to live longer, and evidence suggests that social and productive activities (which include leisure) can be as effective as physical fitness activities in reducing a person's risk of death and enhancing quality of life (Glass et al., 1999; Paganini-Hill et al., 2011). Moreover, greater social integration is linked to a greater likelihood of survival (Holt-Lunstad et al., 2010).

Satisfaction with leisure activities and the quality of social interactions appear more important to quality of life and life satisfaction than frequency of leisure participation (Kielhofner, 2008; Odawara, 2005). Moreover, whereas spending time with family contributes to a general sense of life satisfaction, spending time with friends engenders immediate day-to-day happiness and generates more positive feelings and is associated with greater quality of life, well-being, and morale than spending time with family (Figs. 17.1 and 17.2) (Dedding et al., 2004; Kahana et al., 2013). Engagement in leisure pursuits helps develop social support networks (Heasman & Salhotra, 2008), and the prospect of establishing social connections is a primary reason why adults may choose to pursue an activity (Odawara, 2005). Most pointedly, when older adults discuss activities in their lives that have the most meaning, they rarely mention basic ADL tasks (Odawara, 2005). Rather, leisure and social activities are viewed as having the most meaning in their everyday lives.

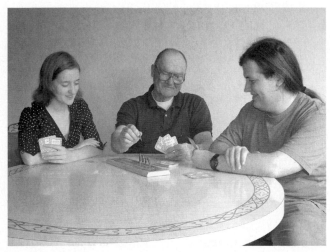

Fig. 17.1 Spending time with family contributes to general life satisfaction.

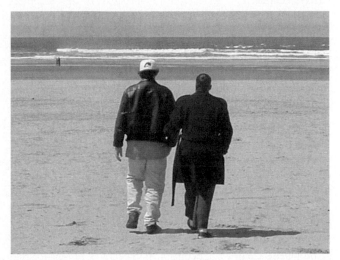

Fig. 17.2 Spending time with friends contributes to immediate day-to-day happiness.

IMPORTANCE FOR PEOPLE WITH DISABILITIES

Research also highlights the importance of leisure and social activities in the everyday lives of adults experiencing physical disabilities. Individuals with varying disabilities report reduced leisure and social participation. For example, advances in medical care have resulted in more polytrauma patients surviving their injuries and living with significant disabilities. These patients experience reduced societal participation, which is associated with decreased health-related quality of life (HRQoL) 1 to 2 years posttrauma (Leijdesdorff et al., 2019). For these individuals, the most important contributors to overall life satisfaction are family life, a sufficient social network, satisfaction with leisure, and vocation (Anke & Fugl-Meyer, 2003). A strong relationship appears to exist between well-being and involvement in leisure and social activities for persons with stroke, more so than

other factors (Akbaraly et al., 2009; Sveen et al., 2004). Adults with congenital disabilities report the importance of leisure in their lives, believing that leisure participation contributes to their physical and mental health (Specht et al., 2002). They describe the pure joy of engaging in leisure activities and the sense of belonging and self-worth that leisure and social activities promote.

Diminished Participation for People With Disabilities

Although adults with physical disabilities can experience the benefits of leisure and social activities (similar to people without disabilities), considerable evidence suggests that many do not. Many adults with physical disabilities are unhappy with their reduced participation in leisure and social activities and experience a subsequent decline in well-being and quality of life. Research confirms that persons who have experienced a stroke do not participate in as many leisure and social activities, particularly outside the home, and they identify this as a significant concern (Akbaraly et al., 2009; Hartman-Maeir et al., 2007; O'Sullivan & Chard, 2010; Rochette et al., 2007; Yi et al., 2015). One study found that 4 months after discharge from outpatient therapy for stroke rehabilitation, 50% of these individuals experienced diminished leisure and social participation (van der Zee et al., 2013). Similarly, reduced leisure and social participation occurs with adults who have arthritis (Hawker et al., 2008; Reinseth & Espnes, 2007; Stack et al., 2015; Theis et al., 2013; Wilkie et al., 2007), spinal cord injuries (Barclay et al., 2015; Bedell, 2012; Price et al., 2011), traumatic brain injuries (Bier et al., 2009; Goverover et al., 2017; Malone et al., 2019; Wise et al., 2010), Parkinson disease (Price et al., 2011; Thordardottir et al., 2014), and multiple sclerosis (Fakolade et al., 2018; Plow, Finlayson, Gunzler, & Heinemann, 2015). For older residents living in assisted living centers, concerns exist about their leisure and social participation: (1) engaging in center-sponsored activities because they are convenient and available, not because they are meaningful; (2) occupying their time with predominantly group activities designed to promote socialization; and (3) missing the opportunity to engage in activities more on their own (Crenshaw et al., 2001). These and other research studies demonstrate that participation in leisure and social activities is a significant concern for adults experiencing physical disabilities, indicating OT practitioners can provide a needed service in this area.

FACILITATING LEISURE AND SOCIAL PARTICIPATION

 QUOTES

Leisure is an occupational performance area, a state of mind, time to be filled, and a tangible activity through which therapeutic goals are met. Melinda Suto (Suto, 2004)

Adults experiencing physical disabilities advocate for leisure and social activities to be an integral part of their rehabilitation. Persons with stroke receiving inpatient rehabilitation services report that leisure activities are a means to their recovery and a lifeline to regain a sense of control over their situations (Cowdell & Garrett, 2003). They strongly desire more leisure and social activities during inpatient rehabilitation and believe this may speed their recovery, alleviate boredom, and ward off potential depression. However, occupational therapy and rehabilitation services (particularly inpatient services) place greater emphasis on physical independence in mobility, basic ADL, and household tasks and limited emphasis on leisure and social participation (Barclay et al., 2015; Korner-Bitensky et al., 2008; Reinseth & Espnes, 2007; Specht et al., 2002; Turner et al., 2000). Leisure should be included as an equally important intervention goal. As Radomski so pointedly stated after reviewing the stroke rehabilitation literature, "We have succeeded in facilitating the recovery of patients' physical skills after stroke but not in advancing their resumption of the social, leisure, and productive activities that make life worth living" (Radomski, 1995).

Although helping clients achieve greater ADL independence can be important, exclusive focus on this outcome ignores what is important to everyone—disability or not. Engagement in leisure and social activities brings greater life satisfaction, quality of life, and well-being than does independent performance of basic ADL tasks (Ball et al., 2007; Sellar & Boshoff, 2006; Suto, 1998). Leisure engagement is valued and recognized by society at large for these benefits (Chen & Chippendale, 2018). Although people with disabilities recognize the significance of leisure and social activities, rehabilitation clients sometimes may not recognize this importance (Barclay et al., 2015; Suto, 1998). They may be so focused on goals related to mobility and ADLs that they choose not to engage in leisure goals and social activities. The client's preference should always be respected with education provided to explain the role of leisure and social participation in the recovery process.

Overview of Occupational Therapy Process

OT practitioners begin the evaluation process by creating an occupational profile (Almborg et al., 2010) that includes gathering information about the meaning of leisure and social activities in the client's life. The evaluation process includes an analysis of occupational performance and should examine the client's ability to engage in desired leisure and social activities, including what supports and hinders his or her participation. Once this information is gathered, OT practitioners develop the intervention plan, collaborating with the client to develop realistic and achievable goals that focus on leisure and social participation, and selecting methods appropriate to the goals and the situation. The plan is then implemented; after a period of intervention, the client, the OT, and the OTA evaluate whether the desired outcome was achieved—that is, whether the client's leisure and social participation improved. The following sections illustrate this process.

Evaluation Process

Following a **client-centered** approach, OTs and OTAs seek to understand the client's perspective on important and meaningful leisure and social activities, particularly those of current concern. The evaluation process is the same as for other areas of occupation; interviews, observations, and standardized assessments are used to gather needed information (American Occupational Therapy Association, 2014). Although the OT begins and completes the initial evaluation, the OTA may perform specific evaluation procedures once service competency is established (Almborg et al., 2010). The OTA may conduct an interview, observe a client, or administer a standardized assessment and then share the information with the OT, who is responsible for its interpretation.

An important consideration during the information gathering process is the client's sociocultural background and beliefs regarding leisure and social participation that influence his or her perceptions about the value, choice, and degree of desired engagement in specific leisure and social activities (Bonder et al., 2004; Odawara, 2005). Through understanding the client's sociocultural perspectives on leisure and social activities (which can be different from one's own), OTs and OTAs can ensure any proposed intervention is in accord with the client's sociocultural background and preferences (Whiteford & Wilcock, 2000) (see Case Study: Gabriella). This often necessitates examining one's own sociocultural background and beliefs in regard to leisure and social activities to

CASE STUDY

Gabriella

Gabriella, a 79-year-old and grandmother to 12, recently fell and broke her hip. She is undergoing rehabilitation at a local skilled nursing facility (SNF). Her youngest grandson, Miguel, will be 8 years old in 3 weeks, and she wants to go on a weekend pass to join her family in the traditional birthday celebration. Gabriella always made her "famous" tamales for family celebrations, for which her extended family will travel miles. Recognizing the importance to Gabriella to retain her role in the family, the OTA broached the possibility of making tamales in the SNF kitchen. Gabriella told her, however, it would be difficult to make them in a kitchen that does not have all the cooking equipment that she has at home and cooking from a wheelchair seems like a lot of work. She also confided, "It's time someone else stepped up and made the tamales," an acknowledgment that Gabriella's matriarchal role within the family was changing. However, the OTA continued to talk with Gabriella about what her family celebrations usually entailed, and Gabriella mentioned that the highlight of the party is always the breaking of the piñata. The OTA proceeded to ask Gabriella if she might consider making a papier-mâché piñata for the party, particularly as the SNF had the supplies and they could enlist the help of other residents if she desired. Gabriella thought it was a great idea and started to make plans to create a large sun, filled with candy for her grandson and birthday guests to enjoy.

ensure that one's own values and beliefs are not unintentionally imposed on a client (Awaad, 2003; Odawara, 2005).

Interviewing Clients. The purpose of interviewing is to gather essential information to begin intervention, but not all information needs to be gathered during one session. Working collaboratively, the OT and the OTA may decide that the OT will briefly review leisure and social activities with a client at initiation of the evaluation and that the OTA will follow with a more in-depth interview. An informal, conversational style that prompts the client to tell stories about his or her leisure and social activities will better elicit the type of information desired—the meaning of leisure and social participation in the client's life (Fig. 17.3). To ensure a client-centered approach, the OTA should begin by asking the client what he or she considers leisure and explore the client's thoughts and feelings about leisure and social participation (Primeau, 2014; Suto, 1998).

The OTA should not continue on to another question after receiving only a brief response to a previous one. The meaning of and benefits received from leisure and social activities cannot be communicated adequately, nor understood by the interviewer, with a one-word or one-sentence response. Follow-up questions can fully illuminate the meaning of activities (Table 17.1). A conversation with careful follow-up questions elicits rich narrative data useful to plan intervention (Bundy & Clemson, 2009). By the end of the conversation the OTA should understand (1) the meaning of leisure and social activities in the client's life, and (2) specific leisure and social activities of most importance and concern to the client that could be addressed during therapy. If a client has difficulty communicating, a similar conversation with family members should occur.

Information about leisure and social activities should be gathered throughout intervention, reflected upon, and used to modify the intervention plan (American Occupational Therapy Association, 2014). The OTA should be sensitive to when a client might be ready to explore new pursuits. The client who cannot resume previous activities is confronted with a loss of self, a particularly distressing feeling. When a client

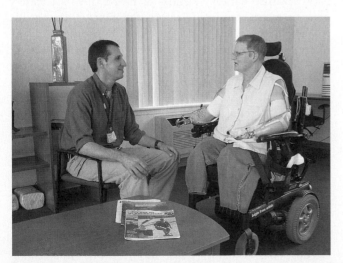

Fig. 17.3 An informal conversation best elicits the meaning of leisure and social participation.

shows readiness to consider new interests, the client and OTA can explore potential activities that have features similar to those in which the client previously engaged and in which the client may be successful and satisfied (see Case Study: Dimitri) (Suto, 1998).

CASE STUDY

Dimitri

Dimitri, a 28-year-old carpet layer, experienced multiple physical traumas from an auto accident. He was admitted to inpatient rehabilitation for a short stay. Although leisure was mentioned during the initial evaluation, Dimitri's priority was to get stronger to manage his basic ADL tasks and return to work. Three days before discharge, Dimitri began to acknowledge that he could not return to work as soon as he hoped and that he would have a lot of free time on his hands. At this time, he and the OTA began exploring his interests and how he might occupy his time at home, focusing on those leisure and social activities of interest that were within his capabilities.

Observing Clients. Whenever feasible, the OTA should observe a client engage in specific desired leisure and social activities, noting the effectiveness of the client's performance skills (American Occupational Therapy Association, 2014) (see Case Study: Stella). Turner and colleagues (Turner et al., 2000) note that OT practitioners, when gathering information about leisure, may be focusing primarily on general information about the client's leisure interests rather than the actual performance of leisure activities, indicating a greater need to focus on the performance of leisure activities during the evaluation process.

CASE STUDY

Stella

Stella was recently diagnosed with Parkinson disease and began outpatient occupational therapy. The OT conducted the initial evaluation, during which she learned that Stella enjoyed creating greeting cards for friends and family on the computer but had stopped because of the difficulty and frustration she experienced as a result of the disease. The OT discussed the evaluation results and intervention plan with the OTA, who then assumed responsibility for intervention. The OTA began by asking Stella if she could observe her using the computer in the clinic, explaining this would provide her with a clearer understanding of Stella's performance skills that supported and hindered her ability to use the computer and to perform other ADL.

Administering Standardized Assessments. Standardized assessments that focus on leisure and social activities may complement the evaluation process, although usage reported by OTs and OTAs is low (Turner et al., 2000). Standardized interest checklists such as the original Neuropsychiatric Institute (NPI) Interest Checklist (Matsutsuyu, 1969) and updated versions such as the Modified Interest Checklist (University of Illinois Board of Trustees, 2020) and Interest

TABLE 17.1 Interview Questions Regarding Client's Leisure and Social Participation	
General Questions	**Follow-Up Questions**
What do you consider leisure in your life?	What makes it leisure for you?
What do you like to do with friends? With family?	What is important about spending time with friends? With family?
What do you particularly enjoy doing?	What makes those things enjoyable?
What type of leisure activities do you prefer?	Creative? Intellectual? Physical? Relaxing? Competitive? Social? Solitary?
What do you like to do because you want to do it, not because you feel you have to do it?	What are those times like when you do things you don't necessarily have to do?
Are there times when you forget about everything else and time seems to fly?	What makes time fly? What is it that makes you forget about everything else?
Are there things you do that you feel you can do the way you want?	What allows you to do it the way you want? What is it that appeals to you about doing it the way you want?
What is (or has been) your routine of engaging in enjoyable activities? Getting together with friends? Family?	What is important about routinely engaging in enjoyable activities? Getting together regularly with friends? With family?
Are there leisure and social activities of concern to you right now?	What is of most concern? What is most important to you?

Modified from Bundy AC. Assessment of play and leisure: delineation of the problem. *Am J Occup Ther* 1993;47(3):217–219.

Checklist (UK) (Heasman & Salhotra, 2008) provide an overview of a client's interest in specific leisure and social activities. These types of checklists provide a variety of activities for which the client identifies those he or she pursued in the past, is currently participating in, or might want to pursue in the future, as well as his or her degree of interest (e.g., none, some, strong). These checklists typically do not ask the client to add to the list other activities he or she considers as leisure or social, nor do they explore the meaning of the activities to the client. A conversation is required to solicit this information. Moreover, interest checklists need to be updated periodically to reflect sociocultural changes in how people typically occupy leisure and social time. A more interactive assessment than written interest checklists, the Activity Card Sort (Baum & Edwards, 2008) uses a set of 89 photographs to help clients identify instrumental, low physical-demand leisure, high physical-demand leisure, and social activities in which the client participates. Lastly, recognizing the importance of distinguishing participating in leisure versus social activities and engaging with friends versus family, the Maastricht Social Participation Profile (Mars et al., 2009) assesses the frequency with which a person engages in 26 different activities, providing a profile of engagement over a 4-week period.

Other standardized assessments ask the client to identify activities that he or she considers leisure or social and identifies the client's performance pattern for those and other activities. The Occupational Questionnaire (OQ) (Smith et al., 1986) is a self-report assessment based on the model of human occupation (Kielhofner, 2008). The OQ requires the client to document the main activity in which he or she engages for each half-hour throughout a morning, day, and evening and identify each activity as work, daily living task, recreation, or rest (Fig. 17.4). For each activity, the client rates how well he or she does the activity, how important it is, and how much he or she enjoys it. Using the OQ allows the OTA to understand which activities the client considers leisure (if any) and to explore the meaning of leisure

from the client's perspective. The Canadian Occupational Performance Measure (COPM) (Law et al., 2005) is another standardized assessment that allows a client to identify activities that he or she considers leisure and social. During this interview-based assessment, the OT or OTA asks a client to identify self-care, productive, and leisure activities considered important and that the client needs, wants, or is expected to do. The COPM also prompts the interviewer to ask about quiet, active, and social activities. Interestingly, research indicates that use of the COPM identifies additional leisure concerns for people with physical disabilities beyond those identified in typical interview procedures (Dedding et al., 2004; McColl et al., 2000; Ward et al., 1996).

Other self-report standardized assessments focus on the meaning and experience of leisure and social activities. Instead of asking the client to identify specific activities in his or her daily life, the client rates his or her perspective on specific qualities associated with leisure (Box 17.3). The Idyll Arbor Leisure Battery (Ragheb & Beard, 1992), a battery of assessments developed within the field of therapeutic recreation, contains the Leisure Attitude Measure, Leisure Interest Measure, Leisure Satisfaction Measure, and Leisure Motivation Scale—all self-report questionnaires that explore various leisure qualities. Although standardized assessments may appear to be a quick and easy method to gather information, the OTA should typically start with an interview and use a standardized assessment to supplement the information gathered during the interview.

Intervention

The intervention process for leisure and social participation is the same as for other areas of occupation—that is, an intervention plan is developed (including the establishment of goals), implemented, monitored, and reviewed (American Occupational Therapy Association, 2014). Intervention should occur in collaboration with the client and should be tailored to each client, focusing on promoting, restoring,

Typical Activities	I consider this activity to be:	I think that I do this:	For me this activity is:	How much do you enjoy this activity:
	1= Work 2= Daily living task 3= Recreation 4= Rest	1= Very well 2= Well 3= Above average 4= Poorly 5= Very poorly	1= Extremely important 2= Important 3= Take it or leave it 4= Rather not do it 5= Total waste of time	1= Like it very much 2= Like it 3= Neither like it nor dislike it 4= Dislike it 5= Strongly dislike it
For the half hour beginning at:				
5.00 a.m.	1 2 3 4	1 2 3 4 5	1 2 3 4 5	1 2 3 4 5
5.30	1 2 3 4	1 2 3 4 5	1 2 3 4 5	1 2 3 4 5
6.00	1 2 3 4	1 2 3 4 5	1 2 3 4 5	1 2 3 4 5
6.30	1 2 3 4	1 2 3 4 5	1 2 3 4 5	1 2 3 4 5
7.00	1 2 3 4	1 2 3 4 5	1 2 3 4 5	1 2 3 4 5
7.30	1 2 3 4	1 2 3 4 5	1 2 3 4 5	1 2 3 4 5
8.00 a.m.	1 2 3 4	1 2 3 4 5	1 2 3 4 5	1 2 3 4 5
8.30	1 2 3 4	1 2 3 4 5	1 2 3 4 5	1 2 3 4 5
9.00 a.m.	1 2 3 4	1 2 3 4 5	1 2 3 4 5	1 2 3 4 5
9.30	1 2 3 4	1 2 3 4 5	1 2 3 4 5	1 2 3 4 5

Fig. 17.4 The Occupational Questionnaire: a sample selection. (From Smith NR, Kielhofner G, Watts J: *Occupational questionnaire*, Chicago, 1986, Model of Human Occupation Clearinghouse.)

BOX 17.3 Sample Questions From the Leisure Interest Measure

Domain	Question	Answers
Physical	I like leisure activities that require physical challenge. _____	Never true
Outdoor	I like the fresh air of outdoor settings. _____	Seldom true
Mechanical	I like repairing or building things in my leisure time. _____	Somewhat true
Artistic	I like to be original in my leisure activities. _____	Often true
Service	I often participate in service activities in my leisure time. _____	Always true
Social	I prefer to engage in leisure activities that require social interaction. _____	
Cultural	I have a strong attraction to the cultural arts. _____	
Reading	I like to read in my free time. _____	

Modified from Ragheb MG, Beard JG. *Leisure Interest Measure*. Ravensdale, WA: Idyll Arbor; 1991.

maintaining, and/or modifying a client's current and future participation in leisure and social activities, and/or preventing a loss of participation. Strategies to enhance a client's well-being, life satisfaction, and quality of life should not focus exclusively on engaging clients in just any leisure or social activities. Engaging in activities just to keep busy does not produce the same results as engaging in activities because they are personally meaningful (Crenshaw et al., 2001). Thus incorporating leisure and social activities into the therapy process should be client centered and unique to each client.

Because activities are both the means and end of occupational therapy intervention, leisure and social activities could be the process by which a client regains performance skills to support his or her participation in daily life activities (American Occupational Therapy Association, 2014; Chen & Chippendale, 2018). For example, by engaging in a favored woodworking project, a client could develop greater skill in grasping, manipulating, and using tools and materials—necessities for many daily activities. However, this approach accounts neither for the fact a client may experience therapy as work (even when engaged in favored leisure pursuits) nor for the inherent benefits of engaging in leisure and social activities. The greater good of leisure and social participation resides in its contribution to a client's quality of life, well-being, and life satisfaction rather than the performance skills he or she may be learning. For example, after a lower limb amputation, a young woman's achievement of going to the movies for the first time with her friends, thoroughly enjoying the time, and feeling great about it afterward far outweighs whether she can effectively and independently negotiate curbs and steps during a community outing. A client's sense of satisfaction, enjoyment, competence, camaraderie, and other qualities associated with engagement in leisure and social activities should be valued equally to the achievement of specific performance skills.

OTs and OTAs have raised concerns regarding payment, sometimes believing insurance will not reimburse for leisure or social activities (Schweitzer et al., 1999). Although each insurance plan is different, Medicare will reimburse for services when leisure or social activities are included (Centers for Medicare & Medicaid Services, 2019; Chen & Chippendale, 2018). As long as reimbursement criteria are complied with and documented accordingly, leisure and social activities may be incorporated into and become the focus of occupational therapy intervention, particularly as a means to achieve greater "independent functioning." In doing so, OTs and OTAs communicate the contribution of all activities to a person's functioning and his or her well-being, life satisfaction, quality of life, and health.

Familiarity with a variety of leisure and social activities and knowledge of how to adapt activities to improve a client's performance provide the OTA with the skills to promote a client's engagement in those activities. The OTA can assist a client's increased participation by helping him or her learn to engage in previous activities using adapted methods and/or explore new activity interests. Additionally, the OTA can create a therapeutic context that capitalizes on the inherent joy and satisfaction of engagement in leisure and social activities.

Intervention Guidelines

An inability to resume a leisure or social activity is seldom attributable solely to physical factors (Morgan & Jongbloed, 1990). Less obvious and more complex reasons are usually involved. OTs and OTAs need to consider all elements that

---

CASE STUDY

Winnie, Part 2: Focusing on Valued Activities After Her Stroke

While in the hospital, Winnie also developed bronchitis. Because of her limited cardiopulmonary endurance, she was subsequently transferred to a SNF for extended (and less intensive) rehabilitation. On admission, she needed maximal assistance to get in and out of bed, complete basic ADL tasks, and propel her wheelchair. She could barely raise her affected right arm to shoulder level or grasp objects; she was frustrated that she could not write her name or use a fork properly. She experienced episodes of eyestrain, difficulty concentrating, and fatigue, particularly at the end of days when her family and friends visited.

Winnie currently struggles to accept her condition and is concerned she might not recover in time for the "May Babies" annual birthday celebration, which is 7 weeks away. The OT interviewed Winnie on admission and identified that leisure and social activities were particularly important. The OT and OTA decided Jodi (the OTA) would conduct a more extensive interview. Because Jodi had demonstrated competency with in-depth interviews, they considered this an efficient use of time.

Using client-centered questions as a guide (see Table 17.1), Jodi obtained more detail about the meaning of leisure and social activities in Winnie's life. Throughout their conversation, Winnie conveyed that leisure and social activities are an integral aspect of who she is, not just something she does for the sake of keeping busy. She related the importance of maintaining her long-time friendships with the "May Babies" and teared up while talking about their annual birthday celebration,

a few months away. She mentioned that when she plays board games with her children and grandchildren the time seems to fly, and before they know it, her grandchildren's bedtime has passed. She commented on the raucous laughter that permeates the house during every family board game. Winnie shared that her daughter-in-law is involved in making quilts for families of soldiers who died in Iraq and Afghanistan and is disappointed she can't help because of her stroke. Maintaining her physical fitness is also important, with swimming being her top priority. Most of all, she is happy when she spends any time with her family, commenting she considers this time a blessing rather than a responsibility. As the conversation with Winnie progressed, Jodi realized she was gathering the information she needed, decided against incorporating an interest checklist, and continued the conversation.

When discussing her valued activities, Winnie repeatedly commented, "I don't see how I'm ever going to do them again." Jodi recognized the extent to which Winnie valued leisure and social activities and gently presented the possibility Winnie would again be able to engage in leisure and social pursuits. Jodi explained they could explore ways she could still be involved in valued leisure and social activities with her family and friends, perhaps engaging in old ones and also considering new ones. By being thoughtful and considerate of Winnie's perspective and gently advocating for Winnie to consider leisure and social activities at this stage of her recovery from stroke, Jodi set the stage for Winnie to begin reclaiming her well-being and quality of life. They were now ready to plan and begin intervention.

support and hinder a client's engagement (i.e., the client's performance skills, performance patterns, client factors, and context and environment) (American Occupational Therapy Association, 2014). The following guidelines are based on research and reflect those issues particularly relevant to leisure and social activities for people with disabilities and older adults. To fully address clients' leisure and social concerns, OTAs will need to draw on the entire breadth of knowledge and skills they possess.

Consider Client's Previous Level of Engagement. If a client engaged in many leisure and social activities before the onset of a health condition, a wider range of options for intervention is possible. People who have a wide range of interests are more likely to continue engaging in a previous leisure activity than those with a narrow range (Jongbloed & Morgan, 1991). This situation was certainly the case for Winnie. Given Winnie's wide range of leisure and social interests, the OTA can draw from more choices and thus is more likely to achieve engagement in some activities, although perhaps in an adapted manner.

Clients who previously participated in a limited range of leisure and social activities and who cannot perform or are not interested in previous activities are likely to need to develop new interests (Jongbloed & Morgan, 1991). In these situations, the OTA may gently propose new leisure and social options that are within the person's capability (see Case Study: Edwin).

CASE STUDY

Edwin
Edwin, 54 years old, is in inpatient rehabilitation after falling from his roof and sustaining a back injury and mild traumatic brain injury. Before his accident, according to his wife, he spent all his spare time restoring old cars with his two brothers and playing golf. This information presented a dilemma for the OTA. She recognized that Edwin would not be able to return to these activities any time soon, yet she was unaware of any other leisure or social pursuits Edwin previously enjoyed. During one session learning bathroom transfers, the OTA asked Edwin whether there was anything that he ever dreamed of doing. Edwin recalled he once thought about becoming a pastry chef but did not think it a particularly masculine career. The OTA suggested he might want to explore this idea and bake something for his wife. Edwin agreed, and the OTA recommended he choose a recipe from among the easy ones in the department recipe file. During their next kitchen session that focused on safe mobility, Edwin made a banana cream pie for his wife. Edwin was pleased with how it turned out, despite dropping some of the filling on the floor. Edwin began to recognize that it was possible to replace his former interests with ones that were within his current capacity and that he enjoyed.

If leisure and/or social activities are not a top priority in the client's life, the OTA should not press a client to accept that such activities will be good for him or her. For example, if a client experiences a condition that prevents him or her from returning to work, the client is less likely to want to substitute leisure and social pursuits for previous productive activities (Morgan & Jongbloed, 1990). In these situations, the OTA should acknowledge and work with the client's desire for productive, not leisure or social, activities. However, the OTA may want to share that engaging in leisure and social activities after a disability significantly contributes to life satisfaction, quality of life, and well-being. The choice to pursue leisure and social activities, however, is always the client's.

Consider Client's Personal Standards of Performance. The quality of performance considered acceptable by a client may determine whether he or she wants to pursue a leisure or social activity. Some clients are willing to resume activities at a lesser level of competence; others are not interested if they cannot perform to their previous standard (Jongbloed & Morgan, 1991; Schweitzer et al., 1999; Wise et al., 2010), particularly if they considered themselves proficient (see Case Study: Jean).

Encouraging a client to engage in previously enjoyed activities may have the undesired effect of making the client feel less than adequate (Morgan & Jongbloed, 1990). In these situations, the OTA may prefer to introduce new activities for which the client, not having a previous standard, may be less likely to judge his or her performance negatively. Other clients choose not to engage in an activity because they cannot do it the way they did it before their new health condition (see Case Study: Catherine).

CASE STUDY

Jean
Jean, 68 years old, loved to play word games and took great pride in her skill. She was diagnosed with early-onset dementia and began attending an adult day program in which the OTA, learning from her family that Jean liked games, tried to involve her in simple word games. Jean refused. Only after carefully observing Jean's reluctance did the OTA realize Jean refused because she recognized she could not play to her previous skill level.

CASE STUDY

Catherine
Catherine, 82 years old, is receiving outpatient occupational therapy to learn more about joint protection techniques after a severe exacerbation of rheumatoid arthritis. She identified her favorite activity, which she feels free to do in her own way, as making her special chocolate chip cookies. She takes great joy in adding various surprise ingredients such as dried cranberries or crushed mints and looks forward to her great-granddaughter's reaction when she babysits her each weekend. The OTA suggested that instead of making cookies from scratch, Catherine could save energy by using prepackaged dough and preserve her joints by cutting the tube of dough with a rocker knife. Catherine immediately rejected the idea because it was not the way she makes cookies. The OTA needed to shift focus and collaborate with Catherine on ways to save energy and protect her joints while still engaging in valued activities in a manner acceptable to Catherine.

In other cases, clients might not want to engage in activities for fear of family members' (and others') disapproval (or the perception of disapproval) of less than perfect performance (Jongbloed & Morgan, 1991) (see Case Study: Marie). If a client is frustrated with his or her diminished ability to engage in a specific leisure or social activity, he or she is less likely to consider using adaptive equipment (Schweitzer et al., 1999). OTAs must respect client choices and rejection of activities, particularly if the client is frustrated. Collaboration with the client can identify other leisure and social activities in which he or she might feel more comfortable and competent.

Emphasize Choice and Control During Activities. When activities are chosen for them and they do not feel in control, clients are less likely to want to participate (Morgan & Jongbloed, 1990). Results from the Well Elderly Program (Clark et al., 1997; Jackson et al., 1998) and a wellness program based on the model of human occupation (MOHO) for healthy older adults (Yamada et al., 2010) indicate that life satisfaction, well-being, and quality of life are enhanced when older adults are given the opportunity to explore and choose what they would like to do and when opportunities are provided that are challenging yet within their capabilities (see Case Study: Community Residence).

CASE STUDY

Marie

Marie, 32 years old, was scheduled for an overnight home visit during her final week of rehabilitation after the onset of Guillain-Barré syndrome. Marie's husband wanted to surprise her with reservations at her favorite restaurant and consulted with the OTA. During their conversation, the OTA shared that Marie had mentioned several times she thought other people were embarrassed when she spilled food and drinks. The OTA carefully suggested that her husband consider a quiet dinner alone at home because some people are uncomfortable going out in public the first time; he agreed. She also suggested to Marie that she might consider discussing her feelings with her husband. On Monday, Marie reported she and her husband had enjoyed two nice dinners at home and had talked a lot over the weekend. She said she was relieved the OTA had addressed the issue of her embarrassment with handling food and utensils with both her husband and her.

CASE STUDY

Community Residence

An OTA working at a community residence for persons with HIV disease is responsible for assisting weekly activities with residents. During one session, the residents said they wanted a barbecue at the end of the month. The OTA helped them develop a plan and decide who would do what. The day of the barbecue, the OTA arrived a few hours early to help with preparations and was pleasantly surprised. Several residents had taken it upon themselves to ask neighbors for donations of flowers and plants and had decorated

the residence. Other residents had already prepared their dishes and were helping others to make theirs. Two residents were busy rehearsing a funny poem they wrote for the invited volunteer staff, a spur-of-the-moment decision on their part. Through assisting self-choice and promoting self-control, the OTA contributed to increased enjoyment and satisfaction in the residents' daily lives.

Emphasize Exploration, Not Only Performance. For many clients, participating in structured leisure exploration programs may be of benefit to assist their eventual engagement in leisure and social activities (Desrosiers et al., 2007; Nour et al., 2002). These types of programs (similar to the previously mentioned programs but developed from a leisure perspective) help clients explore the importance of leisure, develop greater awareness of their perceptions in regard to leisure, identify leisure activities of interest, and develop competence to eventually engage in leisure activities.

Consider Attitudes of Family Members, Friends, and Others. Support from family, friends, and others is an important environmental factor with leisure and social activities (Jongbloed & Morgan, 1991; Specht et al., 2002). Family members' positive attitudes and beliefs, particularly those of spouses and partners, can encourage and support a client to resume prior activities or begin new pursuits. The OTA should also be aware if family members provide only minimal encouragement or even actively discourage leisure and social endeavors (Jongbloed & Morgan, 1991). The OTA could share with a client's family and friends that their support and encouragement are particularly important in regard to engagement in leisure and social activity. As seen later, this encouragement was a key factor during Winnie's occupational therapy. Moreover, when family and friends support the use of adaptive equipment, the client is more likely to accept and use it successfully (Schweitzer et al., 1999). The OTA should involve the client and appropriate family members and friends actively while identifying options for adaptive equipment and skills training (see Case Study: Velda).

CASE STUDY

Velda

Velda is 69 years old. She had polio when she was 3 years old and now lives in an assisted living complex. The OTA is responsible for fostering the residents' participation in valued leisure and social activities. Once every 2 months, the OTA introduces a new handicraft for residents to try. Velda's "gaggle of friends" (as Velda refers to them) look forward to this activity, but Velda often says "if it involves a new-fangled device, I just won't learn it." One month, the OTA introduced rake-knitting and suggested to Velda's friends that they playfully tease Velda into trying this "new-fangled device." It worked; Velda liked it and purchased the required wooden frame so that she could make scarves whenever she wanted (Fig. 17.5).

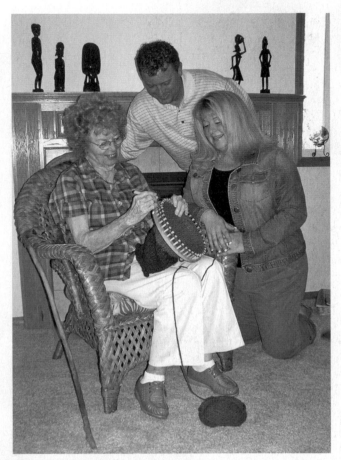

Fig. 17.5 Support of family and friends is important when learning different ways to engage in leisure activities.

Suggest Activities That Appeal to a Client's Altruistic Nature.

Because older adults particularly want to engage in responsible roles and feel depended on (Kahana et al., 2013), the OTA should explore options for leisure and social activities that appeal to a client's altruistic nature. Evidence suggests that when older adults are invited to participate in activities primarily for the benefit of others, such as decorating Valentine cookies for preschool children rather than just decorating Valentine cookies, they are more motivated and likely to participate (Cipriani, 2007; Cipriani et al., 2010; Kahana et al., 2013). When clients are reluctant to consider leisure activities during therapy because they believe it is not "real work" or "frivolous," they are more likely to agree and participate if the activity is presented as something that would benefit someone else. Most importantly, such reasons help a client believe he or she is worthwhile and doing something of value and help establish a sense of community and connectedness (Cipriani et al., 2010). As seen later, this incentive was another key factor during Winnie's occupational therapy intervention.

Identify Barriers to Transportation and Accessibility in the Community.

One of the biggest barriers to engaging in leisure and social pursuits is difficulty with transportation and accessibility in the community (Barclay et al., 2015;

Specht et al., 2002). Given the tendency for adults with physical disabilities to participate in substantially more home-based, sedentary, and solitary leisure and social activities (Almborg et al., 2010; Bier et al., 2009; Wise et al., 2010), OTAs should be familiar with community resources, including feasible means of transportation that might support a client's engagement in activities, particularly social, outside the home. They can then help educate clients and families how best to access and use suitable community resources (see Case Study: Jason). Moreover, helping clients to engage in enjoyable and social activities outside the home may also provide needed respite for family members (Ward et al., 1996).

CASE STUDY

Jason

Before his T-8 spinal cord injury, Jason, who is 33 years old, enjoyed a wide variety of social and leisure activities in the community. He played music with friends once a week, coached his daughter's soccer team, and typically ended the workweek with a date with his partner. The OTA who worked with him at the outpatient clinic knew of community resources and was familiar with the accessibility challenges people using wheelchairs face. She supported Jason's desire to get out of the house and explored with him community options that would be interesting, practical, and accessible. Jason could participate in his community and was no longer a captive in his home.

Consider the Leisure and Social Participation Desires of Family Caregivers.

Although the primary focus of intervention is the client, OTAs should also consider the leisure and social participation desires of family members who care for the client, particularly as many caregivers express diminished satisfaction with their own participation in leisure and social activities (Stevens et al., 2004). Some caregivers (particularly those with a strong family orientation) may find it hard to understand or accept that leisure is important simply because it is good for them. Here it is valuable to educate caregivers and encourage reflection on results to help them see that taking the time to engage in chosen leisure and social activities (outside of their caregiving services) can enhance their own ability to take care of clients (Rogers, 1999).

Focus on Social Participation and Leisure.

When identifying activities, the OTA should consider options beyond typical leisure pursuits such as arts, crafts, and hobbies. Because the primary motivation to engage in leisure activities may be to meet new people, establish friendships, and feel a sense of belonging (Specht et al., 2002), social activities should be identified. For adults with chronic disabilities (Hand et al., 2014) and moderate to severe traumatic brain injury (McLean et al., 2014), social interaction support is related to subjective quality of life and is as important to the individual as providing support for daily living needs. Older adults report that relationships with others are important; one of their strategies to establish social relationships is attendance at more formal gatherings (Clark et al., 1996) such as civic groups or volunteer organizations. Thus the OTA should consider options within the community to meet a client's social needs, particularly those that may not involve family members. One innovative idea involved a group of older adults who could not leave their homes (The Next Big Thing, 2005). A local agency arranged, once a week, a conference call

---

CASE STUDY

Winnie, Part 3: Engaging in Valued Activities After Her Stroke

In addition to targeting Winnie's ability to perform ADL tasks safely and more independently and setting goals to that effect, Jodi, Winnie, and the OT agreed that leisure and social participation should also be a primary focus and outcome during Winnie's anticipated 6-week rehabilitation stay. When asked, Winnie identified her activities of concern as the following:

1. Preparing food for her family
2. Attending the "May Babies" birthday celebration
3. Having fun with her children and grandchildren
4. Volunteering with her daughter-in-law to make quilts
5. Getting back to swimming

Jodi explained that although they would address all her concerns, only one would become an official goal and documented with her ADL and mobility goals. When asked which concern was most important, Winnie chose making quilts for families of soldiers. When asked for clarification, Winnie said she was feeling useless and would feel better if she was doing something for someone else. Thus a goal was documented: "By discharge, patient will satisfactorily engage in her valued leisure pursuit of making quilts for soldiers' families as a volunteer activity." Jodi assured Winnie that her other leisure and social concerns would be addressed and incorporated into therapy sessions that focused on improving Winnie's ability to perform ADL and IADL tasks such as preparing treats and meals for her family and learning to safely move about the community to attend the "May Babies" celebration and get back to swimming.

During Winnie's first week, intervention focused primarily on basic ADL and mobility tasks. However, as Winnie identified that spending time with her family was important, Jodi asked if it would be a good idea if some family members visited during lunch when Winnie was less fatigued. She agreed but felt uncomfortable about asking them and requested Jodi to do this. When Jodi discussed this with Winnie's son, he took charge and arranged a flexible schedule for family and friends to visit throughout the week. Jodi also mentioned to him the importance of Winnie maintaining her role as family matriarch by making choices and feeling a sense of control. Jodi emphasized that although family members were concerned about Winnie, they shouldn't be overprotective; instead, they could encourage her to be as active as she wanted. For example, they could ask Winnie if she preferred to visit in her room, in the lounge, or outside, even if this required her family's help with mobility. Further, knowing that Winnie's eyestrain and limited concentration were troubling, Jodi suggested short and simple board games that Winnie could choose to play with family members, particularly when her grandchildren visited.

Several "May Babies" visited Winnie. One dropped by at the end of a session when Winnie was working on safe transfers in the bathroom. Winnie's friend happened to mention that they were starting to plan the meals for their birthday beach celebration. Jodi immediately recognized Winnie might feel left out and skillfully steered the conversation such that by the end, Winnie and her friend planned to get all the "May Babies" together at the SNF that weekend so that Winnie could help plan the celebration, a role important to her.

As the weeks progressed, Jodi and Winnie considered Winnie's interests and leisure activities and incorporated them into her intervention sessions. They spent several sessions a week in the kitchen, developing her performance skills while preparing muffins for her husband, bread for her children, and cookies for her grandchildren. Jodi asked whether Winnie wanted to give anything special to the "May Babies" for their birthdays. Winnie mentioned that they all enjoyed cooking and thought potted fresh herbs would be a nice gift. To develop her performance skills for all daily life activities, Winnie transplanted several herbs into pots and began sponge painting each one. After Winnie completed the first one, Jodi made arrangements with staff so that Winnie and her grandchildren could complete these together on the weekend in the therapy room.

During the latter part of her stay, Winnie was getting better at moving around the room and could walk with minimal support of her husband down the hallway, albeit a bit slowly and unsteadily. As discharge was getting closer, Jody and Winnie began to consider how she would spend her time once she returned home. Jodi ensured that all team members were aware that many of Winnie's leisure and social interests occurred outside the home and were working with Winnie to help her gain as much independence as possible. Taxis and public transportation were options for her. Although Winnie could see herself eventually returning to swimming, she was hesitant about being around others in public. She wasn't sure how accessible the pool might be and didn't know whether someone could help her if she got into trouble, both in the locker room and in the pool. Jodi gently suggested that it might be good for Winnie to advocate for herself. To do so, she suggested Winnie keep track of her concerns, develop a list of questions, and then call the swim center.

From the beginning, Winnie's official goal was to work together with her daughter-in-law to embroider quilts for soldiers' families and feel satisfied doing so. Jodi initially scheduled a time with Winnie and her daughter-in-law to discuss their original plans and explore ways in which Winnie could continue to participate. Listening to Winnie describe the process of quilt making, Jodi used activity analysis to identify aspects of the activity within Winnie's current ability and to note those for which she would need to further develop her skills or adapt the method. To begin, Jodi recommended that Winnie and her daughter-in-law plan which fabrics they wanted to use and that her daughter-in-law bring them to the SNF. Because this week was the second of rehabilitation, Jodi surmised that Winnie would be frustrated with using scissors because she was not using her right hand to feed herself. Instead, Jodie suggested Winnie solicit her grandchildren's help and direct them to cut the fabric squares. They could do it together during the evenings, thus giving Winnie a reason to be a bit active in the evening, spend time with her grandchildren, and improve her endurance. The original plan was for Winnie to embroider some of the quilt squares after they were cut. Because embroidering would be difficult with Winnie's continued eyestrain and diminished hand control, Jodi inquired whether she was willing to forego embroidery and focus on creating a simpler yet still beautiful quilt. Winnie concurred and began to plan the quilt's design.

By the third week, the last fabric squares were cut, and Jodi scheduled an afternoon session for Winnie to focus on improving her standing balance while using her right arm for balance as she ironed the squares with her left. This process took several sessions, and by the fourth week, the fabric squares were ready to be sewn together. Jodi showed Winnie a method whereby Winnie could pin the fabric with her left hand (which was awkward at first) while using her affected right hand to stabilize the fabric while she pinned. Jodi mentioned that this would foster better control and quality of movement. Jodi also knew that if Winnie made a mistake during the pinning, it could easily be corrected. After their first practice session, Winnie again took charge and solicited the help of her grandchildren during the evenings and weekends. She insisted, however, that she would do all the pinning; her grandchildren would serve only as assistants.

Pinning half of the squares took until the next week to complete, and Winnie mentioned to everyone that she did it all (perhaps "forgetting" that her grandchildren did help a bit!). At this point, discharge was 1 week away, and Jodi made plans for Winnie and her daughter-in-law to begin sewing the squares together. Winnie was reluctant to use the sewing machine, fearing a mistake. Jodi and Winnie tried different methods and discovered an effective technique for Winnie to help her daughter-in-law with the performance skills Winnie had been developing. Although Winnie did not have time to complete the quilt before discharge, when she and Jodi reviewed her goal to engage in a favored leisure activity to her satisfaction, Winnie agreed the goal had been met and acknowledged that although it was not the way she used to do it, she felt good that she was doing something useful. When Winnie was discharged home, she still required slight assistance with some mobility and ADL tasks but reported more self-worth and joy in her daily life, in part from engaging in leisure and social activities again.

during which each adult sang a song with (and for) everyone else. Invariably, each performance was followed by applause and compliments. The agency also arranged other conference calls, tailored to their individual interests, for other clients. For older adults with Internet access, usage of social network sites is on the rise, for sharing photos, news, and other information among a network of contacts (Madden, 2010). These and other innovations can provide valuable social engagement for many older adults and persons experiencing physical disabilities.

Focus on Developing a Routine of Leisure and Social Activities. The final guideline reinforces the importance of establishing and engaging in a routine of activities (the client's performance patterns) (Thordardottir et al., 2014). Older adults report that it is important to keep active in a variety of activities and to set aside time for quiet periods and rest (Clark et al., 1996). Although pattern and routine are useful, a routine of leisure and social activities should be flexible to allow for spontaneity. For example, people with arthritis may reduce the expression of symptoms by pacing and planning of activities throughout the day and week. However, these strategies may constrain spontaneity because of less flexible scheduling (Stack et al., 2015). Because spontaneity can be a key quality of leisure, the OTA should encourage clients to plan daily or weekly routines that allow room for spontaneous decisions.

Given the benefits of participating in leisure and social activities, all OTs and OTAs should recommend, particularly for those who are older and experiencing greater challenges resulting from physical impairments (Glass et al., 1999), engagement in a broad range of relaxing, physical, and social activities. If OTs and OTAs believe a balance of activities is important, a routine of activities should be promoted in which leisure and social participation is valued and balanced in relation to other activities in a client's life.

SUMMARY

With the current focus on patient-driven outcomes, more OTs and OTAs are advocating that occupational therapy services increase the time devoted to leisure and social activities and decrease the time devoted to basic ADL tasks, particularly for clients living in the community (Bier et al., 2009; Cowdell & Garrett, 2003; Parker et al., 1997; Zoerink, 2001). Given the benefits of participating in leisure and social activities for all persons, OTs and OTAs need to address leisure and social participation throughout all phases of their practice. To relegate leisure and social activities to the back burner or consider leisure and social activities only as a means to regain performance skills will diminish the opportunity for clients to experience joy and satisfaction in their daily lives. By implementing intervention that promotes the benefits of leisure and social participation, OTs and OTAs can help their clients enjoy walking the family dog, laughing with a best friend, making a quilt for a first grandchild, and watching sunsets at the beach with a loved one. By engagement in these activities, clients and others can recognize that how one occupies one's daily life is truly related to one's health, well-being, life satisfaction, and quality of life.

> ### QUOTES
>
> The experience of leisure neither cures nor removes the effects of aging, mental health disorders, and chronic health problems. It does, however, have the potential to change the quality of life for many individuals. Melinda Suto (Suto, 1998)

SELECTED READING GUIDE QUESTIONS

1. When meeting a client for the first time to discuss leisure and social activities, how would you solicit the client's perspective?
2. What are the specific benefits associated with participating in leisure and social activities for all adults, disability or not?
3. What are the concerns of people with disabilities with respect to participating in leisure and social activities?
4. Why is it important for an OTA to consider the timing of when to introduce leisure and social participation during therapy? What could happen that might have a negative impact on a client if activities are introduced too soon, too late, or not at all?

LEARNING ACTIVITIES

1. Conduct a mock interview with a classmate or family member using the questions from Table 17.1 as a guide. Audiotape or videotape yourself during the interview and evaluate your skills in eliciting the person's meaning of and experience with leisure and social activities.
2. Keep track of your leisure and social activities for a week. Identify which activities you consider leisure or social, how often you engage in them, their relative value to you according to preference, and the qualities you experience during each activity that make it more leisurely or social. If you could no longer engage in these activities because of a physical disability, which might you give up if you could not do them to your performance standards? Which would you consider continuing even if you had to use an adapted manner?

CASE STUDY

Winnie, Part 4: A Postscript

Winnie was discharged 17 days before the "May Babies" celebration. Although she was grateful to be home at last with her husband, she looked forward to the weekend get-away and to reclaiming some semblance of her life before her stroke. Three days before the celebration, Winnie suffered a second stroke and died. After the funeral, Winnie's family sent a letter to the SNF staff expressing their gratitude and sharing that although Winnie never realized her dream to attend the "May Babies" celebration, hope and joy were a part of her life until the end because of the attention paid to who she was and to what was important in her life.

REFERENCES

Akbaraly, T. N., Portet, F., Fustinoni, S., Dartigues, J. F., Artero, S., Rouaud, O., et al. (2009). Leisure activities and the risk of dementia in the elderly: results from the three-city study. *Neurology, 73*, 854–861. Available from http://doi.org/10.1212/WNL.0b013e3181b7849b.

Almborg, A. H., Ulander, K., Thulin, A., & Berg, S. (2010). Discharged after stroke—important factors for health-related quality of life. *Journal of Clinical Nursing, 19*(15-16), 2196–2206.

American Occupational Therapy Association. (2014). Occupational therapy practice framework: domain & process. 3rd ed. *The American Journal of Occupational Therapy, 68*(1), S1–S48. Available from http://doi.org/10.5014/ajot.2014.682006.

Anke, A. G. W., & Fugl-Meyer, A. R. (2003). Life satisfaction several years after severe multiple trauma—a retrospective investigation. *Clinical Rehabilitation, 17*(4), 431–442.

Awaad, T. (2003). Culture, cultural competency and occupational therapy: a review of the literature. *British Journal of Occupational Therapy, 66*(8), 356–362.

Ball, V., Corr, S., Knight, J., & Lowis, M. J. (2007). An investigation into the leisure occupations of older adults. *British Journal of Occupational Therapy, 70*(9), 393–400.

Barclay, L., McDonald, R., & Lentin, P. (2015). Social and community participation following spinal cord injury: a critical review. *International Journal of Rehabilitation Research, 38*, 1–19. Available from http://doi.org/10.1097/MRR.0000000000000085.

Baum, C. M., & Edwards, D. (2008). *Activity Card Sort* (2nd ed.) Bethesda, MD: AOTA Press.

Bedell, G. M. (2012). Measurement of social participation. In V. Anderson, & M. H. Beauchamp (Eds.), *Developmental social neuroscience and childhood brain insult: theory and practice* (pp. 184–206). New York, NY: Guilford Press.

Bier, N., Dutil, E., & Couture, M. (2009). Factors affecting leisure participation after a traumatic brain injury: an exploratory study. *Journal of Head Trauma Rehabilitation, 24*(3), 187–194.

Bonder, B. R., Martin, L., & Miracle, A. W. (2004). Culture emergent in occupation. *The American Journal of Occupational Therapy, 58*(2), 159–168.

Bundy, A. C. (1993). Assessment of play and leisure: delineation of the problem. *The American Journal of Occupational Therapy, 47*(3), 217–222.

Bundy, A. C., & Clemson, L. (2009). Leisure. In B. Bonder, & V. Dal Bello-Haas (Eds.), *Functional performance in older adults* (3rd ed., pp. 290–306). Philadelphia, PA: F.A. Davis.

Caldwell, L. L. (2005). Leisure and health: why is leisure therapeutic? *British Journal of Guidance & Counselling, 33*(1), 7–26.

Centers for Medicare & Medicaid Services. Medicare benefit policy manual: chapter 15: covered medical and other health services. <https://www.cms.gov/Regulations-and-Guidance/Guidance/Manuals/downloads/bp102c15.pdf>. Accessed 12.07.19.

Chen, S.-W., & Chippendale, T. (2018). Leisure as an end, not just a means, in occupational therapy intervention. *The American Journal of Occupational Therapy, 72*(4), 7204347010. Available from http://doi.org/10.5014/ajot.2018.028316.

Cipriani, J. (2007). Altruistic activities of older adults living in long term care facilities: a literature review. *Physical & Occupational Therapy in Geriatrics, 26*(1), 19–28.

Cipriani, J., Haley, R., Moravec, E., & Young, H. (2010). Experience and meaning of group altruistic activities among long-term care residents. *British Journal of Occupational Therapy, 73*(6), 269–276.

Clark, F., Azen, S. P., Zemke, R., Jackson, J., Carlson, M., Mandel, D., et al. (1997). Occupational therapy for independent-living older adults: a randomized controlled trial. *JAMA, 278*(16), 1321–1326.

Clark, F., Carlson, M., Zemke, R., Frank, G., Patterson, K., Ennevor, B. L., et al. (1996). Life domains and adaptive strategies of a group of low-income, well older adults. *The American Journal of Occupational Therapy, 50*(2), 99—108.

Cowdell, F., & Garrett, D. (2003). Recreation in stroke rehabilitation part two: exploring patients' views. *International Journal of Therapy Rehabilitation, 10*(10), 456—462.

Crenshaw, W., Gillian, M. L., Kidd, N., Olivo, J., & Schell, B. A. B. (2001). Assisted living residents' perspectives of their occupational performance concerns. *Activities, Adaptation & Aging, 26*(1), 41—55.

Cromwell, F. S. (1977). Eleanor Clarke Slagle, the leader, the woman. *The American Journal of Occupational Therapy, 31*(10), 645—648.

Dahan-Oliel, N., Gelinas, I., & Mazer, B. (2008). Social participation in the elderly: what does the literature tell us? *Critical Reviews in Physical and Rehabilitation Medicine, 20*(2), 159—176.

Dedding, C., Cardol, M., Eyssen, I. C., Dekker, J., & Beelen, A. (2004). Validity of the Canadian Occupational Performance Measure: a client-centred outcome measurement. *Clinical Rehabilitation, 18*(6), 660—667.

Desrosiers, J., Noreau, L., Rochette, A., Carbonneau, H., Fontaine, L., Viscogliosi, C., et al. (2007). Effect of a home leisure education program after stroke: a randomized controlled trial. *Archives of Physical Medicine and Rehabilitation, 88*(9), 1095—1100.

Fakolade, A., Lamarre, J., Latimer-Cheung, A., Parsons, T., Morrow, S. A., & Finlayson, M. (2018). Understanding leisure-time physical activity: voices of people with MS who have moderate-to-severe disability and their family caregivers. *Health Expectations: an International Journal of Public Participation in Health Care and Health Policy, 21*(1), 181—191. Available from http://doi.org/10.1111/hex.12600.

Gabriel, Z., & Bowling, A. (2004). Quality of life from the perspectives of older people. *Ageing and Society, 24*(5), 675—691.

Gillen, G., & Boyt Schell, B. (2014). Introduction to evaluation, intervention, and outcomes for occupations. In B. A. Boyt Schell, G. Gillen, & M. Scaffa (Eds.), *Willard and Spackman's occupational therapy* (12th ed., pp. 606—609). Philadelphia, PA: Lippincott Williams & Wilkins.

Glass, T. A., de Leon, C. M., Marottoli, R. A., & Berkman, L. F. (1999). Population-based study of social and productive activities as predictors of survival among elderly Americans. *British Medical Journal, 319*(7208), 478—483.

Goverover, Y., Genova, H., Smith, A., Chiaravalloti, N., & Lengenfelder, J. (2017). Changes in activity participation following traumatic brain injury. *Neuropsychological Rehabilitation, 27*(4), 472—485. Available from http://doi.org/10.1080/09602011.2016.1168746.

Hand, C., Law, M., McColl, M., Hanna, S., & Elliott, S. (2014). An examination of social support influences on participation for older adults with chronic health conditions. *Disability and Rehabilitation, 36*(17), 1439—1444. Available from http://doi.org/10.3109/09638288.2013.845258.

Hartman-Maeir, A., Soroker, N., Ring, H., Avni, N., & Katz, N. (2007). Activities, participation and satisfaction one-year post stroke. *Disability and Rehabilitation, 29*(7), 559—566.

Hawker, G., Stewart, L., French, M., Cibere, J., Jordan, J. M., March, L., et al. (2008). Understanding pain experience in hip and knee osteoarthritis—an OARSI/OMERACT initiative. *Osteoarthritis and Cartilage, 16*, 415—422.

Herzog, A. R., Ofstedal, M. B., & Wheeler, L. M. (2002). Social engagement and its relationship to health. *Clinics in Geriatric Medicine, 18*(3), 593—609.

Holt-Lunstad, J., Smith, T. B., & Layton, J. B. (2010). Social relationships and mortality risk: a meta-analytic review. *PLoS Medicine, 7*(7), e1000316. Available from https://doi.org/10.1371/journal.pmed.1000316.

Horowitz, B. P., & Vanner, E. (2010). Relationships among active engagement in life activities and quality of life for assisted-living residents. *Journal of Housing for the Elderly, 24*(2), 130—150.

< https://doi.org/10.9738/INTSURG-D-17-00104.1 > .

Heasman, D. & Salhotra, G. Interest Checklist (UK). (2008). Model of human occupation theory and application. Web site. < https://www.moho.uic.edu/productDetails.aspx?aid=39 > .

Jackson, J., Carlson, M., Mandel, D., Zemke, R., & Clark, F. (1998). Occupation in lifestyle redesign: the well elderly study occupational therapy program. *The American Journal of Occupational Therapy, 52*(5), 326—336.

Jongbloed, L., & Morgan, D. (1991). An investigation of involvement in leisure activities after a stroke. *The American Journal of Occupational Therapy, 45*(5), 420—427.

Kahana, E., Bhatta, T., Lovegreen, L. D., Kahana, B., & Midlarsky, E. (2013). Altruism, helping, and volunteering: pathways to well-being in late life. *Journal of Aging and Health, 25*(1), 159—187. Available from http://doi.org/10.1177/0898264312469665.

Kielhofner, G. (2008). *Model of human occupation: theory and application* (4th ed.). Baltimore, MD: Lippincott Williams & Wilkins.

Korner-Bitensky, N., Desrosiers, J., & Rochette, A. (2008). A national survey of occupational therapists' practices related to participation post-stroke. *Journal of Rehabilitation Medicine, 40*(4), 291—297.

Kuykendall, L., Tay, L., & Ng, V. (2015). Leisure engagement and subjective well-being: a meta-analysis. *Psychological Bulletin, 141*, 364—403. Available from http://doi.org/10.1037/a0038508.

Law, M. (2002). Participation in the occupations of everyday life. *The American Journal of Occupational Therapy, 56*(6), 640—649.

Law, M., Baptiste, S., Carswell, A., McColl M. A., Polatajko, H., Pollock, N. (2005). *Canadian Occupational Performance Measure.* (4th ed.). Toronto: Canadian Association of Occupational Therapists.

Leijdesdorff, H. A., Krijnen, P., van Rooyen, L., Marang—van de Mheen, P., Rhemrev, S., & Schipper, I. B. (2019). Reduced quality of life, fatigue, and societal participation after polytrauma. *International Surgery, 103*(3-4), 158—166.

Madden, M. (2010). *Older Adults and Social Media* [report]. Washington, DC: Pew Research Center.

Magasi, S., & Hammel, J. (2004). Social support and social network mobilization in African American woman who have experienced strokes. *Disability Studies Quarterly: DSQ, 24*(4). Available from http://dsq-sds.org/article/view/878/1053.

Malone, C., Erler, K. S., Giacino, J. T., Hammond, F. M., Juengst, S. B., Locascio, J. J., et al. (2019). Participation following inpatient rehabilitation for traumatic disorders of consciousness: a TBI model systems study. *Frontiers in Neurology, 10*, 1314. Available from http://doi.org/10.3389/fneur.2019.01314.

Mars, G. M. J., Kempen, G. I. J. M., Post, M. W. M., Proot, I. M., Mesters, I., & Van Eijk, J. T. M. (2009). The Maastricht social participation profile: development and clinimetric properties in older adults with a chronic physical illness. *Quality of Life Research, 18*(9), 1207—1218.

Matsutsuyu, J. S. (1969). The interest check list. *The American Journal of Occupational Therapy, 23*(4), 323—328.

McColl, M. A., Paterson, M., Davies, D., Doubt, L., & Law, M. (2000). Validity and community utility of the Canadian Occupational Performance Measure. *Canadian Journal of Occupational Therapy, 67*(1), 22–30.

McLean, A. M., Jarus, T., Hubley, A. M., & Jongbloed, L. (2014). Associations between social participation and subjective quality of life for adults with moderate to severe traumatic brain injury. *Disability and Rehabilitation, 36*(17), 1409–1418. Available from http://doi.org/10.3109/09638288.2013.834986.

Meyer, A. (1922). The philosophy of occupation therapy. *Archives of Occupational Therapy, 1*(1), 1–10.

Morgan, D., & Jongbloed, L. (1990). Factors influencing leisure activities following a stroke: an exploratory study. *Canadian Journal of Occupational Therapy, 57*(4), 223–229.

Mosey, A. C. (1992). *Applied scientific inquiry in the health professions: an epistemological orientation.* (2nd ed.). Bethesda, MD: American Occupational Therapy Association.

Nour, K., Desrosiers, J., Gauthier, P., & Carbonneau, H. (2002). Impact of a home leisure educational program for older adults who have had a stroke (Home Leisure Educational Program). *Therapeutic Recreation Journal, 36*(1), 48–64.

O'Sullivan, C., & Chard, G. (2010). An exploration of participation in leisure activities post-stroke. *Australian Occupational Therapy Journal, 57*(3), 159–166.

Odawara, E. (2005). Cultural competency in occupational therapy: beyond a cross-cultural view of practice. *The American Journal of Occupational Therapy, 59*(3), 325–334.

Paganini-Hill, A., Kawas, C. H., & Corrada, M. M. (2011). Activities and mortality in the elderly: the Leisure World cohort study. *Journals of Gerontology Series A: Biomedical Sciences and Medical Sciences, 66*, 559–567. Available from http://doi.org/10.1093/gerona/glq237.

Parham, L. D., & Fazio, L. S. (1997). *Play in occupational therapy for children.* St. Louis, MO: Mosby.

Parker, C., Gladman, J., & Drummond, A. (1997). The role of leisure in stroke rehabilitation. *Disability and Rehabilitation, 19*(1), 1–5.

Peloquin, S. M. (1991). Occupational therapy service: individual and collective understandings of the founders, part 1. *The American Journal of Occupational Therapy, 45*(4), 352–360.

Pereira, R. B., & Stagnitti, K. (2008). The meaning of leisure for well-elderly Italians in an Australian community: implications for occupational therapy. *Australian Occupational Therapy Journal, 55*(1), 39–46.

Plow, M. A., Finlayson, M., Gunzler, D., & Heinemann, A. W. (2015). Correlates of participation in meaningful activities among people with multiple sclerosis. *Journal of Rehabilitation Medicine, 47*(6), 538–545. Available from http://doi.org/10.2340/16501977-1948.

Price, P., Stephenson, S., Krantz, L., & Ward, K. (2011). Beyond my front door: the occupational and social participation of adults with spinal cord Injury. *OTJR: Occupation, Participation and Health, 31*(2), 81–88. Available from http://doi.org/10.3928/15394492-20100521-01.

Primeau, L. A. (2014). Play and leisure. In B. A. B. Schell, G. Gillen, & M. Scaffa (Eds.), *Willard & Spackman's occupational therapy* (12th ed., pp. 697–713). Philadelphia, PA: Lippincott.

Radomski, M. V. (1995). There is more to life than putting on your pants. *The American Journal of Occupational Therapy, 49*(6), 487–490.

Ragheb, M. G., & Beard, J. G. (1992). *Idyll Arbor Leisure Battery.* Enumclaw, WA: Idyll Arbor.

Reinseth, L., & Espnes, G. A. (2007). Women with rheumatoid arthritis: non-vocational activities and quality of life. *Scandinavian Journal of Occupational Therapy, 14*(2), 108–115.

Rochette, A., Desrosiers, J., Bravo, G., St-Cyr-Tribble, D., & Bourget, A. (2007). Changes in participation after a mild stroke: quantitative and qualitative perspectives. *Topics in Stroke Rehabilitation, 14*(3), 59–68.

Rogers, N. (1999). Family obligation, caregiving, and loss of leisure: the experiences of three caregivers. *Activities, Adaptation & Aging, 24*(2), 35–49.

Schwartz, K. B. (2009). Reclaiming our heritage: connecting the founding vision to the centennial vision. *The American Journal of Occupational Therapy, 63*(6), 681–690.

Schweitzer, J. A., Mann, W. C., Nochajski, S., & Tomita, M. (1999). Patterns of engagement in leisure activity by older adults using assistive devices. *Technology and Disability, 11*(1/2), 103–117.

Sellar, B., & Boshoff, K. (2006). Subjective leisure experiences of older Australians. *Australian Occupational Therapy Journal, 53*(3), 211–219.

Smith, N. R., Kielhofner, G., & Watts, J. H. (1986). The relationships between volition, activity pattern, and life satisfaction in the elderly. *The American Journal of Occupational Therapy, 40*(4), 278–283.

Specht, J., King, G., Brown, E., & Foris, C. (2002). The importance of leisure in the lives of persons with congenital physical disabilities. *The American Journal of Occupational Therapy, 56*(4), 436–445.

Stack, E. L., Hayward, T., & Roberts, H. C. (2015). Why do people with Parkinson's maintain or stop leisure activities? *Age and Ageing, 44*, i17. Available from http://doi.org/10.1093/ageing/afv036.

Stevens, A. B., Coon, D., Wisniewski, S., Vance, D., Arguelles, S., Belle, S., et al. (2004). Measurement of leisure time satisfaction in family caregivers. *Aging Mental Health, 8*(5), 450–459.

Suto, M. (1998). Leisure in occupational therapy. *Canadian Journal of Occupational Therapy, 65*(5), 271–278.

Suto, M. (2004). Exploring leisure meanings that inform client-centred practice. In C. Carpenter (Ed.), *Qualitative research in evidence-based rehabilitation* (pp. 27–39). Edinburgh: Churchill Livingstone.

Sveen, U., Thommessen, B., Bautz-Holter, E., Wyller, T. B., & Laake, K. (2004). Well-being and instrumental activities of daily living after stroke. *Clinical Rehabilitation, 18*(3), 267–274.

The Next Big Thing. Heard on the phone. Public Radio International; January 21, 2005.

Theis, K. A., Murphy, L., Hootman, J. M., & Wilkie, R. (2013). Social participation restriction among US adults with arthritis: a population-based study using the International Classification of Functioning, Disability and Health. *Arthritis Care & Research, 65*(7), 1059–1069. Available from http://doi.org/10.1002/acr.21977.

Thordardottir, B., Nilsson, M. H., Iwarsson, S., & Haak, M. (2014). You plan, but you never know" — participation among people with different levels of severity of Parkinson's disease. *Disability and Rehabilitation, 36*(26), 2216–2224. Available from http://doi.org/10.3109/09638288.2014.898807.

Turner, H., Chapman, S., McSherry, A., Krishnagiri, S., & Watts, J. (2000). Leisure assessment in occupational therapy: an exploratory study. *Occupational Therapy in Health Care, 12*(2-3), 73–85.

University of Illinois Board of Trustees (2020). Modified Interest Checklist. http://moho.uic.edu/resources/files/Modified%20Interest%20Checklist.pdf.

van der Zee, C. H., Visser-Meily, J. M., Lindeman, E., Kappelle, J. L., & Post, M. W. (2013). Participation in the chronic phase of stroke. *Top Stroke Rehab, 20,* 52−61.

Ward, G. E., Jagger, C., & Harper, W. M. (1996). The Canadian occupational performance measure: what do users consider important? *British Journal of Therapy and Rehabilitation, 3*(8), 448−452.

Whiteford, G. E., & Wilcock, A. A. (2000). Cultural relativism: occupation and independence reconsidered. *Canadian Journal of Occupational Therapy, 67*(5), 324−336.

Wilkie, R., Peat, G., Thomas, E., & Croft, P. (2007). Factors associated with restricted mobility outside the home in community-dwelling adults ages fifty years and older with knee pain: an example of use of the ICF to investigate participation restriction. *Arthritis & Rheumatology, 57*(8), 1381−1389.

Wise, E. K., Mathews-Dalton, C., Dikmen, S., Temkin, N., MacHamer, J., Bell, K., et al. (2010). Impact of traumatic brain injury on participation in leisure activities. *Archives of Physical Medicine and Rehabilitation, 91*(9), 1357−1362.

Yamada, T., Kawamata, H., Kobayashi, N., Kielhofner, G., & Taylor, R. R. (2010). A randomised clinical trial of a wellness programme for healthy older people. *British Journal of Occupational Therapy, 73*(11), 540−548.

Yi, T. I., Han, J. S., Lee, K. E., & Ha, S. A. (2015). Participation in leisure activity and exercise of chronic stroke survivors using community-based rehabilitation services in Seongnam City.

Annals of Rehabilitation Medicine, 39(2), 234−242. Available from http://doi.org/10.5535/arm.2015.39.2.234.

Zoerink, D. A. (2001). Exploring the relationship between leisure and health of senior adults with orthopedic disabilities living in rural areas. *Activities, Adaptation & Aging, 26*(2), 61−73.

RESOURCES

Activity Card Sort (ACS). https://myaota.aota.org/shop_aota/product/1247

Canadian Occupational Performance Measure (COPM). http://www.thecopm.ca/about/

Interest Checklist (UK). https://www.moho.uic.edu/productDetails.aspx?aid=39

Leisure Attitude Measure (LAM). https://www.idyllarbor.com/agora.cgi?p_id=A148&xm=on

Leisure Interest Measure (LIM). https://www.idyllarbor.com/agora.cgi?p_id=A147&xm=on

Leisure Satisfaction Measure (LSM). https://www.idyllarbor.com/agora.cgi?p_id=A146&xm=on

Leisure Motivation Scale (LMS). https://www.idyllarbor.com/agora.cgi?p_id=A149&xm=on

https://www.lrcs.uqam.ca/wp-content/uploads/2017/08/eml28_en.pdf

Modified Interest Checklist. http://moho.uic.edu/resources/files/Modified%20Interest%20Checklist.pdf

Occupational Questionnaire (OQ). http://moho.uic.edu/resources/files/Occupational%20%20Questionnaire.pdf

PART VI

Interventions for Performance Skills and Client Factors

18

The Older Adult

Anne Graikoski

OBJECTIVES

After reading this chapter, the student or the occupational therapy practitioner will be able to do the following:

1. Describe the stages of aging.
2. Understand the various theories of how and why we age.
3. Recognize physical, mental, and social age-related changes the older adult experiences.
4. Recognize the functional abilities of the older adult.
5. Discuss the common conditions that influence health and function in the older adult.
6. Understand the prevalence of major neurocognitive disorders in older adults and how decreased cognition impacts function.
7. Identify the practice settings where services are provided to older adults.
8. Become familiar with evidence-based interventions to promote function and quality of life for older adults.
9. Describe the methods used in a fall prevention program.
10. Explain the federal regulation concerning restraint-free environments.
11. Understand the potential effect of medication on the functioning of the older adult.

KEY TERMS

Major neurocognitive disorder
Acute care hospital
Home health
Adult day services

Assisted living facilities
Polypharmacy
Physical restraints
Chemical restraints

INTRODUCTION

America is getting older; our nation is undergoing a profound demographic transformation. It has been projected that in less than two decades persons 65 and older will outnumber children for the first time in US history (The week staff, 2009). Furthermore, the 2010 US census reported more Americans over the age of 65 than any previous census (The older population, 2011). The aging of our population is due in large part to aging baby boomers, a generation of people born between 1946 and 1964. Beginning in 2030, when all baby boomers will be older than 65, older adults will make up 21% of the American population, increased from 15% today. The US Census Bureau recognizes the impact of a graying population on our health care system. Increased needs for in-home caregiving and assisted living facilities are potential outcomes of the increased number of older adults (The week staff, 2009).

For occupational therapy practitioners, this demographic shift provides an opportunity to demonstrate our unique value as facilitators of functional independence and advocates for continued participation in occupation into older age. This will require an understanding of the strengths of older adults as well as changes and challenges felt by persons as they age. This chapter provides a summary of the physical, mental, and social changes associated with aging, common practice settings for occupational therapy practitioners working with older adults, and an overview of specific intervention practices utilized to enhance function and quality of life for older adults. The aim of this chapter is to increase the occupational therapy assistant (OTA) student's working knowledge of the needs of our aging population.

THE STAGES OF AGING

Aging is a complex and variable process that begins from the moment we are born. Aging is inevitable but also individual. Aging persons are part of a heterogeneous population in which each individual experiences the process of getting older differently. It is imperative for occupational therapy practitioners to remember that aging alone does not necessarily precipitate an increase in disease and dysfunction. Like all other age groups, aging persons are mixed in needs, abilities, and resources with health factors greatly influencing how a person will experience older age (Stalworth & Sloane, 2007).

Lewis described four stages of aging (Lewis, 2003). Stage I, from age 50 to 65 years, is classified as the preretirement age. During this stage, persons typically begin to plan for retirement and use of their leisure time. These individuals may begin to assume new roles, such as grandparent or caretaker of their own elderly parents. Stage II, from age 65 to 74 years, is when individuals may begin to encounter increased health problems. Unfortunately they may experience grief due to the death of a spouse, friends, and/or siblings. Stage III, from age 75 to 84 years, is when independent living is jeopardized. A person in stage III of aging may begin to require assistance with daily life tasks. In stage IV, age 85 years and older, individuals may become increasingly dependent on others. Institutional living arrangements may be required, or they may need to live with a family member (Lewis, 2003).

THEORETICAL APPROACHES TO AGING

Why do we age? As our population gets older, the pursuit for a deeper understanding of why and how we age is critical. Despite aging being inevitable to all persons, science continues to have a relatively poor understanding of the exact mechanisms of aging and whether aging is a beneficial or harmful phenomenon to our population (Lipsky & King, 2015). Understanding the diverse theories of aging may help an occupational therapy practitioner in understanding what is happening to clients as they grow older and hold better expectations of how function will be impacted by the aging process.

Biologic Theories of Aging

Early theories of aging argue that aging is a process of natural selection, meaning that as a species we age in order to eliminate older members of our population, so they do not compete for resources with the younger, more viable, persons. Such theories postulate that aging is for the benefit of the species and should be distinguished from an individual's experience with aging. Evolutionary theories of aging further support the notion that cell death is preprogrammed in our genes; somatic cells will undergo a specified number of divisions based on the individual, causing the individual to age and eventually die. The Hayflick limit theory is an example of a genetic theory that postulates that healthy cells can only divide a finite number of times and that the human lifespan is unsurpassable at just over 120 years (Tierney, 2009). Although evolutionary theories of aging support modern ideology that aging is an individual process, advances in science and technology have disaccredited certain aspects of these theories (Lipsky & King, 2015; Ljubuncic & Reznick, 2009).

Free radical theory of aging assumes that free radicals, highly reactive and toxic forms of oxygen known as reactive oxygen species (ROS), produced by the cell mitochondria, are causational to the aging process. Free radicals cause numerous problems for cells, including damage to the cell membrane, impact on deoxyribonucleic acid (DNA) cell replication, interference with cell transfusion of oxygen causing tissue death, and decreased enzymatic activity, and may trigger pathologic changes resulting in cell mutations. Data continue to support viable aspects of free radical theory, but overall this theory is not a commonly utilized explanation of how and why we age in modern times (Liochev, 2013).

Hormonal aging theories consider the impact of neurons and their associated hormones on aging, considering how the functional decrements in neurons lead to dysfunction in the activity of endocrine glands and their target organs. Hormone theory argues that biologic clocks controlled by our neuroendocrine system control how and when we age. Immunologic theories of aging are similar to evolutionary theories in that they stipulate that our immune system is programmed to decline with age. Our immune systems peak around the age of puberty, and gradually decline from that age. As we get older, our immune antibodies become less effective and increasingly dysregulated. The outcome of this is lessened ability to fight new diseases and increased cellular stress. Research supports the notion that dysregulation of the immune system is correlated to chronic inflammation, cardiovascular disease, Alzheimer disease, and cancer (Jin, 2010).

Biologic environmental influences have also been accredited to aging. Accumulation of harm from environmental factors such as ultraviolet (UV) rays from the sun, exposure to toxic chemicals, viruses, and genetic cross-linking factors, such as nonsaturated fats, have all been considered as potential factors in the aging process. Exposure to such agents may result in errors in protein synthesis and DNA sequencing, causing mutation and dysfunction. Photoaging, changes in the skin's appearance and function due to repeated exposure to UV rays, is a classic example of environmental influence on the way in which one ages (Vierkötter & Krutmann, 2012).

Several additional biologic theories of aging exist; with further advances in medical understanding of aging, updates to existing theories and construction of new ideologies will emerge. However, no one biologic theory of aging is satisfactory in providing a full explanation of the question, How and why do we age?

Psychologic Theory of Aging

Psychologic theories of aging attempt to understand the process of aging through the lens of psychologic attainment. Erik Erikson's theory of human development includes a model of eight stages of psychosocial development a healthy individual will traverse throughout his or her life span. From infancy to mature adulthood, the person passes through stages, meeting new challenges and requiring the person to confront and master new skills. The last two stages of Erikson's model represent middle to mature adulthood. Generativity versus stagnation, the stage of middle adulthood (ages 35–65), focuses on the individual's understanding about his or her value in society. Ego integrity versus despair, the stage of later adulthood (65 years and beyond), involves a retrospective review of life. This last stage requires the older adult to evaluate his or her accomplishments and consider unachieved goals (Schuster & Ashburn, 1992).

Activity Theory

Activity theory is especially pertinent for occupational therapy practitioner awareness given its theoretical similarities to the core values of our profession. Activity theory, a sociologic theory, considers lifestyle as influential to the aging process. Activity theory, an opposition to disengagement theory, proposes that successful aging is the result of maintaining an activity lifestyle and healthy social interaction. Activity theory theorizes that older adults who remain active socially demonstrate improved adjustment to aging, and continued participation in roles leads to improved self-image and life satisfaction (Paúl & Lopes, 2016). *Active aging* is defined as "the process of optimizing opportunities for health, participation and security in order to enhance quality of life as people age" (World Health Organization, 2002, p. 12). Active aging is no longer considered simply the absence of pathology; instead, psychologic, social, economic, and community perspectives are considered when determining an actively aging older adult (World Health Organization, 2002). Activity theory seeks to understand why some people are more adaptive and successful to age-related changes, while others are not. Disengagement theory calls attention to decline, frailty, and dependence that comes with increased age, whereas activity theory follows a strengths-based approach, focusing on the positive and healthy aspects of aging (Paúl & Lopes, 2016).

AGE-RELATED CHANGES

Biopsychosocial changes are expected as we age and have been well documented in literature. As age increases, various body functions decrease, impacting the way in which an older adult participates in meaningful activities. However, the type of changes and the rate of change vary among individuals. Furthermore, many age-related changes do not necessarily affect an older adult's ability to function except when illness or disease occurs (Mills & Coulanges, 2013).

Vision

Normal aging impacts the visual system at varying degrees depending on genetic factors and lifestyle. Visual changes related to aging are marked by the following:
- Gradual decline in visual acuity
- Decreased ability to adapt to light and dark
- Loss of contrast sensitivity
- Increased sensitivity to glare
- Diminished oculomotor responses
- Loss of peripheral fields

Changes in the visual function are related both to the eye structure and to the mechanisms of visual processing. Aging has profound impact on the functionality of the structure of the eye as well as the central nervous system that supports the eye. Age-related vision changes impact an individual's ability to perform visually guided activities and vision-related cognitive tasks, such as driving a car or reading a recipe and then cooking a meal (Dagnelie, 2009).

Loss of visual acuity leads to increased challenge with activities that require ability to see in fine detail. Reading, writing, and all occupations requiring use of small objects and instruments are expected to be impacted with decreased visual acuity associated with normal aging (Dagnelie, 2009).

Occupational therapy practitioners may provide visual aids, such as a magnifying glass, or make adaptions to the task, such as increasing the size of print and lighting in the environment, to assist older adults in maintaining their ability to perform activities despite age-related vision changes.

Difficulties with light and dark adaption may be distinguishable when an older adult finds increased difficulty with navigating poorly lit environments. All persons experience temporary vision loss when transitioning between a brightly lit versus darker environment; a common example of this is the experience of leaving a movie theater on a bright, sunny day. However, with age, sensitivity to this transition is increased (Dagnelie, 2009). Therefore it is important to ensure consistency of lighting in an older adult's environment and educate about compensatory strategies to better adapt to light versus dark.

Reduced sensitivity to contrast will likely impact activities that require an older adult to make distinctions of color or gray scale (Dagnelie, 2009). Loss of contrast sensitivity is specifically relevant to occupational therapy practice, as it often impacts social functioning and safety. These visual changes make it more difficult for the older adult to recognize faces, attend to curbs and drop-offs in the environment, and put together a matching outfit.

Peripheral field loss has profound impact on safety for older adults. With decreased ability to attend to objects in the periphery, an older adult demonstrates decreased safety when driving or navigating obstacles in the environment and may lead to distortions or "disappearing" objects in the visual field (Dagnelie, 2009). Occupational therapy practitioners working with older adults across all settings should be aware and evaluate peripheral field vision and provide environmental or task modifications to ensure the safety of the older adult while performing daily activities.

With age, the cornea becomes thicker and more opaque, while the lens becomes less elastic. These changes decrease the older adult's ability to perform accommodation, the ability to change from distance to near vision. This condition is called presbyopia; it is so common that nearly all persons over the age of 55 require corrective lenses to read (Sandmire, 2010).

Hearing

Presbycusis, age-related hearing loss, affects one in three older adults between the ages of 65 and 74. Hearing loss and changes to the auditory system are expected with increasing age. Typically, hearing loss is gradual; therefore older adults may be less aware that they are not able to hear as well. This becomes problematic as it impacts safety, such as the inability to hear alarms or the presence of harmful stimuli in the environment, and social participation, such as the inability to hear and interact in conversations (National Institute on Deafness and Other Communication Disorders (NIDCD), 2018).

Decreased hearing may result from changes to the different structures of the ear (i.e., the outer, middle, and inner ear structures). Buildup of ear wax in the outer ear impacting a person's ability to hear should be considered by the occupational therapy practitioner to ensure safety and function.

Significant changes to inner ear structures also exist. Sound sensitivity decreases, and loss of neurons results in decreased understanding of speech and reduced ability to attend to auditory stimuli in the environment. The case of middle ear structures causing hearing loss is rare but possible. Abnormalities leading to reduced function of the tympanic membrane, the eardrum, and the ossicle bones may result in loss of hearing (National Institute on Deafness and Other Communication Disorders (NIDCD), 2018). Most commonly, long-term exposure to loud sounds or long-lasting sounds in the environment cause presbycusis. This exposure damages the stereocilia, hairlike cells that translate noise into an electrical signal for neurons to send to the brain in order to hear. Other factors, such as exposure to toxic medications, high blood pressure, and diabetes, damage stereocilia and decrease one's ability to hear (National Institute on Deafness and Other Communication Disorders (NIDCD), 2018). An occupational therapy practitioner should be aware of how hearing loss may impact older adults' ability to have social interactions, engage with their physical environment, and perform meaningful daily occupations.

Musculoskeletal

Although changes to the musculoskeletal system exist, getting older does not mean getting weaker. Loss of muscle strength and power can be present; however, exercise is an effective strategy to mitigate these changes (Jackson et al., 1998). Older adults have decreased bone mass and density secondary to loss of bone marrow and red blood cell production. Decalcification causes bones to become more porous, reducing the quantity and quality of the bone structure. As this demineralization of the bones persists, they become more brittle, increasing likelihood of fracture (Flynn & Mabry, 1992). Composition of cartilage additionally undergoes changes, including decreased water content, increased stiffness, and fragmentation. This is especially important when considering flattening of intervertebral discs, which become less resistant to external weight due to decreased water content. Due to flattening of discs, the overall height of the older adult decreases. These variations in musculoskeletal function result in slower movements, decreased activity tolerance, and loss of range of motion. Senile postural changes are also evident, presenting as:
- Forward head and excessive extension of the cervical spine
- Kyphosis of the thoracic spine
- Flattening of the lumbar spine

Neurologic

The aging body becomes less efficient in receiving, processing, and responding to stimuli. An older adult experiences neurologic changes related to temperature regulation and ability to perceive pain. The older adult may feel cold more easily, which is why it may be common to see an older person wrapped in blankets and requesting to keep personal space warmer than younger persons. Pain perception and reaction to painful stimuli also decrease with age; the number and sensitivity of receptors are reduced in the aging process. Therefore it is increasingly important for an occupational therapy practitioner working with older adults to be aware of and attuned to the presence of painful stimuli (Flynn & Mabry, 1992).

Sexual

Sexual function should not be ignored when establishing interventions with the older adult. Sexual activity, engaging in activities that result in sexual satisfaction, is classified as a basic activity of daily living. Mills and Coulanges (2013) describe sexual changes an older adult experiences: "It is important to be mindful that many older adults maintain desire (libido), sexual capacity, and satisfaction as long as they have their health and a capable partner. The older adult continues to experience the same four stages of human sexual response during sexual stimulation: excitement phase, plateau phase, orgasmic phase, and resolution phase. Common physiological changes in the sexual function of the older adult usually manifest as a gradual slowing. For instance, men may experience a longer time needed for arousal (erection) and women may require more time to develop lubrication. Unlike women, healthy men remain fertile until the end of life. Declining medical status, physiological concerns, and social obstacles are common barriers to sexual activity in later life" (p. 374).

Rest and Sleep

Mills and Coulanges (2013) further describe the importance of rest and sleep for the older adult: "Rest and sleep are influential when exploring an individual's physiological functioning and psychosocial well-being. Both older and younger adults spend an average of 6.5 to 7.5 hours sleeping during a 24-hour period, but older adults spend an additional 3 to 4 hours resting in order to achieve the same amount of sleep attained by younger adults. Poor quality of sleep puts the older adult at risk for depression, adverse effects to medication, and pathological conditions. Rather than being viewed as a consequence of aging, poor sleep should be addressed to improve sleep quality in older adults" (p. 374).

PHYSIOLOGIC CONDITIONS COMPLICATED BY THE AGING PROCESS

The presence of abnormal disease states has profound impact on how an older adult experiences aging. Occupational therapy practitioners must be aware of how normal aging, as well as disease and comorbid conditions, affect the individual, to develop an occupational therapy intervention that:
1. Does not aggravate the condition
2. Promotes remediation of functional limitation
3. Provides compensatory strategies for participation in occupation
4. Respects individual and familial goals, roles, and values

This section of the chapter summarizes the conditions most commonly experienced by older adults that impact function and quality of life.

Cardiovascular Conditions

Cardiovascular disease accounts for a large number of adult deaths in the United States with the greatest percentage attributed to atherosclerosis, deposition of fatty material on the inner walls of the arteries. Although change of function in the cardiovascular system is expected, gerontologists and exercise physiologists suggest that physiologic deconditioning is the major causative factor for heart disease in the older adult (Miller, 2012). Common pathologic cardiovascular conditions an occupational therapy practitioner may encounter working with older adults include hypertension, congestive heart failure (CHF), arteriosclerotic heart disease (ASHD), valvular malfunction necessitating a pacemaker, peripheral vascular disease (PVD), and cardiac arrest (Mills & Coulanges, 2013).

Pulmonary Conditions

The most common pulmonary condition associated with aging is chronic obstructive pulmonary disease (COPD). COPD is an umbrella term for a multitude of pulmonary conditions that result in airflow obstruction. COPD is a functional diagnosis and affects upper and lower respiratory tracts with characterized cough, expectoration, wheezing, and dyspnea. Initially these symptoms are present with exercise, and with further progression, even at rest. These conditions may severely limit a person's stamina and endurance and the ability to tolerate activity thus impairing the ability to participate in self-care, work, and leisure activities (Miller, 2012; Wise, 2018).

Endocrine System Disorder

The most prevalent disorder of the endocrine system in older adults is diabetes. Diabetes mellitus (DM) is an endocrine disorder characterized by abnormally high glucose levels in blood due to the lack of or insufficient production of insulin by the pancreas. Diagnostic criteria for DM require elevation of blood glucose levels during fasting or at 2 hours following a meal. Levels of glucose in the blood vary normally throughout the day, with increase after mealtimes and return to premeal levels within about 2 hours for a healthy person. However, if a person's body does not produce enough insulin to transport glucose into the cells, or if the cell stops responding normally to insulin (insulin resistance), the increased resting level of glucose in the blood versus the cells produces the symptoms associated with diabetes. Type 1 diabetes is characterized by abnormal immune response in which the body attacks insulin-producing cells of the pancreas. Therefore the pancreas produces little to no insulin. Type 1 diabetes was formally referred to as insulin-dependent diabetes or juvenile diabetes. Most persons with type 1 diabetes develop the disease before age 30; however, it can develop later in life. Type 2 diabetes is characterized by continued production of insulin by the pancreas with subsequent resistance to the effects of insulin resulting in insufficient insulin to meet the body's needs. As type 2 diabetes progresses, a decrease in the insulin-producing abilities of the pancreas is noted. Obesity is a chief risk factor for developing type 2 diabetes because obesity causes insulin resistance; obese persons require very large amounts of insulin to maintain normal blood glucose levels (Brutsaert, 2019).

Nervous System Disorders

Nervous system disorders commonly affecting older adults include cerebrovascular accidents (CVAs, or strokes), multiple sclerosis, and Parkinson disease (Mills & Coulanges, 2013). These conditions significantly affect the person's ability to engage in occupation and participate in society, regardless if the person is also experiencing age-related changes. Nervous system disorders are inherently complex and will only be briefly introduced in this chapter. Please see alternative chapters for further details of how these conditions affect a person's ability to participate in meaningful occupations.

Musculoskeletal Conditions

Pathologic changes that develop with aging include osteoarthritis and osteoporosis. These conditions affect the bones and joints. Decreased mobility, joint stiffness, and deformities related to osteoarthritis and osteoporosis increase to difficulty with participation in occupation (Mills & Coulanges, 2013). Although exceedingly common, it is important for occupational therapy practitioners to delineate normal changes to the musculoskeletal system from these conditions.

CASE STUDY

Isadore is an 81-year-old woman with a diagnosis of DM, ASHD, and hypertension. She was recently hospitalized for CHF and has been discharged to a nursing home for rehabilitation. She now requires assistance with self-care activities because of generalized weakness. Isadore is expected to return to the community. She reports interest in returning to an independent self-care status.

After the occupational therapist (OT) and OT assistant (OTA) gathered an occupational profile, analyzed Isadore's occupational performance, and collaborated effectively with their client, the following occupational therapy goals were determined:

1. Isadore will be independent in dressing, grooming, and bathing.
2. Isadore will be able to select, don, and doff her dress independently.
3. Isadore will be able to brush her hair independently.
4. Isadore will be able to reach for her clothing in the closet and grooming supplies in the cabinet independently.

The intervention plan includes the following:

1. Practice sessions in dressing, grooming, and bathing
2. Therapeutic activities to address client factors interfering with occupational performance (i.e., range of motion, muscular endurance, respiratory capacity)
3. Problem solving and active client participation in forming strategies during occupational performance
4. Incorporating energy conservation and work simplification techniques during occupational performance

Outcomes of Intervention

1. Participation in meaningful occupations to support participation in society
2. Client participation in assessment of intervention outcomes

COGNITIVE CHANGES

Major Neurocognitive Disorder

Major neurocognitive disorder (NCD), formally termed *dementia*, is an umbrella term used to describe a collection of neurologic conditions and diseases of which the major symptom is global decline in brain function. Major NCD is marked by an overall decline in memory, language, and problem solving that affects an individual's ability to perform daily activities. Brain changes associated with dementia may also affect behavior, emotions, perceptual-motor skills, and social relationships. NCD is designated as mild or major and requires an acquired deficit in at least one specific area of cognition for diagnosis (see Chapter 22, Intervention for People with Cognitive and Perceptual Deficits). It is critical to note that although dementia affects millions of older adults, it is not a normal process of aging and should not be considered inevitable (Alzheimer's Association, 2019; Verrier Piersol & Jensen, 2017). (Note that this chapter will utilize the terms *major NCD* and *dementia* interchangeably, as dementia is the terminology continuously used in clinical practice.)

Mild NCD refers to slight decline in at least one cognitive domain; however, symptoms are not severe enough to interfere with independence in daily occupations. Major NCD occurs when symptoms of cognitive decline begin to impact an individual's ability to perform daily activities. Major NCD is further designated into mild, moderate, or severe NCD. Mild presentation of major NCD affects participation in instrumental activities of daily living (IADL) such as driving or care of household. Moderate presentation of major NCD affects both IADL and basic activities of daily living (BADL), impacting on a person's ability to perform self-care, such as dressing or grooming tasks, at a previous level of independence. Severe presentation of major NCD indicates dependence in both IADL and BADL (Verrier Piersol & Jensen, 2017).

Many forms of dementia exist, each with a distinctive pathology and presentation. Alzheimer disease (AD) is the most common type of dementia, accounting for 60% to 80% of cases. Vascular dementia is the second most common cause of major NCD. Vascular dementia may occur secondary to a CVA/stroke or other conditions that result in reduced circulation of blood, depriving the brain of essential oxygen and nutrients (Alzheimer's Association, 2019; Mayo Foundation for Medical Education and Research, 2018).

Alzheimer Disease. AD affects approximately 5.4 million Americans, the vast majority being adults 65 years of age and older. It is estimated that one in nine adults age 65 years and older have AD, and in adults age 85 and older the ratio increases to one in three (Verrier Piersol & Jensen, 2017). A degenerative brain disease, AD presents as a slow, progressive decline in mental functioning significantly reducing a person's independence and quality of life. The greatest risk factor for AD is advancing age; however, AD demonstrates familial linkages. Marked neurologic changes associated with AD include shrinking of the cortex, the region of the brain involved in memory, judgment, and language, as well as deposits known as plaques and neurofibrillary tangles. Plaques impair synapses impacting the brain's ability to pass signals between cells. Neurofibrillary tangles kill brain cells through prevention of transportation of food and energy around the brain cells. The cortex is affected first with AD, thus memory loss is one of the first symptoms of the disease (National Institutes of Health (NIH), 2017).

Vascular Dementia. Vascular dementia refers to decline in cognitive function caused by damage to the brain secondary to impaired blood flow. Conditions such as diabetes, high blood pressure and cholesterol, smoking, and CVAs increase risk of vascular dementia. Presentation of vascular dementia differs from AD, which is characterized by a steady decline in function. Vascular dementia, on the other hand, typically presents in a steplike decline with periods of stability in function followed by large episodes of loss of function (Mayo Foundation for Medical Education and Research, 2018). An OT or OTA treating a person with vascular dementia must be prepared for fluctuating levels of functional cognition dependent on amount of blood flow to varying presentation based on area of brain impacted by impaired blood flow.

Environment-Based Interventions for Persons With NCD. An occupational therapy practitioner providing services to persons with major NCD must pay special attention to person–environment interaction, as the environment can have significant effect on engagement in occupations and overall performance of daily tasks (Verrier Piersol & Jensen, 2017). The following section of this chapter examines empirical evidence to support use of environment-based interventions to reduce problematic behaviors associated with dementia and improve perception of environmental stimuli.

Specialized environments, such as special care units and dementia-specific wings of nursing homes, have been examined to determine effectiveness of modification to the environment as a whole to improve function and quality of life (QoL) for persons with dementia. Major takeaways from this research indicate that presenting an environment similar to a home, with private and personalized rooms and variance of ambiance in common areas, is effective in decreasing aggressive behaviors and reducing confusion (Chaudhury et al., 2013; Fleming & Purandare, 2010). A comparison of special care units and traditional nursing homes demonstrates that specialized environments are not necessarily superior, validating the importance of a personalized environment rather than the classification of setting (Verrier Piersol & Jensen, 2017).

Perception-Based Interventions for Persons With NCD. Perception is the use of the senses to interpret information from the environment. Major NCD impacts a person's ability to accurately perceive and encode sensory information; thus OTs and OTAs must be aware of strategies to improve perception and ability to function within a given environment. Perceptual interventions include use of optical devices, visual barriers, and environmental cues and design to reduce problems related to reduced perception (i.e., wandering, getting lost, hallucinations, exit-seeking behavior) (Verrier Piersol & Jensen, 2017). Review of research indicates that interventions designed to compensate, rather than remediate, loss of perception are best practice to improve an interaction with the environment (Letts et al., 2011). Visual barriers and safety measures, such as camouflaged doors and electric locks, have been indicated as effective in reduction in exit-seeking behavior and wandering (Fleming & Purandare, 2010; Hodgkinson et al., 2007; Letts et al., 2011). Use of optical devices or environmental cues, such as printed signs and personal items, demonstrates insufficient evidence for effectiveness at reducing visual hallucinations, agitated behaviors, and wandering behavior (Verrier Piersol & Jensen, 2017).

Limited evidence exists for remediating perception in persons with dementia; however, use of the senses has been found as beneficial for reducing problematic behaviors and improving QoL (Verrier Piersol & Jensen, 2017). There is strong evidence for use of multisensory interventions to improve behavior (Verrier Piersol & Jensen, 2017). Multisensory stimulation environments provide a person with dementia multiple forms of sensory stimulation simultaneously with outcomes in improved behavior, decreased agitation, and improved interaction with caregivers (Verrier Piersol & Jensen, 2017). Empirical evidence exists for use of music to improve behaviors such as agitation, wandering, anxiety, and repetitive vocalizations (Padilla, 2011). Conversely, ambient music played during mealtimes did not demonstrate sufficient evidence for reducing agitation (Lui et al., 2014). Furthermore, moderate evidence exists for regulation of noise in the environment to improve behaviors in persons with dementia. OTs and OTAs should use clinical judgment and careful consideration in terms of use of noise and auditory stimuli in setting, including persons with major NCD (Verrier Piersol & Jensen, 2017).

Conditions such as drug intoxication, hyperthyroidism, and insulin shock may result in symptoms of dementia. When these conditions are treated, the symptoms of dementia usually resolve. Delirium is characterized by extreme disturbances of arousal, attention, orientation, intellectual function, and affect (Mills & Coulanges, 2013). An OT or OTA must be aware of how rapid changes in environment or medical status can induce systems of dementia that may be caused by secondary conditions such as those discussed.

PRACTICE SETTINGS

Occupational therapy practitioners provide services to older adults across the continuum of care. Although the majority of OTAs work in a long-term care setting, care may be provided

TABLE 18.1 Continuum of Care for Older Adults

Acute Care	Inpatient hospitals
	Long-term acute care (LTAC)
Subacute Care	Subacute rehabilitation
	Skilled nursing facilities (SNFs)
Extended Care	Assisted living facilities (ALFs)
Community-Based Care	Home health
	Adult day services
	Senior centers and housing
	Senior wellness programs
	Community mental health centers
	Home modification and accessibility consultants

in a variety of settings. Table 18.1 shows the continuum of care provided to older adults by OTs and OTAs.

Acute Care

Older adults who get injured, are sick, or have exacerbations of chronic conditions may require admission to an **acute care hospital**. Acute care OTs and OTAs must have working knowledge of the treatment of acute conditions, such as a hip fracture or traumatic brain injury, as well as acute or chronic exacerbations (e.g., an exacerbation of COPD). Providing interventions to older adults in acute care settings requires additional considerations as older adults often have an increased number of comorbid conditions as compared to younger adults. Long-term acute care (LTAC) settings offer acute-level care to persons for a myriad of reasons and require discharge from a traditional acute care hospital. Older adults in LTACs are typically additionally frail, requiring increased level of attention and medical care.

Subacute Care

Subacute care is defined as a comprehensive inpatient program designed for the individual who has had an acute event as a result of an illness, injury, or exacerbation of a disease process. Subacute treatment has a determined course of action; however, it does not require intensive diagnostic and invasive procedures that would require acute hospitalization. The severity of the individual's condition requires an outcome-focused interdisciplinary approach that employs a professional team to deliver complex clinical medical interventions and rehabilitation. The majority of individuals in subacute care settings have conditions with diagnoses associated with rehabilitation such as stroke, cardiac conditions, orthopedic conditions (including joint replacements and fractures), general and degenerative neurologic disorders (including multiple sclerosis, muscular dystrophy, Parkinson disease), amputations, severe arthritis, neuromuscular disorders, and general debilitation. The goal of rehabilitation is to return the individual to his or her previous level of function and natural setting (Mills & Coulanges, 2013).

Skilled Nursing Facilities

Skilled nursing facilities (SNFs), formerly known as nursing homes, are residential facilities that provide skilled nursing care, rehabilitative services, or health-related care on a daily basis to individuals who are injured, disabled, or sick. Services include daily basic nursing care or other rehabilitative services that reasonably can be provided only in a nursing facility. These include nursing and related services; specialized rehabilitative services; medically related social services; and activities to attain or maintain to the fullest extent possible the physical, mental, and psychosocial well-being of each individual. An individual may return to his or her natural living environment or remain as a resident based on safety concerns or limited functional ability (Mills & Coulanges, 2013).

Community Settings

Home health services occur in the client's home for those who are unable to get to outpatient appointments. The primary goal for OTs and OTAs working in home health care is to demonstrate outcomes of functional independence and improved QoL for clients in their home environment. Care begins with an initial evaluation from a registered OT compromising of a full assessment of occupational functioning. OTs working in home health care have increased administrative responsibilities related to demonstrating a client's eligibility for services. OTAs have a significant role in providing skilled interventions in the home environment and assisting the OT with demonstration of continuing need for services until desired outcomes are achieved. Intervention is concerned with ensuring clients' ability to safely manage themselves and their homes. OTs and OTAs in home-based settings use their skills in understanding person–environment fit to match the abilities of the person to the demands of the home. Management of chronic conditions and medications is another crucial aspect of home health care (American Occupational Therapy Association (AOTA), 2013).

Adult day services are programs that offer care during the day for the adult with declining function. Services are provided in a group setting. Mills and Coulanges (2013) provide description of services offered by adult day health: "These older adults are often affected by physical, mental, or social problems and sometimes require medical and rehabilitation services that are not offered in senior centers available to the general population" (p. 379). Many well older adults seek these services to support participation in occupation. Occupational therapy practitioners provide valuable, individualized programs (education, leisure management, and consulting services) to this growing population (Mills & Coulanges, 2013).

Extended Care Facilities

Assisted living facilities (ALFs) are centers that offer a combination of housing, support services, and health care.

Assisted living is an innovative approach to meeting the housing and care needs of older adults in a residential rather than an institutional environment. ALFs aim to maximize independence, choice, and privacy. ALFs are meant for older adults who require limited assistance with daily activities; these adults are typically high functioning in BADL and IADL. OTs and OTAs working in assisted living facilities have a primary role in identifying decline in function and providing services to help clients return to prior abilities or to make recommendations for modifications to ensure optimal participation in occupation. OTs and OTAs can also play a role in preventative programming in ALFs, such as fall prevention programs, education in regard to benefit of participation in meaningful activities, and strategies to support person–environment fit (American Occupational Therapy Association (AOTA), 2013).

Aging in Place Initiative—Call to Action for Occupational Therapy Practitioners

Given the significant demographic shift in the United States, there is a call to action for change in health care structure. Previously and currently, our system has been based inside brick-and-mortar facilities, such as assisted living and skilled nursing homes. Conversely, with increased number of aging adults and exorbitant cost of in-facility living, our nation is looking to shift toward a value-based care system in which persons are able to remain living, working, and playing within their current communities. OTs and OTAs should seek to be a part of initiatives with the aim to improve quality of health care, reduce cost of care, and improve our population's health by addressing more than just medical factors. This is a unique time for occupational therapy practitioners to demonstrate the ability to assist older adults with aging in place and maintaining a strong sense of functional independence within their communities.

The Centers for Disease Control and Prevention (CDC) defines the term *aging in place* as "the ability to live in one's own home and community safely, independently, and comfortability, regardless of age, income, or ability level" (Centers for Disease Control and Prevention (CDC), 2009). Furthermore, greater than 90% of older adults want to age in place (Lerner, 2016). This indicates significant need for health care practitioners to understand strategies to facilitate the values and desires of those they treat. As experts in evaluating, treating, and demonstrating outcomes for persons of all ages and abilities to obtain a highest level of independence, OTs and OTAs must also understand the factors contributing to older adults' ability to age in place. It is important for OTs and OTAs to integrate conversations about aging in place early, and across all settings, to support the wants and needs of those they treat and to support a progressive health care system to better support the needs of the US population. Health promotion and prevention are the future of our health care system, so we must be a part of this.

CASE STUDY

Carmen is a 73-year-old widow with diagnoses of COPD, arthritis, hypertension, and depression. She lives in a two-story home with her daughter, two grandchildren, and her mother who lives in the second-floor apartment. Her mother is homebound and receives full-time home care. Carmen's daughter Alicia works full time, cares for her children, and assists with her mother's and grandmother's care. Carmen stopped working as a bookkeeper 8 years ago and retired this year from her part-time job at the library. Carmen presents with +2 edema in both ankles, range of motion (ROM) within functional limits for all joints, and 3/3+ muscle strength in both upper extremities. At this time she exhibits a significant decrease in ADL participation. Carmen rarely goes outside the house and makes infrequent visits to her mother due to shortness of breath and joint pain when climbing the stairs. She no longer participates in housekeeping activities. Carmen has become fearful about her declining independence. She would like to regain active participation within her immediate environment (including modified independence in self-care and ability to perform light home maintenance tasks).

After gathering an occupational profile, analyzing her occupational performance, and collaborating on goals with Carmen and her family, the OT, OTA, and Carmen arrived at the following occupational therapy goals:

1. Carmen will engage in grooming, dressing, and bathing activities with modified independence on a daily basis.
2. She will retrieve clothing from the closet and drawers.
3. She will don/doff clothing with adaptive devices.
4. She will enter the bathtub and shower with adaptive equipment.
5. Carmen will engage in light home maintenance while using energy conservation techniques on a daily basis.
6. She will be out of bed for at least 3 hours in the morning and 3 hours in the afternoon.
7. She will make the bed in the morning on a daily basis.
8. She will engage in light meal preparation.
9. She will wash and put away dishes at least one time per day.
10. Carmen will engage in an exercise routine at least four times per week.
11. She will walk to the front stoop and pick up the mail daily.
12. She will visit with her mother, going up one flight of stairs, at least once per day.
13. She will walk to the neighborhood senior center at least three times per week with another person.
14. She will engage in modified yoga exercises using paced breathing techniques three times per week.

The intervention plan includes the following:

Practice Sessions in Self-Care Skills

1. Problem solving and active client participation in strategy formation during occupational performance
2. Client participation in adaptive equipment, device, and home modification choices
3. Client education and provision of adaptive equipment to assist with housekeeping, bathing, and dressing
4. Client education and training in energy conservation and work simplification activities
5. Client education and instruction in health maintenance and safety

Outcomes of Intervention

1. Participation in meaningful occupations to support participation in society
2. Client participation in assessment of intervention outcomes
3. Familial support to decrease caregiver burden and preserve familial roles and values

INTERVENTIONS TO PROMOTE QUALITY OF LIFE FOR OLDER ADULTS

Fall Prevention

According to the National Safety Council, falls are the third leading cause of injury-related death (Burns et al., 2016). With every 20 minutes that pass, an older adult will die from a fall (Burns et al., 2016). An estimated 3 million older adults are treated in the emergency department subsequent to a fall, with an estimated 5% of falls resulting in a fracture (Burns et al., 2016; Mills & Coulanges, 2013). Falls lead to serious health consequences, including hip fracture, traumatic brain injury, and reduced ability to perform daily tasks. Furthermore, falls create strain on the US health care system. Direct medical costs of fall-related injuries exceed $31 billion each year (Burns et al., 2016).

Often, older adults who have fallen develop a fear of falling and avoid activity performance to avoid falling again. Compared with older adults who have not experienced a fall, those who have fallen tend to experience more functional decline in ADL and social activity. Falls have been shown to be a strong predictor of nursing home placement (Mills & Coulanges, 2013).

Older adults are highly susceptible to falls because of health problems such as arthritis, poor eyesight and hearing, frailty, poor balance and coordination, senility, dementia, and weakness or dizziness secondary to medications. Most falls are multifactorial in nature, resulting due to the intersection of multiple risk factors. Falls may also result from risk factors in the environment such as improper footwear, tripping hazards, or improper fit between person and environment. Strategies to prevent falls among older adults are imperative to promoting successful aging and maintaining ability to participate in desired occupations.

OTs and OTAs participate in fall prevention interventions through assessment of the individual and specific risk factors and developing a client-centered plan of care for individuals to prevent injury and loss of function from falling. The occupational therapy assessment includes information on the sensorimotor, cognitive, and psychologic functions. The OTA, in conjunction with the OT, assists in developing a plan of care geared toward the remediation of deficits or compensation for any loss of function. OTs and OTAs may provide intervention aimed to modify the person, the person's

CASE STUDY

George is an 86-year-old man who sustained a hip fracture 2 weeks ago while changing a light bulb and was admitted to the nursing home for rehabilitative care. George's family hopes to be able to take him home as soon as he is able to walk again. George and his family hope that he will be able to continue to participate in social activities such as going to the senior center and independently performing ADL such as dressing, grooming, bathing, and light meal preparation. George lives alone in a barrier-free (i.e., no steps) senior citizen building. Before the fall he was independent in all self-care activities, attended tai chi classes, and regularly traveled by bus.

He also met with friends weekly at the senior center and attended community events with his girlfriend. During his hospitalization, George underwent a right total hip replacement. Because of his diabetes, healing was slow. During his hospitalization, George spent the days alone and was visited by family and friends in the late afternoon and evening.

On admission to the nursing home, George was assessed as being disoriented (a reaction to anesthesia and pain medication), unable to participate in any self-care activity except eating, and unable to transfer from the bed independently. He had decreased ROM on the right hip and exhibited poor endurance and impaired postural control. He was incontinent and nonambulatory. Because of his disorientation, George made several attempts to climb out of bed, and staff feared that he might fall and reinjure himself. George's behavior triggered a care area assessment (CAA), and a fall risk assessment was performed by the interdisciplinary team.

Each discipline assessed George, and a plan of care was instituted. The recreational staff formulated and implemented an activity plan that included a variety of social activities. The occupational therapy staff was able to suggest mentally and physically stimulating activities that were identified in his occupational profile. The nursing and social service staff provided reality orientation and encouragement for continued participation in therapy and activities.

The occupational therapy evaluation included the gathering of an occupational profile and assessment of George's basic ADL, including dressing, grooming, bathing, and transfer skills. The evaluation of client factors and performance skills included assessment of ROM, muscle strength, endurance, mobility, orientation, ability to follow directions, and ability to conceptualize safety issues. The interview included familial and client discussions about George's goals, interests, and expectations.

The occupational therapy intervention plan included increasing ROM, muscle strength and endurance, topographic orientation, and mobility while providing practice sessions in self-care activities such as dressing, bathing, grooming, and transfer training. The anticipated outcome of George's intervention plan was to promote participation in meaningful occupation with reentry into the community.

As George's mental and physical status improved, he increasingly could make his own decisions and could collaborate with the occupational therapy staff to develop an activity schedule for home. George expressed concern about his ability to return to his prior level of functioning without becoming a burden on his family. He could describe his apartment and where his furniture was located and was able to make decisions about what could and could not be moved. He participated in the rearrangement of the home to eliminate obstacles and increase safety. George was discharged from the nursing home and was referred to a home health service that provided occupational therapy. The home care OT assisted George in readjusting to community life by assessing his ability to perform self-care activities and use public transportation and by offering suggestions for modifying his home.

---

environment, or task demands of desired occupations to prevent falling (Mills & Coulanges, 2013).

Fall prevention interventions aimed to influence personal client factors include balance and strength training, specific coordination training, neuromuscular reeducation, addressing nutrition and hydration, stabilizing disease state, and management of medications. Person–environment fit is also a strong indicator of fall risk. Therefore OTs and OTAs provide intervention to reduce hazards and barriers in a person's environment that may result in falls, including removal of obstacles such as throw rugs, the rearrangement of cabinets to place heavier things on the bottom rather than top shelves, and bathroom aids (e.g., call bell, bathtub seat, grab bars, raised toilet seat Fig. 18.1). To prevent falls, OTs and OTAs may also need to modify the means in which a client performs an occupation and make recommendations for task modifications to improve safety. Provision of assistive technology (e.g., mobility devices) and completion of occupations in a seated position are examples of modification of the task demands to prevent falls. Table 18.2 provides a systematic review of effective fall prevention techniques for community-dwelling older adults.

Polypharmacy

Older adults in the United States use a disproportionate amount of prescription and nonprescription medications. Use of prescription drugs tends to increase with age, with many older adults taking more than one prescription drug. Older adults are at a higher risk for adverse drug reactions than other groups because of age-related changes in physiology, decrements due to chronic diseases, and use of multiple drugs (Ferrini & Ferrini, 2000).

The practice of using multiple medications simultaneously is termed **polypharmacy**. Polypharmacy is common among both institutionalized and community-dwelling older adults. Polypharmacy is the outcome of the presence of multiple comorbid conditions and chronic diseases. Multiple co-conditions are common in older adults; two thirds of persons over 65 years of age have two or more chronic illnesses (Brown, 2016).

Pharmacokinetics is the study of what happens to a drug after it enters the body: its absorption into the bloodstream, its distribution to the body tissues, its metabolism by the liver, and its excretion by the liver or kidney. The physiologic changes of the body associated with aging are hypothesized

Patient _____ Age _____ Room _____

Triggered problems _____

Assessment goals are (1) to ensure that a treatment plan is in place for patients with history of falls, and (2) to identify patients who are at risk for falls and are not currently enrolled in a fall prevention program.

1. Is there a previous history of falls?   Yes_____ No_____
2. Was the fall an isolated event?   Yes_____ No_____

Internal risk factors

Does patient have?	Yes	No
Cardiovascular abnormalities		
Cardiac dysrhythmia		
Hypotension		
Syncope		
Neuromuscular impairments		
Cerebrovascular accident		
Hemiplegia		
Unsteady gait		
Incontinence		
Seizure disorder		
Parkinson's disease		
Chronic/acute condition causing instability		
Loss of leg or arm movement		
Decline in functional status		
Orthopedic impairments		
Arthritis		
Osteoporosis		
Joint pain		
Hip fracture		
Perceptual abnormalities		
Impaired hearing		
Dizziness or vertigo		
Psychiatric or cognitive impairments		
Alzheimer's/dementia		
Decline in cognitive skills		
Delirium		
Manic depression or other affective disorder		
Other dementia		

Fig. 18.1 Sample of falls protocol worksheet.

to influence drug absorption, distribution, metabolism, and excretion. Polypharmacy is correlated to intensification of syndromes associated with aging, such as decreased cognition and mobility status, and decline in functional outcomes. For this reason, it is imperative that older adults and their caregivers pay close attention to medication dosage and frequency to avoid toxic effects (Brown, 2016).

Medication used to treat medical conditions can significantly influence occupation and the older adult's safe participation in society. The client's actual functional capacity may

External factors

	Yes	No
Medications		
Psychotropic medications		
Cardiovascular medications		
Diuretics		
Was medication administered before the fall?		
Was medication administered after the fall?		

If medications were administered before the fall, how much time before the fall were they first administered? _____

List all medications and note possible side effects _____

_____

_____

Appliances and devices

	Yes	No
Pacemaker		
Walker or cane		
Physical restraints		
Other		
Restraints before fall		

Observe patient's use of the device for possible problems and describe performance _____

_____

Environmental and situational hazards

	Yes	No
Glare		
Poor illumination		
Slippery floors		
Uneven floors		
Patterned carpets		
Objects in walkway		
Recent move		
New arrangement of objects		
Proximity of aggressive residents		
Type of activity		
Standing still/walking		
In a crowded area		
Responding to bladder/bowel urgency		
Reaching/not reaching		

Fig. 18.1 (Continued).

Is there a pattern of falls in any of the above circumstances (environmental and situational hazards)? _____

_____

_____

_____

If you know what the resident was doing immediately leading to the fall, have resident repeat the activity and observe _____

_____

_____

_____

Vital signs
  Measure patient's blood pressure and heart rate:

  Supine _____

  1 minute after standing _____

  3 minutes after standing _____

Resident interaction with the environment
Observe resident and check "able" or "not able" and "safe" or "unsafe."

Activity	Able	Not able	Safe	Unsafe
Moving in and out of bed				
Walking				
Turning				
Transferring				
Toileting				

Identified problems _____

_____

_____

_____

_____

_____

_____

_____

Suggested multidisciplinary treatment interventions

Nursing _____

_____

_____

OT/PT _____

_____

_____

_____

_____

Fig. 18.1 (Continued).

be altered by adverse medication effects. Polypharmacy significantly increases risk of falls, specifically medications commonly prescribed to older adults, including benzodiazepines, antidepressants, antipsychotics, antihypertensives, and diuretics (Brown, 2016).

Use of Restraints

The Omnibus Budget Reconciliation Act of 1987 (OBRA 87) made restraint use the exception rather than the rule. The law requires nursing homes to provide quality care and QoL for each individual. This includes maintaining the well-being of

Activities _____

_____

_____

Medical _____

_____

_____

_____

Social services _____

_____

_____

_____

Fig. 18.1 (Continued).

TABLE 18.2 **Fall Prevention in the Older Adult**
Summary of Evidence
• **Mixed evidence** for single-component approaches to fall prevention (i.e., only addressing balance deficits)
• Increased support for dual-task or multitask exercises, such as inclusion of both motor and cognitive components when providing interventions to prevent falls
• **Strong evidence** for group-based, multicomponent interventions (i.e., interventions addressing multiple factors of fall risk in group settings). Programs varied, however, included both exercise and education:
• Exercise: balance, strength, completion of functional tasks, dual-task activities, obstacle course training, and training in fall techniques
• Education: proper footwear, energy conservation, assistive device training, home modification recommendations, fall recovery, medication management, nutrition and hydration, relaxation, and stress management
• Education also focused on increased awareness of risk factors: reduced cognition, postural hypotension, low vision, continence

Elliot S, Leland NE. Occupational therapy fall prevention interventions for community-dwelling older adults: a systematic review. *Am J Occup Ther.* 2018;72:7204190040. https://doi.org/10.5014/ajot.2018.030494.

each individual and ensuring to the greatest practical extent a good QoL by providing services and activities.

Physical restraints are any manual method or any physical or mechanical device, material, or equipment attached or adjacent to the individual's body that the individual cannot remove independently; they restrict freedom of movement or normal access to the body. Physical restraints include vests, belts, wheelchair seat belts, wheelchairs, hand mitts, wheelchair safety bars, bed rails, and other devices used to position an individual.

Chemical restraints are also a method for restricting an individual's movement (Lewis, 2003). Chemical restraints are medications that restrict an individual's interaction with the environment. For the older adult certain medications can produce the effect of chemical restraint. Since the 1990s there have been widespread efforts to reduce the use of physical and chemical restraints and to find alternatives to prevent falls in nursing homes (Padilla, 2011).

Risks of Restraint Use. Ljubuncic and Reznick (2009) described several risks of restraint use. The individual may become agitated and more disoriented. The individual might be embarrassed, which would diminish self-esteem. Restrained individuals may experience increased injuries while attempting to break free from the restraints. The individual may suffer the effects of immobility, including skin breakdown, decreased circulation, and incontinence. The nursing staff may end up with more work, not less, if the individual becomes injured while trying to remove the restraints or develops skin and other problems from restraints.

Most practitioners who work in long-term care settings would agree that these risks continue to be associated with restraint use.

Occupational Therapy Role. Today long-term care facilities are required to provide a restraint-free environment. Restraints are used in only the most extreme cases. These patients require constant monitoring and reassessment of the individual, family notification, and multidisciplinary case management to limit or eliminate the use of a restraint. Long-term care facilities are required to use a multidisciplinary team approach to limit and/or eliminate the use of restraints.

Among the varied multidisciplinary assessments that are performed to reduce or eliminate use of a restraint, most facilities require that an occupational therapy evaluation be completed to determine alternatives to physical restraint. The evaluation will determine the individual's positioning needs and transfer skills, as well as other needs associated with the individual's ability to negotiate the environment safely. In many instances, individuals are restrained because they slide out of their wheelchair. The clinician will need to assess whether this problem is caused by an inappropriate seating and positioning system, an inappropriate type of wheelchair, or other physiologic, neurologic, or orthopedic factors.

In evaluating and determining alternatives to physical restraint, the practitioner must consider the needs of the individual as well as any problems, conditions, and risk factors. If a restraint must be used, the clinician must explain why the restraint is being used; the type of restraint being used; and when, where, for how long, and under what circumstances the restraint is used. Once the underlying problem is identified and resolved, it is the obligation of the multidisciplinary team to eliminate the restraint. If the restraint is used to control a behavior, the clinician must bear in mind that many behaviors are caused by unmet needs and can often be eliminated by meeting those needs. The OT or OTA will be expected to participate as a team contributor to aid in managing the individual's behavior without restraints. The Minimum Data Set (MDS) restraint protocol guidelines include a review of the individual's record and the conditions that seem to precipitate restraint use, including problem behaviors, risk of falls, and treatment regimens (Schuster & Ashburn, 1992). The MDS protocol also includes conditions under which a restraint may be used. These include enhancement of independent ADL performance. For example, although a full-length rail on an individual's bed is intended to reduce the risk of injury by preventing him from getting out of bed, it would nonetheless be considered a restraint. Although still a restraint, a half bed rail that assists an individual with performance of independent transfers would be considered an ADL enhancement. Table 18.3 provides alternatives to restraint use.

Each member of the interdisciplinary team should be trained to support the individual. Team members should learn about the individual's interests and desires. Some staff will be better at

interacting with certain individuals than others will be (Padilla, 2011). Family and significant others who are close to the individual can be questioned (within the allowable boundaries of client confidentiality) to assist with gaining an understanding of the individual's values, interests, and desires.

Communicating With Older Adults and Their Caregivers

The presence multiple comorbid conditions, changes to biopsychosocial functioning, and inherent differences in the culture, values, and beliefs derived from a lifetime of experiences makes communication with older adults and their caregivers especially important (Mills & Coulanges, 2013). Verbal communication provides directions, explains a treatment method, or expresses an idea. Nonverbal communication, such as smiles, frowns, and posture, reinforces or discourages a behavior or provides information regarding pleasure or displeasure (Mills & Coulanges, 2013).

The OT's or OTA's mode of communication can enhance the intervention process by providing the client, the family, and other caregivers with information regarding the expected outcome of the intervention. Mode of communication is also critical when discussing questions, fears, or apprehensions toward intervention methods in a nonthreatening environment (Mills & Coulanges, 2013). By explaining methods, suggesting alternatives, and promoting client/practitioner collaboration, we empower the older adult, the family, and the caregiver to be an active participant in the intervention process. (See Chapter 2 for more information regarding communication.)

Communicating With Family and Significant Others

For many older adults, family members and significant others are the most trusted people in their lives. This trust is based on a common history. OTs and OTAs should consider

TABLE 18.3	Alternatives to Restraints		
Type of Program	**Intervention Approach**	**Skills Addressed**	**Intervention Strategies**
Restorative programs	Remediation of underlying impairment	Proprioceptive deficits Balance impairments Mobility concerns Positioning for safety Participation in activities of daily living (ADL)	ADL Community outings Home modification
Maintenance programs	Maintain optimal functional level	Cognition Physical strength and endurance	Social skills groups Therapeutic recreation/activities Exercise programs
Enhanced environments	Decrease agitation/maximize function	Social participation Arousal Emotional stability Cognition	Home modification (reducing glare, noise reduction) Familiarizing environment (bringing objects from home)
Adaptive equipment	Decrease restraint use	Safety	Bed and chair alarms Low bed height Floor mats Hip protectors

CASE STUDY

Lesson Learned About Client–Practitioner Collaboration

Olivia is an 82-year-old woman who lived alone in a small, one-bedroom, walk-up apartment. As part of a fall prevention study, Marsha, an OT, was assigned to visit Olivia to perform a home safety assessment and assessment of select ADL and IADL. The goal of assessment was to determine environmental modification recommendations, assistive devices, and equipment that would promote Olivia's occupational performance and personal safety within her home.

The study allowed for Marsha to recommend, order, and train her clients with varied devices and equipment to prevent falls. Marsha was excited to participate as an occupational therapy consultant within the study knowing that she could recommend and order equipment for a study participant without cost to the individual. Previously, affordability of adaptive equipment and devices had been a concern to Marsha's clients.

After the assessment, Marsha informed Olivia of the devices and equipment that support her independence and safety in her home. Unexpectedly, Olivia proceeded to cry upon completion of Marsha's report. Marsha was not prepared for the expression of emotion that poured from Olivia. Amidst the tears, Olivia cried out, "All of these things… I can't believe that I need all of these things. I feel so old!"

This experience helped Marsha realize the significance and importance of client–practitioner collaboration. It became apparent to Marsha that she had informed Olivia about her device and equipment needs, but had not included Olivia in the decision-making process.

Marsha's experience with Olivia was invaluable, influencing all aspects of her clinical practice and service delivery. Marsha learned the value of providing client education, listening to the client, providing choices, listening again, providing education, and recommending respectful and realistic solutions.

The significance of client–practitioner collaboration can be easily missed, even in the case of an experienced practitioner, when the practitioner does not initiate the interaction using a client-centered approach. This revelation led Marsha to formulate a systemized method for introducing environmental modifications, adaptive equipment and devices, and tips for promoting person–environment fit.

how trusted individuals can encourage the older adult to participate in the intervention process and to monitor follow-through. Literature also demonstrates support for collaborating with both the client and the caregiver when making environmental modification and assistive device recommendations (Ferrini & Ferrini, 2000). Health care regulations require that both the client and specified family members or significant others be informed about the type of intervention the client receives (Schuster & Ashburn, 1992).

When communicating with families and significant others, the practitioner should be reported in simple terms. Jargon and medical terminology should be minimized and clearly explained. Respectful explanations are crucial, hence the practitioner must find balance in conveying vital information while also facilitating trust and space for constant feedback from the older adult. The therapist must remember that the purpose of communicating with the family is to enhance the intervention process.

OTs and OTAs must also understand the potential impact of a client's functional limitation on the family unit (i.e., familial role changes) (National Institute on Deafness and Other Communication Disorders (NIDCD), 2018). Caregiving is defined as a co-occupation that involves active participation on the part of the caregiver and the recipient of care (Brown, 2016). Caregiver burden has been recognized as a major concern for the families and significant others of older adults with significant functional limitations (i.e., community dwelling older adults). Through effective communication and inclusion of the family and significant others in intervention the practitioner can significantly reduce caregiver burden (Lee et al., 2013; Lin et al., 2010; National Institute on Deafness and Other Communication Disorders (NIDCD), 2018).

One of the challenges of working with the older adult is developing an intervention plan that addresses normal aging when it is accompanied by several pathologic and/or chronic medical conditions; communication is key to overcoming these challenges. As noted earlier in this chapter, the practitioner who is developing intervention plans for persons with multiple diagnoses must be aware of how one diagnosis will affect another and of how one medication may affect or cause symptoms that interfere with functional abilities. For example, someone who is recovering from a CVA may also have a diagnosis of ASHD, CHF, and DM. If the person is to perform light cooking or meal preparation, the intervention plan may require diabetes education for meal planning and compensatory strategies for sensory loss. Rest periods and energy conservation techniques are necessary to minimize CHF-related shortness of breath. The individual must be taught to recognize additional adverse symptoms such as swelling of the feet. Moreover, safety precautions with the use of kitchen knives are essential; a simple cut may take a longer period to heal because of the DM, thereby increasing the risk of infection.

SUMMARY

Aging is a complex process that begins at birth. Health and lifestyle are strong determinants of quality of life as individuals reach maturity. Illness must be viewed separately from reduced abilities. Although some diseases are more common in the older adult, the disease process should not be confused with normal aging.

OTs and OTAs must understand the developmental needs of the older person. In addition, practitioners must be aware of what constitutes normal aging and how superimposed pathologic conditions and adverse medication reactions affect the older person. The practitioner must appreciate values and cultural differences and take care to communicate information clearly to older adults, their families, and other persons involved in their care. OTs and OTAs must be prepared to initiate their interactions and interventions from a client-centered approach that incorporates client—practitioner collaboration throughout all aspects of the service delivery process.

Certified occupational therapy assistants (COTAs) collaborate with the OT in developing intervention plans for the older adult. When developing intervention plans for older clients with multiple diagnoses, the practitioner must be aware of how one diagnosis will affect another and of how one medication may affect or cause symptoms that interfere with functional abilities.

SELECTED READING GUIDE QUESTIONS

1. List three theories that describe how and why we age.
2. Describe four common age-related changes.
3. List four pathologic conditions that are commonly seen in the older adult.
4. List four sensory changes common in the older adult.
5. Discuss potential effects of medication on the function of the older adult.
6. Describe three practice models used when working with clients with multiple diagnoses.
7. Describe four intervention settings in which the OTA may provide services to the older adult.
8. Describe one method that may be used to prevent falls in the older adult.
9. Define restraints.
10. List the risks of restraint use.
11. Describe three interventions that may be used to prevent restraint use.
12. Describe the importance of communicating with the family.
13. Name and discuss techniques that can be used to communicate with patients.
14. Name the components of the comprehensive care plan.

REFERENCES

Alzheimer's Association. (2019). What is dementia? https://www.alz.org/alzheimers-dementia/what-is-dementia.

American Occupational Therapy Association (AOTA). (2013). Occupational therapy's role in home health [Fact Sheet]. https://www.aota.org/~/media/Corporate/Files/AboutOT/Professionals/WhatIsOT/PA/Home-Health.pdf.

American Occupational Therapy Association (AOTA). (2016). Occupational therapy's role in assisted living facilities [Fact Sheet]. https://www.aota.org/~/media/Corporate/Files/AboutOT/Professionals/WhatIsOT/PA/Facts/Assisted%20Living%20fact%20sheet.pdf.

Brown, L. G. (2016). Untangling polypharmacy in older adults. *Medsurg Nursing, 25*(6), 408—412.

Brutsaert, E.F. (2019). Diabetes mellitus (DM). Merck Manuals. https://www.merckmanuals.com/professional/endocrine-and-metabolic-disorders/diabetes-mellitus-and-disorders-of-carbohydrate-metabolism/diabetes-mellitus-dm?query=diabetes%20mellitus.

Burns, E. R., Stevens, J. A., & Lee, R. (2016). The direct costs of fatal and non-fatal falls among older adults—United States. *Journal of Safety Research, 58,* 99—103. Available from https://doi.org/10.1016/j.jsr.2016.05.001.

Centers for Disease Control and Prevention (CDC). (2009). Healthy Places Terminology. https://www.cdc.gov/healthy-places/terminology.htm#a.

Chaudhury, H., Hung, L., & Badger, M. (2013). The role of physical environment in supporting person-centered dining in long-term care: a review of the literature. *American Journal of Alzheimer's Disease & Other Dementias, 28*(5), 491—500. Available from https://doi-org.une.idm.oclc.org/10.1177/1533317513488923.

Cooper, C., Mukadam, N., Katona, C., Lyketsos, C. G., Ames, D., Rabins, P., et al. (2012). Systematic review of the effectiveness of non-pharmacological interventions to improve quality of life of people with dementia. *International Psychogeriatrics / IPA, 24*(6), 856—870. Available from https://doi.org/10.1017/s1041610211002614.

Dagnelie, G. (2009). Age-related psychophysical changes and low vision. *Investigative Ophthalmology & Visual Science, 54*(14). Available from https://doi.org/10.1167/iovs.3-12934.

Dechamps, A., Fasotti, L., Jungheim, J., Leone, E., Dood, E., Allioux, A., et al. (2011). Effects of different learning methods for instrumental activities of daily living in patients with Alzheimer's dementia: a pilot study. *American Journal of Alzheimer's Disease & Other Dementias, 26,* 273—281. Available from https://doi.org/10.1177/1533317511404394.

Ferrini, A. F., & Ferrini, R. L. (2000). *Health in later years.* Boston, MA: McGraw-Hill.

Fleming, R., & Purandare, N. (2010). Long-term care for people with dementia: environmental design guidelines. *International Psychogeriatrics, 22*(7), 1084—1096. Available from https://doi-org.une.idm.oclc.org/10.1017/S1041610210000438.

Flynn, J. E., & Mabry, E. R. (1992). Biophysical development of later adulthood. In C. S. Schuster, & S. S. Ashburn (Eds.), *The process of human development: a holistic life-span approach* (2nd ed.). Philadelphia, PA: Lippincott Company.

Hodgkinson, B., Koch, S., Nay, R., & Lewis, M. (2007). Managing the wandering behaviors of people living in a residential aged care facility. *International Journal of Evidence-Based Healthcare, 5*(4), 406—436. Available from https://doi-org.une.idm.oclc.org/10.1111/j.1479-6988.2007.00078.x.

Jackson, J., Carlson, M., Mandel, D., Zemke, R., & Clark, F. (1998). Occupation in lifestyle redesign: the well elderly study occupational therapy program. *The American Journal of Occupational Therapy, 52*(5), 326—336.

Jin, K. (2010). Modern biological theories of aging. *Aging and Disease, 1*(2), 72—74.

Lee, G., Yip, C. C. K., Yu, E. C. S., & Man, D. W. K. (2013). Evaluation of a computer-assisted errorless learning-based memory training program for patients with early Alzheimer's disease in Hong Kong: a pilot study. *Clinical Interventions in Aging,* 623—633. Available from https://doi.org/10.2147/CIA.S45726.

Lerner, M. (2016). New online service targets aging-in-place residents. *Washington Post.* https://www.washingtonpost.com/news/where-we-live/wp/2016/01/19/new-online-services-targets-aging-in-place-residents/.

Letts, L., Minezes, J., Edwards, M., Berenyi, J., Moros, K., O'Neill, C., et al. (2011). Effectiveness of interventions designed to modify and maintain perceptual abilities in people with Alzheimer's disease and related dementias. *The American Journal of Occupational Therapy*, 65(5), 505–513. Available from https://doi.org/10.5014/ajot.2011.002592.

Lewis, S. C. (2003). *Elder care in occupational therapy*. Thorofare, NJ: Slack.

Lin, L.-C., Huang, Y.-J., Su, S.-G., Watson, R., Tsai, B. W.-J., & Wu, S.-C. (2010). Using spaced retrieval and Montessori-based activities in improving eating ability for residents with dementia. *International Journal of Geriatric Psychiatry*, 25(10), 953–959. Available from https://doi.org/10.1002/gps.2433.

Liochev, S. I. (2013). Reactive oxygen species and the free radical theory of aging. *Free Radical Biology & Medicine*, 60, 1–4. Available from https://doi.org/10.1016/j.freeradbiomed.2013.02.011.

Lipsky, M. S., & King, M. (2015). Biological theories of aging. *Disease-a-Month: DM*, 61(11), 460–466. Available from https://doi.org/10.1016/j.disamonth.2015.09.005.

Lui, W., Cheon, J., & Thomas, S. A. (2014). Interventions on mealtime difficulties in older adults with dementia: a systematic review. *International Journal of Nursing Studies*, 51(1), 14–27. Available from https://doi.org/10.1016/j.ijnurstu.2012.12.021.

Ljubuncic, P., & Reznick, A. Z. (2009). The evolutionary theories of aging revisited—a mini-review. *Gerontology*, 55(2), 205–216. Available from https://doi.org/10.1159/000200772.

Mayo Foundation for Medical Education and Research. (2018). Vascular dementia. Mayo Clinic. https://www.mayoclinic.org/diseases-conditions/vascular-dementia/symptoms-causes/syc-20378793?p=1.

Miller, C. A. (2012). *Nursing for wellness in older adults: theory and practice*. Philadelphia, PA: Lippincott Williams & Wilkins.

Mills, M. D., & Coulanges, K. (2013). The older adult. In M. B. Early (Ed.), *Physical dysfunction practice skills for the occupational therapy assistant* (3rd ed). St. Louis, MO: Elsevier.

National Institute on Deafness and Other Communication Disorders (NIDCD). (2018). Age-related hearing loss. https://www.nidcd.nih.gov/health/age-related-hearing-loss.

National Institutes of Health (NIH). (2017). What happens to the brain in Alzheimer's disease? https://www.nia.nih.gov/health/what-happens-brain-alzheimers-disease.

Olazarán, J., Reisburg, B., Clare, L., Cruz, I., Peña-Casanova, J., Del Ser, T., et al. (2010). Nonpharmacological therapies in Alzheimer's disease: a systematic review of efficacy. *Dementia and Geriatric Cognitive Disorders*, 30, 161–178. Available from https://doi.org/10.1159/000316119.

Padilla, R. (2011). Effectiveness of interventions designed to modify the activity demands of the occupations of self-care and leisure for people with Alzheimer's disease and related dementias. *The American Journal of Occupational Therapy*, 65(5), 523–531. Available from https://doi.org/10.5014/ajot.2011.002618.

Paúl, C., & Lopes, A. (2016). Active aging. In N. Pachana (Ed.), *Encyclopedia of geropsychology*. Singapore: Springer.

Sandmire, D. A. (2010). The physiology and pathology of aging. In R. H. Robnett, & W. C. Chop (Eds.), *Gerontology for the health care professional* (5th ed.). Boston, MA: Jones & Bartlett.

Schuster, C. S., & Ashburn, S. S. (1992). *The process of human development: a holistic life-span approach*. Philadelphia, PA: Lippincott Company.

Stalworth, M., & Sloane, P. D. (2007). Clinical implications of normal aging. *Primary Care Geriatrics*, 14–24. Available from https://doi.org/10.1016/b978-032303930-7.50009-2.

The older population. 2010 Census Briefs. 2011. https://www.census.gov/prod/cen2010/briefs/c2010br-09.pdf

The week staff (2009). The graying of America. *The Week*; 2009. https://theweek.com/articles/859185/graying-america.

Tierney, M. (2009). *The Hayflick Limit*. Toronto: Coach House Books; ProQuest Ebook Central. https://ebookcentral.proquest.com/lib/uneedu/detail.action?docID=760394.

Verrier Piersol, C., & Jensen, L. (2017). *Occupational therapy practice guidelines for adults with Alzheimer's disease and related major neurocognitive disorders*. Bethesda, MD: The American Occupational Therapy Association, Inc.

Vierkötter, A., & Krutmann, J. (2012). Environmental influences on skin aging and ethnic-specific manifestations. *Dermato-Endocrinology*, 4(3), 227–231. Available from https://doi.org/10.4161/derm.19858.

Wise, R. A. (2018). Chronic obstructive pulmonary disease (COPD). Merck Manuals. https://www.merckmanuals.com/professional/pulmonary-disorders/chronic-obstructive-pulmonary-disease-and-related-disorders/chronic-obstructive-pulmonary-disease-copd?query=copd.

World Health Organization. (2002). *Active aging: a policy framework*. Geneva: WHO.

Woods, B., Aguirre, E., Spector, A. E., & Orrell, M. (2012). Cognitive stimulation to improve cognitive functioning in people with dementia. *Cochrane Database of Systematic Reviews*. Available from https://doi.org/10.1002/14651858.cd005562.pub2.

19

Principles of Orthotic Fabrication

Peter Dasilva and Josh McAuliffe

OBJECTIVES

After reading this chapter, the student or the occupational therapy practitioner will be able to do the following:

1. Locate important landmarks in the anatomy of the hand, including arches and other structural elements that contribute to hand function.
2. Identify normal prehension and grasp patterns and describe the three basic positions of the hand.
3. Understand the primary purposes for orthotic use of the upper extremity.
4. Understand the biomechanical, physiologic, and client compliance considerations involved in orthotic selection and fabrication.

5. Determine what low-temperature thermoplastic handling and performance characteristics are useful for fabricating different orthoses.
6. Recognize indications for soft-support orthoses.
7. Explain basic patternmaking, fabrication, and strapping principles and techniques.
8. Draw patterns for and fabricate three basic upper extremity orthoses.

KEY TERMS

Orthosis
Arches
Radial
Ulnar
Creases
Distal
Proximal
Dorsal
Volar

Extrinsic muscles
Intrinsic muscles
Thenar
Hypothenar
Phalanx
Tenodesis action
Low-temperature thermoplastics
Performance characteristics

INTRODUCTION

The hand serves to obtain information, execute motor activities, and express emotions. The hand requires sensation, mobility, and stability to interact effectively with the environment. Any defect in sensory, neuromuscular, skeletal, articular, vascular, or soft-tissue structures affects the functioning of the hand and its appearance (Fess et al., 1981; Gillen, 2010). The function of the proximal joints (shoulder, elbow, forearm) is to place and stabilize the hand for functional activities. Thus the hand must be assessed in relation to function of the entire arm.

Because of its primary role in daily activities and interaction, the appearance of the hand is important. Use of skin moisturizers, manicures, and jewelry testifies to the importance of its attractiveness in interpersonal contact. The exquisite sensibility of the hand permits an amazing level of coordinated activity, and it transmits enormous amounts of

information about the environment to the brain. People use their hands to prepare for and perform all activities of daily living (ADL) and to express themselves. The hearing-impaired person uses the hand to speak, and the blind person uses it to see.

Psychosocial problems may be associated with dysfunction or injury that disrupts the hand's primary role in daily interactions with both the physical world and other people (Tubiana, 1984). Orthotic fabrication/management is one of several treatment modalities used to restore normal function and appearance of the hand. The occupational therapy assistant (OTA) fabricates **orthoses** (i.e., orthopedic devices used to immobilize, mobilize, or protect a body part) and to assist with the assessment of client positioning. This chapter briefly reviews the structure and function of the hand, introduces basic principles and goals of orthotic fabrication, and provides basic instruction on fabrication of three common hand orthoses.

STRUCTURES OF THE HAND

Bones

The wrist and hand are composed of 27 bones: 8 carpals (wrist), 5 metacarpals (palm), and 14 phalanges (fingers). The proximal row of carpals articulates with the radius and ulna of the forearm. Combined movements of hand, wrist, and forearm permit an amazing variety of positions during activity. Fractured bones conversely require rest and stability to heal correctly.

Alignment

The precise relationship of length, mobility, and position of each finger and between the thumb and fingers is the key to functional use. The fingertips converge toward the pad of the thumb during palmar prehension. When individually flexed, they converge toward the center of the wrist (capitate bone), but when simultaneously flexed they contact the palm parallel to each other. Alignment of the digits must be respected during orthotic design and fabrication.

Arches

Three **arches** (curves) are present in the hand: the longitudinal, the proximal transverse, and the distal transverse. The longitudinal arch follows the lines of the carpal and metacarpal bones down along the third finger. The ability to flex and extend the digits occurs along this arch. The proximal transverse arch is a bony, fixed arch formed by the proximal row of carpal bones and annular ligaments. This arch is deep; through it pass all the nerves, blood supply, and tendons of the extrinsic hand muscles. This arch also acts as a fulcrum for the finger flexors, preventing them from bowing during flexion. The distal transverse arch (also called the *metacarpal arch*) lies across the metacarpal heads (knuckles). The dexterity and functional use of the hand rely on the mobility of this arch.

Place your left thumb on the palm side of the fourth and fifth metacarpal heads of your right hand and push them back to where they are flat across with the second and third metacarpal heads. When you attempt to make a fist with your right hand, you will see that it is not possible. Flattening of the distal transverse arch is not a functional position. Flattening may be caused by many conditions, including intrinsic muscle paralysis, edema, scarring, contractures, or poor positioning in an orthosis. The distal transverse arch must be maintained in the orthosis to ensure maximal functional use of the hand while the orthosis is on or off.

Dual Obliquity

The dual obliquity (or two nonparallel lines) (Fig. 19.1) in the hand occurs because the length of the second to fifth metacarpals gradually decreases from the radial (thumb) side of the hand to the ulnar side of the hand. A line drawn through the metacarpal heads forms an oblique angle with a line drawn through the wrist. A second oblique angle occurs at the distal transverse arch. The second and third metacarpals are relatively fixed, stable bones, whereas the fourth and fifth move more freely. Functionally, this means that an object, when

grasped cylindrically, is higher on the radial side of the hand and not parallel to the floor when the hand is in full pronation. An easy way to remember this is simply that the **radial** (thumb) side of the hand is longer and higher than the **ulnar** (small finger) side. Any hand or forearm-based orthosis must respect this anatomy.

Creases

The skin **creases** (folds) (Fig. 19.2) act as guides when the occupational therapist (OT) or the OTA is designing and fitting orthoses. The creases indicate where the axes of motion for the joints occur. The wrist, palmar, thenar, and proximal, middle, and distal finger creases deepen when the associated joint is moved. For the palmar creases the **distal** crease is associated with metacarpophalangeal (MP) flexion of digits III, IV, and V, and the **proximal** crease with digits II and III.

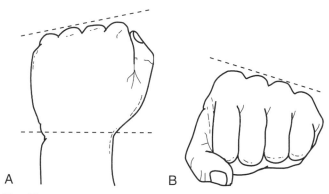

Fig. 19.1 Dual obliquity of hand. (A) Oblique angle of metacarpal heads in relation to axis of wrist joint. (B) Oblique angle of metacarpal heads from radial to ulnar side of hand. (From Fess EE, Gettle KS, Philips CA, et al. *Hand and Upper Extremity Splinting: Principles and Methods.* 3rd ed. St. Louis, MO: Mosby; 2005.)

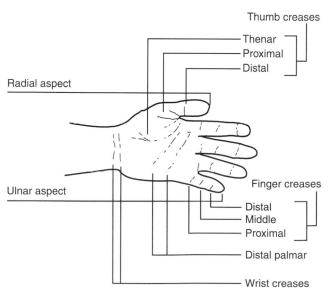

Fig. 19.2 Palmar creases of hand. (From Malick MH. *Manual on Static Hand Splinting: For Use by Physicians, Occupational Therapists and Physical Therapists.* Pittsburgh, PA: Harmarville Rehabilitation Center; 1972.)

Dorsal (back of the hand) orthoses should be constructed so that the orthosis extends to the midpoint of the next proximal joint. The **volar** (palm side) orthosis extends up to but does not include the next distal crease.

 CLINICAL PEARL

The orthosis pattern is drawn to the crease and then shortened approximately 1/8 inch (0.3 cm) to accommodate skin folds.

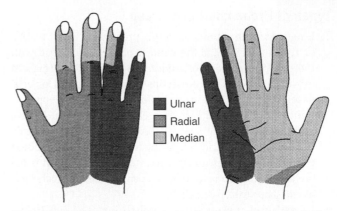

Ulnar
Radial
Median

Fig. 19.3 Sensory distribution in hand. Median nerve distribution includes most of the prehensile surface of the palm.

Skin

The dorsal skin of the hand on the extensor surface is fine, supple, and mobile to allow it to move freely during flexion and extension of the fingers. Scarring and edema limit hand function by hindering skin mobility. The palmar skin (on the flexor surface) by comparison is tough, thick, and inelastic. It protects and supports the underlying structures and prevents slippage between the skeleton and an object grasped (Tubiana, 1984). Multiple factors affect skin integrity, including medical and neurologic conditions, hydration, and job tasks.

Muscles

Movement of the hand and wrist involves 39 muscles: 20 extrinsic (outside the hand) muscles and 19 intrinsic (inside the hand) muscles (Tubiana, 1984). The 20 **extrinsic muscles** originate in the forearm and include the long flexors and extensors of the wrist and fingers, the pronators, and the supinator. The 19 **intrinsic muscles** include those of the **thenar** (thumb side) and **hypothenar** (little finger side) eminences, the lumbricals, and the interossei (Fess et al., 1981). An elaborate ligamentous system in the hand and wrist helps bony alignment by providing stability and mobility. A pulley system improves the mechanical advantage of the long finger muscles by keeping the tendons close to the bones as they glide.

Nerve Supply

Three peripheral nerves supply the hand: the radial, median, and ulnar nerves. In general, the radial nerve supplies the extensor/supinator muscle group and sensation to the dorsal surface of the radial side of the hand. The median nerve supplies the flexor/pronator muscles, the thenar group, and the first and second lumbricals. This nerve provides sensation to the radial side of the palm and thumb. The median nerve therefore is crucial in grasp, prehension, and tactile discrimination functions. The ulnar nerve innervates most of the intrinsic muscles and supplies sensory fibers to the ulnar side of the hand and digits. Fig. 19.3 shows the sensory distribution.

HAND FUNCTION

Understanding the normal functions of the hand is fundamental to designing and fabricating effective orthoses. The hand is the terminal point of the arm. Adequate range of motion (ROM) and sufficient muscle strength in the upper extremity is necessary for full use of the hand. Shoulder motions are critical for reaching and for hand-to-body activities, such as eating, performing personal hygiene, and grooming tasks. Elbow motion and supination/pronation of the forearm permit hand-to-face activities. The wrist, which is used chiefly to stabilize the hand during activity, contributes significantly to functional grip strength (see later section on tenodesis).

MP and interphalangeal (IP) joint flexion and stabilization are critical to grasp and prehension, and joint extension is necessary for release. The distal palmar arch formed by the metacarpals ensures the motion and opposition of the thumb and little finger, the ability to grasp round or large objects, convergence of the fingers during flexion, and the ability to press with the palm against resistance.

Opposition of the thumb is the basis of all prehension patterns. Thumb opposition at the carpometacarpal (CMC) joint is necessary to perform pad-to-pad prehension. Hand orthoses are typically fabricated to stabilize and position the thumb so that grasp and prehension can occur.

The normal hand is capable of mobility and stability at all joints. An orthosis can provide one or the other but rarely both (Coppard & Lohman, 2015; Kiel, 1983). An orthosis may aid in the recovery of dexterity, but hand function is hindered while it is worn due to decreased sensory input and limited mobility.

The normal hand can perform a variety of prehension and grasp patterns. Orthoses can assist these patterns when muscle function is impaired or deformity is present (Coppard & Lohman, 2015).

Prehension and Grasp Patterns

Hand movements are complex and occur in smooth sequence and combinations; however, they can be reduced to six basic patterns of prehension and grasp (Coppard & Lohman, 2015; Kiel, 1983; Malick, 1982). Orthoses can help facilitate prehension and grasp. For example, positioning the thumb in opposition to the index or middle finger can provide stability with pinching tasks in clients with arthritic joints or weak pinch strength.[2] This position is also utilized when possible after surgery to keep the thumb in a functional position.

Types of Prehension and Grasp

1. **Fingertip prehension:** Fingertip prehension (Fig. 19.4A), or tip-to-tip pinch, is the contact of the thumb pad with the pad of the index or middle finger. Fine, coordinated movement allows the fingertips to pick up small objects, fasten snaps and buttons, or hold a needle for sewing.
2. **Palmar prehension:** Palmar prehension (see Fig. 19.4B), also known as three jaw chuck, is contact of the thumb, middle, and index fingers. It is the most common prehension pattern and requires a high degree of coordination. It is the prehension pattern used to hold a pen, utensil, or small object of any shape (e.g., paper clip).
3. **Lateral prehension:** Lateral prehension (see Fig. 19.4C) is contact of the thumb pad with the lateral surface of the distal or middle **phalanx** of the index finger. The other digits may support the index finger, but the stability provided by the contraction of the first dorsal interosseus is essential. This pattern requires less coordination than the others but is stronger. Examples include turning a key or carrying a mug by its handle.

4. **Cylindrical grasp.** Cylindrical grasp (see Fig. 19.4D) occurs when an object is stabilized against the palm by finger flexion. Intrinsic and thenar muscles are essential to the power of this grasp. Examples include holding a drinking glass, hammer, or pot handle.
5. **Spherical grasp.** Spherical grasp (see Fig. 19.4E), or ball grasp, is used to hold round objects against an arched palm. Wrist stability and intrinsic and extrinsic hand muscle strength contribute to the ability to hold an apple, a ball, or a round doorknob.
6. **Hook grasp.** Hook grasp (see Fig. 19.4F) can be accomplished using the fingers only. It requires flexor strength and stability of the IP joints, MP joints, and neutral wrist positioning. Examples include carrying a briefcase or shopping bag or pulling open a drawer.

Tenodesis

In the normal hand when the wrist is flexed, the fingers are passively pulled into extension resulting in **tenodesis action** (Fig. 19.5). The tendons of finger extensors are too short to permit simultaneous flexion of all the joints that the finger extensors cross: wrist, MP, proximal IP, and distal IP. The opposite is also true. With wrist extension the fingers are slightly pulled into flexion (see Fig. 19.5A). This tenodesis action (wrist flexion with finger extension, wrist extension with finger flexion) is easily seen if you relax your fingers and move your wrist into flexion and extension rapidly. Tenodesis action results in a passive prehension pattern.

For a client with quadriparesis, a tenodesis orthosis may cause passive finger flexion through active wrist extension. Release is accomplished by relaxation of wrist extension. (See upcoming case study of Raul.) For a client with radial nerve palsy, a dynamic orthosis may take advantage of tenodesis to increase wrist extension passively during active finger flexion.

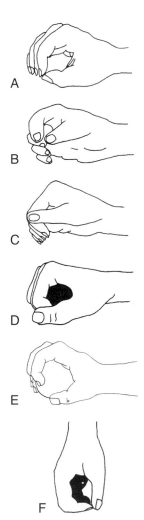

Fig. 19.4 Basic types of prehension and grasp. (A) Fingertip prehension. (B) Palmar prehension. (C) Lateral prehension. (D) Cylindric grasp. (E) Spherical grasp. (F) Hook grasp.

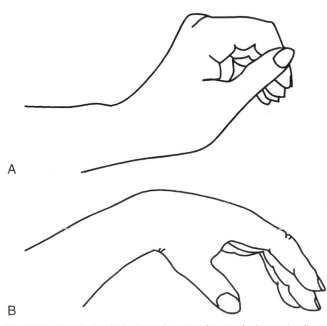

Fig. 19.5 Tenodesis. (A) Active wrist extension results in passive finger flexion. (B) Active wrist flexion results in passive finger extension.

Hand Positions

Functional. The functional position (Fig. 19.6) is the hand position most often used during activity. It is similar to holding a soda can or ball. The wrist is in 20 to 30 degrees of extension; the thumb is abducted and opposed to the pad of the middle finger; metacarpals are flexed to approximately 30 degrees; and IP joints are flexed to approximately 45 degrees. In this position, tension is equal in all muscles; the hand is in its mechanically most efficient posture.

Resting. The resting position (Fig. 19.7) is the position a normal hand assumes when resting passively. In this position the wrist is in 10 to 20 degrees of extension. All finger joints are slightly flexed, and the thumb is midway between opposition and abduction, with the thumb's pad facing the side of the index finger. The proximal, distal, and longitudinal arches are maintained in this position. Orthoses are often fabricated in this position to rest joints or to prevent deformity.

> ### CLINICAL PEARL
>
> When fabricating an orthosis for an older adult who has arthritic changes of the CMC joint the OT often uses the resting position to provide better comfort.

Safe Positioning. The safe position minimizes stress on metacarpal, phalangeal, and IP collateral ligaments, thereby

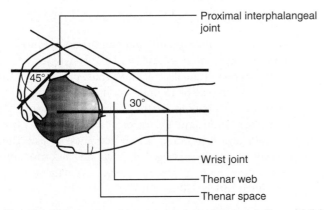

Fig. 19.6 Functional position, lateral view, right hand. (From Malick MH. *Manual on Static Hand Splinting: For Use by Physicians, Occupational Therapists and Physical Therapists.* Pittsburgh, PA: Harmarville Rehabilitation Center; 1972.)

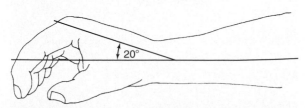

Fig. 19.7 Resting position. (From Malick MH. *Manual on Static Hand Splinting: For Use by Physicians, Occupational Therapists and Physical Therapists.* Pittsburgh, PA: Harmarville Rehabilitation Center; 1972.)

"saving" the hand for eventual motion (Fess et al., 1981). In this position the MP joints are flexed, IP joints are in full extension, and the wrist is in 10 to 30 degrees of extension. This position is common after thermal injuries (burns), trauma, and invasive surgery.

PRINCIPLES OF ORTHOTIC FABRICATION

Types of Orthoses

In the past, orthoses were often classified according to form rather than function. These classifications were called static, dynamic, and static progressive. The Splint (orthotic) Classification System (SCS), which was created by the American Society of Hand Therapists (ASHT) in 1992, "describes splints through a series of six predefined divisions that guide and progressively refine splints' technical names, working from broad concepts to individual splint specifications" (Fess et al., 2005). In 2004 Fess and colleagues further expanded and refined the SCS to create the Expanded Splint Classification System (ESCS) (Fess et al., 2005). Some settings, particularly chronic care and general physical disability settings, continue to use the older system of terms.

The four ESCS purpose classifications for orthoses are immobilization, mobilization, restriction, and torque transmission. The main objective of immobilization orthoses is to immobilize the primary joints in the orthosis; mobilization orthoses move the primary joints. Restriction orthoses restrict motion of the primary joints, whereas torque transmission orthoses (also referred to as exercise orthoses) transmit torque to place primary joint(s) on stretch (Coppard & Lohman, 2015).

> ### CASE STUDY
>
> **Raul**
>
> Raul, a 32-year-old male, has a history of substance abuse. After a night out, he awakes the next evening, unable to move his right wrist or hand, having slept with his head on his arm for nearly 24 hours. The next day, he goes to a medical clinic and is diagnosed with radial nerve palsy, confirmed by electromyography. He is unable to extend his wrist or fingers actively. He is immediately referred to occupational therapy. Over the months of his recovery, three orthoses will be fabricated for him to preserve the orthopedic integrity of his hand, as well as to improve his function.
>
> A safe position orthosis will be fabricated for Raul at his first appointment. The goal of using this orthosis is to preserve the structural integrity of his wrist and hand due to the unopposed active flexion of his wrist and fingers. The client will be instructed in ROM; however, his reliability about positioning and performing his home exercise program is questionable at this time. The client has agreed to wear the orthosis at night to prevent overstretching of his extensor muscles, which in the long term will limit his hand function on nerve recovery. The anatomy of the wrist and hand must be maintained during the many months it will take for nerve regeneration to achieve active ROM.

These ESCS classifications eliminate the ambiguity of the old system, in which the classifications referred to the structure of the orthosis components. Under the new ESCS, a single orthosis can have more than one purpose, thus allowing accurate and precise naming of orthoses according to the specific functions they perform. An example of an orthosis with a dual purpose is a flexion restriction orthosis, which can be used for trigger finger.

Indications for Use of Orthoses

The goal of all orthoses is to enable the client to perform daily life tasks as easily as possible. Static, dynamic, and static progressive orthoses may be used to achieve any combination of the following (Coppard & Lohman, 2015; Fess et al., 1981):

1. To protect, support, or immobilize joints to permit healing after inflammation or injury to the tendons, bones joint, soft tissue, or vascular/nerve supply. An arthritis resting mitt, which immobilizes the MP and wrist joints (of an inflamed arthritic hand), permits IP movement to allow for function (Fig. 19.9).

2. To position and maintain alignment to keep the integrity of the arches, ligamentous structures, and joint relationships. This goal can be accomplished with resting, functional, and safe positions. An adjustable outrigger on an orthosis ensures alignment of the MP joints after surgical replacement (Fig. 19.8).

3. To correct deformity or to prevent further deformity. An ulnar drift positioning orthosis is used to align the fingers of a client with rheumatoid arthritis in a neutral position. In the early stages of the disease the orthosis acts to prevent the rapid progression of the deformity. Later on, it positions the digits for more effective functional use.

4. To substitute for weak or absent muscle function caused by neuromuscular disease and spinal cord or peripheral nerve injury. A radial nerve orthosis (Fig. 19.10) amplifies the strength of the tenodesis action for the client who cannot actively extend the wrist or fingers. With active finger flexion the wrist is passively extended, thus functionally increasing prehensile strength.

5. To maximize ROM by preventing contractures caused by adhesion formation. A dorsal blocking orthosis assists flexion yet blocks extension to decrease stress and stretch on the surgical repair side while permitting tendon excursion.

6. To increase ADL independence by acting as a base for the attachment of devices or compensating for decreased hand function. It is easier for the client, for example, to have an orthosis attached to a razor to allow him or her to hold it or use a walker orthosis (Fig. 19.11) to compensate for weakness or sensory loss.

7. To exercise, which can be accomplished with mobilization or torque transmission orthoses that either assist or strengthen the client's own active motion, depending on the direction of pull of the orthosis.

8. To enhance positioning and functional performance in clients with abnormal tone (Fig. 19.12). This may serve two different purposes, generally not at the same time—either to prevent malalignment or to improve function through low load stress or positioning. There is significant controversy over the fabrication and use of orthoses for clients after stroke, with regard to timing and effectiveness of use. The supervising therapist is obliged to keep well informed on current intervention strategies before deciding on an orthotic intervention (Gillen, 2010).

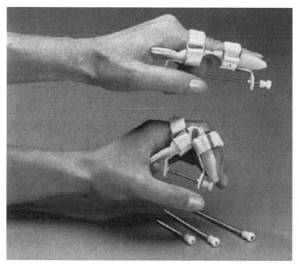

Fig. 19.8 Rolyan proximal interphalangeal joint extension splint for static progressive splinting. (Courtesy Smith and Nephew Rolyan.)

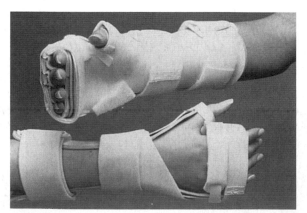

Fig. 19.9 Arthritis resting mitt splint. (Courtesy Smith and Nephew Rolyan.)

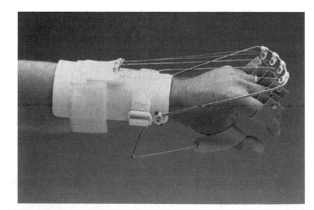

Fig. 19.10 Rolyan static radial nerve splint. (Courtesy Smith and Nephew Rolyan.)

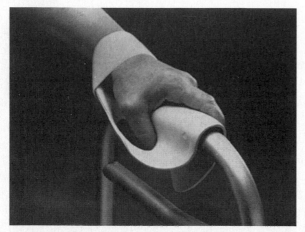

Fig. 19.11 Rolyan walker splint. (Courtesy Smith and Nephew Rolyan.)

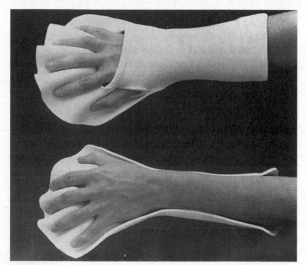

Fig. 19.12 Antispasticity ball splint-dorsal *(top)* and volar *(bottom)* versions. (Courtesy Smith and Nephew Rolyan.)

Biomechanical Considerations

The OT or OTA must bear in mind the following factors when constructing an orthosis.

Bony Prominences. Soft tissue is particularly thin over bony prominences such as the radial and ulnar styloids, the pisiform, the metacarpal heads, and the base of the thumb's metacarpal. Because of the lack of natural padding over these areas, significant potential for skin breakdown due to pressure exists (Malick, 1972). If possible, the practitioner should avoid orthotic contact with bony prominences by trimming and flaring the thermoplastic material.

> ### CLINICAL PEARL
>
> If the OTA chooses to pad an area, a self-stick circle of closed-cell padding is placed on the bone before molding the orthosis so that the OTA can either put the padding back onto the material, to ensure consistent pressure, or leave a "bubble" where the material will be flared out, to avoid the prominence. A circle of sticky-back foam may be used when padded consistent contact is indicated (Fig. 19.13).

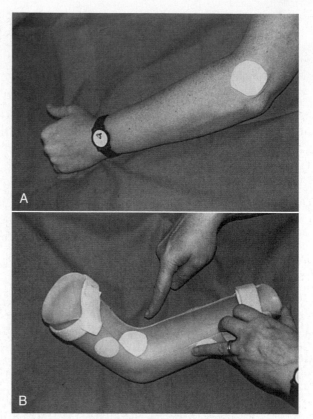

Fig. 19.13 Prepadding technique for bony prominence. (A) Circle of self-adhesive foam applied to client before application of thermoplastic. (B) Self-adhesive foam pad in splint ensures consistent pressure.

Alignment. The normal alignment of the digits should be maintained in the orthosis. The digits, when flexed, are parallel across the palm. At the wrist, 10 degrees of ulnar deviation is the normal resting posture.

Dual Obliquity. The radial side of the orthosis is longer and higher than the ulnar side to match the hand's anatomy (Fig. 19.14).

Joints. Exact positioning of the joints varies and depends on the client's diagnosis and the purpose for which the orthosis is fabricated. For example, the wrist is usually placed at -7 to 9 degrees of extension for carpal tunnel syndrome, at 30 degrees of extension for functional position, or at 20 degrees of extension for resting (Fess et al., 2005). For the client with increased flexor tone, wrist extension is sometimes compromised to permit adequate finger extension. The angle of the wrist also affects tone (Gillen et al., 2008). Diagnosis, common sense, and physician preference all enter into the decision. The OTA should consult the supervising OT to ensure that positioning is as desired.

Prefabricated and soft orthoses are commonly set at 30 degrees of wrist extension, making them an inappropriate choice for a client with carpal tunnel syndrome. You must modify these should a client purchase one or be provided one by his or her physician/insurance carrier.

Preventing the adverse effects of immobilization is extremely important. To a joint, motion is lotion. A static orthosis can

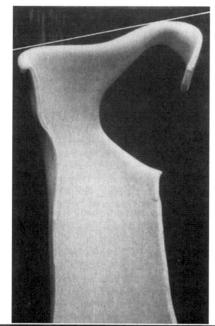

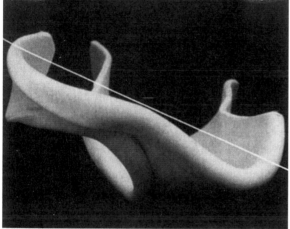

Fig. 19.14 Distal end of cock-up splint demonstrates dual obliquity.

cause joint stiffness, resulting in decreased ROM. Thus two important points are (1) static orthoses must be removed periodically for active or passive exercise unless contraindicated by surgery, infection, or trauma; and (2) unless absolutely unavoidable, joints that do not require immobilization should not be included in or restricted by the orthosis.

Creases. Orthotics should only block skin crease when necessary. Exceptions to this rule are (1) when including a joint because a muscle or tendon passes over it (e.g., immobilization of the wrist after flexor tendon repair in the digit), and (2) when the orthosis physically needs to be made longer to counterbalance the distal force.

In a healthy, nonrestricted hand, joints have an amazing capacity for stability or mobility. An orthosis cannot provide both; therefore the supervising OT must choose between stability and mobility based on the client's dysfunction, purpose of the orthosis, potential deformity, and functional use of the hand. The client may be given both dynamic and static orthoses for the same diagnosis.

Collateral Ligaments. Maintaining the maximal length of finger collateral ligaments whenever possible is important. Proximal interphalangeal (PIP) extension and MP flexion preserve this length (referred to as the intrinsic plus position). If the ligaments are allowed to shorten, restrictions in ROM may occur.

Skin. The volar surface of the hand and forearm has more mass; therefore it is the preferred surface for orthotic fabrication if skin conditions and functional needs can be met. The sensory input received through cutaneous receptors is the key to functional use of the hand. A secretary might prefer a dorsal wrist immobilization orthosis for carpal tunnel syndrome, so that writing is not inhibited by decreased sensory input from the wrist and the ulnar border of the hand.

Open wounds and incision sites should be avoided whenever possible. Pressure or friction results in microtrauma to underlying structures. This trauma increases circulation to the area, and a red spot is seen after the client has worn the orthosis for approximately 20 minutes. All orthoses should be checked for fit after 20 minutes of wear in the clinic to assess potential pressure areas.

It is normal for the client's arm to feel warm or look pink after wearing the orthosis. The OTA or OT can provide stockinette to wear under the orthosis to absorb perspiration. Thermoplastic materials have limited ventilation. Perforated material may improve air exchange. Antimicrobial-coated materials may also be useful for some clients. Pressure is the greatest problem to keep in mind when fabricating an orthosis. In addition to potential spots over bony prominences, pressure may also be caused by poor fit and design. Wider, longer orthoses fit better than short, narrow ones. These steps can lead to less pressure on the skin by an orthosis:

1. Fabricate it to two thirds the length of the forearm.
2. Cover approximately half the circumference of the extremity (midbone trim marks work well) with the orthosis.
3. Fabricate the orthosis proximal to the next skin crease in the wrist/hand area, to leave room for skin folds during ROM.
4. Fold or flare proximal and distal edges so they are rounded.
5. Round all internal and external corners. Sharp corners wear poorly and will dig into the client's skin.
6. Reduce unequal pressure by means of a more conforming fit. The more conforming the orthosis, the better the pressure is distributed.

CLINICAL PEARL

To check for hot spots on clients with dark skin pigmentation, the OTA can run a finger over the bony prominences and then make modifications as needed. Should a pressure spot be evident, place a dab of dark lipstick on the area and reapply the orthosis. This will mark the spot for adjustment (flaring).

Sensorimotor Function. Sensory information and feedback are essential components of normal movement. Orthoses reduce sensory input from the area covered with material and therefore may contribute to the client's discomfort. Many clients requiring an orthosis have decreased sensation because of central or peripheral nerve deficits, and their risk of developing pressure areas with resulting skin breakdown is greater. Because their sensation is diminished, they may not complain that the orthosis is uncomfortable. These clients must be taught to compensate visually and to frequently check for areas of irritation or skin breakdown. Not uncommonly, a caregiver must be instructed to assess ongoing fit if the client is unable to do so.

Precautions

Skin integrity can be compromised by poorly fitting orthoses. It is also influenced by systemic medical conditions such as diabetes (sensory loss and atrophy), dehydration, and congestive heart failure (vascular compromise and edema). Edema increases with immobilization because the orthosis prohibits active motion. During active motion muscles provide the pump that keeps fluids moving. However, immobilization of an edematous extremity is often necessary. Significant edema can occur after trauma and in clients with compromised cardiac status. The orthosis must be large enough to accommodate the edema. The client is instructed to keep the arm elevated whenever possible by placing it up on a pillow when resting or by using a sling when standing for extended periods. As edema in the upper extremity changes, the fit of the orthosis will change. Clients should follow up with the OT or OTA to have their orthosis adjusted or remolded as necessary.

Client compliance is essential, but many reasons for noncompliance exist. The OTA should address these from the start. First, the orthosis must fit well; no one wants to wear something that is uncomfortable. Second, it must be cosmetically acceptable. Orthoses should be clean and neat, not marred by ragged edges and fingerprints. Many clients pay a significant amount of money for the orthosis, and the orthosis is a reflection of the practitioner and the clinic. Third, orthoses are generally an inconvenience to the client. They limit motion and sensation, are warm, and often seem "in the way." The OTA must explain that the temporary inconvenience is necessary for long-term gain in function. A carpal tunnel splint that sits atop a computer does no one any good.

CLINICAL PEARL

If the client has increased edema during the course of the day, the OT or OTA should fabricate the orthosis later in the day. If this is not possible, the practitioner can allow for the anticipated swelling by using multiple layers of stockinette on the arm during fabrication.

Material Selection

A tremendous variety of material is available in the market today for orthotic fabrication. **Low-temperature thermoplastics** are generally used for rigid orthoses. Flexible materials such as heavy fabric, neoprene, knitted elastics, and foam laminates may be used alone or in combination with rigid metal or thermoplastic stays. A quick overview of these soft orthoses follows later in this chapter.

Low-temperature thermoplastics are generally heated in a water bath (splint pan, hydrocollator, electric fry pan). Their molding temperature is 160°F (71.1°C). The heated thermoplastic is applied to the client dry (by blotting the material prior to applying to the client). Low-temperature thermoplastic selection is based on two primary criteria: (1) how it handles during the forming (fabrication) process, and (2) how it performs as a finished product.

Handling characteristics when the material has been heated to the recommended molding temperature include the following:

1. Moldability refers to how the material shapes around contours, or how easy it is to form. Moldability allows the OT or OTA to have the material take a specific shape.
2. Drapability refers to how easily the warm material forms to the client with only gravity to mold it down. The more drapability the material has, the gentler the clinician's touch must be. These materials must be stroked—not poked or pushed—into place. The clinician will not leave fingerprint marks behind if handling the material gently. Material with a great deal of drapability should not be used for larger orthoses. Practitioners with less experience fabricating orthotics generally prefer a low to moderate drape material. *Rebound* is the term used for a material that does not drape but springs back slightly during molding.
3. Elasticity refers to how much the material resists stretch. The clinician should note whether the material resists pulling or tugging.
4. Material with memory returns to its original size and shape when reheated. It is more elastic than nonmemory materials. This material works well for serial orthoses. Serial orthoses are those that are remolded as the client progresses, such as one to increase wrist or digit extension.
5. The time required in the water bath for the material to reach molding temperature is dependant on the type of material and its thickness. One to 3 minutes will usually be sufficient to heat material ⅛ inch (0.3 cm) thick.
6. Edge finishing is the ease with which smooth edges can be formed on materials. Synthetic (all-plastic) materials edge more easily than rubber-based thermoplastics.
7. Self-bonding materials bond to each other when they are warm and dry. Coated materials tack together at the edges, but once the material hardens, they can be popped apart. For a more permanent bond, the coating must be scraped off or removed with a solvent before bonding. A coated material, once stretched, is tackier and more likely to self-bond.
8. Shrinkage may occur in some materials during the cooling process. The final adjustments must compensate for shrinkage.

9. Working time, or the time allowed for molding before the material cools, averages 3 to 5 minutes for solid ⅛-inch thick material. Thinner or perforated material cools faster than thicker, nonperforated material does. Some materials slowly lose conformability during cooling, others lose it quickly. The temperature of the room influences cooling rates and conformability.

> ### 🔶 CLINICAL PEARL
>
> Materials with a lot of drapability should only be used on clients who can hold their extremity in the appropriate position so that gravity can assist the practitioner during forming.

Performance characteristics relate to the end results or how the orthotic works once it has hardened. Performance characteristics include the following:

1. Conformability is how intimately the orthosis fits into contoured areas. Material with a great deal of drapability is prone to be imprinted with the client's fingerprints and hand creases. Orthosis with a lot of conformability is usually more comfortable and less likely to migrate during use.
2. Rigidity is the strength of the orthosis. A rigid orthosis will not bend under stress (from the client's weight, muscle tone, or strength). Rigidity of the orthosis can be improved with a greater number of arches and contours built in. Rigidity and drape are not the same. If formed properly, a material with a lot of drapability may produce a very rigid end product.
3. Flexibility refers to the amount of repeated stress an orthosis can take. It is important in a circumferential (going around the arm) design that needs to be pulled open for donning and doffing. Flexibility is important for a thumb spica orthosis (see Fig. 19.31 later in the chapter).
4. Durability refers to how long an orthosis will last. Natural rubber-based materials are less durable than all-plastic materials because they are more likely to become brittle with age. Low-temperature thermoplastic orthoses are most often used for a temporary condition.
5. Finish on the material may be smooth or slightly textured. Coated materials are slightly easier to keep clean.
6. Moisture permeability (air exchange) is affected solely by the amount of perforation (if any). Memory materials are available in superperforated versions for maximum air exchange.
7. The color of the orthosis affects client compliance. Darker thermoplastic colors show less dirt, and patterned materials are less likely to become lost in institutional bed sheets. Therefore they may be preferred by clients.
8. Thickness is usually measured in inches (e.g., 1/16 inch thick). Thicker materials are usually stronger than thinner ones. Thin material is more responsive to being handled during the forming process and is lighter. Ultrathin materials are not recommended for novice orthotic fabricators. Material 1/8 inch thick is generally used for most orthoses.

Manufacturers' catalogs assist the clinician in selecting appropriate materials for specific orthosis types and for the fabricator's level of skill. Materials change, new ones appear, former ones are retired, features change, and a clinician must keep up to date. The practitioner should mold a sample of material before using it to fabricate an orthosis so that he or she can acquire some experience with its handling characteristics.

Soft-Support Orthoses. Soft-support orthoses are fabricated from more flexible materials and permit partial motion at a joint. These semiflexible orthoses are used to limit motion, protect an area, or ease chronic pain. They may be used for clients who cannot tolerate a rigid immobilization orthosis. Soft-support orthoses can be beneficial for older adult clients whose fragile skin may be more susceptible to breakdown (Fig. 19.15).

Strapping and Padding Principles

Straps hold the orthosis in place and are fastened with hook and loop material, adhesive, or rivets. Most orthoses are

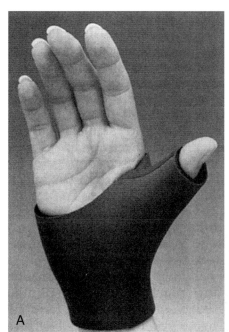
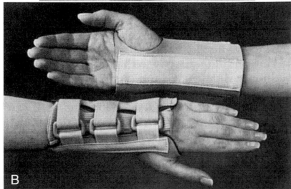

Fig. 19.15 (A) Rolyan neoprene pull-on-thumb support. Warmth and compression of neoprene help reduce pain due to overuse of thumb and wrist. (B) Rolyan D-ring wrist brace with metal support bar in a sleeve on flexor surface. (Courtesy Smith and Nephew Rolyan.)

fastened with a hook and loop at three points to ensure that they do not migrate or rotate on the extremity. Hook fasteners and loop strapping (Velcro) are available with and without self-adhesive backing. The loop strapping is always applied facing the skin to prevent abrasion. Soft straps with foam laminate are used when increased softness is necessary and are compatible with hook fasteners. They can collapse somewhat to accommodate edema. Stretchy strapping may be used to reduce constriction.

D-ring straps may be used for a more secure fit or for a client with decreased coordination. A variety of colors and widths of strapping materials is available. Wider straps may help distribute pressure more evenly. When acute edema is present, an orthosis may be bandaged on, to ensure even pressure distribution.

> **CLINICAL PEARL**
>
> Straps in which a self-adhesive hook is sewn onto the loop strap decrease the risk of losing the strap, which is beneficial in institutional settings.

Padding is available in two basic types: closed cell or open cell. Closed-cell padding does not absorb moisture or bacteria, can be wiped clean, and can be dried. It may be applied directly to the thermoplastic before heating (the material floats in the heat pan, foam side up). This technique is desirable for clients who need insulation from heat, such as burn clients or babies. Polycushion padding is soft, stretchable, and easily molded around contours. Self-adhesive padding (Plastazote) is less stretchable. The clinician should use padding that resists bottoming out (completely compressing) under pressure.

Open-cell cushioning absorbs moisture like a sponge. It is susceptible to bacterial growth and needs to be changed regularly to ensure adequate hygiene. Slow-recovery foams that "mold" to the extremity are often used to compensate for lack of orthotic contour. Moleskin and molestick are thin paddings used to reduce the risk of migration when a noncontouring thermoplastic is used. PPT foam padding is a durable, shock-absorbing padding. Although it is open cell, it has a nylon top skin that allows for easy washing (Performance Health).

Most padding materials are available in thickness of 1/16, 1/8, 1/4, and 1/2 inch (0.15–1.25 cm), with or without self-adhesive backing. The 1/16-inch and 1/8-inch sticky-back paddings are the most commonly used. To ensure a secure adherence on the material around the edges of the padding (and self-adhesive Velcro), the glue surface is heated with a heat gun before applying to the orthosis. Before applying padding directly to the client's skin, the OT or OTA should stick and unstick the glued side on a towel to decrease its adhesive power; thus it will not stick too firmly to the client's skin and can be removed easily.

> **CLINICAL PEARL**
>
> When applying sticky-back foam directly to a bony prominence, one should use a circular shape; it is easier to replace the foam in the indentation left in the thermoplastic.

Client Education on Orthotic Care and Use

Instruction handouts given to clients should include wearing schedules, care instructions, and a precaution statement. When possible, wearing time should be increased over a period of a few days so that the client can become accustomed to it. The clinician must perform frequent skin checks and ensure that the client knows how to clean the orthosis with mild soap and warm—not hot—water and knows to dry it thoroughly before reapplying. The client should be cautioned not to put orthoses in the washing machine or dishwasher or leave them in a hot car in the summer or on a radiator. The orthosis will begin to melt at 135°F (57.2°C) (Jacobs et al., 2003; Jacobs & Austin, 2013). Correct positioning is crucial and should be reviewed with the client. Straps should be snug, not tight. The client should be able to insert a finger under the strap once it is fastened.

After instruction, the client (or caregiver) should be able to do the following: (1) Tell the clinician the purpose of the orthosis and when it should be worn, (2) demonstrate the home exercise program (see Chapter 30), (3) don and doff the orthosis independently, (4) perform skin checks, and (5) explain how to care for the orthosis (Jacobs et al., 2003; Jacobs & Austin, 2013).

> **CLINICAL PEARL**
>
> Instruct the client to secure the strap "watchband tight."

Other Considerations

OTs and OTAs use clinical reasoning to ensure that each client's individual needs are met. Treatment goals and lifestyle considerations (age, dominance, medical/social history, home and work environments) help the clinician determine the best orthotic option. Some examples of this reasoning include using black material for a construction worker or perforated material for someone in a warm climate. Ease of donning and doffing and caregiver instructions are essential for those who rely on others for their care. Weakness, diminished dexterity, and visual acuity issues in the geriatric client will influence the weight of material selected, as well as the type of strapping and closures. Vitality of the skin must also be considered (Amini, 2004).

ORTHOTIC FABRICATION

Specific patternmaking techniques, material suggestions, fabrication instructions, and strapping patterns are provided for each of the three orthoses discussed in this chapter. To start, the following supplies are necessary: (1) heat pan, (2) plastic spatula, (3) towel, (4) sharp, clean scissors, (5) paper towels, (6) grease pen or awl, and (7) heat gun. The heat pan needs a minimum of 2 to 3 inches of water heated to 160°F (71.1°C) (just beyond the simmer setting). It should have an unscratched, nonstick coating.

The following general technical tips will aid the reader in cutting, molding, and finishing various types of orthoses.

Patternmaking

Patterns are usually made on a paper towel. The OTA or OT cuts out and checks the fit on the client, then traces the pattern onto the thermoplastic. Precut orthosis blanks are popular because they significantly decrease fabrication time and cost.

Cutting

Place the pattern on the thermoplastic. Trace it with an awl or marker slightly wider than the pattern itself. You want to be able to cut inside your pattern lines so that the markings are not on the actual orthosis.

1. Using a utility knife, score a rectangular shape around the pattern and snap off the piece.
2. Heat the thermoplastic to the correct temperature by leaving it in the heat pan until it is uniformly flexible.
3. Remove the thermoplastic from the heat pan using the spatula. A plastic spatula will help prevent marring the nonstick coating of the pan.
4. Place the material promptly on the towel and gently swipe it dry. Repeatedly flip the stickier materials over during drying so that they do not adhere to the towel.
5. Support the excess material with one hand and the working surface to prevent stretching. Cut out the marked orthosis. Use the scissors as if you were cutting paper, leaving the blades slightly open between cuts and perpendicular to the material. Round all the corners (Fig. 19.16).

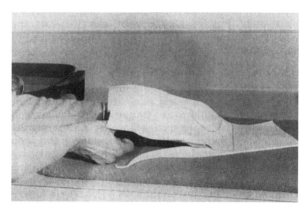
Fig. 19.16 Cutting splint out of heated thermoplastic.

Molding

1. Heat a thermoplastic precut orthosis blank (or reheat the custom-cut orthosis) to the appropriate temperature. Remove the material from the heat pan, dry it, and let it cool for several seconds until it is comfortable to touch.
2. Position the client, preferably so that gravity will assist the thermoplastic draping.
3. Place the thermoplastic material on the arm/hand. Be sure to align the pattern properly. Stroke it into place. Use firm yet gentle strokes with the pads of the fingers or the side of the hand to mold the plastic. Do not poke at the material or grasp it because this may leave behind fingerprints and affect the contour of the orthosis as well. Keep your hands moving when they are on the thermoplastic to prevent imprinting. Make sure to acknowledge the arches and to contour them into the orthosis carefully.
4. Flare the proximal edges of the orthosis and any other edges where pressure might occur. Flared or folded edges are more comfortable and increase the strength of the orthosis.
5. Allow the orthosis to set until it is rigid. Total working time is usually 3 to 5 minutes. Make sure to maintain the client's position while the material sets.
6. If the orthosis was molded in supination, pronate the client's forearm and check the fit.
7. Mark any trim lines that are indicated (e.g., midbone on the forearm, crease clearance, two thirds of the length of the forearm).
8. Thermoplastics with memory need to be consistently molded until the material is firm because of their tendency to return to their original flat shape.

CLINICAL PEARL

If the forearm trough is not centered, grasp the dorsal end and twist it to center the trough. (Off-centering occurs because the contour of the forearm changes as gravity pulls on the flexor muscles.)

 CLINICAL PEARL

Make your pattern marks slightly wide and cut them off when trimming so that no ink stains remain on the orthosis.

Finishing

1. Hold the orthosis up vertically and dip the area to be trimmed repeatedly in and out of the heat pan. When slightly softened, trim to the marked length and gently flare the proximal end toward the outside of the orthosis with a sweeping stroke using the palm of the hand. This flare prevents the proximal end from digging into the forearm musculature.
2. To trim the sides or top, heat the side or top edge either by dipping the material in and out of the heat pan, pouring warm water over the spot to be trimmed, or using a heat gun. Once the material is slightly warm, cut along the trim lines. Do not heat the material to full molding temperature to do this step because it may disfigure the edge.
3. If necessary, smooth rough or jagged edges, again by dipping in and out of the water to slightly heat the material. Polish carefully with the fingertip or palm while the material is still wet.
4. If major fit changes are required, reheat the entire orthosis and remold it. Do not attempt to spot-heat large areas such as the wrist or thumb.

 CLINICAL PEARL

Consider placing moleskin over difficult edges if the client has sensitive skin or had difficulty tolerating orthoses.

Beware of the heat gun. It is difficult to control the flow of hot air with a heat gun, and it is easy to accidentally heat a portion of the orthosis that does not need adjustment.

Strapping

Straps are applied last. Refer to strapping methods and technical information discussed earlier in this chapter. Remember that three points of control are usually necessary to hold an orthosis in place, so at least three straps are customarily used on a forearm-based orthosis (see Fig. 19.26 later in the chapter).

Evaluation

When complete, the orthosis must be analyzed for function, fit, and appearance.

Function

1. Are the arches of the hand maintained? Looking at the orthosis directly on, is the metacarpal area properly arched? Is the radial side of the palm higher than the ulnar side? Looking at the orthosis from the side, is the longitudinal arch obvious?
2. Is the hand positioned properly in the orthosis? Use a goniometer to check joint angles.

Fit

1. Are the straps correctly placed to promote stability and to avoid pressure points?
2. Do the sides of the orthosis extend at least to the midpoint of the bone?
3. Is the orthosis long enough to effectively support the body parts involved? Are the appropriate joint creases visible to permit full joint ROM?
4. Could any edges or corners press into the client's skin? Do any potential pressure sites over bony prominences, such as the ulnar styloid, exist? Check for reddened or warmer areas on the skin after 20 minutes of wearing time.

Appearance

1. Is the surface of the orthosis smooth and free of marks, dents, and rough edges?
2. Are all the corners rounded, edges smooth, and proximal and distal ends flared where appropriate?
3. Are the straps neat and aligned correctly? Is the self-adhesive hook fully covered by the strap?
4. Is it cosmetically acceptable to the clinician and the client?

Directions

Radial Bar Wrist Immobilization Orthosis. A wrist immobilization orthosis is used to support and/or position the wrist. For functional positioning the wrist is aligned at 20 to 30 degrees of extension. In clients with carpal tunnel syndrome the wrist is positioned at −7 to 9 degrees. Use a material with a good deal of drapability and a moderate resistance to stretch.

Pattern.
1. Mark the following landmarks: the MP heads on the radial and ulnar sides of the hand, the base of the web space, the wrist joint on the radial side, and two thirds of the length of the forearm.
2. Draw the pattern as shown in Fig. 19.18, allowing sufficient material so the width of the orthosis can wrap halfway around the forearm.
3. Remove the client's arm and connect, with a circular arc, the web space and wrist markings as seen in Fig. 19.17.
4. Cut out the pattern and check the fit on the client. Adjust as needed.

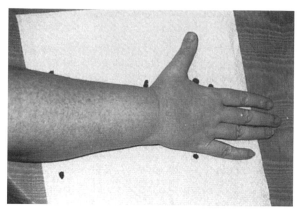

Fig. 19.17 Marking bony landmarks for radial bar cock-up splint on paper towel.

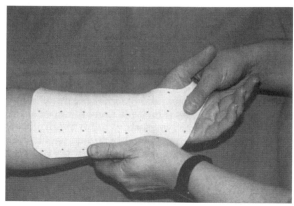

Fig. 19.19 Align splint with palmar arch and begin to mold in contours.

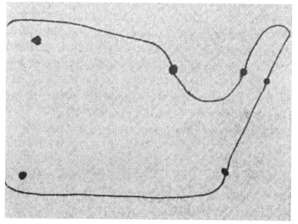

Fig. 19.18 Radial bar cock-up splint pattern.

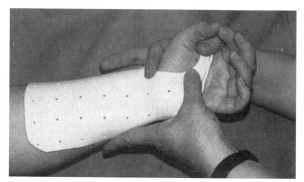

Fig. 19.20 With client in opposition, fold splint at palmar and thenar creases.

Fabrication.

1. Trace the pattern onto the thermoplastic material and heat it. Cut out the orthosis blank and reheat to molding temperature if necessary.
2. With the client's forearm supinated, position the wrist at the appropriate angle of extension and ulnar deviation. Drape the material over the hand/forearm, taking care to line up the distal end with the palmar crease. Wrap the radial bar through the web space around to the dorsum of the hand.
3. Smooth the wrist area of the material by stroking it into place laterally and continue proximally up the forearm, taking care not to twist the trough to either side (Fig. 19.19).
4. Place the thumb gently in the palmar arch area to ensure contour and stroke into place. Flare or fold the distal edge so that the palmar crease (proximal crease at the second MP, distal crease for third to fifth MP) is visible and continues through the web space. Have the client oppose the thumb to the tip of the index or middle finger. This position will cause a fold at the thenar eminence. Flatten this fold down and continue along the radial bar into the web space area as seen in Fig. 19.20.

5. Allow the orthosis to set.
6. Apply straps (Fig. 19.21) to the orthosis proximally, across the wrist and across the dorsum of the hand to the radial bar tab.

CASE STUDY

Raul, Part 2

A radial bar wrist cock-up orthosis will be fabricated for Raul early in his treatment. It will support his wrist, and it is easier to wear "all day," as when putting your hand in a shirt or coat sleeve. It is both cosmetically and socially more acceptable to Raul as he goes through his day. At work he is also using a dynamic outrigger that has been fabricated on a similar base orthosis. The dynamic portion of the orthosis is used for finger extension, so he is better able to use his keyboard at work. The client has stated that he "would not be soon wearing this thing in public." Nonetheless, he is willing to use it for keyboarding so that he can function better at work. He is managing his other ADL using his nondominant hand. As the nerve regenerates over several months, he will no longer need the dynamic orthosis but will continue to use the radial bar cock-up as he waits for his wrist extensor muscles to regain innervation and strength enough to support the weight of his hand.

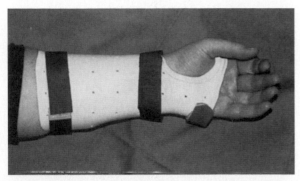

Fig. 19.21 Completed radial bar cock-up splint.

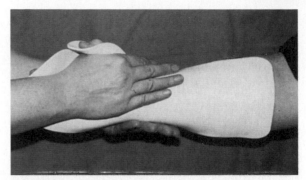

Fig. 19.23 Place warm thermoplastic on client, ensuring that thumb/web space area is properly seated and trough is aligned with forearm.

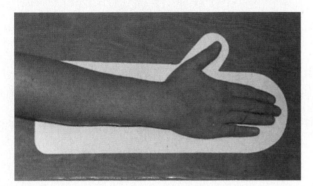

Fig. 19.22 Resting mitt splint with precut splint blank/pattern.

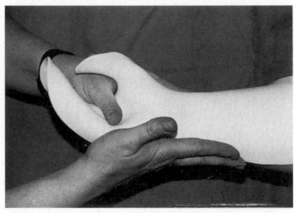

Fig. 19.24 Stroke material into place. Create flanges in hand/thumb/wrist areas. Practitioner's thumb is used to help form palmar arch.

Forearm-Based Hand Immobilization Orthosis (Resting Hand Splint). This splint provides support and positioning for the wrist and fingers. Common goals for using resting orthoses are to decrease joint inflammation and to prevent joint contractures. Use a material with moderate drape and rigid performance.

Pattern.
1. Trace the hand, leaving approximately ½-inch excess width around the hand area and 1½ inches in the forearm area. Mark two thirds of the length of the forearm. Your pattern should resemble a mitten (Fig. 19.22).
2. Cut it out of the paper towel and check the fit on the client before transferring the pattern to the thermoplastic. Once the orthosis blank is cut out of the thermoplastic, reheat to molding temperature if necessary.

Fabrication.
1. Place the warmed material on the client (Fig. 19.23), preferably with the client's forearm in a supinated position so that gravity assists in holding the material in place. Make sure the thumb/web space area is seated properly and flare the thermoplastic to create the flange on the orthosis in the thumb/web area.
2. Stroke the material into position at the wrist. This technique creates a waist in the material and helps keep it from sliding. Continue molding up the forearm.
3. Using two hands, one to ensure correct anatomic position of the wrist/hand and the other to mold, gently form the

material. Create a flange along the sides of the fingers to increase material strength in the hand area (Fig. 19.24). Use alternate hands: one to position, the other to mold. Use your thumb to ensure proper forming in the palmar arch area.
4. Once the material is semirigid, pronate the forearm (Fig. 19.25) and proceed as previously described to trim and finish.
5. Apply straps proximally, at the wrist, across the dorsum of the hand or proximal phalanges, and at the thumb (Fig. 19.26).

Short Opponens Immobilization Orthosis. A short opponens orthosis supports the CMC joint of the thumb when it is inflamed from overuse or arthritic changes. A forearm-based version of this orthosis is used for de Quervain syndrome, a commonly seen tendonitis of the long extensor and abductor tendons of the thumb, which cross the wrist (Fig. 19.32). Use a material with moderate drape and a high degree of contour. In some cases, because of an enlarged IP joint or a bulbous distal phalanx, opening the thumb spica area may be necessary to allow donning and doffing of the orthosis. For such clients, a resilient memory material would be a good choice. Such materials are slightly flexible and hold up well under the repeated stress of being pulled open.

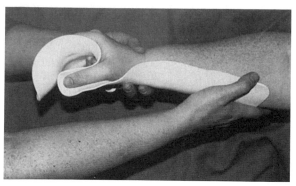

Fig. 19.25 With forearm in pronation, grasp proximal end of splint and twist it to center the trough.

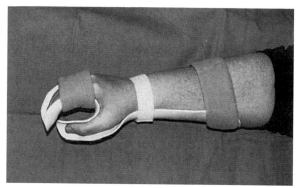

Fig. 19.26 Completed resting splint.

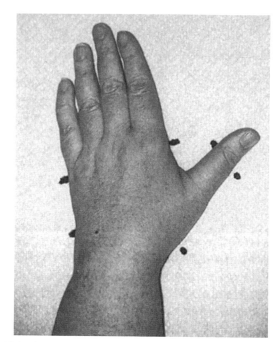

Fig. 19.27 Mark bony landmarks for short opponens splint on paper towel.

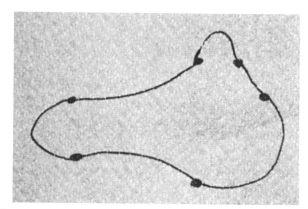

Fig. 19.28 Draw pattern for short opponens splint.

Pattern.
1. Mark the following landmarks on the paper towel: the MP heads on the radial and ulnar sides of the hand, the radial and ulnar sides of the wrist, and the IP crease of the thumb (Fig. 19.27).
2. Draw and cut out the pattern (Fig. 19.28). Check the fit on the client. The bulbous end of the pattern wraps circumferentially around the thumb. Trace the pattern onto the material and proceed as described earlier.

Fabrication.
1. Reheat the material to molding temperature. Position the client's elbow on the table with the forearm straight up. Align the edge of the material with the IP crease and wrap the material snugly around the thumb (Fig. 19.29).
2. Wrap the narrow end of the material around the ulnar border of the hand (Fig. 19.30). Keep this part centered. Ask the client to oppose the thumb to the second digit while you smooth the material into place. Make sure the orthosis contours well into the web space.
3. Have the client flex and extend the wrist as the fit is checked. Wrist motion should not be restricted. If necessary, trim to allow full ROM.
4. Once the orthosis is set, trim if it restricts movement around the thenar crease.
5. Apply a strap to secure the ulnar border to the thenar area (Fig. 19.31).

> **CLINICAL PEARL**
>
> To ensure that the material contours well into the web space, give the client a quarter to pinch. This technique prevents the thumb from moving out of alignment while the material hardens.

> **CLINICAL PEARL**
>
> If the client has difficulty inserting and removing the thumb through the orthosis, pop the overlapped area open by twisting it once the material is completely cool. Secure with hook-and-loop strapping material to allow for an adjustable thumb hole.

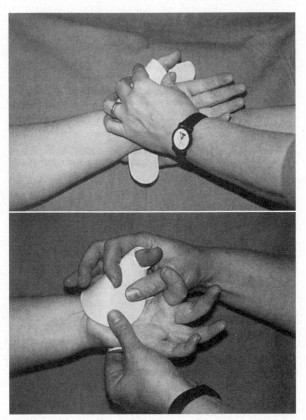

Fig. 19.29 Align edge of splint with interphalangeal crease and wrap snugly around thumb.

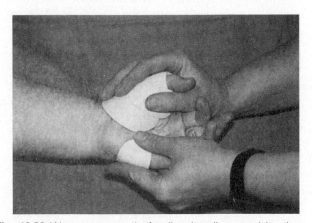

Fig. 19.30 Wrap narrow end of splint dorsally around hand, over ulnar border.

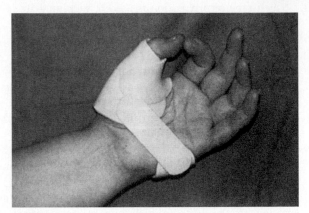

Fig. 19.31 Completed short opponens splint.

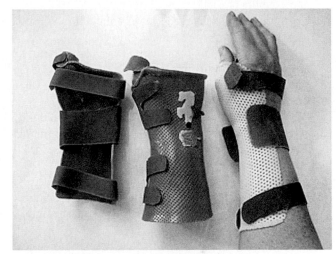

Fig. 19.32 The author's cache of long opponens splints.

SUMMARY

The goal of orthotic fabrication is to preserve or enhance the use of the hand. The construction of every orthosis must respect the hand's natural arches, contours, and mechanics.

The OTA who has achieved service competency may independently construct resting and other static orthoses. Effective orthotic construction requires an understanding of the performance and handling characteristics of the materials, an awareness of precautions, and expertise in patternmaking and use of

materials. The actual physical skill of fabricating orthoses is acquired with patience and practice.

When possible, the orthosis should be designed to best ensure the client's maximal participation in his or her purposeful activities and occupations. The clinician should address any functional issues that wearing the orthosis will create. The orthosis affects the appearance of the hand and should be as neat and attractive as possible.

It is often difficult for clients with repetitive stress injuries to be restricted in the use of their hands by an orthosis. This temporary inconvenience can lead to healing and long-term gain. The outcomes achieved by clients support the use of them as effective tools in occupational therapy practice when used appropriately.

REVIEW QUESTIONS

1. What is the role of the OTA in orthotic fabrication?
2. List five functions of the normal hand.
3. Describe the relationship of shoulder, elbow, and wrist function to hand use.

4. Which type of prehension is used to pick up a straight pin?

5. Which type of prehension is used to turn a key in a lock?

6. Which type of grasp is used to hold a soda can?

7. What happens to the hand if the metacarpal transverse arch is flattened?

8. In which position are the muscles of the hand at the best mechanical advantage to function efficiently?

9. Describe and demonstrate the dual obliquity of the hand. Why is it an important consideration in hand orthotic fabrication?

10. Name the three nerves that supply sensation and motion to the hand. Which one is most critical to tactile discriminative function?

11. Name the three major classifications of orthoses. Give one example of each.

12. How are the adverse effects of immobilization best prevented?

13. What is the optimal position when fabricating an orthosis for wrist for function?

14. What is the optimal position for the orthosis when treating the wrist for carpal tunnel syndrome?

15. What effect does wrist flexion have on hand function?

16. Why is it important to fabricate an orthosis with the MP joints in flexion if these joints are to be immobilized?

17. State six purposes of orthotics.

18. List and discuss three limitations of orthoses.

19. What are the two main characteristics that influence selection of thermoplastic material? Give several examples of each.

20. List six general guidelines for achieving optimal fit and function of the orthosis.

REFERENCES

Amini, D. (2004). Splinting the geriatric hand. *OT Pract, 9*(3), CEU Article.

Coppard, B. M., & Lohman, H. (2015). *Introduction to orthotics: A clinical reasoning and problem-solving approach* (4th ed.). St. Louis, MO: Elsevier Health Sciences.

Fess, E. E., Gettle, K., & Strictland, J. (Eds.), (1981). *Hand splinting: Principles and methods*. St. Louis, MO: Mosby.

Fess, E. E., Gettle, K. S., Philips, C. A., & Janson, J. R. (Eds.), (2005). *Hand and upper extremity splinting: Principles & methods* (3rd ed.). St. Louis, MO: Mosby.

Gillen, G. (2010). *Stroke rehabilitation, a function-based approach* (3rd ed.). St. Louis, MO: Elsevier Health Sciences.

Gillen, G., Goldberg, R., Muller, S., & Straus, J. (2008). The effect of wrist position on upper extremity function while wearing a wrist immobilizing splint. *JPO, 20*(1), 19–23. https://doi.org/10.1097/jpo.0b013e31815f013f.

Jacobs, M. A., & Austin, N. M. (2013). *Orthotic intervention for the hand and upper extremity: Splinting principles and process*. Philadelphia, PA: Lippincott Williams & Wilkins.

Jacobs, M., & Austin, N. (2003). *Splinting the hand and upper extremity: Principles and process*. Philadelphia, PA: Lippincott Williams & Wilkins.

Kiel, J. H. (1983). *Basic hand splinting: A pattern designing approach*. Boston, MA: Little, Brown.

Malick, M. H. (1972). *Manual on static hand splinting: For use by physicians, occupational therapists and physical therapists*. Pittsburgh, PA: Harmarville Rehabilitation Center.

Malick, M. H. (1982). *Manual on dynamic hand splinting with thermoplastic materials: Low temperature materials and techniques*. Pittsburgh, PA: Harmarville Rehabilitation Center.

Performance Health. PPT foam padding, self-adhesive back. <https://www.performancehealth.com/ppt-foam-padding-self-adhesive-back>.

Tubiana, R. (1984). Architecture and functions of the hand. In R. Tubiana, J. Thomine, & E. Mackin (Eds.), *Examination of the hand and upper limb*. Philadelphia, PA: WB Saunders.

RECOMMENDED READING

Bell, J., & Breger-Stanton, D. (2011). The forces of dynamic orthotic positioning: ten questions to ask before applying a dynamic orthosis to the hand. In T. M. Skirven, A. L. Osterman, J. Fedorczyk, & P. C. Amadio (Eds.), *Rehabilitation of the hand and upper extremity* (6th ed.). St. Louis, MO: Elsevier Health Sciences.

Hardy, M. A. (1986). Preserving function in the inflamed and acutely injured hand. In C. A. Moran (Ed.), *Hand rehabilitation*. New York, NY: Churchill Livingstone.

Jacobs, M. A., & Austin, N. M. (2013). *Orthotic intervention for the hand and upper extremity: Splinting principles and process*. Philadelphia, PA: Lippincott Williams & Wilkins.

Lede, P. V., & Veldhoven, G. (1998). *Therapeutic hand splints: A rational approach* (Vol. 1). Antwerp, Belgium: Provan.

McKee, P., & Morgan, L. (1998). *Orthotics in rehabilitation: Splinting the hand and body*. Philadelphia, PA: FA Davis Company.

Melvin, J. L. (1982). *Rheumatic disease: Occupational therapy and rehabilitation*. Worcester, MA: Davis Publications.

20

Neurotherapeutic Approaches to Treatment

*Mary Elizabeth Patnaude**

*Mary Elizabeth Patnaude**

OBJECTIVES

After reading this chapter, the student or the occupational therapy practitioner will be able to do the following:

1. Describe in general terms what is meant by a neurotherapeutic treatment approach.
2. Name the four traditional neurotherapeutic treatment approaches.
3. Describe the basic goals and focus of each of the four neurotherapeutic treatment approaches.
4. Discuss common sensorimotor deficits seen in clients with neurologic dysfunction, and provide examples of how these problems can interfere with function.
5. Provide an example of how each of the neurotherapeutic treatment approaches can be incorporated into activities of daily living training.

KEY TERMS

Cerebrovascular accident (CVA)
Muscle tone
Spasticity
Flaccidity
Proprioceptive stimulation
Cutaneous stimulation
Rood approach
Brunnstrom approach
Proprioceptive neuromuscular facilitation (PNF)

Neurodevelopmental treatment approach (NDT/Bobath)
Approximation
Limb synergy
Manual contacts
Repeated contraction
Rhythmic initiation
Relaxation techniques
Facilitation techniques
Inhibition techniques

INTRODUCTION

Occupational therapists (OTs) and occupational therapy assistants (OTAs) direct treatment for clients who have sustained damage to the central nervous system (CNS) toward promoting and maximizing functional movement to facilitate occupational engagement. Neurotherapeutic treatment approaches are adjunctive techniques directed toward motor performance skills that can assist in achieving this outcome. This chapter introduces practical information about the neurotherapeutic approaches used in occupational therapy treatment for clients facing CNS dysfunction.

The CNS consists of the brain and spinal cord. The brain contains a primary motor and primary somatosensory cortex (Fig. 20.1). This area of the brain is most often damaged when blood supply to the brain is interrupted, such as during a **cerebrovascular accident** (**CVA**) (see Chapter 23). Damage to these structures often causes a dysfunction in motor skills that leads to a decreased ability to produce controlled, coordinated movement. This occurs due to abnormal changes in

muscle tone, balance, posture, and reflexive movement. **Muscle tone**, which refers to the natural tension within a muscle, can become either too high (**spasticity**) or too low (**flaccidity**).

Muscle tone adjusts to the demands of the task, so abnormal muscle tone can affect the ability to move. When the sensorimotor cortex is damaged, muscle tone does not accommodate to the demands of a task and may stay at a constant state of spasticity or flaccidity. Spasticity may lead to a decrease in movement or an inability to initiate movement. Joint contractures may result from lack of movement. On the other hand, if muscle tone is too low (flaccid), a client may have difficulty maintaining an upright position or lifting an arm or leg against gravity.

Damage to the sensorimotor cortex may also adversely affect posture and balance. Posture may become asymmetric because of an imbalance in tone of the trunk muscles. Some may be low tone and some may be high tone, causing the client to lean toward one side or asymmetrically bear weight through the pelvis. This may lead to an inability to complete functional weight shifts. Balance depends on the ability to shift weight and react to changes in positioning, so it may also

* The author would like to acknowledge the previous contribution of Elza Guzman to this chapter.

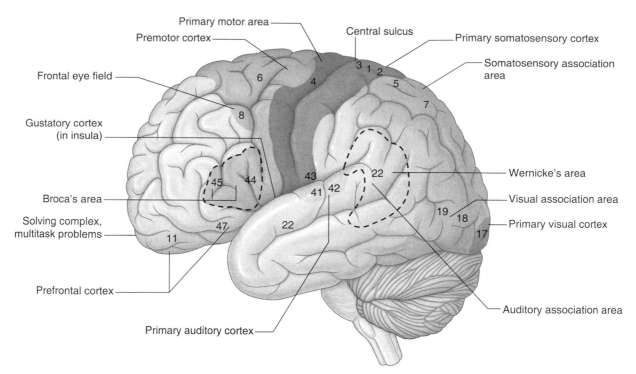

Fig. 20.1 Areas of the neocortex intimately involved in planning of and instruction for voluntary movement. Areas 4 and 6 constitute the motor cortex. (*Red* (dark gray): motor cortex; *blue* (light gray): sensory cortex; *pale blue* (light pale gray) *and pale red* (pale gray): association cortex.) (From Pendleton HM, Schultz-Krohn W. *Pedretti's Occupational Therapy*. 8th ed. St Louis, MO: Elsevier; 2018.)

be adversely affected. This decreased ability to maintain balance while sitting or standing leads to difficulties in performing self-care activities and puts clients at risk for falling.

Reflexes are stereotypical, automatic movements present in all individuals. During normal motor development, reflexes become integrated, allowing an individual to perform controlled movements. After an event that causes CNS damage, reflexes that have previously been well integrated may reappear and become more powerful, limiting the available types of movement. For example, placing an object in the palm of the hand may result in automatic closing of the fingers and the inability to open the hand. This reflex action can affect task-oriented movement.

Finally, damage to the sensorimotor cortex can adversely affect sensation. Some clients may report no feeling in the affected limbs or may describe the arm or leg as feeling heavy and clumsy. Others may not be able to distinguish where the arm is in relationship to objects or other body parts, resulting in decreased coordination.

The goals of neurotherapeutic treatment approaches are to normalize muscle tone, reduce abnormal postural reactions, and induce changes in the sensorimotor cortex. This will lead to more functional motor responses. OTs and OTAs utilizing neurotherapeutic treatment approaches introduce proprioceptive, cutaneous, and sensory stimuli to influence motor responses. **Proprioceptive stimulation** involves stimulating joint and muscle receptors through techniques such as stretching, weight bearing, and resistance (Crepeau et al., 2004). **Cutaneous stimulation** provides input through the

exteroceptors of the skin (Alpern, Lawrence, & Wolsk, 1976; Barr, 1974; Vallbo et al., 1979). *Exteroceptors*, located immediately under the skin, respond to stimuli such as touch, temperature, and pain (Nolte, 2002; Williams & Warwick, 1975). Cutaneous stimuli can be used to facilitate or inhibit muscle responses. Combined with proprioceptive stimulation, cutaneous stimulation may be used to elicit voluntary control of specific muscles.

Some approaches rely on the elicitation of primitive reflexes (automatic, stereotypical motor responses) to produce movement. For example, when a client with poor balance is encouraged to lean toward the weak side, the person may demonstrate a reflexive extension of the affected arm to prevent falling. This situation is an example of a specific reflexive response known as a protective extension.

The OT utilizes a comprehensive evaluation to establish a baseline of the client's level of function and to identify strengths and weaknesses. This baseline allows the OT, with input from the OTA, to identify the neurotherapeutic approach that will best lead to an improvement in motor performance. These approaches should occur in the context of function and lead to an improvement in the motor skills needed for participation in occupation. For example, to assess balance, the OT or OTA may observe a client's ability to maintain balance and upright trunk posture while coordinating forward reach to retrieve a shirt from the closet.

The OTA should be familiar with the various neurotherapeutic approaches and their basic principles and be proficient with the specific techniques used in each to effectively implement treatment. Training and supervision can be provided by the OT. Four neurotherapeutic treatment approaches are most commonly used in practice: the **Rood approach**, the **Brunnstrom (movement therapy) approach**, the **proprioceptive neuromuscular facilitation approach** (PNF), and the **neurodevelopmental treatment approach** (NDT/Bobath).

ROOD APPROACH

Margaret S. Rood was both an OT and a physical therapist (PT) in the 1940s. Although quite dated, her theory was based on the developmental and neurophysiologic literature of the previous decade and provides a foundation for neurotherapeutic approaches used today (Williams & Warwick, 1975). Rood integrated the literature with her own clinical observations to create an approach based on the use of sensory stimulation to effect motor responses.

Rood did not write extensively, seeming to prefer clinical teaching to disseminate her ideas. Most of the literature that describes the Rood approach is based on interpretations by accomplished PTs and OTs such as Ayres (Ayres, 1972; Ayres, 1974), Farber (Farber, 1967; Farber, 1974), Heininger and Randolph (Heininger & Randolph, 1981), Huss (Huss, 1983), and Stockmeyer (Stockmeyer, 1967). Despite some controversy about the efficacy of Rood's techniques, current neuroscience research continues to support the importance of sensory stimulation.

The basic assumption of Rood's theory is that appropriate sensory stimulation can elicit specific motor responses. Rood combined controlled sensory stimulation with a sequence of positions and activities that replicate normal ontogenic motor development (i.e., the normal progression of motor skills) to achieve purposeful muscular responses (Eggars, 1984).

Basic Assumptions

The basic assumptions of Rood's theory are as follows:
1. Normal muscle tone is a prerequisite to movement.

    Clients with CNS dysfunction may exhibit changes in muscle tone, ranging from hypertonicity (too much tone) to hypotonicity (too little tone). This abnormal tone interferes with movement, and the achievement of normalized muscle tone is essential for controlled movement.

    Normal muscle tone flows smoothly and is constantly changing, depending on the demands of a motor act. For example, to turn on the ignition of a car, a person must have good eye–hand coordination, postural control of the trunk muscles, coinnervation of the proximal arm muscles, forearm pronation and supination, and moderately fine prehension and dexterity in the hands.

    In addition, the demands placed on the various muscle groups are different. Rood recognized this when she stated, "Muscles have different duties" (Rood, 1954). Some muscles are used predominantly for heavy work and others for light work. Light-work muscles are called

mobilizers and are primarily the flexors and adductors. The primary function of the light-work muscles is directed toward skilled movement patterns. Heavy-work muscles, however, act as stabilizers and consist of the extensors and abductors (Goff, 1985). The primary function of heavy-work muscles is to allow maintenance of posture and holding patterns of movement. Heavy-work and light-work muscles act together to allow coordinated movements to occur. For example, when a person is putting on a necklace, the heavy-work muscles are responsible for co-contraction proximally at the trunk, shoulder, and forearm, thereby maintaining the arm up against gravity. The light-work muscles, located more distally, are responsible for the coordination and dexterity needed to manipulate the clasp.

Rood (Rood, 1954) also believed that reflexes are the foundation of any voluntary motor act. These reflexes are modified, controlled, and integrated by the CNS. She began therapy by eliciting motor responses on a reflex level and using developmental patterns to improve the motor response.

2. Treatment begins at the developmental level of functioning.

    Rood believed that movement occurs in a developmental sequence. Clients are evaluated developmentally, and treatment follows a developmental sequence. Because one skill builds on the other, clients do not proceed to the next level of sensorimotor development until some degree of voluntary control is achieved. This principle follows the cephalocaudal rule; that is, treatment begins from the head and proceeds downward segment by segment, from proximal to distal, to the sacral area. When adhering to this rule in treatment (e.g., when working with a client on feeding), the clinician would first direct treatment on controlled reaching for the utensil before focusing on holding the utensil (Alpern et al., 1976).

3. Motivation enhances purposeful movement.

    Rood realized that motivation plays an important role in rehabilitation. Activities that are meaningful for the client encourage practice of desired movements. This results in greater client participation in treatment.

4. Repetition is necessary for the reeducation of muscular responses (Barr, 1974).

    Repetition helps develop coordination (Kotte, 1980; Kotte & Lehmann, 1990). Repetition assists the brain in developing an internal "memory" of a specific motor activity. Repetition, however, can be monotonous. To avoid boredom, the OT should provide various activities that incorporate similar motor patterns.

Principles of Treatment

Rood suggested the following four general principles in the treatment of neuromuscular dysfunction: (Rood, 1956)
1. Reflexes can be used to assist or retard the effects of sensory stimulation.

According to Rood, reflexes can be used to influence muscle tone. Two commonly mentioned mechanisms are the tonic neck reflexes (TNRs) and tonic labyrinthine reflexes (TLRs). The TNRs are triggered by changes in the relationship of the head to the neck; TLRs occur with changes in the relationship of the head to gravity. Consequently, any changes in the position of the head to the neck, or in relationship of the head to gravity, can result in increases or decreases in muscle tone. Clinicians must therefore be aware of the position of the head and neck and the potential effects of gravity on the body. For example, in wheelchair seating, symmetric alignment of the head and neck will promote normal muscle tone in the arms and legs.

2. Sensory stimulation of receptors can produce predictable responses.

   Responses to sensory stimulation to specific receptors are predictable. Clinicians using sensory stimulation can use this predictability to achieve a desired outcome. For example, a slow rocking stimulus produces a calming effect and may be beneficial for clients with high tone or agitation.

3. Muscles have different duties.

   As discussed earlier, some muscles predominate as stabilizers (heavy-work muscles), whereas others undertake the duties of mobilization (light-work muscles). According to Rood, each group has distinct functions and characteristics.

4. Heavy-work muscles should be integrated before light-work muscles.

   The principle of integrating heavy-work muscles before light-work muscles refers primarily to the use of the upper extremities (UEs). For example, fine fingertip manipulation (which involves light-work muscles) is not functional if the proximal muscles (heavy-work muscles) are not strong enough to lift or stabilize the position of the arms.

Sequence of Motor Development

Rood proposed the following four sequential phases related to the development of motor control: (Ayres, 1974; Rood, 1956; Rood, 1962)

1. *Reciprocal inhibition (innervation).* Reciprocal inhibition is an early mobility phase that serves a protective function. The muscle acting on one side of a joint *(agonist)* quickly contracts while its opposite *(antagonist)* relaxes. An example of reciprocal innervation is seen in infants who randomly flex and extend their arms and legs.

2. *Co-contraction.* Co-contraction occurs when opposing muscles (usually those surrounding a joint) contract simultaneously, resulting in stabilization of the joint. The co-contraction phase allows an individual to hold a position or an object for a longer time. Standing upright is a result of co-contraction of the trunk muscles, as well as muscles acting on the hips, knees, and ankles.

3. *Heavy work.* The heavy-work phase has been defined as "mobility on stability" (Schmidt, 1991). In this phase the proximal muscles move, and the distal segments are fixed. An example of this phase is creeping. During creeping the infant is in a quadruped (all-fours) position.

The hands and feet are in a fixed position, but the shoulders and hips move.

4. *Skill.* Skill is the highest level of control and combines the efforts of mobility and stability. In a skilled movement pattern, the proximal segment is stabilized while the distal segment moves freely. Reaching overhead to unscrew a light bulb is an example of this pattern.

Ontogenic Movement Patterns

The sequence of motor development described previously occurs as the client is put through a specific sequence that Rood described as ontogenic motor patterns (Goff, 1985). Fig. 20.2 illustrates the eight ontogenic motor patterns.

Supine Withdrawal (Supine Flexion). Supine withdrawal is a total flexion response toward the navel. This position is protective. Supine withdrawal is a mobility posture that requires reciprocal innervation; it also requires heavy work of the proximal muscles and trunk (Rood, 1956). Rood recommended this pattern for clients who do not have the reciprocal flexion pattern and for those dominated by extensor tone (see Fig. 20.2A).

Roll Over (Toward Side-Lying). When the client rolls over, the arm and leg flex on the same side of the body (see Fig. 20.2B). Rolling over is a mobility pattern for the UEs and lower extremities (LEs) and activates the lateral trunk musculature (Stockmeyer, 1967). This pattern is encouraged for clients who are dominated by reflexes or who need segmental movements of the extremities.

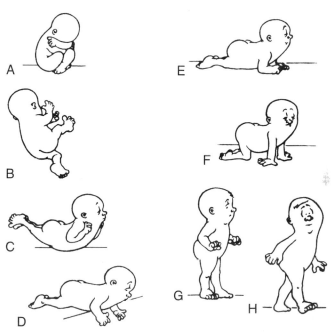

Fig. 20.2 Ontogenic movement patterns. (A) Supine withdrawal. (B) Roll over toward side lying. (C) Pivot prone. (D) Neck contraction. (E) Prone on elbows. (F) Quadruped pattern. (G) Static standing. (H) Walking.

Pivot Prone (Prone Extension). The pivot-prone position demands a full range of extension of the neck, shoulders, trunk, and LEs (see Fig. 20.2C). This pattern has been called both a mobility pattern and a stability pattern. The position is difficult to assume and hold. It plays an important role in preparation for stability in the upright position.

Neck Co-Contraction (Coinnervation). Neck co-contraction is the first real stability pattern. It is used to develop head control and stability of the neck (see Fig. 20.2D). This pattern is necessary to raise the head against gravity.

On Elbows (Prone on Elbow). Following co-contraction of the neck and prone extension, weight bearing on the elbows is the next pattern to achieve. This pattern helps develop stability in the scapular and glenohumeral (shoulder) regions. This position gives the person a better view of the environment and an opportunity to shift weight from side to side (see Fig. 20.2E).

All Fours (Quadruped Position). The quadruped position develops stability of the lower trunk and legs. Initially the client holds the position. Eventually, weight shifting forward, backward, side to side, and diagonally is added. The weight shifting may be preparatory for balance responses (see Fig. 20.2F).

Static Standing. Static standing is thought to be a skill of the upper trunk because it frees the UEs for prehension and manipulation (Stockmeyer, 1967). At first, weight is equally distributed on both legs; then weight shifting begins. This position requires higher-level integration such as maintaining and achieving balance (see Fig. 20.2G).

Walking. Walking unites skill, mobility, and stability. Walking is a complicated process that requires coordinated movement patterns of the various parts of the body (see Fig. 20.2H).

Specific Techniques for Intervention

Rood described in detail the use of cutaneous and proprioceptive stimulation in treatment. Stimuli typically used in clinical practice are briefly described next. Emphasis should be on safe application, precautions, and awareness of the expected outcome of the technique.

When applying any of the cutaneous or proprioceptive techniques, the OTA should always remember that these techniques are adjunctive treatment techniques and are preparatory to functional activity. Whenever possible, the application should be followed immediately by the client's involvement in an activity performed in a functional context. For example, applying deep pressure to the tendon of the biceps may help relax the elbow so that the client can place his or her arm in the sleeve of a shirt with less difficulty.

Cutaneous Stimulation. Cutaneous stimulation is applied to the skin. Light-moving touch, fast brushing, and icing are examples of cutaneous stimulation. Light-moving touch, or slow stroking of the skin, has been used to activate superficial

muscles. The clinical result is a reflexive withdrawal response. Fast brushing, applied through a battery-operated brush, can be performed over the muscle belly of the muscles to be facilitated (Goff, 1985; Stockmeyer, 1967). The results of fast brushing are delayed and do not have a maximal effect until 30 minutes after application.

Icing, a thermal stimulus, has also been used for facilitation of muscle activity (Rood, 1954). Icing is a powerful stimulus, and the results can be unpredictable. Icing can facilitate a flexor withdrawal response in superficial muscles (Stockmeyer, 1967). Icing can also facilitate opening and closing of the mouth and induce swallowing (Huss, 1983).

Strict precautions must be followed for icing or fast brushing; improper use can adversely affect the client. All clinicians using these techniques must be familiar with and strictly adhere to these precautions.

Proprioceptive Stimulation. Proprioceptive stimulation refers to the facilitation of joint and muscle receptors and the vestibular system (Loeb & Hoffer, 1981; McCloskey, 1978; Schmidt, 1991). In general, proprioceptive stimulation gives the clinician more control over the motor response. The motor response lasts if the stimulus continues to be applied (Eldred, 1967; Schmidt, 1991). Several proprioceptive stimulation techniques are used.

Heavy joint compression (Fig. 20.3) facilitates contraction at the joint undergoing compression. This technique can be combined with developmental patterns such as prone on elbows, quadruped (Fig. 20.4), sitting, and standing. Joint compression is clinically most effective when applied through the longitudinal axis of long bones such as the humerus (glenohumeral joint) and the femur (acetabulum).

Quick stretch is applied by holding the proximal bony prominences of the limb to be stretched while moving the distal joint in one direction. For example, the triceps is stretched by securing the elbow while the forearm is pushed into flexion. The response is immediate and short lived.

The tapping technique involves tapping over the belly of a muscle with the fingertips. The OT or OTA percusses (taps)

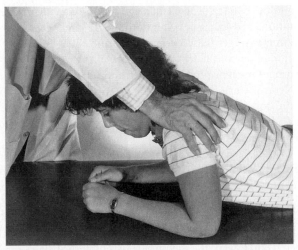

Fig. 20.3 Heavy joint compression.

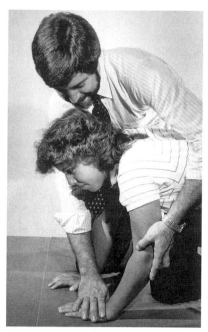

Fig. 20.4 Joint compression in quadruped position.

three to five times over the muscle to be facilitated. This technique may be done before or during the time a client is voluntarily contracting the muscle. Tapping on spastic muscles, or muscles that are likely to develop spasticity, should be avoided. Prolonged or excessive tapping can also result in spasticity and should be avoided.

Vestibular stimulation is another type of proprioceptive input (Clark, 1970). Extreme caution should be taken with vestibular stimulation because it can have a profound effect on the body. Any clinician planning to use vestibular stimulation must be adequately trained and must monitor the client closely during treatment. The OTA who has been instructed in vestibular stimulation by the OT must receive close supervision to ensure the client's safety.

Vibration, applied with a handheld vibrator, has been used to produce tonal changes in muscles (Farber, 1974; Heininger & Randolph, 1981; Huss, 1983). Vibration over spastic muscles, or muscles prone to developing spasticity, should be avoided. The client's age may be a factor in using vibration. For example, vibration should not be used with children younger than 3 years of age and must be used with caution in persons older than age 65. OTAs using vibration in treatment must be properly trained and supervised.

Neutral warmth, an inhibitory technique, has been successful for general relaxation and to reduce muscle tone. It may also be helpful for children with attention deficit disorders (Farber, 1974).

To inhibit spastic or tight muscle groups in which the tendons are accessible, the practitioner can apply manual pressure to the tendinous insertion of a muscle or across long tendons (Ayres, 1974; Heininger & Randolph, 1981). Pressure provided by hard surfaces is more effective than that provided by soft surfaces (Dayhoof, 1975). In the hand a hard cone with the tapered end toward the thumb side to inhibit the flexors can be

used (Farber, 1974). This principle has been used in various orthotic devices to manage muscle imbalance and contracture resulting from spasticity.

To inhibit spastic muscles around a joint, the OT can use light joint compression (**approximation**) with clients who are hemiplegic to alleviate pain and to offset muscle imbalance temporarily around the shoulder joint (Farber, 1974).

Rood also recommended positioning hypertonic extremities in the elongated position for various periods (Matthews, 1978; Rood, 1962). Maintaining stretch in this position has an inhibitory effect. This principle is the basis for inhibitory casting, which is often used with clients who demonstrate severe spasticity of the extremities.

Finally, Rood suggested the use of olfactory and gustatory stimuli to facilitate cranial nerves and to influence the autonomic nervous system (Rood, 1962; Voss, Ionta, & Mayers, 1972). Odors could be used to facilitate a response. Pleasant odors such as vanilla may have a calming effect. Unpleasant and noxious substances such as sulfa and ammonia could trigger protective responses, including coughing and sneezing (Goff, 1985). Rood did not provide specific guidelines for the stimulation of special senses.

Sensory stimulation in clients with neurologic dysfunction can have a powerful effect. OTAs must be properly trained and appropriately supervised when using any of the cutaneous or proprioceptive modalities described in this chapter. Clients to whom these modalities are applied must be closely monitored.

Occupational Therapy Application

The occupational therapy treatment process begins with the OT's evaluation. The evaluation identifies the client's level of motor development. Treatment starts at this level and is directed toward progressing the individual along the developmental continuum. Initially, if severe neurologic damage is present, the client may need to begin with reflexive movements. The OT then progresses the client along the ontogenic development patterns. Sensory stimulation can reinforce these patterns and can be used to inhibit or facilitate specific muscle activity as needed. The sensory stimulation techniques described are used primarily to prepare the client for purposeful activities.

In treatment the OTA should consider ontogenic patterns when positioning clients for activities. For example, the rollover pattern can be reinforced by having the client turn in bed to reach bed controls. Prone-on-elbows positioning can be adapted for tabletop use by having the client sit at a table and lean on his or her elbow and forearm while playing a recreational game. Grooming activities such as shaving or makeup application can also be positioned so that the client must lean on the affected elbow and forearm while reaching for objects. The standing position often provides the best position for activities of daily living (ADL) and purposeful activities. While standing, the client can use the arms to explore and manipulate the environment. For example, while performing a homemaking activity, the individual can reach up to place objects in a cabinet. As the client develops stability in standing, activities that require more weight shifting and balance reactions can be provided.

MOVEMENT THERAPY: BRUNNSTROM APPROACH TO TREATMENT OF HEMIPLEGIA

Signe Brunnstrom was a PT from Sweden. Her practice, teaching, and theory development in the United States extended from the World War II years through the 1970s. Her clinical observations and research led to the development of her treatment approach called movement therapy. Her book, *Movement Therapy in Hemiplegia (*Brunnstrom, 1970*)*, was published in 1970 and applied movement therapy, also known as the Brunnstrom approach, to the treatment of hemiplegia.

Theoretic Foundations

Brunnstrom evolved her treatment approach after study of the literature in neurophysiology, CNS mechanisms, effects of CNS damage, sensory systems and related topics, and clinical observations and application of training procedures (Brunnstrom, 1970). Brunnstrom based her intervention on the concept that the damaged CNS has undergone an "evolution in reverse" and regressed to former patterns of movement. These patterns include the **limb synergies**, which are gross patterns of limb flexion and extension that originate in primitive spinal cord patterns and primitive reflexes (Brunnstrom, 1970). In the normal individual these primitive movement patterns are thought to be modified through the influence of higher centers of CNS control. After a CVA, because the influence of higher centers is disturbed or destroyed, motor function reverts to this primitive state (Brunnstrom, 1970). Reflexes present in early life reappear, and normal reflexes become exaggerated.

The Brunnstrom approach to the treatment of hemiplegia uses the motor patterns available to the client at any point in the recovery process. The goal is to allow progress through the stages of recovery toward more normal and complex movement patterns. Brunnstrom saw synergies, reflexes, and other abnormal movement patterns as a normal part of the process through which an individual with CNS dysfunction must go before normal voluntary movement can occur. Brunnstrom noted that able-bodied people use synergistic movements all the time, but with control and in a variety of patterns that can be modified or stopped at will. Brunnstrom maintained that the synergies appear to constitute a necessary intermediate stage for further recovery. She believed that the gross movement synergies of flexion and extension always precede the restoration of advanced motor functioning after hemiplegia (Brunnstrom, 1970). During the early stage of recovery, Brunnstrom recommended that the client should be aided to gain control of the limb synergies and that selected sensory stimuli can help the client initiate and gain control of movement. Once the synergies can be performed voluntarily, they are modified and movement combinations that deviate from the synergy pattern can be performed (Myers, 1980).

Limb Synergies. A **limb synergy** of flexion or extension, seen in hemiplegia, is a group of muscles acting as a bound unit in a primitive and stereotypical manner (Brunnstrom, 1970). The muscles acting in synergy are linked and cannot act alone. If one muscle in the synergy is activated, each muscle in the synergy responds partially or completely. As a result, the client cannot perform isolated movements when bound by these synergies.

The flexor synergy of the UE consists of scapular adduction and elevation, shoulder abduction and external rotation, elbow flexion, forearm supination, wrist flexion, and finger flexion. Hypertonicity (spasticity) is usually greatest in the elbow flexion component and least in shoulder abduction and external rotation (Fig. 20.5). The extensor synergy consists of scapular abduction and depression, shoulder adduction and internal rotation, elbow extension, forearm pronation, and wrist and finger flexion or extension. Shoulder adduction and internal rotation are usually the most hypertonic components of the extensor synergy, with much less tone in the elbow extension component (Fig. 20.6).

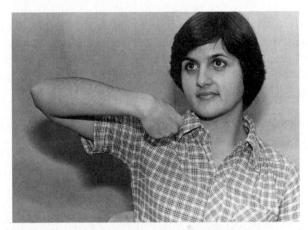

Fig. 20.5 Flexor synergy of upper extremity in hemiplegia.

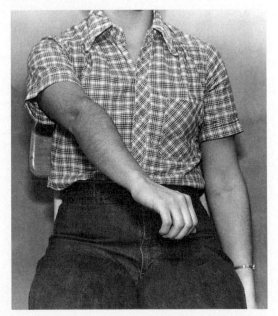

Fig. 20.6 Extensor synergy of upper extremity in hemiplegia.

In the lower extremity (LE) the flexor synergy consists of hip flexion, abduction, and external rotation; knee flexion; ankle dorsiflexion and inversion; and toe extension. Hip flexion is usually the component with the highest tone, and hip abduction and external rotation are the components with the least tone. The extensor synergy is composed of hip abduction, extension, and internal rotation; knee extension; ankle plantar flexion and inversion; and toe flexion. Hip abduction, knee extension, and ankle plantar flexion are usually the most hypertonic components, whereas hip extension and internal rotation are usually less hypertonic.

Characteristics of Synergistic Movement. The flexor synergy is more often seen in the arm, and the extensor synergy is more common in the leg. When the client performs the synergy, the components with the greatest degree of hypertonicity are often most apparent, rather than the entire classic patterns just described. Moreover, the resting posture of the limb, particularly the arm, is usually characterized by a position that represents the most hypertonic components of both flexor and extensor synergies (i.e., shoulder abduction, elbow flexion, forearm pronation, and wrist and finger flexion). With facilitation or voluntary effort, however, the more classic synergy pattern can usually be evoked (Brunnstrom, 1970).

Motor Recovery Process. After a CVA resulting in hemiplegia, Brunnstrom observed that the client progresses through a series of recovery steps or stages in stereotypic fashion (Table 20.1). The progress through these stages may be rapid or slow.

The recovery follows an ontogenic process, usually proximal to distal, so that shoulder movement can be expected before hand movement. Flexion patterns occur before controlled volitional movement, and gross movement patterns can be performed before isolated, selective movement (Brunnstrom, 1970).

Clients' recoveries vary and are influenced by factors such as cognitive deficits, visual-perceptual deficits, family support, motivation, and mood. Few clients make a good recovery of arm function, and the greatest loss is usually in the wrist and hand. Also, no two clients are exactly alike; much individual variation occurs in the recovery process. The motor behavior and recovery process described represent common characteristics that may be observed in most persons after CVA occurs (Myers, 1980).

Principles of Treatment

The goal of Brunnstrom's movement therapy is to facilitate progress through the recovery stages that occur after the onset of hemiplegia (see Table 20.1). Because reflexes represent normal stages of development, they can be used to assist and/or initiate movement. Associated reactions, which are movements seen on the hemiplegic side in response to forceful movements on the normal side, can be used to initiate or elicit synergies by giving resistance to the contralateral (opposite-side) muscle group on the unaffected side. With the asymmetric tonic neck reflex (ATNR), head rotation to the left causes extension of the left arm and leg and flexion of the right arm and leg. With the symmetric tonic neck reflex (STNR), flexion of the neck results in extension of the arm and flexion of the legs.

TABLE 20.1 Motor Recovery After Cerebrovascular Accident (CVA)

CHARACTERISTICS

Stage	Leg	Arm	Hand[a]
1	Flaccidity	Flaccidity; inability to perform any movements	No hand function
2	Spasticity develops; minimal voluntary movements	Beginning development of spasticity; limb synergies or some of their components begin to appear as associated reactions	Gross grasp beginning; minimal finger flexion possible
3	Spasticity peaks; flexion and extension synergy present; hip-knee-ankle flexion in sitting and standing	Spasticity increasing; synergy patterns or some of their components can be performed voluntarily	Gross grasp, hook grasp possible; no release
4	Knee flexion past 90 degrees in sitting, with foot sliding backward on floor; dorsiflexion with heel on floor and knee flexed to 90 degrees	Spasticity declining; movement combinations deviating from synergies are now possible	Gross grasp present; lateral prehension developing; small amount of finger extension and some thumb movement possible
5	Knee flexion with hip extended in standing; ankle dorsiflexion with hip and knee extended	Synergies no longer dominant; more movement combinations deviating from synergies performed with greater ease	Palmar prehension, spherical and cylindric grasp and release possible
6	Hip abduction in sitting or standing; reciprocal internal and external rotation of hip combined with inversion and eversion of ankle in sitting	Spasticity absent except when performing rapid movements; isolated joint movements performed with ease	All types of prehension, individual finger motion, and full range of voluntary extension possible

Data from Brunnstrom S. *Movement Therapy in Hemiplegia.* New York, NY: Harper & Row; 1970.
[a]Recovery of hand function is variable and may not parallel six recovery stages of arm.

Proprioceptive stimuli can also be used to evoke desired motion or tonal changes (Hellebrandt, Schacle, & Carns, 1962). To facilitate a synergy pattern, the therapist can rub skin over the muscle belly with his or her fingertips, thus producing a contraction of the muscle and eliciting the synergy pattern to which the muscle belongs. For example, briskly rubbing the triceps muscle while the client attempts to push the arm through the sleeve of a shirt can promote extensor synergy.

Synergistic movement may be reinforced by the client's voluntary efforts through visual feedback such as mirrors or videotapes or auditory stimuli such as loud and repetitive commands.

Intervention Goals and Treatment Methods

Before initiating any intervention strategies, the OT performs a thorough evaluation of the client's motor, sensory, perceptual, and cognitive functions. The motor evaluation yields information about stage of recovery, muscle tone, passive motion sense, hand function, and sitting and standing balance (Brunnstrom, 1970).

The OT outlines a treatment plan based on the results of this evaluation. The OTA can easily incorporate many of Brunnstrom's techniques into this plan. The treatment goals and methods summarized in this chapter are directed primarily to the rehabilitation of the UE. The treatment goals and techniques chosen depend on the stage of recovery and muscle tone of the individual client.

Bed Positioning. The OTA often instructs the client and caregivers on positioning strategies. Proper bed positioning begins immediately when the client is in the flaccid stage (Brunnstrom, 1970). Proper positioning promotes normal alignment and can decrease the influence of hypertonic muscles. This is important in the prevention of contractures and deformity. For example, the LE often tends to assume a position of hip external rotation and abduction and knee flexion. This position mimics the LE's flexor synergy. If the extensor synergy is developed in the LE, a different position may be present. In this case the LE's posture is characterized by extension and adduction at the hip, knee extension, and ankle plantar flexion.

If the extensor synergy dominates in the LE, the recommended bed position for clients in the supine position is slight hip and knee flexion maintained by a small pillow under the knee. Lateral support of the leg at the knee with pillows or a rolled blanket or bolster should be provided to prevent abduction and external rotation.

If the flexor synergy dominates in the LE, the knee must be maintained in extension. Hip external rotation can be prevented with supports as described.

To position the affected UE, the practitioner supports the arm on a pillow in a position comfortable for the client. Abduction of the UE should be avoided because this position can contribute to shoulder subluxation. While moving the client, the OTA avoids pulling on the affected UE. The client is instructed to use the unaffected hand to support the affected arm when moving in bed.

Bed Mobility. Turning toward the affected side is easier than turning toward the unaffected side. For turning in bed, the OTA can instruct the client to raise the affected arm to a position of forward shoulder flexion with the elbow in extension. The affected LE is then positioned in partial flexion at the knee and hip; the clinician may need to stabilize it in this position. The client turns by swinging the arms and the affected knee across the body toward the unaffected side. As control improves, the client may perform this technique independently to roll toward both sides of the bed.

Balance and Trunk Control. Early in treatment the client needs to develop balance, a prerequisite for functional activities. Clients with hemiplegia may have poor postural/trunk control, often demonstrating a listing (leaning) toward the affected side. To facilitate upright posture, treatment should focus on improving trunk control through a variety of sitting balance exercises with focus on anterior and posterior pelvic tilts and lateral weight shifting. The clinician should support the affected arm to protect the shoulder during these balance-challenging activities. Supporting the arm also prevents the client from grasping the supporting surface during the activity. As trunk control improves, the clinician initiates and assists the client to bend the trunk in various directions. If balance is poor, the clinician can stabilize the client's knees. In this position the clinician can guide the client while moving the trunk in various directions. The clinician can also incorporate passive range of motion (ROM) at the shoulder by raising the client's arms up as the trunk bends forward.

Shoulder Range of Motion. The maintenance of pain-free shoulder ROM is important in clients with hemiplegia. Brunnstrom believed that traditional passive exercises may contribute to pain in these clients (Brunnstrom, 1970). Instead, the shoulder joint should be mobilized through guided trunk motion without forceful stretching.

To accomplish this motion, the client sits erect, cradling the affected arm. The clinician supports the arm under the elbows while the client leans forward. The more the client leans, the greater the range of shoulder flexion that can be obtained. The clinician guides the arm gently and passively into shoulder flexion while the client's attention is focused on the trunk motion. In a similar manner the clinician can guide the arms into abduction and adduction while the client rotates the trunk from side to side. Later, active-assistive movements of the arm in relation to the trunk can begin.

Shoulder Subluxation. Glenohumeral subluxation appears to be a result of dysfunction of the rotator cuff muscles. These muscles maintain the humeral head in the glenoid fossa. Activation of the rotator cuff muscles is necessary if subluxation is to be minimized or prevented. Slings have been used in an effort to hold the humeral head in the glenoid fossa, but they do not activate the muscles needed to protect the integrity of the shoulder joint (Brunnstrom, 1970). Slings have been found to be of little value and may be harmful (Calliet,

1980). Therapeutic taping (kinesiotaping) has also been used to lift the shoulder into alignment.

Methods of Treatment. The training procedures for improving arm function are geared to the client's recovery stage. These procedures are performed primarily by the OT. During stages 1 and 2, when the arm is essentially flaccid or when some components of the synergy patterns are beginning to appear, the aim is to elicit muscle tone and the synergy patterns on a reflex basis. This aim is met through a variety of facilitation procedures.

The OT does not employ treatment methods in any set order but varies them depending on the client's needs. Because the flexor synergy usually appears first, it may be useful to begin trying to elicit the flexor patterns. This attempt should be followed immediately with facilitation of the extensor synergy components, which tend to be weaker and more difficult to perform in later stages of recovery (Brunnstrom, 1970; Perry, 1967). Overtraining of either synergy should be avoided.

When the client has recovered to stages 2 and 3, the synergies are present, and components can be performed voluntarily. During this period, the goal is for the client to achieve voluntary control of the synergy patterns.

The goal of treatment during stages 4 and 5 is to move away from the synergies by mixing components from both synergies to perform new and complex patterns of movement.

In the final recovery period, stage 6, the goal is to achieve ease in performance of movement combinations, to increase isolated motions, and to increase speed of movement. Activities that encourage varying motions and increasing speed of performance can be introduced during this stage.

Brunnstrom described a specific technique to retrain hand function. As in treatment of the rest of the UE, the concept of helping the client progress through the stages of hand recovery is the same. For example, clients are first provided with activities to promote gross grasp, followed by wrist fixation for grasp, then active release (Brunnstrom, 1970).

Occupational Therapy Application

The focus of occupational therapy intervention using the Brunnstrom technique is to assist the client in using newly learned movement patterns for functional and purposeful activities. Using this principle, the OTA can consider incorporating whatever movement the client demonstrates into treatment activities. For instance, during stage 3, when the client can perform synergy voluntarily, the extensor synergy can be used to stabilize an object on a table while the unaffected arm is performing a task. During stage 4 the OTA can provide activities that encourage movements deviating from synergy such as skateboard activities (Fig. 20.7), sponging off tabletops, or finger painting.

Practice in functional movement patterns for self-care can also be performed. They might include hand-to-mouth motions used in eating finger foods, combing hair, washing the face, washing the unaffected arm, and reaching the opposite axilla for washing or application of deodorant (Brunnstrom, 1970).

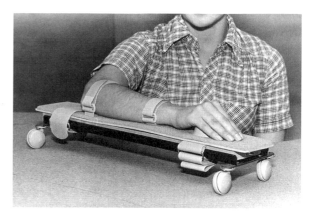

Fig. 20.7 Skateboard activities for synergy or combined movement patterns.

The clinician's role is to analyze activities for movement patterns the client can perform and to select meaningful and interesting activities with the client.

The OTA should always reinforce and encourage any voluntary movement of the affected limb during the performance of self-care activities. Using the arm for dressing and hygiene skills translates the movements to purposeful use. If the client moves beyond stage 4, the number of activities that can be performed increases and more movement combinations are possible. The involvement of the affected limbs in ADL should be encouraged. Gardening, rolling out dough, sweeping, dusting, and washing dishes are a few of the activities that may enlist the affected arm purposefully if hand recovery is adequate.

PROPRIOCEPTIVE NEUROMUSCULAR FACILITATION

PNF originated with Dr. Herman Kabat, a physician and neurophysiologist, in the 1940s. Kabat applied neurophysiologic principles to the treatment of paralysis resulting from poliomyelitis and multiple sclerosis. In 1948 Kabat and Henry Kaiser founded the Kabat-Kaiser Institute in Vallejo, California. At the institute Kabat worked with PT Margaret Knott to develop the PNF method of treatment. By 1951 the diagonal patterns and several PNF techniques were established. In 1952 PT Dorothy Voss joined the staff at the Kabat-Kaiser Institute. She and Knott undertook the teaching and supervision of staff therapists. In 1956 the first edition of Knott and Voss's *Proprioceptive Neuromuscular Facilitation* was published (Voss, 1959a, 1959b).

PNF is based on normal movement and motor development. In normal motor activity the brain registers total movement, not individual muscle action (Jackson, 1931). The PNF approaches use mass movement patterns that resemble normal movement during functional activities. **Facilitation techniques** are superimposed on these movement patterns and postures through **manual contacts**, verbal commands, and visual cues.

Intervention Principles of PNF

Voss presented specific principles of treatment at the Northwestern University Special Therapeutic Exercise Project in 1966. These principles were developed from concepts in the fields of neurophysiology, motor learning, and motor behavior. Examples of some core concepts from these principles are as follows: (Hellebrandt et al., 1962)

1. *Normal motor development proceeds in a cephalocaudal and proximodistal direction.* During evaluation and treatment, the cephalocaudal (head to tailbone) and proximodistal (body center to extremities) directions are followed. Attention is given first to the head, followed by the neck, trunk, and finally the extremities. For clinicians, this order is of importance in treatment that facilitates fine motor coordination in the UEs. Without adequate control of the head, neck, and trunk region, fine motor skills cannot be developed effectively.

2. *Early motor behavior is dominated by reflex activity.* Mature motor behavior is supported or reinforced by postural reflexes. As a person matures, primitive reflexes are integrated and available for reinforcement to allow for progressive development such as rolling, crawling, and sitting. Reflexes also affect tone and movement in the extremities, and head and neck movements affect arm and leg movements (Heininger & Randolph, 1981). For example, reaching for an object can be reinforced by having the head turned toward the object.

3. *Motor behavior is expressed in an orderly sequence of total patterns of movements and posture.* Motor skills develop progressively. For example, an infant learns to roll, to crawl, to creep, and finally to stand and walk. Throughout these stages the infant also learns to use the extremities in different patterns and postures. Initially the hands are used for reaching and grasping within the most supported postures such as supine and prone. As control in these postures develops, the infant begins to use the hands in side-lying, sitting, and standing. Coordination develops as a result.

4. *The growth of motor behavior has a rhythmic and cyclical trend, as evidenced by shifts between flexor and extensor dominance.* These shifts help to develop muscle balance and control. One of the main goals of the PNF treatment approach is to establish a balance among opposing (antagonistic) muscle groups. In treatment the clinician must establish a balance between muscles by first observing where imbalance exists and then facilitating the weaker component. For example, if a client demonstrates a flexor synergy, extension should be facilitated.

5. *Normal motor development has an orderly sequence but lacks a step-by-step quality.* Overlapping occurs; the child does not perfect performance of one activity before beginning another, more advanced activity. Normal motor development follows a predictable pattern, which the practitioner must consider when positioning a client. If one posture technique is not effective in obtaining a desired result, the OTA may need to attempt the activity in another developmental posture. For example, if a client with ataxia cannot write while sitting, the person may practice writing in a more supported posture such as prone on elbows. If the client has not perfected a motor activity such as walking on level surfaces, however, the person may benefit from attempting a higher-level activity such as walking up or down stairs. This activity in turn can improve ambulation on level surfaces. Moving up and down the developmental sequence is a natural occurrence that allows for multiple, varied opportunities for practicing motor activities.

6. *Establishing a balance between antagonists is a main objective of PNF.* As movement and posture change, continuous adjustments in balance are made. When these adjustments are not made, an imbalance in muscles occurs, such as seen in the client with a head injury who cannot maintain adequate sitting balance during a table-top activity because of a dominance of trunk extensor tone. In treatment, emphasis would be placed on correcting the imbalance. In the presence of spasticity, this correction may have to be done by first inhibiting (reducing) the spasticity, then facilitating the antagonistic muscles, evoking reflexes, and promoting stable posture.

7. *Improvement in motor ability depends on motor learning.* Multisensory input facilitates the client's motor learning and is an integral part of the PNF approach. For example, when working with a client on a shoulder flexion activity such as reaching into the cabinet for a cup, the clinician may say, "Reach for the cup." This verbal input encourages the client to look in the direction of the movement to allow vision to enhance the motor response. Thus tactile, auditory, and visual inputs are used. Motor learning has occurred when these external cues are no longer necessary for adequate performance. Practice and repetition enhance motor learning. In treatment, opportunities for practice must be afforded to clients. Practice should be varied and occur in different positions and patterns. This repetition builds skill and coordination.

8. *Goal-directed activities coupled with techniques of facilitation are used to hasten learning of total patterns of walking and self-care activities.* When facilitation techniques are applied to ADL, the objective is improved functional ability. This improvement requires more than instruction and practice alone. Correction of deficiencies is accomplished by directly applying manual contacts and techniques to facilitate the desired response (Voss, 1959b). Examples include applying stretch to finger extensors to release an object and providing joint approximation through the shoulders and pelvis of a client with ataxia to provide stability while standing to wash dishes.

Motor Learning

Motor learning requires a multisensory approach; auditory, visual, and tactile systems are all used to achieve the desired response. The correct combination of sensory input for each client should be identified and altered as the person progresses.

Verbal commands should be brief and clear. Timing of the command is important. Tone of voice may influence the quality of the client's response. Strong, sharp commands are used when maximal stimulation of motor response is desired. A soft tone of voice is used to encourage a smooth movement (e.g., in the presence of pain). Verbal mediation, whereby clients say aloud the steps of an activity, has also been found to enhance learning (Loomis & Boersma, 1982).

Visual stimuli help to initiate and coordinate movement. Visual input should be monitored to ensure that the client is tracking in the direction of movement. The clinician's position and the treatment activity must be considered. For example, if the treatment goal is to increase head, neck, and trunk rotation to the left, the activity should be in front and to the left of the client.

The use of tactile input is essential to guide and reinforce the desired patterns of movement. Manual contacts by the clinician provide this input.

Finally, to increase speed and accuracy in motor performance, the client needs the opportunity to practice. Practice should include part-task and whole-task practice. In part task, emphasis is placed on the parts of the task that the client is unable to perform independently. For example, the client learning to transfer from a wheelchair to a tub bench may have difficulty lifting the leg over the tub rim. This part of the task should be practiced with repetition and facilitation techniques to the hip flexors during performance of the transfer. When the transfer becomes smooth and coordinated, it is no longer necessary to practice parts individually.

Evaluation

The OT, using a PNF approach, completes an initial evaluation to identify the client's abilities, deficiencies, and potential. After the treatment plan is established, ongoing assessment is necessary to determine the effectiveness of treatment; modifications are made as the client changes. The PNF evaluation follows a sequence from proximal to distal. Special attention is given to muscle tone, alignment (midline or a shift to one side), and stability/mobility (Myers, 1980).

When examining the trunk and extremities, the clinician evaluates each segment individually in specific movement patterns, as well as in developmental activities that use interaction of body segments. For example, shoulder flexion can be observed in an individual UE movement pattern, as well as during a total developmental pattern such as rolling.

During the evaluation the OT should note the facilitation techniques and sensory inputs (auditory, visual, tactile) to which the client responds most effectively. Once identified, these techniques and sensory inputs are used to promote controlled movements.

Evaluation should be performed during self-care and other ADL to determine whether performance patterns are adequate within the context of a functional activity. Because

performance may vary from one setting to another, the treatment plan must allow for practice of motor skills in a variety of settings and in locations appropriate to the specific activity.

Intervention Goals and Treatment Methods

Once the evaluation is complete, an intervention plan is developed, including goals the client hopes to accomplish. The clinician uses the techniques and procedures identified in the evaluation as having favorably influenced movement and posture. Similarly, appropriate total patterns and patterns of facilitation are selected to enhance performance.

The treatment techniques used in the PNF approach are diagonal patterns, total patterns, and facilitation techniques.

Diagonal Patterns. The diagonal patterns used in the PNF approach are mass movement patterns observed in most functional activities. Part of the challenge in using this approach is recognizing the diagonal patterns in ADL. Two diagonal motions (D_1, D_2) are present for each major part of the body: head and neck, upper and lower trunk, and extremities. Each diagonal pattern has a flexion and extension component together with rotation and movement away from or toward the midline. Both unilateral and bilateral diagonal patterns are described for the extremities. Only UE patterns are discussed in this chapter.

The movements associated with each diagonal pattern and examples of these patterns seen in ADL are described next. Not all components of the pattern or full ROM are necessarily seen during functional activities. Furthermore, the diagonals interact during functional movement, changing from one pattern or combination to another (Myers, 1982).

Upper extremity unilateral patterns.

1. *UE D_1 flexion (antagonist of D_1 extension).* Scapular elevation, abduction, and rotation; shoulder flexion, adduction, and external rotation; elbow in flexion or extension; forearm supination; wrist flexion to the radial side; finger flexion and adduction; thumb adduction (Fig. 20.8A). Examples in functional activity: hand-to-mouth motion in feeding, combing hair on left side of head with right hand (Fig. 20.9A).
2. *UE D_1 extension (antagonist of D_1 flexion).* Scapular depression, adduction, and rotation; shoulder extension, abduction, and internal rotation; elbow in flexion or extension; forearm pronation; wrist extension to the ulnar side; finger extension and abduction; thumb in palmar abduction (see Fig. 20.8B). Examples in functional activity: pushing car door open from inside (see Fig. 20.9B).
3. *UE D_2 flexion (antagonist of D_2 extension).* Scapular elevation, adduction, and rotation; shoulder flexion, abduction, and external rotation; elbow in flexion or extension; forearm supination; wrist extension to radial side; finger extension and abduction; thumb extension (Fig. 20.10A). Examples in functional activity: combing hair on right side of head with right hand (Fig. 20.11A), swimming the backstroke.

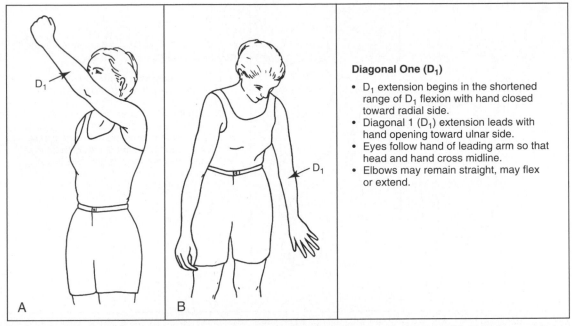

Fig. 20.8 (A) Upper extremity D$_1$ flexion pattern. (B) Upper extremity D$_1$ extension pattern. (From Myers BJ. *PNF: Diagonal Patterns and Their Application to Functional Activities.* Chicago, IL: Rehabilitation Institute of Chicago; 1982, videotape.)

The diagram includes the following text labels:

Diagonal One (D₁)
- D$_1$ extension begins in the shortened range of D$_1$ flexion with hand closed toward radial side.
- Diagonal 1 (D$_1$) extension leads with hand opening toward ulnar side.
- Eyes follow hand of leading arm so that head and hand cross midline.
- Elbows may remain straight, may flex or extend.

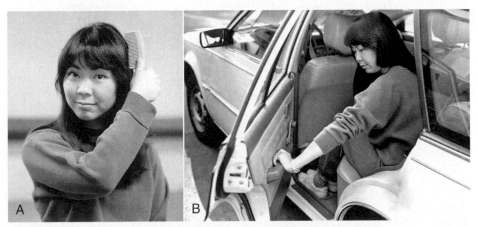

Fig. 20.9 (A) Upper extremity D$_1$ flexion pattern used in combing hair, opposite side. (B) Upper extremity D$_1$ extension pattern used in pushing car door open.

4. *UE D$_2$ extension (antagonist of D$_2$ flexion).* Scapular depression, abduction, and rotation; shoulder extension, adduction, and internal rotation; elbow in flexion or extension; forearm pronation; wrist flexion to the ulnar side; finger flexion and adduction; thumb opposition (see Fig. 20.10B). Examples in functional activity: pitching baseball; buttoning pants on left side with right hand (see Fig. 20.11B).

Bilateral patterns. Movements in the extremities can be reinforced by combining diagonals in the following bilateral patterns:

1. *Symmetric patterns.* Paired extremities perform like movements at the same time (Fig. 20.12). Examples are bilateral symmetrical D$_2$ extension such as starting to take off a pullover sweater (Fig. 20.13A) and bilateral

symmetric D$_2$ flexion such as reaching to lift a large item off a high shelf (see Fig. 20.13B).

2. *Asymmetric patterns.* Paired extremities perform movements toward one side of the body at the same time. Asymmetric patterns facilitate trunk rotation. The asymmetric patterns can be performed with the arms in contact or not (Figs. 20.14 and 20.15). Examples are bilateral asymmetric flexion to the left, with the left arm in D$_2$ flexion and the right arm in D$_1$ flexion such as putting on a left earring (Fig. 20.16) or bilateral asymmetric extension to the left, with the right arm in D$_2$ extension and the left arm in D1 extension such as zipping a left-sided skirt zipper.

3. *Reciprocal patterns.* Paired extremities perform movements in opposite directions at the same time. Reciprocal

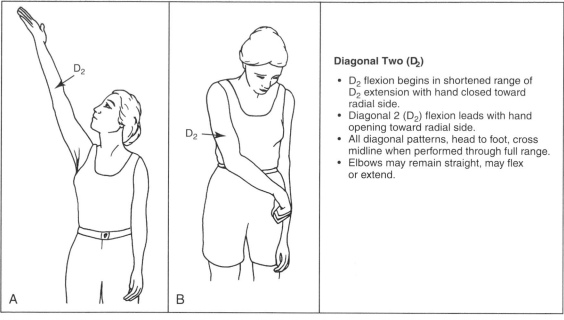

Fig. 20.10 (A) Upper extremity D$_2$ flexion pattern. (B) Upper extremity D$_2$ extension pattern. (From Myers BJ. *PNF: Diagonal Patterns and Their Application to Functional Activities.* Chicago, IL: Rehabilitation Institute of Chicago; 1982, videotape.)

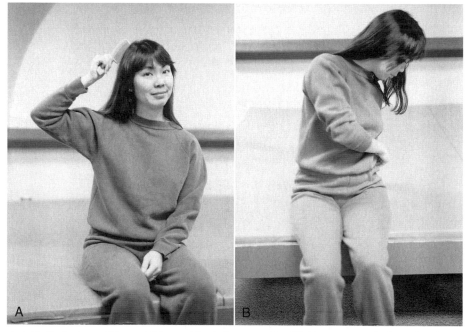

Fig. 20.11 (A) Upper extremity D$_2$ flexion pattern used in combing hair, same side. (B) Upper extremity D$_2$ extension pattern used in buttoning trousers, opposite side.

patterns have a stabilizing effect on the head, neck, and trunk. Examples are pitching in baseball or walking on a balance beam with one extremity in a diagonal flexion pattern and the other in a diagonal extension pattern (Fig. 20.17). During activities requiring high-level balance, reciprocal patterns come into play to maintain balance and prevent a fall.

Diagonal patterns offer several advantages in OT treatment. First, crossing of the midline of the body occurs. Most

functional activities require crossing the midline, which can also be important in the remediation of visual perceptual deficits such as unilateral neglect, in which integration of both sides of the body and awareness of the neglected side are treatment goals. Second, because each muscle has an optimal pattern in which it functions, the total pattern can be used to strengthen weaker ones. Third, the diagonal patterns use groups of muscles; this movement is typical of functional activities. Finally, rotation is always a component in the diagonals. With an injury or the aging process, rotation is often impaired and can be facilitated with movement in the diagonals.

In treatment the OT or OTA would place activities so that movement occurs in a diagonal. For example, if the client is working on a simple homemaking task such as preparing a meal, trunk rotation with extension can be facilitated by placing all the ingredients and utensils on a cupboard located above and diagonal from the client.

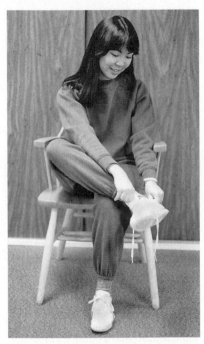

Fig. 20.12 Upper extremity symmetric pattern.

Total Patterns. In PNF, developmental postures are called total patterns of movement and posture (Myers, 1980). Total patterns require interaction between proximal (head, neck, trunk) and distal (extremity) components. Maintenance of postures is important. When posture cannot be maintained, emphasis is placed on the assumption of posture (Voss, 1959b). The active assumption of postures can be incorporated into functional activities. For example, a reaching and placing activity could be designed so that the client must reach for the object while in a supine posture and then move into a side-lying posture to place the object. The use of total patterns also can reinforce individual extremity movements. For example, in an activity such as wiping a tabletop, wrist extension is reinforced while the client leans forward over the supporting arm.

Procedures. PNF techniques are superimposed on diagonal movements and posture. Two procedures, verbal commands and visual cues, have been discussed previously. Other common procedures include manual contact, stretch, traction, and approximation.

Manual contact refers to the placement of the clinician's hands on the client. Pressure from the clinician's touch is used as a facilitating mechanism and provides a sensory cue to help the client understand the direction of the anticipated movement (Voss, 1959b). The amount of pressure applied depends on the specific technique and the desired response. Location of manual contacts is chosen according to the groups of muscles, tendons, and joints responsible for the desired movement patterns. For example, if a client is having difficulty reaching to comb the back of the hair because of scapular weakness, the desired movement pattern would be D_2 flexion. Manual contacts would be on the posterior surface

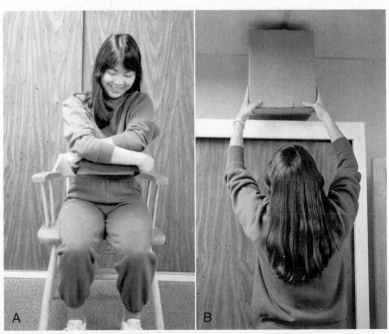

Fig. 20.13 (A) Upper extremity bilateral symmetric pattern used when starting to take off pullover shirt. (B) Upper extremity bilateral symmetric pattern used when reaching to lift box off high shelf.

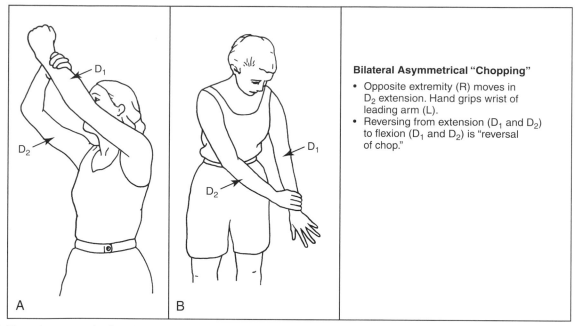

Bilateral Asymmetrical "Chopping"

- Opposite extremity (R) moves in D_2 extension. Hand grips wrist of leading arm (L).
- Reversing from extension (D_1 and D_2) to flexion (D_1 and D_2) is "reversal of chop."

Fig. 20.14 Bilateral asymmetric chopping. (From Myers BJ. *PNF: Diagonal Patterns and Their Application to Functional Activities.* Chicago, IL: Rehabilitation Institute of Chicago; 1982, videotape.)

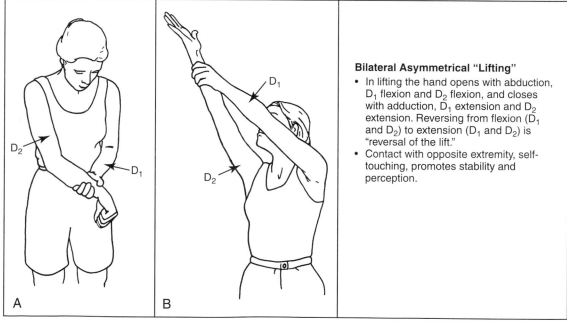

Bilateral Asymmetrical "Lifting"

- In lifting the hand opens with abduction, D_1 flexion and D_2 flexion, and closes with adduction, D_1 extension and D_2 extension. Reversing from flexion (D_1 and D_2) to extension (D_1 and D_2) is "reversal of the lift."
- Contact with opposite extremity, self-touching, promotes stability and perception.

Fig. 20.15 Bilateral asymmetric lifting. (From Myers BJ. *PNF: Diagonal Patterns and Their Application to Functional Activities.* Chicago, IL: Rehabilitation Institute of Chicago; 1982, videotape.)

of the scapula to reinforce the muscles that elevate, adduct, and rotate the scapula.

Stretch is used to initiate voluntary movement and enhance speed of response and strength in weak muscles. When stretch is used in this approach, the part to be facilitated is placed in the extreme lengthened range of the desired pattern (or where tension is felt on all muscle components of a given pattern). After the correct position for the stretch stimulus has been achieved, stretch is superimposed on the pattern. The client should attempt the movement at the exact time that the stretch reflex is elicited. Verbal commands should coincide with the application of stretch to reinforce the movement. Using stretch, the OTA must take care to prevent increasing pain or muscle imbalances. The OTA who plans to use the stretch technique must be thoroughly trained in proper application and precautions.

Traction facilitates the joint receptors by separating the joint surfaces. Traction promotes movement and occurs in

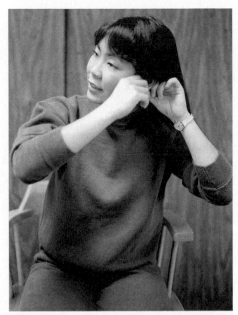

Fig. 20.16 Putting on earring requires use of upper extremity bilateral asymmetric flexion pattern.

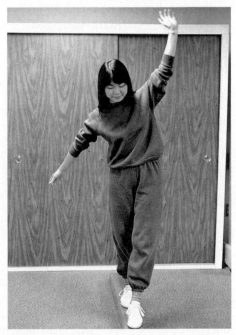

Fig. 20.17 Bilateral reciprocal pattern of upper extremities used to walk balance beam.

pulling motion (Voss et al., 1972). In an activity such as carrying a heavy suitcase, traction can be felt on joint surfaces. Traction may be contraindicated in clients after surgery or fractures or in clients with shoulder subluxation.

Approximation facilitates joint receptors by creating a compression of joint surfaces. It promotes stability and postural control and occurs in pushing motion (McCloskey, 1978). Approximation is usually superimposed on a weight-bearing posture. For example, to enhance postural control in

the prone on elbow position, approximation may be given through the shoulders in a downward direction.

Techniques. Several specific techniques are used with these basic procedures; a few have been selected for mention here. Before incorporating any of these techniques into treatment, both the OT and the OTA must be trained in safe applications and precautions and must demonstrate the appropriate level of competence. Improper application can result in spasticity, pain, and abnormal movement patterns.

Repeated contraction is a technique based on the assumption that repetition of an activity is necessary for motor learning and helps develop strength, ROM, and endurance.

Rhythmic initiation is used to improve the ability to initiate movement, a problem that may be seen in clients with Parkinson disease or apraxia.

Relaxation techniques are an effective means of increasing ROM, particularly when pain or spasticity increases with passive stretch. Two examples of PNF relaxation techniques are contract-relax and hold-relax. Contract-relax techniques involve a holding contraction of the antagonistic pattern against maximal resistance, followed by relaxation and then passive movement into the agonistic pattern. This procedure is repeated at each point during the ROM in which limitation is felt to occur (Voss et al., 1972). Contract-relax is used when no active ROM in the agonistic pattern is present. Hold-relax techniques are performed in the same sequence as contract-relax techniques but involve an isometric (holding) contraction of the antagonist, followed by relaxation and then active movement into the agonistic pattern. This technique may benefit clients with pain.

Occupational Therapy Applications

The PNF approach can be incorporated into occupational therapy practice in a variety of ways. Whenever feasible, the OT or OTA should incorporate appropriate diagonal patterns into functional treatment activities. Tasks can be positioned so that a client can perform the diagonal needed for function. During homemaking, for example, the process of reaching into a bag to retrieve items that are placed on a kitchen shelf could be set up to incorporate the D_1 flexion and D_2 extension patterns. Verbal and tactile cues should be used to promote functional movement patterns. Specific treatment techniques and procedures could be used with these activities to further enhance function.

NEURODEVELOPMENTAL TREATMENT OF ADULT HEMIPLEGIA: BOBATH APPROACH

The NDT/Bobath approach was first developed in the 1940s by Bertha Bobath, a PT, and her husband, Dr. Karel Bobath, a neurologist (Bobath, 1978). The Bobaths coined the term "neurodevelopmental treatment" to describe their work with children with cerebral palsy. Also known as the Bobath approach, NDT has been used successfully by OTs and PTs to treat adult hemiplegia.

The Bobaths believed strongly in the potential of the hemiplegic side for normal function. Based on this belief, they established a treatment program that focused on relearning normal movement. NDT is geared toward encouraging the use of both sides of the body. Development of alignment and symmetry of the trunk and pelvis are emphasized; these conditions are thought to be necessary for normal function of the extremities. When therapists use an NDT approach, clients should be trained to use methods other than compensatory techniques. Relying only on compensatory techniques may lead to overuse of the uninvolved side and underuse of the involved side. This pattern will ultimately interfere with functional recovery of the hemiplegic side.

Common Impairments Associated With Hemiplegia

Motor Impairments. The Bobaths suggested the motor impairments associated with hemiplegia resulted from decreased motor control affecting voluntary movement. Flaccidity (low tone), often seen in the early stages of a CVA, leads to low endurance and low activity tolerance. This period may last a few days to several months. Although no movement in the affected extremities is displayed at this time, a proper treatment program can strongly alter the eventual functional outcome (Bobath, 1978).

After the flaccid stage, the client enters a stage of mixed tone, displaying a combination of flaccidity and spasticity. For example, the UE might have an increase in tone proximally at the scapula and shoulder but a decrease in tone distally at the wrist and hand. If treatment does not address the problems of high tone at this stage, the client progresses to the next stage of spasticity.

Spasticity (increased tone) is the most common problem and the most difficult motor problem to manage after a CVA. If not treated correctly, spasticity can severely compromise functional mobility and ADL performance. Spasticity produces abnormal sensory feedback and contributes to weakness of antagonist muscles. It can cause contractures, pain, and an all-consuming fear in many clients. Fear, pain, and spasticity are often so intertwined that a vicious cycle appears. The spasticity can cause an increase in pain, which can cause an increase in fear, which in turn increases the amount of spasticity (Davis, 1985). Conversely, a reduction in pain and fear can reduce spasticity. Other factors that may influence the amount of spasticity are emotional stress, physical effort, temperature, and the rate of activity.

The typical posture in the adult hemiplegic client (Fig. 20.18) can be described as follows:
- Head—Lateral flexion is toward the involved side with rotation away from the involved side.
- UE—Combination of the strongest components of the flexion and extension synergies appears.
  1. Scapula—depression, retraction
  2. Shoulder—adduction, internal rotation
  3. Elbow—flexion
  4. Forearm—pronation
  5. Wrist—flexion, ulnar deviation
  6. Fingers—flexion

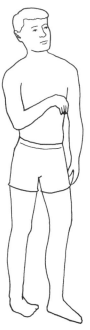

Fig. 20.18 Typical posture of adult with hemiplegia in standing position.

- Trunk—Lateral flexion is toward the involved side.
- LE—Typical extensor posture.
  7. Pelvis—posterior elevation, retraction
  8. Hip—internal rotation, adduction, extension
  9. Knee—extension
  10. Ankle—plantar flexion, supination, inversion
  11. Toes—flexion

Additional Deficits. With these motor problems, clients often have other deficits that can affect function, including diminished weight bearing on the hemiplegic side, sensory loss, neglect, and fear.

Clients with hemiplegia commonly avoid bearing weight on the affected side. When sitting or standing, the client shifts weight to the nonhemiplegic side, thus causing an asymmetric posture that cues the client to lean toward the side. Sensory loss, visual perceptual impairments, and cognitive deficits can contribute to this problem.

Sensory loss varies and may include the loss of stereognosis, kinesthetic awareness, light touch, and light pressure. Abnormal sensation in an extremity, even with good motor control, can render that extremity useless (Bobath, 1978; Davis, 1985). Unilateral body or unilateral spatial neglect can occur after a CVA. It is defined as an inattention to or neglect of visual stimuli presented to the body side contralateral to a lesion (Gillen, 2011). It can result from defective sensory processing or attention deficit, which causes neglect or impaired use of extremities (Gillen, 2011). For example, the client does not dress affected body parts, the client forgets to shave or wash one side of the face, or the client may run into furniture, doorways, or walls located on the affected side.

Fear can also be a major limiting factor for many clients. Fear can be related to loss of sensory awareness, poor balance reactions, lack of protective extension resulting in a fear of falling, and perceptual or cognitive problems (Davis, 1985).

Many other problems related to CVA, including aphasia, apraxia, and visual-perceptual problems, may occur and affect a client's functional abilities.

Evaluation

When evaluating a client using the NDT approach, the OT emphasizes the quality of movement (i.e., how the client moves). During evaluation of coordination, changes in overall muscle tone and postural reactions (rather than specific muscles and joints) are the focus of observation (Bobath, 1978). During the evaluation and treatment the clinician must understand normal posture and movement to identify abnormal patterns. Each client may have a different clinical picture based on age, premorbid physical condition, and normal degenerative changes. Observations should be performed in a functional context because muscle tone may change based on specific task demands.

Observation is a key component in an NDT evaluation. The client is observed from the front, back, and both sides. Comparison of the body's affected and unaffected sides provides information about the client's symmetry. The clinician should observe the client at rest; during sitting, standing, and lying; and while the client is performing various functional activities. During movement any changes in posture and muscle tone of the head, neck, trunk, and extremities should be noted.

When asymmetries are noted, the OT begins to identify possible underlying causes. The practitioner moves the body part through the normal ROM, noting pain and deviations from movement. If resistance is felt, it is likely the result of abnormally high tone. If no resistance is felt but the arm feels heavy, abnormally low tone is the probable cause.

The OT also observes any movement initiated by the client on the weak side. Associated movements, which are normal, may occur when the client attempts to move the weak side and the strong side responds by making the same movement. Associated reactions, in which the client moves using compensatory movements or movements influenced by abnormal synergy patterns, are abnormal and should be avoided. The client should also avoid excessive effort because the exertion can trigger abnormal reactions and movement patterns.

Comparison of the client's movement pattern to the normal movement required for the same task reveals problem areas. For example, when a client reaches for an object, the OT may note that the hemiplegic arm elevates and retracts at the shoulder, flexes at the elbow, supinates at the forearm, and flexes at the wrist and fingers. The trunk may also flex forward to position the hand nearer the object (Fig. 20.19A). In comparison, a normal pattern of movement might include trunk stability with scapular protraction, selective elbow extension with pronation, wrist extension, and finger flexion (see Fig. 20.19B). When comparing the two sides, the OT practitioner can identify elements of abnormal patterns of movement. Understanding the components of normal movement, both in isolation and within the context of an activity, is essential to identifying abnormal patterns.

In NDT the evaluation and treatment processes are intertwined and integrated. While evaluating the client's movement patterns, the clinician performs techniques to promote normal tone and facilitate controlled patterns of movement. The OT continuously assesses the effects of these techniques on the client's movement pattern and adjusts treatment accordingly. The OTA receives information from the OT's evaluation so that activities that reinforce normal movement patterns can be provided in treatment. In addition, the OTA's observation skills should be developed so that adjustments in treatment can be made in the moment, based on actual client performance.

Intervention Goals and Treatment Methods

The goals of NDT are to normalize tone, inhibit primitive patterns of movement, and facilitate automatic, voluntary

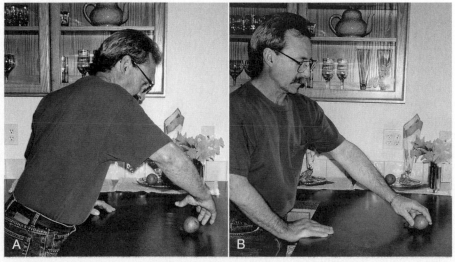

Fig. 20.19 (A) Client reaching forward with abnormal movement patterns. (B) Client using normal movement patterns while reaching forward with uninvolved side.

reactions and subsequent normal movement patterns. The amount of movement a client demonstrates is not as important as the quality of movement performed. The quality of the movement evoked is more important than the amount of movement. During an examination of the quality of movement, the primary concerns are whether the client exhibits good trunk control while moving, whether the movement is free from abnormal muscle tone and synergies, and whether the movement is coordinated.

Facilitation techniques and **inhibition techniques** are important tools in NDT. These techniques are used to normalize, or balance, tone. Normal tone fluctuates based on activity demands; however, if tone is abnormally high or abnormally low, tone problems in movement can occur. The clinician must determine where tone is too high or too low and use techniques to normalize the tone. Therefore abnormally high tone is reduced (inhibited) and abnormally low tone is increased (facilitated). Once normalization of tone occurs, patterns of movement are used to allow the client to experience the sensation of normal movement. These normal movement patterns are guided from proximal points of the body, primarily at the shoulder and pelvis (i.e., key points of control). The reduction of abnormal patterns of movement must be accomplished before normal, selective isolated movements can occur. Normal movement is impossible in the presence of abnormal tone (Brunnstrom, 1970).

According to the Bobaths, normalization of muscle tone can be accomplished by using one or more of the following techniques (Bobath, 1978; Davis, 1985; Eggars, 1984):
- Weight bearing over the affected side
- Trunk rotation
- Scapular protraction
- Anterior pelvic tilt/forward positioning of pelvis
- Facilitation of slow, controlled movements
- Proper positioning
- Incorporating the UE into activities

These techniques provide the foundation for NDT treatment. The techniques are most effective in rehabilitation when initiated in the acute (early) phase but can be used at any time in the treatment regimen.

Weight bearing over the hemiplegic side is an effective way to help regulate or normalize tone and is one of the most common techniques seen in the clinic. Weight bearing can be either facilitory or inhibitory. Weight bearing also provides sensory input to the hemiplegic side, which can increase the client's awareness of the hemiplegic side.

Weight bearing through the UE while sitting or standing helps to normalize tone throughout the arm. Weight bearing is most effective with clients who display a flexor synergy of the UE. The client can be brought into a weight-bearing position in preparation for a functional task during a treatment session.

Before weight bearing through the UE, the OT or OTA must prepare the UE and shoulder girdle. Preparations include scapular mobilization (gliding scapula into abduction, adduction, elevation, depression, and upward rotation). During UE weight-bearing activities, the client's hand should be placed on a mat or bench several inches away from the hip

to prevent wrist hyperextension. The humerus is placed in external rotation, with the elbow in extension. As the client shifts weight over the hemiplegic side, the clinician should not allow the UE to rotate internally or the elbow to collapse. The client should not hang on the arm during weight bearing but instead should move the body over the arm. This position will avoid undue stress on the elbow joint (Fig. 20.20). Weight bearing should not be painful to the client and should be avoided when hand pain or edema is present.

Trunk rotation, or the disassociation of the upper and lower trunk, is another effective way of normalizing tone and facilitating normal movement. Clients with hemiplegia often have a difficult time separating shoulder movements from the pelvic girdle, thus exhibiting a blocklike pattern. To promote disassociation, the clinician should introduce activities that incorporate or facilitate trunk rotation. This activates trunk musculature and aids in trunk stability, which will enhance UE movement.

Trunk rotation performed in the sitting or standing position promotes weight shifting to the hemiplegic side. Additional benefits from trunk rotation activities include increased sensory input and improved awareness of the hemiplegic side and trained compensation for visual field deficits (Fig. 20.21). Often the easiest and most effective way to facilitate trunk rotation is during functional daily activities.

Scapular protraction (scapular abduction) benefits clients who display a flexor synergy of the UE. Following the rule of working proximal to distal, the scapula should always be guided into forward protraction before the client attempts to raise the hemiplegic arm or open the hand. The scapula can be protracted if the clinician cradles the arm with one hand while placing the other hand along the scapula's medial border and then brings the arm forward. Once it is forward, this

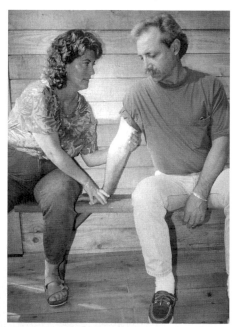

Fig. 20.20 Proper position for weight bearing over hemiplegic side during functional activity.

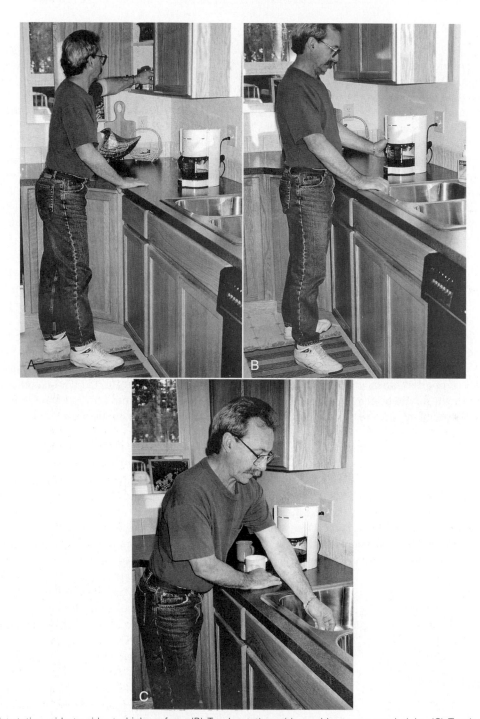

Fig. 20.21 (A) Trunk rotation, side to side, to high surface. (B) Trunk rotation, side to side, to counter height. (C) Trunk rotation, side to side, to lower surface.

position should be maintained for a few seconds before returning to the starting position. Care should be taken not to glide the scapula back into retraction. The pelvis in anterior pelvic tilt position is the optimal sitting position for clients with hemiplegia. This position provides proper alignment of the pelvis, shoulder, and head. Clients often assume a posterior pelvic tilt, which promotes abnormal posture such as thoracic spine flexion, scapular abduction, and cervical flexion. Such a posture has an adverse effect on swallowing, breathing, and visual-perceptual input. It also promotes misalignment

of the shoulder girdle and encourages the flexor synergy of the UE. When performing reaching activities in sitting, the clinician may help the client adjust the pelvis into a greater anterior tilt to promote more effective reaching patterns.

Slow, controlled movements should be facilitated in clients with high tone. Quick movements increase tone and tend to trigger an associated reaction, thus resulting in a flexor synergy of the UE; they should be avoided. Clients with high muscle tone should be instructed to perform activities slowly and in a controlled manner. The OT or OTA should provide feedback to help the client recognize when an activity is performed well.

Proper positioning of the client in bed, sitting, or standing facilitates the development of normal movement throughout the recovery process. It also helps to normalize muscle tone and provide normal sensory input to the body. For example, the preferred position for lying in bed is on the hemiplegic side (Brunnstrom, 1970; Eldred, 1967) (Fig. 20.22), with the client's back positioned parallel to the edge of the bed; head placed on a pillow, avoiding extreme flexion; shoulder fully protracted with at least 90 degrees of shoulder flexion; forearm supinated and elbow flexed; and hand placed under the pillow. An alternate position is with the elbow extended and the wrist either supported on the bed or slightly off the bed. The unaffected leg should be placed on a pillow. The affected leg is slightly flexed at the knee, with hip extended. To prevent the client from rolling onto the back, a pillow is placed behind the back and buttocks for support.

The proper position for sitting is with the client placing both feet flat on the floor, the hips near 90 degrees of flexion, the knees and ankles at less than 90 degrees of flexion, and the trunk extended. The head should be in midline and the affected arm fully supported when working at a table. During standing, the weight should be equally distributed on both LEs, the trunk symmetrical, and the head in midline (Brunnstrom, 1970).

Incorporating the UE into activity is important in promoting functional use of the involved UE. The involved UE can be incorporated via weight bearing, bilateral activities, or guided use. For example, during a writing activity, the client can use the involved arm to bear weight and stabilize the pad. Also, the client can assume a clasped hand (prayer) position of both UEs to perform bilateral, assisted self-ROM, or

therapists can guide and place the UE onto the arm of the chair when the client is pushing up to stand. Incorporating the involved UE into the activity will help develop selective use and bring NDT strategies into daily activities.

Occupational Therapy Application

In the NDT approach the OTA should design activities that can incorporate the hemiplegic UE into routine daily activities. This practice helps to reinforce techniques and interventions that the OT uses in designing the treatment plan. As previously discussed, the OTA can incorporate the hemiplegic UE into activities in three ways: (1) weight bearing through the involved UE during functional activities (Fig. 20.23A), (2) bilateral activities (see Fig. 20.23B), and (3) guided use (see Fig. 20.23C).

Bilateral activity (see Fig. 20.23B) and guiding the affected UE (see Fig. 20.23C) help to discourage the flexion synergy and allow the hemiplegic arm to participate in purposeful activities. In addition, when performing bilateral activities, the client experiences sensory input to the hemiplegic side, and the hemiplegic UE is brought into the visual field. Seeing the UE can be beneficial to clients who have unilateral neglect or visual inattention. Guiding the affected UE is another way to incorporate the hemiplegic UE into activities and can help the client experience normal movement patterns during purposeful activities.

When engaging clients in treatment activities using the NDT approach, the OTA should offer meaningful and practical tasks to enhance carryover from selected normal movement patterns to functional performance. Clients can more easily attend to and be motivated by activities that relate to real-life situations.

Dressing Activities. Dressing and grooming activities are a part of almost every occupational therapy program. These activities are familiar, purposeful, and necessary for independent functioning. The following methods illustrate how NDT principles can be used in ADL training.

The client should sit in a chair with a firm back when dressing. The chair provides stability and can improve balance. The same sequence should be followed to enhance learning.
   Donning shirt.
1. Position shirt across the client's knees with armhole visible and sleeve between knees (Fig. 20.24A).
2. Client bends forward at hips (inhibiting extensor synergy of LE), placing the affected hand in sleeve (see Fig. 20.24B).
3. Arm drops into sleeve; shoulder protraction and gravity inhibit UE flexor synergy.
4. Bring collar to neck.
5. Sit upright; dress nonhemiplegic side.
6. Button shirt from bottom to top.
   Donning underclothes and pants.
1. Clasp hands, and cross affected leg over nonhemiplegic leg (Fig. 20.25). (Clinician helps when needed.)
2. Release hands. Hemiplegic arm can dangle and should not be trapped in lap. When able, client can use affected hand as needed.
3. Pull pant leg over hemiplegic foot.

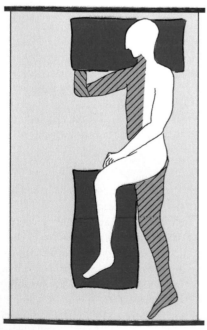

Fig. 20.22 Bed position when lying on affected side.

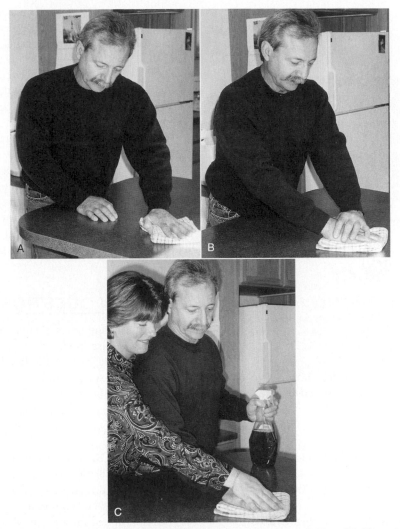

Fig. 20.23 (A) Proper position for weight bearing over hemiplegic side during functional activities. (B) Bilateral use of upper extremity (UE) during functional activities. (C) Guiding UE during functional activities.

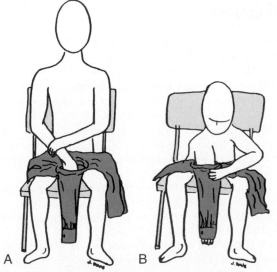

Fig. 20.24 (A) Dressing training. Shirt positioned across client's knees; armhole visible; sleeve dropped between knees. (B) Client bends forward at hips (inhibiting extension synergy of lower extremity) and places affected hand into sleeve.

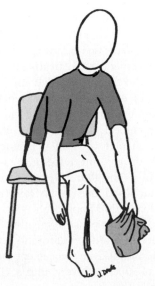

Fig. 20.25 Proper position for putting on undergarments and pants.

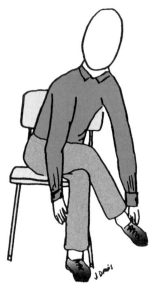

Fig. 20.26 Proper position for putting on socks and shoes.

4. Clasp hands to uncross leg.
5. Place nonhemiplegic foot in pant leg (no need to cross legs). This step is difficult because client must bear weight on hemiplegic side.
6. Pull pants to knees.
7. While holding onto waistband, client stands with clinician's help.
8. Zip and snap pants.
9. Clinician helps client return to sitting position.
   Donning socks and shoes.
1. Clasp hands and cross legs (as before) (Fig. 20.26).
2. Put sock and shoe on hemiplegic foot.
3. Cross nonhemiplegic leg; put on sock and shoe.

SUMMARY

Dysfunction of the sensorimotor cortex, caused by CNS damage due to conditions such as a CVA or traumatic brain injury, can result in muscle imbalance and abnormal muscle tone, poor posture, decreased balance, and loss of controlled movements. Neurotherapeutic treatment approaches are used with clients who exhibit these deficits. These approaches link neurophysiologic principles to the rehabilitation of clients with CNS dysfunction by targeting motor performance skills. In today's clinical practice, many of the techniques described in this chapter are used as adjunctive or preliminary techniques or are integrated into occupation-based treatment activities. The four traditional neurotherapeutic approaches are the Rood, the Brunnstrom (movement therapy), PNF, and Bobath/NDT approach.

The Rood approach emphasizes the use of controlled sensory stimulation to achieve purposeful motor responses (Huss, 1983). The Brunnstrom (movement therapy) approach describes stages of motor recovery after a CVA and applies treatment methods that help a client progress through the recovery stages. PNF uses a multisensory approach in which mass patterns of movement, usually performed in diagonals, help strengthen weak components of movements. The NDT (Bobath) approach emphasizes relearning normal movement while avoiding abnormal movement patterns. Principles include the normalization of muscle tone, avoidance of synergistic movement, and incorporation of the affected side into purposeful activities.

These neurotherapeutic treatment approaches are valuable tools for the OT and OTA. When possible, these techniques should be applied within an occupational context. OTAs planning to use these approaches should be trained and supervised until they achieve service competency. The challenge for all clinicians who use these approaches is to apply them in contexts that are meaningful and purposeful for the client and that will promote independent functioning.

▌REVIEW QUESTIONS

1. Give two examples of clients for whom neurotherapeutic approaches are used.
2. List two basic goals of the Rood approach.
3. List the stages of recovery of arm function after a CVA, as described by Brunnstrom.
4. Describe the UE flexor and extensor synergy patterns.
5. Describe how tone of voice can be used in PNF treatment.
6. Identify the UE PNF diagonal used to bring the hand to the mouth during feeding.
7. Identify the primary goal of the NDT approach.
8. Based on the NDT approach, identify the recommended position in bed for a client with hemiplegia.
9. Describe how the NDT techniques can be incorporated into a basic daily living task.

REFERENCES

Alpern, M., Lawrence, N., & Wolsk, D. (1976). *Sensory processes.* Belmont, CA: Brooks/Cole.

Ayres, J. (1972). *Sensory integration and learning disorders.* Los Angeles, CA: Western Psychological Services.

Ayres, J. (1974). *The development of sensory integration theory and practice.* Dubuque, IA: Kendall/Hunt.

Barr, M. L. (1974). *The human nervous system.* (2nd ed.). New York, NY: Harper & Row.

Bobath, B. (1978). *Adult hemiplegia: evaluation and treatment.* London: Heinemann.

Brunnstrom, S. (1970). *Movement therapy in hemiplegia.* New York, NY: Harper & Row.

Calliet, R. (1980). *The shoulder in hemiplegia.* Philadelphia, PA: FA Davis.

Clark, B. (1970). The vestibular system. In P. H. Mussen & M. R. Rosenweig (Eds.), *Annual review of psychology.* New York, NY: Harper & Row.

Crepeau, E. B, Cohn, E. S, Boyt Schell, B. (Eds.), (2004). *Willard & Spackman's occupational therapy.* (10th ed.). Philadelphia, PA: Lippincott Williams & Wilkins.

Davis, P. (1985). *Steps to follow.* Berlin: Springer-Verlag.

Dayhoof, N. (1975). Re-thinking stroke: soft or hard devices to position hands? *The American Journal of Nursing, 7,* 1142–1144.

Eggars, O. (1984). *Occupational therapy in the treatment of adult hemiplegia.* Rockville, MD: Aspen.

Eldred, E. (1967). Peripheral receptors: their excitation and relation to reflex patterns. *American Journal of Physical Medicine, 46,* 69–87.

Farber, S. (1967). *Neurorehabilitation: a multisensory approach.* Philadelphia, PA: WB Saunders.

Farber, S. (1974). *Sensorimotor evaluation and treatment procedures for allied health personnel.* Indianapolis, IN: Indiana University–Purdue University Medical Center.

Gillen, G. (2011). *Stroke rehabilitation: a function-based approach.* (3rd ed.). New York, NY: Mosby.

Goff, B. (1986). The Rood approach. In *Cash's textbook of neurology for physiotherapists.* (4th ed.). Philadelphia, PA: Lippincott.

Heininger, M., & Randolph, S. (1981). *Neurophysiological concepts in human behavior.* St Louis, MO: Mosby.

Hellebrandt, F. A., Schacle, M., & Carns, M. L. (1962). Methods of evoking the tonic neck reflexes in normal human subjects. *American Journal of Physical Medicine, 41,* 90–139.

Huss, J. (1983). Sensorimotor treatment approaches. In H. L. Hopkins, & H. D. Smith (Eds.). *Willard and Spackman's occupational therapy.* (6th ed.). Philadelphia, PA: Lippincott.

Jackson, J. H. (1931). Selected writings. (Vol. 1). London: Hodder & Stoughton.

Kotte, F. (1980). From reflex to skill: the training of coordination. *Archives of Physical Medicine and Rehabilitation, 61,* 551–561.

Kotte, F., & Lehmann, J. (1990). *Krusen's handbook of physical medicine and rehabilitation.* (4th ed.). Philadelphia, PA: WB Saunders.

Loeb, G. E., & Hoffer, J. A. (1981). *Muscle spindle function in muscle receptors in movement control.* London: Macmillan.

Loomis, J. E., & Boersma, F. J. (1982). Training right brain damaged clients in a wheelchair task: case studies using verbal mediation. *Physiotherapy Canada. Physiotherapie Canada, 34,* 204.

Matthews, P. B. C. (1978). Muscle spindles and their motor control. *Physiological Reviews, 58,* 763.

McCloskey, D. I. (1978). Kinesthetic sensibility. *Physiological Reviews, 58,* 764.

Myers, B. J. (1980). *Proprioceptive neuromuscular facilitation: concepts and application in occupational therapy as taught by Voss.* Chicago, IL: Rehabilitation Institute of Chicago, course notes.

Myers, B. J. (1982). *PNF: Patterns and application in occupational therapy.* Chicago, IL: Rehabilitation Institute of Chicago, videotape.

Nolte, J. (2002). *The human brain: an introduction to its functional anatomy.* (5th ed.). St Louis, MO: Mosby.

Perry, C. (1967). Principles and techniques of the Brunnstrom approach to the treatment of hemiplegia. *American Journal of Physical Medicine, 46,* 789–815.

Rood, M. (1954). Neurophysiological reactions as a basis for physical therapy. *The Physical Therapy Review, 34,* 444–449.

Rood, M. (1956). Neurophysiological mechanisms utilized in the treatment of neuromuscular dysfunction. *The American Journal of Occupational Therapy, 10,* 4.

Rood, M. (1962). The use of sensory receptors to activate, facilitate and inhibit motor response, automatic and somatic, in developmental sequence. In C. Sattely (Ed.), *Approaches to the treatment of clients with neuromuscular dysfunction.* Dubuque, IA: Brown.

Schmidt, R. A. (1991). Motor learning principles for physical therapy. In M. J. Lister (Ed.), *Contemporary management of motor control problems, proceedings of the 11 Step Conference.* Alexandria, VA: Foundation for Physical Therapy.

Stockmeyer, S. A. (1967). An interpretation of the approach of Rood to the treatment of neuromuscular dysfunction. *American Journal of Physical Medicine, 46,* 900–961.

Vallbo, A. B., Hagbarth, K. E., Torebjörk, H. E., & Wallin, B. G. (1979). Somatosensory, proprioception sympathetic activity in human peripheral nerves. *Physiological Reviews, 59,* 919–957.

Voss, D. E. (1959a). Application of patterns and techniques in occupational therapy. *The American Journal of Occupational Therapy, 8,* 191–194.

Voss, D. E. (1959b). Proprioceptive neuromuscular facilitation: the PNF method. In P. H. Pearson & L. E. Williams (Eds.), *Physical therapy services in the developmental disabilities.* Springfield, IL: Thomas.

Voss, D. E., Ionta, M. K., & Myers, B. J. (1972). *Proprioceptive neuromuscular facilitation.* (3rd ed.). Philadelphia, PA: Harper & Row.

Williams, P., & Warwick, R. (1975). *Functional neuroanatomy of man.* Philadelphia, PA: WB Saunders.

21

Interventions for Visual and Other Sensory Dysfunction

Lori M. Shiffman

OBJECTIVES

After reading this chapter, the student or the occupational therapy practitioner will be able to do the following:

1. Explain how sensory dysfunction or the absence of sensation affects areas of occupation.
2. Understand the process of recovery from peripheral nerve dysfunction.
3. Give examples of compensatory strategies for clients with sensory loss caused by central nervous system or peripheral nervous system lesions.
4. Describe how the OTA would educate the client and significant other(s) on injury prevention for a client who lacks protective sensation.
5. Understand the importance of the client's visual history and the functional effects of common visual conditions and diseases.
6. Identify some remedial and compensatory strategies used for treatment of visual dysfunction.
7. Explain the role of the OTA when working with clients with visual-perceptual dysfunction.
8. Identify the primary objectives of occupational therapy treatment of clients with balance dysfunction.

KEY TERMS

Somatosensory
Special sensory systems
Visual perception
Visual acuity
Oculomotor control
Visual fields
Visual attention
Visual scanning
Pattern recognition

Visual memory
Visual cognition
Age-related macular degeneration (ARMD or AMD)
Cataracts
Diabetic retinopathy
Glaucoma
Homonymous hemianopsia
Unilateral neglect
Visuovestibular integration

INTRODUCTION

Engagement in occupation relies on the ability to see, hear, feel, smell, taste, and balance; to organize sensations into meaningful representations of the world; and to plan and sequence responses (American Occupational Therapy Association, 2008). Impairments in client factors (body functions and body structures) can affect functional performance to varying degrees (American Occupational Therapy Association, 2008; World Health Organization, 2001). Levels include none, mild, moderate, severe, and complete impairment (World Health Organization, 2001). Sensation is unique to each person (Dunn, 2001). The occupational therapist (OT) assesses all areas of occupation for each client's unique context (American Occupational Therapy Association, 2008) and establishes a treatment plan to address all problem areas in conjunction with the client. The occupational therapy assistant (OTA) should be aware of the results to thus provide the planned therapeutic interventions in treatment. This chapter presents techniques the OTA might employ at entry level and introduces interventions the more experienced OTA practitioner, who has acquired service competency under qualified supervision, would provide.

This chapter focuses on the treatment of client factors of specific mental functions and sensory functions, including sensation, vision, visual-perception, and balance. The OTA should integrate information from this chapter (and from Chapters 9, 20, and 25) to understand how to provide the most effective interventions specific to each client, especially in more complex cases, such as the case study of James. The OTA should also be familiar with any and all precautions, strategies, and devices for each client; understand how to involve family, significant others, and caregivers; and coordinate treatment with other health care professionals.

CASE STUDY

James

James is a left-handed, 48-year-old man diagnosed 10 years ago with multiple sclerosis. He was recently discharged home, following an acute care hospital stay, due to a recent exacerbation (flareup). At discharge, James showed reduced attention and concentration, blurred vision, numbness and mild spasticity of all extremities, mild intention tremors of both upper extremities, lack of protective sensation of the right hand, mild weakness overall, balance issues, and limited endurance. James is married and has two sons, ages 9 and 11. James's wife, Maura, works full time as a dental hygienist. The referral for home health services included occupational therapy for evaluation and treatment, which the client completed at home. The OT recommended treatment twice weekly for 6 to 8 weeks. James and his family live in a one-floor ranch-style home, designed to accommodate his functional and mobility needs.

The occupational profile showed before his most recent flareup, James was responsible for his own personal activities of daily living (ADL) and selected instrumental activities of daily living (IADL). He prepared breakfast and dinner for his family, made lunch for himself, worked as a website designer 16 to 20 hours a week from his home office, edited his church's monthly newsletter, cared for his sons after school, and played sports videogames with them.

Maura performs the majority of household tasks. The children help with some of the chores. Immediate family members provide assistance with lawn care, home maintenance, home repair, and transportation. The occupational performance analysis showed James feeds himself but spills his food and drink, washes and dresses his upper body, and transfers with minimal to moderate assistance. He is no longer able to stand and uses a power scooter for all mobility. James requires moderate to maximal assistance for all lower body ADL. Regarding IADL, James microwaves leftovers for lunch and cares for his sons after school, including helping them with their homework. He takes more time to complete all ADL and IADL tasks.

Regarding performance skills, James showed reduced visual attention and concentration, blurred vision even with glasses, double vision, decreased light touch and proprioception of both sides (left greater than right), lack of protective sensation of his left hand, impaired memory, impaired body scheme, and visual agnosia. James stays out of bed and performs tasks for about 60 minutes before needing to rest in bed for at least 2 hours afterward. He stated that he values all of his life roles. Short-term goals include preparing breakfast for the family and after-school snacks for his sons, playing games with them, dressing himself with "a little help," and reading computer magazines. Maura returned to work 8 a.m. to 4 p.m. weekdays because she has used all of her time off. The client is also receiving physical therapy in the home twice a week for management of increased tone, weakness, balance, endurance, and functional mobility.

THE SENSORY SYSTEM

The sensory system of the brain processes all sensory information from internal and external sources (Gutman & Schonfeld, 2019). The sensory receptors receive information from a person's internal body structures and the external environment and sends it to the brain for interpretation. When the sensory system is functioning in an optimal way, the process works quickly and smoothly. Individuals are usually unaware of the importance of sensation until it is impaired or absent. When there is dysfunction in the sensory system, the process of receiving information can be slowed and disorganized, causing impairment (World Health Organization, 2001). Sensation is divided into the **somatosensory** and **special sensory systems** (Gutman & Schonfeld, 2019). The somatosensory components include the primary senses (i.e., tactile, deep pressure, pain, proprioception, kinesthesia) and the cortical senses (i.e., two-point discrimination, stereognosis) (Gutman & Schonfeld, 2019). The special sensory system includes vision, hearing, smell, taste, and balance (Gutman & Schonfeld, 2019).

INTERVENTIONS FOR SENSORY DYSFUNCTION

Sensory dysfunction can result from damage to or diseases of the central nervous system (CNS), peripheral nervous system (PNS), or cranial nerves. Lesions in any parts of the nervous system can cause dulled or absent sensation in affected areas.

Sensory dysfunction of CNS origin can cause sensory changes affecting the entire body, as occurs with multiple sclerosis (MS), traumatic brain injury (TBI), and cerebrovascular accident (CVA).

There are many terms used to identify sensory dysfunction. Some of them include *anesthesia* (complete loss of sensation), *paresthesia* (abnormal sensation such as tingling or "pins and needles"), *hypoesthesia* (decreased or dulled sensation or hyposensitivity), *hyperesthesia* (increased tactile sensitivity or hypersensitivity), *analgesia* (complete loss of pain sensation), and *hypoanalgesia* (diminished pain sensation). Clients with hyposensitivity or analgesia are at higher risk for injury because protective sensation is lacking, as in James's case. Clients with hypersensitivity such as those with Guillain-Barré syndrome (GBS) may find touch so painful they avoid it.

Sensory impairments severe enough to require treatment can make performing everyday occupations difficult (American Occupational Therapy Association, 2008; World Health Organization, 2001). James has decreased sensation in all four extremities. This dysfunction increases the time it takes for him to perform daily tasks and puts him at increased risk for injury. Due to fatigue, he spends more time lying down in bed or resting in one position in a recliner. These two factors cause him to stay in one position too long and make him susceptible to developing skin breakdown. The occupational therapy treatment plan includes client education on the importance of skin protective techniques. These include weight-shifting every 30 minutes when sitting and changing position every 2 hours when lying down.

OT and OTA collaboration plays a large role in improving the performance of persons with sensory changes or loss. This includes providing interventions to facilitate recovery of sensory function in clients for whom the nervous system will heal. It includes implementing compensatory strategies for permanent sensory loss. OTs and OTAs provide client education for both of these groups.

Treatment Guidelines

Before evaluation of sensory dysfunction can begin, the OT clinicians must know the medical diagnoses, cause of sensory impairments, prognosis for return of sensation, and current nerve function recovery. Information from review of the client's medical chart and the occupational therapy evaluation will indicate whether the treatment plan approach should be remedial, compensatory, or both.

Remedial treatment targets the plasticity of the human nervous system to restore the sensory cortical map (Scheiman, 2011). This approach works more successfully in clients with reversible conditions (usually involving the PNS). Candidates for sensory reeducation programming should understand the purpose of repeated practice and incorporating use of the involved body part in functional tasks (Callahan, 1995).

Compensatory treatment employs strategies for adjusting and adapting to sensory changes or losses. Such strategies include precautions to avoid injury, use of other senses, and environmental modifications.

The next section considers treatment approaches for the two major types of sensory dysfunction: CNS and PNS.

Central Nervous System Dysfunction

Effects of sensory changes. CNS damage can occur from trauma to the brain, conditions such as CVA, and diseases such as MS or Parkinson disease (PD). Sensory dysfunction can create functional difficulties in some or all of the areas of occupation (American Occupational Therapy Association, 2008; World Health Organization, 2001). The inclination to move is based on how well sensory information is received and interpreted by the brain. Persons with poor or no sensation have little or no urge to change position or move. James, for example, has less urge to move. Attempted movement may be clumsy or uncoordinated, even when muscle recovery is good. An example is trying to walk on a leg that has "fallen asleep." The leg muscles are still working, but the sensation has changed, and the movements feel awkward. Clients with sensory dysfunction are at much higher risk for injury, especially if they have cognitive deficits such as impulsivity, reduced safety awareness, or impaired memory. Such clients will require supervision for all tasks to prevent injury.

Sensory dysfunction may compound the effects of other deficits such reduced motor control or coordination. James has shown impairments in ADL, IADL, work, play, leisure, and social participation. These impairments are caused by several deficits in body function, including sensory function (American Occupational Therapy Association, 2008; World Health Organization, 2001). He requires assistance in self-care, can perform only minimal caregiver and home management chores, has suspended his work role, and has reduced leisure roles.

Client education. Sensory recovery can be a slow process. It may stop before full recovery is achieved. Because safety is primary, the clinician must teach clients, family members, caregivers, and others about the sensory changes and how to protect the affected body parts while the client is performing all tasks. First, the OTA helps the client increase self-awareness by recognizing sensory symptoms, learning to self-monitor, and maintaining vigilance to prevent injury. The clinician reinforces safety factors in every training session. For example, James would include whole-body skin checks to prevent pressure sores in his daily routine. The client should have many opportunities to practice skills and use them in daily tasks. The client who cannot self-monitor because of cognitive dysfunction will require constant supervision. In this case, the OT and OTA must educate the caregiver(s) on strategies to modify the environment to help the client function safely despite sensory dysfunction.

The OTA should be aware of the type of sensory impairment for each individual client. These may include absent, dulled, hypersensitive, or mixed impairment. To plan effective interventions, promote function, and prevent injury requires an understanding of all safety precautions and contraindications for treatment.

Intervention Approaches for Sensory Dysfunction

Remedial treatment. Remedial treatment changes client factors with the goal of restoring function (American Occupational Therapy Association, 2008). Remedial treatment for sensory loss, due to CNS lesions, is designed to promote recovery of sensory processing to allow a client to engage in purposeful, occupation-based activity. Traditional sensorimotor approaches have focused on promoting the return of muscle function of involved extremities using various forms of sensory input such as light touch, deep pressure, weight bearing, and the like (Bobath, 1990; Brunnstrom, 1970; Rood, 1956; Voss, 1959).

Carr and Shepherd (Carr & Shepherd, 1987) used task performance to promote motor relearning and assist sensory integration. Other practitioners have adapted sensory reeducation techniques to treat clients with sensory changes from CNS dysfunction using a graded approach. The client learns how to incorporate the involved body part(s) in purposeful activities such as leaning on the involved arm while seated at table (passive sensory training) followed by a progressive program to discriminate object by size (Dunn, 2001), temperature, texture, weight, and shape (Borstad et al., 2013). The client would increase use of the involved side as sensory and motor function recover. Some research supports the effectiveness of passive sensory training, but evidence for the effectiveness of active sensory retraining is limited (Borstad et al., 2013; Schabrun & Hillier, 2009).

OTAs should receive training in sensory reeducation techniques before utilizing them. After receiving the proper training, the OTA may perform sensory retraining techniques, such as modified constraint movement therapy (Page, Sisto, Levine, & McGrath, 2004), mirror therapy (Altschuler et al., 1999), sensory glove (Knutson, Gunzler, Wilson, & Chae, 2016), or task-specific training (Lang & Birkenmeier, 2014) to improve performance in functional tasks. Care should be given to ensure any sensory input does not cause unintentional consequences such injury or increased spasticity.

Compensatory treatment. Compensatory treatment focuses on modifying the context or activity to support occupational engagement (American Occupational Therapy Association, 2008). For clients with sensory deficits, compensatory strategies help the client maximize safe performance in occupation by working around problems associated with sensory dysfunction. Callahan (Callahan, 1995) proposed guidelines for clients with missing or impaired protective sensation of the hand: (1) Avoid or limit exposure of the involved body part(s) to hot, cold, and sharp objects; (2) distribute forces evenly when using tools or objects, by enlarging the handle; (3) take regular rest breaks; (4) use vision to guide movement and observe positioning of body parts; (5) check the skin for signs of stress (redness, edema, warmth) from excessive force or repetitive pressure, and rest the area if these signs occur; and (6) perform skin care as recommended by the physician to keep skin soft and pliant. Using these principles would lead to a recommendation for the modification of shaving for James. This would include having him shave with an electric razor, strapped to his dominant hand, rather than using a razor with blades.

Peripheral Nervous System Dysfunction

Effects of sensory changes. Peripheral nerve injury (PNI) may affect the nerve "cell body, the myelin sheath, axons, or neuromuscular junction" (Rubin, 2008). In the mildest and most temporary form of PNI, nerve fiber damage usually results from reduced circulation (Gutman & Schonfeld, 2019). Clinicians should always know the type of peripheral nerve damage and the expected recovery period. When the myelin (the outer coating of the nerve that insulates the axon) is damaged, regeneration occurs at a rate of about 1 mm per day (Rubin, 2008). The most severe injury involves the nerve cell body and results from penetrating wounds, crushing, or stretching (Gutman & Schonfeld, 2019). Cell body regrowth is slow (~ 8 mm/day (Rubin, 2010) [~ 0.33 inch/day]), and because several of the branches from the nerve trunks can be over 1 m in length (~ 40 inches), recovery may take several months to 1 year (Rubin, 2010). During recovery, clients often experience increased sensitivity of the affected parts, may guard sensitive areas, and avoid using them.

PNS dysfunction caused by PNI can result from a variety of causes: nerve injury (carpal tunnel syndrome), entrapment (spinal stenosis), metabolic disease (diabetes), or inflammation (GBS). Damage can occur in one set of nerves or in several, depending on the cause. Symptoms of PNI include muscle weakness, hyperesthesia, hypoesthesia, lack of sensation, pain, muscle atrophy, loss of the ability to perspire, and changes in the quality of the skin and nails innervated by the affected nerves (Gutman & Schonfeld, 2019). The skin can dry out and may be more easily injured. If the client has no open wounds or infection, early treatment of hypersensitivity

is best—before sensory reeducation begins (Sharma-Abbott & Larson, 2015). Specific techniques for sensory reeducation are beyond the scope of this chapter. OTAs should refer to specific state practice guidelines to determine the level appropriate for their scope of practice.

Client education. Education focuses on injury prevention and function. Clients usually perform better and experience less pain when they are in control and can move the involved body parts on their own with their uninvolved arm (rather than having someone else moving them). The OTA can teach clients how to instruct others to help them move without causing discomfort or injury. If cognitive dysfunction prevents a client from using an involved part safely, then the clinician would recommend constant supervision.

Remedial treatment. Remedial treatment or sensory reeducation is introduced after desensitization treatment is completed (Waylett-Rendell, 2004). The purpose is to promote recovery of dulled or absent sensation via specific sensory input. When nerves in the hand are repaired or recover after injury, the messages to the brain are altered. The new pattern of neural impulses may be so different that the brain fails to identify the sensory stimulus, and the client may incorrectly interpret the sensory information. Sensory reeducation introduced immediately after surgical nerve repairs can help the client "maintain the cortical representation of the injured hand and upper extremity in the brain" (Lundborg & Rosen, 2011) and enhances the client's potential for functional recovery after nerve injury (Dellon, 1981). The OT generally provides sensory reeducation. The OTA with proven advanced proficiency may perform it under the OT's direct supervision. Box 21.1 shows some of the elements of a sensory reeducation program for PNI (Dellon, 1981).

Compensatory treatment. Increasing clients' awareness of the specific sensory deficits associated with PNS dysfunction, especially protective sensation, is key to ensuring safety during occupational performance. Education for both client and

---

> **BOX 21.1 Elements of a Sensory Reeducation Program for Impairments of the Peripheral Nervous System (Dellon, 1981; Sharma-Abbott & Larson 2015)**
>
> **Early phase:** Education on protecting the involved body part. The client observes the therapist touching the involved area once a day progressing to several times a day. The client watches the uninvolved body part move in a mirror, visualizing movement of the involved part.
>
> **Second phase:** First with eyes open and then with eyes closed, the OT moves an object such as a pencil eraser up and down the affected area to enhance sensation of moving touch. As this sense recovers, the clinician introduces constant touch, then gentle pressure.
>
> **Late phase:** Graded exercises targeting object recognition tactilely by discriminating "size, shape, weight, temperature, and texture." (Sharma-Abbott & Larson, 2015)
>
> **Frequency of training:** Training occurs two to four times daily for sessions of 10 to 15 minutes.

family is necessary to effectively utilize compensatory training for clients with reduced or absent sensation. The OT and OTA would determine recommendations for each client, based on the client's goals and life situation. In some cases, recommendations may be made for the client to avoid using the involved limb during functional activities that are potentially unsafe, especially if the person is impulsive, inattentive, or lacks safety awareness. The client with permanent sensory dysfunction must learn how to function safely in all environments with the assistance of others.

SUMMARY OF INTERVENTIONS FOR SENSORY DYSFUNCTION

The skin receptors and sensory organs send information from the environment to the brain through the peripheral and spinal nerves. Sensation provides information about the external environment necessary to guide purposeful and effective motor actions. Sensory dysfunction disrupts the link between sensation and movement. The clinician should be aware of the type and extent of sensory dysfunction and expected recovery for each client. Lack of protective sensation can increase the client's risk for injury. OTs and OTAs can help improve the daily lives of persons with sensory impairments by maximizing safe, functional use of the involved extremity and by providing remedial and compensatory interventions. Lifelong changes in sensation will require the client with sensory loss to adapt. Sensory reeducation and remediation require advanced training and should not be performed by the entry-level OTA.

INTERVENTIONS FOR VISION DEFICITS AND VISUAL-PERCEPTUAL DYSFUNCTION

Understanding and using visual information requires vision and **visual perception**. Vision is a sensory function involving the reception of sensory information through the visual receptors (American Occupational Therapy Association, 2008; World Health Organization, 2001). Visual perception is the process by which information from visual receptors is integrated with information from the other senses and interpreted by the brain. This process requires the brain to combine information from all of the senses: visual, proprioceptive (pressure), kinesthetic (sense of movement), tactile (touch), vestibular (balance and equilibrium), olfactory (smell), and auditory (hearing). In adapting to the environment, the brain puts together the separate pieces of sensory information it receives, integrating them to form a visual image of the environment. Because sensory information coming into the CNS is constantly changing, the picture is dynamic and constantly changing, too.

James's visual dysfunction includes blurred and double vision. His perceptual dysfunction includes impaired body scheme and visual agnosia (reduced ability to recognize objects by sight). Visual, physical, and cognitive problems

increase James's performance time for ADL. The OTA could incorporate compensatory strategies into ADL training. Examples include allowing more time to perform tasks, spreading out the supplies (increasing contrast by placing a white washcloth on a dark countertop when performing upper body bathing, using the same sequence each time when using his body parts while dressing to improve body scheme awareness, or using large-print waterproof labels to address visual agnosia).

Visual acuity can be defined as how clearly the human eye can discriminate detail and contrast. It can be affected by nearsightedness, farsightedness, presbyopia, astigmatism, eye diseases, trauma to the eye, or CNS dysfunction. These eye conditions may result in damage to the eye structure or function (World Health Organization, 2001). Vision impairment affects 1.3 billion people worldwide, and is expected to increase (World Health Organization, 2018).

Refractive errors are the most common cause of vision problems in the United States (Vision Health Initiative, 2015). More than 30 million adults older than 40 are nearsighted; more than 11.5 million are farsighted (Congdon et al., 2004). About 3.3 million people over age 40 are legally blind or have low vision (Vision Health Initiative, 2015). Individuals with best corrected vision of 20/200 in the "better seeing eye" are considered legally blind (Vision Health Initiative, 2015). Low vision is defined as having best corrected vision of 20/40 or worse (Vision Health Initiative, 2015). The most common causes of blindness or low vision are associated with aging, which include "age-related macular degeneration, cataract, diabetic retinopathy, and glaucoma" (Vision Health Initiative, 2015).

The OT practitioner should be aware of the client's preexisting visual acuity and if the client uses glasses or contacts, and what type. Nearsightedness, farsightedness, and astigmatism are often easily corrected with prescription corrective lenses (i.e., eyeglasses or contact lenses). As adults age, they typically require glasses to read because of presbyopia (farsightedness associated with age-related changes of the lens). Many use over-the-counter glasses, which do not account for any differences between each eye or astigmatism. Clients who require correction for both nearsightedness and farsightedness wear bifocal, trifocal, or progressive lenses. Some clients may wear two different contact lenses, one for distance and one for near. The lenses of the eyeglasses may show a distinct demarcation(s) of the different corrections such as with bifocals or trifocals or may be unnoticeable, as with progressive lenses. Many modifications such as ultraviolet (UV) protection from UVC/UVB/UBA radiation, blue light blocking, progressives (lenses that are clear indoors and darken in the sunlight), and glare-proofing are available. Some individuals choose to get laser eye surgery to correct nearsightedness. Everyone should always wear sunglasses with UV protection outside to protect the retina from the damaging UV rays of the sun.

The occupational therapy evaluation includes exploring the client's visual history, identifying the presence of visual symptoms, whether corrective lenses are used and for what purpose, the age the client began wearing glasses and for what purpose, age of current glasses and their condition, date of the last professional vision examination by a vision specialist, name of the vision specialist, the presence of eye diseases, and any history of eye injury or eye surgery. The OT then assesses visual functions, including visual acuity, **oculomotor control**, and **visual field** testing. All clients who use or need corrective lenses should have current eyeglasses or contact lenses that provide optimal corrected vision. Some clients who used contact lenses prior to their illness or injury may no longer be able to; they may have to return to wearing eyeglasses. It is not unusual for clients to have lost their glasses or to wear outdated or ill-fitting glasses. The OT may request a referral for a vision examination from the client's physician. The OT and OTA would include use of devices recommended by the vision specialist in treatment. Examples include magnifying devices such as glasses, a telemicroscope or a handheld electromagnifier such as closed-circuit television [CCTV], among others (Freeman, 2011). The OT and the OTA assist the client in determining environmental modifications for safe mobility and function within the home. Some examples of this include removing clutter to clear pathways and maintaining good lighting in all areas (American Occupational Therapy Association, 2013). Because James has blurred and double vision with his glasses, he might benefit from a current vision assessment.

The OT and OTA may assist clients in establishing routines related to proper use (e.g., wearing them for functional mobility, reading, all tasks) and care. Clients may need reminders to remember to wear glasses, practice putting them on and taking off, cleaning them, and putting them in and out of their case. A headband can secure glasses and prevent loss. Eye glass chains that go around the neck can be a safety hazard and are not usually recommended. All clients function better when vision is properly corrected.

Visual Perception, Organization, and Processing

Visual-perceptual skills are organized in a hierarchy of levels that work together (Fig. 21.1) (Warren, 1993). The ability to use visual-perceptual skills to adapt to the environment depends on the interaction of all of these skills. One should read the hierarchy from the bottom up. First, at the foundation level, the brain must receive clear, concise visual information from the environment through the three primary visual functions: visual acuity, oculomotor control, and the visual fields.

Visual acuity ensures visual information sent to the brain is sharp, clear, and accurate. Oculomotor control occurs by effective coordination of eye movements by the eye muscles. The visual fields represent reception of complete information from the environment in all areas of vision. These primary visual functions act together so that humans can focus on, see, and follow moving targets in the environment. These functions also provide the basis for all higher-level skills. James has blurred vision, thus indicating reduced visual acuity. He also has double vision that may indicate problems with eye coordination, which commonly occurs in individuals with MS. He does not show any visual field deficits.

Visual attention, the next level in the hierarchy, involves fixating gaze on an image for as long as required and shifting to other objects as needed. When processing speed is reduced, the client must attend visually long enough to process all of

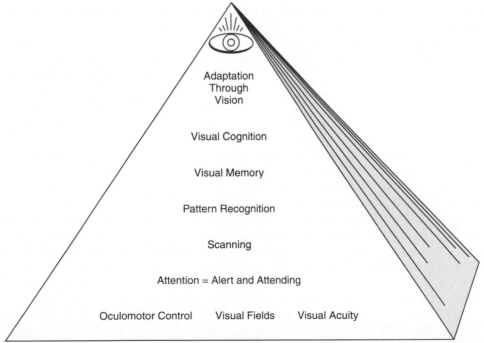

Fig. 21.1 Hierarchy of visual perceptual skill development in the central nervous system. (Courtesy Josephine C. Moore. From Warren M. A hierarchical model for evaluation and treatment of visual perceptual dysfunction in adult-acquired brain injury. Part I. *American Journal of Occupational Therapy.* 1993;47:42.)

the information. James has reduced attention and concentration, which may affect visual attention as well.

Visual scanning consists of shifting attention from one visual target to another in smooth succession while the image is seen clearly. Scanning allows a person to focus visual gaze on a chosen object on the area of the retina with the greatest ability to process detail, even when the eyes, the head, or the object is moving. Adults scan in an organized, systematic, and efficient pattern (National Eye Institute, 2016; Warren, 1990). James's reduced attention and blurred/double vision would slow scanning speed.

Pattern recognition is the ability to identify the important features of objects and the environment and to use these features to distinguish an object from its surroundings and objects from each other (Gianutsos, Ramsey, & Perlin, 1988). James has visual agnosia, which is a facet of pattern recognition.

Visual memory is the next skill level in the hierarchy. The brain must be able to create and retain a mental image of the observed object in the mind's eye and process visual information in short-term memory. The brain must also be able to store the image in long-term memory and then remember the information from a selection of choices (recognition) or retrieve it from memory (recall) when needed.

The highest skill in the hierarchy is **visual cognition**, the ability to manipulate visual information mentally, understand the mental image, and integrate it with other sensory information, using all the other skills described in the hierarchy. Visual cognition serves as a foundation for all learning.

The brain works most efficiently when all systems work together. A disruption of any of the skills at any level in the hierarchy will reduce performance at that level and all the levels above, as seen with James.

Understanding the role of vision at each level is key to treatment planning. The following information is provided to prepare the OTA to provide treatment under supervision of the OT.

Primary Visual Dysfunction

Visual Acuity. Visual acuity is more than just the ability to read a line on the letter chart. It represents a complex interaction between the optical system, which focuses light at the back of the eye on the retina, and the CNS processing, which transforms that light into the visual images seen. CNS visual processing begins at the cornea where light comes in and passes through the lens to the retina, where the sensory photoreceptors respond and send those signals through the optic nerves for interpretation in the brain. Visual images must be focused precisely. The retinal field contains an estimated 1 million discretely coded photoreceptors, which enable the CNS to detect minute differences between patterns.

The four most common optical deficits reducing acuity are myopia, hyperopia, presbyopia, and astigmatism. These conditions usually affect both eyes, causing blurred vision and are usually corrected with glasses or contacts. In myopia (nearsightedness), the image of an object is focused in front of the retina. In hyperopia, the image comes into focus behind the retina (National Eye Institute, 2016). Presbyopia is caused by age-related changes or reduced elasticity of the lens of the eyes. It affects most adults age 40 years and older. Astigmatism is an irregular curvature of the cornea. Persons with two or more of these optical defects together require bifocal, trifocal, or progressive lenses, containing correction for each problem.

The health and integrity of the retina influences the image quality sent on to the brain. The macular area of the retina is particularly critical for identification of visual detail. Unfortunately, this structure is also vulnerable to eye or systemic diseases that can damage its function. The clinician may treat clients with eye conditions or diseases such as **age-related macular degeneration** (**ARMD** or **AMD**), **cataracts**, **diabetic retinopathy**, and **glaucoma**. Preexisting vision conditions, which previously may have affected visual function minimally, may become a bigger factor affecting functional performance such as after experiencing a CVA or TBI.

ARMD affects acuity of central vision and is the leading cause of "irreversible loss of central vision of the elderly" (Mehta, 2019a), as well as permanent impairment of reading and closeup vision for older adults (Khazaeni, 2019b). It affects 1.8 million adults aged 40 and older in the United States, and is expected to increase to 3 million by 2020 (Friedman et al., 2004; Khazaeni, 2019b). Risk factors include hypertension and smoking (Khazaeni, 2019b). There are two types of ARMD, dry and wet. ARMD always starts as dry. About 10% of individuals with the dry type will become wet (Khazaeni, 2019b). Central visual loss occurs gradually over years and is painless (Khazaeni, 2019b). Peripheral vision stays intact but the central loss can lead to legal blindness (Kitchel, 2004) (best corrected vison in one eye to 20/200). Macular damage of the retina significantly reduces the ability to distinguish visual details and color, such as identifying faces of family members (Sokol-McKay, 2005). Individuals with ARMD can ambulate using their residual vision but do not have sufficient vision to drive (Sokol-McKay, 2005). There is no cure for ARMD, but control of hypertension, cessation of smoking, dietary supplements, drug treatment, and laser treatment may slow its progression (Khazaeni, 2019b). Clients with ARMD who require occupational therapy would likely be seen by the OT with advanced training in low-vision rehabilitation (Sokol-McKay, 2005).

The leading cause of blindness worldwide is cataracts (Khazaeni, 2019a). Cataracts reduce the quality of the image projected onto the retina by clouding the lens of one or both eyes. More than 20 million adults in the United States older than 40 have one or more cataracts (Khazaeni, 2019a). They are caused by aging, trauma, smoking, alcohol use, systemic diseases such as diabetes, and exposure to UV light (Khazaeni, 2019a). The incidence of cataracts is increasing as the population ages. Cataracts result in a gradual, painless loss of vision (Khazaeni, 2019b). Early symptoms of cataracts are cloudiness of vision, which mimics seeing through plastic wrap. Other early symptoms include decreased contrast, issues with glare, difficulty differentiating blue from black, and needing more light to see (Khazaeni, 2019b). Treatment involves surgical removal of the affected lens(es), replaced with an intraocular lens implant, which usually improves vision to 20/40 (Khazaeni, 2019b). Although the implanted lenses have some UV protection, clients should always wear sunshades with UV protection before and after surgery.

Diabetic retinopathy affects both eyes. It is caused by damage to the retinas due to dilation and leakage of retinal blood vessels or the growth of abnormal retinal blood vessels (Congdon et al., 2004; National Eye Institute-National Institutes of Health, 2015). Spots of missing vision (blind spots) occur first, progressing to blurred vision and then more widespread visual loss (Mehta, 2019b). About 4.1 million Americans (40−45% with diabetes) have diabetic retinopathy, 50% of which are unaware they have the condition (National Eye Institute-National Institutes of Health, 2015). It is a "major cause of blindness, particularly of working-age adults" (Mehta, 2019b). Severity of disease is dependent on the "duration of diabetes, blood glucose levels, and blood pressure levels" (Mehta, 2019b). Control of these symptoms can delay the onset and lessen the severity of the disease. Medications, laser therapy, or surgery can be effective in reducing symptoms (Mehta, 2019b; Vision Health Initiative, 2015). Individuals with diabetes "should get a comprehensive dilated eye exam at least once a year" and individuals with diabetic retinopathy more frequently as indicated (Mehta, 2019c). Low-vision rehabilitation might be provided by the OT with advanced training.

Glaucoma is the second leading cause of blindness in the United States and worldwide. It is a progressive, usually bilateral disease affecting more than 3 million American adults. It is caused when increased pressure in the eye damages the optic nerve (Rhee, 2017a; Rhee, 2017b). Glaucoma is six times more common in adults over age 60 (Rhee, 2017b). The two types of glaucoma are closed angle and open angle. Closed-angle glaucoma has a sudden painful onset and is a medical emergency (Rhee, 2017b). Open-angle glaucoma is the most common. It is a slowly progressive, painless type causing optic nerve damage due to increasing eye pressure (Rhee, 2017b). Blind spots occur first, then gradually progress to loss of peripheral vision causing tunnel vision (Rhee, 2017b). Risk factors include a family history of glaucoma, diabetes, African American and Hispanic descent, and age 40 and older (Rhee, 2017a). Medical treatment includes the lifelong use of eyedrops, laser surgery, or incisional surgery (Rhee, 2017b). Although glaucoma can be treated effectively, any visual loss is permanent. Some clients with glaucoma may require low-vision rehabilitation provided by the OT with advanced training.

The conditions discussed in this section are progressive to varying degrees and may be treated by medications or surgery. These interventions are provided by a vision specialist such as an ophthalmologist (MD) or an optometrist (OD). Only ophthalmologists can perform eye surgery. Treatment can also include use of prescriptions lenses. Clients may be candidates for low-vision assessment and interventions through local health care systems or state/national resources. Optometrists certified in vision development (COVD) or

fellows in vision development (FCOVD) are specially trained in evaluating and treating children and adults with the full spectrum of visual issues and impairments.

OTs and OTAs may work with other professionals with specialized training in the rehabilitation of visually impaired clients. These include "teachers of visually impaired (TVIs), orientation and mobility specialists (O&Ms)" (Duffy, Huebner, & Wormsley, 2011), vision rehabilitation therapists (VRT), and low-vision therapists (CLVT). These specialists complete certificate, bachelor's, or master's degree programs. OTs and OTAs coordinate treatment with vision specialists to maximize function and safety in all relevant areas of occupation. Any OT or OTA can complete certification as an O&M specialist. The OT can achieve Board Certification in Low Vision (SCLV) and the OTA can achieve Specialty Certification in Low Vision (SCLV-A) through the American Occupational Therapy Association.

Treatment Interventions for Visual Acuity Deficits. There are many conditions in which visual acuity loss is progressive or permanent. The OT can teach clients how to adapt the environment and/or the activity to increase function. This can be done by modifying the background contrast, illumination, background pattern, size, and spacing.

The key to using contrast effectively is to identify the items the clients need to see and to increase the contrast with surrounding features. Individuals with low vision have difficulty distinguishing groups of colors that fall in the same value range such as the dark colors (navy blue, brown, and black) or light or pastel colors when used with each other (VisionAware, 2019a). Light lettering on a dark background is sometimes easier to read (Duffy, 2019c). Mixing colors of different shades (light to dark) is more effective. James would see dark food containers on a light shelf much better.

CLINICAL PEARL

To experience the dark−light value range, place several objects similar in shape but different in color next to each other on a table. Step back and squint. You will see darker colors are harder to tell apart and lighter colors tend to blend together. To achieve high contrast for a person with vision impairment, choose colors that look different when you squint (e.g., black print on a matte [not shiny] background, white on navy blue, or yellow on black). You can then individualize treatment based on each client's needs.

Increasing light intensity and illumination better enables objects and environmental features to be seen more clearly. For example, using a portable flashlight would make it easier to read a menu in a restaurant. The challenge is to increase illumination without increasing glare. Natural and white lighting are better for this than standard fluorescent lighting.

Patterned backgrounds camouflage objects lying on them. Even people with excellent vision have trouble finding a paper clip or earring on a patterned carpet. Solid colors are recommended for background surfaces such as bedspreads, bed sheets, placemats, dishes, countertops, rugs, towels, carpets, and furniture coverings, as they are optimal for clients with vision impairment.

Individuals with reduced visual acuity can see items such as maps, photos, and print more easily if the size is increased. Standard font size of print for the sighted population varies from 8 to 13 point (Kitchel, 2004). Print size of 18 point is considered large, but clients may require print that large or larger, depending on their needs (Duffy, 2019c). Font styles without serifs (additional strokes) such as Arial are easier for individuals with low vision to read (Duffy, 2019b). An example would be **Apples** (18-point font and easier to read without serifs) versus Apples (18-point font but more difficult to read with serifs). Specific changes in print proportions, character thickness, edging, or style can improve readability, which can be found in the Accessibility features on all electronic devices (Khazaeni, 2019a). E-readers are also easily adaptable to meet the needs of users with visual impairment (American Occupational Therapy Association, 2013). The OTA could help James select the optimal features, including font or color coding, which can be used to customize large-print reading materials and therapy instructions using an e-reader or perhaps audiobooks.

Clutter in an environment causes the same problems as pattern. Spacing objects farther apart can further improve visibility. A person who has difficulty identifying objects will perform better when asked to scan a kitchen shelf with a few orderly items, rather than one with dozens of items. The same is true of closets, drawers, desks, bookshelves, countertops, and clinic areas.

Oculomotor Control. The process by which the eye muscles control eye movements is oculomotor control. Oculomotor skills include eye alignment, range of motion (ROM), speed, and coordination. Impaired oculomotor control can cause several problems. To maintain a single visual image, the eyes must line up evenly and move together. If the muscles of one eye are paretic (weakened), the eye may drift toward one side of the eye socket (i.e., drift either in or out). When the movement of one eye does not match the other, the person often sees a double image (called diplopia or double vision) (Scheiman, 2011). To eliminate the double image, the client often tilts the head or closes one eye, which reduces depth perception. If ROM is affected, the person may not be able to move the eyes in all planes as well, causing difficulty with using the eyes together in a coordinated manner, reducing scanning speed. The client may complain of headaches, eye strain, or neck pain. Treatment for oculomotor dysfunction should be coordinated by the OT with the guidance of vision specialists (Gianutsos & Matheson, 1987). This may include vision therapy or partial occlusion or blocking of eyeglass lens (es). Eye patching is much less used than in the past and would only be used currently when recommended by a vision specialist.

Visual Field Deficits. Clients may experience a number of visual field deficits or field cuts. These can greatly limit the client's function in near (i.e., reading) and far (i.e., functional mobility) tasks. **Homonymous hemianopsia**, the loss of visual field in the corresponding right or left halves of each eye, is the most common visual impairment occurring after a CVA (Warren, 2009), but may occur after TBI. The physician or vision specialist would diagnose hemianopsia. The OTA should be familiar with signs such as (1) placing objects in one visual field, (2) problems finding easily seen items in the environment, (3) consistently bumping into objects, and (4) making consistent errors in reading. The most significant change occurs in visual scanning. Instead of spontaneously using a wider scanning strategy, clients tend to shorten their scope of scanning (Windsor, Ford, & Windsor, 2020d). The person experiencing visual field loss is often unaware of any absence of vision and may not be aware of the boundary between the seeing and nonseeing field. Instead, they (incorrectly) perceive a complete visual scene. Objects seem to disappear and reappear without warning. The client tends to miss or misidentify details when viewing objects. Writing and reading can be a challenge, causing frustration for the client.

Intervention strategies for visual field deficits. Interventions for clients with visual field deficits involve education combined with strategies. First, the clinician educates the client on becoming aware of field cuts and the effect they have on functional performance. Under the direction of the OT, the OTA then incorporates recommended techniques and devices into meaningful activities, to improve scanning and saccades in all visual fields. Families and caregivers should be included in this. Remedial strategies focus on increasing the accuracy, speed, scope, and effectiveness of the scanning and saccadic patterns. The client learns to use head movements to compensate for any limitations in the visual field.

Additional compensatory strategies include modification of the client's environment. These include things such as adding color and contrast to borders (door frames, furniture, edges of steps, etc.), reducing patterns in the environment, decluttering it, and increasing contrast of objects. Field expansion prism lenses prescribed by a vision specialist can be effective at improving functional mobility in those with homonymous hemianopsia (Bowers, Keeney, & Peli, 2008). An example of this would be to wear them when shopping in the grocery store.

The OT would address visual-perceptual and motor skills first because these are necessary for normal visual reading skills (Leff et al., 2000). The OT and OTA would work in conjunction with speech-language pathologists to address reading and writing issues. When reading, clients with visual field deficits have difficulty locating the correct line of print, staying on the line, and seeing all of the words. A left visual field deficit impairs the ability of clients to move their eyes to the far left hand margin of the reading material when beginning a new line of text. Clients with right field cuts may not read all the way to the end of each sentence. Compensatory techniques such as red line boundary markers, L-shaped print blockers (Scheiman, 2011), turning the reading material at a 45-degree angle to a 90-degree angle, and looking for the last letter of a word (rather than the first) are effective (Rummel, 2020; Scheiman, 2011). The client is taught to move the eyes to find the red line to avoid missing any of the material. A ruler, an index card, or print blocker can be held under the line being read to assist clients to stay in line while reading. The client can also check off each line to help keep his or her place. To learn how to stay on the line when writing, the client can learn to watch the pen tip and maintain visual fixation as the hand moves across the page and into the area of visual field loss.

Driving "is a complex task requiring the integration of visual-perceptual stimuli, information processing, good judgment and decision making, and the performance of appropriate motor responses" (Classen et al., 2009). Driving is highly valued because it enables individuals to participate in a variety of areas of occupation (Classen et al., 2009). Each US state has specific guidelines regarding the amount of vision required for driving. A client with impairments needs to be evaluated and cleared by a physician. Certified driving rehabilitation specialists (CDRS), who are OTs (see Chapter 15), specialize in driving evaluation. Clients may be referred to them for testing. These tests have three outcomes: (1) Pass the evaluation without restrictions, (2) pass with restrictions, or (3) fail to meet the criteria and have to discontinue driving. Restrictions may include driving during daylight hours, limiting distance, and avoiding driving in inclement weather. Those who fail to meet the criteria must surrender their driver's license resulting in loss of driving privileges. There are many other additional factors that would determine continuation of driving such as medications, orientation, memory, reaction time, and safety awareness.

Deficits in Visual Skills Resulting From CNS Dysfunction

Visual Attention and Scanning. Visual attention can be divided into two categories that work together: focused or selective visual attention and ambient or peripheral visual attention (Rensink, 2010). Focused or selective attention enables persons to discriminate visual details accurately, recognize persons, and identify objects (Rensink, 2010). Ambient or peripheral attention allows people to use peripheral vision to detect and locate moving items in the environment (Rensink, 2010).

Injury to the brain can disrupt normal scanning patterns and awareness resulting in **unilateral neglect** (or hemi-inattention, hemispatial neglect, spatial neglect, hemispatial inattention). Right-sided brain lesions result in left unilateral neglect. About 20% of adults with lesions of the left brain show right unilateral neglect (Vahlberg & Hellstrom, 2008). Ways in which neglect manifests are clients not showing awareness of the involved side of their body, not dressing the involved side, missing food on half of their plate, and bumping into objects on the involved side (Goff, 2010). The OTA can use recommendations made by the OT to identify strategies to address each client's unique unilateral neglect in treatment.

Unilateral neglect differs from visual field deficits, such as hemianopsia. They seem similar but have differing effects on performance. A visual field deficit causes vision loss, impairing the ability to gather visual information in the field by not moving the eyes far enough to see the visual information. In contrast, the client with unilateral neglect makes no attempt to search for information on the involved side (opposite of the brain lesion) (Heilman, Valenstein, & Watson, 2000).

Clients with visual field loss may have more awareness of their deficits than those with unilateral neglect, but they still have difficulty completing tasks requiring awareness and scanning, such as walking through a mall (Yang, Chung, Li-Tsang, & Fong, 2013). Those who experience both visual field deficits and neglect miss visual information on the side of the field deficit and are not able to direct their attention toward there to compensate. This leads to a greater degree of functional impairment.

Pattern Recognition. Decreased pattern recognition results when a person does not thoroughly and efficiently scan the environment for objects. Clients with right-sided brain injury may fail to recognize an object or pattern because they do not perceive or see all of it. Clients with left-sided brain injuries may be aware of objects but have difficulty identifying them. James has visual agnosia (inability to recognize and name objects), suggesting that he has left-sided brain involvement. Treatment would include incorporating graded pattern recognition into functional tasks the client would usually do.

Visual Memory. Visual memory depends on accurate pattern recognition. When an important aspect of an object is not perceived, the brain generates an inaccurate representation. If the representation is not accurate, the CNS may not recognize the object or may misidentify it. When this occurs, the CNS has difficulty establishing an accurate visual memory of the object.

Because we do not store information through vision alone, information stored in memory can be retrieved through other senses. If a person does not recognize an object by looking at it, the person can pick it up and feel it or repeat its name aloud. Thus a client with a visual deficit that results in inaccurate pattern recognition may still function reasonably well in ADL provided a variety of sensory information is available.

Visual Cognition. Visual cognition is the result of the integration of all the foundation skills—visual attention, visual scanning, pattern recognition, and memory. Any deficit in these lower-level skills reduces the person's ability to apply these skills and adapt to environmental demands.

Deficits in visual cognition result in problems identifying the spatial properties of objects and mentally manipulating these properties in thought. Many terms are used to describe the deficits that occur in visual cognition. They include *spatial agnosia, impaired visual closure, spatial relations,* and *figure-ground discrimination.*

Intervention Strategies for Visual-Perceptual Deficits. Interventions for visual-perceptual deficits focus on teaching the client to take in visual information in a consistent, systematic, and organized manner. Clients with left unilateral neglect tend to avoid going into the involved space, performing saccades that are too short (hypometric) (Windsor, Ford, & Windsor, 2020a). They may start reading in the middle of the sentence, miss seeing items, or not hear someone speaking to them on their involved side. To improve function, they learn to reorganize their scanning pattern by starting the process of scanning in the impaired space (or left side) first (Windsor, Ford, & Windsor, 2020b). They may benefit from visual field expansion prism lenses as determined by the vision specialist.

The OT would incorporate two scanning strategies: a left-to-right rectilinear pattern for reading and a left-to-right circular pattern for scanning an unstructured array (such as looking for the TV remote). Any therapeutic activity chosen to reestablish an organized scanning pattern through exploratory saccadic eye movements is more effective if the client is required to physically manipulate the objects scanned (Windsor et al., 2020a). Research has shown that a stronger mental representation of a visual image is formed if what is seen is verified by tactile exploration (Congdon et al., 2004). The working field should be large enough to require the client to either turn the head or change body positions to accomplish the task. The OTA can incorporate the training of systematic scanning into near tasks such as sorting mail and using a smartphone, and tasks requiring far vision and functional mobility such as selecting clothing in a closet or navigating in the home. James could address his visual agnosia through sorting and organizing his oral hygiene items or playing videogames with his sons.

Clients with left-sided brain injuries benefit from engaging in activities emphasizing conscious attention to detail, careful review, and comparison of objects. These include any type of matching or sorting activity such as laundry, matching socks, and putting together an outfit.

To improve selective attention, the OTA teaches clients to study objects consciously, especially items placed in the involved space. Matching activities that require discrimination of subtle details are especially effective. Treatment may begin by using pairs of common objects such as spoons, combs, or pens, which may be easier to match because they are familiar. Also effective are games such as in apps, Connect Four, and word search puzzles. The client learns to double check his or her work to ensure that critical details are not missed.

Many clients with brain involvement may overestimate their abilities, believing they are unaffected by injury and may even deny they have the problem (Toglia, 1991; Windsor, Ford, & Windsor, 2020c). They may not fully appreciate the purpose of treatment. These issues may contribute to reduced safety awareness, necessitating constant supervision for safety. To increase insight, Abreu and Toglia advocate teaching clients how to monitor and control performance by learning to recognize and correct for errors (Abreu & Toglia, 1987). The clinician gives the client immediate feedback about performance and learns self-monitoring techniques such as activity prediction. This involves the client predicting how successfully an activity will be performed and identifies

aspects of the activity in which errors are likely to occur. The client then compares actual performance with predicted performance. Employing this technique helps the client become aware and anticipate how the deficit will affect functional performance.

Research has shown clients with brain injury may not transfer skills spontaneously from one learning situation to the next. A final treatment guideline is to practice the skill within context to ensure better carryover to functional activities. Repetition and practice in a variety of circumstances help the client generalize the skill and transfer it to new situations. Real-life situations, preferably in the home or community, are most likely to help the client develop insight into abilities and learn compensation for limitations. Cafeterias, gift shops, restaurants, and shops near the treatment facility can be used to expose the client to more realistic and demanding visual environments.

James has several deficits within the visual-perceptual hierarchy. These changes can cause him to make errors in viewing and manipulating simple and complex visual information. James could participate in a graded dressing program, beginning with the aspects he can perform without assistance and progressing to aspects in which he requires minimal assistance. Because of visual impairments, incoordination, and sensory deficits, he would not be a candidate for using a buttonhook to fasten buttons because of incoordination; he would more likely benefit from wearing loose-fitting pullover shirts. He could space out his clothing so that he can see the items to identify them more easily. Initially, the OT practitioner would limit ADL training time to just over James's attention span to reduce frustration and fatigue, gradually increasing training time with progress. He could play easier videogames without time limits with his sons.

Vision Loss: Compensatory Techniques for ADL

Performing ADL may be overwhelming for the person with a new vision loss. Clients should be encouraged to use the remaining vision and senses to gather and filter information. The OT and OTA teach safety techniques first, breaking each activity into small parts and organizing all materials before beginning each activity.

Eating. Clients with gradual or new visual impairments may experience a lack of confidence eating foods requiring multiple steps such as cutting, seasoning, self-serving, or using utensils. Initially, self-feeding with finger foods is recommended progressing to eating food with a spoon, then the use of other utensils, as indicated so the client gains confidence through success.

General suggestions for clients to use are as follows:
1. Place the plate with a nonskid bottom on a contrasting colored placemat. Some clients may benefit from using a plate guard on a regular plate or scoop dish (Duffy et al., 2011).
2. Use the dinner plate as point of reference on the table and place the other items around it. The place

setting should be the same at every meal. Using the plate as a sample clock can help clients recall the location of food items from meal to meal (e.g., in the 1-o'clock position).

3. Maintain tactile contact with the table and bend forward while eating (if there are no swallowing or balance problems) so food falling from the utensil will land on the plate (Duffy et al., 2011).

4. Use a thermal cup with a lid with spout or cutout and straw for hot and cold liquids.

Simple Food Preparation. Using a large tray different in color than the dishes, cups, and utensils keeps all items together, minimizes the area to be cleaned, and reduces the need to carry items. Storing items on the same shelves within reach makes it easier to locate and handle the items (American Occupational Therapy Association, 2013). Using precut foods such as fruit, salad items, sliced deli meats or cheese, and sliced bread can eliminate the need to use a knife and can reduce risk of accidental injury.

Mobility and Safe Travel. Many clients with significantly impaired vision learn safe mobility techniques through working with an O&M specialist. They may use mobility aids such as a probing (white cane) or support cane, a guide dog, smartphone GPS apps geared for visually impaired individuals, and sensor-based assistive devices. All OTs and OTAs working with visually impaired clients should understand the basics of functional mobility. Trailing helps the client "locate a door, walk in a straight line, or detect the position of objects" to navigate indoors (VisionAware, 2019b). It involves the use of the hands to trail along a smooth, stationary object in a straight line such as a wall or table edge. The client uses the arm closest to the trailing surface, extended diagonally, about 12 inches from the body (VisionAware, 2019b). The hand should lightly touch the trailing surface, with the fingers slightly bent toward the palm "slightly cupped," the fingers acting as "bumpers" to "warn about objects" that may be encountered (VisionAware, 2019b). Sighted guiding involves the sighted person guiding a vision-impaired person to navigate in the environment (Sight Connection, 2011). The guide should always ask the client to take his or her arm (Sight Connection, 2011). The client grasps the guide's arm lightly above the elbow, with thumb outside and fingers wrapped, holding his or her own arm relaxed, with elbow bent (Sight Connection, 2011). The guide stands beside the client and walks in front with the client following a half step ahead, to ensure safety (Sight Connection, 2011). The guide should try to set a comfortable pace. Additional training for the guide is required for going through doorways, using steps, getting in and out of a car, among other activities.

Money Management. Managing money independently is an important functional skill. The client would learn to differentiate coins by the size and texture of edges. Because US paper money denominations are the same size and color, there is a system based on folding to distinguish them. Singles should

remain flat in the wallet unfolded (Willings, 2017). Fives can be folded in half to make a square (Willings, 2017). Tens can be folded in half vertically with the folded side up so the client avoids putting other bills inside the fold (Willings, 2017). Twenties can be folded twice into fourths (Willings, 2017). The iBill Talking Money Identifier, a battery operated device, or smartphone app such as EyeNote can be used to identify bills (Willings, 2017).

Clothing and Accessories Identification. Adequate lighting in dressing areas (where lighting tends to be poorer) is important. Various strategies can be useful for those with visual impairments to organize and differentiate different articles of clothing with or without the use of labels (Dellon, 1981). Examples of strategies include using texture or features (e.g., fasteners, trimmings) to identify certain garments (gray sweater with six buttons and no collar), matching outfits to group together on one hanger, or using containers with compartments such as egg cartons to store small items such as jewelry (Duffy, 2019a).

Writing. Some visually impaired clients may require training and/or use of devices in order to write. It may be easier for those who learned when they had better vision (Duffy, 2019b). Large-tip pens, pens such as Boldwriter 20/20 with easier to read ink that does not bleed through paper, and rigid or flexible writing guides are commercially available (Duffy, 2019b). Clients learn how to write in a straight line, use correct spacing, cross and dot letters (Duffy, 2019b), among other skills. Using the forefinger of the nonwriting hand can help guide the pen and helps with spacing of the writing and with changing lines (Duffy, 2019b).

VESTIBULAR FUNCTION

Vestibular function is defined as "sensation related to position, balance and secure movement against gravity" (American Occupational Therapy Association, 2008). It includes the inner ear (semicircular canals and otoliths or crystals), the eighth cranial nerve (vestibulocochlear), and the vestibular nuclei in the brainstem and the cerebellum (Kaylie, 2019). Normal balance incorporates vestibular input, visual input from the eyes (**visuovestibular integration**), and proprioceptive input from the joints (Kaylie, 2019). Deficits in any of these components will likely result in balance issues causing symptoms such as dizziness, lightheadedness, unsteadiness, vertigo (room spinning), nausea, and feelings of fogginess or a sense of being "off" (Kaylie, 2019). Causes of vestibular dysfunction are varied: brainstem or cerebellar hemorrhage, MS, Meniere's disease, migraines, medication side effects (Kaylie, 2019), CVA, and TBI. Physicians specializing in otorhinolaryngology (ENT), neurology, or rehabilitation medication would evaluate the client with balance problems to determine the diagnosis and medical treatment plan. This might include medications (oral or skin patches), vestibular rehabilitation (including specific physical maneuvers such as Epely (Kaylie, 2019)), or balance retraining (remedial and compensatory). Vestibular rehabilitation requires advanced knowledge (Cohen, Burkhardt, Gronin, & McGuire, 2006) performed by an OT or a physical therapist. The OTA may address balance issues when service competency is demonstrated.

Interventions for Balance Dysfunction

The primary objective of occupational therapy treatment of clients with balance dysfunction is maximizing performance in occupations while maintaining safety, especially fall and injury prevention. Clients tend to be more visually dependent and may experience symptoms when there is lower lighting or when closing their eyes such as when shampooing their hair in the shower. Intervention might include mobility training using devices (seatbelts for wheelchairs, gait belts, canes, walkers), the use of a tub seat when showering, safety education for the client and significant others, and environmental and task modifications (Kannenberg, 2014). The OT would fully assess James's "balance issues." Treatment for James by the OTA, with demonstrated service competency, would include fall prevention, safe transfers, and maintaining sitting balance while performing functional tasks such as dressing and food preparation.

SUMMARY

A variety of structures in the eye, cranial nerves, and brain are responsible for the processing of visual information. A deficit in visual processing requires therapeutic intervention when it prevents successful participation in functional tasks or causes permanent disability (American Occupational Therapy Association, 2008; World Health Organization, 2001). Occupational therapy evaluation and treatment of visual perception is based on a hierarchy of skill levels that are so interrelated that a skill function cannot be disrupted at one level without negatively affecting all perceptual processing. Intervention focuses on increasing the accuracy and organization of the sensory input into the system by remediating skills, adapting the environment, and teaching clients compensatory strategies to minimize the effect of deficits on functional performance. The experienced OTA might teach compensatory techniques to persons with vision loss to maximize functional performance and mobility or choose to achieve SCLV-A or O&M certification. The list of SCLV practitioners by state is on the AOTA.org website, Education and Careers tab, Ready to Advance Your Career tab, Board and Specialty Certifications tab. The OTA should also be familiar with the many resources clients with impaired vision might be using or might benefit from, through information, services, or assistive devices such as the American Academy of Ophthalmology Smart Sight, American Optometric Association, College of Optometrists in Vision Development, Blind Rehabilitation Services, National Library Service, the Lighthouse Guild, Lions Club, VisionAware, Maxi-Aids, Apple store apps, among others.

Treatment of clients with visual, visual-perceptual, and vestibular dysfunction requires clinical reasoning skills,

experience, and expertise. Although clients with these conditions can recover, they may have residual lifelong functional impairments to which they will need to adapt. Some clients, such as James, may have additional deficits that may further reduce their ability to participate in some areas of occupation (American Occupational Therapy Association, 2008). The OT and OTA play an important role in helping clients set and meet achievable short-term and long-term goals (see Quotes box) to maximize health and participation through engagement in meaningful occupations (American Occupational Therapy Association, 2008; World Health Organization, 2001).

QUOTES

Long-Term Occupational Therapy Goal Identified by Case Study Client James

"Most important to me is taking care of my boys, helping out around the house, doing more for myself, then maybe the church website. I think I could work in a few months when I'm not so tired all the time."

REVIEW QUESTIONS

1. Describe how sensory changes cause problems in performance skills and body functions.
2. Compare and contrast the roles of the OT and the OTA in the treatment of clients with CNS and PNS dysfunction.
3. List some safety precautions used for clients with total sensory loss of one hand.
4. Explain how the OTA would treat a client with sensory changes on the left side of the body and poor self-awareness of deficit areas. How would the OTA instruct the client's significant other(s)?
5. List three environmental modifications that would help a client with a severe deficit in visual acuity make a sandwich.
6. Explain what techniques a client with ARMD might use to play cards. How would this client's performance differ from a client who has advanced diabetic retinopathy?
7. A client tells the OTA that his glasses "don't work anymore." How might the OTA best handle the situation?
8. Describe how the OT practitioner would coordinate treatment with the client's vision specialist(s).
9. Contrast the effects of a visual field loss with the effects of left unilateral neglect.
10. Describe the scanning strategies used to train clients with right-sided brain injuries to compensate for unilateral neglect.
11. Identify some strategies the client with 20/200 best corrected vision of both eyes would use on a trip to the grocery store.
12. Explain the effect visual acuity loss would have on a client who already has balance impairment.

REFERENCES

Abreu, B. C., & Toglia, J. P. (1987). Cognitive rehabilitation: a model for occupational therapy. *The American Journal of Occupational Therapy, 41*(7), 439–448.

Altschuler, E. L., Wisdom, S. B., Stone, L., Foster, C., Galasko, D., Llewellyn, D. M., et al. (1999). Rehabilitation of hemiparesis after stroke with a mirror. *Lancet, 353,* 2035–2036.

American Occupational Therapy Association. (2008). Occupational therapy practice framework: domain and process (2nd ed.). *American Journal of Occupational Therapy, 62,* 625–683.

American Occupational Therapy Association. (2013). Living with low vision. <https://www.aota.org/-/media/Corporate/Files/AboutOT/consumers/Adults/LowVision/Low%20Vision%20Tip%20Sheet.pdf>.

Bobath, B. (1990). *Adult hemiplegia: Evaluation and treatment* (3rd ed.). Oxford: Butterworth-Heinemann, Ltd.

Borstad, A. L., Bird, T., Choi, S., Goodman, L., Schmalbrock, P., & Nichols-Larsen, D. S. (2013). Sensory motor training and neural reorganization after stroke: a case series. *Journal of Neurologic Physical Therapy, 37*(1), 27–36.

Bowers, A. R., Keeney, K., & Peli, E. (2008). Community-based trial of a peripheral prism visual field expansion device for hemianopia. *Archives of Ophthalmology, 126*(5), 657–684.

Brunnstrom, S. (1970). *Movement therapy in hemiplegia: A neurophysiological approach.* New York, NY: Harper & Row.

Callahan, A. D. (1995). Methods of compensation and re-education for sensory dysfunction. In J. M. Hunter, E. J. Mackin, & A. D. Callahan (Eds.), *Rehabilitation of the hand* (4th ed.). St Louis, MO: Mosby.

Carr, J. H., & Shepherd, R. B. (1987). *A motor relearning programme for stroke* (2nd ed.). London: Heinemann Medical Books.

Classen, S., Levy, C., McCarthy, D., Mann, W. C., Lanford, D., & Waid-Ebbs, J. K. (2009). Traumatic brain injury and driving assessment: an evidence-based literature review. *American Journal of Occupational Therapy, 64,* 580–591.

Cohen, H. S., Burkhardt, A., Gronin, G. W., & McGuire, M. J. (2006). Specialized knowledge and skills in adult vestibular rehabilitation for occupational therapy practice. *American Journal of Occupational Therapy, 60*(6), 669–678.

Congdon, N., O'Colmain, B., Klaver, C. C., Klein, R. Z., Munoz, B., Friedman, D. S., et al. (2004). Causes and prevalence of visual impairment among adults in the United States. *Archives of Ophthalmology, 122*(4), 477–485.

Dellon, A. L. (1981). *Evaluation of sensibility and reeducation of sensation in the hand* (3rd ed.). Baltimore: Williams & Wilkins.

Duffy, M. A. (2019a). Organizing and labeling clothing when you are blind or have low vision. Vision Aware. <https://visionaware.org/everyday-living/home-modification/room-by-room/bedroom-and-closets/>.

Duffy, M. A. (2019b). Signing your name and handwriting if you are blind or have low vision. Vision Aware. <https://visionaware.org/everyday-living/essential-skills/reading-writing-and-vision-loss/signing-your-name-and-handwriting/>.

Duffy, M. A. (2019c). Using large print. Vision Aware. <www.visionaware.org>.

Duffy, M. A., Huebner, K. M., & Wormsley, D. P. (2011). Activities of daily living and individuals with low vision. In M. Scheiman (Ed.), *Understanding and managing vision deficits: A guide for occupational therapists* (3rd ed.). Thorofare, NJ: Slack.

Dunn, W. (2001). The sensations of everyday life: empirical, theoretical, and pragmatic considerations (Eleanor Clarke Slagle Lecture). *American Journal of Occupational Therapy, 55,* 608–620.

Freeman, P. B. (2011). Low vision: overview and review of low vision evaluation and treatment. In M. Scheiman (Ed.), *Understanding and managing vision deficits: A guide for occupational therapists* (3rd ed.). Thorofare, NJ: Slack.

Friedman, D. S., O'Colmain, B. J., Muñoz, B., Tomany, S. C., McCarty, C., deJong, P. T., et al. (2004). Prevalence of age-related macular degeneration in the United States. *Archives of Ophthalmology, 122,* 564–572.

Gianutsos, R., & Matheson, P. (1987). The rehabilitation of visual perceptual disorders attributable to brain injury. In M. J. Meier, A. L. Benton, & L. Diller (Eds.), *Neuropsychological rehabilitation.* New York, NY: Guilford.

Gianutsos, R., Ramsey, G., & Perlin, R. R. (1988). Rehabilitative optometric services for survivors of acquired brain injury. *Archives of Physical Medicine and Rehabilitation, 69*(8), 573–578.

Goff, J. E. (2010). Assessing unilateral neglect in acute care—raising clinician awareness. *OT Practice, 15*(22), 14–17.

Gutman, S. A., & Schonfeld, A. B. (2019). *Screening adult neurologic populations* (2nd ed.). Bethesda, MD: AOTA Press.

Heilman, K. M., Valenstein, E., & Watson, R. T. (2000). Neglect and related disorders. *Sem Neurology, 20*(4), 463–470.

Kannenberg, K. (2014). Vestibular rehabilitation in occupational therapy practice. *OT Practice, 5.* Available from www.AOTA.org.

Kaylie, D. M. (2019). The Merck manual professional version. <https://www.merckmanuals.com/professional>.

Khazaeni, L. M. (2019a). Cataracts. The Merck manual consumer version. <www.merckmanuals.com>. Accessed 16.08.19.

Khazaeni, L. M. (2019b). Cataracts. The Merck manual professional version. <www.merckmanuals.com>.

Kitchel, J. E. (2004). Large print: guidelines for optimal readability and APHont™, a font for low vision. <https://www.aph.org/aph-guidelines-for-print-document-design/>.

Knutson, J. S., Gunzler, D. D., Wilson, R. D., & Chae, J. (2016). Contralaterally controlled functional electrical stimulation improves hand dexterity in chronic hemiparesis—a randomized trial. *Stroke, 47,* 2596–2602.

Lang, C. E., & Birkenmeier, R. L. (2014). *Upper-extremity task specific training after stroke or disability: A manual for occupational and physical therapy.* Bethesda, MD: AOTA Press.

Leff, A. P., Scott, S. K., Crewes, H., Hodgson, T. L., Cowey, A., Howard, D., et al. (2000). Impaired reading in patients with right hemianopia. *Ann Neurology, 47,* 171–178.

Lundborg, G., & Rosen, B. (2011). Sensory reeducation. In T. M. Skirven, A. I. Osterman, J. Fedorczyk, & P. C. Amadio (Eds.), *Rehabilitation of the hand and upper extremity* (6th ed.). Philadelphia, PA: Elsevier Mosby.

Mehta, S. (2019a). Age-related macular degeneration (AMD or ARMD). The Merck manual professional version. <https://www.merckmanuals.com/professional/eye-disorders/retinal-disorders/age-related-macular-degeneration-amd-or-armd?query=age%20related%20macular>.

Mehta, S. (2019b). Diabetic retinopathy. The Merck manual consumer version. <https://www.merckmanuals.com/home/eye-disorders/retinal-disorders/diabetic-retinopathy?query=diabetic%20retinopathy>.

Mehta, S. (2019c) Diabetic retinopathy. The Merck manual professional version. <https://www.merckmanuals.com/professional/eye-disorders/retinal-disorders/diabetic-retinopathy?query=diabetic%20retinopathy>.

National Eye Institute. (2016). Facts about hyperopia. <https://www.nei.nih.gov/learn-about-eye-health/resources-for-health-educators/eye-health-data-and-statistics/farsightedness-hyperopia-data-and-statistics>.

National Eye Institute-National Institutes of Health. (2015). Facts about diabetic retinopathy. <https://www.nei.nih.gov/learn-about-eye-health/eye-conditions-and-diseases/diabetic-retinopathy>.

Page, S. J., Sisto, S., Levine, P., & McGrath, R. E. (2004). Efficacy of modified constraint movement therapy in chronic stroke: a single-blinded randomized control trial. *Archives of Physical Medicine and Rehabilitation, 85*(1), 14−18.

Rensink, R. A. (2010). Seeing seeing. *Psyche, 16*(1), 68−78.

Rhee, D. J. (2017a). Glaucoma. The Merck manual consumer version. <www.merckmanuals.com>.

Rhee, D. J. (2017b). Overview of glaucoma. The Merck manual professional version. <www.merckmanuals.com>.

Rood, M. (1956). Neurophysiological mechanisms utilized in the treatment of neuromuscular dysfunction. *American Journal of Occupational Therapy, 10*(4), 220−225.

Rubin, M. (2010). Overview of peripheral nervous systems disorders. The Merck manual professional version. <https://www.merckmanuals.com/professional/neurologic-disorders/peripheral-nervous-system-and-motor-unit-disorders/overview-of-peripheral-nervous-system-disorders?query=peripheral%20nervous%20system%20disorders>.

Rubin, M. (2008). Peripheral nervous system and motor unit disorders—introduction. <http://www.merckandcoinc.net/mmpe/sec16/ch223/ch223a.html>.

Rummel, E. (2020) Loss of visual field due to brain injury hemianopsia and neglect. Brain Injuries. <https://www.braininjuries.org/hemianopsia_field_loss.html>.

Schabrun, S. M., & Hillier, S. (2009). Evidence for the retraining of sensation after stroke: a systematic review. *Clinical Rehabilitation, 23*(1), 27−39.

Scheiman, M. (2011). Management of refractive, visual efficiency, and visual information processing disorders. In M. Scheiman (Ed.), *Understanding and managing vision deficits: A guide for occupational therapists* (3rd ed.). Thorofare, NJ: Slack.

Sharma-Abbott, R., & Larson, R. N. (2015). Sensory reeducation and sensitization. In R. J. Saunders, R. P. Astifdis, S. L. Burke, J. P. Higgins, & M. A. McClinton (Eds.), *Hand and upper extremity rehabilitation—a practical guide*. London: Elsevier Science.

Sight Connection. (2011). Sighted guide technique. <www.sight-connection.org>.

Sokol-McKay, D. A. (2005). Facing the challenge of macular degeneration: therapeutic interventions for low vision. *OT Practice, 10*(9), 10−15.

Toglia, J. P. (1991). Generalization of treatment: a multicontext approach to cognitive perceptual impairment in adults with brain injury. *American Journal of Occupational Therapy, 45*(6), 505−516.

Vahlberg, B., & Hellstrom, K. (2008). Treatment and assessment of neglect after stroke—from a physiotherapy perspective: a systematic review. *Adv Physiother, 10*, 178−187.

VisionAware. (2019a). Home modifications for people who are blind or have low vision. <https://visionaware.org/everyday-living/home-modification/>.

VisionAware. (2019b). Using the trailing technique. <www.visionaware.org>.

Vision Health Initiative. (2015). Common eye disorders and diseases. <https://www.cdc.gov/visionhealth/basics/ced/>.

Voss, D. E. (1959). Applications in patterns and techniques in occupational therapy. *American Journal of Occupational Therapy, 8*(4), 191.

Warren, M. (1990). Identification of visual scanning deficits in adults after cerebrovascular accident. *American Journal of Occupational Therapy, 44*(5), 391−399.

Warren, M. (1993). A hierarchical model for evaluation and treatment of visual perceptual dysfunction in adult acquired brain injury, parts 1 and 2. *American Journal of Occupational Therapy, 47*(1), 42−66.

Warren, M. (2009). Pilot study on activities of daily living limitations in adults with hemianopsia. *American Journal of Occupational Therapy, 63*, 626−633.

Waylett-Rendell, J. (2004). Sensory reeducation. In E. Crepeau, E. Cohn, & B. Boyt Schell (Eds.), *Willard & Spackman's Occupational Therapy* (10th ed.). Baltimore: Lippincott Williams & Wilkins.

Willings, C. (2017). Money identification & management. Teaching Visually Impaired. <https://www.teachingvisuallyimpaired.com/money.html>.

Windsor, R. L., Ford, C. A., & Windsor, L. K. (2020a). Explorative saccadic training. <http://www.hemianopsia.net/scanning-therapy/>.

Windsor, R. L., Ford, CA, & Windsor, L. K. (2020b). Hemianosia treatment. <http://www.hemianopsia.net/hemianopsia-treatment/>.

Windsor, R. L., Ford, C. A, & Windsor, L. K. (2020c). Hemispatial inattention (visual neglect). <http://www.hemianopsia.net/visual-neglect/>.

Windsor, R. L. , Ford, C. A. & Windsor, L. K. (2020d). Scanning therapy—hemianopsia.net. Everything you need to know about hemianopsia. <http://hemianopsia.net/scanning-therapy/>.

World Health Organization. (2001). *International classification of functioning, Disability and Health (ICF)*. Geneva, Switzerland: World Health Organization.

World Health Organization. (2018). Blindness and vision impairment. <https://www.who.int/news-room/fact-sheets/detail/blindness-and-visual-impairment>.

Yang, N. Y. H., Chung, R. C. K., Li-Tsang, C. W. P., & Fong, K. N. K. (2013). Rehabilitation Interventions for unilateral neglect after stroke: a systematic review from 1997 to 2012. *Front Human Neuroscience, 7*, 1−11.

22

Intervention for People with Cognitive and Perceptual Deficits

Regula H. Robnett

OBJECTIVES

After reading this chapter, the student or the occupational therapy practitioner will be able to do the following:

1. Describe basic cognitive deficits and how they may affect functional performance.
2. Compare and contrast evidence-based (or commonly used) remedial and adaptive approaches for cognitive impairments that affect occupational performance.
3. Describe strategies for specific cognitive deficits, including executive skills dysfunction.
4. Understand the advantages of focusing on strength-based intervention for cognition and perception.
5. Identify the effects of visual perceptual deficits on functional skills.
6. Compare and contrast evidence-based remedial and adaptive approaches for perceptual impairments affecting occupational performance.
7. Articulate managing the challenges of working with clients who have cognitive and perceptual impairments.

KEY TERMS

Orientation
Higher-level cognitive functions
Attention
Memory
Remediation approach
Adaptation/adaptive approach
Transfer-of-training approach
Categorization
Functional approach

Compensation
Domain-specific training
Executive functions
Astereognosis
Apraxia
Ideomotor apraxia
Ideational apraxia
Charles Bonnet syndrome

"The human brain is the most magnificent system in the universe." (Nussbaum, 2003)

INTRODUCTION

Our brains control everything we do, from breathing, to simple and complex movement sequences, to solving complicated problems. Cognition (i.e., thinking, learning, and memory) and perception (i.e., the interpretation of incoming sensory information) are challenging client factors to address in occupational therapy practice. Whereas physical client factors such as decreased range of motion or strength can be observed directly, impaired cognitive or perceptual skills can only be *inferred* through the client's behavior. Performance skills are "observable elements of action that have an implicit functional purpose" (p. S25) (American Occupational Therapy Association, 2014a). These skills form the building blocks of tasks within various occupations. The occupational therapist (OT) evaluates each client and focuses on cognitive and perceptual performance skills (bottom-up approach) and/or engagement in occupations (top-down approach). The goals are often related to remediating or accommodating for client factor and performance skill deficits, while promoting one's retained strengths.

The occupational therapy assistant (OTA) has a distinct role working with clients who have cognitive and perceptual impairments. The range of services provided within this role depends on various factors: the OTA's level of experience and service competencies, familiarity and skill level in this area of practice, the intervention setting (including the geographic location), facility guidelines, and state practice laws. Where a shortage of medical personnel exists (e.g., in rural communities and general medical settings), the OTA may work with people who have cognitive and perceptual disorders more frequently. Clients present with cognitive and/or perceptual deficits in all intervention settings. Therefore all OTAs need to be familiar with these aspects of occupational performance and learn appropriate cognitive and perceptual intervention techniques to enhance overall occupational performance.

Recognizing the OTA's crucial role, this chapter presents a number of important concepts and techniques for OTAs to implement during interventions. However, before taking action, the responsible OTA will acquire the necessary service competencies under qualified supervision and gain the required knowledge through educational opportunities. Settings and jurisdictions differ in their guidelines for OTA services; the OTA is responsible for learning these relevant guidelines and for following them to ensure compliance with state and national regulatory entities (American Occupational Therapy Association, 2014b; American Occupational Therapy Association, 2018; American Occupational Therapy Association, 2019).

This chapter is divided into two separate sections: one on cognition and one on perception (specifically visual perception). Although these are not isolated from one another (and often are intertwined), they are separated in the chapter for ease of understanding. Each section examines foundational concepts and intervention techniques related to client factors, performance skills, and occupations in varied contexts. The section on perception includes a discussion of the interaction between perception of sensory input and subsequent motor actions because these are intricately linked in producing occupational performance outcomes.

OCCUPATIONAL THERAPY INTERVENTION PROCESS

Impairments in Cognition

The goal of cognitive rehabilitation is positive functional change. Interventions might include education about strengths and deficits, process training and ongoing practice to relearn former skills, strategy training to compensate for ongoing deficits, and training in functional activities to improve daily life skills and improve levels of independence (Malia, Law, & Sidebottom, 2003). The OTA would not be expected to design an individualized cognitive retraining program but certainly will assist in its implementation. An understanding of basic intervention techniques is essential.

According to the *OT Practice Framework, 3rd ed* (American Occupational Therapy Association, 2014a), client factors related to cognitive performance skills include the following:

- *Global mental functions* such as consciousness (awareness and alertness**), orientation** (to self, others, place, and time), personality (the big five factors model of personality (McCrae & Costa, 1997)), temperament and impulse control, energy and drive (motivation, appetite, and craving), and sleep.
- *Specific mental functions* such as **higher-level cognitive functions** (insight/judgment, concept formation, metacognition, and cognitive flexibility), **attention** (sustained, selective, alternating, and divided), **memory** (short- to long-term and working memory, as well as various types such as procedural, prospective, semantic, and episodic), and thought functions (awareness of reality and logical thought), and the mental component of complex movement sequencing.

The OTA might consider cognition in relation to the underlying skills necessary for planning and carrying out performance in occupations of relevance to the client, be these activities of daily living (ADL), instrumental ADL (IADL), rest and sleep, education, work, play, leisure, and/or social participation (American Occupational Therapy Association, 2014a). These underlying performance process skills (American Occupational Therapy Association, 2014a) include, but are not limited to, the following:

- *Choosing* such as selecting appropriate clothing for the weather or the correct kitchen gadgets for cooking
- *Attending* such as paying attention throughout a task (not getting distracted, for example, while cooking)
- *Sequencing* such as determining the correct or logical order of dressing (e.g., socks before shoes) or repairing a broken faucet
- *Organizing* such as placing needed items in an orderly spatial fashion (e.g., items needed for a project placed where one can see them and within easy reach)
- *Adjusting* such as coming up with alternate ways to complete the task more effectively (e.g., different grip, taking a break, changing the temperature of the oven to keep something from burning)

OTs and OTAs primarily utilize two intervention approaches with clients experiencing deficits in cognition. The **remediation approach** (establishing, restoring (American Occupational Therapy Association, 2014a)) focuses on restoring cognition to its former level (or as close as possible), and the **adaptation or adaptive approach** (modifying, compensating (American Occupational Therapy Association, 2014a)) focuses on modifying or adapting the task and/or the environment to enhance occupational performance. The OT who is designing the intervention for the specific client may decide to use one or the other or both approaches simultaneously. OTs and OTAs may also use health promotion, maintenance, and prevention approaches.

Remediation Approach. "Cognitive rehabilitation is goal oriented, and while problem focused, builds on strengths" (Sohlberg & Mateer, 2001, p. 21). The remediation approach seeks to improve or restore cognitive skills. Remediation involves engagement in tasks that are intended to enhance recovery from an acquired brain injury (ABI) or other cognitive impairments. These activities may involve occupations requiring cognitive or process skills, or specific brain exercises (often online) used to promote cognitive performance. The evidence that computer-based cognitive exercises improve cognitive performance after brain injury is weak and needs further research (Fetta, Starkweather, & Gill, 2017). The underlying assumption is that the brain can reorganize itself after ABI, and new learning can take place. Sometimes this approach is also referred to as the **transfer-of-training approach** (Gillen, 2009). Pencil-and-paper, tabletop, and computer-based activities may include various cognition-based exercises such as word problems, crossword puzzles, word/letter finds, mazes, math computations/problems, copying designs, sequencing tasks, and figure replications (Fig. 22.1). These activities are intended to be introduced at a

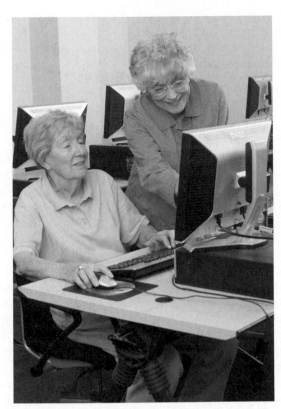

Fig. 22.1 Various computer games or activities target cognitive skills such as problem solving, memory, puzzles, and attention. (From Birchenall J, Streight E. *Mosby's Textbook for the Home Care Aide.* 3rd ed. St Louis, MO: Elsevier; 2013.)

level just above the client's present cognitive level. Given encouragement and support from the practitioner as needed, the clients are encouraged to challenge their current level of thinking and responding and thus aspire to a higher level of performance (e.g., more accurate or quicker). The activity is scored for accuracy; deficits or improvements in the areas of motivation, attention, and concept formation are noted. Additional distractions may be added during the activities as improvement occurs, to test the extent to which the client can continue to perform in a more distracting context. The key to success with remedial cognitive approaches such as listed is the ability of the client to transfer this improving ability with paper and pencil or computer-based exercises to real-life situations. For example, doing math computations would be expected to also help in calculating the amount of money needed to purchase items at a store. Computer-based activities provide a means to practice cognitive skills and may be a valuable tool for rehabilitation. However, evidence indicates that cognitive retraining exercises used in isolation, rather than under the direction of a skilled professional, may not be an effective means to enhance life skills (Cicerone, Goldin, & Ganci, 2019). Nonetheless there are myriad opportunities for online games and exercises. Commercial educational programs and specialized software can provide graded treatment modules focusing on specific areas of cognition such as remediation of arithmetic skills, attention, concentration, concept formation, memory, reasoning, association, **categorization**

(sorting into classes or groups as same or different), cause-and-effect reasoning, problem solving, organization, generalization, level of abstraction, judgment, safety awareness, spatial orientation, sequencing, and verbal memory. Software programs can be used in the clinic as an adjunct to therapy or as a home program but should be used with the oversight of skilled intervention (Cicerone et al., 2019).

The remediation approach is also used when the client is engaged in meaningful, real-life tasks (rather than contrived cognitive exercises). For example, intervention to improve money management would involve shopping: perhaps deciding what to buy, purchasing items, and counting change. In this case the assumption is that repeated practice on a task at a level that is challenging (the just-right challenge—i.e., not overwhelming but also not boring due to being too simple) can also lead to improvements in the cognitive performance of that task. Neistadt (1994) long ago promoted the use of occupational tasks such as meal preparation as superior to contrived but related activities. More recently in a small qualitative study involving 14 people who had sustained ABIs, Doig and colleagues (2011) compared the participants' opinions about the use of simulated occupations in a day hospital setting to home-based occupational therapy. These researchers found that the participants preferred the home therapy due to it being more "real life," more satisfying, and more effective (Doig et al., 2011). Whenever possible, client-centered daily occupations should be used rather than rote client-factor—based exercises. The OTA carries through these interventions and can give input into the planning process by sharing the client's interests and responses. Details of the client's successes or difficulties are intended to be shared among the occupational therapy team as well as the broader rehabilitation team on an as-needed basis.

> ### CLINICAL PEARL
> To improve cognitive functioning, "the ideal time to intervene is throughout the entire lifespan before functional problems emerge" (Vance, Roberson, & McGuinness, 2010, p. 24).

Adaptation Approach. The adaptation or adaptive approach (also called the **functional approach**) can use intact cognitive skills to compensate for deficits. Variations of this approach focus on context, activity demands, and performance patterns such as habits and routines. Engaging in occupations that are meaningful to the client is fundamental to the adaptive approach (Gillen, 2009). The assumption is that impairments are likely to be long term so the goal is to maximize performance by adapting to, or working around, the deficits. Using the adaptive approach in the realm of cognitive intervention can involve many aspects, individualized for the client by the treating OT. General examples include written reminders for decreased memory, sequence lists/pictures for enhancing ADL performance, and working on what-if scenarios to handle emergencies. In providing intervention, the OT or OTA considers the context in which the individuals will ultimately perform tasks (e.g., where they will work or live). Many adaptations are likely to be situation specific and may need to be reassessed and adapted each time the client's context changes (Table 22.1).

Successful outcomes may involve shifting roles, altering or reducing demands placed on clients, or giving them fewer challenging responsibilities in relation to other members of the family or coworkers. Maintaining their participation to the fullest extent possible is also important. For example, a client who can no longer safely sequence the steps for making a family dinner using the current kitchen appliances may benefit from a shift of responsibility for meal preparation to another family member. Perhaps the client can still be involved by completing components that contribute to the overall meal preparation activity (e.g., stirring, washing produce, measuring ingredients, and setting the table, possibly all with supervision). Family members may report that it is easier and quicker to do the task themselves, but if this is the case, family education about the importance of remaining engaged and productive is warranted (to avoid learned helplessness and to promote occupational performance). Programs such as Meals on Wheels may provide a nutritious alternative for those who do not have familial support. Clients may work diligently with occupational therapy practitioners just to set up a routine to heat up certain meals (e.g., microwave meals) in the client's kitchen (the specific context). Remediation involving returning to former

cooking skills is possible if cognitive skills are expected to improve. Again, using the adaptive approach does not preclude using remediation for some skills at the same time or at some point in the intervention process.

Habits and Routines

Habits "hold together the patterns of ordinary life that help make life more effortless and help define one's character" (p. 60) (Tham, Fallaphour, & Erikson, 2017). Habits are "specific, automatic behaviors performed repeatedly, relatively automatically, and with little variation" (American Occupational Therapy Association, 2014a, p. S27). After they have been repeated enough so that a pattern has been established, much of what we do is guided by this self-perpetuating behavior. Some habits are adaptive (e.g., brushing our teeth after breakfast) while others are dysfunctional or ineffective (Tham et al., 2017). Consider how chaotic life may be after a brain injury; little in life may make sense. The use of familiar habits, especially those that are less demanding and more automatic in well-known contexts, can provide the foundation for positive, albeit specific, routines. Individualized-for-this-client, meaningful occupations are the key to successful outcomes (Tham et al., 2017).

Establishing new habits and routines can provide order and consistency in the flow of activities and will reduce demands for decision making by the client, thus promoting successful participation in daily tasks. This type of intervention is especially important for those with decreased cognition (e.g., neurocognitive disorders such as Alzheimer disease [AD]) who tend to need to rely on structure and routines. To assist in establishing routines, the OTA may use daily checklists, introduce a systematic filing system, set up a regular and perhaps simplified ADL schedule, help the person organize tools or supplies, and/or set up the environment for the client to easily complete specific tasks in a predetermined sequence (Figs. 22.2 and 22.3). Routines are "patterns of behavior that are observable, regular, repetitive, and that provide structure for daily life" (p. S27) (American Occupational Therapy Association, 2014a). Repetition and consistency over time are necessary for a routine to become fully established into a set of automatic behaviors. Sometimes the needed repetition is much greater than one might expect; those with cognitive impairments will likely need more time. As the routine and habits become ingrained (again in whatever timeframe needed, within reason), the client may be able to complete the task with greater ease, accuracy, speed, and better overall performance. The occupational therapy team can determine which client-centered habits and routines should be addressed.

Cognitive Strategies

Cognitive strategies are tools to improve learning, thinking, remembering, and problem solving. They are used on a regular basis by most people to improve occupational performance. For example, to improve the chances of remembering someone's name when being introduced, one may say the name a few times (either aloud or silently) or may connect the person's name to someone with the same name or try to make another connection (Toglia, Rodger, & Polatajko, 2012). The client with enough self-awareness and who is

TABLE 22.1	Examples of Treatment Approaches
Approach	**Activity Example: Buttoning**
Adaptive approach (also known as *functional, adaptation,* or *compensatory*)	Change physical object (use contrasting or bigger buttons); change performance pattern by simplifying the routine (e.g., fewer buttons or alternate fasteners such as Velcro); grade the task down into a simpler perceptual sequence by starting to button at the bottom of the shirt; change activity demands or modify the intervention (sewing up part of a button shirt to eliminate buttoning); bigger buttons may be easier to manage.
Remedial approach	Practicing the task of buttoning with OTA providing the necessary assistance; try backward chaining or challenging client with a *slightly* more difficult buttoning task.
Transfer-of-learning	Use a button board or buttoning game before learning buttoning on self.

OTA, Occupational therapy assistant.

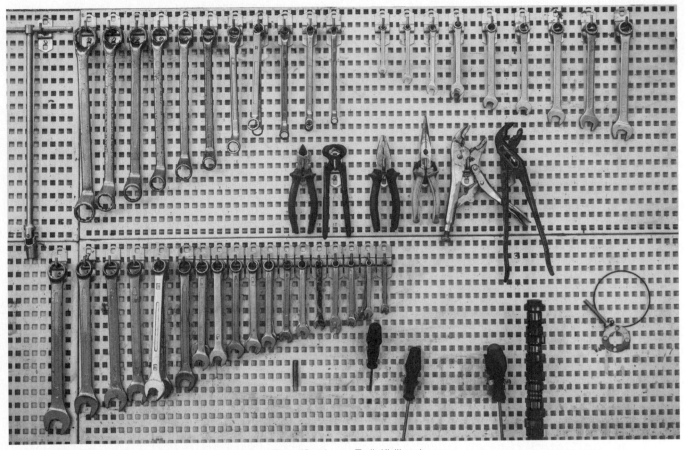

Fig. 22.2 Well-organized tools promote ease of access. (From iStock.com/Tarik Kizilkaya)

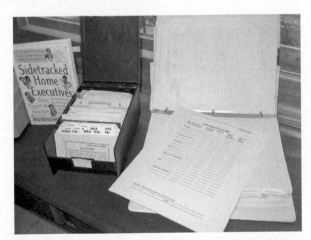

Fig. 22.3 A file system listing daily activities and logs of important documents and their location maintains the client's participation in higher-level cognitive function.

motivated to improve performance can be taught these types of internal strategies (Parenté & Herrmann, 2010; Toglia et al., 2012). The OTA can assist the client by reinforcing these strategies. For example, to enhance memory performance the client may use visual imagery, mental rehearsal, mnemonics, chunking, association, and repetition (Gillen, 2009; Wilson, 2010). To improve attention to task, the client may use sensory strategies such as wearing

earplugs or headphones, taking sensory breaks, or reading the material aloud to enhance concentration.

Clients with cognitive impairments may find these strategies difficult to initiate on their own. If this is the case, external strategies initiated by others such as the OT, OTA, or a family member may be more effective. For example, ensuring that the intervention (or any activity) takes place in a low-key environment, or reminding the client to use noise-reducing headphones when needed, may be helpful. For the interested reader, a helpful review of cognitive strategies (with many examples), theoretical underpinnings, and a detailed framework of their use is available (Toglia et al., 2012).

Interventions for Cognitive Impairments

In the *Occupational Therapy Practice Framework* (American Occupational Therapy Association, 2014a) mental functions are separated into global and specific. Global mental functions include consciousness and orientation. Specific mental functions include attention, memory, thought, and higher-level cognitive functions. Under mental functions the *Framework* also includes personality, drive, and sleep. While these are important, the reader is referred directly to the document for further examples in these realms.

Consciousness and Orientation Functions. Consciousness relates to being awake and alert. Someone in a coma is unconscious. Orientation builds on the foundation of being conscious of one's surroundings and is classified as being:

1. Alert and oriented to self (A & O × 1)
2. Oriented to self and place (A & O × 2)
3. Oriented to self, place, and time (A & O × 3)

Time is the most conceptually abstract construct and is therefore most easily lost. Orientation can be viewed as a developmental construct; we first learn who we are (the self), then we incorporate others (context). Finally, we understand the concept of time (e.g., telling time; understanding days, weeks, years; and grasping the amorphous nature of time in our memory bank).

Staff and family members who encounter a person who is not oriented can assist in orienting the person to self, others, place, time, and situation (e.g., "Hi, Mrs. A. I'm Nancy your occupational therapist, and today we are going to make lunch together. It's a wonderful sunny Thursday. . .."). This suggestion is based on the work of Inouye et al. (2006), who designed the evidence-based Hospital Elder Life Program (HELP) to prevent delirium in older hospital patients. Generally it is not helpful to quiz the person about information related to orientation (e.g., "Do you know what day it is?") because this can easily make the person feel defensive and lead to frustration and possibly fear (of being tested).

External aids such as calendars, bulletin boards, and orientation boards with pertinent information (e.g., the facility's name, the date, the season, and current events) are often used in long-term settings or rehabilitation centers. These must be kept up to date or they can directly contribute to further disorientation (Inouye et al., 2006). A helpful strategy for orienting someone is to use familiar photographs, especially with captions (either for those who can read or for professional caregivers who can use these to start conversations) (Bourgeois, 2007). For example, a photo of a young child might have the caption: "Ted Jones, my son, at age 3, in 1958." Sometimes just looking at family photos can help orient and calm the person. Limited evidence exists supporting the use of structured orientation groups as being helpful in delaying institutionalization and cognitive decline in people with dementia (Metitieri, Zanetti, & Geroldi, 2001). Tanaka et al. (2017) found group intervention to be preferable to individual intervention (or control group intervention) for improving orientation and cognitive test performance. However, definitive guidelines for providing orientation information, either on an individual or group basis, are lacking. Even when gains are made in cognitive functioning test scores based on orientation drills, improvements may not carry over to daily functional performance (Patton, 2006).

CLINICAL PEARL

Never argue or debate with someone who is confused or disoriented. You cannot win the argument, and frustration on both sides will surely ensue. Instead, try redirecting attention to another topic that is less distressing. If redirecting does not work, leave for a minute or two and then return.

Attention Functions. Attention functions are included in the *Framework* (American Occupational Therapy Association, 2014a) as specific mental functions. Attention as a construct includes sustained attention to task (focusing), alternating attention between two or more tasks, divided attention (attending to more than one task simultaneously), concentration (focusing), and attending to a task under distracting circumstances (American Occupational Therapy Association, 2014a). Attention difficulties occur more frequently in disruptive environments, especially for older adults who have more difficulties inhibiting responses. However, they may do just as well when focusing on one task and may benefit from mindfulness-based attention training (Whitmoyer, Fountain-Zaragoza, & Andridge, 2018). Most people find it easier to focus their attention when the environment is not overloaded with various types of auditory, visual, or other sensory stimuli. For example, if someone needs to concentrate on maintaining balance while walking, do not chat with the person about other issues. Carrying on even normal, everyday conversations while walking may distract the client enough to cause a fall.

The initial goal of treating attention impairments is to identify the optimal environment that enables the client to attend to task for the longest time possible. As attention and level of concentration improve, the person will be able to focus longer under more distracting (or more natural) conditions. Therefore, at some point, chatting while the person is walking may be a therapeutic intervention to challenge the client (and push the limits of the just-right challenge). Not all people can improve (or remediate) their level of attention. Those who cannot improve are likely to function more effectively in a low-stimulus environment or an environment individualized for level of stimulus and conducive to their specific needs. Music of interest to the individual may be used to promote attentional skills (Shih, Huang, & Chiang, 2009). Formalized attention training models are available both electronically and through specific learning systems. Gillen (2009) offers a patient handout with the following recommendations: avoiding distractions or interruptions, keeping away from crowds, taking a break as soon as one begins to feel fatigued, getting enough exercise, and being sure to ask for help when needed. Cicerone et al. (2019) recommend direct attention training along with metacognitive strategy training to promote generalization of the training to daily task performance for those with ABI such as traumatic brain injury or stroke. Also, their systematic review stresses the importance of therapist involvement to promote the carryover of training (Cicerone et al., 2019).

Memory Functions. Memory is not one simple construct. Often when people talk about poor memory they are referring to short-term memory or the ability to remember facts for a brief time period (e.g., names, grocery lists, telephone numbers). An important consideration about short-term memory is that it relies heavily on adequate attention. One cannot remember what one did not attend to initially (Gillen, 2009; Levy, 2011) (Fig. 22.4). Asking someone if he or she has good memory skills yields little reliable information precisely

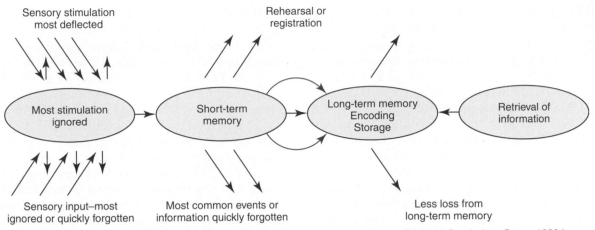

Fig. 22.4 Path of memory. (Modified from Baddeley AD. *Essentials of Human Memory*. Hove, England: Psychology Press; 1999.)

because people with memory difficulties have difficulty remembering (Baddeley, 2014; Knight & Godfrey, 2002). One aspect to keep in mind is that recall (outright remembering something "out of the blue") is more difficult than being able to identify something that was seen or encountered in the past (e.g., multiple-choice questions). This is important when considering the best way to present the just-right challenge.

In general, people can remember seven digits for a short period of time (with a standard deviation of $\pm$ 2). This is based on Miller's research in the 1950s and still holds true today (Gillen, 2009; Miller, 1956). Most people can remember a phone number long enough to dial it. This kind of remembering activates the working memory system, which involves remembering while doing a task. For example, besides remembering a phone number as one dials a phone, a person also remembers rules to a game while playing or what cards have been played during a strategic card game. One actively uses, interacts with, or manipulates the information with the intention of retaining the information for the duration of the task. Other examples of activities that require intact working memory include cooking (especially using recipes without repeatedly looking back) and recalling and implementing multistep driving directions just obtained from a helpful person on the street.

Procedural memory concerns recall of procedures or motor skills such as driving (the motoric aspects), riding a bicycle, or dressing. Procedural memory is often retained in persons who have ABI or even AD and may be able to be used as a basis to reestablish habits (Levy, 2011; Sohlberg & Mateer, 2001; Sohlberg & Turkstra, 2011). Unfortunately intact procedural memory may be a detriment at times. A person with AD, for instance, may recall the procedures of driving (turning the key, steering, putting the right foot on the gas pedal), but procedural memory does not assist the person in being a defensive driver—that is, one who effectively problem solves and manages unexpected but common circumstances that occur while on the road (e.g., inclement weather, other bad drivers, children/pets running into the road).

Prospective memory refers to memory utilized for future tasks (Sohlberg & Turkstra, 2011). Prospective memory tasks are common in everyday life: When we make appointments we need to arrive on time, medication needs to be taken at prescribed times, and deadlines need to be met at work. Fortunately there are an abundance of compensatory measures for decreased prospective memory. These include low-tech calendars and lists as well as high-tech reminders from smartphone applications or home assistant prompts. Sometimes working with the client in developing techniques to assist in remembering these essential tasks can be helpful (e.g., linking taking medications with another established routine such as brushing teeth or eating breakfast or leaving the keys on a hook right by the door).

Episodic memory is simply memory for episodes or events in one's life (e.g., first day of school, birthday parties, weddings). As people get older, episodic memory may decrease to a degree, although in typical aging this change does not generally interfere with day-to-day functioning. Semantic memory concerns our deep-seated memory of language and basic facts that most of us know (e.g., multiplication tables, grammar, geographic facts). In typical aging this type of memory tends to be maintained or may even improve into one's 80s, even though verbal fluency may decline slightly (Laver, 2016).

These differing types of memory are related to one another, but a client may have more difficulties with one type than another. The OTA may want to consider the pathways involved in developing and using memories because clients may have difficulty at any point in the formation of memory progression. (See Fig. 22.4 for a schematic of the process.) The person must first pay attention to the incoming stimulus, then store the information (if it is important), and ultimately retrieve it. People generally have more success recognizing information than recalling it outright. Retention of information improves when the person repeats and manipulates it (Levy, 2011). For example, if a client needs to remember hip precautions following hip surgery, involving the person in practicing these precautions during daily tasks (first under your supervision), writing them down, and talking about them (vs just hearing or reading about them once) will promote improved recall and adherence.

Thought Functions. Thought, or the process of thinking, is an activity that is almost constant in the human brain (even during sleep). Generally, when engaged in a specific task, our thoughts are logical, organized, and relate to the current task or topic. Deficits in this realm (such as disorganized thinking) hinder effective task completion or topic understanding. Thomas (2015) describes appropriate thought functions as "mentally utilizing information that relates to the concept or activity at hand" (p. 92). Awareness of reality (knowing truth from fiction) is also important and may not always be clear cut.

The *Framework* (American Occupational Therapy Association, 2014a) considers higher-level cognitive functions, which include executive functions such as planning, cognitive flexibility, insight, judgment, and organizing. Many of our daily tasks, especially those that are more involved (complicated or complex), require higher-level thought. Examples of occupations involving higher-level thought functions include planning a birthday party, budgeting a monthly household with limited funds, or cooking a several-course meal so that everything is ready at the same time.

PRINCIPLES OF COGNITIVE RETRAINING TO ENHANCE LEARNING AND MEMORY

Interventions related to cognitive functioning involve several different aspects:
- *Promoting improved performance* of thinking, learning, and memory (create/promote/establish/restore) (Thomas, 2015)
- *Prevention* of cognitive losses (preferred, if possible) (prevent)
- *Maintaining* cognition to the highest degree possible (maintain)
- *Compensating* for deficits in thinking and memory (modify) (American Occupational Therapy Association, 2014a)

Learning

Challenging the brain to think harder (e.g., problem solving or promoting new learning) can help the brain to continue in a growth pattern (rather than decline) even into old age. Typical children and adults who are motivated to challenge themselves do not usually need occupational therapy; they just need to find new learning opportunities (e.g., taking a course, reading, challenging gaming). New learning may be the best prevention method in avoiding cognitive losses (Niechcial, Vaportzis, & Gow, 2019; Nussbaum, 2003). Prevention also includes engagement in activities that stimulate learning and thinking, either in real-life or simulated situations. Maintaining cognitive performance could involve practicing pertinent cognitive activities akin to the ongoing practice of a sport. Examples of **compensation** or adaptation (thus promoting the best cognitive performance possible) include simplifying the environment (e.g., fewer distractions or choices) or making the task simpler (e.g., fewer steps) and using strategies (e.g., writing lists, phone reminders).

One of the more recent developments in cognitive rehabilitation involves the use of the Cognitive Orientation to Daily Occupational Performance (CO-OP) approach, which focuses on the use of task-specific training on repeated problem-solving strategies following the "Goal-Plan-Do-Check" analyses. When compared to standard occupational therapy treatment in a small group of stroke survivors in the community, the CO-OP approach was associated with greater improvements (although both groups did improve) (Polatajko, McEwen, & Ryan, 2012). Using the CO-OP approach, the client comes up with a goal (e.g., making muffins), and the practitioner works with the person to develop a specific plan to meet that goal. After enacting the plan, the client checks the success of the plan and with guidance adjusts the goal to increase the probability of success. For example, if adding an egg to the mixture was problematic due to the client only having use of one hand, the therapist/client team would try a different physical approach, check back on its success, and adjust the plan as needed upon completion. More details on this approach are available (Polatajko & Mandich, 2004).

CLINICAL PEARL

The field of neuro-occupation supports the idea that engaging in meaningful occupations (i.e., as perceived by the client) can promote brain development and health (Royeen, 2003). The process of synapse development and growth is "not only sensitive to experience, it is driven by experience" (Metz & Robnett, 2011, p. 117).

Grading

Intervention activities can be graded by changing some aspect of the activity or the occupational demands. Many possibilities are presented in the *Framework* (American Occupational Therapy Association, 2014a). One example would be to alter the social demands of the task, either by easing the social expectations placed on the client to interact with others or to challenge the client socially by encouraging increased group participation. Other aspects of the activity demand that might be altered may include space demands (e.g., enlarging the space may make the task easier or more difficult), the objects used (e.g., familiar vs unfamiliar appliances), or the number of steps of a task. The OTA and the OT can collaborate to optimize learning and cognition by considering how aspects of any pertinent activity support or hinder occupational performance.

Cueing

During intervention, the OT or OTA systematically provides verbal and physical cues and can modify the cueing according to the client's responses. Cues can be external (provided by the practitioner), directive (e.g., "Put your right arm in the sleeve first" or "Do what I do"), used to direct attention to a particular aspect of a task (e.g., "What is not quite right here?"), promote problem solving (e.g., "What do *you* think comes next?"), or to facilitate recall (e.g., "What's the next step?") (Toglia, 2011). The OT and OTA must keep the outcome goals at the forefront. If remediation or improvement is expected, the cues should become more general and internalized (evolve into self-cueing) as the person can begin to handle this challenge. Ensuring successful performance with the least assistance (including cueing) is the art and the science of occupational therapy intervention.

Learning Style

To promote learning and memory of important information, the practitioner needs to consider the client's preferred learning style. To understand more about learning styles in general, the VARK website (Fleming, 2019) is helpful as it offers a questionnaire that will help readers determine their own learning style or learning style combination (visual, aural, reading/writing, or kinesthetic). Although the VARK questionnaire is considered an instructional tool rather than a test, preliminary psychometric analysis shows limited but positive results. By identifying the client's optimal learning style, as a practitioner you may be able to enhance learning. Visual learners prefer visual stimulation to promote learning (e.g., pictures, photos, videos), whereas aural learners prefer to listen to instructions or hear other needed information. Aural learners enjoy stories and examples to enhance their retention, and they often want to talk about what they have learned in therapy. Those who prefer reading and writing may also choose to take notes and write down what they want to remember from the therapy session. For these avid readers, suggesting websites for further information can be beneficial, and they value written handouts (Hamilton, 2005).

Kinesthetic learners use a hands-on approach to learning (Hamilton, 2005). They benefit from engaging in the tasks to be learned. Demonstrations, the use of models, and interacting with the material to be learned through their various senses are all helpful to promote long-term learning. Indeed, Benjamin Franklin already understood this when he said, "Tell me and I forget, teach me and I may remember, involve me and I learn." OTs and OTAs are, after all, "doing" therapists.

As the characteristics of the optimal teaching/learning methods (most often multimodal) are uncovered, this information can be communicated to the client, to others who work with the client, and to the client's family. For example, in working with a specific client who was diagnosed with moderate dementia to learn how to incorporate hip precautions, a simple song about them was both delightfully repeated and eventually integrated into daily tasks, whereas written and verbal instructions did not stick.

In addition, providing multimodal input can be helpful for retention. When the input stimuli spans more than one sense modality (e.g., reading about hip precautions, talking about them, and practicing these during everyday tasks [seeing and feeling how they are done]), ease and depth of learning can be enhanced (Piccirilli, Pigliautile, & Arcelli, 2019). Always strive for creative engagement, which is likely to enhance everyone's experience (including your own).

When considering written and spoken information, the readability of this material must match the skills of the client. Handouts need to be written in plain, direct, and concise language, using bullets and figures, when appropriate, to convey information. The use of medical jargon and complicated words will decrease the level of understanding. The intention is not for the information to be "dumbed down," the informer should only keep in mind that every day or "living room language" is more comprehensible and acceptable. Make the effort to communicate at the right level for each client (Riffenburgh & Stableford, 2020).

Memory

Memory performance can sometimes be remediated for those with only mild impairments, although remediation has not been shown to be effective for those with moderate or severe memory losses (Cicerone et al., 2019; Cicerone, Langenbahn, & Braden, 2011). Remediation often involves practicing memory tasks such as learning word lists or remembering names. These exercises seem to work most effectively if the person is motivated to improve his or her performance and if the items to be remembered are meaningful to the person (e.g., a grocery list vs a random list of meaningless words) (Levy, 2011). Memory training, perhaps in the form of group mental aerobics, may have potential for increasing memory functioning and other cognitive skills (Hayslip, Paggi, & Poole, 2009). If the person is not able to improve memory performance, various external strategies such as smartphone applications, cue cards, or signs around the home may be used (Table 22.2).

Domain-specific training, or task-specific training, may be used for the client who has global memory deficits. This client may be able to learn new skills to be used in a particular situation (usually after much repetition) but the client may not be expected to transfer or generalize these learning processes or skills to a new environment. An example is the client who is taught one-handed cooking skills in the occupational therapy department's kitchen but cannot transfer these skills to the home environment. In this case, home instruction would be preferable. If home occupational therapy is not an option, then the problem of learning transfer must be addressed during intervention. Gillen (2009) suggests the following techniques: practicing techniques in various settings, especially in the client's natural environments; practicing strategies (e.g., for remembering) during multiple meaningful tasks; and making the client aware of the intention of the intervention (e.g., using self-awareness or metacognition). Transfer of learning will occur more easily if the new setting or altered task is only slightly different (known as a "near transfer of learning") (Gillen, 2009; Toglia, 2011). Again, given that the client does not have typical cognition, more repetition than initially anticipated may be needed. Job coaching, a type of supported employment in which OTAs may provide on-the-job therapy services, is based on promoting new learning through these techniques. For best results, the skills needed for the job are taught to the client at the client's job site (Wehman, 1991).

Higher-Level Cognitive Functions

Higher-level cognitive functions include insight and judgment, awareness, concept formation, time management, organization, problem solving, and decision making (American Occupational Therapy Association, 2014a). Sometimes these skills are called **executive functions** because they are used to manage and control other less complex cognitive processes. The client's level of awareness of higher-level cognitive

TABLE 22.2	Examples of Adaptive and Compensatory Strategies	
Task	**Impairment**	**Strategy**
Dressing	Sequencing deficit	Consistently place garments in the sequence to be donned, provide laminated checklist, develop routine
Bathing	Sequencing deficit	Provide a pictorial of the sequence of washing—starting distally and progressing proximally (laminated if necessary in shower)
Feeding	Sequencing deficit or lack of judgment	Provide smaller utensils that assist the intake of smaller portions with each bite; encourage putting down utensil between bites
Safety and emergency maintenance	Judgment deficit	Provide step-by-step instructions for handling emergency by phone or wherever needed; obtain and encourage use of electronic device to summon assistance
Job performance	Impaired short-term memory	Employ calendars or day-to-day planners; use smart device for reminders
Meal preparation	Impaired short-term memory or decreased attention	Purchase appliances that shut off automatically; set timers; use recipes; check off what has been completed (can use laminated sheets with dry erase markers)
	Figure-ground impairment	Use high contrast between foreground and background (e.g., plates vs placemats, drinks vs mugs), simplify and organize
Social participation	Disorientation	Have people wear name tags; start conversation with statement of who the visitor is; display schedule boards that include who will visit; use calendars
Reading	Visual field loss	Use a red marker or ribbon to mark the edge of the page; place written material on the unaffected side
Bathing	Unilateral neglect	Make sure water heater is turned down to 120°F or lower, for safety, because the hot water knob is generally on the left

function strengths and deficits will determine the type of intervention to be used. At one extreme is the client who has a high degree of awareness. This type of client may learn to respond to internal strategies for self-monitoring or to environmental compensatory cues. For example, the client may develop a mnemonic or jingle to assist in organizing and remembering information or keep a notebook, calendar, to-do lists, and other reminders to stimulate initiation of activity. One mnemonic to use for remembering to take all the necessary items when one changes locations is STOP—Stop, Think, Observe (all around you), Proceed.

OTs and OTAs may use various intervention approaches to address awareness impairments. Remediation of awareness deficits may be appropriate for those with mild impairments who have the capacity to learn new information. Awareness level may be increased through the use of self-estimation by asking the client to predict the outcome of a question or task performance and then together processing the discrepancies that may exist between what was expected and what actually occurred (Katz & Maeir, 2011). The practitioner and client can also reverse roles within the context of intervention to promote increased awareness of safety issues. Toglia (2011) suggests using self-evaluation both before a task and following the completion of the task to problem-solve errors in performance and to build self-awareness. This not only gives the practitioner a sense of the client's self-awareness level but also imparts information about the person's level of self-confidence. Intervention may focus on the client's ability to question and evaluate his or her own or others' performance.

Feedback using videos of occupational performance can be helpful for remediation. To be effective it must be based on a foundation of trust, given with timeliness in a private setting, allow the client opportunity for self-reflection related to errors, and involve occupations meaningful to the client (Schmidt, Fleming, & Ownsworth, 2015). A peer group approach can also be useful in obtaining feedback from others to build the client's self-awareness (Toglia, 2011). Videotaping behavior is objective and can provide a visual record, which can be used by the OT or OTA to discuss performance with clients to assist them in learning to use techniques to effectively control their behaviors. Those with impairments in self-awareness may not fully understand or be able to admit that any deficits exist. These clients may need cueing from nonjudgmental others they trust.

CLINICAL PEARL

When a problem seems difficult to solve, breaking it down into pieces may make the solution obvious. It also will allow for more careful analysis (Whimbey, Lochhead, & Narode, 2013). One of the most highly regarded characteristics of OTs and OTAs is the ability to break tasks and goals down to manageable, doable steps.

The focus of intervention for higher-level cognitive dysfunction is generally to promote effective reasoning, organizing, and problem solving. Learning proficient problem solving is a worthwhile goal when it is a reasonable expectation, although this type of learning is not generally easy for those with higher-level cognitive dysfunction. The OTA should model the step-by-step process and help the client to use the sequence of problem solving when challenges occur during daily tasks.

The steps are:

1. Defining the main points of the problem in relevant terms
2. Organizing or structuring the information into easy and difficult portions of the problem (e.g., breaking down the problem)
3. Developing possible solutions
4. Choosing one best solution
5. Executing the solution
6. Evaluating the outcome (Beyer, 1987; Ylvisaker, Jacobs, & Feeney, 2003), and then perhaps starting again

The client may be able to learn this sequence along with instructions to follow the steps when a problem is encountered in therapy or during day-to-day tasks. Along a similar vein, Parenté and Herrmann (Parenté & Herrmann, 2010) offer steps in decision making, which also may be impaired in those with cognitive deficits.

They use the mnemonic of DECIDE in the following way:

D = Deciding to get going and to not procrastinate

E = Evaluating options (looking for options that offer win-win solutions)

C = Creating new options if none are found to be suitable

I = Investigating the best options

D = Discussing potential choices with others (initially avoiding sharing one's own opinion) and listening to their advice

E = Evaluating your feelings (thinking twice before taking action)

The OTA can use these sequences to assist clients to transfer and apply decision making and problem solving to a variety of situations. These may include the context of occupational therapy intervention and their everyday lives. The bottom line is to gather as much information as possible, make a decision, and move on from there (Michaud & Wild, 1991).

> **CLINICAL PEARL**
>
> The occupational therapy practitioner can assist with decision making by encouraging the client to consider all feasible options. Rarely is either "yes" or "no" the only way to go.

Intervention for Behavioral Impairments. A deficit in higher-level cognitive functioning (including decreased self-awareness) may result in behavioral or social impairments due to the client's lack of insight or judgment and deficient problem-solving skills. These deficits may occur during recovery in persons who have experienced an ABI or who have other neurocognitive impairments. Behavioral management strategies may be helpful to control or restrict behavioral outbursts. Team members may need to give the client consistent, client-specific, direct feedback regarding the inappropriateness of the behavior. If the client's level of insight and self-control warrant, internal strategies (such as personal timeout or actively removing oneself from the situation) can be incorporated into the client's plan. External controls also may be used as needed. For example, a team member may escort clients to a quiet area until they are able to feel in control of their behavior. The team member must remain calm and provide consistent verbal cues related to the situation. Strong emotional response, including yelling or arguing with the client, can exacerbate the situation. Training programs to provide positive behavior support such as the Mandt System (https://www.mandtsystem.com/) may be helpful in facilities and at worksites where behavioral issues are more common.

SUMMARY OF INTERVENTION FOR THOSE WITH COGNITIVE IMPAIRMENTS

Cognitive performance and capacity always need to be considered during occupational therapy interventions because the brain controls all voluntary, and most involuntary, actions. For those who are functioning at a high cognitive level, learning new tasks and problem solving comes easily. For those who have impairments, the challenge is to make the most of their cognitive strengths while managing their deficits. Due to the complexity of factors and the compounding effect of multiple impairments in cognition, interventions involving cognitive training or retraining can be convoluted and time consuming. Those with impaired cognition may require more time to learn new skills or to consistently use compensatory measures. Clients with significant cognitive impairments specifically require integrated team-based interventions to promote optimal functioning.

When working with adults (or anyone) with cognitive deficits, the occupational therapy practitioner is encouraged to maintain hope for and with the person. Focus on the person's strengths, even if these are hidden under a few layers of what seems negative and perhaps does not remotely engender hope. Dunn (2017) encourages all of us to reevaluate what we call "deficits," to see them in another light, perhaps as an "uber strength" (p. 395). For example, anxiety can be the impetus for us to put energy into organizing and structuring our lives; displaying too much emotion can be revisioned as being an extremely caring and warm-hearted person. Strengths and deficits are not opposite, they are both sides of the same coin. As a practitioner, always consider focus on the person's self-defined authentic life. Support people to "live their own version of a satisfying life" (not yours) (Dunn, 2017, p. 395). We can learn from positive psychology to help promote flourishing (eudaimonia) instead of simple pleasure (hedonia; see https://www.psychologytoday.com/us/basics/positive-psychology).

Flourishing fits well with engagement in meaningful occupations. Nurturing strengths and positivity (even for imperfect persons in an imperfect world) is more likely to lead to the evolvement of therapeutic, genuine rapport and successful outcomes.

> **CLINICAL PEARL**
>
> Always think biopsychosocially—do what you can to make sure that the client's environment, physical condition (including positioning and level of pain), and emotional state are optimally primed for learning.

INTERVENTION FOR PERCEPTUAL DEFICITS

"Perception is not simply the registration and evaluation of sense data, but rather an active taking hold of the world" (Kielhofner, 2008, p. 72). Perception is the interpretation of incoming sensory data. Intact perceptual skills allow the person to interpret and impart logical meaning to the input arriving through their sensory systems, including auditory, tactile, olfactory, gustatory, vestibular (primarily head position), proprioceptive (body in space and bodily movement), and visual information (Thomas, 2015). Accurate understanding of this information is a necessary (although insufficient) element to promote correct responses to the environment and subsequent successful engagement in occupations. Adept performance of daily tasks in just about all areas of occupation requires intact perceptual and cognitive skills. Accurate perceptual processing (based on incoming sensory data) provides a foundation for appropriate motor actions. Due to the direct impact on motor actions, remediation or compensation for perceptual deficits (specifically visual) may result in improved functional performance (Neistadt, 1994). OTs and OTAs can focus on retraining specific perceptual skills and/or incorporating perceptual retraining into functional tasks such as ADL, IADL, education, and work.

As with intervention for cognitive deficits, the two most common approaches are the remediation and adaptation approaches. The remediation approach uses transfer-of-training or perceptual retraining, through practice, exercises, and engagement in meaningful activities that relate to the deficient areas (Gillen, 2009). Typically these practice drills have involved tabletop, pencil-and-paper, and computer activities. The adaptive approach uses client skills that are intact or relatively intact to compensate for skills that are deficient. Adaptation and compensation may also use extrinsic or environmental measures that help enable or improve performance. Intervention activities should be client centered and involve functional, real-life, and meaningful tasks (Gillen, 2009; Neistadt, 1994).

Body Schema Related Perceptual Deficits: Descriptions and Interventions

Perceptual and cognitive impairments are intricately related. Perceptual deficits may be misinterpreted as cognitive deficits by the casual observer who observes flawed motor responses brought on by impaired perception and assumes this means that clients cannot understand what is being asked of them. Fascinating reading that explores the sometimes devastating impact of perceptual difficulties is presented in the book by Oliver Sacks, *The Man Who Mistook His Wife for a Hat and Other Clinical Tales* (Sacks, 1998). Even highly experienced OTs and OTAs can find perceptual deficits extremely challenging to address, and yet to achieve successful occupational performance they must be tackled.

Postural body geometry, which is necessary to keep our bodies in alignment gravitationally, seems to be more often impaired after right-side brain damage (Lafosse, Kerckhofs,

& Vereeck, 2007). This impairment is often associated with spatial neglect (generally left) and can result in poor postural control, loss of balance, and pushing syndrome, in which the person pushes contralateral to the side with the lesion. These body scheme deficits, if severe, can greatly affect the person's potential for rehabilitation. Researchers (Corbin & Unsworth, 1999; Zoltan, 2007) offer a number of intervention strategies for body scheme disorders, including the following:

- Providing tactile stimulation to the body parts affected. Stimulation may be given by the practitioner, or preferably clients can learn to attend to the body parts by themselves (perhaps starting with body lotion, which can be soothing).
- Facilitating normal bilateral movements when possible during everyday tasks, by encouraging and through verbal and physical guidance.
- Using a mirror (especially a full-length mirror) to augment the visual awareness of the neglected body parts.
- Educating clients (and their families) about the disorder to the level they can understand, with an emphasis on safety, and especially letting clients/families know that visual perceptual impairments are the result of the brain injury, not their fault.

Kempler (2005) suggests avoiding use of the words *right* and *left* in giving directions if these are confusing to the client, but rather providing a visual cue (e.g., colored tape) on one side or the other to remind the client the difference between the two sides (e.g., shoes).

CLINICAL PEARL

With visual perceptual disturbances, as with other neurologic disturbances such as dementia, it is crucial to blame the disease, not the person. At times this is an easier concept for the practitioner to learn than the family or the clients as they may get impatient with the person (or themselves) who is no longer the same as he or she was.

Astereognosis. Stereognosis is the perceptual skill of identifying familiar objects and geometric shapes through touch, proprioception, and cognition without the aid of vision (e.g., finding a nickel among the coins in your pocket by feel). **Astereognosis**, or tactile agnosia, is a deficit of this skill. The person is unable to perceive identity of objects due to the loss of capacity to sense or organize shape, texture, temperature, or weight (Bradshaw & Mattingly, 1995). Vision is often used to compensate. In the example mentioned, the person could take all the coins out of the pocket and lay them on the table to see which one is a nickel. Astereognosis may occur after a lesion on either side of the brain in the somatosensory perception areas, which is a common lesion site in cerebrovascular accident (CVA) and in neurologic conditions such as cerebral palsy (Connell, Lincoln, & Radford, 2008). Stereognosis, or seeing with the hands, is integral to the typical performance of everyday activities.

Interventions to remediate astereognosis include practicing identifying objects first using vision and then, with vision occluded, describing the object and carefully exploring its tactile features (Fig. 22.5). Practicing stereognosis should occur during tasks that are meaningful for the client. A sample task for a homemaker might be finding specific utensils while doing the dishes in soapy water (with sharp knives removed for safety). Similar games or object-finding activities can be devised for whatever task the client claims is difficult. More scientific scrutiny of visual perceptual interventions would be helpful.

Apraxia. Praxis is a Latin word that refers to "doing or acting." Praxis is a complex, ongoing, evolving process that involves cognitive planning and physical coordination to accurately carry through the person's motor plans. **Apraxia**, then, is the inability to plan and perform the motor acts necessary to complete ordinary tasks such as dressing or brushing teeth, even though there are no obvious motoric deficits or significant muscular weaknesses. Apraxia is a common condition occurring in nearly half of those who have sustained a stroke on the left side of the brain, and in approximately one-third of those diagnosed with AD with corticobasal degeneration (Pazzaglia & Galli, 2019).

Gillen (2009) reviewed the evidence regarding interventions to overcome apraxia. Similar to cognitive rehabilitation, interventions fall into two categories: remediation to "decrease the apraxic impairment" (p. 122) or adaptation, which focuses on learning strategies to improve occupational performance in spite of apraxia. Although the evidence for remediation is still scant, tactile, kinesthetic stimulation in addition to "visual and verbal mediation input" (p. 123) and the practicing of gestures (not entire tasks) have been undertaken. Recently Pazzaglia and Galli (2019) reviewed several studies on the interventions used to remediate or manage apraxia. No definitive treatment recommendations have been forthcoming.

Occupational therapy intervention for apraxia involves compensating for associated impairments. In the case of apraxia involving problems with dressing, for example, the OT or OTA can teach the client to develop a set routine for dressing by providing cues to assist the client in distinguishing clothing item features such as right arm from left arm or front from back (Zoltan, 2007). The client can be encouraged to look for distinctive features such as the collar or label to orient the clothing item correctly. The client may position the garment the same way each time, as in laying out a shirt with the buttons face down and top away from the client to promote the development of a specific routine. To assist a client who has difficulty buttoning a shirt, different tactics might work; individualized trial and error is often necessary. The shirt could be partially buttoned and the client could finish the task of buttoning (as in backward chaining), or the buttoned-down shirt could be worn as a pullover shirt, which is likely to be easier for the client (Neistadt, 1994). Another technique could be to cue the client to start buttoning at the bottom of the shirt or sweater because it is easier to match the right and left halves when the garment can be seen and the edges are distinct (Fig. 22.6). Rarely is only one occupation impacted when apraxia manifests itself. The practitioner always needs to provide the type of instructions, assistance, and feedback that is most appropriate for the client. The occupational therapy team can collaborate to find the most effective techniques for each client. While one person may need direct step-by-step directions and physical assistance, another may need only a verbal cue to get the task done. For examples of instructional, assistance level, and feedback strategies see Table 22.3.

Two primary types of apraxia, **ideomotor** and **ideational apraxia**, may occur as a consequence of having had a stroke. Both significantly affect occupational performance. Ideomotor apraxia is an inability to plan or perform a motor skill. The patient may understand the concept, may even be able to describe the intended motion and attempt to carry out the task, but cannot execute the motor act at will. Some skills such as waving goodbye or brushing teeth may be performed spontaneously, but not on demand. Ideational or conceptual apraxia is the "breakdown of knowledge of what is to be done to perform" or the loss of "a mental representation of the concept required for performance" (Gillen, 2009, p. 110). Clients may seem confused and display hesitant motor actions, or they may not be able to initiate the task at all. While it may be difficult to distinguish

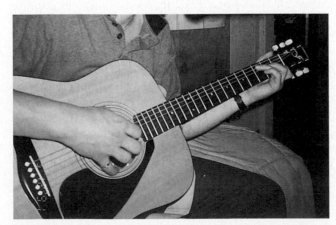

Fig. 22.5 Playing an instrument can require a good sense of stereognosis. For example, one cannot constantly watch while one plays the guitar. (From Leifer G. *Introduction to Maternity and Pediatric Nursing.* 8th ed. St Louis, MO: Elsevier; 2019.)

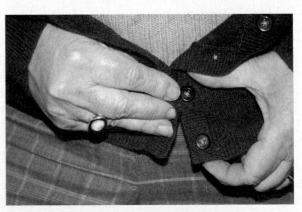

Fig. 22.6 Buttoning starting from the bottom is easiest because one can see and line up the bottom edges of the sweater.

TABLE 22.3   Potential Strategies[a] for Working With Those Who Have Apraxia (Presented in Hierarchic Fashion)

Instructions	• Be sure to do intervention in relevant environment for client, if needed
	• Try verbal prompts first (multistep or single step)
	• Alert the client through touch
	• Use gestures and point to objects
	• Demonstrate task (whole or part)
	• Use pictures
	• Write down instructions
	• Put objects in proper sequence and hand them to client one at a time
	• Start the task together
Assistance level (in order of need)	• No assistance needed
	• Verbal prompts (to review steps or direct attention), vary intonation as needed
	• Use gestures
	• Use sequential pictures
	• Provide physical assistance as needed
Feedback to client	• No feedback needed
	• Verbal feedback about results
	• Provide information related to sensory evaluation of results (e.g., ask clients what they see, hear, feel)
	• Provide physical feedback (posture, support, and positioning)
	• Feedback provided about objects for task (pointing to or giving client object)
	• Verbal feedback at level of understanding about level of performance
	• Use mirror during task
	• Provide video feedback

[a]If none of these techniques work, client is likely dependent in task.

Adapted from Gillen G. *Cognitive and Perceptual Rehabilitation: Optimizing Function.* St Louis, MO: Mosby Elsevier; 2009:126; originally from Van Heugten CM, Dekker J, Deelman BG, et al. Outcome of strategy training in stroke patients with apraxia: a phase II study. *Clin Rehab.* 1998;12(4):294–303.

between ideational and ideomotor apraxia in individual clients, those who have not lost the concept of the task (i.e., those with ideomotor apraxia) may be able to complete tasks, especially those that are automatic. Thus ideomotor is the less debilitating form of apraxia. For those with ideomotor apraxia, practicing automatic (formerly familiar) routines may enable the client to return to simplified versions of their daily tasks. Those displaying ideomotor apraxia may do better attempting the entire task rather than the individual components, especially if this is a familiar habitual task that is completed in a typical context (e.g., environment, time of day, with familiar items). To complete a toothbrushing task, the practitioner may try handing the toothbrush with toothpaste on it to the client while he or she is in the bathroom standing in front of the sink with the intention of promoting the spontaneous completion of this task.

Intervention for those with apraxia can be particularly challenging for clients who have concurrent aphasia or communication difficulties. The practitioner should use clear, concise, concrete instructions, repeated as needed. Breaking down tasks into component steps and teaching each step separately may be effective. Guiding the client through the correct movements, while giving intermittent tactile and proprioceptive input, may be more successful than verbal or demonstrated instructions. After the client has performed each step of the task separately, the clinician can begin to combine the steps, grading the complexity and number of steps as the client is able (Okkema, 1993).

An example of a complete task is combing hair. The OT or OTA can break the task into a motor sequence with or without hand-over-hand guidance: pick up comb; bring comb to hair; move comb across top of head, down left side, down right side, and down back; and replace comb on table. Clients verbalizing (or envisioning) each step as they complete it may be helpful. The clinician may instruct the client to watch (in this case using a mirror) as each step is completed (Butler, 1999). Repetition is necessary for effective results. For examples of instructional, assistance level, and feedback strategies, see Table 22.3.

Visual Processing and Visual Perception Intervention Approaches (See Chapter 21)

Visual Agnosia (see Chapter 21). Agnosia is a condition in which a person does not recognize common everyday objects. Visual agnosia is a failure to recognize items that can be seen. The person can see the objects, but the perception is without meaning (Zoltan, 2007). The problem may be specific to one type of item (e.g., faces, utensils, supplies) or more global. Dense agnosia results in a general and extremely debilitating inability to interact appropriately with visually perceived items. Clients may carry out unusual or even bizarre acts such as donning underwear on the head or using a comb as a toothbrush. Visual perceptual functions sometimes improve spontaneously. Zoltan (2007) shares some helpful hints in management of this deficit, including promoting the use of other sensory modalities such as touch to add texture or edge orientation cues, providing labels, and giving verbal cues as needed. More recently, Heutink et al. (2018) conducted a systematic review on interventions for visual agnosia, encompassing 22 published articles, the majority of which were case studies or had very small sample sizes. They discussed both restorative measures (such as visual exercises), which have not yet been determined to be effective, but which do need to be "systematically evaluated" (p. 1506), as well as compensatory measures. They found tactile and auditory (verbal description) measures to be the most helpful.

Impairments in Visual Discrimination

Visual discrimination includes several subskills such as discrimination by form, depth perception, figure-ground perception, and spatial relations. Form discrimination is the ability to group and to differentiate various forms of the same type of item (e.g., various makes of cars are still identified as vehicles) and to identify an item when viewed from various vantage points such as from the side or the back. Helpful techniques may include practice in identifying objects not only by sight but also through tactile manipulation. The therapist must make sure that the item is presented in the most common position (upright, forward facing). Labeling and organizing items are adaptations that may make it easier for the person to recognize items of interest.

Depth perception is the ability to recognize and understand differences in distances between objects. This skill requires vision in both eyes to get the true binocular effect of perceiving three-dimensional space. However, people can and do use other cues besides binocular vision to determine depth or spatial relations between objects. One cue is the relation of size to distance, in that same-sized items that are farther away appear smaller. Learning about the typical relationships between different-sized objects over time is also helpful. In addition, light, shadows, and movement in relation to the observer can play into the understanding of distance and depth.

Figure-ground perception is the ability to distinguish an object from its background such as a fork in a pile of silverware or a certain type of flower in a garden. Practicing finding objects at the level the client is able to, starting with a few objects with a high-level of obvious contrast if necessary, and gradually introducing more complexity to challenge the person to improve, may enhance these perceptual skills, but strong evidence for this type of intervention is lacking. If the client is unable to understand how these perceptual factors affect daily performance and how to compensate for their absence, educating the family and trusted others about adapting the environment and cueing is certainly necessary (Fig. 22.7).

Charles Bonnet syndrome is an unusual yet not uncommon occurrence that also impacts visual perceptual performance. Up to 50% of those diagnosed with macular degeneration (age-related [AMD], one of the most common diagnoses of low vision affecting older adults) experience Charles Bonnet syndrome (Macular Society, 2019). This strange phenomenon involves visual perceptual deficits in the form of hallucinations and can occur in the context of other low-vision diagnoses as well. The phenomenon is similar to phantom limb sensation; however, instead of the loss of a limb, the person has lost visual capacity, and the brain is simply trying to fill in the sensory gaps (Strong, 2019). These disturbances (as those affected would certainly describe them as "disturbing") may involve the simple sensation of movement among visual stimuli or light flashes to full-blown visual misrepresentations (Macular Society, 2019; Strong, 2019). As one client described it, "the flowered curtains became a detailed circus scene." Addressing Charles Bonnet syndrome is important when working with adults who have the diagnosis of AMD (or other visual diagnoses such as diabetic retinopathy,

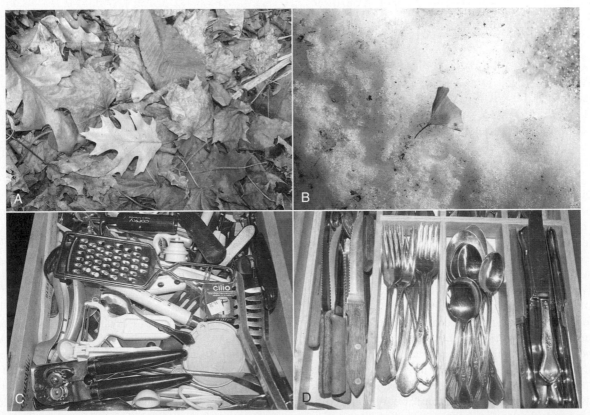

Fig. 22.7 Figure-ground examples. (A) Finding different types of leaves in a pile. (B) Increasing contrast and simplicity makes the task easier. (C) It is difficult to find a soup spoon in a cluttered drawer. (D) Organizing utensils can help the client find needed items.

retinitis pigmentosa, and glaucoma). By simply asking if they think they have experienced seeing things that were unusual or might not have been real, one can determine if this phenomenon is occurring. Educating the person about this syndrome can provide great relief, especially since the topic may not have been brought up by other health care professionals. They may have thought that they experience hallucinations based on a psychiatric disorder, which is not the case. Those with AMD (or other visual diagnoses and no significant cognitive impairments) can easily learn that the interpretation of visual stimuli takes place in the visual processing system (where something goes awry due to the syndrome), and that Charles Bonnet is not an uncommon disorder. While a cure seems to be lacking, some have found blinking during the experience and better lighting (spot lighting with minimal glare) may be helpful (Strong, 2019).

SUMMARY OF INTERVENTIONS FOR COGNITIVE AND PERCEPTUAL DEFICITS

Effective restoration or management of cognitive and perceptual skill impairments requires understanding the underlying mechanisms and identifying the point of breakdown in a particular action or task. A competent OT or OTA has the ability to conduct activity analyses as needed to determine the usual demands of any pertinent task, as well as the specific client factors and performance skills, including the requisite levels of those factors/skills needed to successfully complete the task. Through this analysis process, the OT or OTA can determine what skills are lacking and when during the process performance breaks down. Adaptations can be made to simplify the task or the environment to promote successful performance. A strong foundation of occupational therapy evidence for intervention in cognition and perception has not yet been firmly established. Despite this, OTs and OTAs throughout the world regularly provide successful interventions in the areas of cognition and perception, both restorative and adaptive or compensatory approaches. As the evidence slowly continues to mount, through high-quality, peer-reviewed research projects and subsequent publications, OTs and OTAs will more often be on the team of experts who understand and have learned the science and art of optimally managing cognitive and perceptual impairments that have impacted clients' meaningful occupations.

The practice recommendations, guidelines, and options offered by the in-depth systematic review and analysis of the efficacy of cognitive rehabilitation techniques by Cicerone et al. (2019) can be extremely helpful in designing and carrying through interventions for cognitive and perceptual impairments. While specific recommendations are beyond the scope of this chapter, several general recommendations are worth sharing, even if these merely provide the impetus to explore the topics further. These recommendations were written with treatment planning in mind, but they are worth sharing among the rehabilitation team for intervention implementation as well. The review by Cicerone et al. (2019)

is highly recommended for those who work in the field of cognitive rehabilitation as a journal club selection, as their review is worth discussing. Highlights are as follows:

- Cognitive retraining involving computer exercises should involve goal-directed intervention to increase performance in everyday occupations under the direction of a rehabilitation therapist (e.g., occupational therapy practitioner).
- Evidence supports the use of visual scanning training to mitigate left neglect; computer activities can be used to this end but should not be used in isolation.
- Group and individual-based intervention for those with mild impairments in prospective memory is recommended and includes the use of both internal strategies (visual imagery and association techniques) and external compensatory techniques (such as provided by assistive technology).
- Self-monitoring and self-regulation training may be effective for problem solving and goal management, and video/verbal feedback can be an important aspect of increasing self-awareness.
- Severe deficits may be most effectively managed through specific skills training (as transfer of training is less likely).
- Perhaps most important for occupational therapy clinical practice is for practitioners to ensure "that any evidence-based intervention is relevant to the person's everyday functioning" (Cicerone et al., 2019, p. 1528).

> ### CLINICAL PEARL
>
> As Fine (1991) stated long ago, the following still holds true today: "Personal perceptions and responses to stressful life events are crucial elements to survival, recovery, and rehabilitation, often transcending the reality of the situation or the interventions of others. The inner life (affective and cognitive processes and content) holds the potential for transforming traumas into varying degrees of triumph" (p. 493).

SUMMARY

Cognitive and perceptual impairments are complex and can seem overwhelming to the novice practitioner. They can only be viewed through behaviors, never directly. Working in this realm requires the OTA to develop astute observational skills and an awareness of providing the just-right level of cueing and assistance. Learning to develop one's best version of therapeutic-use-of-self and the ability to appreciate the impact of context on functioning are important aspirations. Breaking down the functional performance deficits through activity analysis (provided by a thorough knowledge base of the *Framework* (American Occupational Therapy Association, 2014a)) is necessary to promote client's skills/strengths while addressing areas of concern through adaptation and compensation. Many theories have been developed to assist practitioners in providing thoughtful and cohesive interventions. The OT is responsible for evaluation, planning, and designing interventions for clients with cognitive and perceptual deficits. The OTA can contribute by carefully observing client behavior and by applying general intervention principles and techniques in consultation with the OT. Detailed intervention methodology in cognition and perception is beyond the scope of this textbook; however, interested OTAs can educate themselves on the possibilities. OTAs are encouraged to obtain continuing education and sufficient clinical experience to refine their skills so that they can competently and confidently work with clients who have cognitive and/or perceptual impairments.

> **CLINICAL PEARL**
>
> Have hope. Convey hope. People are resilient and can work to make positive changes. As a client-centered occupational therapy practitioner, you can be a catalyst for this transformation.

REVIEW QUESTIONS

1. Compare and contrast the roles of the OT and the OTA in the intervention of clients with deficits in cognition and/or perception.
2. Come up with examples of how several different cognitive and perceptual impairments affect daily performance by relating them to areas of occupation in the *Occupational Therapy Practice Framework*.
3. Compare remedial and compensatory/adaptive intervention techniques as to when you would use one rather than the other, or both at the same time. How do these approaches fit into client-centered practice?
4. List three strategies used for patients with deficits in orientation.
5. Give at least three examples (beyond those mentioned in the chapter) of each of the different types of memory described using everyday activities (short term, working, long term, prospective, episodic, and semantic). Explain how these types differ.
6. Describe how context (as many aspects as are pertinent [see the *Occupational Therapy Practice Framework*, p. 28]) would affect the intervention approach for clients with memory deficits, and give two or three examples of interventions that might be helpful.
7. Give examples of strategies and activities used for the client with unilateral neglect.
8. Describe the specific steps you might use in working with a client who has ideomotor apraxia to relearn teeth brushing. Describe why having ideational apraxia would likely make the learning more difficult.
9. Explain how astereognosis might affect the completion of a skill you do every day and suggest intervention techniques.
10. Why is addressing Charles Bonnet syndrome important for those with visual diagnoses such as macular degeneration?

REFERENCES

American Occupational Therapy Association. (2014a). Occupational therapy practice framework: domain and process (3rd ed.). *The American Journal of Occupational Therapy, 68*(Suppl. 1), S1–S48.

American Occupational Therapy Association. (2014b). Guidelines for supervision, roles, and responsibilities during the delivery of occupational therapy services. *The American Journal of Occupational Therapy, 68*, S16–S22. Available from: https://doi.org/10.5014/ajot.2014.686S03.

American Occupational Therapy Association. (2018). Occupational therapy assistant supervision requirements. https://www.aota.org/~/media/Corporate/Files/Secure/Advocacy/Licensure/StateRegs/Supervision/Occupational%20Therapy%20Assistant%20Supervision%20Requirements%20Oct%202016%20FINAL.pdf.

American Occupational Therapy Association. (2019). Occupational therapist–occupational therapy assistant partnerships: achieving high ethical standards in a challenging health care environment. Retrieved from: https://www.aota.org.

Baddeley, A. (2014). *Essentials of human memory: classic edition.* New York: Psychology Press.

Beyer, B. K. (1987). *Practical strategies for the teaching of thinking.* Boston, MA: Allyn & Bacon.

Bourgeois, M. S. (2007). *Memory books and other graphic cuing systems: practical communication and memory aids for adults with dementia.* Baltimore, MD: Health Professions Press.

Bradshaw, J. L., & Mattingly, J. B. (1995). *Clinical neuropsychology: behavioral and brain science.* San Diego, CA: Academic Press.

Butler, J. A. (1999). Evaluation and intervention with apraxia. In C. Unsworth (Ed.), *Cognitive and perceptual dysfunction* (pp. 257–298). Philadelphia, PA: F.A. Davis.

Cicerone, K. D., Goldin, Y., Ganci, K., et al. (2019). Evidence-based cognitive rehabilitation: systematic review of the literature from 2009 through 2014. *Archives of Physical Medicine and Rehabilitation, 100*, 1515–1533. Available from: https://doi.org/10.1016/j.apmr.2019.02.011.

Cicerone, K. D., Langenbahn, D. M., Braden, C., et al. (2011). Evidence-based cognitive rehabilitation: updated review of the literature from 2003 through 2008. *Archives of Physical Medicine and Rehabilitation, 92*(4), 519–530.

Connell, L. A., Lincoln, N. B., & Radford, K. A. (2008). Somatosensory impairment after stroke: frequency of deficits and their recovery. *Clinical Rehabilitation, 2008*(22), 758–767.

Corbin, L., & Unsworth, C. (1999). Evaluation and intervention with unilateral neglect. In C. Unsworth (Ed.), *Cognitive and perceptual dysfunction* (pp. 357–392). Philadelphia, PA: F.A. Davis.

Doig, E., Fleming, J., Cornwell, P., et al. (2011). Comparing the experience of outpatient therapy in home and day hospital settings after traumatic brain injury: patient, significant other and therapist perspectives. *Disability and Rehabilitation, 33*(13-14), 1203–1214.

Dunn, W. (2017). Strengths-based approaches: what if even the 'bad' things are good things? *The British Journal of Occupational Therapy, 80*(7), 395–396. Available from: https://doi.org/10.1177/0308022617702660.

Fetta, J., Starkweather, A., & Gill, J. M. (2017). Computer-based cognitive rehabilitation interventions for traumatic brain injury: a critical review of the literature. *The Journal of Neuroscience Nursing, 49*(4), 235–240.

Fine, S. B. (1991). Resilience and human adaptability: who rises above adversity? 1990 Eleanor Clarke Slagle Lecture. *The American Journal of Occupational Therapy, 45*, 493–503.

Fleming, N. (2019). The Vark questionnaire V8.01. http://vark-learn.com/the-vark-questionnaire/?p = questionnaire.

Gillen, G. (2009). *Cognitive and perceptual rehabilitation: optimizing function.* St Louis, MO: Mosby Elsevier.

Hamilton, S. (2005). How do we assess the learning style of outpatients? *Rehabilitation Nursing Journal, 30*(4), 129–131.

Hayslip, B., Jr., Paggi, K., Poole, M., et al. (2009). The impact of mental aerobics training on memory impaired older adults. *Clinical Gerontologist, 32*(4), 389–394.

Heutink, J., Indorf, D. L., & Cordes, C. (2018). The neuropsychological rehabilitation of visual agnosia and Balint's syndrome. *Neuropsychological Rehabilitation, 1*, 1–20.

Inouye, S. K., Baker, D. I., Fugal, P., et al. (2006). Dissemination of the hospital elder life program: implementation, adaptation, and successes. *Journal of the American Geriatrics Society, 54* (10), 1492–1499.

Katz, N., & Maeir, A. (2011). Higher-level cognitive functions enabling participation: awareness and executive functions. In N. Katz (Ed.), *Cognition, occupation, and participation across the life span* (4th ed., pp. 13–40). Bethesda, MD: AOTA Press.

Kielhofner, G. (2008). *Model of human occupation theory and application* (4th ed.). Baltimore, MD: Lippincott, Williams & Wilkins.

Kempler, D. (2005). *Neurocognitive disorders of aging.* Thousand Oaks, CA: Sage Publications, Inc.

Knight, R. G., & Godfrey, H. P. D. (2002). Behavioral and self-report methods. In A. D. Baddeley, B. A. Wilson, & F. N. Watts (Eds.), *The handbook of memory disorders.* Chichester, UK: John Wiley & Sons Ltd.

Lafosse, C., Kerckhofs, E., Vereeck, L., et al. (2007). Postural abnormalities and contraversive pushing following right hemisphere brain damage. *Neuropsychological Rehabilitation, 17*(3), 374–396.

Laver, G. D. (2016). Aging and semantic memory. In N. Pachana (Ed.), *Encyclopedia of Geropsychology.* Singapore: Springer. Available from: https://doi.org/10.1007/978-981-287-080-3.

Levy, L. (2011). Cognitive aging. In N. Katz (Ed.), *Cognition, occupation, and participation across the life span* (3rd ed., pp. 117–141). Bethesda, MD: AOTA Press.

Macular Society. (2019). Visual hallucinations. https://www.macularsociety.org/visual-hallucinations.

Malia, K., Law, P., Sidebottom, L., et al. (2003). *Recommendations for best practice in cognitive rehabilitation therapy: acquired brain injury.* Exton, PA: The Society for Cognitive Rehabilitation, Inc.

McCrae, R. R., & Costa, P. T., Jr. (1997). Personality trait structure as a human universal. *The American Psychologist, 52*, 509–516.

Metitieri, T., Zanetti, O., Geroldi, C., et al. (2001). Reality orientation therapy to delay outcomes of progression in patients with dementia. A retrospective study. *Clinical Rehabilitation, 15*(5), 471–478.

Metz, A., & Robnett, R. (2011). Engaging in mentally challenging occupations promotes cognitive health throughout life. *Gerontology Special Interest Section Quarterly, 34*(2), 1–4.

Michaud, E., & Wild, R. (1991). *Boost your brain power.* Emmaus, PA: Rodale Press.

Miller, G. (1956). The magical number seven, plus or minus two. *Psychological Review, 63*, 81–97.

Neistadt, M. E. (1994). Perceptual training for adults with diffuse brain injury. *The American Journal of Occupational Therapy, 48*, 225–233.

Niechcial, M. A., Vaportzis, E., & Gow, A. J. (2019). People's views on preserving thinking skills in old age. *Educational Gerontology, 45*(5), 341–352.

Nussbaum, P. (2003). *Brain health and wellness.* Tarentum, PA: Word Association Publishers.

Okkema, K. (1993). *Cognition and perception in the stroke patient: a guide to functional outcomes in occupational therapy.* Gaithersburg, MD: Aspen.

Parenté, R., & Herrmann, D. J. (2010). *Retraining cognition: techniques and applications.* Towson, MD: Towson State University.

Patton, D. (2006). Reality orientation: its use and effectiveness within older person mental health care. *Journal of Clinical Nursing, 15*(11), 1440–1449.

Pazzaglia, M., & Galli, G. (2019). Action observation for neurorehabilitation in apraxia. *Frontiers in Neurology, 10*(309), 1–10.

Piccirilli, M., Pigliautile, M., Arcelli, P., et al. (2019). Improvement in cognitive performance and mood in healthy older adults: a multimodal approach. *European Journal of Ageing, 16*(3), 327–336.

Polatajko, H. J., & Mandich, A. (2004). *Enabling occupation in children: the cognitive approach to occupational performance (CO-OP) approach.* Ottawa, Ontario: COAT Publications ACE.

Polatajko, H. J., McEwen, S. E., Ryan, J. D., et al. (2012). Pilot randomized controlled trial investigating cognitive strategy use to improve goal performance after stroke. *The American Journal of Occupational Therapy, 66*(1), 104–109.

Riffenburgh, A., & Stableford, S. (2020). Health literacy and clear communication: keys to engaging older adults and their families. In R. Robnett, N. Brossoie, & W. Chop (Eds.), *Gerontology for the health care professional* (4th ed., pp. 109–128). Burlington, MA: Jones & Bartlett Learning.

Royeen, C. B. (2003). Chaotic occupational therapy: collective wisdom for a complex profession. *The American Journal of Occupational Therapy, 57*(6), 609–624.

Sacks, O. (1998). *The man who mistook his wife for a hat and other clinical tales.* New York, NY: Harper & Row.

Schmidt, J., Fleming, J., Ownsworth, T., et al. (2015). An occupation-based video feedback intervention for improving self-awareness: protocol and rationale. *Canadian Journal of Occupational Therapy, 82*(1), 54–63.

Shih, Y., Huang, R., & Chiang, H. (2009). Correlation between work concentration level and background music: a pilot study. *Work (Reading, Mass.), 33*, 329–333. Available from: https://doi.org/10.3233/WOR-2009-0880.

Sohlberg, M. M., & Mateer, C. A. (2001). *Cognitive rehabilitation: an integrative neuropsychological approach.* New York, NY: The Guilford Press.

Sohlberg, M. M., & Turkstra, L. S. (2011). *Optimizing cognitive rehabilitation: effective instructional methods.* New York, NY: Guilford Press.

Strong, J. (2019). "Playthings of the brain": phantom visions in Charles Bonnet syndrome. *Journal of Gerontological Social Work, 62*(5), 586–596. Available from: https://doi.org/10.1080/01634372.2019.1631927.

Tanaka, S., Honda, S., Nakano, H., et al. (2017). Comparison between group and personal rehabilitation for dementia in a geriatric health service facility: single-blinded randomized controlled study. *Psychogeriatrics, 17*(3), 177–185.

Tham, K., Fallaphour, M., & Erikson, A. (2017). Performance capacity and the lived body. In R. Taylor (Ed.), *Kielhofner's model of human occupation theory and application* (5th ed., pp. 74–90). Philadelphia, PA: Wolters Kluwer.

Thomas, H. (2015). *Occupation-based activity analysis* (2nd ed.). Thorofare, NJ: Slack Inc.

Toglia, J. P. (2011). A dynamic interactional approach of cognition in cognitive rehabilitation. In N. Katz (Ed.), *Cognition, occupation, and participation across the life span* (3rd ed., pp. 161–201). Bethesda, MD: AOTA Press.

Toglia, J. P., Rodger, S. A., & Polatajko, H. J. (2012). Anatomy of cognitive strategies: a therapist's primer for enabling occupational performance. *Canadian Journal of Occupational Therapy, 79*(4), 225–236.

Vance, D. E., Roberson, A. J., McGuinness, T. M., et al. (2010). How neuroplasticity and cognitive reserve protect cognitive functioning. *Journal of Psychosocial Nursing and Mental Health Services, 48*(4), 23–30.

Wehman, P. H. (1991). Cognitive rehabilitation in the workplace. In J. S. Kreutzer, & P. H. Wehman (Eds.), *Cognitive rehabilitation for persons with traumatic brain injury: a functional approach* (pp. 269–288). Baltimore, MD: Brookes.

Whimbey, A., Lochhead, J., & Narode, R. (2013). *Problem solving & comprehension: a short course in analytical reasoning.* Oxford, UK: Routledge.

Whitmoyer, P., Fountain-Zaragoza, S., Andridge, R., Bredemeier, K., Londerée, A., Kaye, L., & Prakash, R. (2018). Mindfulness training and attentional control in older adults: a randomized controlled trial. https://doi.org/10.31231/osf.io/hmp82.

Wilson, B. A. (2010). *Memory rehabilitation: integrating theory and practice.* New York, NY: Guilford.

Ylvisaker, M., Jacobs, H. E., & Feeney, T. (2003). Positive supports for people who experience behavioral and cognitive disability after brain injury: a review. *The Journal of Head Trauma Rehabilitation, 18*(1), 7–32.

Zoltan, B. (2007). *Vision, perception, and cognition* (4th ed.). Thorofare, NJ: Slack, Inc.

PART VII

Clinical Applications

23

Cerebrovascular Accident

Deborah Greenstein Simmons

OBJECTIVES

After reading this chapter, the student or the occupational therapy practitioner will be able to do the following:

1. Define and list potential causes of cerebrovascular accident (CVA, stroke).
2. Discuss modifiable and nonmodifiable risk factors for CVA.
3. Explain the role of the occupational therapy practitioner in preventing common complications after a CVA.
4. Describe deficits commonly seen following hemispheric, cerebellar, and brainstem CVA and how they impact functional performance during familiar and new tasks.
5. Understand how a CVA may affect performance skills, including motor, sensory-perceptual, cognitive, communication, social (behavioral), and performance patterns to identify appropriate occupational therapy treatment strategies.
6. Identify occupational therapy treatment strategies for clients after a CVA in the following areas of occupation: activities of daily living, instrumental activities of daily living, work, leisure, and social participation.
7. Explain the role of the occupational therapy practitioner in providing client-centered services to stroke survivors across the rehabilitation continuum of care (e.g., from acute management to inpatient rehabilitation, to home care, to outpatient).
8. Understand the importance of educating and involving caregivers in occupational therapy interventions following a CVA.
9. Identify the role of the occupational therapy practitioner in health management and health maintenance as it pertains to CVA prevention.

KEY TERMS

Cerebrovascular accident (CVA, stroke)
Occupational therapy
Hemiplegia/hemiparesis
Transient ischemic attack
Ischemic
Hemorrhagic
Thrombus
Embolus
Aneurysm
Hypertension
Flaccid paralysis/hypotonicity
Aphasia
Apraxia
Neuroplasticity
tPA
Deep venous thrombosis (DVT)
Dysphagia

Cognition
Subluxation
Hypertonicity
Hypotonicity
Synergy pattern
Spasticity
Ataxia
Constraint-induced movement therapy (CIMT)
Robotic-assisted therapy
Agnosia
Hemianopsia
Adynamia
Anosognosia
Impulsivity
Perseveration
Pseudobulbar affect
Dysarthria

INTRODUCTION

Cerebrovascular accident (CVA, stroke) is the leading cause of serious long-term adult disability (Benjamin, Blaha, & Chiuve, 2017). More than 4 million stroke survivors live in the United States alone, and each year approximately 795,000 people experience a new or recurrent CVA. Approximately 30% of these CVAs result in death within 30 days of onset (Benjamin et al., 2017; Centers for Disease Control and Prevention, 2017). At least half of stroke survivors report permanent disability, resulting in complete or partial dependence during basic activities of daily living (ADL) (Brandsater, 2005). There is a profound economic impact of CVA on socioeconomic factors with estimates placing the cost of CVA in the United States at over $34 billion per year, with indirect costs raising this statistic to an astounding $73 billion per year (Benjamin et al., 2017). Adult stroke survivors are the single largest diagnostic group seen by **occupational therapy** practitioners working in the physical dysfunction field (Trombly & Radomski, 2008). Occupation therapy helps to maximize functional independence to return to desired life roles and plays an important role in the rehabilitation of stroke survivors across the continuum of care, beginning in the acute care phase of CVA and continuing through community reintegration.

CVA (or stroke) is a sudden loss of blood supply to the brain resulting in brain cell damage and cell death. The interruption and blood supply can be caused by a hemorrhage or a blockage. The cell damage and death resulting from the interruption in blood supply causes varying levels of neurologic deficits. The extent of the damage and the areas of the brain in which the lesion occurs will influence the functional deficits.

Seventy percent of clients who sustain a CVA will demonstrate **hemiplegia** (motor paralysis on one side of the body) or **hemiparesis** (partial motor loss on one side of the body). Motor loss will occur in the extremities, trunk, and facial muscles. Motor function is controlled by the primary motor cortex (M1) in the frontal lobe of the brain. The M1 on the right side of the brain controls voluntary movement on the left side of the body, and the left side of the brain controls movement on the right side of the body. Therefore lesions in this area of the brain result in motor loss to the opposite (contralateral) side of the body. For example, a lesion in the left M1 area of the brain may result in hemiparesis to the right arm. A CVA that occurs in the cerebellum or brainstem will result in different functional outcomes. For example, a CVA in the cerebellum may cause decreased coordination. (More specific deficits will be discussed later in this chapter.) CVA symptoms caused by a brief and temporary blockage to part of the brain are known as **transient ischemic attacks** (TIAs). The symptoms of a TIA are usually mild, develop suddenly, and resolve within minutes or hours with no ongoing deficits. Approximately one third of persons who experience a TIA will experience a CVA. Therefore it is important to recognize the symptoms of a TIA and seek immediate treatment to reduce the risk of a CVA (Benjamin et al., 2017).

Many adults experience and ignore warning symptoms of CVA because they may be unfamiliar with the fact that they are signs of a CVA (American Stroke Association, 2005; Benjamin et al., 2017). Early detection of warning signs and symptoms can result in early administration of effective and appropriate CVA therapies, which may reduce CVA progression and residual deficits (American Stroke Association, 2005). Early warning signs of CVA are listed in Box 23.1.

Etiology

CVAs occur in two ways: **ischemic** and **hemorrhagic**. An ischemic CVA occurs when a blockage in the blood supply to the brain results in a lack of oxygen to brain tissue. Ischemic CVA, which account for approximately 87% of all CVA (Benjamin et al., 2017), can be caused by a **thrombus** (a blood clot that forms within a vessel) or an **embolus** (blood clot, plaque, or other debris that travels throughout the vessel).

BOX 23.1 Warning Signs of Cerebrovascular Accident (CVA)

Sudden numbness or weakness of the face, arm, or leg, especially on one side of the body
Sudden confusion
Sudden difficulty speaking or understanding, slurred speech
Sudden blurred vision or loss of vision
Sudden difficulty walking, dizziness, loss of balance or coordination
Sudden severe headache with no known cause

A hemorrhagic CVA occurs when a weakened blood vessel to the brain bursts and causes bleeding in the brain. This results in a lack of oxygen to brain tissue. Hemorrhagic CVAs account for approximately 13% of all CVAs but result in a significantly higher mortality rate (Benjamin et al., 2017). Vessels that commonly burst are ballooning (**aneurysm)** or a cluster of abnormal blood vessels (arteriovenous malformation [AVM]).

Risk Factors

Of the many major risk factors that may increase the likelihood of a client sustaining a CVA or TIA, some are not able to be changed (nonmodifiable) and some are (modifiable) (Table 23.1). Nonmodifiable risks include age, gender, and race. The risk of CVA increases with age: Two thirds of all CVAs occur in persons older than age 65, and the risk doubles every decade after age 55 (Benjamin et al., 2017; Goldstein, 2011). Men are at a higher risk than women before age 65; women are at a higher risk after age 75 (Benjamin et al., 2017). African Americans are at two times greater risk than

TABLE 23.1 Risk Factors for CVA

Modifiable/Unmodifiable	Risk Factors
Unmodifiable risk factors	Age
	Gender
	Race and ethnicity
	Genetic predisposition
	Aneurysm and arteriovenous malformation
Modifiable risk factors	Hypertension
	Cardiac disease
	Diabetes mellitus
	Obesity
	Stress
	Diet
	High cholesterol
	Use of contraceptives with high dose of estrogen
	Cigarette smoking
	Alcohol use
	Sedentary lifestyle
	Use of nonsteroidal anti-inflammatory medication (aspirin not included)

other racial groups. This may be due to higher rates of preex-isting conditions such as **hypertension**, diabetes, and sickle-cell anemia (Benjamin et al., 2017; Keenan & Shaw, 2011; Centers for Disease Control and Prevention, 2017).

There are many modifiable risks that will decrease the likeli-hood of experiencing a CVA. These include preventing hyper-tension and diabetes through control of blood pressure and blood sugar, managing cholesterol levels, and making healthy lifestyle choices. Some healthy choices include smoking cessa-tion, weight management, implementation of a healthy diet, and regular participation in exercise. Occupational therapists (OTs) and occupational therapy assistants (OTAs) can provide education about CVA prevention to clients who exhibit modi-fiable and/or nonmodifiable risk factors for CVA.

Effects

Depending on the area of the lesion, a CVA may result in loss of, or damage to, many body functions. This may include mental (cognitive), sensory (visual or proprioceptive), neuro-muscular or movement related (muscle tone and motor reflexes), speech (voice and speech), and autonomic body functions. The area of the brain affected by CVA is deter-mined by the cerebral blood supply involved (Mohr, Wolf, Choi, & Weir, 2004). Motor return and functional improve-ments typically occur primarily within the first 3 months after a CVA but can continue for months or years following (Mohr et al., 2004). Factors such as advanced age, coma, seizures, poor perceptual or cognitive functions, delayed or lack of motor return, absent sensation, prior history of CVA, chronic medical conditions, and depression may result in a less favor-able outcome following a CVA (Brandsater, 2005; Kaplan, Caillet, & Kaplan, 2003; Abbott, Bladin, & Donnan, 2001).

Immediately after a CVA, a client may experience **flaccid paralysis** (absence of muscle tone) or **hypotonicity** (low mus-cle tone) of the affected side with reduced or absent reflexes (Kaplan et al., 2003). Other areas may include impaired pos-tural control, sensory deficits, visual impairments, perceptual dysfunction, cognitive dysfunction, behavioral and personal-ity changes, autonomic dysfunction, and impaired speech and language skills (Brandsater, 2005; Kaplan et al., 2003). The outcome and severity of a CVA depend on the type, size, location, and density of the brain damage; the timing and suc-cess of medical care; other medical or neurologic problems; and the client's state of health before the CVA (Mohr et al., 2004; Stein, Harvey, & Winstein, 2015). Conditions often associated with aging, such as arthritis, diabetes, heart disease, and osteoporosis, can affect outcomes during CVA recovery and must be considered during rehabilitation (Brandsater, 2005; Gillen, 2010).

Left-Sided CVA

The M1 and the primary somatosensory cortex (SS1) areas of the left cerebral hemisphere control right-sided motor and sensory function. The M1 and SS1 also control also controls vision to the right visual field, language and speech, time con-cepts, behavior changes, analytic thinking, and math, reading, and writing skills (Chemerinski, Robinson, & Kosier, 2001;

Gutman, 2008). Clients with left hemispheric CVA often dem-onstrate **aphasia** (dysfunction in language expression and recep-tion) and **apraxia** (dysfunction in the ability to execute motor tasks). They commonly achieve self-care independence earlier than clients with right hemispheric CVA, but they are more likely to experience depression (Rajashekaran, Pai, Thunga, & Unnikrishnan, 2013; Zhang, Zhao, Fang, Wang, & Zhou, 2017).

Right-Sided CVA

The M1 and SS1 of the right cerebral hemisphere control left motor and sensory function. Visual-perceptual skills, imagi-nation and creativity, memory, insight, and attention and problem solving also originate in the right hemisphere. The multimodal association areas, which integrate sensory infor-mation into perceptual experiences, are in this hemisphere so it plays an important part in interpreting information from the environment and one's own body (Gutman, 2008). Damage to this hemisphere results in difficulties with spatial analysis, physical orientation, and praxis (Sterzi et al., 1993). Clients with right hemispheric CVA may retain verbal skills, which may mask perceptual dysfunction. It is important to implement environmental safety precautions when clients with right hemisphere damage demonstrate impulsivity and impaired spatial perception.

Left-Sided Versus Right-Sided CVA

Although the left and right cerebral hemispheres show speciali-zation, both control several of the same functions. The ability of the brain to reorganize its structure and function following new therapeutic experiences is a phenomenon known as **neu-roplasticity** (Mang, Campbell, Ross, & Boyd, 2013). The brain is able to transfer signals that once operated in a region dam-aged to a different location. These neural pathways will strengthen over time as therapy reinforces new learning. Left-hand—dominant adults tend to exhibit less specialization than right-handed adults (Kaplan et al., 2003). Similarities and dif-ferences between left and right CVAs are shown in Table 23.2 (Goldberg, 1990; Gutman, 2008; Sterzi et al., 1993).

Bilateral CVA

CVAs that cause damage to both hemispheres are called bilat-eral CVAs. Deficits to be expected following bilateral strokes may incorporate characteristics from both sides and may vary in severity. Treatment interventions for clients with head injury may be used after bilateral CVA (see Chapter 24).

Cerebellum and Brainstem CVA

The cerebellum receives sensory input from the body via the spinal cord and is responsible for muscle action, coordina-tion, and control needed for balance, posture, and smooth functional movements. Common impairments associated with cerebellar CVA include abnormal reflexes of the head and torso, decreased coordination of fine and gross move-ments, impaired balance, dizziness, difficulty swallowing and articulating, and cranial nerve deficits (Gutman, 2008).

CVAs in the brainstem are often life threatening because the brainstem is the control center for essential life functions

TABLE 23.2 Differences and Similarities Between Left-Sided and Right-Sided Cerebrovascular Accident

Left-Sided Cerebrovascular Accident and Right-Sided Hemiplegia	Skills	Right-Sided Cerebrovascular Accident and Left-Sided Hemiplegia
Right-sided paralysis/paresis, decreased motor control of repetitive movements (dysphagia[a])	Motor	Left-sided paralysis/paresis, more severe motor problems, decreased motor response time (dysphagia)
Right-sided sensory loss	Sensory	Left-sided sensory loss
Right visual field cuts (visual neglect)	Visual	Left field cuts, visual neglect
Impaired right/left discrimination, verbal apraxia (hemi-inattention, motor apraxia)	Perceptual	Unilateral neglect, hemi-inattention, motor apraxia, constructional apraxia, dressing apraxia, agnosia, disorientation for directionality, difficulty crossing midline
Decreased analytic thinking, impaired logic, impaired time concepts, impaired memory associated with language	Cognitive	Impaired attention span, impaired understanding of the whole, decreased creativity, impaired memory for performance, poor insight, poor safety awareness, poor judgment
Slow performance, cautious behavior, depression	Behavioral	Impulsivity, emotional lability
Aphasia, agraphia, dyscalculia, decreased understanding of gestures, impaired reading, decreased ability to learn new information	Speech and language	Decreased ability to differentiate between gestures, decreased learning for familiar (old) information

[a]Conditions in parentheses play a lesser role.

such as breathing, heart rate, blood pressure, and arousal. As with a cerebellum CVA, survivors of a brainstem CVA may also present with dizziness and impaired balance, coordination deficits, difficulty with chewing and swallowing, impaired articulation, cranial nerve deficits, and weakness or paralysis (Gutman, 2008). Additionally, they may experience difficulty with double vision and vital autonomic functions such as consciousness, body temperature regulation, breathing, and heart function (American Heart Association, 2019).

Recurrent CVA

Approximately one third of stroke survivors experience a second CVA within 5 years of the initial CVA (Benjamin et al., 2017). Risk of recurrence increases as age and number of prior CVAs increase (Benjamin et al., 2017). Occupational therapy treatment programs should include education related to health management of modifiable risk factors for CVA. Box 23.2 offers suggestions for incorporating this information into occupational therapy interventions.

MEDICAL MANAGEMENT

Dedicated CVA centers improve survival rates and reduce secondary complications from CVA (American Stroke Association, 2005). Emergency room care provided within 3 hours of symptom onset results in better survival rates and improved functional outcomes. Emergency medical treatment of CVA includes airway maintenance, establishment of proper fluid balance, and management of medical complications. Other medical management for ischemic CVA includes medication and surgery. Tissue plasminogen activator (**tPA**) can prevent or reduce damage to cerebral tissues (American Stroke Association, 2005) by helping

reestablish blood flow to the brain. It is considered the gold standard in emergency treatment for ischemic CVA. The timing of its administration is critical, so individuals should seek immediate medical care when experiencing symptoms. Surgery can repair damaged blood vessels, which reduces bleeding and prevents additional damage to intact cerebral tissues. Endovascular treatment and clot removal procedures facilitate blood flow restoration, which improves

BOX 23.2 Examples of Ways to Incorporate Cerebrovascular Accident (CVA) Health Management and Maintenance into Occupational Therapy Interventions

Diet/Weight Management

Provide client/caregivers information on how to make heart healthy food choices.

Teach client/caregivers how to read food labels to identify low-sodium and low-fat choices.

Work with client/caregiver on how to locate heart healthy recipes online or in magazines.

Provide home exercise and conditioning programs based on client's activity tolerance.

Medication Compliance

Work with medical team on simplifying medication regimen for clients with cognitive impairments.

Teach client/caregivers reasons for medication, side effects, importance of timely refilling of medication.

Train client in use of adaptive devices (e.g., pill splitter, medication organizers, one-handed syringe) when indicated.

Recommend telemonitoring of medication compliance in the home, if necessary.

functional outcomes and decreases mortality. Ongoing treatment for CVA often includes anticoagulation medications to lower risk of recurrent blood clots (Goyal et al., 2015).

Medical Complications

Stroke survivors are prone to a wide range of multiple complications to all body systems, including respiratory, cardiovascular, neurologic, integumentary (skin), and genitourinary. Many of these can be prevented by mobilization, close medical monitoring, and interdisciplinary collaboration during rehabilitation. Prevention is most effective when begun on the day of admission (Brandsater, 2005; Stein et al., 2015).

Cardiovascular complications account for the leading causes of death following a stroke. These include **deep venous thrombosis (DVT)**, which is the most common complication after a CVA. It is most often due to immobilization and typically develops in the veins of the legs (Dorsher & McMichan, 1993; Piambianco, Orchard, & Landau, 1995). Classic signs and symptoms of DVT include fever and redness, pain, and tenderness at the clot site. Some clients never demonstrate any clinical symptoms. Diagnosis of DVT can be done through medical imaging. Once diagnosed, anticoagulation medication is used to dissolve the clot and prevent further development of blood clots. Anticoagulant medications are the most effective at preventing DVTs (Adams et al., 2007; Piambianco et al., 1995). Early mobility and thromboembolic deterrent stockings may also be used concurrently with medication to prevent DVTs.

Damage from a DVT is caused when a blood clot, or thrombus, breaks away and travels to other regions of the body such as the heart, lungs, or brain. Pulmonary emboli (PE) are thromboembolisms that travel to and become lodged in the lungs. They are the most common cause of death within the first month after a CVA (Dorsher & McMichan, 1993; Mohr et al., 2004; Piambianco et al., 1995). Inferior vena cava (IVC) filters may be placed within the vein to catch blood clots and prevent them from traveling to the heart and lungs. Other complications to the lungs following a CVA may include infections such as pneumonia because of impaired mobility, poor inhalation because of weakness of respiratory muscles, and swallowing impairments that result in aspiration (Brandsater, 2005; Jamison & Orchanian, 2007).

Aspiration can occur in clients with CVA who present with difficulty swallowing (**dysphagia**) due to weakened muscle control along the oropharyngeal or gastrointestinal tract, decreased swallow reflexes, and poor tongue control (Brandsater, 2005; Jamison & Orchanian, 2007; Kidd, Lawson, Nesbitt, & MacMahon, 1993). When the tissue that sits over the trachea (called the epiglottis) fails, food and drink can travel to the trachea and subsequently into the lungs rather than continue from the pharynx toward the stomach (Armstrong & Mosher, 2011). Aspiration occurs when food or liquid travels to the lungs rather than the stomach. Common signs of aspiration include coughing, throat clearing, and increased oral secretions. Close monitoring of swallow, modified diets, proper positioning, and effective hand

hygiene can reduce the risk of developing pneumonia after CVA (Armstrong & Mosher, 2011).

A primary consequence of aspiration is pneumonia. About one third of people who have had a CVA develop pneumonia during their recovery. Pneumonia can lead to further complications such as respiratory failure, infection, deconditioning, and death.

Cardiac complications are the second leading cause of death after CVA. Twenty percent of CVA clients have comorbid cardiac disease. (American Stroke Association, 2005). For these clients, comprehensive medical management and individualized treatment must be implemented to avoid further strain on the heart (see Chapter 32).

Neurologic complications following a stroke include seizures. Damage to brain tissue may cause seizures in 10% to 18% of stroke survivors (Abbott et al., 2001). The risk for seizures is highest during the first year after the CVA. Anticonvulsant medications are used to control and prevent seizure activity. Seizure medication may impair occupational performance due to causing drowsiness and impaired **cognition** (Bartels, Duffy, & Belhand, 2011).

Other medical complications due to stroke are impairments in the integumentary, genitourinary, and musculoskeletal systems. A significant complication that arises from the integumentary system is the development of decubitus ulcers (pressure areas that typically develop over bony prominences) due to skin breakdown. Contributing factors to decreased skin integrity include prolonged immobility, contracture, sensory loss, malnutrition, and cognitive impairments. Frequent weight shifting, turning and positioning schedules, regular exercise, frequent skin checks, proper nutrition, and the monitoring of all positioning and pressure relief devices can significantly reduce the risk of pressure damage (Bartels et al., 2011).

Dysfunction of the genitourinary system may result in incontinence following a CVA. This may be caused by physical changes, communication difficulties, or vision challenges. Urgency, physical strain, sleep, or bowel needs may also lead to episodes of incontinence. Urinary retention is also common and can lead to urinary tract infections. Maintenance of continence and prevention of urinary tract infections are common goals in the early care following CVA. These goals may be achieved by regular toileting schedules, bowel and bladder retraining, diet, and fluid control. Medication may aid in regulating digestion and elimination as well as reducing fluid retention (Wyman, Burgio, & Newman, 2009).

A common musculoskeletal complication following a CVA is shoulder **subluxation** due to compromise of the glenohumeral joint. Subluxation occurs when the humerus slips out of the glenoid cavity resulting in a gap between the humeral head and the acromion. Causes of subluxation include weakness of the rotator cuff muscles, direct trauma, or improper positioning. Shoulder subluxation may cause pain in the joint. Without proper treatment, it can also lead to joint deformity, adhesive capsulitis, and long-term range of motion (ROM) deficits.

Diagnosis of shoulder subluxation can be done through palpation or x-ray imaging. Shoulder subluxation can be prevented through supportive positioning and by avoiding traction when handling the affected extremity. Treatment interventions for shoulder subluxation are discussed later in this chapter (Murie-Fernández et al., 2012).

Once medically stable, stroke survivors can transition to an inpatient rehabilitation setting for ongoing therapeutic care and medical management (American Stroke Association, 2005). Effective rehabilitation for the CVA survivor includes a multidisciplinary approach with client and caregivers actively involved in treatment planning and goal setting at each stage.

Occupational Therapy Process

OTs and certified OTAs focus on improving occupational performance through facilitation of independence in ADL and instrumental activities of daily living (IADL). This can be done through improvement in motor function, integration of sensory-perceptual and cognitive functions, and promoting health management and lifestyle modifications to reduce risk of recurrent CVA. All these strategies assist clients in resuming participation in meaningful activities and life roles.

Occupational Profile. An occupational profile is the first step of the intervention process. This allows OTs and OTAs at all levels of care to gather information about the client's occupational history and experiences to provide intervention and make appropriate recommendations for the next level of care. An occupational profile can be developed through informal interview or through a formal assessment, such as the Canadian Occupational Performance Measure (COPM).

Assessment of Occupational Performance. The OT, with input from the OTA, evaluates performance skills (e.g., motor and praxis, sensory-processing, emotional regulation, cognitive function, and communication skills) and areas of occupation (e.g., ADL, IADL, education, work, leisure, and social participation) to formulate an intervention plan. Client factors, including values and beliefs, must be identified during the evaluation process and how they may help direct treatment priorities and planning. The OT uses assessment tools that focus on task performance during different areas of occupation to identify the client's strengths and weaknesses. Occupational therapy assessment of contextual factors, including environmental factors, social supports, and cultural roles, should be considered when developing a plan of care and identifying interventions that will support successful engagement in meaningful occupation. An understanding of the client's needs, goals, priorities, and concerns further enhances the occupational therapy process (American Occupational Therapy Association, 2017). Occupational therapy services for a client with CVA focus on preventive and rehabilitative goals in occupational performance. Overall occupational therapy goals are listed in Box 23.3.

Intervention Process. Occupational therapy intervention occurs throughout the continuum of care for the CVA

BOX 23.3 General Occupational Therapy Goals for Clients With Cerebrovascular Accident (CVA)

1. Preventing of secondary complications and injury
2. Facilitating typical postural and movement patterns
3. Maximizing active and passive range of motion (AROM, PROM), strength, and motor coordination
4. Maximizing functional use of the affected side
5. Remediating and/or compensating for visual perceptual and cognitive dysfunction
6. Maximizing level of independence in all areas of occupation
7. Maximizing safety and independence during functional mobility
8. Maximizing functional cognitive and communication skills
9. Education and training on adaptive techniques for residual deficits
10. Assisting in reintegration into meaningful social participation

survivor. In the acute care setting, intervention may begin at the bedside. Clients in this stage are medically fragile. Treatment must be individualized, and precautions must be followed to ensure safety. Occupational therapy intervention in acute care focuses on early mobility, graded exercise to the client's activity tolerance, prevention of complications, and basic self-care training.

The focus of intervention in acute and subacute rehabilitation is on promoting independence in ADL, IADL (see Chapter 13: Activities of Daily Living), work (see Chapter 16: Work), and leisure skills. It may include a focus on basic life roles and skills needed to transition to the home setting. Once home, home care services integrate these learned skills to maximize safety and independence within the home environment. Additional focus on community reintegration and social participation can occur at this stage. Outpatient services continue rehabilitation goals until maximum functional performance is achieved. Intervention at this stage may involve special programming such as job reentry or driving rehabilitation. Home evaluations and modifications are important components of the rehabilitation process to reinforce a safe and successful return to independent living in the home and community setting.

Grading of intervention. Determining the initial level of difficulty for a client is based on the evaluation results. Once this is determined, intervention can be graded in many ways, to increase or decrease the difficulty to meet the just-right challenge for the client. Activities can be graded by modifying the complexity, allowing more or less time, modifying cues, and/or alternating the amount of assistance provided. Age, medical status, symptoms of disease, or other complications also impact the need to grade intervention. Since clients with CVA often experience fluctuations and changes in their recovery, frequent reassessment of the treatment program is necessary to adjust to changing levels of skill. The OT and OTA continually increase task complexity to match client skills until intervention goals are achieved.

Factors Influencing the Occupational Therapy Process.
Research demonstrates that early initiation of occupational therapy for clients with CVA results in better functional outcomes and shorter lengths of inpatient stays. Due to the frequency of medical complications mentioned earlier, working with clients in the acute stages of recovery requires a high level of clinical competence. OTAs should utilize continuing education and experiences to enhance clinical competency to sharpen clinical reasoning and keep skills up to date (Coleman et al., 2017).

In the early phase of CVA, medical status can change daily. Frequent reassessment by the OT may be necessary to provide direction to the OTA, to make safe and appropriate clinical decisions. The accompanying Alert box provides considerations for practitioners during this initial phase of rehabilitation. All OTs and OTAs treating clients with CVA must know signs and symptoms of all diagnoses, as well as current emergency protocols and procedures. Careful attention must be given in treatment planning to avoid activities that may worsen symptoms. OTAs should monitor clients with CVA carefully during treatment and be ready to modify interventions if the client demonstrates signs of activity intolerance. Interdisciplinary communication with the medical team is essential at this stage to ensure safe treatment and comprehensive monitoring of the client's status.

> **⚠ ALERT**
>
> **Safety Considerations in the Early Phase of Rehabilitation After CVA**
> - Review chart prior to each treatment session and consult with supervising OT whenever there are changes in the client's status or plan of care as well as when new medical orders are written.
> - Be aware of the presence of all monitors, feeding tubes, catheters/ostomies, and peripheral/central line placements and adhere to appropriate precautions.
> - Check and adhere to all precautions related to vital signs (e.g., blood pressure, heart rate, oxygen saturation rates).
> - Begin each session with an assessment of vital signs, mental status, and activity readiness.
> - Monitor vital signs closely throughout treatment session and proceed based on client's tolerance and response to intervention.

The majority of clients with CVA are over age 65 and have higher rates of comorbid diagnoses and chronic medical conditions (Roth & Harvey, 2015; Stroke facts, 2017). While older clients benefit from rehabilitation, advanced age has been associated with more severe symptoms, longer recovery time, and overall greater disability in ADL and thus must be considered when developing plans of care (Kalra, 1994; Stein et al., 2015).

DOMAINS OF OCCUPATIONAL THERAPY INTERVENTION

Movement-Related Functions

Abnormal reflexes (such as asymmetric tonic neck reflex) and impaired postural mechanisms (such as absent protective extension) often manifest following a CVA. Postural reactions such as righting, equilibrium, and protective extension can be impaired, delayed, or absent. This leads to a decreased ability to maintain balance when moving, which compromises stability, body alignment, and mobility. Intervention should focus on the identification of typical movement patterns that have been overpowered by abnormal motor function and the use of new motor rehabilitation techniques to help build new neural pathways (neuroplasticity). These techniques help to integrate and reinforce functional and efficient movement patterns into everyday occupations.

Positioning. Proper positioning after CVA is important to reduce the development of abnormal muscle tone, facilitate healthy circulation, and reduce the risk of pneumonia and other medical complications (Elovic & Bogey, 2010; Ferdinand & Roffe, 2016). Positioning interventions should be individualized to the specific needs of the client. Good positioning promotes proper trunk and extremity alignment, reduces the risk of contracture development, ensures balance of agonist and antagonist muscle groups, and prevents skin breakdown (Skalsky & McDonald, 2012). Good positioning techniques improve functional performance and reduce risk of pressure ulcer development. It is reliant on proper training of clinicians and staff and is less effective when skills are out of date and techniques improperly used (Chitambira & Evans, 2018).

Proper positioning of a limb with **hypertonicity** (increased muscle tone) can reduce the risks of contractures and skin breakdown. Proper positioning of a limb with **hypotonicity** (decreased muscle tone) can reduce the risk of skin breakdown and overstretching muscles (leading to the development of joint laxity and shoulder subluxation). In all positions, the trunk should be aligned symmetrically. Affected extremities should be supported to reduce edema and prevent injury. Muscle tone is dependent on speed of movement, so sudden movement should be avoided during position changes, to decrease activation of abnormal muscle tone on affected muscle groups. Clients may require adaptive devices such as wedges, bolsters, extra pillows, towel rolls, or splints to maintain proper alignment and positioning. Frequent change of position should be incorporated to encourage awareness of both sides of the body and promote good skin integrity.

When sitting upright, the client's trunk should be symmetric and erect. The affected arm should be supported with pillows, a bedside table, or a lap tray. The affected leg should be positioned in flexion at the hip and knee joints. A properly fitting wheelchair significantly improves a client's sitting posture (see Chapter 15). A lumbar support, a solid seat and back, or a custom cushion can maximize comfortable and symmetric sitting. The feet should always be supported while the client is sitting. Wheelchair lap trays or an arm trough may be required (Fig. 23.1) for safe management of the upper extremity (UE).

A hand immobilization orthosis (commonly known as a resting hand) is commonly used to protect the affected forearm, wrist, and hand to reduce the risk of contracture development and to improve skin hygiene (Fig. 23.2)

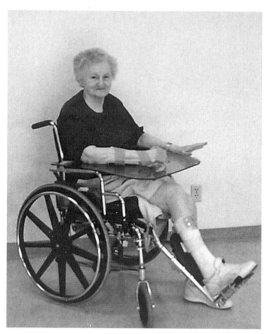

Fig. 23.1 Client using a lapboard to support hemiplegic arm while sitting in a wheelchair. A lapboard promotes proper wheelchair positioning and symmetric trunk alignment.

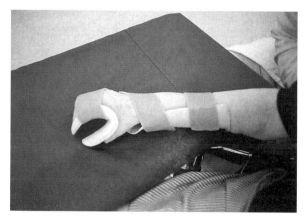

Fig. 23.2 A resting hand splint properly supports hemiplegic forearm, wrist, and hand in a functional position.

(Choi, Yang, & Song, 2017). This orthosis may be used to maintain tissue length and provide a low-load prolonged stretch in a hand with spasticity. Whether prefabricated or custom made, the resting hand splint supports the distal arm in a functional position (see Chapters 20 and 25). The use of this orthosis has been shown to be most effective when promoting functional use and spasticity management after CVA, when used as an adjunct to occupational therapy treatment (Choi et al., 2017). Each client using one of these orthoses should be provided with an individualized wearing schedule that takes into consideration current muscle tone, functional task expectations, functional cognition, and skin integrity. It must be removed at regular intervals during the day to prevent learned nonuse, promote sensory awareness of the hand, and encourage

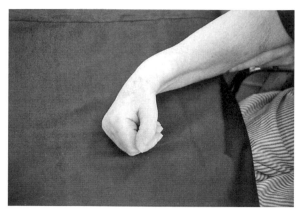

Fig. 23.3 Typical UE flexion synergy.

functional use (Milazzo & Gillen, 2010). Client and caregivers must be educated on proper technique for application and care of the orthosis, including accurate return demonstration.

Abnormal Muscle Tone. A limb may present as flaccid (hypotonic with decreased tone) after CVA; however, over time, the limb may become spastic (hypertonic with increased tone). Spasticity can severely impact the functional performance of a limb. When moving, a client may demonstrate a flexion or extension pattern called **synergy**. A flexor synergy pattern results when spasticity of the flexor muscles (such as elbow and wrist flexors) leads to a strong, involuntary, adducted and flexed position of the UE (Fig. 23.3). Prolonged time spent in this position can shorten muscles leading to contractures and decreased functional use of the limb (Cheung et al., 2015).

Functionally, the influence of synergy patterns is more obvious in movements against gravity, especially those requiring effort and reach. For example, during ambulation, as the client attempts to flex at the hip, knee, and ankle joints to step forward, he or she may experience unintended hip extension and adduction, knee extension, and ankle plantar flexion. Without intervention, synergy patterns can lead to contractures, deformities, and atypical movement patterns in the affected extremities, as well as asymmetries in the trunk.

Spasticity, the velocity-dependent increase in normal muscle tone, can be classified as minimal, moderate, or severe. It fluctuates frequently. It may decrease during sleep or rest and increase in response to stressors such as pain, fatigue, infections, injury, ulcers, bowel dysfunction, and medication reactions (Cheung et al., 2015). A significant increase in tone may indicate that the client has a urinary tract infection, a developing decubitus pressure sore, or bowel obstruction. In these cases, spasticity usually reduces to previous levels after successful medical treatment of the underlying problem. Spasticity may interfere with the client or caregiver's ability to perform hygiene tasks leading to a decrease in skin integrity. For example, spasticity of the finger flexors may result in a clenched fist pattern, leading to skin breakdown in the palm of the hand. Medical interventions for severe spasticity, used in conjunction with therapy, include nerve blocks and oral or injected antispasticity medication (Dobkin, 2004; Elovic & Bogey, 2010).

Motor Deficits. Voluntary motor control, absent immediately following a CVA, may return in stages and may stop at any time. Return of motor function typically occurs proximal to distal, from the trunk to shoulders and hips through to the extremities. Motor recovery often begins with partial activation of muscle groups and progresses to stronger, more coordinated movements against gravity. Although complete recovery may not occur, clients can often regain full functional use of their UE. This is more often experienced when sensation and awareness of the hemiplegic side is intact (Birch, Proctor, Bortner, & Lowenthal, 1960; Bolognini, Russo, & Edwards, 2016). Unilateral and bilateral lesions to the cerebellum lead to deficits in coordination, known as **ataxia**. Ataxia complicates actions such as stepping, reaching, and maintaining posture.

Hemiplegia can cause atypical movements leading to poor movement quality and decreased functional use of the extremity (Bobath, 1990). Typical muscle synergies can change as a result of the type of damage or disruption to the motor pathways in the brain (McMorland, Runnalls, & Byblow, 2015). Gross motor skills typically return before fine motor skills. Movement type and quality are quickly impacted by weakness, fatigue, infection, and certain drugs. As motor function returns, gross and fine motor coordination deficits such as ataxia may occur. Chapters 6 and 21 discuss coordination impairments that can occur in a person after CVA.

Balance Impairment. After a CVA, balance may be impaired due to an imbalance and weakness in trunk muscles, decreased sensory awareness, and postural instability when sitting and standing. Balance impairments increase fall risk, especially in conjunction with other diagnoses such as deconditioning. Decreased balance can affect UE movement by limiting ROM needed to reach, complete self-care tasks, and manage assistive mobility devices. Therefore it is important to incorporate functional positioning and facilitation of proper body mechanics. When sitting, clients may benefit from supportive devices such as lateral trunk supports, seat belts, or lapboards to increase stability and safety as trunk strength and coordination improve. The use of visual feedback during alignment and weight-shifting exercises can significantly improve outcomes related to posture and body mechanics (Pellegrino, Giannoni, Marinelli, & Casadio, 2017). Additionally, balance training that incorporates the affected UE will encourage use of motor and cognitive-perceptual skills (Abreu, 1995).

Intervention for Movement-Related Functions. Treatment of the motor dysfunction focuses on improving ROM, strength, and control of the affected regions to support task performance and maximum function. The prevention of joint deformity is an important goal for OTs and OTAs to focus on for clients following a CVA.

Improvement in ROM

Passive ROM (PROM). PROM exercises maintain full joint ROM and should be performed at least twice daily until enough active movement returns to maintain ROM. It can be limited by fluctuating tone, subluxation, pain, edema, fractures, joint diseases, and reduced scapular and clavicular mobility. Research indicates that early intervention to increase ROM leads to improved functional outcomes in the affected UE during the acute phase of recovery (Hosseini, Peyrovi, & Gohari, 2019; Kim, Lee, & Sohng, 2014).

PROM exercises may be performed by a therapist, caregiver, or the client (self-ROM [SROM]). The client may complete them using the unaffected arm. Clients should take care when completing SROM, to keep the arm supported and to avoid increasing muscle response (Box 23.4).

Active ROM (AROM). AROM is performed by the client and requires voluntary movement of the hemiplegic UE. When there is minimal active movement, active-assisted ROM (AAROM) exercises are performed. These exercises involve initiation of movement from the client and partial assist from the unaffected UE, another person, or an assistive/robotic device to complete the motion. Individually designed home ROM exercise programs have been found to increase motor recovery. Integration of the UE into functional daily activities that encourage ROM helps stimulate neuroplasticity and reinforce motor recovery (Lee et al., 2018; Turton & Fraser, 1990).

Intervention for shoulder subluxation and pain. As discussed previously, when muscles of the hemiplegic shoulder are weakened, the glenohumeral (GH) joint can separate and become subluxed. Factors that contribute to increased risk for subluxation include severe sensory loss, poor UE support, poor alignment of GH joint during ROM exercises, arthritis of the shoulder joint, and incorrect handling of the involved UE by staff or untrained family members (Dobkin, 2004; Gillen, 2010). Thorough education is required to ensure proper techniques, and precautions are utilized when working with clients at risk of subluxation. Overhead pulley exercises past 90 degrees should be avoided for clients with subluxation.

Pain in a subluxed GH joint may or may not be present; however, movement and/or inappropriate rest positions can exacerbate discomfort. Shoulder pain can be prevented through proper positioning, PROM exercises, and education of client, staff, and family on proper handling techniques. The affected UE should always be fully supported. Pillows can be used in bed to maintain proper alignment while lapboard and

---

BOX 23.4 Self-Range of Motion (SROM) of the Spastic Upper Extremity

Should be pain free

Should be performed in a slow, controlled manner; avoid quick movements

Should take each joint through its full ROM; if possible, hold for a few seconds at end of ROM to maintain stretch

arm troughs are helpful when seated in a wheelchair. When upright during functional mobility and activity, the client may benefit from kinesiotaping of the arm at the shoulder to reduce the risk of subluxation and decrease pain in a hemiplegic shoulder. Kinesiotaping involves a hypoallergenic tape applied to the shoulder to lift the head of the humerus back into the glenoid fossa (Chengqi, Jingyi, & Yang, 2018).

The use of arm slings to support the shoulder is controversial because many standard slings encourage a flexed and adducted UE posture while reducing sensory feedback, without reducing the risk for subluxation (Gillen, 2010). Clients who have severe edema, have severe hypotonia in the UE, or are at high risk for injury due to cognition or hemibody neglect may require a sling temporarily during transfers or gait training to maximize safety (Gillen, 2010; Kaplan et al., 2003). If a sling is provided, the client and caregiver must be given clear instructions as to the purpose of the sling, when it should be worn, and proper technique for sling application. Continued assessment of whether the sling is meeting its intended purpose is essential.

Motor retraining. Motor retraining programs encourage normal postural mechanisms, typical movement patterns, and use of the affected side in functional activities. Motor retraining is accomplished with sensorimotor (see Chapter 21) or with task-oriented, function-based approaches (Charness, 2004; Davies, 2000; Dobkin, 2004; Gillen, 2010). Some basic considerations for motor retraining activities are listed in Box 23.5 (Charness, 2004; Dobkin, 2004; Gillen, 2010; Nilsen, Gillen, & Gordon, 2010; Page & Levine, 2005).

Constraint-induced movement therapy (CIMT) techniques have been found to be beneficial in improving arm function and use in clients with CVA with learned nonuse (Dromerick, Edwards, & Hahn, 2000; Gillot, Holder-Walls, Kurtz, & Varley, 2003; Page, Sisto, Johnston, & Levine, 2002; Taub, Uswatte, & Pidikiti, 1999). CIMT combines forced use of the affected arm during intensive training and active participation in specific functional activities while immobilizing the unaffected limb. While research in this area is ongoing, CIMT is multifaceted, can be modified to be client specific, and is shown to elicit improved functional outcomes when

---

BOX 23.5 General Considerations for Motor Retraining Activities After Cerebrovascular Accident (CVA)

- Select and engage client in activities that are goal directed, task oriented, and meaningful.
- Match activities with client's skill level and grade activity up as client improves.
- Teach client to think about movement before and while performing an activity (mental practice).
- Provide opportunities for client to perform activities in different positions (e.g., sitting, standing), at varying speeds and in different contexts.
- Allow client ample opportunities for both mental and motor practice.

---

adjusted to each client (El-Helow et al., 2015; Taub et al., 1999).

Robotic-assisted therapy is also used for retraining upper arm movements after CVA and has been found to improve effectiveness of rehabilitation in selected populations. The use of robotic-assisted devices in therapy provides the opportunity for high-intensity, repetitive, task-specific, and interactive treatment of the impaired upper limb, as well as an objective, reliable means of monitoring patient progress (Kwakkel, Knollen, & Kregs, 2008; Lo et al., 2010; Volpe, Krebs, & Hogan, 2003). Virtual reality systems such as the Wii or Kinect also provide opportunities for motor retraining after CVA by directing automated, real-time feedback to the client (Stein, Krebs, & Hogan, 2009).

Normalization of muscle tone. Active movement of hypotonic muscles can be facilitated through stimulation of specific sensory factors. Inhibition (reduction of tone) of hypertonic muscles can be accomplished through positioning and handling. Tactile and proprioceptive input can help to decrease high tone. In the presence of increased muscle tone, slow and controlled movements should be encouraged, as sudden and extreme movements can elicit a further increase in hypertonicity. Use of robotic-assisted therapy, neuromuscular electrical stimulation, functional mobility and positioning, occupational-based task training, and medication management are used to facilitate typical movement patterns (Belagaje, 2017). Task-specific, repetitive, and novel tasks help to reinforce those neuroplastic principles that are vital to motor recovery. Mirror therapy, where the unaffected limb performs movements and exercises next to a mirror placed perpendicular to midline to give the illusion of typical movement patterns in the affected limb, has shown positive influences on motor return after CVA when used in conjunction with standard therapy protocols. The use of mirror therapy has been associated with improved functional outcomes and higher levels of functional independence during stroke rehabilitation (Baricich, Carda, Cisari, Lanzotti, & Invernizzi, 2013). OTAs looking to address muscle tone in treatment should collaborate closely with the OT, as specialized training in this area is required.

Bilateral integration. Bilateral integration of the UE is an early and important goal in CVA rehabilitation, even if the affected arm does not demonstrate functional movement. Increased tactile and visual input will encourage development of sensory experiences used during movement. The affected UE should always be properly positioned and kept within the client's view, including during one-handed activities (Bobath, 1990). Activities with hands clasped, such as pushing a ball or towel on a tabletop, can incorporate the affected arm into activity (Bobath, 1990; Gillen, 2010). As motor function returns, the affected arm initially serves as a stabilizer and progresses to providing some assistance and may eventually become functionally comparable to the unaffected side in all tasks.

Muscle strengthening and endurance. Stroke survivors often demonstrate a loss of muscle strength and a significant reduction of muscle endurance due to overall weakness

(Gillen, 2010; Gillen, 2010). Therefore therapeutic goals directed toward strength and endurance should be a carefully planned component of the occupational therapy plan of care. Abnormal muscle tone and the inability to isolate desired muscles can make it difficult to accurately assess strength. Complex positioning techniques may be necessary to prevent injury and obtain accurate results. If spasticity is present in the affected UE, resistive exercises should be prescribed with caution as they can increase tone.

Strengthening of the unaffected side is appropriate if increased resistance does not result in increased spasticity of the hemiplegic side. If prescribed, resistive exercises should focus on both agonist (targeted) and antagonist (opposing) muscle groups. Clients should be monitored closely so that exercises can be graded appropriately and modified if increased spasticity is observed. Joint protection techniques, such as type of strengthening tools, should be considered especially when motor control and sensation remain below baseline function. Increasing number of repetitions and/or amount of resistance will target both strength and endurance.

Nearly one half of all stroke survivors report fatigue as a factor that interferes with participation in daily activities and exercise programs (Ivey et al., 2015). Endurance training should be included in every CVA program and should be graded according to each client's abilities and lifestyle needs. Inclusion of intermittent rest periods is essential. Monitoring of vital signs (e.g., blood pressure, pulse, respiration) during exercise may be required for clients with additional cardiovascular considerations (see Chapter 32: Cardiac Dysfunction). For these clients, the OTA should demonstrate clinical competence for monitoring vital signs and ensure adherence to specific parameters prescribed by the referring physician.

Edema management. Edema, or fluid accumulation, is a common but preventable complication after a CVA. Edema can be caused by various factors, including immobility, poor circulation, dependent positioning, poor posture, sensory loss, and excessive exercise (Giang, Ong, Krishnamurthy, & Fong, 2016). Swelling increases the diameter of the skin, which becomes soft and malleable. Prolonged edema can progress to firm skin, stiff joints, pain, and loss of ROM. Ongoing untreated edema can lead to systemic complications such as renal dysfunction and congestive heart failure. Congestive heart failure, where fluid builds up around the heart and causes it to pump inefficiently, can be caused by many factors, including diabetes, hypertension, cardiovascular disease, and obesity. These are all considered common comorbidities of CVA. Understanding early signs and symptoms of these medical conditions is imperative, to be diagnosed and addressed as quickly as possible. See Chapter 29 for detailed edema reduction techniques.

Compensatory techniques. Clients whose hemiplegia effects their dominant side may require dominance retraining to their nondominant side (Bobath, 1990). When a client experiences a significant impairment in motor function on one side of the body, compensation strategies are useful. These include one-handed techniques, use of adaptive equipment, and functional positioning techniques. See Chapter 13

for specific strategies useful for clients experiencing hemiplegia. When performing ADL and IADL, clients should incorporate the affected UE into the activity as much as possible (e.g., as a stabilizer) to reinforce motor return and awareness to the affected side.

Sensory-Related Dysfunction

CVA can cause absent or impaired visual, auditory, olfactory, gustatory, and somatosensory functions. Movement requires integration of sensorimotor input and can be profoundly impacted by diminished or absent sensation (Bolognini et al., 2016).

Visual. Occupational therapy practitioners should be aware of many factors that affect visual performance. Because CVA usually occurs in the elderly, many clients with CVA may exhibit age-related visual deficits such as cataracts, macular degeneration, and glaucoma (see Chapter 21) at baseline (Kalra, 1994). Obtaining information about any preexisting visual deficits can aid in realistic treatment planning and understanding of CVA-related changes. The OT may perform a visual screening after CVA and can work in conjunction with an ophthalmologist or optometrist to identify the presence of visual impairments.

CVA can result in visual deficits that can significantly impact safety and performance during daily activities. Of stroke survivors, 60% experience visual changes immediately following CVA (Hanna, Hepworth, & Rowe, 2017; Rowe et al., 2010). Common visual deficits seen after CVA include decreased acuity, field loss, double vision (diplopia), increased or decreased eye movements and coordination, visual processing, and **agnosia** (the inability to recognize familiar people and objects) (Bolognini et al., 2016). Strategies such as prisms and field expanders, patching, and scanning techniques are common techniques to improve or compensate for visual deficits caused by CVA (Rowe, 2016; Rowe et al., 2010).

Hemianopsia is the loss of vision on the same side of each eye. Homonymous hemianopsia is a loss of the visual field of the lateral (temporal) aspect of the affected side and the medial (nasal) aspect of the unaffected side, resulting in a loss of one half of the visual field. Heteronymous hemianopsia is vision loss on different sides of each eye and is less commonly seen after CVA. Clients with visual field loss are unable to see their environment within the affected area. If inattention or neglect is also present, the client may not be aware of this field loss. Visual deficits related to perceptual dysfunction are discussed later in this chapter (Rowe, 2016).

Auditory. Hearing loss is uncommon but may be seen following a CVA. If hearing deficits exist in clients after CVA, they are most commonly a result of normal aging; however, an elevated risk of sensorineural hearing loss has been linked to people after a CVA compared to persons without CVA (Kuo, Shiao, Wang, Chang, & Lin, 2016; Lavine & Hausler, 2001). To avoid erroneously labeling clients with hearing loss as "confused," clients with suspected hearing loss require thorough evaluation and documentation of hearing loss by an audiologist.

Somatosensory. Changes in the senses of touch, pain, pressure, temperature, vibration, and proprioception are common after CVA (Kaplan et al., 2003). Without tactile feedback, clients experience difficulty using affected extremities even if movement is functional (Meyer, Karttunen, Thijs, Feys, & Verheyden, 2014). Deficits in quality, coordination, and speed of movement due to somatosensory dysfunction increase one's risk for injury.

Olfactory and Gustatory. Olfactory (smell) and gustatory (taste) impairments are less common, but still among senses affected after CVA (Foulkes, 1990). These senses typically occur in conjunction with one another (Green, McGregor, & King, 2008). These senses are very important when considering nutrition and dietary intake. OTs and OTAs can instruct clients about changes in taste or smell that could contribute to poor appetite, ineffective hygiene techniques, safety concerns (e.g., inability to smell dangerous odors), and a reduced enjoyment of pleasurable odors and tastes. These deficits may affect nutrition and quality of life for some clients.

Perceptual Dysfunction

Perception is the complex interaction of a person and the environment used to interpret information. CVA may affect a variety of visual-perceptual and sensorimotor skills (Walker & Lincoln, 1991). Changes in perception after CVA alter the way a person interacts with the environment, both motorically and cognitively, and can impact motor performance, quality of life, and social participation.

Visual Perception and Processing. Visual attention is a purposeful visual response to the environment. Visual scanning, or tracking, is the process of selecting objects on which to focus attention by systematically searching the environment. A common visual-perceptual impairment seen after CVA is inattention where one fails to identify and respond to stimuli in the region opposite the region in the hemisphere affected by CVA. Clients with visual inattention have difficulty transferring their gaze or attending to objects on the affected side (Hepworth et al., 2016; Stone, Halligan, & Green, 1993). Their perceived visual field shifts to exclude large portions of their environment. Their eye movements tend to be slower and may be less coordinated. When clients cannot attend, track, and scan, the ability to identify objects or people is diminished. Hemi-inattention can affect function and safety significantly.

Spatial Relations. The ability to identify shapes and recognize the relationship between different objects and between object and self is known as spatial relations. Clients may have trouble judging the distance between objects or following a familiar route (Zoltan, 2007). Deficits in executing concepts such as *over*, *under*, *through*, and *behind* can cause problems

in ADL tasks (Söderback, Bengtsson, Ginsburg, & Ekholm, 1992).

Visual figure-ground perception is the ability to distinguish forms hidden within a complicated background (Zoltan, 2007). Clients with figure-ground deficits may appear distractible but could in fact be responding to irrelevant visual information and be unable to process and identify the intended object (Jamison & Orchanian, 2007).

Difficulty with vertical or horizontal orientation (directionality) may be present, predominantly in clients with left-sided CVA (Birch et al., 1960). Because visual orientation is important to the righting reactions needed for upright posture and body mechanics, these disturbances interfere with balance, ADL and IADL performance, and ambulation (Birch et al., 1960; Davies, 2000). Since clients with these deficits have a distorted perception of the vertical plane, tactile cues can be more effective than verbal when prompting them to assume an upright position in sitting or standing.

Perceptual Motor Impairments

Perceptual motor skills are the link between processing information from the environment and executing movements in response. These skills rely heavily on the processing of different sensations to develop motor responses. A person who has had a CVA may have perceptual motor deficits that interfere with functional independence.

Unilateral Neglect. As discussed earlier, unilateral neglect is the inability to interpret stimuli from the affected side of the body or environment. Unilateral neglect can occur with or without hemianopsia. Clients may show a gaze preference, keeping the head turned away from the affected side and may not incorporate the affected half of the body or environment into functional tasks. Clients with unilateral neglect often demonstrate difficulties in ADL, functional mobility, and safety awareness. Unilateral neglect that persists past the acute phase of CVA has been associated with a poorer functional outcome in therapy (Clark, 2001).

Apraxia (Dyspraxia). Apraxia or dyspraxia results in difficulty or inability to plan or execute movements. These difficulties are not caused by elemental motor or sensory impairments. Clients can have difficulty performing purposeful movement on command, understanding the concept of a task, or drawing or constructing two-dimensional or three-dimensional designs. Apraxia can cause challenges in clients' ability to perform ADL and IADL tasks necessary for healthy and independent living (Walker & Lincoln, 1991). During occupational therapy intervention the use of errorless learning, blocked repetition, task-specific training, and multimodal cuing have been shown to improve performance in clients with apraxia when provided consistently in a functional environment (Bieńkiewicz, Brandi, Goldenberg, Hughes, & Hermsdörfer, 2014). Step-by-step cues to complete basic self-care tasks can improve understanding of the instructions. Hand-over-hand assistance or cuing may be required to initiate, terminate, or resume an action.

Body Awareness. Body scheme deficits affect understanding of body construction, spatial relationships, awareness of body parts in relation to one another, and right and left discrimination (Ayres, 1962; MacDonald, 1960). Because these skills are basic to all motor function, poor body orientation and postural awareness can cause functional deficits, which are particularly evident in balance and mobility, as well as increase safety concerns such as elevated fall risk (Bang & Cho, 2016; Cela, Álvarez, Bouza, & Breen, 2014; Khader & Tomlin, 1994; MacDonald, 1960). Body awareness training—using slow repetitive movements to increase focus and attention on body mechanics and postural alignment—has been shown to significantly impact static and dynamic balance needed in functional daily tasks (Khader & Tomlin, 1994). Increased body awareness is directly correlated with improved balance and independence in daily activities (Ahn, 2018; Bang & Cho, 2016).

Agnosia. Agnosia refers to the inability to process sensory information. As a result, the ability to recognize objects by vision, hearing, touch, or proprioception (position sense) is compromised despite intact senses. Symptoms are worsened when the client has an impaired body awareness and unilateral neglect (Goldberg, 1990; Maskill & Tempest, 2017). One of the more common challenges is tactile agnosia or astereognosis, which is the inability to recognize familiar objects by touch without vision. Additional information on these and other sensory and perceptual dysfunctions can be found in Chapters 9, 22, and 24.

Interventions for sensory and perceptual dysfunction. Occupational therapy interventions for the client with CVA may include sensory reeducation and compensatory techniques, as described in Chapter 21.

Perceptual deficits: Remediation. Perceptual difficulties are often not well understood by clients, families, or caregivers. Remediation focuses on the goal of skill restoration by addressing the underlying deficits (see Chapters 21 and 22). Clients, families, and caregivers require thorough education about visual perception and perceptual motor impairments to best understand and participate in the rehabilitation process.

Perceptual deficits: Compensation. OTs and OTAs can focus on the client's areas of strength and intact skills to compensate for deficits in perception, which may require an alternate strategy of completion. Since task performance improves when meaningful to the client, treatment activities should be selected based on the client's interests, previous lifestyle, current strengths and needs, living situation, and goals (Arya et al., 2012). Caregivers should be trained in the use of compensatory strategies to allow for carryover outside of therapy times.

The amount of training needed in compensatory strategies varies among clients. Some require minimal or no intervention, whereas others need ongoing blocked practice and cues. Clients with neglect may benefit from implementing scanning techniques, participation in functional tasks, and video feedback to improve awareness (Rubio & Van Deuson, 1995; Söderback et al., 1992; van Vliet & Wulf, 2006). The use of

prisms and field expander lenses has been shown to improve functional balance and task performance in clients with neglect (Nijboer, Olthoff, Van der Stigchel, & Visser-Meily, 2014). (See Chapters 21 and 22.)

The use of consistent organization practices within the home and frequently accessed spaces is crucial for clients with body awareness and spatial relation dysfunction. Some strategies include using clothing labels and learning consistent routes to navigate the environment. See Chapters 21 and 22 for more specific interventions.

Cognitive deficits: Remediation. Cognition deficits affect multiple domains and are commonly experienced after CVA. Occupational therapy intervention for functional cognition requires a comprehensive initial assessment to determine what specific areas have been impacted by CVA so a client-centered plan of care can be developed (Jokinen et al., 2015). Occupational therapy intervention for cognitive deficits focuses on maximizing long-term generalization of learned skills and safety procedures. Providing opportunities for clients to actively work on transferring skills from one task to another is key for true learning and carryover to occur.

After CVA, cognitive deficits may lead to behavioral problems that impair the client's safety, ability to interact with others, and participation in therapy. Clients with behavioral deficits may have a limited understanding of the motives and consequences of their behavior. Please refer to Chapter 22 for a thorough discussion of intervention techniques for clients with the following impairments.

Initiation and motivation. Initiation and motivation (**adynamia**) refer to the difficulty starting and following through with tasks.

Attention and concentration. Attention is the brain's ability to select and concentrate on a task in the environment and ignore other things. Distractibility and difficulty maintaining focus are common after CVA. Challenges in attention are worsened by fatigue, depression, illness, disinterest, and certain medications and can result in cognitive overload.

Disorientation and confusion. Orientation includes awareness of person, place, time, and situation. Using reality orientation prior to activity can help improve cognitive functioning.

Memory. Memory is the ability to receive, retrieve, and integrate information for short-term, delayed, and long-term use.

Sequencing and organization. Sequencing involves planning, organizing, and completing the steps of a task in correct order. Effective organization requires higher level attention, concentration, orientation, memory, and correct sequencing.

Abstract reasoning and problem solving. Concrete, literal thinking occurs when abstract reasoning is impaired. It leads to difficulty planning ahead, recognizing problems, or generating solutions.

Flexibility of thinking. Thinking involves the flow of ideas and using one's mind to reason or consider them. Inflexibility or rigidity is the inability to adapt thinking patterns or behaviors in response to change.

Dysfunction of insight. Anosognosia is lack of insight about deficits, current situation, and lifestyle changes. Poor insight may also reduce a client's safety awareness and increase risk for injury.

Judgment and safety awareness. Poor judgment and decreased safety awareness impair the ability to understand consequences of behavior and actions.

Generalization of learning. Generalization of learning is the ability of the client to transfer skills learned in one situation to another situation.

Cognitive fatigue. Cognitive fatigue leads to decreased attention and concentration, increased lethargy, increased distractibility, decreased quality of performance, decreased performance speed, increased frustration, and complaints of fatigue.

Impulsivity and perseveration. Impulsivity can lead to significant safety concerns and increase risk for falls. Motor **perseveration** is the nonpurposeful repetition of an action without the cognitive ability to cease (Gutman, 2008). Clients with perseveration have difficulty terminating a task and will usually continue until an external cue or physical assist intervenes. Perseveration is more obvious during activities that are repetitive in nature such as writing, combing hair, or shaving.

Mood and emotional impairments. Mood and emotional impairments, including lability, depression, and anxiety, are common in the first year after CVA, but can occur at any time (Carota & Bogousslavsky, 2012; Dennis, O'Rourke, Lewis, Sharpe, & Warlow, 2000; Ivey et al., 2015). There is often overlap between different types of emotional disturbances.

Cognitive deficits: Compensation. Motivation can be facilitated by the use of structure and organization with client-directed activities. Multimodal cues may stimulate clients with decreased initiation to begin an activity. Establishing realistic, meaningful, achievable treatment goals and providing frequent positive feedback improve motivation and provide a just-right challenge. As skills improve, the client and clinician should continuously create and modify treatment goals together. See Chapter 22 for specific remediation strategies.

Clients with impaired attention benefit from short sessions utilizing motivating activities. Stimulation should be limited, concrete instructions should be given, and time and difficulty should be adjusted as needed.

Clients with organization deficits benefit from a gradual increase of task difficulty. A step-by-step training should include recognizing a problem, generating solutions for the problem, selecting and implementing a solution, and then assessing the effectiveness of the solution selected.

Clients who manifest concrete thinking benefit when transitions are eased, which may include longer breaks between activities. Intervention for insight deficits involves gradual introduction to performance problems. Visual feedback, refraining from contradicting confabulated thoughts or ideas, and creating a nonthreatening environment where the client can safely explore the subjective meaning of their concerns are helpful techniques when working with someone with decreased insight. Training should take place in the real-life situations that are relevant and meaningful to the client (Jenkinson, Preston, & Ellis, 2011).

When clients demonstrate difficulty with learning new information, it may be helpful to increase instruction time, repeat instructions, and provide written prompts. Being able to understand and distinguish between the possible causes of functional problems is imperative because it will prompt treatment strategies and guide occupational therapy treatment. For example, when clients experience difficulty with dressing, the OT or OTA must discern if the problem is the result of perceptual dysfunction (apraxia) or cognitive dysfunction (sequencing) to guide remediation, as the solution would look very different (Walker & Lincoln, 1991).

Emotional Dysfunction and Mood Impairments. Damage sustained to the limbic system, where emotion and mood are controlled, may cause emotional lability (**pseudobulbar affect**), which is the inability to control the expression of emotions (Carota & Bogousslavsky, 2012). Inappropriate, uncontrolled outbursts of laughing or weeping are common. Emotionally charged situations, whether pleasant or unpleasant, can cause such responses. Some clients may become combative and agitated often as a result of confusion. Medications and behavior modification programs can reduce these behaviors. In the most severe cases of agitation, some clients may need to be restrained for safety (King & Reiss, 2013; Richter, 2005).

By some estimates, 70% of stroke survivors experience depression (Lökk & Delbari, 2010). Symptoms of depression include lethargy, apathy, excessive sadness, forgetfulness, disorganization, loss of appetite, withdrawn affect, and sleep disturbance. Anxiety often accompanies depression, so it may also need to be addressed (Carota & Bogousslavsky, 2012). Anxiety may result in increased dependence on staff and others as well as a decreased frustration tolerance.

Depression can be a reactive and appropriate grieving response to loss or as a result of cerebral damage (especially of the left hemisphere) (Alajbegovic, Djelilovic-Vranic, Nakicevic, Todorovic, & Tiric-Campara, 2014; Carota & Bogousslavsky, 2012; Herrmann et al., 1995). Poststroke depression can adversely affect long-term functional outcomes as it has a negative correlation with long-term independence (Ahn, Lee, Jeong, Kim, & Park, 2015; Chemerinski et al., 2001; Pohjasvaara, Vataja, Leppävuori, Kaste, & Erkinjuntti, 2001). Early identification and medication management is essential in facilitating participation and engagement in recovery.

Behavioral challenges that result from CVA may reduce a client's ability or willingness to participate in therapy. The OT and OTA can get a better understanding of the current behavior of a client by obtaining a comprehensive history of prior behavior patterns and coping methods. Since family and friends may view changes in behavior as a loss of their loved one, clinicians should provide education to understand why behavioral challenges occur and to teach them to implement effective behavioral strategies. Providing education to significant others and caregivers early and often can help reinforce their understanding and help them to process the behaviors and changes that have occurred.

Psychosocial Adjustment and Adaptation.

OTs and OTAs can play a strong role in helping clients and family to adjust and adapt to disability. A decrease in independence may affect the client's performance patterns and disrupt daily habits and routines. This may in turn impact the daily lives of family, friends, and caregivers. Therefore client-centered treatment approaches are crucial to this process. OTs and OTAs can do this by understanding and incorporating client and caregiver goals and expectations into the treatment. Discharge planning should be directed toward helping clients prepare for the impact of their current needs on prior life roles, habits, and routines (Schlesinger, 1962; Wallenbert & Jonsson, 2005).

Coping with the effects of CVA can be difficult, and clients and families need time to learn how to manage the many personal and social changes. Repetition may be necessary to clarify questions, reduce concerns, and reinforce supports available. Coping with extreme role reversals and changes in functional abilities after the CVA is challenging for all involved. Allowing families and newly appointed caregivers to actively participate in the therapy process is critical, especially in preparation for discharge from a rehabilitation program. Prior to discharge, home visits, formal caregiver training, and dynamic discussions can help with this preparation. Providing client and family education on resources and teaching them how to access information once they return home are both vital.

Caregivers are at risk for stress-related conditions and burnout. OT intervention should include acknowledging the caregiver's contribution, addressing caregiver needs, and offering strategies to reduce the risk of burnout (O'Sullivan, 2007). Options such as alternating family members, hiring professional help in the home, or using respite care can reduce stress. Some stroke survivors and families choose to participate in community or online CVA support groups, often after discharge (online support resources for caregivers can be found at the end of this chapter). Engaging family and friends throughout the rehabilitative process can reduce stress levels and help to improve generalization of skills to the home environment.

Behavioral Dysfunction: Intervention.

Occupational therapy intervention for clients with disruptive behaviors after CVA focuses on the development of appropriate behavior management strategies and integration of these techniques into daily life. An important strategy for managing impulsivity is providing multimodal cues slowly, calmly, and one step at a time in a distraction-free environment. The clinician should use a straightforward approach, providing immediate reinforcement. To improve attention to detail, a graded approach will initially focus on recognizing errors and progress to correcting errors. The end goal is for the client to reflect on performance and use observations to improve quality of performance. Prior to an activity, asking clients to predict their performance and then working with them to compare predictions to actual performance can also help improve insight into abilities.

When treating clients with agitated or combative behaviors, OTs and OTAs should review their current behavioral state prior to each session and decide whether treatment is appropriate at that time. If agitation increases, treatment should be discontinued immediately and reattempted only when symptoms have subsided. Interdisciplinary communication with a psychologist or neuropsychiatrist can also be helpful.

Social skills training. The deficits resulting from CVA can have a major impact on social skills and participation. Common behaviors include exhibiting disruptive behavior and emotional outbursts, interrupting others, seeking constant immediate reinforcement, making sexually inappropriate comments, or performing other attention-seeking behaviors. These behaviors can be minimized with consistent limit setting. Social skills training, individually or in a group setting, where the client can use self-reflection and feedback from the clinician, can be effective in improving appropriate behavior. Different behavioral techniques should be utilized based on the client's specific needs.

Oral-Motor Dysfunction

Oral-motor control is the coordination of movements needed for speech, facial expression, sucking, chewing, and swallowing. It utilizes the muscles and other structures of the face, throat, and tongue.

Dysarthria.

The coordination of facial muscles, lips, tongue, and jaw help produce clear and articulated speech. After CVA, oral-motor dysfunction causes weakness in the muscles required for speech and may present with facial palsy or drooping. Reduced sensation often accompanies muscle weakness. Clients with **dysarthria** present with slurred speech that is often rapid or slowed, uneven, and monotone, making it challenging to understand depending on the severity of symptoms.

Dysphagia.

Dysphagia (difficulty in swallowing or the inability to swallow) is caused by sensory loss and muscle weakness in the structures of the mouth and throat that control swallowing (Buchholz, 1994). Weakness in swallowing is known as oropharyngeal dysphagia and is characterized by dysfunction of the nerves and muscles in the mouth, pharynx, and upper esophageal sphincter. Abnormalities at the level of the esophagus are known as esophageal dysphagia. Typically clients who have sustained damage to the medulla area of the brainstem are the ones who exhibit dysphagia immediately after CVA (Fuller, 2014; Gutman, 2008). Other regions of the brain often linked to dysphagia include the cortical, subcortical, and white matter tracts in the left hemisphere (Wilmskoetter et al., 2019). Common observable clinical signs of dysphagia include drooling, pocketing of food in the cheeks, coughing, and a wet voice. Clients with dysphagia are at a high risk for aspiration of saliva or food, which can lead to aspiration pneumonia (Armstrong & Mosher, 2011; Kidd et al., 1993). The accompanying Alert box contains safety precautions related to clients with oral motor dysfunction. For a thorough discussion of the management of the occupation of eating and feeding, see Chapter 11.

! ALERT

Safe Feeding for Clients With Dysphagia (See Chapter 11)
- Determine proper positioning for mealtime, including necessary equipment to promote the best position for eating.
- Understand and comply with prescribed solid and liquid diet consistencies.
- Observe and monitor client closely during intake.
- Educate and involve client, family, and caregivers in client feeding protocol.
- Demonstrate competence for emergency procedures for choking and aspiration.

Speech and Language Dysfunction. The Broca area, Wernike area, and angular gyrus (which control language) are located in the left hemisphere. Therefore language dysfunction most commonly occurs in clients with left-sided CVA; however, it can sometimes occur with damage to other regions of the brain. Studies have shown that hand dominance can play a role in location of the language centers in the brain and can cause speech and language centers to be located within the right hemisphere or distributed between both hemispheres (Boeree, 2004). Deficits in semantics, pragmatics, and prosody needed in the cognitive operations of language and speech processing typically result from damage to the right hemisphere (Tompkins, 2012). OTs and OTAs promote communication by reinforcing techniques and adapting augmentative communication devices recommended by the speech-language pathologist.

Aphasia. Aphasia is an acquired language disorder that causes a wide variety of deficits in verbal comprehension, written comprehension (alexia), oral expression, written expression (agraphia), ability to interpret gestures, or mathematical skills (acalculia) (Halpern, 2000). Several different types of aphasia exist. Anomia, or word-finding difficulty, can occur in all types. Clients with expressive aphasia (Broca aphasia) have difficulty producing speech but can comprehend it. Clients with receptive aphasia (Wernicke aphasia) have difficulty with language comprehension. These clients may be able to produce fluent speech but cannot comprehend it. Global aphasia is characterized by a loss of both language areas. The ability to form words is often absent or significantly diminished. Clients with global aphasia often may react to gestures, voice intonations, and facial expression but have difficulty responding appropriately to these cues. Careful consideration of what clients comprehend is important to bridge the gap between what clients seem to understand and what they actually understand (Whitworth, Webster, & Howard, 2005).

Most clients with aphasia use a variety of communication methods, including alphabet boards, computers or tablets, picture boards, gestures, and writing. Some can speak single words or phrases. Accuracy may decrease with increased

---

BOX 23.6 Suggestions for Improving Communication With Clients Who Have Aphasia

- Be patient.
- Reduce environmental distractions.
- Use face-to-face communication; establish and maintain eye contact during communications.
- Stress the important words in sentences.
- Speak clearly in simple, direct sentences; do not raise volume unless indicated otherwise.
- Ask yes/no or required choice questions.
- Utilize written cues, drawings, and gestures in addition to speech.
- Allow adequate time for a response to questions; do not interrupt.
- Observe and respond to nonverbal communications from client (body language, gestures).
- Let the client know if you do not understand; if necessary, take a short break to avoid client frustration.
- Encourage independence and reinforce attempts to use speech with positive feedback.

---

fatigue. Box 23.6 provides suggestions for communicating with clients with aphasia (Gillen & Rubio, 2010; Trombly & Radomski, 2008).

AREAS OF OCCUPATION AND OCCUPATIONAL THERAPY TREATMENT TECHNIQUES

Occupational therapy intervention for the client with CVA focuses primarily on areas of occupation, including ADL, IADL, work, leisure, and social participation (American Occupational Therapy Association, 2017). Studies have found that increased physical disability, anxiety, and depression are correlated with decreased quality of life as reported by stroke survivors (De Wit et al., 2017). Multifaceted plans of care that incorporate physical rehabilitation and psychosocial support and improve functional performance with clients' meaningful occupations is imperative when addressing quality of life and level of independence of stroke survivors (van Mierlo, van Heugten, Post, Hoekstra, & Visser-Meily, 2018). Suggestions for functional treatment interventions for these areas are provided in Table 23.3.

ADL and IADL: Intervention

Self-care tasks after a CVA often require extra time to allow for integration of new skills and to reflect on the way bodily changes impact performance (Guidetti, Asaba, & Tham, 2009). Occupational therapy sessions should allow for extra time for learning, practice, and reflection. Interventions to improve self-care skills often begin with basic activities and progress to higher level skills. See Chapters 11 and 13 for specific interventions for mealtime occupations, ADL, and IADL for clients following a CVA.

TABLE 23.3   Areas of Occupation and Suggested Treatment Strategies

Selected Area of Occupation[a]	Treatment Considerations and Activities	Adaptive/Compensatory Strategies and Techniques
Activities of Daily Living		
Bathing and Showering Obtaining and using supplies; soaping, rinsing, and drying body parts; maintaining safe position and balance while bathing; transferring to and from bathing positions	Maintaining balance while reaching to wash body parts, practice turning water on and off and adjusting temperature; transfer training into tub and shower; sequencing activities	Wash mitt, soap-on-a-rope, pump-style soap dispenser, long-handled sponge, bath bench, handheld shower, grab bars; establish routine for bathing regimen
Bowel and Bladder Management Complete, intentional control of bowel movements and urinary bladder and, if necessary, use of equipment for bladder control	Manage and empty leg bag, self-catheterization training, bladder/bowel retraining program	Leg bag straps, catheter clamps, suppository inserter, digital stimulator, panty liners/incontinence pads
Toilet Hygiene Obtaining and using supplies, managing clothing, maintaining toileting position, toilet transfer, cleaning body, caring for menstrual and continence needs	Mobility activities such as rolling side to side, bridging and lifting hips to use bedpan, transfer training onto/off toilet, reaching body parts to clean self, raise/lower and adjust clothing	Use of grab bars, raised toilet seat, bedside commode, bidet to assist with hygiene, toilet tissue aid, loose fitting clothing with elastic fastenings
Dressing Selecting appropriate clothing and accessories; obtaining clothing; dressing/undressing including fastening and adjusting, applying, and removing personal devices, prosthesis, or orthosis	Practice undressing first in loose fitting garments, use full-length mirror while sitting supported in chair and then progress to unsupported sitting (e.g., at edge of bed); use clothing in contrasting colors, select clothing and lay out in advance	Teach adaptive/one-handed dressing techniques, Velcro fastenings, elastic waistbands and shoelaces, shoe horn, provide adaptive straps on splints to improve the client's ability to don and doff them to don and doff
Feeding Setting up food, using utensils, cups (follow direction of dysphagia therapist)	Monitor client for swallowing problems, follow dietary and dysphagia guidelines and restrictions when indicated, oral motor intervention	Use of plate guards or scoop dish, adapted cups with lids or easy grip handles; cup and straw holders, adapted utensils, rocker knife, antiskid placemat, proper positioning at table, teach strategies for one-handed technique to open food containers and packages. For clients with hemianopsia, place food tray in intact visual field.
Functional Mobility Bed mobility, wheelchair mobility, transfers, functional ambulation	Provide progressive mobility training on a variety of surfaces; teach bed mobility, including rolling, bridging, moving from supine to sit; teach indoor wheelchair mobility over even, uneven, and inclined surfaces Transfer training to a variety of surfaces, including the bed, chair, toilet, tub, floor Train on safe indoor functional ambulation, including reinforcing the use of ambulatory device, instruction on how to transport objects during ambulation activities	Use of bedrails, overhead trapeze bars, pull straps to assist with bed mobility, patient lift for dependent clients Specialized wheelchair assessment and training, including hemi-wheelchair that is lower to ground for easier propulsion; wheelchair modifications (e.g., removable armrests, brake extension, swing-away leg rests), recliner; lightweight, one-arm drive; power mobility Use portable ramps/chair lifts for patients unable to manage stairs; use walker basket, backpack, lidded cups while transporting objects during functional ambulation; adaptive wheelchair propulsion (e.g., use of the unaffected upper extremity and lower extremity to propel and steer)
Personal Care Device Using, cleaning, and maintaining personal care items such as hearing aids, glasses, orthotics, adaptive equipment	Practice cleaning, caring for, and learning sources for repair or replacement of eyeglasses, splints, braces, slings, edema gloves, communication devices, and durable medical equipment, such as wheelchairs or bath seats	Wash mitt; magnifying lens; notebook with written directions, address book with phone numbers and contact persons for service and repair

(Continued)

TABLE 23.3 Areas of Occupation and Suggested Treatment Strategies—cont'd

Selected Area of Occupation[a]	Treatment Considerations and Activities	Adaptive/Compensatory Strategies and Techniques
Personal Hygiene and Grooming Shaving, cosmetic application; hair, nail, and skin care; deodorant application; cleaning mouth; brushing and flossing teeth; removing, cleaning, and reinserting dental orthotics and prosthetics	Use mirror during grooming activities Organizing and sequencing activities Promote the proper positioning during hygiene and grooming activities Comb or brush hair, and practice putting on and taking off hair clips, bobby pins, headbands Scrub nails with stationary brush, file nails with stationary nail file, cut nails with stationary nail clipper, and paint nails with stationary nail polish brush Open and close deodorant, adjust deodorant level, and apply deodorant Open and close mouthwash containers and rinse mouth; open and close toothpaste and brush teeth; remove, reinsert, and clean dentures	Small, adjustable double-sided mirror with magnifying and regular sides; angled wall mirror, electric safety razor, razor holder with strap (for higher-level clients using a manual razor); aerosol can dispenser, handles for can such as shaving cream; electric hair trimmers, air dry hair to avoid having to manipulate blow dryer, large or extended-handle comb/brush, comb/brush with Velcro strap, suction nail brush, suction nail file, pump-style toothpaste dispenser, denture brush, denture tablets (reduced need for brushing), suction denture brush, glycerin swabs to clean mouth, use stick or cream deodorant
Toilet Hygiene	Mobility activities such as rolling side to side, bridging and lifting hips to use bedpan, transfer training onto/off toilet, reaching body parts to clean self, raise/lower and adjust clothing	Use of bidet to assist with hygiene, loose fitting garments with elastic fastenings, toilet tissue aid Use of grab bars, raised toilet seat, bedside commode
Instrumental Activities of Daily Living *Care* Care of others, care of pets, child rearing	Direct care of adults may not be possible depending on level of impairment Improve safe ability to care for children and pets Train in assertive techniques to direct and supervise home health aides, attendants, and housekeepers who might assist in care for others	Modified baby doll with added weight cuffs, adapted games and stories to use with children, one-hand release crib and high chair Adapted pet care products (e.g., single packet foods, larger-handle bushes and leashes with solid grips)
Communication Management Use of writing equipment, telephones, computers, communication boards, call lights, emergency systems, Braille writers, telecommunication devices, and augmentative communication devices	Dominancy retraining, if indicated, establish effective pen/marker grip patterns; graded writing exercises; look up and dial phone numbers, one-handed typing Practice emergency training/call light use	Built-up writing utensils, writing aids; clipboards, phone holders, speaker phone and head sets, programmable cell phone, modifications to keyboards and computer adaptations (e.g., touch pads, expanded keyboard, "sticky keys"), smartphones
Community Mobility Moving in the community; using public and private transportation	Outdoor wheelchair/functional ambulation training, including practice going in/out all types of doors; using the elevator; performing car transfers Sequencing and planning activities for taxi rides or getting information regarding the bus/train/paratransit schedules, using public transportation, if appropriate Obtain a wheelchair sticker for car or license plate for disabled from state Department of Motor Vehicles if approved by doctor	Treated wheelchair tires, appropriate footwear for outdoor terrains, transfer board, reachers, notebook/smartphone or tape recorder for information Wheelchair carrier for car, ramp for van Refer for driving evaluation, including assessment for adaptive controls for driving car or van Assist with completion of paratransit application process, if appropriate
Financial Management Using fiscal resources; making financial transactions, including budgeting, paying bills	Perform commercially available budgeting exercise, practice writing checks, paying bills online and balancing accounts	Calculator with large number keyboard, flow chart of monthly bills, computer software for financial management, direct deposit with online and automatic bill-paying systems, smartphones with budgeting applications
Health Management and Maintenance Developing, managing, and maintaining routines for health and wellness promotion, including medication routines	Identify client's risk factors for cerebrovascular accident and strategies to reduce modifiable ones (e.g., smoking cessation, stress reduction groups, walking for weight reduction); improve	Cookbooks/online resources for low-salt, low-fat, and low-sugar recipes; provide individualized home exercise program, which may include Theraband, light

(Continued)

TABLE 23.3 Areas of Occupation and Suggested Treatment Strategies—cont'd

Selected Area of Occupation[a]	Treatment Considerations and Activities	Adaptive/Compensatory Strategies and Techniques
	and apply knowledge of nutrition and of prescribed diet; and develop home exercise programs for self-range of motion, and general conditioning as indicated; use of Wii video games for fitness and mobility training	weights, relaxation tapes, referral to wellness and exercise groups Smartphones with medication schedule applications Telemonitoring for medication management, glucometer use
	Understand medication use and precautions; understand how to adhere to schedule; practice opening and closing medication containers, practice simulated administration; use consumer skills to learn to ask questions about medications, report side effects, and obtain refills	Pill sorters, adaptive insulin synergies, speak with physician regarding single-dose medication regimes, easy-open medication containers
	Introduce activities to maintain cognitive fitness and flexibility (e.g., word puzzles, word searches)	
Home Establishment and Management Developing, managing, and maintaining personal and household possessions and environments, including maintaining and repairing personal possessions (clothing and household items) and knowing how to seek help or whom to contact	Home management activities such as folding clothing, towels, sheets, practicing sorting and measuring laundry detergent, using washer and dryer, putting clothing in closet, vacuuming, making bed, mopping, emptying trashcans and sorting recyclables	Rolling cart to transport heavy items; premeasured laundry detergents, front-loading washer and dryer for wheelchair users, labeling closets to organize storage
	Practice simple household responsibilities such as changing a lightbulb, replacing batteries, watering plants, and cleaning refrigerator—progress as possible; determine capabilities for certain jobs and assistance options for the remaining jobs	Reachers, pull-down ironing board, lightweight iron; work station for laundry; sweep, dust, mop from wheelchair or while ambulating; straighten up room; remove linens from beds; handheld vacuum, lightweight upright vacuum cleaner, long-handled dust pan, wonder-mop (for use with one hand), long-handled cleaning sponge, fitted bed sheet, trash bags with built-in tie, recyclable sorters
Meal Preparation and Cleanup	Graded cooking program beginning with planning and preparing a tabletop, cold snack, moving to hot meals in oven and cleanup	Adaptive one-handed cutting boards, jar openers, pot handle holders, use of rolling cart, one-handed electric can openers, angled wall mirror over stove, built-up utensils, long arm oven mitt
	Full training should incorporate the use of the appliances the client will use at home, as well as kitchen organization and mobility activities	Label drawers and refrigerator; rearrangement of items with those the most used more accessible One-pot meals, timers, preplanning, and organizing meals in advance
Safety and Emergency Management	Practice responding to emergencies, including how to recognize hazards and taking action to reduce threat to safety Brainstorm emergency management plans, prepare a "go" bag for emergencies, recommend clients carry valuables on body rather than in backpack on back of wheelchair to prevent theft, assist clients in identifying "backup" for equipment (e.g., power w/c users) and assistance in event of emergency	Programmable cell phone and emergency call systems; obtain stickers from local firehouse to put on windows indicating that a person with a disability resides in household
Shopping Preparing shopping lists, selecting and purchasing items, selecting method of payment, competing transaction	Perform simulated shopping activities, including online and telephone ordering; money management skills, including counting money, making change	Store money in accessible purse or wallet, use debit card, adaptive shopping cart; automated online grocery ordering (e.g., Fresh Direct)

(Continued)

TABLE 23.3 Areas of Occupation and Suggested Treatment Strategies—cont'd

Selected Area of Occupation[a]	Treatment Considerations and Activities	Adaptive/Compensatory Strategies and Techniques
Work Employment interests and pursuits, seeking and acquisition of employment, job performance, retirement preparation and adjustment, volunteerism	Perform simulated work tasks and work samples; work hardening program as appropriate; explore retirement options and plan for retirement activities, assist with identifying potential community volunteer experiences that might be appropriate	Adapt work environment for wheelchair and ambulatory device user; make recommendations for reasonable accommodations based on specific client needs and job responsibilities (e.g., adaptive keyboard, phone headset)
Leisure Leisure exploration and participation	Identify and practice previous leisure tasks; adapt technique or equipment for these tasks Assist client in developing and exploring alternative leisure tasks	Adaptive book holders, audio books, automatic card shufflers, adaptive games and equipment such as bowling ramps, one-handed needlepoint hoops, large print books and playing cards, Wii games
Social Participation [a]Engaging in characteristic and expected activities with community, family, peers, and friends	Social skill training, role playing, videotaping; identify and make appropriate community referrals Participation in online social networking, blogging, etc. to maintain social interactions	Assist client in exploring and identifying community resources Make referrals to community support groups Identify and offer strategies to address environmental barriers to community groups

[a]AOTA (2014).

CASE STUDY

Luis

Luis is a right-handed 57-year-old man who recently retired from the police force. Luis is divorced and lives in a single-family home that he owns with his daughter Maria. Since his retirement 6 months ago, Luis has been enjoying his new-found free time by completing a variety of small home improvement projects that he had been putting off because of his former work schedule.

Three days ago, Luis woke up with a headache and at breakfast that same morning Maria noticed that his speech was slurred and that he was dragging his left foot when he walked. She immediately took him to the hospital emergency room. Medical workup revealed Luis had suffered a right CVA, and he was admitted to the inpatient stroke unit. His medical history is significant for high blood pressure and cigarette smoking. Maria reported to the medical team that her father has not been compliant with taking his blood pressure medicine and still smokes a pack of cigarettes a day.

The stroke team evaluated Luis and made a referral to rehabilitation. The OT completed an initial evaluation and determined that Luis had significant deficits in all areas of occupation, including eating, personal hygiene, showering, dressing, and functional mobility. Luis was not ambulatory and was using a wheelchair for mobility on the stroke unit.

The OT's assessment of performance skills revealed that Luis had deficits in both motor and process skills. Specifically, he demonstrated decreased balance, which contributed to an asymmetric posture while he was sitting and standing. Luis's left UE had flaccid muscle tone and no active ROM. Tactile sensation was, however, intact throughout his entire left side.

Cognitively, Luis was alert and oriented; he was able to follow multistep directions. When fatigued, however, he became easily distracted. During functional activities, Luis exhibited a decreased awareness of his left side and, as a result, his left arm was often off to his side.

The OT noted that Luis was motivated for therapy and expressed interest in improving his ability to perform personal self-care. When discussing his deficits, Luis became tearful and expressed sadness about the amount of assistance he needed to perform simple tasks such as shaving.

When Luis is ready to be discharged from the hospital, the current plan is for him to return home with home care services. Luis agrees with this plan but is concerned about how he will manage at home while his daughter is at work.

1. How might Luis's balance deficits be affecting his ability to perform self-care activities such as dressing and bathing? What compensatory techniques could he learn to increase independence in these areas?
2. What are some potential complications of Luis having a flaccid arm? What preventive strategies could address these complications? Should he be provided with a sling? Why or why not?
3. How might Luis's decreased awareness of his left arm affect his safety during functional mobility?
4. What information would you need about Luis's home environment to assist with planning for discharge?
5. How would you involve Maria in Luis's occupational therapy plan of care at this time?
6. How might you incorporate health management and CVA prevention education into Luis's occupational therapy plan of care?

CASE STUDY

Malia

Malia is a right-handed 70-year-old woman who sustained a left CVA resulting in right hemiparesis 6 weeks ago. She is currently receiving home care occupational therapy services and has a home health aide 7 days a week for 4 hours a day. The home health aide will not be covered by her insurance once skilled occupational therapy services are completed in 2 weeks.

Malia lives with her husband in a first-floor walkup apartment. Prior to her CVA, she was independent in all basic ADL and IADL tasks and was the primary homemaker for the family. Malia misses this role and is looking forward to resuming her home management tasks as soon as possible.

Currently, Malia presents with mild right weakness and deceased sensory awareness in her right hand. She ambulates at a modified independent level indoors with a cane but needs contact guard when negotiating steps. She is easily fatigued and requires extra time and rest breaks during the day.

Cognitively, Malia is alert, fully oriented, and can follow two-step directions; however, she can become distracted when performing multistep tasks due to stimuli in her environment.

At this time, Malia has achieved independence in all basic ADL. She would like to resume involvement in simple home management tasks and has identified participation in meal preparation and cleanup as short-term goals.

1. What safety concerns are raised by Malia's sensorimotor and attention deficits as they relate to her participation in meal preparation activities?
2. Describe two treatment considerations and/or adaptive strategies for meal preparation and cleanup that can be incorporated into Malia's treatment session.
3. Describe a graded sequence of tasks that might be used during treatment with Malia to work toward increasing her independence in meal preparation.
4. How would you involve Malia's husband and home health aide in her occupational therapy program at this time?

SUMMARY

CVA results in a complex disability that can affect all areas of occupational performance. The ability for clients to reach their goals depends on multiple factors, including region and extent of damage to the brain, client medical comorbidities, client motivation and adjustment, client support systems, and the timely application of appropriate treatment by health professionals. Acute hospital and inpatient rehabilitation emphasize on providing rehabilitation services to clients to get them back to a community level as quickly as possible. Community settings may include the home, adult day programs, and outpatient settings. In addition to providing direct treatment to clients with CVA, OTs and OTAs can also play an important role in designing health maintenance programs directed toward prevention and education in this area.

▌ REVIEW QUESTIONS

1. Explain the difference between a CVA and a TIA.
2. Name three common warning signs of CVA.
3. Explain why stroke survivors are at higher risk for developing medical complications.
4. Describe how occupational therapy treatment would change for a client who develops a DVT of the left extremity.
5. Describe the effects of long-standing edema of the hemiplegic forearm and hand.
6. How are the occupational therapy goals for deformity and injury prevention important to the achievement of rehabilitation goals for the client with a CVA?
7. Discuss the differences in roles of the OT practitioner treating the stroke survivor in acute care and home health settings.

8. What are the effects of abnormal reflexes and impaired postural mechanisms on the sitting balance of the client who has experienced a CVA?
9. State and discuss the important considerations for positioning a client with a CVA in bed and the wheelchair.
10. What factors would prevent a client from using adaptive equipment for dressing?
11. Why is it important in self-care training to allow opportunities for practice?
12. What are the purposes of the lap tray and resting hand splint for the client with hemiplegia?
13. Explain why PROM is recommended for the client with a flaccid upper extremity.
14. Why is scapular mobility required for pain-free ROM activities for the shoulder?
15. What strategies can be implemented to prevent subluxation of the shoulder?
16. Describe some methods of positioning the affected arm and leg to reduce edema.
17. How can a CVA affect vision?
18. Explain how to increase the attention of a client who is easily agitated.
19. Explain why early and frequent inclusion of the family and caregivers is important to occupational therapy treatment planning and implementation.
20. Describe how the OTA could incorporate health maintenance and management into treatment interventions.

REFERENCES

Abbott, A. L., Bladin, C. F., & Donnan, G. A. (2001). Seizures and stroke. In J. Bogousslavsky, & L. R. Caplan (Eds.), *Stroke syndromes* (2nd ed.). New York, NY: Cambridge Press.

Abreu, B. (1995). The effect of environmental regulations on postural control after stroke. *The American Journal of Occupational Therapy*, 49(6), 517–525.

Adams, H. P., Jr., del Zoppo, G., Alberts, M. J., Bhatt, D. L., Brass, L., Furlan, A., et al. (2007). Guidelines for the early management of adults with ischemic stroke: a guideline from the American Heart Association/American Stroke Association Stroke Council, Clinical Cardiology Council, Cardiovascular Radiology and Intervention Council, and the Atherosclerotic Peripheral Vascular Disease and Quality of Care Outcomes in Research Interdisciplinary Working Groups. *Circulation*, 115, e478–e534.

Ahn, D. H., Lee, Y. J., Jeong, J. H., Kim, Y. R., & Park, J. B. (2015). The effect of post-stroke depression on rehabilitation outcome and the impact of caregiver type as a factor of post-stroke depression. *Annals of Rehabilitation Medicine*, 39(1), 74–80.

Ahn, S. N. (2018). Differences in body awareness and its effects on balance function and independence in activities of daily living for stroke. *Journal of Physical Therapy Science*, 30(11), 1386–1389.

Alajbegovic, A., Djelilovic-Vranic, J., Nakicevic, A., Todorovic, L., & Tiric-Campara, M. (2014). Post stroke depression. *Medical Archives*, 68(1), 47–50.

American Heart Association. (2019). Brain stem stroke. <https://www.stroke.org/en/about-stroke/types-of-stroke/brain-stem-stroke>.

American Occupational Therapy Association. (2014). Occupational therapy practice framework: domain and process. (3rd ed.) *The American Journal of Occupational Therapy*, 68, S1–S48.

American Stroke Association. (2005). Recommendations for the establishment of stroke systems of care. *Stroke; a Journal of Cerebral Circulation*, 36, 690–703.

Armstrong, J. R., & Mosher, B. D. (2011). Aspiration pneumonia after stroke: intervention and prevention. *Neurohospitalist*, 1(2), 85–93.

Arya, K. N., Verma, R., Garg, R. K., Sharma, V. P., Agarwal, M., & Aggarwal, G. G. (2012). Meaningful task-specific training (MTST) for stroke rehabilitation: a randomized controlled trial. *Topics in Stroke Rehabilitation*, 19(3), 193–211.

Ayres, A. (1962). *Perceptual motor training for children*. Proceedings of Study Course IV, Third International Congress, World Federation of Occupational Therapists *Approaches to the Treatment of Clients With Neuromuscular Dysfunction*. Dubuque, IA: William C Brown.

Bang, D. H., & Cho, H. S. (2016). Effect of body awareness training on balance and walking ability in chronic stroke patients: a randomized controlled trial. *Journal of Physical Therapy Science*, 28(1), 198–201.

Baricich, A., Carda, S., Cisari, C., Lanzotti, L., & Invernizzi, M. (2013). The value of adding mirror therapy for upper limb motor recovery of subacute stroke patients: a randomized controlled trial. *European Journal of Physical and Rehabilitation Medicine*, 49, 311–317.

Bartels, M. N., Duffy, C. A., & Belhand, H. E. (2011). Pathophysiology and medical management of stroke and acute rehabilitation of stroke survivors. In G. Gillen (Ed.), *Stroke rehabilitation: a function-based approach* (3rd ed.). St Louis, MO: Mosby.

Belagaje, S. R. (2017). Stroke rehabilitation. *Continuum (Minneapolis, Minn.)*, 23(1), 238–253.

Benjamin, E. J., Blaha, M. J., Chiuve, S. E., Cushman, M., Das, S., Deo, R., et al. (2017). Heart disease and stroke statistics—2017 update: a report from the American Heart Association. *Circulation*, 135, e229–e445.

Bieńkiewicz, M. M., Brandi, M. L., Goldenberg, G., Hughes, C. M., & Hermsdörfer, J. (2014). The tool in the brain: apraxia in ADL. Behavioral and neurological correlates of apraxia in daily living. *Frontiers in Psychology*, 5, 353.

Birch, G. H., Proctor, F., Bortner, M., & Lowenthal, M. (1960). Perception in hemiplegia: judgment of the vertical and horizontal by hemiplegic clients. *Archives of Physical Medicine and Rehabilitation*, 41, 19.

Bobath, B. (1990). *Adult hemiplegia: evaluation and treatment* (3rd ed.). Oxford, UK: Butterworth-Heinemann Ltd.

Boeree, C. G. (2004). Speech and the brain. <http://www.ship.edu/~cgboeree/speechbrain.html>.

Bolognini, N., Russo, C., & Edwards, D. J. (2016). The sensory side of post-stroke motor rehabilitation. *Restorative Neurology and Neuroscience*, 34(4), 571–586.

Brandsater, M. E. (2005). Stroke rehabilitation. In J. A. Delisa, B. M. Gans, W. L. Bockenek, W. R. Frontera, L. H. Gerber, S. R. Geiringer., et al. (Eds.), *Physical Medicine and Rehabilitaion: Principles and Practice* (4th ed.). Philadelphia: Lippincott William & Wilkins.

Brandsater, M. E., Roth, E. J., & Siebens, H. C. (1992). Venous thromboembolism in stroke: literature review and implications for clinical practice. *Archives of Physical Medicine and Rehabilitation*, 73(Suppl. 5), S379–S391.

Buchholz, D. W. (1994). Dysphagia associated with neurological disorders. *Acta Otorhinolaryngologica Belgica*, 48(2), 143–155.

Carota, A., & Bogousslavsky, J. (2012). Mood changes after stroke. *Frontiers of Neurology and Neuroscience*, 30, 70–74.

Cela, V. M., Álvarez, A. A., Bouza, M. D., & Breen, P. E. (2014). Perception of body scheme, self-esteem and quality of live on people with acquired brain injury. *The Procedia - Social and Behavioral Sciences*, 132, 135–141.

Centers for Disease Control and Prevention. (2017). Stroke facts. <http://www.cdc.gov/stroke/facts.htm>.

Charness, A. (2004). *Stroke/head injury. Rehabilitation Institute of Chicago procedure manual*. Rockville, MD: Aspen.

Chemerinski, E., Robinson, R. G., & Kosier, J. T. (2001). Improved recovery in activities of daily living associated with remission of post stroke depression. *Stroke; a Journal of Cerebral Circulation*, 32(1), 113–117.

Chengqi, H., Jingyi, Y., & Yang, L. (2018). The effect of kinesiology taping on the hemiplegic shoulder pain: a randomized controlled trial. *Journal of Healthcare Engineering*, 18, 1–11.

Cheung, J., Rancourt, A., Di Poce, S., Levine, A., Hoang, J., Ismail, F., et al. (2015). Patient-identified factors that influence spasticity in people with stroke and multiple sclerosis receiving botulinum toxin injection treatments. *Physiotherapy Canada. Physiotherapie Canada*, 67(2), 157–166.

Chitambira, B., & Evans, S. (2018). Repositioning stroke patients with pusher syndrome to reduce incidence of pressure ulcers. *BJNN*, 14(1), 16–21.

Choi, J. B., Yang, J. E., & Song, B. K. (2017). The effect of different types of resting hand splints on spasticity and hand function among patients with stroke. *Journal of Ecophysiology and Occupational Health*, 16(1-2), 42–51.

Clark, S. (2001). Right hemisphere syndrome. In J. Bogousslavsky, & L. R. Caplan (Eds.), *Stroke syndromes*. (2nd ed.). New York, NY: Cambridge Press.

Coleman, E. R., Moudgal, R., Lang, K., Hyacinth, H. I., Awosika, O. O., Kissela, B. M., et al. (2017). Early rehabilitation after stroke: a narrative review. *Current Atherosclerosis Reports*, 19, 59.

Davies, P. M. (2000). *Steps to follow: the comprehensive treatment of clients with hemiplegia* (2nd ed.). New York, NY: Springer-Verlag.

Dennis, M., O'Rourke, S., Lewis, S., Sharpe, M., & Warlow, C. (2000). Emotional outcomes after stroke: factors associated with poor outcome. *The Journal of Neurology, Neurosurgery, and Psychiatry, 68*, 47–52.

De Wit, L., Theuns, P., Dejaeger, E., Devos, S., Gantenbein, A. R., Kerckhofs, E., et al. (2017). Long-term impact of stroke on patients' health-related quality of life. *Disability and Rehabilitation, 39*(14), 1435–1440.

Dobkin, B. H. (2004). Rehabilitation and recovery of the client with stroke. In J. Mohr, P. Wolf, D. Choi, & B. Weir (Eds.), *Stroke: pathophysiology, diagnosis, and management* (4th ed.). Philadelphia, PA: Churchill Livingstone.

Dorsher, P. T., & McMichan, J. C. (1993). Pulmonary considerations in rehabilitation. In M. Sinaki (Ed.), *Basic clinical rehabilitation medicine* (2nd ed.). St Louis, MO: Mosby.

Dromerick, A. W., Edwards, D. F., & Hahn, M. (2000). Does the application of constraint-induced movement therapy during acute rehabilitation reduce arm impairment after ischemic stroke? *Stroke; a Journal of Cerebral Circulation, 31*(12), 2984–2988.

El-Helow, M. R., Zamzam, M. L., Fathalla, M. M., El-Badawy, M. A., El Nahhas, N., El-Nabil, L. M., et al. (2015). Efficacy of modified constraint-induced movement therapy in acute stroke. *European Journal of Physical and Rehabilitation Medicine, 51*, 371–379.

Elovic, E., & Bogey, R. (2010). Spasticity and movement disorders. In R. L. Braddom (Ed.), *Physical medicine and rehabilitation: principles and practice* (4th ed.). Philadelphia, PA: Lippincott Williams & Wilkins.

Ferdinand, P., & Roffe, C. (2016). Hypoxia after stroke: a review of experimental and clinical evidence. *Experimental & Translational Stroke Medicine, 8*, 9.

Foulkes, M. A. (1990). Design issues in chemosensory trials. *Archives of Otolaryngology--Head & Neck Surgery, 116*(1), 65–68.

Fuller, K. S. (2014). Stroke. In C. C. Goodman, & W. G. Boissonnault (Eds.), *Pathology: implications for the physical therapist* (3rd ed.). Philadelphia, PA: WB Saunders.

Giang, T. A., Ong, A., Krishnamurthy, K., & Fong, K. (2016). Rehabilitation interventions for poststroke hand oedema: a systematic review. *The Hong Kong Journal of Occupational Therapy, 27*(1), 7–17.

Gillen, G. (2010). *Stroke rehabilitation: a function-based approach* (3rd ed.). St Louis, MO: Mosby.

Gillen, G. (2010). Upper extremity function and management. In G. Gillen (Ed.), *Stroke rehabilitation: a function-based approach* (3rd ed.). St Louis, MO: Mosby.

Gillen, G., & Rubio, K. B. (2010). Treatment of cognitive and perceptual deficits: a function-based approach. In G. Gillen (Ed.), *Stroke rehabilitation: a function-based approach* (3rd ed.). St Louis, MO: Mosby.

Gillot, A. J., Holder-Walls, A., Kurtz, J. R., & Varley, N. C. (2003). Perceptions and experiences of two survivors of stroke who participated in constraint-induced movement therapy home programs. *The American Journal of Occupational Therapy, 57*(2), 168–176.

Goldberg, E. (1990). Associative agnosias and the functions of the left hemisphere. *Journal of Clinical and Experimental Neuropsychology, 12*(4), 467–484.

Goldstein, L. B. (2011). *A primer on stroke prevention and treatment: an overview of AHA/ASA.* Hoboken, NJ: Wiley-Blackwell.

Goyal, M., Demchuk, A. M., Menon, B. K., Eesa, M., Rempel, J. L., Thornton, J., et al. (2015). Randomized assessment of rapid endovascular treatment of ischemic stroke. *NEJM, 372*, 1019–1030.

Green, T. L., McGregor, L. D., & King, K. M. (2008). Smell and taste dysfunction following minor stroke: a case report. *Canadian Journal of Neuroscience Nursing, 30*(2), 10–13.

Guidetti, S., Asaba, E., & Tham, K. (2009). The meaning of context in recapturing self-care after stroke and spinal cord injury. *The American Journal of Occupational Therapy, 63*, 323–322.

Gutman, S. (2008). *Quick reference neuroscience for rehabilitation professionals: the essential neurological principles underlying rehabilitation practice* (2nd ed.). Thorofare, NJ: Slack.

Halpern, H. (2000). *Language and motor speech disorders in adults* (2nd ed.). Austin, TX: Pro-Ed.

Hanna, K., Hepworth, L., & Rowe, F. (2017). The treatment methods for post-stroke visual impairment: a systematic review. *Brain Behaviour, 7*(5), e00682.

Hepworth, L. R., Rowe, F. J., Walker, M. F., Rockliffe, J., Noonan, C., Howard, C., et al. (2016). Post-stroke visual impairment: a systematic literature review of types and recovery of visual conditions. *Ophthalmology Research International Journal, 5*(1), 1–43.

Herrmann, M., et al. (1995). Poststroke depression: is there a patho-anatomic correlate for depression in the post-acute stage of stroke? *Stroke; a Journal of Cerebral Circulation, 26*(5), 850–856.

Hosseini, Z. S., Peyrovi, H., & Gohari, M. (2019). The effect of early passive range of motion exercise on motor function of people with stroke: a randomized controlled trial. *Journal of Caring Sciences, 8*(1), 39–44.

Ivey, F. M., & Macko, R. F. (2015). Prevention of deconditioning after stroke. In: J. Stein, R. L. Harvey, & C. J. Winstein (Eds.), *Stroke: Recovery and Rehabilitation* (2nd ed.). New York, NY: Demos.

Jamison, P. W., & Orchanian, D. P. (2007). Cerebrovascular accident. In B. J. Atchison, & D. P. Dirette (Eds.), *Conditions in Occupational Therapy: Effect on Occupational Performance* (3rd ed.). Baltimore, MD: Williams & Wilkins.

Jenkinson, P. M., Preston, C., & Ellis, S. J. (2011). Unawareness after stroke: a review and practical guide to understanding, assessing, and managing anosognosia for hemiplegia. *Journal of Clinical and Experimental Neuropsychology, 33*(10), 1079–1093.

Jokinen, H., Melkas, S., Ylikoski, R., Pohjasvaara, T., Kaste, M., Erkinjuntti, T., et al. (2015). Post-stroke cognitive impairment is common even after successful clinical recovery. *European Journal of Neurology, 22*(9), 1288–1294.

Kalra, L. (1994). Does age affect benefits of stroke unit rehabilitation? *Stroke; a Journal of Cerebral Circulation, 25*(2), 347–351.

Kaplan, P. R., Caillet, R., & Kaplan, C. P. (2003). *Rehabilitation of stroke.* Philadelphia, PA: Butterworth-Heinemann.

Keenan, N. L., & Shaw, K. M. (2011). Coronary heart disease and stroke deaths. *MMWR Supplement, 60*, 62–66. Available from http://www.cdc.gov/mmwr/preview/mmwrhtml/su6001a13.htm.

Khader, M. S., & Tomlin, G. S. (1994). Change in wheelchair transfer performance during rehabilitation of men with cerebrovascular accident. *The American Journal of Occupational Therapy, 48*(10), 899–905.

Kidd, D., Lawson, J., Nesbitt, R., & MacMahon, J. (1993). Aspiration in acute stroke: a clinical study with videofluoroscopy. *QJM: Monthly Journal of the Association of Physicians, 86*(12), 825–829.

Kim, H. J., Lee, Y., & Sohng, K. Y. (2014). Effects of bilateral passive range of motion exercise on the function of upper extremities and activities of daily living in patients with acute stroke. *Journal of Physical Therapy Science, 26*(1), 149–156.

King, R. R., & Reiss, J. P. (2013). The epidemiology and pathophysiology of pseudobulbar affect and its association with neurodegeneration. *Degenerative Neurological and Neuromuscular Disease, 3,* 23–31.

Kuo, C. L., Shiao, A. S., Wang, S. J., Chang, W. P., & Lin, Y. Y. (2016). Risk of sudden sensorineural hearing loss in stroke patients: a 5-year nationwide investigation of 44,460 patients. *Medicine, 95*(36), e4841.

Kwakkel, G., Knollen, B. J., & Kregs, H. I. (2008). Effects of robot-assisted therapy on upper limb recovery after stroke: a systematic review. *Neurorehabilitation and Neural Repair, 22*(2), 111–121.

Lavine, R., & Hausler, R. (2001). Auditory disorders after stroke. In J. Bogousslavsky, and L. R. Caplan (Eds.), *Stroke Syndromes* (2nd ed.). New York, NY: Cambridge Press.

Lee, S. I., Adans-Dester, C. P., Grimaldi, M., Dowling, A. V., Horak, P. C., Black-Schaffer, R. M., et al. (2018). Enabling stroke rehabilitation in home and community settings: a wearable sensor-based approach for upper-limb motor training. *IEEE Journal of Translational Engineering in Health and Medicine, 6,* 1–11.

Lo, A. C., Guarino, P. D., Richards, L. G., Haselkorn, J. K., Wittenberg, G. F., Federman, D. G., et al. (2010). Robot-assisted therapy for long-term upper-limb impairment after stroke. *NEJM., 362,* 1772–1783.

Lökk, J., & Delbari, A. (2010). Management of depression in elderly stroke patients. *Neuropsychiatric Disease and Treatment, 6,* 539–549.

MacDonald, J. C. (1960). An investigation of body scheme in adults with cerebral vascular accidents. *The American Journal of Occupational Therapy, 14,* 75–79.

Mang, C. S., Campbell, K. L., Ross, C. J. D., & Boyd, L. A. (2013). Promoting neuroplasticity for motor rehabilitation after stroke: considering the effects of aerobic exercise and genetic variation on brain-derived neurotrophic factor. *Physical Therapy, 93*(12), 1707–1716.

Maskill, L., & Tempest, S. (2017). Complex perceptual functions: body scheme and agnosia, constructional skills and neglect. In J. Grieve, & L. Gnanasakaran (Eds.), *Neuropsychology for occupational therapists: cognition in occupational performance.* Hoboken, NJ: Wiley-Blackwell.

McMorland, A. J., Runnalls, K. D., & Byblow, W. D. (2015). A neuroanatomical framework for upper limb synergies after stroke. *Frontiers in Human Neuroscience, 9,* 82.

Meyer, S., Karttunen, A. H., Thijs, V., Feys, H., & Verheyden, G. (2014). How do somatosensory deficits in the arm and hand relate to upper limb impairment, activity, and participation problems after stroke? A systematic review. *Physical Therapy, 94*(9), 1220–1231.

Milazzo, S., & Gillen, G. (2010). Splinting applications. In G. Gillen (Ed.), *Stroke rehabilitation: a function-based approach* (3rd ed.). St Louis, MO: Mosby.

Mohr, J. P., Wolf, P., Choi, D., & Weir, B. (2004). *Stroke: pathophysiology, diagnosis, and management* (4th ed.). Philadelphia, PA: Churchill Livingstone.

Murie-Fernández, M., Carmona Iragui, M., Gnanakumar, V., Meyer, M., Foley, N., & Teasell, R. (2012). Painful hemiplegic shoulder in stroke patients: causes and management. *Neurología (English Edition), 27*(4), 234–244.

Nijboer, T. C. W., Olthoff, L., Van der Stigchel, S., & Visser-Meily, J. M. A. (2014). Prism adaptation improves postural imbalance in neglect patients. *Neuroreport, 25*(5), 307–311.

Nilsen, D. M., Gillen, G., & Gordon, A. M. (2010). Use of mental practice to improve upper-limb recovery after stroke: a systematic review. *The American Journal of Occupational Therapy, 64,* 695–708.

O'Sullivan, A. (2007). AOTA's statement on family caregivers. *The American Journal of Occupational Therapy, 61*(6), 710.

Page, S. J., & Levine, P. (2005). Effects of mental practice on affected limb use and function in chronic stroke. *Archives of Physical Medicine and Rehabilitation, 86*(4), 399–402.

Page, S. J., Sisto, S., Johnston, M. V., & Levine, P. (2002). Modified constraint-induced therapy after subacute stroke: a preliminary study. *Neurorehabilitation and Neural Repair, 16*(3), 223–228.

Pellegrino, L., Giannoni, P., Marinelli, L., & Casadio, M. (2017). Effects of continuous visual feedback during sitting balance training in chronic stroke survivors. *Journal of Neuroengineering and Rehabilitation, 14*(1), 107.

Piambianco, G., Orchard, T., & Landau, P. (1995). Deep vein thrombosis: prevention in stroke clients during rehabilitation. *Archives of Physical Medicine and Rehabilitation, 76*(4), 324–330.

Pohjasvaara, T., Vataja, R., Leppävuori, A., Kaste, M., & Erkinjuntti, T. (2001). Depression is an independent predictor of poor long-term functional outcome post stroke. *European Journal of Neurology, 8*(4), 315–319.

Rajashekaran, P., Pai, K., Thunga, R., & Unnikrishnan, B. (2013). Post-stroke depression and lesion location: a hospital based cross-sectional study. *Indian Journal of Psychiatry, 55*(4), 343–348.

Richter, R. W. (2005). The pathophysiology of emotional lability: many paths to a common destination. *The American Journal of Geriatric Pharmacotherapy, 3*(Suppl. 1), 9–11.

Roth, E. R., & Harvey, R. L. (2015). Rehabilitation of stroke syndromes. In R. L. Braddom (Ed.), *Physical medicine and rehabilitation* (3rd ed.). Philadelphia, PA: WB Saunders.

Rowe, F. R. (2016). Visual effects and rehabilitation after stroke. *Community Eye Health/International Centre for Eye Health, 29*(96), 75–76.

Rowe, F. R., Walker, M., Rockliffe, J., Pollock, A., Noonan, C., Howard, C., et al. (2010). Care provision and unmet need for post stroke visual impairment. *Stroke Association Thomas Pocklington Trust,* 1–48.

Rubio, K. B., & Van Deuson, J. (1995). Relation of perceptual and body image dysfunction to activities of daily living of persons after stroke. *The American Journal of Occupational Therapy, 49*(6), 551–559.

Schlesinger, B. (1962). *Higher cerebral functions and their clinical disorders.* New York, NY: Grune & Stratton.

Skalsky, A. J., & McDonald, C. M. (2012). Prevention and management of limb contractures in neuromuscular diseases. *Physical Medicine and Rehabilitation Clinics of North America, 23*(3), 675–687.

Söderback, I., Bengtsson, I., Ginsburg, E., & Ekholm, J. (1992). Video feedback in occupational therapy: its effects in clients with neglect syndrome. *Archives of Physical Medicine and Rehabilitation, 73*(12), 1140–1146.

Stein, J., Harvey, R., Winstein, C., Wittenberg, G., & Zorowitz, R. (2015). *Stroke recovery and rehabilitation* (2nd ed.). New York, NY: Demos Medical.

Stein, J., Krebs, H. I., & Hogan, N. (2009). *Stroke recovery and rehabilitation.* New York, NY: Demos Medical.

Sterzi, R., Bottini, G., Celani, M. G., Righetti, E., Lamassa, M., Ricci, S., et al. (1993). Hemianopsia, hemianesthesia, and hemiplegia after right and left hemisphere damage: a hemispheric difference. *The Journal of Neurology, Neurosurgery, and Psychiatry, 56*(3), 308—310.

Stone, S. P., Halligan, P. W., & Green, R. J. (1993). The incidence of neglect phenomena and related disorders in clients with acute right or left hemisphere stroke. *Age Aging, 22*(1), 46—52.

Taub, E., Uswatte, G., & Pidikiti, R. (1999). Constraint-induced movement therapy: a new family of techniques with broad application to physical rehabilitation—a clinical review. *Journal of Rehabilitation Research and Development, 36*(3), 237—251.

Tompkins, C. A. (2012). Rehabilitation for cognitive-communication disorders in right hemisphere brain damage. *Archives of Physical Medicine and Rehabilitation, 93*(Suppl. 1), S61—S69.

Trombly, C. A., & Radomski, M. V. (2008). *Occupational therapy for physical dysfunction* (6th ed.). Baltimore, MD: Lippincott Williams & Wilkins.

Turton, A., & Fraser, C. (1990). The use of home therapy programmes for improving recovery of the upper limb following stroke. *The British Journal of Occupational Therapy, 53*, 457—462.

van Mierlo, M., van Heugten, C., Post, M. W. M., Hoekstra, T., & Visser-Meily, A. (2018). Trajectories of health-related quality of life after stroke: results from a one-year prospective cohort study. *Disability and Rehabilitation, 40*(9), 997—1006.

van Vliet, P. M., & Wulf, G. (2006). Extrinsic feedback for motor learning after stroke: what is the evidence? *Disability and Rehabilitation, 28*(13-14), 831—840.

Volpe, B. T., Krebs, H. I., & Hogan, N. (2003). Robot-aided sensorimotor training in stroke rehabilitation. *Advances in Neurology, 92*, 429—433.

Walker, M. F., & Lincoln, N. B. (1991). Factors influencing dressing performance after stroke. *The Journal of Neurology, Neurosurgery, and Psychiatry, 54*(8), 699—701.

Wallenbert, I., & Jonsson, H. (2005). Waiting to get better: a dilemma regarding habits in daily occupation after stroke. *The American Journal of Occupational Therapy, 59*, 218—229.

Whitworth, A., Webster, J., & Howard, D. (2005). *A cognitive neuropsychological approach to assessment and intervention in aphasias: a clinician's guide.* New York, NY: Psychology Press.

Wilmskoetter, J., Bonilha, L., Martin-Harris, B., Elm, J. J., Horn, J., & Bonilha, H. S. (2019). Mapping acute lesion locations to physiological swallow impairments after stroke. *NeuroImage Clinical, 22*, 101685.

Wyman, J. F., Burgio, K. L., & Newman, D. K. (2009). Practical aspects of lifestyle modifications and behavioural interventions in the treatment of overactive bladder and urgency urinary incontinence. *International Journal of Clinical Practice, 63*(8), 1177—1191.

Zhang, Y., Zhao, H., Fang, Y., Wang, S., & Zhou, H. (2017). The association between lesion location, sex and poststroke depression: meta-analysis. *Brain Behavior, 7*, e00788.

Zoltan, B. (2007). *Vision, perception, and cognition: a manual for the evaluation and treatment of the adult with acquired brain injury* (4th ed.). Thorofare, NJ: Slack, Inc.

RECOMMENDED READING

Bolte, J. (2006). *My CVA of insight: a brain scientist's personal journey.* New York, NY: Penguin Group.

Carr, J. H., & Shepherd, R. B. (2003). *CVA rehabilitation: guidelines for exercise and training to optimize motor skill* (2nd ed.) Oxford: Butterworth-Heinemann.

Duncun, P. W., Zorowitz, B., Bates, B., Choi, J. Y., Glasberg, J. J., Graham, G. D., et al. (2005). Management of adult CVA rehabilitation care: a clinical practice guideline. *Stroke; a Journal of Cerebral Circulation, 36*(9), e100—e143.

Gillen, G. (2010). *CVA rehabilitation: a function-based approach* (3rd ed) St Louis, MO: Mosby.

Gutman, S. (2008). *Quick reference neuroscience for rehabilitation professionals: the essential neurological principles underlying rehabilitation practice* (2nd ed.). Thorofare, NJ: Slack.

Kime, S. K. (2005). *Compensating for memory deficits: using a systematic approach.* Bethesda, MD: American Occupational Therapy Association.

Sabari, J. (2015). *Occupational therapy practice guidelines for adults with CVA.* Bethesda, MD: American Occupational Therapy Association.

Siebert, C. (2014). *Occupational therapy practice guidelines for home modifications.* Bethesda, MD: American Occupational Therapy Association.

Stein, J., Harvey, R., Macko, R., et al. (2015). *CVA recovery and rehabilitation.* New York, NY: Demos Medical.

ONLINE RESOURCES FOR STROKE SURVIVORS AND CAREGIVERS

American Heart Association: www.americanheart.org.

Caring.com: www.caring.com.

Family Caregiver Alliance: www.caregiver.org.

Medix Health Information, Medical Questions and Patient Community: www.imedix.com.

National Alliance for Caregiving: www.caregiving.org.

National Association of Area Agencies on Aging: www.n4a.org.

National CVA Association: www.CVA.org.

National Family Caregivers Association: https://caringcommunity.org/resources/models-research/national-family-caregivers-association-nfca/#:~:text=The%20National%20Family%20Caregivers%20Association,aged%2C%20or%20disabled%20loved%20one.

The Stroke Network: http://www.stroke-network.com/.

24

Traumatic Brain Injury

Lori M. Shiffman and Rachael Schaier

OBJECTIVES

After reading this chapter, the student or the occupational therapy practitioner will be able to do the following:

1. Define traumatic brain injury (TBI) and identify its common causes.
2. Identify characteristics of and differences between different levels of consciousness (coma, vegetative state, minimally conscious state).
3. Explain the purpose of sensory regulation and how it is addressed in the treatment of the client with mild, moderate, and severe TBI.
4. Identify one to two occupational therapy treatment activities for clients with TBI at each level of the revised Rancho Los Amigos Levels of Cognitive Functioning.
5. Identify how engagement in occupation, participation, and health are affected by TBI.
6. Explain the role of occupational therapy practitioners in working on the interdisciplinary neurorehabilitation team in assisting clients with TBI manage behavioral issues.
7. Identify and describe appropriate remedial, functional, and compensatory treatments for specific client factors caused by TBI.
8. Describe the role of the family and significant others in the recovery process of the client with TBI.

KEY TERMS

Traumatic brain injury (TBI)
Postconcussion syndrome (PCS)
Minimally conscious
Open brain injury
Closed brain injury
Diffuse axonal injury (DAI)
Primary injury
Secondary injury

Posttraumatic amnesia (PTA)
Decorticate posturing
Decerebrate posturing
Posttraumatic vision syndrome (PTVS)
Impaired initiation
Disinhibition
Emotional lability
Sensory regulation

INTRODUCTION

Traumatic brain injury (TBI) is an alteration in brain function or other evidence of brain pathology caused by an external force (Brain Injury Association of America, 2011). TBI is a life-altering experience that causes physical, cognitive, behavioral, and emotional changes affecting the ability to engage in occupations and perform everyday life activities, roles, habits, and routines (American Occupational Therapy Association, 2008). No two clients with TBI show exactly the same symptoms. Some brain injuries are fatal, whereas others result in mild to severe damage. One TBI client may emerge from coma, respond inconsistently, and show no purposeful behavior, eventually requiring lifelong assistance. Another client may be able to complete all activities of daily living (ADL) but have difficulty with instrumental activities of daily living (IADL), rest and sleep, education, work, play/leisure, or social participation (American Occupational Therapy Association, 2008) and require external structure, cues, or assistance from others to function. Another client may regain functional independence in all life roles with some if any modifications. All clients with TBI will learn how to make the necessary adjustments to attain maximum functioning through neurorehabilitation treatment. The occupational therapist (OT) and occupational therapy assistant (OTA) are an integral part of that process.

This chapter begins with an overview of the incidence, pathophysiology, and medical management related to changes in body structures (World Health Organization, 2001) as the result of TBI. The occupational therapy evaluation, performed by the OT, is discussed briefly. The main focus of this chapter is on interventions in which the OTA might be expected to participate. Changes in client factors and performance skills and their effect on performance patterns are presented in more detail to help the reader understand the differences between clients functioning at a lower level from those functioning at intermediate to advanced levels (Table 24.1).

TABLE 24.1 Rancho Los Amigos Levels of Cognitive Functioning

Level of Cognitive Function	Characteristics
I. No Response: Total Assistance	Appears to be in a deep sleep
	Completely unresponsive to any stimuli presented
	Reacts inconsistently and nonpurposefully to stimuli in a nonspecific manner
II. Generalized Response: Total Assistance	Responses are limited in nature and are often the same regardless of stimulus presented
	Responses may be physiologic changes, gross body movements, and/or vocalization
	Earliest response may be to deep pain
	Responses are likely to be delayed
	Reacts specifically but inconsistently to stimuli
III. Localized Response: Total Assistance	Responses are directly related to the type of stimulus presented in the environment such as head turning toward a sound
	Withdrawal of extremity and/or vocalization when presented with a painful stimulus
	May follow simple commands in a delayed and inconsistent manner such as closing eyes or squeezing or extending an extremity
	Responds to auditory and visual stimuli (in the visual fields at near distances)
	After external stimulus is removed, client may lie quietly and may also show a vague awareness of self and body by responding to discomfort by pulling at nasogastric tube or catheter
	May show bias by responding to some persons (especially family, friends) but not to others
	Heightened state of activity with severely decreased ability to process information
IV. Confused-Agitated: Maximal Assistance	Detached from the present and responds primarily to own internal confusion
	Behavior is often bizarre and nonpurposeful relative to immediate environment
	May cry out or scream out of proportion to stimuli even after removal, show aggressive behavior, attempt to remove restraints or tubes, or crawl out of bed in a purposeful manner
	Lack of discrimination between persons or objects
	Unable to cooperate directly with treatment effort
	Verbalization is often incoherent and/or inappropriate to the environment
	Confabulation may be present; patient may be euphoric or hostile
	Attention is very short; selective attention is often minimal at best
	Lack of awareness of present events
	Lacks short-term recall but may react to past events
	Needs maximum assistance to perform basic self-care (feeding, dressing)
	If not disabled physically, the client may be able to perform motor activities as in sitting, reaching, and ambulating as part of agitated state, but not purposefully on request
	May show mood shifts from euphoric to agitated without any relationship to environmental events
	Appears alert
V. Confused-Inappropriate, Nonagitated: Maximal Assistance	Able to respond to simple commands fairly consistently
	Responses are nonpurposeful and random in more complex situations and with less structure
	May be agitated, but not on an internal basis (as in Level IV) but rather as a result of external stimuli—and usually out of proportion to the stimulus
	Gross attention to the environment but is highly distractible
	Lacks ability to focus attention on a specific task without frequent redirection back to it
	With structure, the client may be able to converse on a social, automatic level for short periods of time
	Verbalization is often inappropriate; confabulation may be triggered by present events
	Memory is severely impaired, with confusion of past and present in reaction to ongoing activity
	Lacks initiation of functional tasks and often shows inappropriate use of objects without external direction
	May be able to perform previously learned tasks when structured but cannot learn new information
	Responds best to self, body, comfort—and often family members
	Usually can perform self-care activities with assistance and may accomplish feeding with maximum supervision
	May wander off either randomly or with vague intention of "going home"
	Goal-directed behavior but depends on external input for direction
VI. Confused-Appropriate: Moderate Assistance	Response to discomfort is appropriate and the client tolerates unpleasant stimuli (e.g., nasogastric tube) when need is explained
	Follows simple directions consistently and shows carryover for relearned tasks (such as self-care)
	Needs less supervision with familiar tasks (old learning)
	Shows little or no carryover for new learning
	Responses may be incorrect because of memory problems, but they are appropriate to the situation
	Responses may be delayed
	Decreased ability to process information with little or no anticipation or prediction of events
	More depth and detail in past memories than recent memory
	Beginning awareness of situation by realizing an answer is unknown

(Continued)

TABLE 24.1	**Rancho Los Amigos Levels of Cognitive Functioning—cont'd**
Level of Cognitive Function	**Characteristics**
	No longer wanders and is inconsistently oriented to time and place
	Selective attention to tasks may be impaired, especially with difficult tasks and in unstructured settings, but is now functional for common daily activities (30 minutes with structure)
	Shows at least vague recognition of some staff and has increased awareness of self, family, and basic needs (such as food), again in an appropriate manner as in contrast to Level V
	Appears appropriate and oriented within hospital and home settings
VII. Automatic-Appropriate: Minimal Assistance for Daily Living Skills	Completes daily routine automatically but often does so in an almost robotic way
	Minimal to absent confusion but has shallow recall of what has been done
	Shows increased awareness of self, body, family, foods, people, and interaction in the environment
	Superficial awareness of but lacks insight into own condition, demonstrates decreased judgment and problem solving, lacks realistic planning for the future
	Shows carryover for new learning but at a decreased rate
	Requires at least minimal supervision for learning and for safety purposes
	Independent in self-care activities and supervised in home and community skills for safety
	With structure, can initiate tasks in social and recreational activities of interest
	Unaware of needs and feelings of others
	Oppositional/uncooperative
	Judgment remains impaired, such that client cannot drive a car
	Unable to recognize inappropriate behavior in social interactions
	Completes familiar tasks in a distracting environment for 1 hour
VIII. Purposeful and Appropriate: Standby Assistance	Aware of and responsive to culture
	Shows carryover for new learning if acceptable to life role and needs no supervision after activities are learned
	Within physical capabilities, client is independent in home and community activities, including driving
	Vocational rehabilitation to determine ability to return as a contributor to society (perhaps in a new capacity) is indicated
	Shows continued impairments in comparison to previous level of function in abilities, reasoning, tolerance for stress, judgment in emergencies, or unusual circumstances
	Irritable
	Argumentative
	Self-centered
	Depressed
	Social, emotional, and intellectual capacities may continue to be decreased but are functional for society
	Recognizes and corrects inappropriate behavior in social interactions but needs standby assistance to make corrections
	Alert and oriented
	Recalls and integrates past and recent events
	Can shift back and forth between tasks, complete them accurately for about 2 hours
IX. Purposeful and Appropriate: Standby Assistance on Request	Uses assistive memory devices such as planners, to-do lists
	Performs familiar personal, household, work, and leisure activities, independently
	Performs new personal, household, work, and leisure activities, with assistance as needed
	Aware of problems that interfere with performance after they occur and can take corrective action but may need standby assistance to anticipate problems
	Thinks of consequences of actions with standby assistance
	May become easily irritated and have a low frustration tolerance
	Depression may continue
	Monitors self for appropriateness of social interaction with standby assistance
	Multitasks in all environments and may require periodic rest breaks
X. Purposeful and Appropriate: Modified Independence	Initiates use of assistive memory devices independently
	Performs new personal, household, work, and leisure activities but may need more time and use of compensatory strategies
	Anticipates problems but may need more time and use of compensatory strategies
	Estimates abilities accurately and can make changes as indicated
	Recognizes the needs of others and socially interacts appropriately all of the time
	Periodic episodes of depression
	Irritability and lowered frustration tolerance stressed, fatigued, or ill

Modified from Rancho Los Amigos Medical Center. *Original Scale: Levels of Cognitive Functioning*. Downey, CA: Rancho Los Amigos Medical Center, Adult Brain Injury Service; 1995.

CHANGES IN BODY STRUCTURES AND FUNCTIONS

Incidence of Traumatic Brain Injury

About 10 million people are affected by TBI worldwide, and it is predicted to be the major cause of death and disability by 2020 (Bruns & Hauser, 2003). In the United States, more than 2.8 million persons sustain a new TBI every year (Taylor, Bell, Breiding, & Xu, 2017). About 3% are fatal, 10% of persons with TBI require hospitalization, and 90% are treated and released from the emergency room (Taylor et al., 2017). Overall, young children, adolescents, and the elderly have the highest incidence of TBI (Centers for Disease Control & Prevention, 2019), as well as persons who have had previous brain injuries. Adults older than age 75 have the highest rate of hospitalization and fatalities due to TBI (Taylor et al., 2017). The leading causes of death from TBI are motor vehicle crashes for persons age 5 to 24, intentional self-harm for adults age 25 to 64, and falls for adults age 65 and older (Taylor et al., 2017). Half of TBIs are caused by motor vehicle accidents, 20% to 30% are caused by falls, and about 12% are caused by firearms (Popescu, Anghelescu, Daia, & Onose, 2015). Between 300,000 and 3,800,000 adults (≥18 years) sustain sports-related TBIs every year, 86% of which are mild (Bruns & Hauser, 2003). About one third to one half of persons hospitalized for TBI are found to be legally intoxicated, and it is estimated that nearly two thirds have a history of drug and alcohol abuse (Corrigan, 1995; Weil, Corrigan, & Karelina, 2018). The risk for sustaining a TBI is four times greater for persons who drink alcohol than those who do not imbibe (Bombardier, Rimmele, & Zintel, 2002).

Since the onset of the wars in Iraq and Afghanistan in 2001 and other global venues, there has been an increase in TBI in the US military. About 4.2% of members of all branches of the armed forces have sustained a TBI (VA Health Care, 2008). Over 76% of injuries are considered mild (Frieden & Collins, 2013). Among military personnel serving in combat who experience battle-related injuries, about 30% sustain some form of TBI, most commonly from blast injuries (VA Health Care, 2008). Enhanced protection such as the use of body armor and helmets has improved the survival rate from blast exposure (Wheeler & Acord-Vita, 2016). Service members who experience a loss of consciousness are more likely to experience postconcussive symptoms (Wilk et al., 2010), which could lead to **postconcussive syndrome** (**PCS**), a more persistent set of physical, cognitive and emotional symptoms (Wheeler & Acord-Vita, 2016). In 1992, Congress authorized the development of the Defense and Veterans Brain Injury Center (DVBIC), the first of its kind collaboration between the Department of Defense (DOD), Department of Veterans Affairs (VA), and the Brain Injury Association of America (BIAA) (Martin, Schwab, & Malik, 2018). The purpose of this center is to address the specific needs of injured veterans through "multisite medical care, clinical research, and education centers" (Defense & Veterans Brain Injury Center, 2014; Martin et al., 2018; Wilk et al., 2010).

DVBIC has made enormous contributions to the way members of the medical and rehabilitation teams evaluate and treat brain injury affecting military service members, veterans, and civilians working in the military. OTs and OTAs are an integral part of the brain injury rehabilitation team (Defense & Veterans Brain Injury Center, 2014), providing medically necessary skilled therapy services.

Overall, males sustain TBI about twice as often as females. Interpersonal or self-directed violence with firearms is the leading cause of brain injury—related deaths for males (Centers for Disease Control & Prevention, 2019). However, many more females sustain brain injuries caused by their intimate domestic partners, but there is little research regarding the incidence because such assaults are underreported. Also, TBI may not be as recognized in domestic abuse survivors by medical professionals, law enforcement, family, or even survivors themselves. One study showed 60% of survivors of domestic violence screened positive for TBI (Hetwig, 2003). The OT practitioner should be aware of the risk factors for TBI for all clients.

The mortality rate for TBI has decreased by 20% since 1980, reflecting improvement in prevention (Centers for Disease Control & Prevention, 2019). During the same time period, transportation TBI-related deaths have decreased by 40% due to increased use of seatbelts, airbags, child safety seats, a reduction of impaired driving (Centers for Disease Control & Prevention, 2019), improved automobile safety design, and use of motorcycle helmets.

More than 5.3 million Americans are living with disability related to their brain injury (National Center for Injury Prevention & Control, 2003). The prognosis for younger persons is better than for older persons with similar injuries (Marquez de la Plata et al., 2008); 75% to 80% of brain injuries are mild, 10% are moderate, and 10% are severe (National Center for Injury Prevention & Control, 2003). About 15% to 30% of individuals with a mild TBI are at higher risk for "developing post-concussion syndrome" (Padula & Shapiro, 2000).

Clients with mild TBI may have additional injuries such as lacerations, fractures, or other complications as a result of the trauma. Because mild TBI can be underreported, the OTA who is familiar with these signs and symptoms when seeing clients of any diagnosis should report any such observations to the OT. Improved education of health care professionals concerning the signs and symptoms has also led to increased recognition, diagnosis, and treatment of mild TBI (National Center for Injury Prevention & Control, 2003). The OT and OTA should always be aware of coexisting conditions that will affect treatment of clients with TBI.

Pathophysiology

All TBIs are caused by an external force. The nature and degree of damage determine the type of injury the medical intervention is required to treat the damage. Two mechanisms of injury disrupt body structures (World Health Organization, 2001), traumatic impact and traumatic inertia, causing both primary and secondary damage to the brain.

CASE STUDY

Bruno: A Client Functioning at Low Level

Bruno is a 19-year-old who sustained a severe TBI when he fell off a ladder while painting a house as part of his summer job. Bruno had a positive loss of consciousness and began to experience seizures at the scene of the accident. He had no previous medical problems and did not take any prescription medications. Bruno was immediately transported to the Level I trauma medical center and admitted to the intensive care unit (ICU). A computed tomography (CT) scan of the head showed subdural hematoma (SDH) of the left temporal lobe and fracture of the occipital bone. X-rays also showed a fractured left scapula. His Glasgow Coma Scale (GCS) score was 6. Within 48 hours, Bruno underwent a decompressive craniotomy to remove the left portion of his skull to alleviate the pressure on the brain and prevent further damage. The client was in a coma; he required placement of a Foley catheter due to urinary incontinence and a gastrointestinal tube because he was not able to eat by mouth.

Initial Occupational Therapy Evaluation

The OT reviewed the medical record, evaluated Bruno, interviewed his mother, and reported the following findings:

Bruno lives in a two-story home with his parents and 16-year-old sister. At the time of the injury, he was on summer break from his freshman year at a local community college, where he was majoring in criminal justice. He is left-hand dominant, and has no history of learning disabilities or academic difficulties. Before his injury, Bruno was completely independent in all activities of daily living and instrumental activities of daily living, including his student role. He enjoyed socializing with friends, playing on his club basketball team, and going out with his girlfriend he had been dating since high school.

Acute Care Inpatient Status

Two weeks later, Bruno awoke from his coma and progressed to a **minimally conscious** state. He responded to pain, actively moved his right arm and leg, but did not follow commands or verbalize at all. He would open his eyes during his wake cycle and would occasionally fixate on photos of family or track his mother's movements when she sat bedside. His sleep patterns were abnormal (i.e., sleeping most of the day and night). Bruno could not move his left extremities. His left arm rested with his elbow flexed and fingers flexed into his palm. He grimaced with pain during passive range of motion (ROM) of his left arm. Medications were prescribed to prevent seizures, reduce spasticity, regulate the wake/sleep cycle, reduce gastric discomfort, decrease agitation and pain, and increase alertness. All medications and nutrition were administered through his gastrointestinal tube.

Inpatient Rehabilitation

Once medically stable, Bruno was transferred to the rehabilitation unit. The OT and physical therapist (PT) worked together to get Bruno out of bed and sitting up in a tilt-in-space wheelchair with a pressure relief cushion to prevent pressure sores. Due to his poor head and neck control, the chair was fitted with a contoured headrest and a chest strap applied due to poor trunk control and impulsivity (Fig. 24.1). Bruno wore a helmet at all times to protect his brain while out of bed. He required maximal assistance of two to transfer from the bed to the chair. Initially, occupational therapy treatment focused

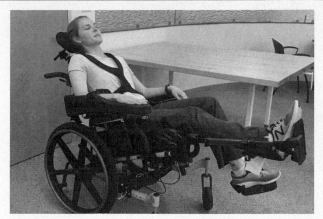

Fig. 24.1 Chair fitted with a contoured head rest and a chest strap applied.

on Bruno's orientation, following simple commands and using familiar objects such as a hairbrush and washcloth. Within 2 weeks he had emerged from a minimally conscious state and was verbally communicating, following most commands, performing some basic self-care tasks, and using objects for their intended purpose such as washing his face with a washcloth.

Bruno required moderate assistance with all ADL and functional mobility. He struggled to use his nondominant right hand for daily activities. Moderate muscle tone limited left elbow, wrist, and finger extension. The OT initiated the dynamic splinting protocol to prevent left elbow contractures and provided a resting hand splint worn when sleeping to keep Bruno's hand in a functional position (wrist neutral and fingers extended). He wore a left ankle foot orthosis (AFO) and used a large based quad cane to walk. During ADL training, Bruno often overreached when performing functional tasks and required maximal cues when walking to avoid bumping into the wall, objects, or people, showing significant visual spatial deficits.

Bruno continued to make progress in walking, no longer needing to use the quad cane. However, he required 24-hour supervision to walk due to persistent impulsivity, poor recall, and impaired visual spatial deficits. He tended to forget to put on his AFO and helmet, often got lost, and sometimes bumped into objects and people. Therefore he was a significant fall risk. Signs posted in his room reminding him to "call for a nurse" and "put on your helmet" eventually proved effective. Bruno dressed himself but needed assistance for his AFO and buttons. He was continent of bowel and bladder, could manage toileting independently, but he needed supervision for safe functional mobility. He required moderate verbal and visual cues to shower due to sequencing and functional memory deficits. Bruno was discharged home under his parents' supervision and referred to outpatient occupational therapy services.

Outpatient Occupational Therapy

Following discharge home, Bruno continued to wear the dynamic elbow splint and resting hand splint at night. He progressed to nearly full functional elbow extension. He could actively move his left arm but was limited by weakness, decreased coordination, and mild to moderate muscle tone.

Bruno initiated the occupational therapy home exercise plan to address these deficits. Because of continued visual spatial and functional memory impairments, he required supervision when he walked in his neighborhood because he tended to get lost. His parents, sister, or other family members monitored him at all times because of continued poor judgment and impulsivity, especially when going outside and using social media. His mother quit her job so she could be at home with him and drive him to all community activities such as his medical appointments. Bruno's girlfriend broke off their relationship while he was in the hospital. He took a year off from college. His friends have taken him out to dinner and movies several times since he has been home but have noticed he has a hard time following group conversations, gets tired, sometimes doesn't "get jokes," and is socially unaware.

In outpatient occupational therapy, Bruno learned to use apps on his phone to help him sequence and remember the steps to perform daily activities such as doing laundry and making breakfast. His therapists and parents cue him to use these compensatory strategies, but his follow-through is inconsistent. At this point in his recovery Bruno demonstrates reduced insight and is not able to recognize his inability to return to his previous life. His goals are to use his left arm for everything and to drive.

Traumatic impact injuries are further categorized by whether the injury is open (penetrating) or closed (nonpenetrating). An **open brain injury** occurs when the skull sustains fracture(s) and breach of the meninges, commonly caused by gunshots, stabbings, falls, vehicular accidents, and sports injuries. A **closed brain injury** occurs when both the skull and brain remain intact. Both open and closed injuries can cause specific or widespread damage within the brain. **Diffuse axonal injury (DAI)** occurs when acceleration, deceleration, and rotational forces are applied to the head and cause brain tissue to shear (stretch). Common causes are blasts, assaults, falls, vehicular accidents, and sports injuries. Since the soft brain sits within a hard skull, during rapid acceleration and deceleration (e.g., in a car crash) the brain is damaged on opposite sides, known as contrecoup injuries. The white matter of the cerebral hemispheres, the corpus callosum, and the brainstem are the most commonly affected areas (Adams et al., 1989). Damage may be severe enough to induce a coma or mild enough to cause a concussion. Brief loss of consciousness may or may not result.

Primary injury results from initial trauma(s) to the brain. Medical intervention plays a key role after the primary injury occurs to prevent secondary injury. **Secondary injury** results from a series of chemical reactions in the brain that can occur immediately after the injury, hours or days later, and can significantly worsen the damage caused by primary injury (Park, Bell, & Baker, 2008). These secondary effects include intracranial hematomas, cerebral edema, increased intracranial pressure, hydrocephalus, intracranial infection, and post-traumatic seizures. They account for the greatest number of deaths associated with TBI in hospitals (Ghajar, 2000). Early diagnosis and medical management of secondary effects during the acute phase of the injury help minimize impairments of bodily structures, reducing the risk of additional brain damage, such as what occurred with Bruno.

Medical Management

The objectives are medical and surgical management of the client with a TBI is to minimize the effects of the immediate injury, reestablish normal bodily functions, and prevent secondary complications (Losiniecki & Shutter, 2010). Establishing medical stability is the first priority. Due to improved rates of survival from severe injuries and shorter stays in acute settings, OTs and OTAs may treat clients in rehabilitation settings with a host of medical issues. A craniotomy, performed by a neurosurgeon, may be necessary to decrease rising intracranial pressure and bleeding during the acute phase of recovery, such as with Bruno. The most common secondary neurologic deficits related to brain injury include seizures, chronic pain, and headaches. All members of the interdisciplinary team, the client, and family/caregivers must be aware of seizure risks and precautions, how to recognize one, and what to do if it occurs. Other medical intervention involves the use of medications for pain, seizures, etc. (Losiniecki & Shutter, 2010). OTs and OTAs should also be familiar with common medical devices, their purpose, use, precautions, and contraindications. Examples of common co-occurring medical conditions after TBI are discussed next.

Cardiopulmonary problems can result from direct trauma to the chest, complications from initial interventions, or damage to the areas of the brain that control heart and lungs. Clients may require ventilators, tracheostomies, or oxygen supplementation. The OTA with demonstrated service competency might be expected to take vitals of clients to monitor medical stability. Musculoskeletal damage may be related to the trauma or accident (i.e., fractures, nerve injuries) or directly related to the brain injury (i.e., spasticity or decreased range). Careful monitoring helps reduce complications such as contractures or heterotopic ossification. OT treatment may include positioning, splinting, orthotics, exercises, and/or modalities.

Bowel and bladder dysfunction caused by damage to the brain or spinal cord have a direct impact on daily functioning and quality of life. Incontinence and urinary tract infections are common. The OTA should be aware of voiding schedule and medical devices for these dysfunctions, such as Foley catheters and suprapubic catheters. It is especially important to be aware of these when the client is transferring, such as during bed mobility and bed to wheelchair transfers.

Initially many clients are unable to take food or fluids orally because they are unconscious or have impaired swallowing (dysphagia). Fluids and medications are provided intravenously. For clients who cannot take anything by mouth (NPO), a nasogastric tube (passed through the nose) or a gastrostomy tube (inserted through the abdominal wall into the stomach) will be inserted to provide hydration and nutrition.

The speech-language pathologist (SLP) is often the team member who evaluates swallowing issues and dysphagia. OTs and OTAs with advanced training may also be involved in this treatment area. See Chapter 11 for specific occupational therapy interventions for mealtime occupations. The OTA should be aware of all eating and drinking precautions and contraindications, know the signs of choking and aspiration (inhaling food or fluids into the lungs, which can lead to pneumonia), and be familiar with the medical devices used by all clients.

The metabolic and endocrine systems control bodily functions and are sensitive to brain trauma, which can result in an imbalance in the body's hormone production, most commonly affecting the pituitary and hypothalamus (West and Sharp, 2014). The pituitary gland regulates the other endocrine glands, also working in conjunction with the hypothalamus. Disruptions of endocrine function can affect attention, concentration, sexual function, and sleep.

Following TBI, clients often have incisions, wounds, abrasions, lacerations, or stitches related to the direct trauma. They may also have secondary complications such as skin breakdown and infections (e.g., methicillin-resistant *Staphylococcus aureus* [MRSA]). Proper positioning in bed and wheelchair is essential to promote healing, protect skin integrity, prevent complications, and maximize comfort and function.

Alterations in sleep and rest patterns occur in 30% to 70% of people with brain injuries (Viola-Saltzman & Watson, 2012). This factor can significantly decrease quality of life, as it did for Rosie in the upcoming case study. Specific sleep disorders include posttraumatic hypersomnia (excessive sleepiness), central and obstructive sleep apnea, restless leg syndrome, and insomnia (Viola-Saltzman & Watson, 2012). The OTA should be aware of sleep hygiene recommendations, including sleep schedule, positioning strategies, and devices for optimal sleep.

All team members would be expected to know what circumstances would require calling for emergency assistance. The OTA would also be expected to know when to call for nonemergency assistance such as nursing when the client's IV pump alarm sounds.

Care for the client after TBI occurs over a time frame that may span from days to years. In some cases, care is needed for the entirety of the remaining lifespan. After the initial medical evaluation and treatment in the emergency room, the client is transferred to the ICU for constant medical care. Once medically stable, the client is transferred to a comprehensive inpatient rehabilitation facility (IRF), long-term acute care hospital (LTACH), subacute rehabilitation or skilled nursing facility (SNF), or a transitional rehabilitation program (Ashley, Masel, & Nagel, 2016). The ultimate goal of recovery is return to home and community in outpatient and day treatment programs, home-based services, and school/vocational services (Ashley et al., 2016). Alternatives include SNFs and long-term residential programs. OTs and OTAs can work in any of these settings. Every client's progression through the care continuum is different, depending on factors such as severity of symptoms, comorbidities, medical complications, behavioral concerns, client/family presence, and financial constraints.

Occupational Therapy in the ICU

Medical stability is the main goal of treatment in the ICU. However, early mobilization and participation in functional activities contribute to better client outcomes (Bartolo et al., 2017). Occupational therapy intervention begins when the client is medically stable. The OT completes the evaluation, modified to accommodate the client's complex medical needs. The initial assessment finds key information such as preinjury occupations (ADL, IADL, education, work, etc.), adaptive equipment needs, and discharge disposition. Interviews with a client's family and/or caregivers help develop a comprehensive history of the client's performance patterns (habits, routines, rituals, and roles) to develop the occupational profile, essential for creating client-centered intervention in the treatment plan. Bruno's mother stayed bedside during his entire acute care stay; she posted photos of him and his girlfriend on prom night and his college basketball teams to show what her son's life was like prior to the accident.

Occupational therapy treatment in acute care may be limited due to short length of stay and the complexity of a client's medical needs, but it is critical for functional recovery (American Occupational Therapy Association, 2017). Interventions address basic ADL, performance skills (coordination and ambulation), and body functions (neuromuscular and movement-related functions, sensory and mental functions) (American Occupational Therapy Association, 2008). Treatment interventions may focus on preparatory methods (tone normalization), purposeful activity (dressing and bathing), and education (adaptive equipment and assistive technology use). The OTA may be expected to optimize proper bed and sitting positioning, maintain ROM, facilitate responses to stimuli, ensure practice of basic hygiene skills, and increase endurance for activity. The OT will evaluate for splints and positioning devices for joint and skin protection. Client and family education are key to ensure carryover of strategies and treatment recommendations for ROM exercises, transfers, safety, and use of durable medical equipment. To facilitate functional object use and self-care, Bruno could practice washing his face in occupational therapy, while sitting upright in bed rather than lying down, since this more closely relates to how he used to do it.

CLASSIFICATION OF INJURY

Indicators of Recovery

The spectrum of deficits from TBI varies and can be characterized as severe, moderate, or mild. Severity is determined by several factors, including duration and depth of loss of consciousness (LOC), ability to visualize brain damage on neuroimaging tests, length of **posttraumatic amnesia** (**PTA**), and the GCS score.

PTA is the length of time from the injury to the moment an individual regains memory of daily events (UAB Traumatic Brain Injury Model System, 2019). There are two

CASE STUDY

Rosie: A Client Functioning at a High Level

Rosie is a 36-year-old, restrained driver of a car involved in a motor vehicle accident (MVA). A truck ran a stop sign and struck her car on the passenger side, injuring her 16-year-old nephew, who was riding in the front passenger seat. Rosie sustained a deep laceration over her left eye and briefly lost consciousness. She was transported by ambulance to the emergency room, where she received 10 stitches for the laceration and complained of a severe headache, dizziness, and neck pain. Her head and neck x-rays and head CT scan were negative. She was diagnosed with whiplash and discharged to home, with recommendations to rest. However, she chose to visit her nephew in the ICU. When her headache, neck pain, and dizziness worsened, she went home. Rosie woke up the next day with a severe headache, light sensitivity, fatigue, severe neck and upper back pain, numerous body aches, dizziness, and difficulty paying attention and concentrating. She stayed home for the next 10 days, leaving her house only to visit her nephew and see her doctor, who diagnosed concussion, sleep disturbance, and cervical muscular strain. She was prescribed medication for pain and sleep, and physical therapy. She reported feeling better after taking medications and attending six physical therapy sessions, so Rosie decided to return to work full time as a fourth-grade teacher. Although she had worked at the same school for 9 years, Rosie noticed the fluorescent lights and noises in the school were difficult to tolerate. By the end of the first day Rosie was so exhausted she had to call her husband for a ride home, after which she slept for 14 hours. Her experience for the remainder of the week was similar, and she chose to find a quiet area in the school to rest in the dark as often as she could to get through the day. Rosie also noticed she had difficulties with focusing, remembering, organizing her schedule, thinking of words to say, and sleeping at night. At times she would forget the lesson she was teaching and started using notes to help. She typed them because her handwriting quality decreased significantly. Without provocation, she was likely to burst into tears. When she stopped doing most household management tasks, daily walks, and leisure reading at home, she could perform slightly better at work. Rosie continued to teach for the next 4 weeks but was always exhausted, made several errors in bill paying, and began falling farther and farther behind in keeping up with her lesson plans. She isolated herself socially except to visit her nephew in the hospital twice a week. She repeatedly expressed remorse to her sister how she felt responsible for her nephew's serious injuries. Rosie noticed she was "always tired," more irritable, less focused, unable to

converse for more than a few minutes, and more emotional than before her injuries. She got up often during the night because she could not stay asleep, kept all the lights off, stopped watching television, bumped into objects in the home, and dropped things. Rosie was referred to a neurologist, who diagnosed a mild TBI with executive dysfunction, posttraumatic headache, postconcussive syndrome, posttraumatic stress syndrome, posttraumatic vision syndrome, depression, disordered sleep, fatigue, and sensory hypersensitivity. The neurologist prescribed medications for headache pain, fatigue, depression, alertness, and sleep. He recommended that Rosie take a 3-month leave of absence from work, effective immediately, and that she only drive locally and during daylight hours until she completed a driving assessment. He also referred her to a licensed professional counselor, occupational therapy, physical therapy, and speech-language pathology for evaluation and treatment.

Outpatient Occupational Therapy

Rosie was independent in self-care but required more time to complete all tasks. She reported feeling dizzy when she closed her eyes in the shower. The OT recommended a shower chair for safety. Rosie required assistance to complete IADL; she relied on her husband and others to help. Rosie's husband worked long hours as a mechanical engineer and has always been responsible for home repairs and yard work. Following his wife's injury, he also took over most of the cooking, grocery shopping, light cleaning, and bill paying. The family hired a cleaning service every 2 weeks. Despite using more prepared foods, Rosie still had difficulty with meal preparation, made errors in timing of different foods, overcooking foods, and leaving the oven on after using it. She became distracted easily and often did not complete tasks such as laundry without reminders from her husband. Despite using a pill organizer, she forgot when to take medications and had difficulty following her smartphone calendar, relying on reminders from her spouse for both. She was easily fatigued and took a long nap (2–3 hours) each afternoon when she could.

Rosie demonstrated reduced visual tracking, reduced convergence, impaired depth perception, double vision, and impaired saccades, causing reading problems. Prior to her injury, she did not wear corrective lenses. At the time of her outpatient treatment, she was only driving on local familiar roads because even using GPS she tended to get lost. Despite being of assistance and emotionally supportive, Rosie's husband reported feeling considerable stress. Rosie had been rated Level VIII on the Ranchos Los Amigos Scale. Her goals were to regain all of her previous life roles.

---

types of PTA. Some clients may experience one or both. Retrograde amnesia is a partial or total loss of the ability to recall memories of events or information learned before the brain injury (Cantu, 2001), and anterograde amnesia is a decreased ability to create new memories after the injury (Cantu, 2001). One of the more accurate predictors in determining the severity of diffuse brain damage is the duration of PTA. When a person with a severe TBI comes out of coma, PTA can last from a few days to months (UAB Traumatic Brain Injury Model System, 2019). Retrograde

memory improves over time, but anterograde is among the last functions to return (Cantu, 2001). This can negatively affect attention and awareness of deficits and greatly impact a client's receptiveness and engagement in treatment.

A person suspected of having a brain injury brought to any major medical facility is typically assessed using the GCS score to rate the level of severity. Regardless of the level of injury, the most significant recovery usually occurs during the first 2 years, especially the first 6 months; however, neurologic recovery can slowly continue for years.

Functional Assessment

A number of assessment scales are used with persons with TBI for clinical evaluation, program evaluation, prediction of outcome, and to produce data for clinical research. The GCS is divided into categories of eye opening, best motor response, and verbal response; 15 items are scored (Teasdale & Jennett, 1974). A score of 13 to 15 indicates mild impairment, 9 to 12 moderate impairment, and under 8 severe impairment (Wilson, Pettigrew, & Teasdale, 1998). Bruno had a GCS score of 6, indicating a severe injury. The client with a TBI can show a variety of symptoms from severe limitations in most of the areas described later in this chapter to subtle deficits evident only in high-level, complex activities.

Other scales and objective measures such as the Disability Rating Scale (Hall, Cope, & Rappaport, 1985; Rappaport, Hall, Hopkins, Belleza, & Cope, 1982), the Functional Independence Measure (Goble, Hier-Wellner, & Lee, 1989), the Glasgow Outcome Scale-Extended (Wilson et al., 1998), the Community Integration Questionnaire (Willer, Rosenthal, Kreutzer, Gordon, & Rempel, 1993), and observational assessments such as the Rancho Los Amigos Scale of Cognitive Functioning (Rancho Los Amigos Medical Center, 1980) (see Table 24.1) are some of those used to evaluate the effects of TBI. The OT would participate with the team in using these assessments, and the OTA should be familiar with the scale(s) used in the rehabilitation setting.

After a TBI, recovery occurs along a continuum. The revised version of the Rancho Los Amigos Scale of Cognitive Functioning (Rancho Los Amigos Medical Center, 1980) divides recovery into 10 stages (see Table 24.1). In addition to identifying cognitive deficits and skills, the revised version also includes behavioral and functional deficits and skills occurring at the various stages of recovery. Becoming familiar with these stages will prove useful to the clinician as one seeks to recognize and understand the various characteristics of recovery from TBI. The information is also useful for educating caregivers and families.

In addition to the assessments discussed earlier, the OT assesses areas of occupation, performance skills, performance patterns, context, activity demands, and client factors (American Occupational Therapy Association, 2008; World Health Organization, 2001). Despite the considerable differences in the severity of their brain injuries, Bruno and Rosie have both experienced changes in their ability to perform valued occupations. Bruno demonstrates deficits in most performance skills and patterns, while Rosie, despite her higher level of function, also shows diminished performance skills (American Occupational Therapy Association, 2008). Bruno requires much more assistance to participate in his occupations, whereas Rosie has changed her habits to accommodate her brain injury (performing fewer chores) and life roles (performs fewer roles, including work) due to her symptoms.

The OT also assesses performance in the context of each client's life, which includes cultural (beliefs, activity patterns), physical (environment), social, personal (age, gender,

socioeconomic status, educational status), spiritual, temporal (stage of life, time of year, duration of problems), and virtual (technology) factors (American Occupational Therapy Association, 2008). At the time of the accident, Bruno was a young adult with limited life experience; he was just starting his college education, living at home, and financially reliant on his parents. Therefore some of the skills he needs to learn will be new and challenging. The OT identifies the activity demands (tools and materials used in tasks, space demands and physical environment, social demands, sequencing and timing, motor skills required, and body parts used in the task) (American Occupational Therapy Association, 2008) and adapts them to promote success for the client. For example, the OT might observe Bruno eating to determine the reason he spills his food. Perhaps he is using his nondominant right hand and could benefit from further practice in improving coordination and possibly a plate guard.

Finally, the OT assesses client factors, including body functions and body structures (American Occupational Therapy Association, 2008; World Health Organization, 2001). Body functions that would be addressed in treatment include all physiologic and psychologic functions such as mental functions (memory, emotional regulation), sensory functions (vision, proprioception), neuromuscular and movement functions (ROM, postural reactions), cardiovascular and respiratory functions (endurance, maintaining vitals), and skin functions (protection) (American Occupational Therapy Association, 2008; World Health Organization, 2001). Rosie has well-established highly valued roles, particularly at work. Since her injury, she has not been able to maintain any habits, roles, or routines consistently. Occupational therapy intervention can help her reestablish roles, beginning with those in the home, a familiar environment. Bruno has deficits in all body functions as listed. Rosie's problems are mostly related to cognitive, specific, and global mental functions. The remainder of this chapter explores occupational therapy interventions in areas relevant to Bruno, Rosie, and other clients who have sustained TBI.

Clinical Picture of Clients With TBI

The following is intended to illustrate what a trained clinician will observe working with this population. Some deficits are visually recognizable and apparent to anyone; however, other deficits are more subtle and require careful, clinical judgment to recognize and intervene. The clinical picture after a TBI encompasses all the physical, cognitive, visual, psychosocial, and behavioral symptoms a client may experience; some are temporary as they recover, and some are long standing and will remain with them for the rest of their lives.

Abnormal Reflexes. Depending on the location of damage, a client could present with impaired reflexes. The most severely injured clients may exhibit primitive reflexes such as the asymmetric tonic neck reflex (ATNR) and the symmetric tonic neck reflex (STNR) (see Chapter 6). Treatment focuses on inhibiting these reflexes and facilitating normal movement patterns. Bruno demonstrated flexor synergistic movement patterning of his left side. The OTA with service competency under the direction of the OT would facilitate normal movement patterns involving the entire body (head, neck, trunk, and extremities) using neurodevelopmental techniques (NDTs) to achieve normalized movement patterns to promote functional use of the left side (see Chapter 20).

Limitations of Joint Motion. Limitations in active and passive ROM are common problems for many clients with TBI caused by increased muscle tone, contractures, heterotopic ossification, fractures or dislocations, and pain. Interventions for loss of range vary depending on the cause. The OT will identify the cause(s) and determine the treatment strategies for the OTA to use when addressing reduced range.

Abnormal Muscle Tone. Abnormal muscle tone may be exhibited by clients following TBI. Lower motor neuron impairment may lead to decreased muscle tone (hypotonicity or flaccidity) and upper motor neuron impairment may lead to increased muscle tone (hypertonicity or spasticity). All skeletal muscles of the head, neck, trunk, and extremities may be affected. Clients experiencing flaccidity lose active movement but have intact passive range, unless limited by other factors such as fractures. The affected body part may appear floppy. In this case it is essential that the limb be positioned carefully to prevent joint damage or subluxation. A client with hypertonicity (spasticity) cannot voluntarily relax the affected extremities, which may limit range. Due to this lack of movement tendons can shorten permanently, leading to contractures (abnormal and often permanent loss of joint mobility).

The client in a coma may develop **decorticate posturing** (sustained contraction of both upper extremities [UEs] in flexion, internal rotation, and adduction; trunk and both lower extremities [LEs] in extension, internal rotation, and adduction). Another presentation, associated with a less favorable prognosis, is **decerebrate posturing** (sustained contraction of the trunk and extremities in extension, adduction, and internal rotation). Abnormal tone can be seen in the first days or weeks after injury or take months to develop. These postures may diminish over time as the client recovers neurologically.

Spasticity will fluctuate with changes in the client's position, voluntary movement, or medication. Infection, illness, pain, an overfilled bladder, impaction of the bowels, menstruation, environmental factors, stress, or resistance to the affected or unaffected muscles on the opposite side can also alter tone. Occupational therapy intervention for abnormal muscle tone begins with proper positioning and maintenance of full active and passive ROM to prevent contractures. Long-term consequences of severe spasticity include reduced ability to perform ADL, difficulty in maintaining proper bed or sitting positioning, reduced functional mobility (difficulty with transfers, gait deviations), painful spasms, disruption of sleep, increased risk for skin breakdown, contractures, reduced breath control, reduced speech, and pneumonia (Ito, 1998). Spasticity may range from minimal to severe. Medical treatment options may include oral medications such as Baclofen,

intramuscular injections, nerve blocks, or neurosurgery (cutting nerves or nerve roots) (Leung, King, & Fereday, 2019). Injections of neurotoxin when combined with serial casting, splinting, and active movement can be effective in treating severe spasticity (Leung et al., 2019). Bruno had moderate increased tone of his left elbow, wrist, and fingers initially, requiring UE rehabilitation, medications, and dynamic splinting. Functional use improved despite residual weakness and mild spasticity.

Muscle Weakness. Muscle weakness (paresis) may be directly related to brain damage or a result of secondary nerve damage or other factors. Weakness may impact any one or many parts of the body necessitating special positioning of the affected body parts. It may also impact one's extremities in a variety of ways and affect functioning such as the ability to use hands for writing and eating.

Postural Dysfunction

Postural deficits result from imbalanced muscle tone; delayed or absent righting reactions; impaired motor control; and deficits in vision, cognition, and perception. Adaptations to compensate for decreased postural control include various seating modifications such as using a rolling walker or a tilt-in-space wheelchair like Bruno used at the beginning of his rehabilitation.

Impaired Motor Control and Motor Speed. Motor control allows for smooth, purposeful movements of body parts during functional tasks. Impairment in voluntary motor control in all the extremities (quadriparesis) or one side of the body (hemiparesis) results from an imbalance in muscle tone and muscle weakness. Impaired fine and gross motor coordination affects performance of basic and advanced ADL. Many clients with TBI also experience reduced gross and fine motor speed. Bruno and Rosie both displayed slower motor speed while performing functional tasks.

Ataxia. Ataxia is abnormal movement and disordered muscle tone seen in clients with TBI due to damage to the cerebellum and/or to the sensory pathways. Ataxia can affect movements of the head, neck, and trunk but usually affects the extremities. The client with ataxia has lost the ability to make minute adjustments that allow for smooth coordination of movements; the movements instead appear jerky or shaky. Ataxia can cause problems in fine motor tasks such as eating, using the features on a smartphone, or typing on a computer keyboard, among other tasks.

Sensory Changes. Clients with TBI may experience decreased or lost sensation. Impairment may occur in perception of light touch, sharp or dull discrimination, proprioception, kinesthesia, temperature sense, pain perception, or stereognosis. Damage to cranial nerves may cause an impaired sense of taste and smell. Hypersensitivity can interfere with one's interaction with the physical and social environment. Rosie is hypersensitive to noise and visual input. She compensates by isolating herself, keeping all overhead lights off at home, and wearing earplugs when she is with other people in the community.

Decreased Functional Endurance. Decreased endurance may be due to the direct brain injury and/or deconditioning. OT intervention involves a graded program to gradually increase the client's ability to actively participate in daily activities. Bruno and Rosie both needed to compensate for their low endurance and fatigue. They did this by pacing themselves during activities by taking frequent breaks, limiting participation in social and work obligations, and practicing good sleep hygiene. Bruno continued to struggle with pacing himself in everyday activities such as when going out with his friends.

Dysphagia

Many clients with TBI have difficulty swallowing food or liquid (dysphagia). Specific deficits include difficulty controlling oral secretions, handling thin liquids, chewing, or managing food with mixed textures. Clients may choke easily, allowing food or liquid into their lungs (aspiration) and increasing their risk for pneumonia. Poor awareness of deficits, impaired judgment, recall, and/or impulsivity contribute to difficulty adhering to dietary restrictions such as only drinking thickened liquids. The OTA with service competency would help train the client using the eating guidelines determined by the OT and/or SLP, such as taking smaller bites, swallowing completely before taking the next bite, sipping liquid after each bite, and using feeding devices such adapted utensils, plates, and cups. Family and/or caregiver education and training are essential to ensure consistency with the dietary guidelines.

Visual Function

Individuals with TBI may sustain trauma to the vision system that can significantly affect a previously intact visual system. (See Chapter 21 for an in-depth discussion of interventions for visual and sensory dysfunction.) The eye and eyelid can also sustain direct injury. Some of the visual problems that may result from a TBI include double vision, blurred vision, reduced ability to follow objects (tracking), visual field defects (seeing only part of an image), dry eyes, and incomplete eyelid closure (ptosis), which can also contribute to dry eye. Some clients with TBI have **posttraumatic vision syndrome** (**PTVS**), which affects visual acuity, oculomotor control (eye coordination), binocular vision (eye teaming), and coordination between the focal (detail oriented) and ambient (peripheral) aspects of the visual and balance systems. Symptoms of PTVS include double vision, reduced gaze stability (perceiving stationary objects as moving), impaired attention and concentration, reduced visual memory, glare sensitivity, impaired balance, visual-spatial misperceptions, and loss of coordination and postural control (Padula & Shapiro, 2000). PTVS causes problems with reading, functional mobility, balance, and visual efficiency. Rosie demonstrated symptoms of PTVS that affected her ability to read. Reading was required for her teaching career and leisure,

both of which she highly valued. The impact of visual impairments on functional performance depends on the type, severity, and presence of deficits in other areas such as sensation and balance.

Perceptual Function

The ability to accurately perceive sensory information and respond to people and objects within the environment is necessary for successful, independent function (Ayres, 1973). Depending on the nature and extent of damage in TBI, impairment may involve visual, tactile, body scheme, language, and motor functions (see Chapters 21 and 22). Clients may experience the following: visual agnosia (inability or slowness in recognizing objects by sight), impaired left/right discrimination, impaired figure-ground perception, reduced topographic orientation (spatial orientation), impaired depth perception, tactile agnosia (astereognosis) or inability or slowness in recognizing objects by touch, impaired body scheme (reduced ability to identify body parts), unilateral neglect (reduced perception of one side), and apraxia (impaired motor planning). These deficits may affect the ability to interpret sensory information accurately and interact with objects, tools, or people in the environment successfully. Impaired depth perception and topographic orientation coupled with cognitive deficits created problems with route finding for Bruno when he walked around his neighborhood and for Rosie when driving.

Cognitive Function

Varying degrees of cognitive deficits may result from TBI and include disorientation, impaired attention, reduced concentration, reduced insight, impaired memory, **impaired initiation** (difficulty in determining and beginning the first actions, steps, or stages of a task), diminished safety awareness, decreased ability to process information accurately, and difficulty with executive functions and abstract reasoning (see Chapter 22 for an in-depth discussion of this).

Disorientation. For clients at a lower level of function, disorientation to varying degrees often occurs in relation to person, place, time, and situation (circumstance). The client appears confused and may need frequent basic reorientation or reassurance through verbal and visual cues during their daily routine until orientation improves consistently.

Reduced Insight

Many clients with TBI have reduced insight and self-awareness, which correlate with the level of cognitive function (see Table 24.1). These specific deficits can be due to actual physiologic brain damage or, in part, denial. The lower-functioning client is much more likely to lack insight and self-awareness, which can have a negative impact on the client's ability to understand strengths, deficits, purpose of therapeutic tasks, and so forth. This may lead to refusal to participate, which could be misinterpreted as noncompliance. The OTA should be aware of how treatment planning takes into consideration each client's level.

Impaired Attention and Concentration

The client with TBI often has deficits in the ability to attend to relevant information and sustain attention for the time needed to complete tasks (concentration). This often leads to difficulty attending in the presence of any type of distraction, internal or external. Lower-level clients are often distracted by somatic (bodily) internal concerns such as discomfort associated with catheterization or intravenous tubing, pain, or urinary urges. These distractions may cause them to try to remove the tubes any time they can reach the devices. Currently medical facilities differ in how they address this problem. OTAs should be aware of the specific intervention to manage this behavior. These may include the use of mitts or 24-hour supervision. Clients with difficulty attending to tasks in a distracting environment often have a reduced ability to tune out irrelevant sounds or visual information. Both Bruno and Rosie have reduced attention spans but manifested them differently. Bruno was more easily distracted in a busy environment; Rosie was more easily overwhelmed, fatigued, and likely to develop a severe headache.

Impaired Initiation. Impaired initiation can significantly affect the ability to function. Reduced initiation is not synonymous with impaired motivation. Clients with initiation problems may often hesitate because they are unsure of the first step of tasks and generally benefit from external written or verbal cues to get going. When they come to a stopping point, they may get stuck again requiring more cues to continue the task. Initiation differs from motivation. Reduced motivation causes the client to lack the incentive to perform tasks. Rosie requires cues for the first step of shorter, more achievable tasks such as making a sandwich.

Impaired Memory. Several types of memory impairments exist and range from the inability to recall a few words just heard (immediate memory), to forgetting what one ate for breakfast (short-term memory), to forgetting events that occurred 24 hours ago or years before the injury (long-term memory). Memory impairment contributes to confusion and is manifested by the inability to learn and carry over new tasks. If the client does not remember personal information accurately or completely, the OT or OTA must seek other sources of information such as family members.

Decreased Safety Awareness. Unsafe behaviors exhibited by some clients with TBI may result from reduced impulse control, decreased insight into deficits, impaired judgment, or a combination of all these. Disorientation and impaired memory can contribute to the inability to recognize risks in a variety of situations or analyze consequences of actions. Bruno and other such clients will require 24-hour supervision for safety. The OT and OTA could work with the client and family to help them learn how to monitor the client (starting in the hospital environment) and how to modify all environments to maximize safety. Examples would include adding railings on all stairs, unplugging kitchen appliances, and removing controls from the stovetop.

Delayed Information Processing. Difficulty with processing visual, auditory, and other sensory information within a normal time frame results in slowed or delayed processing speed. The delay may be a few seconds or minutes. The OT or OTA should allow the client sufficient time to process and respond during treatment, which would likely reduce feelings of being overwhelmed. Bruno demonstrated delayed processing and benefitted more from visual and tactile cues than from auditory cues.

Impairments in Executive Functioning and Abstract Reasoning. Executive functioning is a prerequisite to functioning in adult roles and is key to setting goals, planning, and effectively completing tasks. This requires high-level problem solving, reasoning, and judgment. Clients with brain injuries tend to view situations in concrete terms, interpreting all information at the most literal level. Functional independence, including appropriate social skills and successful return to work, demands mastery and control of executive functions (Goga-Eppenstein, Hill, & Yasukawa, 1999). Clients with executive dysfunction usually require assistance or supervision to function. Bruno demonstrated concrete thinking, reduced thought flexibility, and reduced abstract reasoning. For Bruno, occupational therapy intervention could focus on maximizing his ability to perform basic functional tasks such as use of social media and then progressing to school-related tasks such as introductory college-level mathematics.

Behavioral Impairment

Behavioral impairments often occur during recovery from a TBI and can challenge both the treatment staff and the families. Behavioral management is a key element of rehabilitation. Teamwork is essential, because health care providers or family members should have up-to-date information of the current behavioral problems and the planned strategies to avoid unintentionally reinforcing the client's undesirable behavior.

Common behavioral issues include lowered frustration tolerance, agitation, combativeness, disinhibition, emotional lability, and refusal to cooperate. The client may have a reduced ability to tolerate frustration and may act out when asked to complete tasks. Graded programming using relevant tasks matching the client's current abilities that builds success will help reduce frustration and acting out. The client who cannot filter distractions is sensitive to sensory information, or if asked to perform beyond his or her present capability may become agitated especially in noisy, visually active environments. An agitated client may become verbally abusive or combative and kick, bite, grab, or spit. These behaviors may be directed at the person the client perceives as the source of agitation such as the therapist or toward others in the environment. Clinicians should be aware which clients are more easily prone to agitation and should select a treatment environment that will help minimize the probability of occurrence. Although combative behavior may occur in isolation, some clients go through a period of combativeness that lasts for weeks or months. In such cases, a consistent behavior management program must be immediately determined and used by the entire interdisciplinary team and all others interacting with the client.

A client with **disinhibition** who lacks proper social awareness and understanding of boundaries often acts inappropriately. Disinhibited behavior includes making inappropriate comments, using obscene language, removing clothing, taking food off others' trays, ignoring dietary guidelines, or making sexual comments or advances toward staff members, other clients, or others nearby. The OTA would be part of the rehabilitation team, which determines the best plan and strategies to address these behaviors for each client.

Emotional lability is the display of exaggerated and sometimes inappropriate emotional responses to situations. The client reacts by weeping, giggling, or laughing uncontrollably, which may be misinterpreted as deliberate. The OTA should be aware of the interdisciplinary team plan to address these issues. Rosie can be irritable and frustrated when overwhelmed; therefore incorporating short, successful treatment activities that she finds relevant into occupational therapy sessions would be most therapeutic.

Management of Emotions and Affective Function

The OT and OTA are integral parts of the neurorehabilitation team that helps the client with TBI, the client's family, and all other social support systems to address the numerous emotional changes caused by the injury. They may experience the stages of grieving for their losses: denial, anger, bargaining, depression, and acceptance (Kübler-Ross, 1969). Clients may move back and forth through these stages and may experience several at once. Many clients initially deny their symptoms, which can be considered a coping mechanism, given the serious nature of the losses sustained. Lack of insight and self-awareness can also be misinterpreted as denial. Denial becomes dysfunctional when it lasts for more than 2 years (Gutman, 2001). Anger can occur with or after denial. The client's anger may be directed at health care workers or at family members (Gutman, 2001), which can be very stressful. As emotional recovery progresses, some clients use bargaining as a strategy and may become more cooperative and motivated in therapy (Gutman, 2001). Clients may exhibit depression, believing that hope is lost (Gutman, 2001), especially as insight and self-awareness improve. Clients may experience genuine grieving for the losses resulting from the brain injury. The grieving process and depression can be especially profound. The final stage is acceptance, in which clients accept the residual skills and limitations and are willing to work toward a life with all of these changes (Gutman, 2001). Recovery is a lengthy process, and clients with TBI may experience these stages over many years, which can also be very stressful (Broughton, 2012).

Some clients may have a history of psychiatric or emotional problems, which may be exacerbated by TBI. Other clients may experience new psychiatric or emotional problems as a result of TBI. Some of these, such as reactive depression, are associated with normal reactions to the losses associated with TBI, whereas other conditions are organic or caused by the injury (e.g., depression, lability, reduced frustration tolerance, increased anxiety). Understanding the client's previous methods of coping can assist in the selection of treatment activities. For example, a client may have listened to certain types of music to relax and so may benefit from listening to a favorite song to relax in the same manner. Psychiatric or emotional problems worsened or caused by the TBI are generally responsive to medical and psychiatric treatment.

OCCUPATIONAL THERAPY EVALUATION

The OT initiates the evaluation by explaining the role of occupational therapy and then completes the evaluation of the client with a TBI. The findings establish a baseline for treatment. The OT discusses the results with the OTA and develops the treatment plan in conjunction with the client if cognitively able and/or family members and significant others.

Safety Precautions for Clients With TBI

The OTA should know all precautions and contraindications prior to treating each client with TBI. This includes level of supervision needed, oral intake restrictions, risk for seizures, fall protocol, weight-bearing guidelines, presence of impulsivity or combativeness, and types of assistive devices used.

OCCUPATIONAL THERAPY INTERVENTION FOR CLIENTS AT A LOW FUNCTIONAL LEVEL

Occupational therapy intervention for the client with a severe TBI or for a client with an injury at the lowest levels of cognitive function (Rancho Los Amigos Medical Center, 1980) (Levels I–IV in Table 24.1; see Case Study: Bruno) aims to increase the person's level of overall responsiveness and awareness through structured graded programming, divided into simple steps. Adequate time must be allowed for a response because low arousal causes delays in processing information and performance speed. The following guidelines can be applied to some individuals with moderate brain injury as well.

Intervention can be broken down into six areas: sensory regulation, bed positioning, wheelchair positioning, splinting and casting, management of swallowing problems, neuromuscular intervention, and family/caregiver training. To optimize the client's progress in recovery, all neurorehabilitation treatments occur simultaneously. The OT and OTA must coordinate treatment with the rest of the team so as not to overwhelm the client, such as occurred with Bruno.

General Principles

There are three stages of recovery associated with the Rancho Los Amigos Level of Cognitive Functioning Scale (Rancho Los Amigos Medical Center, 1980; Senelick & Dougherty, 2001;

Wheeler & Acord-Vita, 2016). These stages are useful for guiding occupational therapy treatment planning (see Table 24.1) (Rancho Los Amigos Medical Center, 1980) and are applicable to clients with severe, moderate, and mild TBI.

1. *Acute Care Stage 1.* Coma, persistent vegetative state, or minimally conscious state may occur. The primary objective is to achieve medical stability and prevent medical complications (Wheeler & Acord-Vita, 2016). This stage corresponds to Rancho Los Amigos Levels I to III (Rancho Los Amigos Medical Center, 1980; Wheeler & Acord-Vita, 2016). The OT practitioner focuses on "improving underlying client factors," (Wheeler & Acord-Vita, 2016) (such as "awareness and alertness"), (Wheeler & Acord-Vita, 2016) "preventing the development of secondary impairments" (Wheeler & Acord-Vita, 2016) (contractures, pressure sores, etc.), restoring motor function (Wheeler & Acord-Vita, 2016). Interventions would include "positioning, splinting, range of motion," (Wheeler & Acord-Vita, 2016) orientation, and multimodal stimulation (Padula & Shapiro, 2000). The latter would be performed by the OTA who has demonstrated service competency.

2. *Rehabilitation Stage 2.* Confusion occurs with increasingly goal-directed behavior. This stage corresponds to Rancho Los Amigos Levels IV to VI. The OT practitioner focuses on "occupational performance skills," (Wheeler & Acord-Vita, 2016) including graded ADL and IADL training while minimizing environmental overstimulation (American Occupational Therapy Association, 2008; Rancho Los Amigos Medical Center, 1980; World Health Organization, 2001), maximizing function and especially safety.

3. *Community and Outpatient Stage 3.* Begins after discharge from the acute care or inpatient rehabilitation (Wheeler & Acord-Vita, 2016). Outpatient rehabilitation addresses Rancho Los Amigos Levels VII to X (American Occupational Therapy Association, 2008; Huebner, Johnson, Bennett, & Schneck, 2003; Rancho Los Amigos Medical Center, 1980; Wheeler & Acord-Vita, 2016). Therapy focuses on higher-level performance to reestablish preinjury roles as much as possible, teaching compensatory strategies and techniques to work around remaining impairments (American Occupational Therapy Association, 2008), in the home and community, and might include school, work, leisure, and social roles (Wheeler & Acord-Vita, 2016). Part of the therapeutic process would include educating clients about their skills and deficits because increased self-awareness is important for success in adapting to changes occurring as the result of TBI (Wheeler & Acord-Vita, 2016).

Occupational therapy treatment begins with preparatory methods. Purposeful activities may simulate performance in occupations. The goal is participation in life occupations. Criteria for discharge from occupational therapy for clients with TBI may include the following:
- All goals have been met.
- The client has reached a plateau in therapy and is no longer making progress.
- The client is no longer able to participate in therapy because of other factors.
- Medically necessary skilled occupational therapy services are no longer required or the client no longer wishes to participate (American Occupational Therapy Association, 2008; World Health Organization, 2001).

Sensory Regulation

The most severely injured clients have a deep disruption of consciousness (Padilla & Domina, 2016). Clients in a coma are unconscious and do not respond to the external stimulation or environment in any purposeful way. There is no sleep-wake cycle (Padilla & Domina, 2016). Some clients emerge from a coma into a vegetative state. These clients show reflexive behavior, involuntary movements, sleep-wake cycles where their eyes are open at times, but show a lack of awareness of themselves or the environment (Maiese, 2019). Clients in a minimally conscious state show awareness (Maiese, 2019), but their responses to tactile, auditory, or visual stimuli may be inconsistent.

Sensory regulation is the ability to receive and integrate information from all the senses. Treatment involves visual, auditory, tactile, and other stimuli in specific functional and familiar tasks. The most effective sensory combinations (termed *multimodal*) involve all the senses (Padilla & Domina, 2016). The client is actively engaged to maximize the benefit. Treatment sessions are usually brief (initially about 10 minutes) and incorporate both sides of the body. The OT and OTA use common everyday functional tasks such as grooming, rolling in bed, or using the nurse call system. The OT and OTA continually observe the client during treatment sessions and document any changes such as head turning in response to sounds, visual attention and tracking, vocalizations, and following commands. The OT should select the most meaningful tasks to the client. For example, the client may prefer using a hairbrush rather than a comb. These interventions would only be provided by the OTA with demonstrated service competency under direct supervision of the OT.

Functional Mobility

Mobility training for clients such as Bruno can be subdivided into bed mobility, transfer training, wheelchair mobility, and functional ambulation. The NDT principles of bilateral involvement, weight bearing, rotation, and tone normalization should be incorporated as appropriate. The OT coordinates all programming with other involved team members, including the nurse, PT, and caregiver(s).

Bed Positioning

Clients with TBI with impaired active movement may not be able to automatically reposition their body to relieve pressure, as they would have done automatically prior to the injury. Bed positioning is important to address from the onset of treatment because the client initially spends most of the time in bed. OTs and OTAs, often in conjunction with nursing and physical therapy, focus on developing a treatment program minimizing risk for development of pressure sores, facilitating normal tone, and preventing loss of joint range and mobility. Positions include supine, side-lying, and sitting up in bed. The adjustable features of the bed, bolsters, pillows, or splints are used as needed, whenever in bed and whether the client is awake or asleep. The OT and OTA must be aware of the presence of medical devices and appliances, which limit certain positions. Bed rails and call bells placed within reach should be utilized for safety.

Frequent position changes (every 2 hours) should be completed to prevent skin breakdown (i.e., decubitus ulcers). Decreased body mass and sensory loss both increase risk of skin breakdown. Bed and wheelchair positioning should avoid pressure on bony prominences and other vulnerable areas prone to skin breakdown, including earlobes, scapulae, elbows, hips, ankles, and heels.

Clients at risk for falls may have bed sensors or a pad, which sounds an alarm if the client tries to get out of bed without assistance. The OTA should inform the nursing staff when deactivating the alarm when working on bed mobility or transfers in treatment with the client. Overhead positioning slings may assist the client who requires significant physical assistance or is dependent for bed mobility.

Bed Mobility

Bed mobility training starts with rolling, moving up and down in bed, bridging (lifting hips off the bed), moving from a supine to a sitting position, and the reverse. Safety is stressed throughout all mobility training. Rolling is more difficult toward the stronger side because the weaker side may not be able to initiate the roll; thus the client may require more assistance to one side than the other. Rolling and moving up and down should be practiced when the bed is in the flattened position, which is easier for the client. It should be noted clients with increased intracranial pressure should not lie flat. The head of the bed should be elevated at least 30 degrees. Bed mobility skills are easily adapted using NDT methods (i.e., roll side to side by putting the stronger leg under the weaker leg, clasp hands, bring the arms up to shoulder height, and initiate the roll). The client may require use of the half bed rails to help roll, push up, or bridge the hips in bed. Bridging is an important skill because it helps the client manage lower body hygiene and dressing.

Clients who have been on bed rest for an extended time will require a graded program to transition from lying supine to sitting upright. They begin by sitting upright in bed with the head of the bed elevated, all rails up progressing to the edge of the bed sitting, using a graded approach. Getting up too quickly can drop blood pressure (orthostatic hypotension) causing clients to become dizzy, faint, and fall. The OTA with service competency might be involved in edge-of-bed sitting training, which includes monitoring blood pressure. Clients progress to sitting from supine to the edge of the bed with more assistance when they require full back support to maintain sitting balance and less assistance when able to sit without full back support. Hospital bed height can be adjusted

or a sturdy step stool may be placed under the feet to ensure their feet lie flat on the floor prior to an activity to maintain balance.

Transfer Training

As soon as there is medical clearance, the client may be allowed to transfer out of bed. Transfer training usually begins with the client moving from the bed to the wheelchair. Often the chair is a high-back reclining wheelchair or chair. The medical benefits provided by upright posture include improved respiratory function and circulation, reduced risk for blood clots in the lower extremities, and reduced isolation. The OT assesses the client for factors (such as paralysis, weakness, spasticity, or loss of sensation) that would influence the choice of positioning devices or customized seating. As the client becomes accustomed to sitting upright, sitting time increases, as tolerated. After each sitting session, the skin should be checked for reddened pressure areas, and positioning equipment should be provided if needed.

The amount of assistance and the type of transfer vary with the client. Neuromuscular, visual, visual-perceptual, and cognitive skills determine the selection of the type of transfer to be used in training. The ultimate goal is for the client to transfer as safely and independently as possible, with or without equipment. Some clients may require the use of a mechanical lift, physical assistance of one or more people, or use of a sliding board. Using the same technique each time helps the client learn and remember the process. If possible, it is preferable for transfers to be practiced by moving to both sides so that the client can learn to transfer to either side, which may be required in various settings (e.g., public restrooms). However, during initial training, transferring to the strongest side (e.g., Bruno's right side) is the safest option and recommended until the client is strong enough for the other side.

The OTA would train caregivers with the objective of learning how to assist the client in all types of transfers required for all settings (e.g., wheelchair, commode, car). Practice reduces fear and builds confidence.

Wheelchair Mobility

Many clients with TBI requiring the use of a wheelchair for functional mobility will use a manual type. The first step to wheelchair use is assessing and prescribing proper wheelchair positioning.

1. *Wheelchair Positioning Program.* Effective seating and positioning requires trunk stability, a stable base of support at the pelvis, maintaining the body at midline, and holding the head upright for the client to use UEs in functional activities and visually attend to their environment (see Fig. 24.1).
2. *Graded Seating Program.* Clients who do not have sufficient trunk stability and head control to sit upright will require a reclining wheelchair with a high back and head support. Proper positioning should target postural deficits and facilitate alignment through the choice of

the wheelchair design and positioning devices. Often the client can be positioned using commercially made equipment, but the OT or OTA may need to fabricate or adapt seating devices. The following are guidelines to consider for optimal positioning.

a. *Pelvis.* Wheelchair positioning begins with pelvic alignment because poor hip positioning causes poor head and trunk alignment and influences tone throughout the entire body. Prior to advancing to sitting in a wheelchair, treatment should focus on stretching the hips and back to achieve neutral pelvic alignment. A solid seat insert placed on top of the sling seat of the wheelchair facilitates a neutral to slight anterior tilt of the pelvis. An insert with a slightly wedged seat (with the downward slope pointing toward the back of the wheelchair) can be used to flex the hips to help inhibit extensor tone in the hips and legs, to help prevent the client from sliding forward out of the wheelchair. A lumbar support may help to maintain a natural curve of the spine in the lower back. Wheelchair cushions distribute weight to reduce pressure areas and properly position the client. A seatbelt angled across the pelvis will help to maintain the hips back up against the back of the wheelchair, the desired position. Pressure mapping is a more recent innovative tool that helps identify any areas of concern and determine appropriate cushions for the client (Dillbeck, 2013).

b. *Trunk.* After the pelvis is positioned, the trunk is next. The goal is for the client to achieve trunk stability in midline while sitting, allowing for the use of UEs without losing balance. A solid back insert or solid contoured back behind the client facilitates a more upright position. Lateral trunk supports can be used to eliminate leaning to either side due to weak musculature or abnormal muscle tone; a chest strap or crossed chest straps will decrease leaning forward, pull back the shoulders, and allow for chest expansion. Custom-made trunk support systems ordered by the physician are fabricated by an orthotist for clients with severe positioning problems.

c. *Head.* For clients with minimal or no active head control, achieving an upright midline head position can be difficult. Most head control devices employ static positioning. The head is kept from falling forward by a forehead strap. Caution must always be taken to avoid overstressing the cervical area or giving excessive resistance to spastic neck muscles. Reclining the client back will eliminate this problem but also will reduce weight bearing through the trunk and pelvis and limit visual interaction with the environment. The recommended position is no more than 10 to 15 degrees reclined to prevent the abovementioned problems and limit extensor posturing. Dynamic head positioning is the alternative to static head positioning. The advantages of a dynamic device are good alignment of the head on the trunk, equal distribution of pressure,

and allowing the client to begin initiating head movements actively.

d. *Lower Extremities.* Calf supports attached to elevating leg rests can provide additional support for both legs. Thigh pads placed along the lateral aspect of the thigh may be used to decrease abduction. An abductor wedge may be placed between the legs to eliminate adduction. Proper footwear (e.g., high-top athletic shoes) can serve to help position the feet correctly. Use of a foot wedge placed on top of the foot plate under the feet can prevent plantar flexion contractures for one or both feet. Foot plates also offer proprioceptive input and can help normalize tone. Some clients may require calf or toe straps to help keep the legs solidly on the footrests.

e. *Upper Extremities.* The arms should be positioned with the scapula neutral, shoulders in slight flexion and external rotation, the elbows in slight flexion, forearms pronated, and wrists and fingers in a functional position on the level surface. A lap tray is often used to achieve the optimal positioning of the arms on a level surface. Some clients who require support for one arm may use an arm trough. Wedges can be used to elevate the affected arm, if needed, to manage edema. Some clients may wear splints while sitting upright in the wheelchair.

Wheelchair positioning involves regular reevaluation and modification of equipment to meet the changing needs of the client. The OTA with demonstrated service competency may be involved in this aspect of occupational therapy intervention, possibly in coordination with a PT.

Wheelchair mobility training also involves learning to manage wheelchair parts (e.g., removing footrests, managing wheel locks, placing a lapboard on and off) and propelling the wheelchair both indoors and outdoors on different types and levels of surfaces safely. The client learns and practices each skill until it is mastered. Initially, endurance for pushing the wheelchair may be quite limited, which builds with practice. Some clients may require gloves to protect the hands from blistering caused by the friction on the wheelchair rims. Use of a power wheelchair may be a better option for some clients, but this involves a higher cost and more extensive training.

Functional Ambulation

Functional ambulation refers to the client's ability to walk when completing daily tasks. The PT assesses the individual's ability to ambulate, recommends assistive devices as indicated, and performs ambulation training. The OT or OTA incorporates carryover of ambulation into ADL and IADL tasks, while using proper technique, devices, and precautions. Some functionally mobile clients eventually can walk and carry, hold, move, and use items or tools while performing tasks. An OT or OTA might recommend wearing a waist pack or backpack to carry items if clients have difficulty carrying them while walking.

Splinting (Static and Dynamic) and Casting

Static splints are used to properly position or support a body part with the objective in preparation for functional use. Casting and dynamic splints progressively increase passive ROM when increased muscle tone and contractures (or possible contractures) are present. Both aim to reduce abnormal tone or soft tissue tightness, increase or maintain passive ROM, increase the functional potential of the body part, prevent skin breakdown, and prevent contractures. The OT selects the most appropriate intervention for the client depending on multiple factors, including skin integrity, sensory loss, and opportunities for functional use. Sometimes the OT will need to fabricate the splint, but many times the OT can use commercially available, prefabricated dynamic splinting options to increase ROM as well. The OTA should be familiar with the purpose and use of the specific type of splint selected.

The most commonly used splint is the resting hand splint for clients with flaccidity and mild spasticity (see Chapter 19). This type of splint positions the wrist and fingers into extension and abducts the thumb, providing gentle passive stretch to the wrist and hand. Proper passive positioning of the involved wrist and hand into a functional position is intended to prevent contractures. Other common splints include the wrist cockup splint, which supports the weakened wrist, and the antispasticity splint, which abducts the fingers and inhibits increased tone. It is most effective for mild to moderate tone (Fig. 24.2). Clients with more severe flexor tone of the wrist and fingers are at risk for skin breakdown and may use a cone-shaped resting hand splint.

A typical splint schedule begins with 2 hours on and 2 hours off, but the wearing schedule depends on the individual client's needs. A casting program is implemented when other splinting methods for managing spasticity are ineffective. Casts are made of fiberglass or plaster. Fiberglass is preferred because it is lighter in weight, sets (hardens) more quickly, and is easier to apply than plaster. The most common UE cast is designed to increase elbow extension.

Serial casting uses a sequence of casts to gradually stretch the involved joint contracture, increasing passive ROM. Each cast is worn for up to several days, removed and replaced with the next one in the series, each getting slightly closer to the desired end position if there are no signs of skin breakdown such as redness. Once the desired ROM has been achieved, the final cast is removed, cut in half (bivalve), and the edges of both halves of the cast are finished. The client usually wears the bivalve cast to maintain ROM. Serial casting is performed on only one joint at a time (Goga-Eppenstein et al., 1999). The OTA with demonstrated service competency may assist the OT or OTA in serial casting. Research supports the use of casting and/or splinting in conjunction with botulinum toxin injections and active movement for the management and prevention of contractures (Leung et al., 2019).

Swallowing and Eating Problems

The experienced OTA might train clients with TBI who have impaired swallowing, neuromuscular, visual, cognitive, and/or behavioral deficits impacting their ability to participate in self-feeding. Thickened liquids or liquids in the form of ice chips, ice pops, or flavored gelatin may be the only way these clients can safely take in fluids orally. Some clients may be on eating restrictions temporarily and others permanently.

The client may have other deficits that interfere with eating such as reduced attention, visual changes, left unilateral neglect, impaired memory, reduced sequencing, impulsivity, sensory deficits, weakness, and incoordination. When there is a choking risk, the OTA should ensure nearby emergency medical assistance when working with such clients.

Clients with TBI require a structured, consistent feeding routine to reestablish proper and safe eating. Assistive devices such as a plate guard and a cup with a lid or built-up handles may be useful to increase safe independence in eating.

Neuromuscular Impairments

Clients with severe and moderate TBI can experience a variety of motor impairments. Weakness, spasticity, rigidity, soft tissue contractures, primitive reflexes, reduced or absent postural reactions, impaired sensation, and reduced fine motor coordination will have a negative impact on occupational performance. All treatment should be task oriented and functionally based. The OT may incorporate neurophysiologic techniques such as NDT, proprioceptive neuromuscular facilitation (PNF), and Rood techniques described in Chapter 20 into treatment activities. The common principles of treatment are to (1) progress proximal to distal, (2) establish symmetric posture, (3) integrate both sides of the body into activities, (4) encourage bilateral weight bearing, and (5) introduce a normal sensory experience. Many therapists combine techniques; the OT would determine the selection and timing of these approaches. These and other such

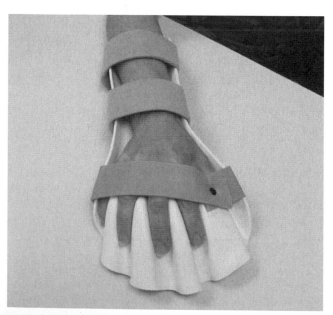

Fig. 24.2 Antispasticity splint. (From Pendleton HM, Schultz-Krohn W. *Pedretti's Occupational Therapy.* 8th ed. St Louis, MO: Elsevier; 2018.)

techniques require specialized training, including hands-on practice and clinical experience. The experienced OTA with service competency using these techniques may incorporate them into functional training under the direct supervision of the OT.

Treatment often begins by addressing trunk instability. Trunk stability is necessary for sitting upright and for effective limb movements. Treatment of postural instability of the trunk should focus on achieving alignment and stimulating muscle responses in the trunk muscles. Alignment will facilitate stability. Once trunk control and stability improve, treatment should progress to functional activities using UEs.

The client with severe TBI may have a reduced sensation and/or feeling of movement, which can impair coordination, restrict functional mobility, and increase risk for injury. Pain can interfere with attention, concentration, sleep, functional mobility, and active participation. Ataxia is a common problem interfering with motor control and can affect one or all four extremities. See Chapter 13 for specific intervention strategies to treat the decreased coordination resulting from ataxia. Overall, neuromuscular impairments can have a significant effect on the physical ability to perform functional tasks, including speed and accuracy.

Caregiver Education

One of the strongest predictors of success in rehabilitation after a TBI is social support. Family, friends, and significant others are integral to the rehabilitation process, especially in the beginning stages, because they may be better able to elicit a response from the client than health care team members. In addition, they often serve as sources of information regarding the client's preinjury roles, habits, routines, and rituals, as well as the coping style.

Education of the family and/or caregivers begins in the initial encounter with an OT or OTA. The OT practitioner grades the caregiver education and training so that basic skills are taught first, with more complex skills introduced after the simpler skills are mastered.

The significant changes in the life of the client with TBI and the impact on the family are important considerations. Family members who serve as primary caregivers experience more stress than less involved family, such as the case with both Rosie and Bruno. Clients and their caregivers may seek counseling to help them cope with the enormity of the situation. The interdisciplinary team, including the OT and OTA, can also help them locate resources to provide transportation, respite care, psychological support, or professional services or groups offered through the local rehabilitation hospital and the national or state BIAA. Taking personal time does reduce caregiver stress and burnout.

Treatment of Clients With TBI at a Higher Functional Level

The recognition of symptoms and diagnosis of mild (and for some moderate) brain injury is sometimes overlooked initially. Because clients appear to be functioning at a higher level, some health care practitioners may assume they have no problems performing their daily routines. It is not unusual for clients with mild TBI to be diagnosed weeks, months, or even years after their initial injury. Concepts discussed in this section are also applicable to clients who sustained a severe TBI and have recovered to a higher functional level. Many clients with TBI are dissatisfied that they cannot perform tasks as they did before the injury. No matter when they are diagnosed, clients with brain injury can often improve their function through neurorehabilitation.

Occupational therapy treatment for clients at Rancho Los Amigos Levels VII to X (see Table 24.1 and both case studies) focuses on areas of occupation, addressing issues with body functions, improving performance skills, adapting performance patterns, and activity. Clients may experience a variety of sensory changes, including pain. There is often hyposensitivity to taste, smell, touch, and proprioception and hypersensitivity to light and sound, as occurred with Rosie. The OT would focus on improving Rosie's ability to increasingly tolerate environmental stimuli.

Vision

Visual dysfunction commonly results from TBI. The OT's evaluation includes a complete vision history, including if the client currently uses or needs corrective lenses, screening of visual acuity, eye coordination, visual field, and visual function (see Chapter 21). In some cases, the glasses may have been lost or broken in the incident causing the TBI or the glasses prescription may not be current. Clients who previously wore contact lenses may not be able to wear them again (due to problems such as eye injury or dry eye), and will have to revert back to using glasses. For clients needing updated corrective lenses, the OT should recommend a referral to a vision specialist. Occupational therapy intervention addresses vision problems through functional activities. The OT and OTA increase the client's awareness and understanding of impairments, maximize the client's use of residual vision, and instruct the client in compensatory strategies and how to incorporate these into daily functioning. Recommendations from the vision specialist for clients with PTVS should be incorporated into the treatment plan. Adaptations used for vision impairments include providing enlarged print (such as with Rosie), spacing objects far apart so that they are easily seen, increasing the illumination on the task, using contrasting colors (e.g., placing a green toothbrush on a white towel), and marking steps, corners of walls, and table edges with reflective tape.

Vision rehabilitation may be effective in alleviating PTVS and other visual deficits caused by TBI. Interventions include remedial exercises and instruction in and use of compensatory strategies, devices, and modification of the environment (Gianutsos, 1997). Optometrists use "lenses, prisms, occlusion, low vision aids and visual therapy" to treat visual disorders (Scheiman, 2011). The American Academy of Optometry, the College of Optometrists in Vision

Development (COVD), and the Optometric Extension Program Foundation list optometrists trained in visual therapy (Scheiman, 2011). A COVD behavioral optometrist specializes in providing visual therapy services. Although some OTs are specially trained in vision therapy, most usually provide interventions for compensation and environmental adaptation.

Visual-Perceptual Training

Visual input is an important component of perceptual processing. Retraining is usually termed *visual-perceptual training*. Rehabilitation approaches to treating perceptual dysfunction are remedial and compensatory, using functional tasks as feasible. The remedial approach asserts that the adult brain is sufficiently plastic to repair; it reorganizes itself after injury (Neistadt, 1994) (neuroplasticity) and involves reestablishing skills. For example, Bruno learned his way about the rehabilitation unit propelling himself to his appointments independently after high repetition using the same daily schedule. To improve route finding, Rosie could practice relearning the configuration of the grocery store where she regularly shops in the actual store. The functional approach is based on the theory that recovery results from the use of intact brain areas to perform adapted functional activities, compensating for lost function (Neistadt, 1990). Rosie had difficulty using the GPS unit in her car. In occupational therapy, she could explore the functions of the GPS unit and make adjustments to compensate for problems with route finding, similar to how Bruno relied on personally meaningful visual cues (basketball) posted outside his therapists' offices to help him navigate the rehabilitation unit.

Cognitive Retraining

The OT and OTA can utilize cognitive retraining for executive dysfunction. It is effective when accomplished through graded programming using a variety of functional tasks relevant to each client with TBI. To begin, the OT and OTA assist the client to determine which functional activities to address first. They then target one or more cognitive deficits in each task, as well as deficits in motor control, visual-perception, or sensory changes. Activities should be age appropriate, matched to the client's current capabilities, and relevant. Clients perform better in ADL and IADL tasks that are familiar and meaningful to them, which they understand and value. Examples would include bathing, folding laundry, and using desktop or laptop computers, tablets, and smartphones. Repetition through practice of skills is important for individuals with cognitive deficits. The following are some treatment guidelines for common cognitive issues for clients with TBI. Chapter 20 includes more detailed interventions.

To address disorientation initially, information should be presented in a matter-of-fact tone, reminding the client of the key basic information such as the day of the week, the time of day, etc. The clinician should avoid repeatedly asking the client to answer questions because doing so may lead to frustration, reduced cooperation, or agitation. The OTA can teach families and significant others how to provide reorientation cues and help determine relevant assistive devices (smartphone) and environmental cues specific and personally relevant to the client. For example, Bruno might be more likely to notice and attend to a large sign in his room with the day of the week written on a large picture of a basketball than a blank piece of paper. The reorientation process can take from weeks to months. Although disorientation resolves with recovery for most clients, for some the disorientation may be permanent.

Occupational therapy programming for clients with impaired attention and concentration would begin with shorter treatment sessions in a distraction-free environment using familiar functional tasks. The OTA would grade therapy by increasing the amount of time the client can attend and concentrate and the presence and type of distractions. Sequencing can be practiced in a variety of tasks such as dressing, assembling a sandwich, writing emails or texts, or using apps to grocery shop and manage banking.

Establishing a routine using a meaningful cueing system can help the client improve functional memory. Bruno had more difficulty with new learning and carryover and benefitted from lower expectations, which were graded as he succeeded. He initially relied on a checklist to help him recall steps to his morning routine, eventually progressing to using reminders on his phone. Rosie may have benefitted from using a family schedule board at home posted in an obvious place, a checklist for chores, and a smartphone daily schedule app. Bruno and Rosie set up well-marked and designated areas in their own home to place frequently used belongings (e.g., a tray for keys, purse, and wallet).

Strategies for Behavioral Management

The use of behavioral intervention strategies is intended to help the client maximize function. This approach is preferable to using medications (chemical restraints) or physical restraints. Consistent behavioral programming by all individuals working with clients with TBI is the most effective. The program would include strategies to limit undesirable behaviors and increase desirable behaviors while ensuring the client's safety as well as others such as treating health care providers and family. This phase can be especially difficult for them, who will require encouragement and support. These strategies are divided into two categories: environmental and interactive.

Environmental strategies involve modifying the environment to facilitate appropriate behaviors, inhibit unwanted behaviors, and help to maintain the safety of the client. The first step is to create a quiet treatment area. The reduction of environmental sensory stimulation helps calm the individual. A single occupant hospital room is preferred. Visual and auditory distractions should be minimized. For example, television and overhead lights should be turned off, walls should be kept plain, extra furniture should be removed, and the door should be closed, if possible and safe.

Agitated clients who are unsafe to be alone may require one-on-one supervision and extra padding on their hospital bed. Some clients require an alarm system to help the rehabilitation team monitor their location at all times and prevent unsafe behaviors such as getting out of bed or the wheelchair, entering prohibited areas, or wandering outside. The transmitter may be attached out of reach to the underside of the wheelchair or worn in bracelet form.

To interact with the agitated client, the clinician should speak in a calm voice with a soothing matter-of-fact tone at eye level. All communication should be brief to prevent overwhelming the client with details, which might cause frustration and increase confusion. Another behavior management technique is diversion. For agitated clients who cannot redirect themselves, the OT or OTA can divert their attention such as by changing the subject. Overall, every person interacting with the client with behavioral issues, including rehabilitation team members, family members, and significant others, should work together using the techniques and strategies identified in the interdisciplinary treatment plan.

Self-Care. ADL retraining is more effective in improving the client's functional independence when occurring in a familiar and meaningful context. Key elements to relearning include structure, grading, and repetition. A self-care program should be structured and consistent, with the client following the same daily routine in the same environment, using the same sequence of steps to accomplish the task. As the client makes improvements, the clinician reduces structure and cues and focuses on improving the client's ability to complete the task when the routine is interrupted or altered in some way. The OT or OTA breaks tasks into smaller segments, a technique known as grading, to facilitate the relearning process. Approaches such as backward chaining, in which the therapist assists the client with the majority of the activity and the client completes the final step, can be easily modified for each individual client's needs. Another strategy is to organize the steps of the activity sequence into a list of visual and written cues, such as with Bruno. Repetition helps clients carry over ADL skills learned, promoting progress, especially when including caregiver participation.

The OT and OTA should employ techniques that increase functional independence by reinforcing normal motor patterns. The experienced OTA with demonstrated service competency might use a specific neurophysiologic approach that helps to normalize tone and integrate both sides of the body into self-care activities (see Chapter 20).

Group Treatment

When the OT determines it to be beneficial, group treatment can be added as a supplement to individual treatment. It provides learning experiences that enrich the client beyond that of individual treatment and structured opportunities in which clients can develop more effective interpersonal interactions, communication, and psychosocial skills.

Group participation, which may be run by OTs alone or with other professionals, allows clients to get feedback from their peers, which can lead to increased self-awareness and problem solving (Rath, Simon, Langenbahn, Sherr, & Diller, 2003). Groups are most effective when functionally based. Goals include improving pragmatics, learning appropriate social interaction and behavior, increasing attention and concentration, and working on skills such as remembering names and taking turns to speak. The group leader must understand each client's individual goals so that the client can achieve optimum value from the experience. For example, Bruno could tolerate a group activity for about 30 to 60 minutes; Rosie, however, could not tolerate group work due to her sensory sensitivity and decreased endurance.

Areas of Occupation

As the client with TBI regains functional skills and independence in basic self-care, occupational therapy treatment expands to include IADL, education, work, play, leisure, and social interaction.

The OTA should be aware of each client's previous level of function and goals before initiating treatment interventions. Training is graded to suit the client's functional level. At the end of each occupational therapy session, the OT should review the session as well as the next day's schedule. Establishing short-term and long-term goals with the client and family (if possible) is important. As the client makes progress, the OT and OTA increase the task demands until all goals are met. Prior to his injury, Bruno did his own laundry. Therefore initial occupational therapy sessions might have included sorting and folding a few items of clothing, increasing the level of difficulty with progress.

Community Reintegration

Community reintegration is a goal that begins being addressed in occupational therapy upon admission. Once the client reaches the maximal independence possible during the inpatient phase, the focus of occupational therapy shifts to assisting the client in regaining as many home and community roles as possible. Since clients initially gain skills in familiar settings, focusing on familiar settings in the therapy process increases the likelihood of successful transfer of training from the rehabilitation setting to the home and community. The OT and OTA can assist the client with TBI and family members in exploring relevant community resources. The BIAA has extensive information and links to resources online at www.biausa.org. Each state has a BIAA chapter that provides information, sponsors support groups and other services, and serves as a resource for the brain-injured person and family.

Clients who participate in treatment incorporating "resilience focused intervention improve psychological health and adjustment after TBI" (Kreutzer et al., 2018). The program would include adopting traits to cope with the challenges, improving an understanding of their symptoms and what to expect in the recovery process, increasing awareness of strengths and weaknesses, improving skills sets such as problem-solving and communication skills, being actively involved in recovery, and learning ways to develop a positive outlook (RAI—Resilience and Adjustment Intervention, 2020). Rosie's depression and lowered self-confidence have caused her to withdraw from the community and her family. She may benefit from an occupational therapy treatment plan beginning with tasks she can more easily accomplish to build confidence.

Outcome After TBI

Studies have shown that clients with brain injury tend to have a better prognosis if they have a higher initial GCS score (Teasdale & Jennett, 1974), shorter duration of PTA, are younger, and have more years of education (Bontke, 1991). The greater the injury to the brain, the more likely there will be residual problems.

After completing inpatient and outpatient rehabilitation for possibly 9 to 12 months, Bruno progressed to Rancho Los Amigos Level VIII. He regained functional use of his left arm. He completed rehabilitation at a modified level of independence for ADL and routine IADL. He continued to require supervision for more complex tasks requiring executive functioning and socialization. He and his family hoped his insight would improve as his recovery continued. This would allow him to utilize the recommended cognitive strategies, including using academic accommodations for which he is eligible through the Americans with Disabilities Act (Americans with Disabilities Act of 1990), to be successful in returning to school.

After 6 months of rehabilitation, Rosie recovered to Rancho Los Amigos Level IX, achieving some aspects of her occupational therapy long-term goal (Quote 24.2). These included completing all ADL independently with time, requiring some assistance for IADL and accommodations for leisure and social roles, and returning to teaching. She continued to require long-term counseling to help with coping and adjustment to the permanent changes in her life caused by the TBI. Overall, both clients made significant progress through the occupational therapy intervention provided to them.

SUMMARY

Occupational therapy is an integral part of neurorehabilitation treatment of the adult client with TBI and requires experience, expertise, and clinical reasoning skills. Most clients have numerous deficits to varying degrees in areas of occupation, as well as issues with mental functions and behavior that may interfere with treatment at times. The main focus of occupational therapy intervention is to engage the client in occupation, making the process dynamic and interactive (American Occupational Therapy Association, 2008).

Occupational therapy goals should be tailored to meet the specific needs of each client. They should be meaningful, functionally based, and structured for the contexts and environments in which each client lives. Primary caregivers, family, and significant others also play a key role in the client's recovery and therefore should be involved in all aspects of the occupational therapy process, from admission to discharge.

> ### QUOTE 24.1
>
> **Long-Term Occupational Therapy Goal Identified by Case Study: Bruno**
>
> *"I want my left arm to get better and drive again."*

> ### QUOTE 24.2
>
> **Long-Term Occupational Therapy Goal Identified by Case Study: Rosie**
>
> *"I want to go back to my old life, when everything was easy to do."*

REVIEW QUESTIONS

1. Define TBI and how it affects participation in meaningful occupations.
2. List some of the most common causes of TBI.
3. Describe the role of the OTA with a low-level client with TBI in the ICU.
4. How would abnormal postures of the right side affect a client's ability to roll in bed?
5. Explain why a client with TBI at Rancho Los Amigos Level IV might hit people. How could the OTA modify the environment to help reduce this behavior?
6. Describe a therapeutic activity the OTA could use during the first caregiver training session for a client with a severe TBI.
7. Explain how the OTA could help a client with disorientation and memory problems remember the day of the week.
8. Family members of a client with TBI inconsistently follow her eating precautions. Explain how the OTA might handle the situation.
9. How much assistance from the OTA might a client at a Rancho Los Amigos Level VII require to identify a long-term occupational therapy goal?
10. What would cause a client with a TBI to refuse to attend a therapy session?
11. Identify three issues a client with a mild TBI might encounter when using his new cell phone.
12. Within the first month of treatment, a family member of a client with a moderate TBI is having difficulty accepting the client's limitations and insists he will have a complete recovery. What could the OTA do to help that family member?
13. For a client with TBI who functions at a concrete level, should the OTA pursue a functional or remedial approach to perceptual training? Explain.
14. The mother of a 20-year-old client with TBI is at the hospital every day. Staff has noticed she has started sleeping in a chair in his room while he is at therapy. What does her behavior indicate?
15. A client with TBI who always wears glasses arrives for his outpatient appointment having forgotten them. What could the OTA do so that the client can still participate in therapy that day?

REFERENCES

Adams, J. H., Doyle, D., Ford, I., Gennarelli, T. A., Graham, D. I., & McLellan, D. R. (1989). Diffuse axonal injury in head injury: definition, diagnosis and grading. *Histopathology, 15*, 49–59.

American Occupational Therapy Association. (2008). Occupational therapy practice framework: domain and process (2nd ed.). *The American Journal of Occupational Therapy, 62*, 625–683.

American Occupational Therapy Association. (2017). Occupational therapy in acute care. <https://www.aota.org/About-Occupational-Therapy/Professionals/RDP/AcuteCare.aspx>.

Americans with Disabilities Act of (1990). (ADA). 42 U.S.C. §§ 12101-12213.

Ashley MJ, Masel BE, Nagel MP. (2016). Brain injury overview. In: *The essential brain injury guide.* (5th ed.) Fairfax, VA: Brain Injury Association of America; 1-27.

Ayres, A. J. (1973). *Sensory integration and learning disorders.* Los Angeles, CA: Western Psychological Services.

Bartolo, M., Bargellesi, S., Castioni, C. A., Intiso, D., Fontana, A., Copetti, F. A., et al. (2017). Mobilization in early rehabilitation in intensive care unit patients with severe acquired brain injury: an observational study. *Archives of Physical Medicine and Rehabilitation, 49*, 715–722.

Bombardier, C. H., Rimmele, C. T., & Zintel, H. (2002). The magnitude and correlates of alcohol and drug use before traumatic brain injury. *Archives of Physical Medicine and Rehabilitation, 83*(12), 185–191.

Bontke, C. F. (1991). Medical advances in the treatment of brain injury. In J. S. Kreutzer, & P. Wehman (Eds.), *Community integration following traumatic brain injury.* Baltimore, MD: Brooke.

Brain Injury Association of America. (2011). BIAA adopts new TBI definition. <https://www.biausa.org/public-affairs/public-awareness/news/biaa-adopts-new-tbi-definition>.

Broughton R. The Kubler-Ross stages of grief are different with TBI. 2012. <https://www.brainline.org/video/kubler-ross-stages-grief-are-different-tbi>.

Bruns, J., Jr, & Hauser, W. A. (2003). The epidemiology of traumatic brain injury: a review. *Epilepsia, 44*(Suppl. 10), S2–S10.

Cantu, R. C. (2001). Posttraumatic retrograde and anterograde amnesia: pathophysiology and implications in grading and safe return to play. *Journal of Athletic Training, 36*(3), 244–248.

Centers for Disease Control and Prevention. (2019). *National Center for Injury Prevention and Control. Traumatic brain injury and concussion: get the facts.* Atlanta, GA.

Corrigan, J. D. (1995). Substance abuse as the mediating factor in the outcome of traumatic brain injury. *Archives of Physical Medicine and Rehabilitation, 76*(4), 302–309.

Defense and Veterans Brain Injury Center. (2014). TBI and the military. <https://dvbic.dcoe.mil/tbi-military>.

Dillbeck A. (2013). Wheelchair seating: obtaining necessary equipment for individuals with complex needs. <http://www.rehab-pub.com/2013/07/wheelchair-seating-obtaining-necessary-equipment-for-individuals-with-complex-needs/>.

Frieden, T. R., & Collins, F. S. (2013). *National Center for Injury Prevention and Control. A Report to Congress on the Traumatic Brain Injury in the United States: Understanding the Public Health Problem Among Current and Former Military Personnel.* Atlanta, GA: Centers for Disease Control and Prevention.

Ghajar, J. (2000). Traumatic brain injury. *Lancet, 356*(9233), 923–929.

Gianutsos, R. (1997). Visual rehabilitation following acquired brain injury. In M. Gentile (Ed.), *Functional vision behavior: a therapist's guide to evaluation and treatment options* (pp. 267–294). Rockville, MD: AOTA Press.

Goble, L., Hier-Wellner, S., & Lee, D. (1989). The role of community reintegration activities in a day treatment service. *Physical Disabilities (Special Interest Section Newsletter), 12*(3), 7–8.

Goga-Eppenstein, P., Hill, J. P., & Yasukawa, A. (1999). *Casting protocols for the upper and lower extremities.* Gaithersburg, MD: Aspen.

Gutman, S. A. (2001). The psychosocial sequelae of traumatic brain injury, part II: identification, AOTA continuing education article. *OT Practice, 6*(5), CE1–CE8.

Hall, K., Cope, D. N., & Rappaport, M. (1985). Glasgow Outcome Scale and Disability Rating Scale: comparative usefulness in following recovery in traumatic head injury. *Archives of Physical Medicine and Rehabilitation, 66*(1), 35–37.

Hetwig M. (2003). Traumatic brain injury in domestic violence programs in Iowa: screening pilot. Des Moines, IA: Department of Health and Human Services (DHHS) Health Resources and Services Administration, Maternal and Child Bureau to the Iowa Department of Public Health.

Huebner, R. A., Johnson, K., Bennett, C., & Schneck, C. (2003). Community participation and quality of life outcomes after adult traumatic brain injury. *The American Journal of Occupational Therapy, 57*(2), 177–185.

Ito, M. (1998). Consciousness from the viewpoint of the structural-functional relationships of the brain. *International Journal of Psychology, 3*, 191–207.

Kreutzer, J. S., Marwitz, J. H., Sima, A. P., Mills, A., Hsu, N. H., & Lukow, H. R. (2018). Efficacy of the resilience and adjustment intervention after traumatic brain injury: a randomized controlled trial. *Brain Injury, 32*(8), 963–971.

Kübler-Ross, E. (1969). *On death and dying.* New York, NY: Macmillan Publishing Company.

Leung, J., King, C., & Fereday, S. (2019). Effectiveness of a programme comprising serial casting, botulinum toxin, splinting and motor training for contracture management: a randomized controlled trial. *Clinical Rehabilitation, 33*(6), 1035–1044. Available from http://doi.org/10.1177/0269215519831337.

Losiniecki, A., & Shutter, L. (2010). Management of traumatic brain injury. *Current Treatment Options in Neurology, 12*(2), 142–154.

Maiese, K. (2019). Vegetative State and Minimally Conscious State. *The Merck manual professional version.* <https://www.merck-manuals.com/professional/neurologic-disorders/coma-and-impaired-consciousness/vegetative-state-and-minimally-conscious-state>.

Marquez de la Plata, C. D., Hart, T., Hammond, F. M., Frol, A. B., Hudak, A., Harper, C. R., et al. (2008). Impact of age on long-term recovery from traumatic brain injury. *Archives of Physical Medicine and Rehabilitation, 89*(5), 896–903.

Martin, E., Schwab, K., & Malik, S. (2018). Defense and veterans brain injury center: the first 25 years. *The Journal of Head Trauma Rehabilitation, 33*(2), 73–80.

National Center for Injury Prevention and Control. (2003). *A report to congress: mild traumatic brain injury in the united states: steps to prevent a serious public health problem.* Atlanta, GA: Centers for Disease Control and Prevention.

Neistadt, M. E. (1990). A critical analysis of occupational therapy approaches for perceptual deficits in adults with brain injury. *The American Journal of Occupational Therapy, 44*(4), 299–304.

Neistadt, M. E. (1994). Perceptual retraining for adults with diffuse brain injury. *The American Journal of Occupational Therapy, 48*(3), 225–233.

Padilla, R., & Domina, A. (2016). Effectiveness of sensory stimulation to improve arousal and alertness of people in a coma or persistent vegetative state after traumatic brain injury: a systematic review. *The American Journal of Occupational Therapy,* *70*(3), 1−8.

Padula, W. V., & Shapiro, J. (2000). Post-trauma vision syndrome following TBI. In W. V. Padula (Ed.), *Neuro-optometric rehabilitation* (3rd ed.). Santa Ana, CA: Optometric Extension Program.

Park, E., Bell, J. D., & Baker, A. J. (2008). Traumatic brain injury: can the consequences be stopped? *Canadian Medical Association Journal, 178*(9), 1163−1170.

Popescu, C., Anghelescu, A., Daia, C., & Onose, G. (2015). Actual data on epidemiological evolution and prevention endeavors regarding traumatic brain injury. *Journal of Medicine and Life, 8*(3), 272−277.

RAI—Resilience and Adjustment Intervention. (2020). Virginia Commonwealth University Family Support Research. Department of Physical Medicine and Rehabilitation; Department of Neuropsychology and Rehabilitation Psychology. <https://tbi.vcu.edu/interventions/>.

Rancho Los Amigos Medical Center. (1980). *Levels of cognitive functioning.* Downey, CA: Rancho Los Amigos Medical Center, Adult Brain Injury Service [Revised by Malkmus, D., Stenderup, K.; 1974. Revised by Hagen, C., 1995].

Rappaport, M., Hall, K. M., Hopkins, K., Belleza, T., & Cope, D. N. (1982). Disability rating scale for severe head trauma: coma to community. *Archives of Physical Medicine and Rehabilitation, 63*(3), 118−123.

Rath, J. F., Simon, D., Langenbahn, D. M., Sherr, R. L., & Diller, L. (2003). Group treatment of problem-solving deficits in outpatients with traumatic brain injury: a randomised outcome study. *Neuropsychological Rehabilitation, 13*(4), 461−488.

Scheiman, M. (2011). Resources [appendix A]. In M. Scheiman (Ed.), *Understanding and managing vision deficits: a guide for occupational therapists* (3rd ed.). Thorofare, NJ: Slack.

Scheiman, M. (2011). Management of refractive, visual efficiency, and visual information processing disorders. In M. Scheiman (Ed.), *Understanding and managing vision deficits: a guide for occupational therapists* (3rd ed.). Thorofare, NJ: Slack.

Senelick, R., & Dougherty, K. (2001). *Living with brain injury.* New York, NY: Guilford Press.

Taylor, C. A., Bell, J. M., Breiding, M. J., & Xu, L. (2017). Traumatic brain injury-related emergency department visits, hospitalizations, and deaths—United States, 2007 and 2013. *MMWR Surveillance Summaries, 66,* 1−16.

Teasdale, G., & Jennett, B. (1974). Assessment of coma and impaired consciousness. A practical scale. *Lancet, 2,* 81−84.

UAB Traumatic Brain Injury Model System. (2019). *Injury control recovery system database.* Washington, DC: National Institute of Disability and Rehabilitation Research, Office of Special Education and Rehabilitative Services. Department of Education. <https://www.uab.edu/medicine/tbi/uab-tbi-information-network/bims-infosheets>.

VA Health Care. (2008). *Mild traumatic brain injury screening and evaluation implemented for OEF/OIF veterans, but challenges remain.* Washington, DC: Government Accountability Office (GAO), GAO-08-276.

Viola-Saltzman, M., & Watson, N. F. (2012). Traumatic brain injury and sleep disorders. *Neurologic Clinics, 30*(4), 1299−1312. Available from http://doi.org/10.1016/j.ncl.2012.08.008.

Weil, Z. M., Corrigan, J. D., & Karelina, K. (2018). Alcohol use disorder and traumatic brain injury. *Alcohol Research, 39*(2), 171−180. <www.arcr.niaaa.nih.gov/arcr392/article06.htm>.

West, T. A., & Sharp, S. (2014). Neuroendocrine dysfunction following TBI: when to screen for it. *The Journal of Family Practice, 63*(1), 11−16.

Wheeler, S., & Acord-Vita, A. (2016). Occupational therapy process for adults with traumatic brain injury [appendix C]. In S. Wheeler, & A. Acord-Vita (Eds.), *Occupational therapy practice guidelines for adults with traumatic brain injury.* Rockville, MD: AOTA Press.

Wilk, J. E., Thomas, J. L., McGurk, D. M., Riviere, L. A., Castro, C. A., & Hoge, C. W. (2010). Mild traumatic brain injury (concussion) during combat: lack of association of blast mechanisms with persistent postconcussive symptoms. *The Journal of Head Trauma Rehabilitation, 25,* 9−14. Available from http://doi.org/10.1097/HTR/0b013ee318bd090f.

Willer, B., Rosenthal, M., Kreutzer, J. S., Gordon, W., & Rempel, R. (1993). Assessment of community integration following rehabilitation for traumatic brain injury. *The Journal of Head Trauma Rehabilitation, 8*(2), 75−87.

Wilson, J. T., Pettigrew, L. E., & Teasdale, G. M. (1998). Structured interviews for the Glasgow Outcome Scale and the extended Glasgow Outcome Scale: guidelines for their use. *Journal of Neurotrauma, 15*(8), 5730585.

World Health Organization. (2001). *International Classification of Functioning, Disability and Health (ICF).* Geneva, Switzerland: WHO.

25

Degenerative Diseases of the Central Nervous System

Megan Samuelson

OBJECTIVES

After reading this chapter, the student or the occupational therapy practitioner will be able to do the following:

1. Describe four degenerative diseases.
2. List the signs and symptoms of these diseases.
3. Understand the focus of occupational therapy related to the treatment of degenerative diseases.
4. Describe the precautions that must be observed in the treatment of these diseases.
5. Recognize and describe evidence-based occupational therapy interventions used to treat clients with degenerative diseases across the various stages of the disease.

KEY TERMS

Degenerative neurologic diseases
Multiple sclerosis (MS)
Parkinson disease (PD)
Amyotrophic lateral sclerosis (ALS)
Alzheimer disease (AD)
Emotional lability
Progressive neurologic diseases

Demyelination
Remission
Exacerbation
Rigidity
Bradykinesia
Dementia
Task segmentation

INTRODUCTION

Degenerative neurologic diseases cause progressive pathologic changes in the central nervous system (CNS), which have an impact on occupational performance. Some have an onset in childhood and others in adulthood. This chapter will focus on the following conditions that typically present in adulthood: **multiple sclerosis (MS)**, **Parkinson disease (PD)**, **amyotrophic lateral sclerosis (ALS)**, and **Alzheimer disease (AD)**. In the cases of these diseases, the CNS functions normally in childhood and adolescence, but begins to deteriorate at the time of disease onset. Changes in the CNS result in loss of functioning in one or more of the following areas: sensation, motor control, and cognition.

No cures exist for these diseases. Effective medical and rehabilitation management can delay and decrease the debilitating effects and allow for better occupational engagement. Occupational therapists (OTs) and occupational therapy assistants (OTAs) optimize quality of life for clients with degenerative neurologic diseases by helping to manage symptoms, compensate for dysfunction, and adapt meaningful daily activities as function declines. Adaptation can occur to the activity, the environment, or the client's skills.

OTs and OTAs consider many factors when working with this population, including the impact of the diagnosis on social, physical, and cultural contexts. They must plan for regularly scheduled reassessment to account for the decline in performance in areas of occupation caused by degeneration, especially in cases where there is limited medical intervention available. They carefully prescribe adaptive devices and/or durable medical equipment based on the length of time it will likely be used. They understand that most client will exhibit inconsistent performance in areas of occupation throughout the day, due to fatigue issues or cognitive changes. For example, clients experiencing cognitive decline may exhibit evening delirium, known as sundowning.

Many psychosocial issues related to coping with a progressive disease need to be taken into account as well. Clients with degenerative conditions deal with end-of-life issues, fear related to probable future decline of function, anxiety, depression, and sense of self while functional independence may be declining. This may lead to **emotional lability**, or uncontrollable periods of crying or laughing. The psychosocial impact of the diagnosis on the family occurs related to role changes, ability to provide care, or potential loss of a loved one.

Working with those presenting with **progressive neurologic diseases** is complex and challenging. Interventions vary based on the stage of the disease and the context in which the OT or OTA is interacting with the client (e.g., acute care vs long-term care vs home). Therefore a client-centered approach, which embraces the autonomy of the individual, the strengths they bring to therapy, the client-therapist interaction, and the decisions they make regarding care, is recommended

---

BOX 25.1 Client-Centered Practice Considerations

1. Recognize that the recipients of occupational therapy are uniquely qualified to make decisions about their occupational functioning.
2. Offer the client a more active role in defining goals and desired outcomes.
3. Make the client-therapist relationship interdependent to enable the solution of performance dysfunction.
4. Shift to a model in which occupational therapists work with clients to enable them to meet their own goals.
5. Focus evaluation (and intervention) on the contexts in which clients live, their roles and interests, and their culture.
6. Allow the client to be the problem definer so that in turn the client will become the problem solver.
7. Allow the client to evaluate his or her own performance and set personal goals.

(Law, Baptiste, & Mills, 1995). Box 25.1 suggests ways to implement client-centered practice. These strategies focus and define the occupational therapy process, empower clients, and allow the practitioner to individually tailor agreed-upon therapy goals.

Occupational Therapy Process

The Canadian Occupational Performance Measure (Law, Baptiste, & Carswell, 2005) is a client-centered, standardized tool that is useful to gather the occupational profile on clients with degenerative conditions due to the multiple and extensive areas in which they may experience disruptions to occupational performance. This assessment allows the client to identify areas of performance difficulty, rate the importance of each, and rate his or her satisfaction with the current performance. It also allows family members and caregivers to give input to prioritize intervention focus.

The occupational profile and analysis of occupational performance provide the OT and the OTA with a thorough understanding of the client's areas of strengths and weaknesses and allows them to establish with the client realistic long-term and short-term goals. These goals focus on maximizing quality of life. This is done by facilitating the client's ability to engage in meaningful occupations as the disease progresses, preventing secondary complications, educating clients on strategies to self-manage the effects of the disease process, and educating caregivers about safe and effective ways to provide assistance to the client while not undermining the client's autonomy.

The degenerative nature of these conditions may lead to the need for various living situations. While clients remain in the home, they benefit from periodic home evaluations. The foci of the home evaluation should be on the following:

- *Elimination of hazardous conditions that could trigger a fall.* One of the main ways to achieve this is to maintain even surfaces whenever possible. This could include leveling doorway thresholds with the floors and replacing gravel or cobblestone walkways. It is also beneficial to remove area rugs, such as throw or scatter rugs. If area rugs need to remain, they should have beveled edges.
- *Consideration of home modifications.* Examples of home modifications include the installation of an elevator, stair-glide, stall shower, or ramp. Accessibility issues may need to be addressed for those clients using a device for gait or wheeled mobility.
- *Education about activity modifications* in the living room includes recommending replacement of deep, low chairs with those with firm cushions, a straight back, and padded armrests. For those clients who cannot get out of the chair independently, automatic lift chairs are available. In the kitchen, commonly used items should be placed so that excessive bending and reaching are not required. The client's walker can be fitted with a bicycle basket to make it easier to carry objects.
- *Assist in the evaluation of necessary assistive devices or durable medical equipment.* In the bathroom, grab bars, a raised toilet seat with a safety frame, and a shower chair or tub transfer bench are recommended. In the bedroom, a sturdy chair with armrests should be used while dressing. A raised bed with a firm mattress and a trapeze over the bed also help with bed mobility. A bedside commode or urinal should be considered when the client makes frequent nighttime trips to the bathroom.

The progressive nature of these diseases requires that treatment goals be established in small increments so that the client may see a measure of progress. The progressive and chronic nature of these diseases may cause clients to require extensive care beyond what is possible within the client's social support system. When the client and family can no longer cope with advancing symptoms in the home, placement in a long-term care facility is indicated. Long-term care facilities provide (1) comprehensive rehabilitation programs, (2) contracture prevention programs (via positioning, splinting, and range of motion [ROM]), (3) decubitus ulcer prevention and treatment, (4) adjunctive medical interventions such as tube feedings, (5) bowel/bladder management strategies, (6) suctioning of respiratory secretions, (7) palliative care, (8) counseling programs, and (9) specialized medical equipment such as mechanical lifts, electric hospital beds, and pressure-relieving mattresses. In addition, they provide the 24-hour supervision needed for client safety, and many have the capacity to provide specialized end-of-life care such as hospice services. Hospice services focus on comfort rather than cure, while emphasizing quality of life, promoting personal choice and dignity, and providing care and support to the bereaved.

CONDITIONS

Multiple Sclerosis (MS)

MS is the most common progressive, disabling neurologic disease in young adults. Its inflammatory process caused by an autoimmune reaction leads to **demyelination** of nerves of the CNS, including the brain, spinal cord, and optic nerves (Reidak, Jackson, & Giovannoni, 2010). Myelin, the tissue surrounding and protecting the nerve fibers of the CNS, helps nerve fibers conduct electrical impulses. In MS, the body mistakenly attacks and destroys the myelin in multiple areas (demyelination), leaving scar tissue known as sclerosis. These damaged areas are also known as plaques or lesions. The two processes of demyelination and plaque formation impede the transmission of nerve impulses to and from the brain. The signs and symptoms that manifest depend on the area(s) that develop plaques (Kalb & Reitman, 2010). Occupational therapy plays a key role in the rehabilitation of those with MS (Finlayson, 2008).

Epidemiology. Seventy percent of individuals with MS manifest symptoms between 20 and 40 years of age, usually around age 30. Almost 70% of individuals manifest symptoms between ages 20 and 40. Although less common, it can occur in children, teens, and older adults. MS affects women more commonly than men (2 women for every 3.1 men).

Some genetic and environmental causes are associated with MS, although there is no strong causation. Individuals who have a close relative with MS have a 1/40 chance of developing it. Those without a relative with it have a 1/750 chance of developing it. Whites are more often affected than in Hispanics or Blacks. It is more prevalent in higher latitudes. MS affects approximately 400,000 in the United States and 2.1 million people worldwide (Calabresi, 2004; DeMaagd & Philip, 2015; Graff, Vernooij-Dassen, & Thijssen, 2006; Hatakeyama, Okamoto, Kamata, & Kasuga, 2000; Kalb & Reitman, 2010; Reidak et al., 2010; Solaro et al., 2015).

Disease Course. Evidence of damage to at least two separate parts of the CNS at two points in time is required for the disease to be diagnosed and others to be ruled out. MS may follow various courses related to progression. There are four specific courses of progression (Calabresi, 2004; Graff et al., 2006; Hatakeyama et al., 2000):

1. *Relapsing/Remitting.* Eighty-five percent of those initially diagnosed with MS present with this course, which is characterized by acute attacks with full or partial recovery. Between attacks the disease does not progress.
2. *Secondary Progressive.* This course progresses at a variable rate after one experienced a relapsing/remitting course. Fifty percent of those initially diagnosed with a relapsing/remitting course develop secondary progressive within 10 years and 90% within 25 years.
3. *Primary Progressive.* Ten percent of diagnosed MS cases follow this course, which causes progressive disability without **remission** from the onset of the disease.
4. *Progressive Relapsing.* Five percent of diagnosed MS cases are progressive from the onset with clear acute relapses.

Impact on Client Factors. Each client with MS will present with a unique set of clinical manifestations depending on the locations of the lesions and the stage of the disease process. Symptoms directly caused by demyelination include fatigue, visual disturbances (Frohman, 2008), cognitive disturbances (Schiffer, 2008) (slowed processing, memory loss [including explicit and episodic memory], decreased attention [including alternating and divided attention], impairment of executive functions), affective disturbances (depression, bipolar disorders, lability, euphoria, antisocial behavior) (Arnett, Higginson, Voss, Randolph, & Grandey, 2002; Kesselring, 2004; Law et al., 2005; Samuel & Cavallo, 2008), sensory changes (numbness, tingling, pain), loss of postural control, dizziness and vertigo, tremor, dysphagia, speech disturbances, heat intolerance, spasticity (Kushner & Brandfass, 2008), weakness, ambulation disturbances, sexual dysfunction, and bowel/bladder dysfunction (Holland, 2008; Holland & Reitman, 2008).

Medical Management. Medical treatment for MS focuses primarily on alleviating symptoms with antidepressants and antispasmodic medications (Calabresi, 2004; Graff et al., 2006; Hatakeyama et al., 2000). High-dose corticosteroids are used to control for acute **exacerbations**. Immunomodulators are used to reduce the number of relapses and limit the development of new lesions. Typical drugs include Avonex, Betaseron, Copaxone, Novantrone, Tysabri, and Rebif. The OTA can assist the physician by reporting changes in the client's behavior and physical status.

During the chronic stages of MS, medical management of the disease may include catheterization for urinary dysfunction, tube feeding for swallowing disorders, and nerve blocks or surgical release of tendons for treatment of severe contractures.

Occupational Therapy Process for Clients With MS. The unpredictable course of the disease can be challenging for OTs and OTAs. The variable and unpredictable course changes a client's functional ability and level of independence at varying times throughout the day, from day to day, and over the course of the disease. For example, a client who uses a sliding board to transfer may require only supervision in the morning but may require physical assistance by the afternoon. These changes require a therapist who is in tune with the client and able to make regular adjustments to the intervention plan.

Precautions. The functional status of an MS client may be affected by a variety of factors such as stress, heat, pain, fatigue, and exacerbations (Multiple Sclerosis Council for Clinical Practice Guidelines, 1998). OTs and OTAs should assist clients with MS to avoid overfatigue. They should also assist them to monitor for safety issues secondary to loss of postural control and/or cognitive impairment and be aware of combined effects of cognitive and physical impairments.

OTs and OTAs should educate clients to guarding against soft tissue injury secondary to sensory loss. They should use caution around potential dangers such as sharp objects and hot water. They should monitor the effects of room temperature on well-being. For example, cooler room temperatures are better than warmer rooms. Finally, thermal modalities, such as hot packs, should be used with caution due to possibilities of sensory loss and heat intolerance.

Evaluation. The initial evaluation process for the MS client sets the tone and prepares both the client and the OT or OTA for the treatment sessions to follow. OTAs should utilize the principles of a client-centered assessment (Pollock, 1993) (see Box 25.1) because of the multiple areas of occupation that are affected. The client and caregivers should determine which occupations are to be addressed first. The results of the evaluation determine the areas appropriate for remediation (deconditioning) and those for compensatory techniques (wheeled mobility). OTs and OTAs should clearly explain the reason for the evaluation and describe what will occur during the evaluation to alleviate anxiety or stress. Rest breaks should be incorporated if the client becomes fatigued. The evaluation process should culminate in an intervention plan agreed upon by both the therapist and the client with an emphasis on the improvement and/or maintenance of meaningful occupations needed for maximal independence.

The evaluation includes assessment of client factors, activity patterns, areas of occupation, and quality-of-life issues. Client factors include strength, muscle tone, sensation, coordination, joint ROM, endurance, balance, vision, and cognitive functions.

Performance in areas of occupation including basic and instrumental activities of daily living (ADL, IADL), work, and play/leisure must be evaluated objectively (Finlayson, 2008). The OT should address sleep patterns, as disrupted sleep can contribute to fatigue levels. The ADL evaluation may be administered by an experienced OTA who has demonstrated competency in these evaluation techniques. The coordination and interpretation of the evaluation results comprise the role of the OT.

Intervention. The treatment methods selected for MS clients are determined by individual goals for the client and are guided by the client's clinical presentation. Due to the progressive nature of MS, interventions and goals should be focused on the client's need to adapt as the disability progresses.

Improving participation via fatigue management. Of clients with MS, 75% to 95% experience fatigue and 50% to 60% report it to be the factor that most limits participation (National Clinical Advisory Board, 2008a). Fatigue-related disruption to participation is caused by comorbid medical conditions, psychological issues (anxiety and stress), disrupted sleep, poor trunk stability, movement disorders, and the environment (increased ambient temperature).

MS-related fatigue has been characterized as primary and secondary fatigue. Primary fatigue is due to the disease process: cortical damage, conduction blocks from demyelinated motor pathways, increased energy demands for muscle activation, and increased energy demands from co-contraction of agonists and antagonists. Secondary fatigue is due to deconditioning, respiratory muscle weakness, and pain (Multiple Sclerosis Council for Clinical Practice Guidelines, 1998).

A two-step process can be used to treat MS-related fatigue (National Clinical Advisory Board, 2008a). The first is to eliminate secondary causes of fatigue (depression, medication imbalance, impaired sleep) and manage fatigue-causing symptoms (tremor, excess energy expenditure). The second is to manage primary fatigue through the combination of pharmacology and energy conservation techniques.

Interventions to counteract fatigue and improve occupational participation include cooling via use of a cooling garment (Multiple Sclerosis Council for Clinical Practice Guidelines, 1998; Schwid et al., 2003), energy conservation techniques (Box 25.2) (Mathiowetz, Matuska, & Murphy, 2001; Multiple Sclerosis Council for Clinical Practice Guidelines, 1998; Vanage, Gilbertson, & Mathiowetz, 2003), and aerobic conditioning (Petajan et al., 1996). Aerobic training can be helpful in reducing fatigue (Petajan et al., 1996). The OT and OTA must carefully determine the correct intensity and duration of the exercise program to prevent exacerbation of symptoms.

Improving participation via control of tremors and movement disorders. Movement disorders such as tremor and ataxia are common problems for people living with MS. Compensatory strategies appear to be the most successful for controlling movement disorders and improve performance despite their presence (Box 25.3) (Gillen, 2000; Gillen, 2002; Jones, Lewis, Harrison, & Wiles, 1996).

Improving participation via cognitive compensations. Decreased cognitive functioning significantly impedes the rehabilitation process because the client is less able to store and receive new information. Cognitive changes may be present throughout the disease and fluctuate with time of day, task difficulty, and environmental distractions; cognitive function may worsen with fatigue (Bobholz & Rao, 2003). Short-term and long-term memory deficits contribute to confusion and agitation. New information should be presented to the client simply and repetitively. Consistency in the therapy program as to day, time, and modalities helps to orient the client and minimize frustration. Compensatory strategies seem

---

BOX 25.2 Energy Conservation Techniques Used by Clients With Multiple Sclerosis

- Pacing
- Successful work/rest ratio
- Use of electronic aids as needed
- Flexible home and work schedules
- Recognition of fatigue warning signals
- Successful use of compensatory strategies
- Acceptance of a request for assistance
- Home/work modifications
- Appropriate ambulatory aids
- Power mobility aids (power wheelchair or scooter)
- Control of spasticity
- Improved trunk control
- Techniques to control tremor
- Activities of daily living assistive devices
- Durable medical equipment
- Heat control
- Pharmacologic interventions

BOX 25.3 Interventions Related to Ataxia and Tremor

- Orthotics/splinting (wrist support, thumb support via opponens splints, cervical collar)
- Using the environment for stability (e.g., leaning on the work surface, high-back chairs)
- Adaptive devices (Dycem, long straw, suction devices, built-up handles)
- Assistive technology (speaker phone, adapted mouse/keyboard)
- Weights (wrist weights, weighted gloves, weighted devices, etc.) may be effective for subtle movement disorders
- Posture/position of activity focused on trunk support
- Minimize the number of joints moving simultaneously during activities
- Keep upper extremities stabilized against the trunk
- Keep the elbow on the work surface (propping)
- Promote a calm/focused emotional state
- Control fatigue
- Adapt activities to eliminate the need to reach into space
- Decrease effort
- Decrease fine motor coordination demands
- Experiment with both slow and fast movements
- Provide exercise for proximal (trunk/scapula) stability
- Pharmacologic management

BOX 25.4 Cognitive Strategies Used by Clients With Multiple Sclerosis

- Use memory aids: timers, watch alarms, personal data assistants, reminder lists, memory books, Post-it notes, computerized organizers, dictation systems.
- Allow extra time for task completion and processing.
- Decrease environmental distractions.
- Avoid multitasking.
- Schedule difficult cognitive tasks during periods of high energy.
- Avoid fatigue.
- Delegate responsibilities.
- Solve problems aloud.
- Check work for accuracy.
- Keep organized and avoid clutter.
- Determine which (visual or auditory) processing system is most effective.

to be the most effective intervention because remediation of cognitive deficits (e.g., memory drills) has little research support (Graff et al., 2006) (Box 25.4).

According to the National Multiple Sclerosis Society, "Interventions should be designed to improve the person's ability to function in all meaningful aspects of family and community life. Intervention should involve systematic, functionally oriented, therapeutic activities that are based on understanding of specific deficits (National Clinical Advisory Board, 2008b; Ghahari & Finlayson, 2018) (Fig. 25.1). Commonly, a compensatory approach is used. This may

include strategies such as cognitive structuring, in which cognitive tasks are learned and practiced as a routine. The client might also be encouraged to substitute intact cognitive abilities to compensate for abilities that are impaired. For example, the client who does not remember the words for certain items might use pictures instead. To reduce fatigue the client might use organizers, employ assistive technology, and schedule activities for times of day when energy is higher. A structured environment and structured routines conserve energy and promote organization. Memory strategies (e.g., lists, mnemonics, clustering, visualization techniques) and recording devices might also be used. To improve attention and reduce distractibility, it is helpful to maintain a quiet environment. The specific strategies and solutions should be individual and client centered, focusing on desired areas of participation and providing increased functioning (National Clinical Advisory Board, 2008b).

Improving participation via managing sensory deficits. A variety of sensory and perceptual disorders affect clients with MS. OTs and OTAs most often focus on educating the client and family to be aware of issues and to use compensatory techniques. Tactile and perceptual dysfunction, such as impaired sensation and astereognosis, interfere with fine motor tasks such as buttoning, managing utensils, money manipulation, computer use, and writing. Clients with intact visual skills may be able to compensate visually. Other adaptations such as built-up handles, use of Velcro, and universal cuffs may help the client compensate (see Chapter 13).

The impaired sense of pain and temperature could cause burns or other injuries. Clients should use caution during kitchen and bathroom activities. Clients with MS may also experience increased pain due to open wounds, muscle imbalance, overuse injuries, and postural malalignment. Some interventions to decrease pain may be helpful and include deep breathing, visualization, biofeedback, correcting muscle imbalance, correcting postural alignment, transcutaneous electrical nerve stimulation (TENS), cryotherapy (cooling), and occupational adaptation to decrease the use of compensatory movement patterns.

Visual deficits such as double vision, blurred vision, decreased acuity, and nystagmus may make even simple ADL difficult. Clients can be taught compensatory techniques such as covering one eye (full or partial visual occlusion) to minimize double vision or using devices for those with low vision such as magnifying glasses, large-print books, and audiobooks. See Chapter 21 for interventions for clients with visual and sensory loss.

Clients with MS are taught by the OTA to plan their day and pace themselves accordingly (see Box 25.1). Planning and energy conservation help the client budget strength and endurance to meet daily needs. Important activities, including exercises, are done in the morning or after a scheduled nap or rest period. Graded resistive exercises increase the strength of key muscle groups and should be targeted to specific muscle groups that are task specific. To increase endurance, emphasis should be placed on increasing repetitions rather than increasing weights. The benefits of aerobic exercise for this

Personal factors	Environmental factors	Occupational factors
Symptoms of MS and other health conditions (e.g., fatigue, pain, balance)	**Physical environment** (e.g., accessibility, use of assistive technology)	**Physical demands of the task or activity** (e.g., need to bend, reach, lift, carry)
Physical capacities (e.g., strength, joint motion)	**Social environment** (e.g., presence and type of social supports)	**Cognitive and perceptual demands of the task/activity** (e.g., need to multi-task, remember complex sequences, visual-spatial demands)
Cognitive and perceptual capacities (e.g., memory, attention, problem solving, visual-spatial abilities)	**Cultural environment** (e.g., values, expectations)	**Steps and sequencing of the activity** (e.g., number of steps, flexibility of sequences)
Psychological and emotional issues (e.g., self-efficacy, mental health)	**Socio-economic issues** (e.g., cost of medication)	**Temporal aspects of the activity** (e.g., when it is performed, for how long)
Specific skills and knowledge relative to performance of the tasks and activities in question (e.g., knowledge of meal preparation)		**Need for or use of specific tools and technology during the activity** (e.g., computer, appliances, adapted devices)

Fig. 25.1 Physical, environmental, and occupational factors related to MS. (From Ghahari S, Finlayson M. *A Resource for Healthcare Professionals: Occupational Therapy in Multiple Sclerosis Rehabilitation.* New York, NY: National Multiple Sclerosis Society; 2018.)

population have been documented in terms of improved fitness and quality of life (Petajan et al., 1996).

Clients with severe loss of muscle strength sometimes can perform functional activities with the help of devices that substitute for weak muscles. For example, the OTA may encourage the client to use an overhead suspension sling or mobile arm support to increase independence (Fig. 25.2).

Contracture prevention and treatment. Clients with severe weakness that prevents full active ROM (AROM), as well as those with spasticity, have the potential to develop soft tissue contractures. Contracture is prevented by deliberate and regular limb movement; active movement is preferred over passive when possible. Moving the client through complete ROM—and not just the middle ranges—is essential. Therapists must determine what a full ROM is for each individual client. A joint that moves or is moved through its full ROM via engagement in daily activities rarely develops deformities. A program of AROM and passive ROM (PROM) combined with a terminal stretch at least twice per day is recommended if contracture is beginning to develop. Low-load prolonged stretch via splints or positioning must be used if a contracture has developed. During the terminal stretch, the proximal body part should be well stabilized.

Whenever possible, the client should perform self-ranging techniques. PROM of each joint through the full range should be done daily. The OT or OTA may be responsible for teaching the family or a nursing assistant the techniques of ROM.

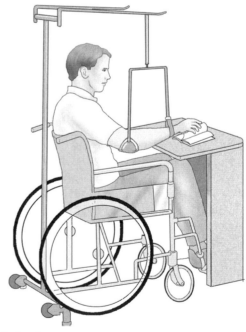

Fig. 25.2 Overhead suspension sling used for those with proximal UE weakness to enhance self-feeding, computer use, etc. (From Gillen G. *Stroke Rehabilitation: A Function-Based Approach.* 3rd ed. St Louis, MO: Elsevier; 2010.)

The OT may administer inhibition techniques (such as icing or positioning to decrease tone before PROM) to clients with severe spasticity. Splints to maintain range or provide sustained stretch may be indicated to treat or prevent contractures of the elbow, wrist, ankle, or hand.

Activities of daily living. Independence in ADL promotes self-esteem and quality of life (Kesselring, 2004). OTs and OTAs may provide assistive devices and adaptive techniques to enable MS clients to be safer, more independent, and more efficient in both ADL and IADL. Cups with lids, scoop dishes, and adapted utensils assist eating. Long-handled shoe horns, reachers, sock aids, and elastic shoelaces are some of the devices that can increase independence and ease of dressing (see Chapter 13). The OTA works with the client to evaluate the effectiveness of equipment and to provide training on an individual basis. As the disease progresses, modifications in equipment and techniques will be necessary. A client with limited strength and severe impairment in mobility may require an environmental control unit (ECU) to operate lights, television, or radio (see Chapter 14).

Communication. Clients with MS may experience disruptions in written and verbal communication. OTs and OTAs can collaborate with the speech therapist to devise a method of improving communication skills. Augmentative and alternative communication devices can be useful to clients with severe disruption in speech. The OTA may provide equipment that enables the client to use these devices, such as splints for upper extremity (UE) stabilization or mouth sticks. Adaptive writing devices (built-up and weighted pens, pen holders, and magnetized wrist stabilizers) compensate for decreased coordination and weakness. Special computer keyboards and large-button and speech-activated telephones assist independent communication for clients with motor deficits. (see Chapter 14).

Seating and wheeled mobility. As the disease progresses, many clients will require the use of a wheelchair (manual or electric) or power scooter for mobility. The primary considerations in recommending a wheelchair for an MS client are as follows:

- Overall endurance
- Trunk control
- Lower extremity (LE) strength, coordination, sensation, and endurance
- UE strength, coordination, sensation, and endurance
- Disease prognosis

Clients with sufficient UE strength and overall endurance should have a lightweight, high-strength manual wheelchair if they are to propel themselves. Clients with a rapidly progressive type of the disease may require wheelchairs with reclining backs or a tilt-in-space (Gillen, 2000) frame to compensate for diminished trunk control. In some cases, an electric wheelchair or electric scooter may be indicated. Wheelchair modifications that can be useful include oblique rim projections, lateral supports, solid back and seat inserts, head positioners, and brake extensions (Gillen, 2000). Training in wheelchair mobility and transfer techniques may be taught as part of the client's occupational therapy program. Geri-chairs may be used in long-term care settings for clients who are unable to propel a chair and who require added postural support.

OTs and OTAs can focus on safe positioning of clients while they are in their wheelchair and on other surfaces.

Impaired sensation, incontinence, and decreased mobility put clients with MS at an increased risk for skin breakdown. Interventions to prevent skin breakdown include pressure-relieving mattresses and wheelchair cushions as well as pressure relief protocols. Wheelchair pushups are effective for clients with adequate strength.

Leisure skills. Leisure skills provide mental and social stimulation and substitute avocational interests for vocational skills. The OTA can assist the client by stressing the importance of activity engagement and by recommending adaptive devices such as card holders, shufflers, and adapted board games. The client should be encouraged to manage time effectively, planning for social events with naps and limited exercise on days when evening activities are scheduled (Lomen-Hoerth et al., 2003).

Work. Clients with MS may be able to maintain their ability to work during various stages of the disease or during **remission**. Through incorporating modifications to their schedule and adaptive devices to increase ease-of-work tasks, they can continue meaningful occupations. Worksite modifications for wheelchair accessibility may be required. The OTA may assist the OT in conducting the vocational evaluation, which may be used to determine a worker's ability to continue the job, and in making recommendations for adaptive equipment. The interventions might include (but are not limited to) use of technology or mobility aids, workstation modification, or change in how the tasks are completed. Throughout the advanced stages of the disease, maintenance of function and compensation for lost function are necessary (Ghahari & Finlayson, 2018).

Psychosocial issues. A diagnosis of MS can lead to shock, denial, and anger. As the disease progresses, the client may become depressed (Joy & Johnston, 2001; Mohr, Classen, & Barrera, 2004; Mohr et al., 1999). Incidence of depression is higher for people living with MS than for the general population or for people with other neurologic diagnoses. Other affective conditions include bipolar disorder, lability, and (less commonly) antisocial behavior. Assets and characteristics of those who cope well with MS (and other diagnoses) include the following (Arnett et al., 2002; Mohr et al., 1999):

- Support
- Connectedness
- Sense of humor
- Spirituality
- Openness

OTs and OTAs may assist in fostering adaptive coping strategies such as active coping, seeking emotional support, seeking instrumental support, positive reframing, planning, humor, acceptance, and religion (Meyer, 2001).

The OTA can offer emotional support to both the client and family. The client should be encouraged to maintain a daily schedule of activity. Referral to MS support groups sponsored by the local Multiple Sclerosis Society may be helpful in dealing with the daily stress of having a chronic progressive disease. Additional support and information are available online at the reference and health sites and in chat groups.

The members of the rehabilitation team, including the OTA, have an obligation to help the family and the client adjust to the disease and to provide encouragement, emotional support, training, and exercise programs. Occupational therapy can help the MS client function as productively as possible within the limits of the disease.

Parkinson Disease

PD is a slow, chronic, progressive disease of the nervous system that was first described by James Parkinson in 1817 as "shaking palsy" (Solaro et al., 2015). Four cardinal signs of PD include resting tremor, **rigidity** in skeletal muscle, **bradykinesia** (slow movements), and postural instability. Pathology is characterized by degeneration in dopaminergic pathways in the basal ganglia, particularly in the substantia nigra. The function of the substantia nigra is to produce dopamine, the neurotransmitter that transports signals to motor control areas such as the caudate and putamen. In PD, dopaminergic neurons deteriorate at a fast rate, and the amount of dopamine that is produced decreases, resulting in initial impairments. When signs and symptoms are noticed, 80% of the dopaminergic neurons have already deteriorated. Diagnosis is made by the presence of at least two of the cardinal signs and the client's response to levodopa, a dopamine precursor (Clarke & Moore, 2004; National Institute of Neurological Disorders and Stroke, 2006).

The symptom complex of PD is termed parkinsonism. Not all clients with parkinsonism have PD. Besides the formal diagnoses of PD, other pathologies that result in parkinsonism include drug-induced parkinsonism (i.e., parkinsonism caused by antipsychotic medications), progressive supranuclear palsy, corticobasal degeneration, multiple system atrophy, and vascular parkinsonism (i.e., multiple small strokes) (National Institute of Neurological Disorders and Stroke, 2006).

Epidemiology. At least 500,000 Americans are living with diagnosed PD. Approximately 50,000 individuals are diagnosed each year, and thousands of people live with the disease undiagnosed. PD has a male to female ratio of 3 to 2. Although the average age of diagnosis is 60, approximately 15% of those living with PD are diagnosed before age 40 (Clarke & Moore, 2004; National Institute of Neurological Disorders and Stroke, 2006; Walter & Vitek, 2004).

Disease Course. The cause of PD is not clear. Researchers hypothesize that causes include a combination of genetic and environmental factors. Approximately 15% to 25% of people living with PD have a relative with the disease. Risk of developing PD is increased twofold to threefold if a first-degree relative is affected. Those who sustain serious and recurrent traumatic brain injuries (e.g., professional boxers) may develop a form of PD, as may those living in rural conditions and those exposed to herbicides, pesticides, or some synthetic narcotic agents. Further research continues to attempt to establish the cause of the disease (Clarke & Moore, 2004; National Institute of Neurological Disorders and Stroke, 2006).

Impact on Client Factors. PD primarily affects motor skills. Research suggests that pathophysiologic changes associated with PD, such as sleep disorders, depression, and cognitive changes, may start before the onset of motor features (Schrag, Horsfall, Walters, Noyce, & Petersen, 2015; Solaro et al., 2015). The four primary symptoms, according to the National Institute of Neurological Disorders and Stroke, are as follows (National Institute of Neurological Disorders and Stroke, 2006):

- *Tremor.* Typically this is a pill-rolling tremor involving the thumb and forefinger, which move rhythmically back and forth at a rate of four to six beats per second (National Institute of Neurological Disorders and Stroke, 2006). Although tremor often begins in a hand, it may in some people first affect another body part such as a foot. Generally, the tremor increases with stress and is visible when the person is awake and the body is at rest (not moving). Intentional movement reduces the tremor, which also disappears during sleep.
- *Rigidity.* Most people with PD experience some rigidity (resistance to movement). This rigidity is caused by an imbalance in the innervation of agonist-antagonist coordination. Antagonist muscles remain contracted instead of relaxing when the agonist (primary mover) contracts. Muscular rigidity classically manifests as cogwheel rigidity (short, jerky movements caused with passive range).
- *Bradykinesia.* Bradykinesia manifests as a slowing of voluntary and automatic movements, resulting in difficulty performing ordinary daily activities with ease. Bathing, dressing, and other daily activities take much longer to perform.
- *Postural instability.* Balance is impaired and clients are at risk of falling. A stooped posture with forward head position may be present (National Institute of Neurological Disorders and Stroke, 2006). Clients may also fall backwards during standing activities (retropulsion) (Winogrodzka, Wagenaar, Booij, & Wolters, 2005).

Rigidity and postural instability result in typical gait patterns that are characterized by a stooped-forward posture; loose arm swing; a slow, shuffling gait; or a festinating gait (small, fast steps, which propel forward with ever-increasing speed). The client has difficulty in stopping the forward motion. Episodes of freezing (Panisset, 2004) (sudden difficulty walking through doorways or making turns) are experienced during gait. In addition, other motor impairments such as a small and crowded writing style (micrographia) and decreased facial expression (mask face) may be present.

Dysfunction in oral musculature may result in drooling, dysphagia, and monotone speech with low volume as PD progresses (Solaro et al., 2015). The client may also demonstrate disorders in bowel and bladder control. Depression is common in this population (Lemke et al., 2004). **Dementia** and other cognitive problems are common. "Some, but not all, people with PD may develop memory problems and slow thinking. In some of these cases, cognitive problems become more severe, leading to a condition called Parkinson's dementia late in the course of the disease. This dementia may affect memory, social judgment, language, reasoning, or other mental skills" (National Institute of Neurological Disorders and Stroke, 2006). Other impairments include emotional changes, urinary problems or constipation, skin problems, sleep problems, orthostatic hypotension, muscle cramps and dystonia, pain, fatigue and loss of energy, and sexual dysfunction (National Institute of Neurological Disorders and Stroke, 2006). Occupational therapy intervention can be tailored to the stage of progression the client is experiencing (Box 25.5) (Hoehn & Yahr, 1967).

Medical Management. PD cannot be cured. The focus of medical management is the relief of symptoms through medication and surgery. Sinemet, a combined carbidopa-levodopa formula, is a common formula of the most frequently prescribed PD medication (Calabresi, 2004), levodopa (a drug converted to dopamine in the brain) (National Institute of Neurological Disorders and Stroke, 2006). Sinemet leads to on-off periods that result in a fluctuation in motor and functional status. Working with clients during times when the medication is at both an optimal and suboptimal level provides OTs and OTAs with a full overview of the client's functioning throughout the day. Required levels of assistance vary greatly depending on the timing of drug administration (Dixon et al., 2007). Other commonly prescribed medications (apomorphine, bromocriptine, pramipexole, ropinirole) are dopamine agonists (i.e., they mimic dopamine in the brain) (National Institute of Neurological Disorders and Stroke, 2006). Dopamine drugs may cause nausea and decreased blood pressure; therefore clients should be monitored closely. In older adults, dopamine agonists may result in hallucinations. The OTA should report any adverse reactions to the physician as soon as possible.

In the early stages of PD, milder dopamine agonist medications and anticholinergic drugs are prescribed to reduce rigidity and tremor. As symptoms progress, levodopa is added to control them. Medications to treat depression and pain, as well as nutritional supplements, may also be prescribed.

Surgical options to manage symptoms include deep brain stimulation, pallidotomy, and thalamotomy (Walter & Vitek,

2004). These may be used more frequently in those for whom medication is not effective. Surgical interventions are most effective to control tremor, bradykinesia, and rigidity. They do not directly prevent loss of balance, slow gait, speech impairments, and postural deficits.

Occupational Therapy Process for Clients With PD. Those living with PD experience substantial restrictions to participation and limitations in activity. Multiple client factors adversely affect their performance in many areas of occupation. In addition, those living with PD may limit their involvement in life situations because of fear of falling and concerns related to continence, drooling, or the time and energy expenditure required to participate in meaningful occupations. A decreased ability to participate in daily life will lead to a referral for occupational therapy services (Gillen, 2009; Murphy & Tickle-Degnen, 2001).

Precautions. Safety during ambulation is very important for clients with PD. They are at an increased risk for falls due to impairments in postural control orthostatic hypotension. In addition, doorways, elevators, crowds, and surface changes may trigger freezing behavior (Panisset, 2004). Dysphagia is a risk so all eating and swallowing precautions should be followed. Impairments in mobility and incontinence increase the risk of skin breakdown. Pressure-relieving wheelchair cushions and mattresses and pressure relief protocols should be encouraged to decrease the risk of skin breakdown.

Evaluation. The OT, with input from the OTA, will evaluate functional performance levels related to work, leisure, ADL, and IADL. In addition, measurement of flexibility, strength, quality of movement, rigidity, standing and sitting balance, cognitive skills, and coordination will be completed.

Occupational therapy intervention. Evidence-based reviews of rehabilitation strategies, including occupational therapy interventions, have demonstrated a positive effect on both client factors and areas of occupation (de Goede, Keus, Kwakkel, & Wagenaar, 2001; Dixon et al., 2007; Murphy & Tickle-Degnen, 2001; Patti, Reggio, Nicoletti, Sellaroli, & Nicoletti, 1996; Steultjens, Dekker, Bouter, Leemrijse, & van den Ende, 2005; Trend, Kaye, Gage, Owen, & Wade, 2002). In addition, they have demonstrated the need for further research to solidify the evidence base for occupational therapy intervention. In general, reviews have concluded that people living with PD can effectively learn new tasks and improve their functional performance through focused practice of meaningful tasks (Murphy & Tickle-Degnen, 2001).

Improving participation in areas of occupation. Clients with PD benefit from learning strategies designed to increase efficiency, safety, and independence (Corr, Frost, Traynor, & Hardiman, 1998). Strategies may be learned via graded task-specific practice and may include the use of adaptive devices and environmental modifications (Box 25.6) (Gillen, 2009; Patti et al., 1996; Ward & Robertson, 2003).

The client should attend physical therapy for gait training as a foundation for functional mobility. The OT can supplement this training by using verbal cues to remind the client to stand erect, lift the feet, and follow the prescribed gait pattern.

BOX 25.5 Staging the Advancement of Parkinson Disease

Hoehn and Yahr Scale

Stage 1: Unilateral tremor, rigidity, bradykinesia, minimal or no functional impairment

Stage 2: Bilateral tremor, rigidity, bradykinesia, with or without axial signs such as facial involvement, independent with activities of daily living (ADL), no balance impairment

Stage 3: Worsening of symptoms, impaired righting reactions, disability related to ADL, balance changes, may still maintain independence with interventions

Stage 4: Requires help with some or all ADL, cannot live alone without assistance, able to walk and stand

Stage 5: Confined to a bed or wheelchair, maximal assistance required

Bed mobility skills, transfer training, and wheelchair mobility skills should be taught by the OTA if indicated. As the client's ambulation status declines, a power or manual wheelchair may be required. The client should be advised to purchase a lightweight wheelchair. Oblique rim projections, a pressure-relieving cushion, elevating swing-away leg rests, and reclining backs should be considered.

Community mobility is often impaired during the middle and late stages of PD. Addressing transportation options and creating a plan for engaging in community mobility should be part of the occupational therapy intervention plan. Clients with PD oftentimes require assistance from others for transportation. It is important to be aware of community mobility services and support programs to decrease caregiver burden and dependence on family members for daily errands.

PD often impacts participation in individuals' hobbies and interests. The OT and OTA should collaborate with their client on intervention priorities to retain a sense of self and normalcy. Adaptive devices for playing cards and board games, gardening, and doing crafts are available through various vendors. The OTA may have to encourage the client and family to develop new interests.

Motor skills/prevention of deformities. The increased rigidity and tendency toward immobility increase the risk of contracture development and general deconditioning. The client with PD requires a daily home exercise program for AROM and stretching, as well as clinic appointments in which the exercise program can be closely supervised by the OTA or OT. The frequency of therapy is determined by the physician in consultation with the OT. AROM exercises may be done individually or in a group setting. Passive and/or active stretching exercises are indicated to maintain flexibility. Typical muscle groups and individual muscles that become limited and are a focus for stretching include the following:

- Hip flexors
- Knee flexors
- Gastrocnemius
- Pectoralis major and minor
- Anterior trunk/neck musculature

In the later stages of the disease, splinting may be indicated to maintain joint ranges and skin integrity. Verbal prompting and visual cues (sitting client in front of mirror) can be used to promote improved postural control. It is common for clients with PD to experience shallow breathing. Encourage the client to take deep breaths and offer breathing exercises if indicated.

Clinicians can use visual, tactile, and auditory cues to help clients initiate movement (Ma, Trombly, Tickle-Degnen, & Wagenaar, 2004; Tse & Spaulding, 1998). Auditory cues should be short, firmly spoken commands such as "stop" and "step up." Rhythmic music and counting can also help to initiate movement. Auditory commands coupled with counting are especially helpful in teaching the client transfer techniques and during functional mobility tasks.

Graded resistive exercises and gross motor activities, particularly sports activities, are used to develop strength and general mobility. Functional fine motor tasks such as jewelry making, manipulating money, and picking up small objects may assist in developing and maintaining hand function and coordination. These tasks can be graded by changing the size of the objects. The clinician should monitor and record the time it takes for the client to complete the task. Hand-strengthening modalities include repetitions with hand grippers and therapeutic putty exercises.

Communication. Clients with PD often experience disruptions to communication such as monotone, low-volume speech. OTs and OTAs can increase the benefits of speech therapy by providing breathing and postural exercises.

BOX 25.6 Examples of Modifications in Activities of Daily Living for People Living With Parkinson Disease

Feeding skills may be improved with weighted utensils (for subtle tremors), scoop dishes, Dycem products, long straws, rocker knives, and cups with lids. Because of the control required for this task, meals should be timed with peak medication effects. See Box 25.3 for suggestions related to tremor control during feeding. Consider safe swallow strategies such as small bites/sips, alternating solids/liquids, staying upright after a meal, and avoiding taking thin liquids by straw. Food consistencies and the thickness of liquids should be considered.

Dressing skills may be enhanced with easy-to-use front fasteners (Velcro closures, elastic shoelaces, elastic waist bands, zipper pulls). Because of balance deficits, clients should be discouraged from bending down to don shoes and socks. Clients should instead be taught to sit and use long-handled shoehorns, reachers, sock aids, and dressing sticks and always to be seated when dressing. Clients with a shuffling gait should not wear rubber-soled or crepe-soled shoes because they may cause tripping. Flat leather soles are preferred. Ordering clothing one size larger may also ease donning and doffing procedures. Increased time should be scheduled for dressing.

Grooming tasks are simplified with electric toothbrushes, electric razors, and hands-free hair dryers. Bimanual oral care and shaving may be helpful. Suction brushes and soap holders may increase ease of grooming. Grooming tasks should be performed while seated. See Box 25.3 for suggestions about controlling tremors that interfere with grooming.

Bathing can be performed safely and more independently using long-handled brushes, soap on a rope, soap pumps, and bath mitts. Durable medical equipment such as a bath bench or seat, grab bars, and a handheld shower will decrease fall risks and increase independence as well. No-slip bathmats (inside and outside the tub) should be considered. Sliding doors should be replaced with curtains.

Toileting ability is enhanced and made safer via raised toilet seats, 3:1 commode, or toilet frames in conjunction with grab bars. Bedside commodes, male/female urinals, or condom-style catheters for men may be options for nighttime toileting needs.

Written communication may be enhanced by rhythmic writing programs, lined paper, or built-up pens. Printing may be easier than cursive writing. Word processors may be an option for some.

Diminished blinking responses and disturbances of the ocular muscles may impair the client's ability to read and write. Adaptations and modifications for writing/reading tasks include:

- Large-print books and audiobooks
- Computers and word processors
- Felt-tip markers
- Signature stamp for in the workplace
- Cordless and automatic dialing telephones
- Switch-operated devices
  - Voice-activated or sound-activated devices may not be useful due to decreased vocal volume

Psychosocial issues. Clients with PD often withdraw from society because of embarrassment, difficulty in mobility, and depression (Welsh, 2004). A daily schedule to encourage exercise, outside activity, and social contacts may be helpful to both clients and families. Information and support groups for clients with PD and their families are available through local chapters of the Parkinson's Disease Foundation. The National Parkinson Foundation and the online computer network for PD offer advice and education. Group counseling and day treatment programs provide emotional and social outlets.

Advanced PD. In the late stages of the disease, clients have severe deficits in communication, mobility, balance, swallowing, and cognition. It is typical for the client to need a wheelchair for mobility and be dependent in ADL tasks. Environmental modifications can increase access and control to maintain a positive quality of life. Social isolation becomes a serious problem. Complications due to severe impairment in mobility include skin breakdown, aspiration pneumonia, fractures from falls, and joint contractures. These impairments can be prevented or lessened through the use of pressure-relieving surfaces, proper head alignment, use of a flow control cup at meals (see Chapter 11), daily passive range of motion (PROM) exercises, and orthotic application (see Chapter 19). Group activities can be helpful in minimizing the social isolation often experienced by those with advanced PD.

Amyotrophic Lateral Sclerosis

ALS, or Lou Gehrig disease, is a progressive disease characterized by the degeneration of the motor neurons in the anterior horn cells of the spinal cord, brainstem, and corticospinal tracts. ALS is classified as a motor neuron disease, in which motor neurons gradually degenerate and die (National Institute of Neurological Disorders and Stroke, 2003). Both upper motor neurons and lower motor neurons are affected, eventually losing any ability to send messages to muscles. Consequently, muscles weaken and atrophy. Fasciculations or small twitch movements occur. Death is inevitable once the brain is affected and voluntary movement ceases (National Institute of Neurological Disorders and Stroke, 2003). OTs and OTAs working with ALS clients should be aware of the following:

- Clients lose the ability to breathe without ventilatory support once the muscles in the diaphragm and chest wall lose innervation (National Institute of Neurological Disorders and Stroke, 2003).

- Some individuals may become depressed and experience problems with memory and executive functions (National Institute of Neurological Disorders and Stroke, 2003).
- ALS does not affect a person's ability to see, smell, taste, hear, or recognize touch. Clients usually maintain control of eye muscles and bladder and bowel functions, although in the late stages of the disease most clients need help getting to and from the bathroom (National Institute of Neurological Disorders and Stroke, 2003).
- Focal weakness typically begins in the arm, leg, or bulbar muscles.

Epidemiology. ALS is the most common form of motor neuron disease. Men are 20% more likely to have the disease than women. ALS is most commonly diagnosed between the ages of 40 and 70, with an average age of 55. Some cases occur in persons in their 20s and 30s. People of all races and ethnic backgrounds are affected. Approximately 30,000 Americans live with ALS, and an estimated 5600 are diagnosed each year (ALS Association, n.d).

Cause. The cause of ALS is unknown. The majority of cases (90–95%) occur randomly (sporadic), whereas 5% to 10% of cases are considered familial. The pattern of inheritance requires only one parent to carry the gene that causes the disease. Approximately 20% of familial cases result from a gene defect. Environmental factors such as exposure to metal toxicity and viral infection are also being researched (National Institute of Neurological Disorders and Stroke, 2003).

Impact on Client Factors. ALS affects voluntary muscles. Because ALS involves both the upper and lower motor neurons, motor involvement includes both spasticity and stiffness (upper motor neuron) and weakness, low tone, and atrophy (lower motor neuron). In addition, bulbar signs such as speech deficits, swallowing difficulties, and respiratory involvement occur. Although prognosis is difficult to predict, individuals with early bulbar involvement have a poorer prognosis (Fujimura-Kiyono et al., 2011). Eye muscles, external sphincters controlling bowel and bladder management, the five senses, and the heart, liver, and kidneys are usually spared (National Institute of Neurological Disorders and Stroke, 2003).

Early symptoms of the disease include difficulty walking and/or picking up objects, and/or performing fine motor tasks. The number and side of the limbs affected vary from person to person. The client typically complains of weakness, stiffness, and cramping. There is atrophy of the intrinsic muscles of the hands. The client exhibits hyperactive reflexes and fasciculations (twitching) that can be observed under the skin. The weakness spreads to other muscle groups relatively quickly and involves all the limbs and the neck and trunk muscles (National Institute of Neurological Disorders and Stroke, 2003). Eventually the client's muscles become flaccid, resulting in severe disabilities (i.e., requiring total care) in performance in areas of occupation. ALS is primarily a disease of the motor system, but emerging evidence suggests that cognitive impairment that mimics frontal and temporal lobe **dementia** may exist (Abe, 2000; Hanagasi et al., 2002; Lomen-Hoerth et al., 2003). Signs of this include impaired reasoning, judgment, decision making, sequencing, and regulation of emotions, which negatively impact behavior.

Clients with ALS may consider themselves prisoners of their bodies due to the severe pattern of weakness that emerges. As the disease progresses and respiratory muscles fail, clients, families, and the team must decide whether to provide ventilator assistance. Most individuals with ALS experience respiratory failure 2 to 5 years after the onset of symptoms (if no tracheostomy or ventilation is provided). Death generally results from respiratory complications (National Institute of Neurological Disorders and Stroke, 2003).

Medical Management of ALS. There is no cure for ALS, so treatment is considered palliative. The US Food and Drug Administration has approved the drug riluzole (Rilutek) to slow progression of the disease (National Institute of Neurological Disorders and Stroke, 2003). Medication is also prescribed to reduce uncomfortable symptoms and improve quality of life through control of muscle spasms and pain, minimization of drooling, and treatment of depression. Respiratory and swallowing problems may require tracheotomy and gastrostomy procedures. Frequent suctioning to clear the airway may be necessary. Because of the client's compromised respiratory system, care should be taken to avoid exposure to respiratory infections. Frequent reevaluation of the client's respiratory status is necessary to determine ventilator support options.

Occupational Therapy Intervention Process. OTs and OTAs enable clients with ALS to adapt and maintain the maximal level of functioning throughout the course of the disease, as well as to assist care providers with the necessary skills to safely and effectively assist with daily care issues (Casey, 2001; Corr et al., 1998; van den Berg et al., 2004).

During the initial evaluation the OT, with input from the OTA, establishes a baseline of functional abilities and limitations related to areas of occupation, ROM, muscle strength and tone, pain, and chewing and swallowing abilities. In addition, they gather information regarding the home layout. Frequent reevaluation of the client's status is required as the disease progresses. Evaluation procedures include standardized evaluations, interviews, and performance-based observations. The ALS Functional Rating Scale (Miano, Stoddard, Davis, & Bromberg, 2004) is used throughout the country to monitor disease progression in this population (Francis, Bach, & DeLisa, 1999; Han et al., 2003). It measures the following areas: speech, salivation, swallowing, handwriting, cutting food and handling utensils, dressing and hygiene, turning in bed and adjusting bed clothes, walking, climbing stairs, and respiratory insufficiency. The OTA may assist in the evaluation of occupational performance areas.

Intervention

Improving participation in areas of occupation. Intervention will vary depending on the stage of the disease. Early

symptoms may include loss of fine motor coordination and hand weakness. Assistive devices such as built-up utensils and writing devices, Dycem, suction devices, scoop dishes, plate guards, key holders, and devices to open containers may help improve function (see Chapters 11 and 13). Early balance changes due to weakness (i.e., foot drop) may necessitate adaptive ambulation devices or braces (e.g., an ankle foot orthotic) to prevent falls and improve upright function. The OTA should focus on using ambulation devices in functional situations such as kitchen activities and train the client in relation to daily living problems such as transporting and carrying items (Casey, 2001). Walker baskets or trays may be useful. Energy conservation techniques (see earlier) should be taught in the early stages of the disease.

As the disease progresses and UE weakness continues to progress, further adaptations are necessary. Functional splints may be necessary to maintain the ability to eat, use a computer, write, use a communication device or environmental control unit, or turn pages. Typical splints that are used to maintain or increase function in this population are wrist extension splints, short or long opponens splints, universal cuff, or dorsal wrist extension splints with a universal pocket (Fig. 25.3). In addition, head and neck stability may be compromised, thus requiring a cervical collar. Splints may be used in conjunction with an overhead suspension sling or deltoid aid to compensate for proximal weakness (see Fig. 25.2).

Trunk and/or LE weakness will affect the client's functional mobility skills. Transfers may be made easier for both clients and caregivers by teaching the use of a sliding board or mechanical lift.

Depending on financial means, home modifications such as ramps, elevators, stair-glides, and ceiling lifts may be necessary. Similarly, bathroom modifications and equipment such as roll-in showers, rolling commodes, pocket doors, offset hinges, removal of glass shower doors, and/or adapted bath seats help maintain independence, increase safety, and facilitate caregiver assistance.

Motor skills and prevention of deformities. When using gentle therapeutic exercises with this population, the OT and OTA should take care to avoid fatiguing the client. Gentle exercise matched to the client's current condition will help maintain functional abilities and improve mood. Nonresistive, gradable exercise such as water activities or walking, tai chi, or gentle yoga is appropriate. PROM is provided when the client cannot move the joint actively to the end of the range; PROM may be used in conjunction with positioning and splints to prevent contracture and control spasticity. Relaxation and deep breathing exercises should be taught. If exercise is an important occupation for the client, it should be done over several short periods throughout the day, rather than in one long session so as to avoid fatigue. Exercise will not result in increased muscle bulk but may improve aerobic function, decrease fatigue, or help control depression. In the latter stages of the disease more intensive passive stretching/ranging and splinting (i.e., resting hand splints) are required to prevent contracture development (Mitsumoto & Shockley, 1998).

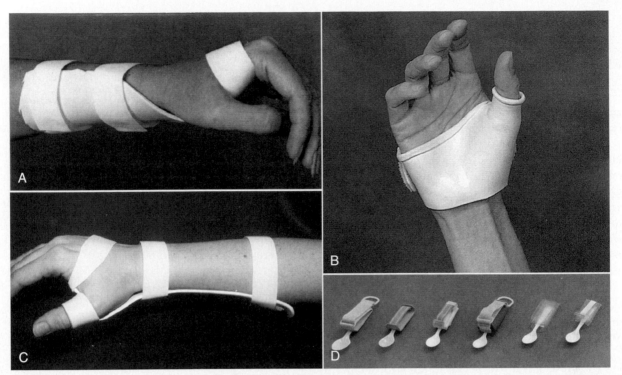

Fig. 25.3 Typical splints used to increase or maintain function in those living with amyotrophic lateral sclerosis. The splints provide stability for unstable joints secondary to weakness and place the wrist or hand in a functional position. (A) Wrist extension splint. (B) Short opponens splint. (C) Long opponens splint. (D) Universal cuff. The universal cuff can be used in conjunction with a wrist support as well. (A-C, From Fess EE, Gettle KS, Philips CA, et al. *Hand and Upper Extremity Splinting: Principles and Methods*. 3rd ed. St Louis, MO: Mosby; 2005. D, Courtesy Sammons Preston, Bolingbrook, IL.)

Communication. The trauma associated with the loss of verbal communication skills is compounded by the fact that the client retains significant mental capacity. The OT and OTA may work jointly with a speech therapist to establish an alternative method to help the client communicate thoughts and needs. Initially the client may be able to write. A communication board, an electronic communication aid, and a computer with a voice module offer other alternatives. The OTA may be involved in positioning the client and fabricating the UE equipment and switches that enable use of these devices. It is important that the client be able to call for help. Call bells that can be controlled with any part of the body with a minimal amount of pressure are available and will become necessary when the client can no longer speak.

Assistive technology. Computers and ECUs enable the ALS client to perform a variety of tasks, from speech to turning on lights and appliances. Computers can be activated by a variety of different types of keyboards and switches. The OTA can assist in determining the client's functional capacity to operate these devices and may be called on to make recommendations as to the type of device to purchase or borrow (Hatakeyama et al., 2000). See Chapter 14 for an in-depth discussion of assistive technology.

Mobility and positioning. In the early stages of the disease, the client may ambulate with a cane or walker. In later stages the client will require wheeled mobility. Due to the progressive nature of the disease a motorized wheelchair with a reclining or tilt-in-space function will eventually be needed (Trail, Nelson, Van, Appel, & Lai, 2001). This should be taken into account when consulting on a wheelchair purchase. In late stages, proper positioning of the head and trunk can be provided with head and lateral supports. Pressure-relieving cushions are indicated to prevent skin breakdown. Local ALS centers may be helpful in terms of procuring equipment via a lending program or suggesting ways to obtain financial assistance.

Psychosocial issues. Reactive depression and anxiety disorders are common among those living with terminal diseases such as ALS. Medication and counseling may help ameliorate depression. The rehabilitation team needs to provide psychological support to help in coping with the devastating effects of the disease. Independence in meaningful activities may increase the client's self-esteem in addition to improving functional status. Support groups or individual counseling for clients and their families should be recommended.

Alzheimer Disease

AD is a progressive, slow deterioration of brain tissue that results in impaired cognition and functional deficits. Deficits include impairments in language and memory, disturbances in the sense of time and place, personality changes, and emotional instability (National Institute of Neurological Disorders and Stroke, 2004; Srinivas, 1999; Weiner, 1999).

Dementia is not a disease itself but a set of symptoms that accompanies a disease. Dementia refers to the loss of mental function in two or more areas such as language, memory, visual abilities, spatial abilities, or judgment that is severe enough to affect daily life. Many diseases cause dementia, including multi-infarct dementia, PD, Huntington disease, Pick disease, and Creutzfeldt-Jakob disease. Other conditions such as acquired immunodeficiency syndrome (AIDS), traumatic brain injury, and tertiary syphilis may result in symptoms of dementia. The most commonly known cause of irreversible dementia in adults is AD. Also known as senile dementia of the Alzheimer type (SDAT), this disease was first described by Dr. Alors Alzheimer in 1907.

Epidemiology. AD affects approximately 4.5 million Americans. It is estimated that by the year 2050 the number of individuals living with AD could range from 11 to 16 million. One in 10 Americans has a family member with AD, and one in three has an acquaintance with it. Of individuals over age 65, 10% are affected by AD; 50% of individuals over age 85 are affected. Inherited forms of the disease can sometimes affect individuals in their 30s and 40s (National Institute of Neurological Disorders and Stroke, 2004; Srinivas, 1999; Weiner, 1999). Lifespan following the initial diagnosis of AD ranges from 8 to 20 years, which is half of the expected lifespan of individuals without dementia.

Cause. The cause of AD remains unclear, but the following may be potential causes and risks (National Institute of Neurological Disorders and Stroke, 2004; Srinivas, 1999; Weiner, 1999):

- *Increased age.* The likelihood of developing AD doubles every 5 years after age 65.
- *Family history.* The likelihood of developing AD increases as the number of family members with AD increases.
- *Genetic link.* Familial AD usually occurs before age 60 and has been linked to specific genes. Variations in certain genes are being studied to determine whether they make some individuals more or less susceptible to the disease.

Signs and Symptoms. Early warning signs of AD include memory loss, difficulty performing familiar tasks, problems with language (i.e., as in word finding or word substitutions), disorientation, impaired judgment, decreased abstract thinking, misplacing items, mood or behavior changes, personality changes, and loss of initiative. The stages of the disease have been documented from early, middle, to late stage (Box 25.7) (Reisberg, Ferris, de Leon, & Crook, 1982). Understanding the stage of AD will assist in setting goals and planning treatment.

Medical Management. No cure or treatment will slow the progression of the disease so medical management is focused on decreasing problematic symptoms. Medications that target behavioral and psychiatric symptoms are most effective in conjunction with behavioral interventions and environmental modifications. Celexa, Prozac, Paxil, and Zoloft improve mood and decrease irritability. Ativan or Serax decrease anxiety and restlessness. Seroquel, Risperdal, and Clozaril may be beneficial for management of hallucinations and delusions (National Institute of Neurological Disorders and Stroke, 2004; Srinivas, 1999; Weiner, 1999).

BOX 25.7 Stages of Alzheimer Disease

Stage 1: No cognitive impairment
Stage 2: Very mild cognitive decline; subjective complaints of memory loss or word finding, not detected on formal examination

Mild/Early-Stage Alzheimer Disease

Stage 3: Mild decline: word-finding deficits, naming objects, misplacing objects, decrease in planning
Stage 4: Moderate cognitive decline: decreased knowledge of recent events, decreased ability to perform higher-level mental calculations, decreased memory for personal information, inability to participate in complex tasks, socially withdrawn

Moderate Stage/Midstage Alzheimer Disease

Stage 5: Moderately severe cognitive decline: major memory gaps, assistance needed for complex daily living tasks, confusion related to orientation, inability to perform simple calculations, still knows own name and names of spouse and children, needs help picking out clothing based on the season and weather
Stage 6: Severe cognitive decline: memory worsens, personality changes emerge, extensive help required for activities for daily living, occasionally forgets name of spouse, decreased dressing ability, dysfunction of sleep-wake cycle, assistance required for toileting, incontinence, delusions, hallucinations occur, compulsion/repetition of behaviors

Severe/Late-Stage Alzheimer Disease

Stage 7: Very severe cognitive decline: does not respond to environment, mutism, inability to control movement, requires feeding assist, loses ability to walk and sit without assistance, dysphagia, skeletal muscle rigidity

---

Occupational Therapy Process. At all stages of AD, OTs and OTAs focus on maximizing independence and providing guidance and support to the family and caregivers (Corcoran, 2002).

Evaluation. A thorough history and occupational profile should be gathered from the client and family as the first step. The OT, with input from the OTA, then evaluates the client to establish a baseline related to performance in areas of occupation and to determine the level of care and supervision necessary for the client. This includes the assessment of client factors such as cognitive, motor, and sensory skills. An intervention plan is developed to provide guidelines and goals to guide the process. Information from the evaluation may assist the family to make the best decision regarding the most appropriate and safe living situation for the client. This may be in the home or a facility such as assisted living long-term care.

Cognition should be evaluated using occupation-based, standardized assessment tools. Motor functioning should be assessed and include measurement of active and passive ROM, coordination, balance, transfer skills, and praxis. Self-care assessment should be gathered during eating, dressing, grooming, and toileting. In the early stages of the disease

IADL (e.g., housekeeping, leisure skills, work-related tasks) should also be assessed (Corcoran, 2002).

Intervention. Box 25.8 provides evidence for interventions provided to clients with AD.

Activities of daily living. In the middle stages of AD, the client begins to demonstrate difficulty performing simple ADL. Frequent reminders to initiate a task, such as "wash your face" or "put on your shirt" may be required. As the disease progresses, the client has problems sequencing multistep tasks and benefits from help with breaking the tasks down into one-step segments. This process, known as **task segmentation**, guides the client to complete ADL tasks with the verbal prompting of the therapist and helps to train and refocus on the task at hand. Instead of saying, "Wash your face," the client is instructed, "Pick up the washcloth. Put the washcloth in the water. Now put some soap on the washcloth. Wash around your mouth." These instructions are offered in a calm, reassuring manner. Positive feedback in the form of praise is provided after each step. Physical prompts (hand-over-hand assistance) may also be given if the client permits it. The OT and OTA should instruct clients' caregivers in these task segmentation methods and remind them of the importance of allowing clients to perform as much of their own daily care as possible.

A client with AD typically demonstrates poor frustration tolerance. It is important to avoid situations that may trigger behavioral outbursts. Activities should be analyzed and graded to ensure that the client has the physical and cognitive skills necessary to perform the task.

Impairments in mobility, strength, and safety awareness may pose a safety risk in the home. A home safety assessment can provide the family and/or caregivers with information regarding possible hazards in the home or community environments that need to be removed or adapted. The bathroom is an area where adaptive equipment and environmental adaptations can increase safety. Other areas include the removal or securing of power tools, electric appliances, medications, household cleansers, and smoking materials. Clients should be restricted from accessing stairways, open windows, balconies, and the stove as they can present a potential hazard to the client.

Clients with AD often experience disruptions to mealtime occupations. Mealtime intervention can improve the experience for both the client and the caregiver. See Chapter 11 for intervention suggestions and adaptive devices to improve occupational performance during mealtime.

Environmental design. The OTA can help the caregiver structure the environment to help maximize the client's functioning. Eliminating clutter in the environment helps to minimize confusion and risk for falls. Contrasting colors allow the client to differentiate an object from the background. Simple changes such as eliminating the condiments from the kitchen table and ensuring contrast of color between the plate and table (and the plate and the food) simplify mealtime. Contrasting the color of the toilet seat and bowl with the bathroom floor helps to aid in toileting. Minimizing the amount of furniture and maintaining traffic areas free of

> ### BOX 25.8 Evidence Briefs and Alzheimer Disease/Dementia
>
> - Dooley and Hinojosa (2004): This study examined the extent to which adherence to occupational therapy recommendations would increase the quality of life of persons with Alzheimer disease living in the community and decrease the burden felt by family members caring for them. Caregivers completed measures of their feelings of burden and the quality of life, including level of function of the persons with Alzheimer disease. The authors concluded that individualized occupational therapy intervention based on the person-environment fit model appears effective for both caregivers and clients.
> - Graff et al., (2006): This study set out to determine the effectiveness of community-based occupational therapy on daily functioning of clients with dementia and the sense of competence of their caregivers. The intervention consisted of 10 sessions of occupational therapy over 5 weeks, including cognitive and behavioral interventions to train clients in the use of aids to compensate for cognitive decline and caregivers in coping behaviors and supervision. The authors concluded that occupational therapy improved clients' daily functioning and reduced the burden on the caregiver, despite the clients' limited learning ability. Effects were still present at 12 weeks.
> - Graff et al. (2007): This study set out to investigate effects of community occupational therapy on dementia clients' and caregivers' quality of life, mood, and health status and caregivers' sense of control over life. The intervention (as described earlier) consisted of 10 sessions of occupational therapy over 5 weeks or no intervention. Cognitive and behavioral interventions were used to train clients in the use of aids to compensate for cognitive decline and caregivers in coping behaviors and supervision. The authors concluded that community occupational therapy should be advocated both for dementia clients and their caregivers because it improves their mood, quality of life, and health status and caregivers' sense of control over life. Effects were still present at follow-up.

obstacles decrease the risk of falls in the home. Gates and locks on stairways and doors may need to be installed for safety. Signs identifying the client's room and bathroom may be helpful. These design features should also be implemented in clinical settings (Josephsson, Backman, Borell, & Nygård, 1995; Painter, 1996; Sheldon & Teaford, 2002).

Adult day care and group activities. Programs at adult day care facilities offer the caregiver a respite from the daily pressure and stress of taking care of a loved one with AD. These programs offer a variety of group activities within a structured environment, striving to provide the client with positive social opportunities. OTs and OTAs may provide group intervention in community-based adult day care settings or in long-term care facilities. The clients often enjoy music-based activities, simple and familiar games, crafts, sensory stimulation, reminiscing games, and pet visits. Clients often have the most success with familiar activities and more difficulty with new activities. Activities should be focused on adults and not children, so as not to demean clients. See Chapter 22 for more suggestions for interventions for clients impaired cognition.

Reality orientation. As AD progresses, clients experience impairment in orientation. Formal daily orientation programs to review the client's name, the date, the weather, and the location may be helpful. In addition, the client should always be addressed by name, and all staff should introduce themselves and tell the client their function regularly, as if they have just met. The OT and OTA should regularly review the names of the clients' close family members and show them their rooms, the dining room, etc. Clocks and calendars should be clearly displayed. Memory books may also be used (Hafler, 2004).

Exercise programs. Exercise, whether offered as a group or individual activity, is important to maintain strength, coordination, and ROM. Simple group calisthenics can be done in a standing or sitting position. The addition of rhythmic music helps to keep the client involved in the activity. Parachute activities and ball, scarf, or balloon tosses may provide beneficial group exercise. Dancing and walking are activities that the caretaker can easily do with the client. If the client cannot participate in group exercise programs or if he or she has joint contractures, the client should be involved in a daily PROM program. It is recommended that exercise programs be offered at the same time each day to help establish a routine.

Psychosocial issues. Clients with AD may demonstrate decreased participation due to impaired behavior. These include agitation, physical aggression, depression, inappropriate sexual behaviors, stealing, paranoia, and hallucinations. Although some of these may be managed with medication, behavioral interventions increase the effectiveness of medications and may allow for a decrease in dosages that may have serious side effects (van den Berg et al., 2004). OTs and OTAs should approach clients with a calm, reassuring voice and should never manifest anger or argue with the client. Gentle redirection and refocus should be used. Clear instructions should be given on the most appropriate behaviors. Using the name of the client's spouse in the request often helps to achieve the desired behavior (e.g., "Mary wants you to take a bath now."). Reducing the amount of stimulation, noise, or unstructured time sometimes helps to decrease agitation and antisocial behavior (Rogers et al., 1999). Occupational therapy intervention will be most effective when provided in a quiet, distraction-free environment.

In the final stages of the disease, the burden of care caused by dependence in daily tasks often requires long-term and skilled nursing care. Occupational therapy services may be provided to decrease the burden of care on nursing staff and maintain health. Some interventions to achieve this include toileting programs to decrease the need for a two-person dependent transfer, stretching and positioning recommendations to prevent skin breakdown, orthotic prescriptions to prevent joint contractures, and sensory stimulation to increase periods of wakefulness.

Throughout the course of the disease, the family will need guidance and support to help cope with the effect of the AD on the client, the family, and other caregivers (Hogan et al., 2003). The impairments caused by the disease cause disruptions in roles, leading to the client taking on the role of child and the adult child taking on the role of parent. OTs, OTAs, and other team members can provide support for these difficult transitions. Support groups, chat rooms, and the Alzheimer's Disease and Related Disorders Association may provide advice and information.

SUMMARY

This chapter focused on four degenerative diseases: multiple sclerosis, Parkinson disease, amyotrophic lateral sclerosis, and Alzheimer disease. These four conditions share many factors with other neurologic diseases that cause a progressive loss of function. The treatment goals and interventions provided in this chapter can provide useful guidelines for providing occupational therapy treatment to clients experiencing many different degenerative disorders.

Providing care to clients with degenerative and often fatal conditions is difficult and can take an emotional toll on clients, therapists, and caregivers. Close collaboration between the OT and OTA can be effective in providing the complex interventions necessary to treat the many disruptions in client factors caused by degenerative conditions. Optimal outcomes can be achieved through the collaboration of the OT and OTA with other health care providers.

REVIEW QUESTIONS

1. List the precautions that need to be observed when treating a client with MS.
2. Briefly describe the three clinical signs associated with PD and explain how these signs affect the treatment process.
3. Discuss the psychosocial aspects of treating clients with degenerative diseases.
4. Describe how assistive technology can be used to increase the functional level of the client with ALS.
5. Describe the treatment goals associated with each of the diseases discussed in this chapter: MS, PD, ALS, and AD.
6. Describe the ways the OTA can help the MS client cope with fatigue.
7. Explain how the OTA can use adaptive devices to promote independence in feeding skills for clients with degenerative diseases.
8. Describe the techniques used by the OT practitioner to promote proper positioning and the prevention of decubitus ulcers in clients with degenerative diseases.
9. Describe the role of the OTA in the treatment and prevention of contractures with clients with MS, PD, ALS, and AD.
10. List some of the environmental changes that the OTA may recommend in the home of a client with AD.

CASE STUDY

Peter

Peter is a 30-year-old loan officer who enjoys movies, fishing, eating out, and concerts. He was recently engaged to be married. Peter was diagnosed with MS 5 years ago. One week ago, he experienced an exacerbation of symptoms. He is motivated, alert, and oriented × 3. He can follow complex directions but lacks concentration on tasks as presented. His speech is understandable. He often loses his train of thought.

Motor function: Peter demonstrates 4/5 strength in both UEs. The greatest limiting factor is fatigue. His LEs are graded as 2/5 on manual muscle testing (MMT).

Sensory: He has intact sensation in his bilateral UEs. Light touch pain sensation is absent below the umbilicus.

Postural control: Peter requires close supervision for static sitting and moderate assistance for all weight shifting and reaching activities beyond his arm span. He falls laterally and posteriorly while seated.

Neurobehavioral deficits: Peter's greatest complaint is loss of short-term memory and feeling "disorganized." He also reports feeling "blue and tired." His greatest fear is that this exacerbation will limit his ability to work. In addition, the OT notes that he presents with deficits related to sustained attention and short-term memory.

ADL: Peter requires moderate assist for dressing, bathing, and toileting. In addition, all sliding board transfers require minimal assistance. He feels that his dependency in these areas is "humiliating."

Peter has just been transferred to the rehabilitation unit, and you will be the primary OTA working with him. Peter's desire is to return home and to work as soon as possible.

1. Reread the case study material. Underline and star the problems of most concern to the client.
2. Place problems in order of priority and select the first three. State a short-term goal for each. Describe one or more treatment methods the OTA could use to address this goal.
3. Describe the type of wheelchair and the wheelchair features that would be appropriate for Peter at this time.
4. Describe how you would respond to Peter's desire to return to work.

REFERENCES

Abe, K. (2000). Cognitive function in amyotrophic lateral sclerosis. *Amyotrophic Lateral Sclerosis and other Motor Neuron Disorders, 1*(5), 343–347.

ALS Association. About ALS, who gets ALS. (n.d.). <https://www.als.org/understanding-als/who-gets-als>.

Arnett, P. A., Higginson, C. I., Voss, W. D., Randolph, J. J., & Grandey, A. A. (2002). Relationship between coping, cognitive dysfunction and depression in multiple sclerosis. *The Clinical Neuropsychologist, 16*(3), 341–355.

Bobholz, J. A., & Rao, S. M. (2003). Cognitive dysfunction in multiple sclerosis: a review of recent developments. *Current Opinion in Neurology, 16*(3), 283–288.

Calabresi, P. A. (2004). Diagnosis and management of multiple sclerosis. *American Family Physician, 70*(10), 1935–1944.

Casey, P. (2001). Occupational therapy. In: H. M. Mitsumoto (Ed.), *Amyotrophic lateral sclerosis: A comprehensive guide to management.* New York, NY: Demos Medical Publishing.

Clarke, C., & Moore, A. P. (2004). Parkinson's disease update. *Clinical Evidence, 11*, 1736–1754.

Corcoran, M. A. (2002). Occupational therapy intervention for persons with dementia and their families. *OT Practice, 7*(20).

Corr, B., Frost, E., Traynor, B. J., & Hardiman, O. (1998). Service provision for clients with ALS/MND: a cost-effective multidisciplinary approach. *Journal of Neurological Sciences, 160*(Suppl. 1), S141–S145.

de Goede, C. J. T., Keus, S. H. J., Kwakkel, G., & Wagenaar, R. C. (2001). The effects of physical therapy in Parkinson's disease: a research synthesis. *Archives of Physical Medicine and Rehabilitation, 82*(4), 509–515.

DeMaagd, G., & Philip, A. (2015). Parkinson's disease and its management: part 1: disease entity, risk factors, pathophysiology, clinical presentation, and diagnosis. *P and T, 40*(8), 504–532.

Dixon, L., Duncan, D. C., Johnson, P., Kirkby, L., O'Connell, H., Taylor, H. J., et al. (2007). Occupational therapy for clients with Parkinson's disease. *Cochrane Database of Systematic Reviews, 3*, CD002813.

Dooley, N. R., & Hinojosa, J. (2004). Improving quality of life for persons with Alzheimer's disease and their family caregivers: brief occupational therapy intervention. *The American Journal of Occupational Therapy, 58*(5), 561–569.

Finlayson, M. (2008). *Occupational therapy in multiple sclerosis rehabilitation.* New York, NY: National Multiple Sclerosis Society.

Francis, K., Bach, J. R., & DeLisa, J. A. (1999). Evaluation and rehabilitation of clients with adult motor neuron disease. *Archives of Physical Medicine and Rehabilitation, 80*(8), 951–963.

Frohman, E. M. (2008). *Diagnosis and management of vision problems in MS.* New York, NY: National Multiple Sclerosis Society.

Fujimura-Kiyono, C., Kimura, F., Ishida, S., Nakajima, H., Hosokawa, T., Sugino, M., et al. (2011). Onset and spreading patterns of lower motor neuron involvements predict survival in sporadic amyotrophic lateral sclerosis. *Journal of Neurology, Neurosurgery, and Psychiatry, 82*, 1244–1249.

Ghahari, S., & Finlayson, M. (2018). *A resource for healthcare professionals: Occupational therapy in multiple sclerosis rehabilitation.* New York, NY: National Multiple Sclerosis Society.

Gillen, G. (2009). *Cognitive and perceptual rehabilitation: Optimizing function.* St Louis, MO; Elsevier.

Gillen, G. (2000a). Maximizing independence: occupational therapy intervention for clients with Parkinson's disease. *Loss Grief Care Journal of Professional Practice, 8*(3-4), 65–67.

Gillen, G. (2000b). Improving activities of daily living performance in an adult with ataxia. *The American Journal of Occupational Therapy, 54*(1), 89–96.

Gillen, G. (2002). Improving mobility and community access in an adult with ataxia. *The American Journal of Occupational Therapy, 56*(4), 462–466.

Graff, M. J. L., Vernooij-Dassen, M. J. M., & Thijssen, M. (2006). Community-based occupational therapy for clients with dementia and their care givers: randomised controlled trial. *BMJ, 333*(7580), 1196.

Graff, M. J. L., Vernooij-Dassen, M. J. M., Thijssen, M., Dekker, J., Hoefnagels, W. H. L., & Olderikkert, M. G. M. (2007). Effects of community occupational therapy on quality of life, mood, and health status in dementia clients and their caregivers: a randomized controlled trial. *The Journals of Gerontology. Series A, Biological Sciences and Medical Sciences, 62*(9), 1002–1009.

Hafler, D. A. (2004). Multiple sclerosis. *Journal of Clinical Investigation, 113*(6), 788–794.

Han, J. J., Carter, G. T., Hecht, T. W., Schuman, N. E., Weiss, M. D., & Krivickas, L. S. (2003). The Amyotrophic Lateral Sclerosis Center: a model of multidisciplinary management. *Critical Reviews Physics Rehabilitation Medicine, 15*(1), 21–40.

Hanagasi, H. A., Gurvit, I. H., Ermutlu, N., Kaptanoglu, G., Karamursel, S., Idrisoglu, H. A., et al. (2002). Cognitive impairment in amyotrophic lateral sclerosis: evidence from neuro-psychological investigation and event-related potentials. *Cognitive Brain Research, 14*(2), 234–244.

Hatakeyama, T., Okamoto, A., Kamata, K., & Kasuga, M. (2000). Assistive technology for people with amyotrophic lateral sclerosis in Japan: present status, analysis of problem and proposal for the future. *Technology Disability, 13*(1), 9–15.

Hoehn, M., & Yahr, M. (1967). Parkinsonism: onset, progression, and mortality. *Neurology, 17*(5), 427–442.

Hogan, V. M., Lisy, E. D., Savannah, R. L., Henry, L., Kuo, F., & Fisher, G. C. (2003). Role change experienced by family caregivers of adults with Alzheimer's disease: implications for occupational therapy. *Physical Occupational Therapy in Geriatrics, 22*(1), 21–43.

Holland, N. J. (2008). *Bowel management in multiple sclerosis.* New York, NY: National Multiple Sclerosis Society.

Holland, N. J., & Reitman, N. C. (2008). *Bladder dysfunction in multiple sclerosis.* New York, NY: National Multiple Sclerosis Society.

Jones, L., Lewis, Y., Harrison, J., & Wiles, C. M. (1996). The effectiveness of occupational therapy and physiotherapy in multiple sclerosis clients with ataxia of the upper limb and trunk. *Clinical Rehabilitation, 10*(4), 277–282.

Josephsson, S., Backman, L., Borell, L., & Nygård, L. (1995). Effectiveness of an intervention to improve occupational performance in dementia. *Occupational Therapy Journal Research, 15*(1), 36–49.

Joy, J. E., & Johnston, R. B. (2001). Multiple sclerosis: current status and strategies for the future. In: *Committee on multiple sclerosis: Current status and strategies for the future.* Washington, DC: National Academic Press.

Kalb, R., & Reitman, N. (2010). *Overview of multiple sclerosis.* New York, NY: National Multiple Sclerosis Society.

Kesselring, J. (2004). Neurorehabilitation in multiple sclerosis: what is the evidence-base? *Journal of Neurology, 251*(Suppl. 4), S25–S29.

Kushner, S., & Brandfass, K. (2008). *Spasticity.* New York, NY: National Multiple Sclerosis Society.

Law, M., Baptiste, S., & Carswell, A., et al. (2005). *The Canadian Occupational Performance Measure.* 4th ed. Ottawa: CAOT Publications ACE.

Law, M., Baptiste, S., & Mills, J. (1995). Client-centered practice: what does it mean and does it make a difference? *Canadian Journal of Occupational Therapy, 62*(5), 250–257.

Lemke, M. R., Fuchs, G., Gemende, I., Herting, B., Oehlwein, C., Reichmann, H., et al. (2004). Depression and Parkinson's disease. *Journal of Neurology, 251*(Suppl. 6), SI24–S27.

Lomen-Hoerth, C., Murphy, J., Langmore, S., Kramer, J. H., Olney, R. K., & Miller, B. (2003). Are amyotrophic lateral sclerosis clients cognitively normal? *Neurology, 60*(7), 1094–1097.

Ma, H., Trombly, C. A., Tickle-Degnen, L., & Wagenaar, R. C. (2004). Effect of one single auditory cue on movement kinematics in clients with Parkinson's disease. *American Journal of Physical Medicine & Rehabilitation, 83*(7), 530–536.

Mathiowetz, V., Matuska, K. M., & Murphy, M. E. (2001). Efficacy of an energy conservation course for persons with multiple sclerosis. *Archives of Physical Medicine and Rehabilitation, 82*(4), 449–456.

Meyer, B. (2001). Coping with severe mental illness: relations of the Brief COPE with symptoms, functioning, and well-being. *Journal of Psychopathology and Behavioral Assessment, 23*, 265–277.

Miano, B., Stoddard, G. J., Davis, S., & Bromberg, M. B. (2004). Inter-evaluator reliability of the ALS functional rating scale. *Amyotrophic Lateral Sclerosis Other Motor Neuron Disorders, 5*(4), 235–239.

Mitsumoto, H., & Shockley, L. (1998). Amyotrophic lateral sclerosis: continuum of care from diagnosis through hospice. *Home HealthCare Consulting, 5*(6), 20–29.

Mohr, D. C., Classen, C., & Barrera, M., Jr. (2004). The relationship between social support, depression and treatment for depression in people with multiple sclerosis. *Psychological Medicine, 34*(3), 533–541.

Mohr, D. C., Dick, L. P., Russo, D., Pinn, J., Boudewyn, A. C., Likosky, W., et al. (1999). The psychosocial impact of multiple sclerosis: exploring the client's perspective. *Health Psychology, 18*(4), 376–382.

Multiple Sclerosis Council for Clinical Practice Guidelines. (1998). *Fatigue and multiple sclerosis: Evidence-based management strategies for fatigue in multiple sclerosis.* Washington, DC: Paralyzed Veterans of America.

Murphy, S., & Tickle-Degnen, L. (2001). The effectiveness of occupational therapy-related treatments for persons with Parkinson's disease: a meta-analytic review. *The American Journal of Occupational Therapy, 55*(4), 385–392.

National Clinical Advisory Board. (2008a). *Management of MS-related fatigue.* New York, NY: National Multiple Sclerosis Society.

National Clinical Advisory Board. (2008b). *Assessment and management of cognitive impairment in multiple sclerosis.* New York, NY: National Multiple Sclerosis Society.

National Institute of Neurological Disorders and Stroke. (2006). *Parkinson's disease: Hope through research.* Bethesda, MD: National Institutes of Health.

National Institute of Neurological Disorders and Stroke. (2003). *Amyotrophic Lateral Sclerosis Fact Sheet.* Bethesda, MD: National Institutes of Health.

National Institute of Neurological Disorders and Stroke. (2004). *The Dementias: Hope Through Research.* Bethesda, MD: National Institutes of Health.

Painter, J. (1996). Home environment considerations for people with Alzheimer's disease. *Occupational Therapy Health Care, 10*(3), 45–63.

Panisset, M. (2004). Freezing of gait in Parkinson's disease. *Neurologic Clinics, 22*(Suppl. 3), 53–62.

Patti, F., Reggio, A., Nicoletti, F., Sellaroli, T., & Nicoletti, D. (1996). Effects of rehabilitation therapy on Parkinson's disability and functional independence. *Journal of Neurologic Rehabilitation, 10*(4), 223–231.

Petajan, J. H., Gappmaier, E., White, A. T., Spencer, M. K., Mino, L., & Hicks, R. W. (1996). Impact of aerobic training on fitness and quality of life in multiple sclerosis. *Annals of Neurology, 39*(4), 432–441.

Pollock, N. (1993). Client-centered assessment. *The American Journal of Occupational Therapy, 47*(4), 298–301.

Reidak, K., Jackson, S., & Giovannoni, G. (2010). Multiple sclerosis: a practical overview for clinicians. *British Medical Bulletin, 95,* 79–104.

Reisberg, B., Ferris, S. H., de Leon, M. J., & Crook, T. (1982). The Global Deterioration Scale for assessment of primary degenerative dementia. *The American Journal of Psychiatry, 139*(9), 1136–1139.

Rogers, J. C., Holm, M. B., Burgio, L. D., Granieri, E., Hsu, C., Hardin, J. M., et al. (1999). Improving morning care routines of nursing home residents with dementia. *Journal of the American Geriatrics Society, 47*(9), 1049–1057.

Samuel, L, & Cavallo, P. (2008). *Emotional issues of the person with MS.* New York, NY: National Multiple Sclerosis Society.

Schiffer, R. B. (2008). *Cognitive loss in multiple sclerosis.* New York, NY: National Multiple Sclerosis Society.

Schrag, A., Horsfall, L., Walters, K., Noyce, A., & Petersen, I. (2015). Prediagnostic presentations of Parkinson's disease in primary care: a case-control study. *Lancet Neurology, 1,* 57–64.

Schwid, S. R., Petrie, M. D., Murray, R., Leitch, J., Bowen, J., Alquist, A., et al. (2003). A randomized controlled study of the acute and chronic effects of cooling therapy for MS. *Neurology, 60*(12), 1955–1960.

Sheldon, M. M., & Teaford, M. H. (2002). Caregivers of people with Alzheimer's dementia: an analysis of their compliance with recommended home modifications. *Alzheimer Care Q, 3*(1), 78–81.

Solaro, C., Ponzio, M., Moran, E., Tanganelli, P., Pizio, R., Ribizzi, G., et al. (2015). The changing face of multiple sclerosis: prevalence and incidence in an aging population. *MS Journal, 21*(10), 1244–1250.

Srinivas, P. (1999). Diagnosis and management of Alzheimer's disease: an update. *Medical Journal of Malaysia, 54*(4), 541–549.

Steultjens, E. M. J., Dekker, J., Bouter, L. M., Leemrijse, C. J., & van den Ende, C. H. M. (2005). Evidence of the efficacy of occupational therapy in different conditions: an overview of systematic reviews. *Clinical Rehabilitation, 19*(3), 247–254.

Trail, M., Nelson, N., Van, J. N., Appel, S. H., & Lai, E. C. (2001). Wheelchair use by clients with amyotrophic lateral sclerosis: a survey of user characteristics and selection preferences. *Archives of Physical Medicine and Rehabilitation, 82*(1), 98–102.

Trend, P., Kaye, J., Gage, H., Owen, C., & Wade, D. (2002). Short-term effectiveness of intensive multidisciplinary rehabilitation for people with Parkinson's disease and their carers. *Clinical Rehabilitation, 16*(7), 717–725.

Tse, D. W., & Spaulding, S. J. (1998). Review of motor control and motor learning: implications for occupational therapy with individuals with Parkinson's disease. *Physical Occupational Therapy in Geriatrics, 15*(3), 19–38.

van den Berg, J. P., de Groot, I. J., Joha, B. C., van Haelst, J. M., van Gorcom, P., & Kalmijn, S. (2004). Development and implementation of the Dutch protocol for rehabilitative management in amyotrophic lateral sclerosis. *Amyotrophic Lateral Sclerosis Other Motor Neuron Disorders, 5*(4), 226–229.

Vanage, S. M., Gilbertson, K. K., & Mathiowetz, V. (2003). Effects of an energy conservation course on fatigue impact for persons with progressive multiple sclerosis. *The American Journal of Occupational Therapy, 57*(3), 315–323.

Walter, B. L., & Vitek, J. L. (2004). Surgical treatment for Parkinson's disease. *Lancet Neurology, 3*(12), 719–728.

Ward, C. D., & Robertson, D. (2003). Rehabilitation in Parkinson's disease. *Reviews in Clinical Gerontology, 13*(3), 223–239.

Weiner, M. F. (1999). Alzheimer's disease update: using what we now know to help clients. *Consultant, 39*(3), 675–678.

Welsh, M. (2004). Parkinson's disease and quality of life: issues and challenges beyond motor symptoms. *Neurologic Clinics, 22* (Suppl. 3), S141–S148.

Winogrodzka, A., Wagenaar, R. C., Booij, J., & Wolters, E. C. (2005). Rigidity and bradykinesia reduce interlimb coordination in Parkinsonian gait. *Archives of Physical Medicine and Rehabilitation, 86*(2), 183–189.

26

Spinal Cord Injury

Erin Kelly Speeches

OBJECTIVES

After reading this chapter, the student or the occupational therapy practitioner will be able to do the following:

1. Understand the difference between complete and incomplete spinal cord injury and the classification system used to describe such levels of injury.
2. Recognize and identify the various spinal cord injury syndromes.
3. Briefly describe the medical and surgical management of the individual who has experienced a traumatic spinal cord injury.
4. Identify some of the complications that can limit optimal functional potential.
5. Describe the changes in sexual functioning in males and females after spinal cord injury.
6. Identify the specific assessment tools employed by the occupational therapist before developing treatment objectives.
7. Analyze the critical issues faced by the occupational therapy practitioner in developing treatment objectives during the acute, active, and discharge phases of the rehabilitation process.
8. Identify in detail the functional outcomes, including equipment considerations and personal and home care needs, that can be reached at each level of complete injury under optimal circumstances.
9. Describe how the normal aging process is accelerated by the effects of spinal cord injury and explain how functional status may change.

KEY TERMS

Quadriplegia
Tetraplegia
Paraplegia
ASIA impairment scale
Vital capacity
Hypotension

Autonomic dysreflexia
Spasticity
Heterotopic ossification
Tenodesis
Decubitus ulcers

CASE STUDY

Stephen

Stephen is a 44-year-old Caucasian man who sustained a C7–8 complete (ASIA A) spinal cord injury (SCI) as a result of a fall. He also sustained facial lacerations and bilateral radial wrist fractures, which necessitated casting without internal fixation. Stephen is divorced with no biologic children. He is a firefighter and an auto mechanic. Stephen is athletic; he is a triathlete and marathon runner. Just before his accident, Stephen had moved into a second-story apartment.

Stephen was referred to occupational therapy on the day of his injury and initially was evaluated in the intensive care unit within 24 hours of injury. He was immobilized in cervical traction and bilateral wrist casts on a kinetic bed. His specific manual muscle test revealed 3+ to 4 strength in deltoids, biceps, and triceps. Wrists could not be tested secondary to bilateral wrist casts, and finger and thumb flexion and extension were noted to be at least 2− bilaterally.

Sensory examination was intact to the C7 dermatome. Vital capacity was low secondary to the absence of innervation of

intercostal and abdominal musculature, and Stephen required respiratory treatments four times daily to mobilize lung secretions. Because of his immobilization, he required assistance for all aspects of his self-care and mobility.

Occupational therapy treatment objectives included (1) maintaining optimal range of motion (ROM) in all joints for optimal upper extremity (UE) function and seated positioning; (2) achieving optimal strength and endurance in available musculature; (3) achieving optimal independence in all self-care skills, including bathing, toileting, and skin care; (4) achieving independent wheelchair mobility on all indoor and outdoor surfaces; (5) receiving appropriate durable medical equipment (DME) to meet both short-term and long-term needs (e.g., manual and power wheelchair, cushion, and bathing and toileting equipment); (6) returning to safe and accessible housing; and (7) being educated in all aspects of care and independently instructing caregivers in assistance needed.

Stephen has had a difficult time accepting that he has a complete SCI. He could not imagine how he could function at work and in his community as an individual with quadriplegia. His college and church community offered a tremendous amount of support, yet he continued to be depressed and angry over his loss of mobility and independence. He received regular psychological counseling and attended a weekly peer support group.

Upon discharge from acute rehabilitation, Stephen returned to a newly rented single-story home that required bathroom modifications and ramps at the front and back entrances. Stephen initially received 4 hours of attendant care daily. He required assistance only for completion of his daily bath and bowel program, as well as for some homemaking tasks. After

Stephen received in-home occupational therapy services for home setup and community transition issues, his need for personal care diminished; he now requires only homemaking assistance. He regularly visits a neighborhood gym to maintain UE strength and endurance, and he will soon be driving a modified van. His vocational plans are on hold until his van and driving training are completed.

Throughout this chapter, consider the muscles that are sufficiently innervated to be clinically functional, the areas of dysfunction, the optimal equipment to enhance mobility, and the long-term consequences of Stephen's injury in relation to his lifestyle.

INTRODUCTION

Rehabilitation of an individual with SCI is a lifelong process that requires readjustment to nearly every aspect of life. The occupational therapy assistant (OTA) and the occupational therapist (OT) each play a significant role in physical and psychosocial restoration and in helping the individual achieve maximum independence. Through accurate assessment, retraining, and adaptive techniques and equipment, OTs and OTAs provide their clients with the tools and resources needed to achieve their maximal physical and functional potential.

SCIs occur for many reasons; trauma is the most common. Trauma can result from motor vehicle accidents, falls, sports accidents, diving accidents, and violent injuries such as gunshot and stab wounds (Consortium for Spinal Cord Medicine, Paralyzed Veterans of America, 1999; Spencer, 1993). Normal spinal cord function may also be disturbed by diseases such as tumors, myelomeningocele, syringomyelia, multiple sclerosis, cancer, and amyotrophic lateral sclerosis. Some of the treatment principles outlined in this chapter may have application to these conditions; however, the emphasis is on rehabilitation of the individual with a traumatic SCI.

SPINAL CORD INJURY PRESENTATION AND IMPLICATIONS

SCI results in **quadriplegia** (more recently labeled tetraplegia by the American Spinal Injury Association [ASIA]) or paraplegia. **Tetraplegia** is any degree of paralysis of the four limbs and trunk musculature. There may be partial UE function, depending on the level of the cervical lesion. **Paraplegia** is paralysis of the lower extremities (LEs) with some involvement of the trunk and hips depending on the level of the lesion (Consortium for Spinal Cord Medicine, Paralyzed Veterans of America, 1999; Spencer, 1993).

SCIs are discussed in terms of the regions (C, cervical; T, thoracic; L, lumbar; and S, sacral) of the spinal cord in which they occur and the numerical order of the neurologic segments (Bashar & Hughes, 2018). The level of SCI designates the last fully functioning neurologic segment of the cord. For example, C6 refers to the sixth neurologic segment of the cervical region of the spinal cord as the last fully intact neurologic segment (Freed, 1990; Pierce & Nickel, 1977).

Complete Versus Incomplete Neurologic Classifications

The extent of neurologic damage depends on the location and severity of the injury (Fig. 26.1). A complete injury or lesion causes loss of both motor and sensory functions resulting in total paralysis and loss of all sensation from the complete interruption of the ascending and descending nerve tracts below the level of the lesion.

In an incomplete injury some of the sensory or motor nerve pathways below the level of the lesion are preserved partially or completely intact (Bromley, 1998; Pierce & Nickel, 1977).

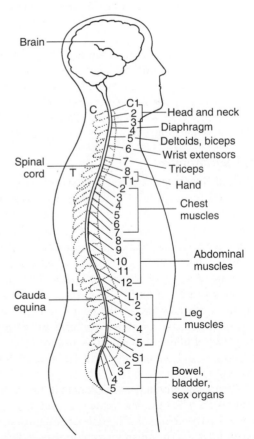

Fig. 26.1 Spinal nerves and major areas of body they supply. (From Paulson S, ed. *Santa Clara Valley Medical Center Spinal Cord Injury Home Care Manual.* 2nd ed. San Jose, CA: Santa Clara Valley Medical Center; 1994.)

Pathways must be preserved in the sacral segments to qualify as incomplete. Segments at which normal function is found often differ on the two sides of the body; further, a given segment may have differences between sensory and motor function as revealed by testing. Incomplete lesions may involve several neurologic segments, such as a C5 injury may have the last intact neurologic level at C5 with a zone of partial preservation (ZPP) to C7, with absence of neurologic function below C7.

A very careful neurologic examination, performed by trained clinicians, is essential to determine whether an injury is complete or incomplete. The **ASIA impairment scale** uses the findings from the neurologic examination to categorize injury types into specific categories (Box 26.1) (American Spinal Injury Association, 1992).

Clinical Syndromes

Central Cord Syndrome. Central cord syndrome (CCS), the most common incomplete SCI, occurs when there is more cellular destruction in the center of the cord than in the periphery (Bashar & Hughes, 2018). It is most often caused by cervical hyperextension (e.g., from a fall) and often seen in older adults with arthritic changes or developing stenosis that have caused a narrowing of the spinal canal. Paralysis and sensory loss are greater in the UEs because these nerve tracts are more centrally located than nerve tracts for the LEs. Other symptoms include bladder dysfunction, sensory loss below the level of injury, and painful sensations such as tingling, burning, or dull aching (Bashar & Hughes, 2018).

Brown-Séquard Syndrome (Lateral Damage). Brown-Séquard syndrome results when trauma to the cord results in damage on one side. This is often caused by stabbing or gunshot injury, ischemia, or infectious or inflammatory diseases suchas multiple sclerosis (National Institute of Neurological Disorders and Stroke, 2019). Motor paralysis and loss of proprioception occur below the level of injury, on the ipsilateral side. Loss of pain, temperature, and touch sensation occurs on the contralateral side.

Anterior Spinal Cord Syndrome. Anterior spinal cord syndrome results from injury that damages the anterior aspect of the cord or anterior spinal artery. This syndrome involves paralysis and loss of pain, temperature, and touch sensation, while proprioception is preserved (Bashar & Hughes, 2018).

Conus Medullaris Syndrome. Conus medullaris syndrome is a type of incomplete SCI resulting from damage of the sacral cord (conus) and lumbar nerve roots within the neural canal. This usually results in loss of reflexes (areflexia) to the bladder, bowel, and lower extremities (Bashar & Hughes, 2018).

Cauda Equina Syndrome. The cauda equina means "horse's tail" and is made up of the nerves at the end of the spinal cord. Damage to it occurs with fractures below the L2 level. Cauda equina syndrome is a condition that describes injury to it. These nerves are peripheral and lead to flaccid paralysis. Unlike the spinal cord, peripheral nerves regenerate at a rate of 1 to 2 mm per day (Bashar & Hughes, 2018). Therefore this injury may lead to a better recovery than one to the spinal cord. However, patterns of sensory and motor deficits are highly variable and asymmetric in this syndrome (Bashar & Hughes, 2018).

Prognosis for Recovery

Prognosis following a SCI depends on whether the lesion is complete or incomplete. If no motor or sensory recovery is demonstrated below the lesion in the first 72 hours to 1 week postinjury, there is less likelihood of it returning (Bashar & Hughes, 2018). However, partial to full return of neurologic function one spinal nerve root level below the fracture may occur in the first 6 to 9 months after injury. The majority of improvements occur within 1 year postinjury. Motor function is more likely to occur in incomplete lesions, but determining exactly how much and how quickly it will return is difficult (Penrod, Hegde, & Ditunno, 1990). Recovery becomes less likely the farther postinjury that a client gets.

Spinal Shock

A stage of spinal shock occurs immediately postinjury that may last 24 hours to 6 weeks. In this stage reflex activity ceases below the level of the injury (Pierce & Nickel, 1977). The bladder and bowel are atonic or flaccid. Deep tendon reflexes are decreased, and sympathetic functions are disturbed. This disturbance results in decreased constriction of blood vessels, low blood pressure, a slower heart rate, and no perspiration below the level of injury (Spencer, 1993).

The spinal cord is usually not damaged below the level of the lesion. Therefore muscles that are innervated by the neurologic segments below the level of injury usually develop spasticity because the monosynaptic reflex arc is intact but separated from higher inhibitory influences. Deep tendon reflexes become hyperactive, and spasticity may be evident. Sensory loss continues, and the bladder and bowel usually become spastic ("upper motor neuron" bladder) in clients whose injuries are above T12. The bladder and bowel usually remain flaccid ("lower motor neuron" bladder) in clients whose lesions are at L1 and below. Sympathetic functions become hyperactive. Spinal reflex activity (mass muscle spasms) usually becomes evident in the areas below the level of the lesion (Bromley, 1998; Paulson, 1994; Penrod et al., 1990).

MEDICAL AND SURGICAL MANAGEMENT OF SPINAL CORD INJURY

After a traumatic event in which SCI is likely, the conscious victim should be questioned carefully about cutaneous numbness and skeletal muscle paralysis before being moved. Emergency medical technicians, paramedics, and air transport personnel are trained in SCI precautions and extrication techniques for moving a possible SCI victim from an accident site. Movement of the spine must be prevented during the transfer procedures. A firm stretcher or board to which the victim's head and back can be strapped should be procured before moving the victim. Axial traction on the neck should be maintained, and any movement of the spine and neck should be prevented during this process (Bashar & Hughes, 2018). Careful examination, stabilization, and transportation of the client may prevent a temporary or minimal SCI from becoming more severe or permanent. Initial care is directed toward preventing further damage to the spinal cord and, if possible, reversing any neurologic damage by stabilization or decompression of the injured neurologic structures (Freed, 1990; Malick & Meyer, 1978; Pierce & Nickel, 1977).

Steroids are administered in the first 24 to 48 hours postinjury to reduce swelling at the lesion site and minimize further damage to the cord. However, this protocol is still being researched and not definitively recommended (Miękisiak et al., 2019). Other emerging acute therapies, still in the experimental phases, include the induction of hypothermia and administration of pharmacologic neuroprotective agents (Bashar & Hughes, 2018).

The examining physician performs a careful neurologic examination to aid in determining both the orthopedic and neurologic extent of injury. Anteroposterior and lateral x-rays are taken, with the client's head, neck, or spine immobilized, to help determine the type of injury. A computed tomography (CT) scan or magnetic resonance imaging (MRI) can be used for further evaluation. The acute medical goals are restoration of normal spinal alignment, stabilization of the injured area, and decompression of neurologic structures under pressure due to fracture or swelling. Surgical interventions to decompress the spinal cord and achieve spinal stability and normal bony alignment include open reduction with internal fixation (ORIF) and spinal fusion (Bashar & Hughes, 2018; Freed, 1990; Pierce & Nickel, 1977). When adequate immobilization can be achieved nonoperatively, surgery is not indicated. Bony realignment and stabilization can be achieved

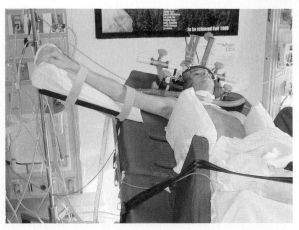

Fig. 26.2 Kinetic bed with custom arm positioner. Designed and fabricated by the Occupational Therapy Department, Santa Clara Valley Medical Center of San Jose, CA. (Courtesy Luis Gonzalez, Media Resource Department, Santa Clara Valley Medical Center.)

by immobilization and skeletal traction. A rotating kinetic bed can be used for this (Fig. 26.2). It provides constant rotation that allows for continuous pressure relief, mobilization of respiratory secretions, and easy access to the client's entire body for bowel, bladder, and hygiene care. These specialized beds are recommended for clients with an unstable spine who need to be immobilized for an extended time.

It is best for clients to be provided with portable immobilization as soon as possible. This can be provided by a halo vest or cervical collar for cervical injuries (Fig. 26.3A) and a thoracic brace or body jacket for thoracic injuries (see Fig. 26.3B) (Bashar & Hughes, 2018). Portable immobilization allows the client to be transferred to a standard hospital bed, to maintain upright posture in a wheelchair and to be involved in an active therapy program (Bashar & Hughes, 2018). Initiating an upright sitting tolerance program shortly after injury can significantly reduce the incidence and severity of further medical complications, including deep vein thrombosis (DVT), joint contractures, skin breakdown, and the general deconditioning that can result from prolonged bed rest (Bashar & Hughes, 2018).

The benefits of early transport to a specialized SCI center have been documented and include improved outcomes and fewer complications (Bashar & Hughes, 2018; Hanak & Scott, 1983). Spinal cord centers offer a complete and multidisciplinary team of professionals who specialize in SCI. Clients treated in specialized SCI centers have reduced total lengths of stay, decreased incidence of pressure ulcers, lower rates of joint contractures, and increased neurologic recovery. Additionally, individuals sent to specialized rehabilitation SCI centers were found to make functional gains with greater efficiency (Bashar & Hughes, 2018).

Complications of SCI

Skin Breakdown. Injury to the skin or underlying tissue is caused by a loss of blood supply due to prolonged pressure. These pressure injuries result in skin damage that ranges from a reddened area to a wound involving full thickness skin

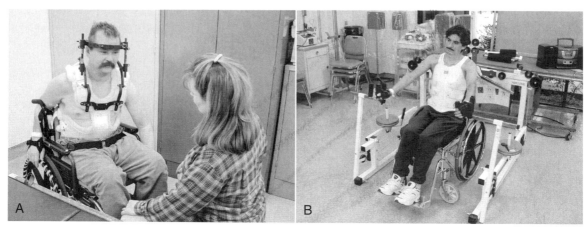

Fig. 26.3 (A) Halo vest, one type of cervical neck immobilization device for clients with quadriplegia and high-level paraplegia (T1–4). (B) Body jacket, one type of immobilization device for paraplegia. (Courtesy Luis Gonzalez, Media Resource Department, Santa Clara Valley Medical Center.)

damage. This occurs because the client is either unable to feel messages of pain or discomfort or unable to move in response to them if they are felt. Prolonged sitting or lying in one position decreases blood flow and increasing skin temperature, which leads to tissue breakdown. Heat can burn and destroy tissues while shearing forces destroy underlying tissue. The areas over bony prominences, such as the sacrum, ischium, trochanters, elbows, heels, iliac crest, scapula, knees, toes, and rib cage, are most at risk for skin breakdown (Bashar & Hughes, 2018).

Skin breakdown can lead to serious infections, which may become life threatening. Preventative measures can greatly reduce the risk. It is important to be aware of the signs of developing skin problems, to reduce the risk of breakdown. The staging of pressure ulcers is as follows:

- Stage 1: Skin is hyperpigmented (reddened) and blanches to the touch.
- Stage 2: Skin is hyperpigmented but does not blanch to the touch, indicating necrosis (or tissue death) has begun.
- Stage 3: Skin is open, and a blister or ulceration has developed.
- Stage 4: Skin is open, and underlying fascia (muscle, tendon, bone) is visible.

Skin breakdown can be prevented by relieving and eliminating pressure points and protecting vulnerable areas from excessive shearing, moisture, and heat. OTAs can help the client perform measures to prevent pressure injuries. These include performing scheduled pressure relief and skin inspections, maintaining good skin hygiene (including keeping it clean and dry) and adequate hydration and nutrition, and wearing properly fitting clothing. During activities of daily living (ADL) sessions, OTAs can teach clients to perform skin examinations using adaptive equipment, such as a mirror, and how to integrate skin inspection into their daily routines. OTAs can also direct others and teach caregivers to watch for signs of developing skin problems or introduce technology, such as smartphone apps for pressure relief and skin inspection reminders (Bashar & Hughes, 2018). Skin damage can occur within 30 minutes, so frequent weight shifting,

repositioning, and vigilance are essential for preventing skin breakdown (Pierce & Nickel, 1977; Wilson, McKenzie, & Barber, 1984).

Decreased Vital Capacity. Those who have sustained cervical and high thoracic lesions experience acute respiratory compromise and decreased **vital capacity**. Clients with injuries at C4 and above will require mechanical ventilation to breathe due to paralysis of the diaphragm, intercostal muscles, and abdominal muscles and will require assistance to maintain a clear airway free of secretions (Bashar & Hughes, 2018). Those with injuries between C4 and T6 may have a tracheostomy and will be able to breathe on their own but will have markedly limited chest expansion and decreased ability to cough because of weakness or paralysis of the intercostal and abdominal muscles, which can cause respiratory tract infections. Reduced vital capacity affects the overall endurance level for activity. Endurance can be improved by assisted breathing and by vigorous respiratory and physical therapy. Strengthening of the sternocleidomastoids and the diaphragm, manually assisted coughing, and deep breathing exercises are essential to maintain optimal vital capacity (Paulson, 1994; Penrod et al., 1990).

Osteoporosis. Osteoporosis develops in clients with SCIs because of disuse of long bones, particularly of the lower extremities. Osteoporosis may be sufficiently advanced for pathologic fractures to occur 1 year after the injury (Soleyman-Jahi, Soleyman-Jahi, & Yousefian, 2018). Pathologic fractures are most common in the supracondylar area of the femur, the proximal tibia, the distal tibia, the intertrochanteric area of the femur, and the neck of the femur. Pathologic fractures are usually not seen in UEs. Daily standing with a standing frame may slow the onset of osteoporosis; however, this method is controversial and is not embraced in all rehabilitation programs (Pierce & Nickel, 1977; Wilson et al., 1984). A standing program must fit into the client's ADL routine after discharge to be effective on an ongoing basis. Not all reimbursement sources will cover the cost of standing equipment. Research has also shown that more than 5 hours of standing per week could preserve tibial bone mass density in those with SCIs within 1 year or less (Soleyman-Jahi et al., 2018).

Orthostatic Hypotension. A lack of muscle tone in the abdomen and lower extremities causes blood pooling in these areas, resulting in decreased blood pressure (**hypotension**). Orthostatic hypotension occurs when the client moves from supine to upright or changes body position too quickly. Symptoms are dizziness, nausea, and loss of consciousness (Freed, 1990). When this occurs, the client must be reclined quickly and, if sitting in a wheelchair, tipped back with legs elevated until symptoms subside (Bashar & Hughes, 2018). As sitting tolerance and level of activity increase, this problem can diminish, but some people may continue to experience hypotensive episodes. Abdominal binders, compression garments, antiembolism stockings, and medications can aid in increasing blood flow and reducing symptoms.

Autonomic Dysreflexia. **Autonomic dysreflexia** is a life-threatening complication experienced with injuries at T6 or above. It is caused by reflex action of the autonomic nervous system in response to noxious stimuli such as a distended bladder or bowel, kidney or bladder stone, constipation or bowel impaction, infection, pressure sore, DVT, ingrown toenail, broken bone, thermal or pain stimuli, or visceral distention. The symptoms are immediate pounding headache, anxiety, perspiration, flushing, chills, nasal congestion, sudden onset of hypertension, and bradycardia. The most dangerous sign of autonomic dysreflexia is a rapid rise in systolic blood pressure that is 20 to 40 mmHg higher than the individual's baseline blood pressure.

Autonomic dysreflexia is a life-threatening medical emergency, and the client should not be left alone (Freed, 1990; Pierce & Nickel, 1977; Wilson et al., 1984). The condition is treated by placing the client in an upright position and removing anything restrictive, such as abdominal binders or antiembolism stockings. The bladder should be drained or the legbag tubing should be checked for obstruction. Blood pressure and other symptoms should be monitored until they return to normal. The OTA must be aware of symptoms and treatment because autonomic dysreflexia can occur at any time after the injury.

Spasticity. **Spasticity** is a common complication of SCI (Yarkony, 1994). It is an involuntary muscle contraction below the level of injury that results from lack of inhibition from the brain. Patterns of spasticity change over the first year, gradually increasing in the first 6 months and reaching a plateau about 1 year postinjury (Yarkony, 1994). A moderate amount of spasticity can be helpful in the overall rehabilitation of the client with SCI, as it helps to maintain muscle mass, facilitates blood circulation to help prevent pressure sores, and can assist in ROM and bed mobility. A sudden increase in spasticity can alert the client to other medical problems such as bladder infections, skin breakdown, or fever.

Severe spasticity can be frustrating to both the client and the therapist because it can interfere with function such as self-feeding and transfers. It may also cause pain, loss of ROM, and disrupted sleep (Bashar & Hughes, 2018). Therapeutic interventions such as consistent ROM exercises and stretching can help maintain flexibility while splints, braces, or serial casting can be used to provide continuous stretch to the muscle (Bashar & Hughes, 2018).

Severe spasticity may be treated more aggressively with a variety of medications or with nerve or motor point blocks using chemodenervative agents such as strains of botulinum toxin (Botox) (Bashar & Hughes, 2018). In more severe cases intrathecal medication therapy (e.g., baclofen pump) or neurosurgical procedures can be performed (Freed, 1990; Paulson, 1994; Penrod et al., 1990).

Heterotopic Ossification. **Heterotopic ossification** (HO), also called ectopic bone, is bone that develops in abnormal anatomic locations and occurs in 16% to 53% of individuals with SCI (Yarkony, 1994). It most often occurs in the muscles around the hip and knee, but can develop at the elbow and shoulder as well (Bashar & Hughes, 2018). The onset of HO is generally 1 to 6 months after injury; the initial symptoms are swelling, warmth, and decreased joint ROM. These symptoms are often discovered during physical or occupational therapy treatments despite negative radiologic findings. Early diagnosis and initiation of treatment can minimize complications. Treatment consists of medication and the maintenance of joint ROM during the early stage of active bone formation to preserve the functional ROM necessary for good wheelchair positioning, symmetric position of the pelvis, and maximal functional mobility. If HO progresses and substantially limits hip flexion, it can cause a pelvic obliquity while sitting. The obliquity can cause trunk deformities, such as scoliosis and kyphosis, and skin breakdown at the ischial tuberosities, trochanters, and sacrum (Freed, 1990; Pierce & Nickel, 1977).

Sexual Function. The sexual drive and the need for physical and emotional intimacy are not altered by SCI. However, problems of mobility, functional dependency, altered body image, complicating medical problems, and the attitudes of partners and society affect social and sexual roles, access, interest, and satisfaction.

Lack of sensation over one part of the body is accompanied by increased or altered sensation over other parts of the body. The sexual response of the body after a SCI needs to be explored in the same way a person learns what muscles are working and where he or she can feel.

In males, erections and ejaculations are often affected by SCI. However, this problem is variable and needs to be evaluated individually. Often the motility of sperm in men with SCI is decreased even when other function is near normal (Amador, Lynne, & Brackett, 1998). Significant advances in treatment are identifying the possible sources of infertility associated with SCI and exploring ways to address the problem.

In women, menstruation usually ceases for an interval of weeks to months after injury and will usually return normally in time. Vaginal lubrication during sexual activity may change, but fertility is not affected, so females with SCI can still conceive and give birth. Special attention must be given to the interaction of pregnancy and childbirth with SCI, especially in regard to blood clots, respiratory function, bladder infections, dysreflexia, the use of medications during pregnancy, and breastfeeding.

Awareness and acceptance by professionals are increasing, and sexual counseling and education are a regular part of many rehabilitation programs for all types of physical disabilities. While some clients lack basic sex education, others may feel asexual because of their disability, altered self-esteem, and isolation from peers; therefore they may feel uncomfortable with any type of sexual interaction. For these reasons sexual education and counseling must be geared to the needs of the individual client and his or her significant other.

Occupational therapy practitioners can address sexuality and help individuals overcome difficulties in expressing their sexuality in social contexts through use of the PLISSIT model. PLISSIT is an acronym that stands for permission, limited information, specific suggestions, and intensive therapy (Krantz, Tolan, Pontarelli, & Cahill, 2016). The PLISSIT model helps practitioners discuss sexual functioning with people with disabilities in four phases: (1) giving permission to ask about sexual issues and letting their clients know it is safe and appropriate to ask questions, (2) providing limited information in response to direct questions, (3) making specific suggestions based on problems presented, and (4) making a referral to intensive therapy if a practitioner is not able to meet a client's needs (Krantz et al., 2016).

OCCUPATIONAL THERAPY PROCESS

Rehabilitation will not determine the degree of recovery. The goals of rehabilitation include prevention and minimization of further medical complications through education, maintenance and improvement of strengths and skills that are present, maximizing function in self-care activities, facilitating mobility, and optimizing lifestyle options for the client and his or her family. The overall goal is maintaining the body and general well-being in a "recovery-ready" mode.

Evaluation

Assessment of the client is an ongoing process that begins on the day of admission and continues long after discharge on an outpatient follow-up basis to gauge the client's functional progress and the appropriateness of treatment and equipment. A comprehensive initial evaluation is essential to determine baseline neurologic, clinical, and functional status to formulate a treatment program and substantiate progress. Initial data gathered from the medical chart will provide personal information, medical diagnoses, and other pertinent medical information. Input from the multidisciplinary team will enhance the occupational therapy practitioner's ability to accurately predict realistic outcomes.

Discharge planning begins during the initial evaluation. Therefore the client's social and vocational history and past and expected living situations are necessary for planning a treatment program that meets the client's ongoing needs.

Physical Status. While the OT performs the evaluation, the OTA is responsible for selecting appropriate treatment options to meet the client's needs based on the evaluation results. Before contact with the client, the OT obtains specific medical precautions from the primary and consulting physicians. Skeletal instability, related injuries, or medical complications will affect how the client should be moved and the allowed active or resistive movements.

Passive ROM (PROM) is measured before an ASIA neurologic examination or specific manual muscle testing to determine available pain-free movement. Evaluation of PROM identifies the presence of or potential for joint contractures, which could suggest the need for preventive or corrective splinting and positioning.

Shoulder pain that leads to decreased shoulder and scapular ROM is extremely common in clients with C4–7 tetraplegia. Prolonged bed rest and nerve root compression subsequent to the injury also results in scapular immobilization. Shoulder pain must be thoroughly assessed for proper treatment to be provided before the onset of chronic discomfort and functional loss.

Accurate assessment of the client's muscle strength is critical in determining the precise neurologic level of impairment and establishing a baseline for physical recovery and functional progress. Using accepted ASIA motor examination and muscle testing protocols ensures accurate and consistent techniques for this complex evaluation. The motor examination should be repeated as often as needed to provide an ongoing picture of the client's strength and progress.

Sensation is evaluated for light touch, superficial pain, and kinesthesia and determining the areas of absent, impaired, and intact sensation. These findings are useful in establishing the level of injury and determining functional limitations (Fig. 26.4) (Consortium for Spinal Cord Medicine, Paralyzed Veterans of America, 1999).

If the client is evaluated in the acute stage, spasticity is rarely noted because the client is still in spinal shock. When spinal shock subsides, increased muscle tone may be present in response to stimuli. The therapist will then determine whether the spasticity interferes with or enhances function.

An evaluation of wrist and hand function will determine the degree to which a client can manipulate objects, which is used to determine the need for equipment such as positioning splints or universal cuffs or, later, for a tenodesis orthosis (wrist-driven flexor hinge splint) (see Chapter 13). Gross grasp and pinch measurements indicate functional abilities and may be used as an adjunct to muscle testing to provide objective measurements of baseline status and progress for clients who have active hand musculature (Heinemann, Magiera-Planey, Schiro-Geist, & Gimines, 1987).

Clinical observation is used to assess endurance, oral motor control, head and trunk control, LE functional muscle strength, and total body function. More specific assessment in any of these areas may be required, depending on the individual.

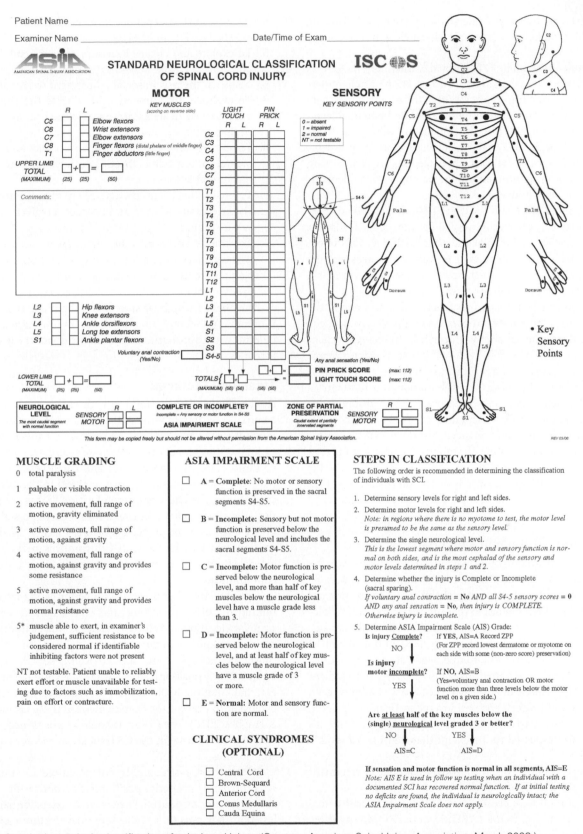

Fig. 26.4 Standard neurologic classification of spinal cord injury. (Courtesy American Spinal Injury Association, March 2006.)

The OTA's observation skills in these areas will assist the other team members in their treatment progressions.

An increased number of combined traumatic SCI—head injury diagnoses suggests that a specific cognitive and perceptual evaluation may be necessary (Hill, 1987). Assessing a client's ability to initiate tasks, follow directions, carry over learning day to day, and complete simple to complex problem-solving tasks contributes to the information base needed for appropriate and realistic goal setting. Understanding the client's learning style, coping skills, and communication style is also essential.

Functional Status. The OTA provides treatment in ADL as a primary area practice. Therefore observation of a client performing ADL is an important aspect of the occupational therapy evaluation, which determines present and potential levels of functional ability. The evaluation and simultaneous treatment should begin as soon as the client is cleared for out-of-bed activity. Light activities such as feeding, hygiene at sink level, and object manipulation may be appropriate, depending on the level of injury.

Direct interaction with the client's family and friends provides valuable information regarding the client's support systems while in the hospital and after discharge. This information is relevant to later caregiver training in areas that the client may require the assistance of others to accomplish, such as self-care and mobility tasks.

In addition to physical and functional assessments, the OTA has the opportunity to observe the client's psychosocial adjustment to the disability through activities the client participates in (Pierce & Nickel, 1977). Establishing rapport and mutual trust is important to facilitate participation and progress in all phases of rehabilitation. An individual's motivation, determination, socioeconomic background, education, family support, acceptance of disability, executive functioning abilities, and financial resources can be invaluable assets or limitations in determining the outcome of rehabilitation. The OTA must clearly observe each client's status and communicate the observations to the primary OT in order for effective treatment approaches to be established.

Establishing Treatment Objectives

Establishing treatment objectives in collaboration with the client, family, and rehabilitation team is important, especially when primary objectives of the rehabilitation team may not align with the client's goals. Psychosocial factors, cultural factors, cognition, environment, and individual financial considerations must be identified and integrated into a treatment program that will meet the unique needs of each individual. Every client and injury are different, so a variety of treatment approaches and alternatives may be necessary to address each factor that may affect goal achievement (Hanak & Scott, 1983). Increased participation can be expected if the client's priorities are respected to the extent that they are achievable and realistic.

The general objectives for occupational therapy treatment of the client with SCI are as follows:

1. To maintain or increase joint ROM and prevent deformity via active ROM (AROM) and PROM, splinting, and positioning
2. To increase the strength of all innervated and partially innervated muscles through the use of enabling and purposeful activities
3. To increase physical endurance and activity tolerance via enabling and purposeful activities

4. To maximize independence in all areas of occupation, especially ADL and IADL
5. To explore and engage in leisure interests and vocational potential
6. To aid in the psychosocial adjustment to disability
7. To evaluate, recommend, and educate the client in the use and care of necessary durable medical and adaptive equipment
8. To ensure safe and independent home and environmental accessibility through safety and accessibility recommendations
9. To assist the client in developing the communication skills necessary to train and instruct caregivers to provide safe assistance
10. To educate clients and their families of the benefits and consequences in relation to long-term function and the aging process of maintaining healthy and responsible lifestyle habits

The client's length of stay in the inpatient rehabilitation program and ability to participate in outpatient therapy determine the appropriateness and priority of the just-named activities.

Treatment Methods

Acute Phase. When working with clients with SCI in the acute care setting, the role of the OT and OTA is to preserve joint integrity and mobility with positioning and early mobilization, restore function through self-care training, initiate education and training families and caregivers, and coordinate care such as preparing for transition to the next level of care. During the acute, or immobilization, phase of rehabilitation, the client may be in traction or wearing a stabilization device such as a cervical collar or body jacket. Medical precautions must be implemented during this period. Flexion, extension, and rotary movements of the spine and neck are contraindicated.

Optimal joint alignment should be initiated through positioning and orthotics at this time. In clients with tetraplegia, scapular elevation and elbow flexion (as well as limited shoulder flexion and abduction while on bed rest) can potentially cause shoulder pain and limited ROM, so UEs should be intermittently positioned in 80 degrees of shoulder abduction, external rotation with scapular depression, and full elbow extension to prevent the development of these issues (Bashar & Hughes, 2018). The forearm should be positioned in pronation because injuries at the C5 level are at risk for supination contractures.

When muscle strength is not adequate to support the wrist or hands properly, positioning orthotics for the hand and wrist are introduced. When wrist extension strength is less than fair plus (3 + /5), a supportive orthotic should be fabricated that maintains a neutral wrist, an opposed thumb, an open thumb web space, and natural finger flexion at the metacarpophalangeal (MP) and proximal interphalangeal (PIP) joints (Bashar & Hughes, 2018). If wrist extension strength is fair plus (3/5) or greater, a short opponens soft or thermoplastic splint should be considered to maintain the web space and support the thumb in opposition. This splint can be used functionally while the client is trained to use a **tenodesis** grasp. Splints should be dorsal rather than volar in design to allow maximal sensory feedback while the client's hand is resting on any surface. PROM, AROM, and active-assisted ROM (AAROM) of all joints should be performed within strength, ability, and tolerance levels. Muscle reeducation techniques for wrists and elbows should be employed when indicated, and light progressive resistive exercises for wrists and hands may be carried out (Bashar & Hughes, 2018).

The client should be encouraged to engage in self-care activities such as feeding and hygiene by using simple devices such as a universal cuff or built-up handles. Although the client may be immobilized in bed, discussion of anticipated DME, home modifications, and caregiver training should be initiated to allow sufficient time to prepare for discharge.

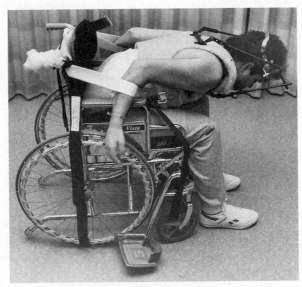

Fig. 26.5 Forward weight shift using loops attached to wheelchair frame. This client has C6 quadriplegia with symmetric grade 4 deltoids and biceps and wrist extensors.

Active Phase. During the active, or mobilization, phase of the rehabilitation program, the client can sit in a wheelchair and should begin developing upright tolerance. At this time, a high priority is determining a method of relieving sitting pressure for the purpose of preventing **decubitus ulcers** on the ischial, trochanteric, and sacral bony prominences (Bashar & Hughes, 2018). If the client has quadriplegia yet has at least a muscle grade of fair (3) for bilateral shoulder and elbow strength, leaning forward over the feet will relieve pressure on the buttocks. Simple cotton webbing loops are secured to the back frame of the wheelchair (Fig. 26.5). A person with low quadriplegia (C7) or a person with paraplegia with intact UE musculature can perform a full depression weight shift off the arms or wheels of the wheelchair. Weight shifts should be performed every 30 to 60 minutes until skin tolerance is determined.

AROM and PROM exercises should be continued regularly to prevent contractures, and orthotics or casts of the elbows may be indicated to correct contractures that are developing. Clients who have wrist extension can learn to use a functional tenodesis grasp: When the wrist is extended, the fingers automatically flex and allow them to grasp objects (Bashar & Hughes, 2018). Some tightness in the wrist extensors and long finger flexor tendons is desirable to give tension in the tenodesis grasp and maintain the thumb interphalangeal (IP) joint in extension for alignment of the thumb to the index finger (Bashar & Hughes, 2018). The desirable contracture is developed by ranging finger flexion with the wrist fully extended and finger extension with the wrist flexed, thus never allowing the flexors or extensors to be in full stretch over all of the joints that they cross (Fig. 26.6) (Wilson et al., 1984).

Elbow contractures should be prevented as often as possible because full elbow extension is necessary for the client to prop oneself to maintain balance during static sitting and to assist in transfers. In the absence of triceps innervation, a person with C6 quadriplegia can maintain forward sitting balance by shoulder depression and protraction, external rotation, full elbow extension, and full wrist extension (Fig. 26.7).

Progressive resistive exercise and resistive activities can be applied to fully and partially innervated muscles. Shoulder

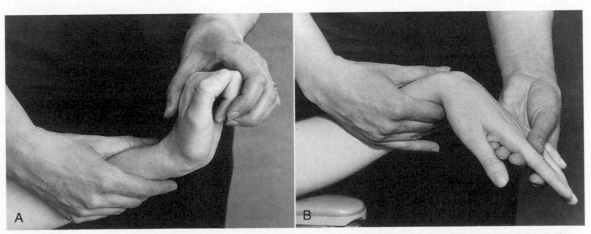

Fig. 26.6 Tenodesis action. (A) Wrist is extended when fingers are passively flexed. (B) Wrist is flexed when fingers are passively extended.

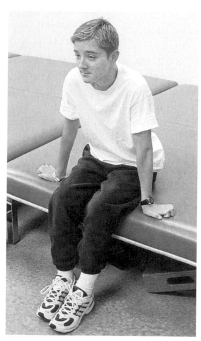

Fig. 26.7 A client with C6 quadriplegia; forward sitting balance is maintained (without triceps) by locking elbows. This technique is valuable for maintaining sitting balance, bed mobility, and transfers. (Courtesy Luis Gonzalez, Media Resource Department, Santa Clara Valley Medical Center.)

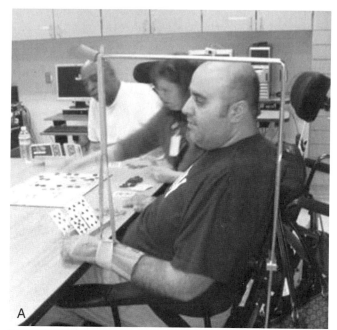

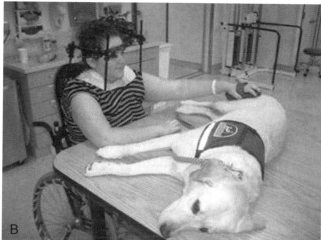

Fig. 26.8 (A) Client with injury at C5 utilizing overhead sling for tabletop activity. (B) Use of a service dog as a treatment option to facilitate bilateral upper extremity (UE) use. (Courtesy Luis Gonzalez, Media Resource Department, Santa Clara Valley Medical Center.)

musculature should be exercised so as to promote proximal stability, with emphasis on the latissimus dorsi (shoulder depressors), deltoids (shoulder flexors, abductors, and extensors), and the remainder of the shoulder girdle and scapular muscles. The triceps, pectoralis, and latissimus dorsi muscles are necessary for transfers and for weight shifting when seated. Wrist extensors should be strengthened to enhance natural tenodesis function, thereby maximizing the necessary prehension pattern in the hand for functional grasp and release (Bashar & Hughes, 2018).

The treatment program should be graded to increase the amount of resistance that can be tolerated during activity. As muscle power and endurance improve, increasing the amount of time in wheelchair activities will help the client participate in activities throughout the day.

Many assistive devices and equipment items can be useful to the person with SCI. However, every attempt should be made to have the client perform the task with the least restrictive device or no equipment, if possible.

When appropriate, the universal cuff for holding eating utensils, toothbrushes, pens, and typing sticks offers increased independence. A wrist cock-up splint to stabilize the wrist with attachment of the universal cuff may be useful for persons with little or no wrist extension. A plate guard, cup holder, extended straw with straw clip, and nonskid table mat can facilitate independent feeding. A wash mitt and liquid soap appear to make bathing easier; however, the added difficulty of donning and doffing such equipment must be considered. Many people with quadriplegia can use a button hook to fasten clothing while pull-over shirts and Velcro closures may

be easier to don and doff. A transfer board may facilitate safe transfers. Clients may outgrow the use of initially necessary equipment as they acquire greater strength and coordination (Bashar & Hughes, 2018).

The ADL program may be expanded to include independent feeding with devices, oral and facial hygiene, and upper-body bathing, bowel and bladder care (such as digital stimulation and intermittent catheterization), UE dressing, and transfers using the slide board (Bashar & Hughes, 2018). Developing communication skills in writing, using the telephone, electronic devices, and computer keyboard should be an important part of the treatment program (Fig. 26.8). Training in the use of the mobile arm support, overhead slings, wrist-hand orthosis (flexor hinge or tenodesis splint), and assistive devices is also part of the occupational therapy program.

The OTA should continue to provide psychological support by allowing and encouraging the client to express frustration, anger, fears, and concerns (Spencer, 1993). The occupational therapy clinic in a spinal cord center should provide an atmosphere where clients can establish support groups with other inpatients and outpatients who can offer their experiences and problem-solving advice to those in earlier phases of their rehabilitation.

The assessment, ordering, and fitting of DME such as wheelchairs, seating and positioning equipment, mechanical lifts, beds, and bathing equipment is extremely important. Such equipment will be specifically evaluated by the OT, the physical therapist, or the interdisciplinary team and would be ordered only when definite goals and expectations are known. Inappropriate equipment can impair function and cause further medical problems such as skin breakdown or trunk deformity; the therapist must take into account all functional, positioning, environmental, psychological, and financial considerations that affect the client's equipment needs. The desired equipment, especially wheelchairs, seat cushions, back supports, positioning devices, and bathing equipment, should be available for demonstration and trial by the client before final ordering (Bashar & Hughes, 2018). The OTA involved in the treatment of an individual with SCI must be familiar with what has been recommended for the client because the OTA will be training with similar equipment to simulate the discharge setting.

In addition to enhancing respiratory function by supporting the client in an erect, well-aligned position that maximizes sitting tolerance and optimizes UE function, wheelchair seating must assist in the prevention of joint deformity and skin breakdown. An appropriate and adequate wheelchair cushion helps distribute sitting pressure, assists in the prevention of skin breakdown, stabilizes the pelvis as needed for proper trunk alignment, and provides comfort (Bashar & Hughes, 2018). The OT and OTA can help prevent fixed trunk and pelvic deformities such as kyphosis and scoliosis, which can lead to considerable skin problems and later uncorrectable cosmetic deformities, by making good trunk alignment and seating a priority from the outset. The OTA should work closely with the entire treating team to ensure consistent training and use of the seating system to support each client.

An increasing number of individuals with high-level spinal cord injuries at C4 and above are surviving and participating in active rehabilitation programs. The treatment and equipment needs of these individuals are unique and extremely specialized, ranging from mouthsticks and assistive technology to ventilators and sophisticated electric wheelchairs and drive systems (Table 26.1) (levels C1−3 and C3−4). Commercially available assistive technology such as cell phones, electronic readers, and notebook computers has greatly enhanced the options available to high-level tetraplegics (Fig. 26.9).

A home evaluation will be performed once the client's place of discharge is determined and they can tolerate leaving the hospital for a few hours. The OT, client, and family members can then assess the home environment and engage in home activities in anticipation of return to a safe and accessible environment. The OTA must be knowledgeable about safety and accessibility options for a variety of environments and often must reinforce the necessity of having appropriate modifications completed before discharge. The OTA should be aware of accessibility requirements in the home, as well as those required in the workplace by the Americans with Disabilities Act of 1990 (ADA) (see Chapter 16).

Shorter inpatient rehabilitation stays have moved the extended phase of treatment to outpatient or home care. Adaptive driving, home management, leisure activities, or workshop skill assessments using hand-based or power-based tools are feasible and appropriate treatment modalities for evaluating and increasing UE strength, coordination, and trunk balance. While these skills may not be a priority during inpatient hospitalization, such activities can improve socialization and assess problem-solving skills and potential work habits.

OTs and OTAs may assist in the exploration of vocational potential of persons with SCI. High-level injuries cause dysfunction in many areas of occupation. Therefore clients may need to explore a change in vocation or alternative methods of accessing former vocations. Vocational rehabilitation can be complicated by decreased motivation and feelings of hopelessness and by loss of health benefits. The psychosocial aspects of lost and altered roles and identities, vocational and otherwise, should be considered throughout the rehabilitation process.

The OTA can assist in determining the client's level of motivation, functional aptitudes, attitudes, interests, and personal vocational aspirations throughout the treatment program, particularly in ADL, mobility, and work simulation activities. The OTA can observe the client's executive functioning skills such as attention and memory, manual ability with splints and devices, accuracy, speed, perseverance, work habits, and work tolerance level. The OTA can offer valuable information from observations during activities. When suitable vocational objectives have been selected, they may be pursued in an educational setting or in a work setting, usually out of the realm of occupational therapy.

Aging With SCI. After survival of an acute SCI, the primary goal of rehabilitation is independence. Independence as the measure of quality of life for people with disabilities is an idea accepted and often perpetuated by survivors and health care professionals alike (Whiteneck & Charlifue, 1993).

OTs and OTAs treating clients with SCI have considerable responsibility in influencing the level of independence from the acute setting and active rehabilitation, through outpatient and follow-up care over the course of the individual's lifespan. Understanding the aging process in both able-bodied and disabled individuals is necessary for providing appropriate options and fostering attitudes that prevent further injury and enhance the quality of the client's life at any age.

When SCI is compounded by the increased fatigue and weakness often associated with normal aging, the functional status of the individual may decline. The OTA may note these

TABLE 26.1 Expected Functional Outcomes

Expected Functional Outcome		Equipment	FIM/ASSISTANCE DATA		
			Exp	Med	IR

Level C1–3
Functionally relevant muscles innervated: sternocleidomastoid, cervical paraspinal, neck accessories
Movement possible: neck flexion, extension, rotation
Patterns of weakness: total paralysis of trunk, upper extremities, lower extremities; dependent on ventilator
NSCISC sample size: FIM = 15/assist = 12

Expected Functional Outcome		Equipment	Exp	Med	IR
Respiratory	Ventilator dependent	Two ventilators (bedside, portable)			
	Inability to clear secretions	Suction equipment or other suction management device			
		Generator/battery backup			
Bowel	Total assist	Padded reclining shower/ commode chair (if roll-in shower available)	1	1	1
Bladder	Total assist		1	1	1
Bed mobility	Total assist	Full electric hospital bed with Trendelenburg feature and side rails	1	1	1
Bed/wheelchair transfers	Total assist	Transfer board Power or mechanical lift with sling	1	1	1
Pressure relief/ positioning	Total assist	Power recline and/or tilt wheelchair Wheelchair pressure-relief cushion Postural support and head control devices as indicated Hand splints may be indicated Specialty bed or pressure-relief mattress may be indicated			
Eating	Total assist		1	1	1
Dressing	Total assist		1	1	1
Grooming	Total assist		1	1	1
Bathing	Total assist	Handheld shower Shampoo tray Padded reclining shower/commode chair (if roll-in shower available)	1	1	1
Wheelchair propulsion	Manual: total assist Power: independent with equipment	Power recline and/or tilt wheelchair with head, chin, or breath control and manual recliner Vent tray	6	1	1–6
Standing/ambulation	Standing: total assist Ambulation: not indicated				
Communication	Total assist to independent, depending on workstation setup and equipment availability	Mouthstick, high-tech computer access, environmental control unit Adaptive devices everywhere as indicated			
Transportation	Total assist	Attendant-operated van (e.g., lift, tie-downs) or accessible public transportation			
Homemaking	Total assist				
Assist required	24-hour attendant to include homemaking Able to instruct in all aspects of care		24[a]	24[a]	12–24[a]

Level C4
Functionally relevant muscles innervated: upper trapezius, diaphragm, cervical paraspinal muscles
Movement possible: neck flexion, extension, rotation; scapular elevation; inspiration
Patterns of weakness: paralysis of trunk, upper extremities, lower extremities; inability to cough, endurance and respiratory reserve low secondary to paralysis of intercostals
NSCISC sample size: FIM = 28/assist = 12

(Continued)

TABLE 26.1 Expected Functional Outcomes—cont'd

Expected Functional Outcome		Equipment	FIM/ASSISTANCE DATA		
			Exp	Med	IR
Respiratory	May be able to breathe without a ventilator	If not ventilator-free, see C1–3 for equipment requirements			
Bowel	Total assist	Reclining shower/commode chair (if roll-in shower available)	1	1	1
Bladder	Total assist		1	1	1
Bed mobility	Total assist	Full electric hospital bed with Trendelenburg feature and side rails			
Bed/wheelchair transfers	Total assist	Transfer board	1	1	1
Pressure relief/ positioning	Total assist; may be independent with equipment	Power or mechanical lift with sling Power recline and/or tilt wheelchair Wheelchair pressure-relief cushion Postural support and head control devices as indicated Hand splints may be indicated Specialty bed or pressure-relief mattress may be indicated			
Eating	Total assist		1	1	1
Dressing	Total assist		1	1	1
Grooming	Total assist		1	1	1
Bathing	Total assist	Handheld shower Shampoo tray Padded reclining shower/commode chair (if roll-in shower available)	1	1	1
Wheelchair propulsion	Manual: total assist Power: independent	Power recline and/or tilt wheelchair with head, chin, or breath control and manual recliner Vent tray	6	1	1–6
Standing/ambulation	Standing: total assist Ambulation: not usually indicated	Tilt table Hydraulic standing table			
Communication	Total assist to independent, depending on workstation setup and equipment availability	Mouthstick, high-tech computer access, environmental control unit			
Transportation	Total assist	Attendant-operated van (e.g., lift, tie-downs) or accessible public transportation			
Homemaking	Total assist				
Assist required	24-hour attendant to include homemaking Able to instruct in all aspects of care		24[a]	24[a]	16–24[a]

Level C5

Functionally relevant muscles innervated: deltoid, biceps, brachialis, brachioradialis, rhomboids, serratus anterior (partially innervated)

Movement possible: shoulder flexion, abduction, and extension; elbow flexion and supination; scapular adduction and abduction

Patterns of weakness: absence of elbow extension, pronation, all wrist and hand movement; total paralysis of trunk and lower extremities

NSCISC sample size: FIM = 41/assist = 35

Respiratory	Low endurance and vital capacity caused by paralysis of intercostals; may require assist to clear secretions				
Bowel	Total assist	Padded shower/commode chair or padded transfer tub bench with commode cutout	1	1	1
Bladder	Total assist	Adaptive devices may be indicated (electric leg bag emptier)	1	1	1

(Continued)

TABLE 26.1 Expected Functional Outcomes—cont'd

Expected Functional Outcome		Equipment	FIM/ASSISTANCE DATA		
			Exp	Med	IR
Bed mobility	Some assist	Full electric hospital bed with Trendelenburg feature with client controls			
Bed/wheelchair transfers	Total assist	Transfer board	1	1	1
		Power or mechanical lift			
Pressure relief/ positioning	Independent with equipment	Power recline and/or tilt wheelchair			
		Wheelchair pressure-relief cushion			
		Hand splints			
		Specialty bed or pressure-relief mattress may be indicated			
		Postural support devices			
Eating	Total assist for setup, then independent eating with equipment	Long opponens splint	5	5	2.5–5.5
		Adaptive devices as indicated			
Dressing	Lower extremity: total assist	Long opponens splint	1	1	1–4
	Upper extremity: some assist	Adaptive devices as indicated			
Grooming	Some to total assist	Long opponens splint	1–3	1	1–5
		Adaptive devices as indicated			
Bathing	Total assist	Padded tub transfer bench or shower/ commode chair	1	1	1–3
		Handheld shower			
Wheelchair propulsion	Power: independent	Power recline and/or tilt wheelchair with harm drive control	6	1	1–6
	Manual: independent to some assist indoors on noncarpeted, level surface; some to total assist outdoors	Manual: lightweight rigid or folding frame with handrim modification			
Standing/ambulation	Total assist	Hydraulic standing table			
Communication	Independent to some assist after setup with equipment	Long opponens splint			
		Adaptive devices as needed for page turning, writing, button pushing			
Transportation	Independent with highly specialized equipment; some assist with accessible public transportation; total assist for attendant-operated vehicle	Highly specialized modified van with lift			
Homemaking	Total assist				
Assist required	Personal care: 10 hr/day		16[a]	23[a]	10–24[a]
	Homecare: 6 hr/day				
	Able to instruct in all aspects of care				

Level C6

Functionally relevant muscles innervated: clavicular; pectoralis; supinator; extensor carpi radialis longus and brevis; serratus anterior; latissimus dorsi
Movement possible: scapular protraction; some horizontal adduction, forearm supination, radial wrist extension
Patterns of weakness: absence of wrist flexion, elbow extension, hand movement; total paralysis of trunk and lower extremities
NSCISC sample size: FIM = 43/assist = 35

Respiratory	Low endurance and vital capacity secondary to paralysis of intercostals; may require assist to clear secretions				
Bowel	Some total assist	Padded tub bench with commode cutout or padded shower/commode chair	1–2	1	1
		Other adaptive devices as indicated			
Bladder	Some total assist with equipment; may be independent with legbag emptying	Adaptive devices as indicated	1–2	1	1

(Continued)

TABLE 26.1   Expected Functional Outcomes—cont'd

Expected Functional Outcome		Equipment	FIM/ASSISTANCE DATA		
			Exp	Med	IR
Bed mobility	Some assist	Full electric hospital bed Side rails Full to king standard bed may be indicated			
Bed/wheelchair transfers	Level: some assist to independent Uneven: some to total assist	Transfer board Mechanical lift	3	1	1–3
Pressure relief/ positioning	Independent with equipment and/or adaptive techniques	Power recline and/or tilt wheelchair Wheelchair pressure-relief cushion Pressure-relief mattress or overlay may be indicated Postural support devices			

Eating	Independent with or without
	equipment; except cutting,
	which is total assist
		Adaptive devices as indicated
		   (e.g., U-cuff, tendinosis splint,
		   adapted utensils, plate guard)
			5–6	5	4–6

Dressing	Independent upper extremity;
	some assist to total assist for
	lower extremities
		Adaptive devices as indicated
		   (e.g., buttonhook; loops on
		   zippers, pants; socks, Velcro on
		   shoes)
			1–3	2	1–5

Grooming	Some assist to independent with equipment	Adaptive devices as indicated (e.g., U-cuff, adapted handles)	3–6	4	2–6
Bathing	Upper body: independent Lower body: some to total assist	Padded tub transfer bench or shower/ commode chair Adaptive devices as needed Handheld shower	1–3	1	1–3

Wheelchair
propulsion
	Power: independent with standard
	arm drive on all surfaces
	Manual: independent indoors; some
	total assist outdoors
		Manual: lightweight rigid or folding
		   frame with modified rims
		Power: may require power recline or
		   standard upright power wheelchair
			6	6	4–6

Standing/ambulation	Standing: total assist Ambulation: not indicated	Hydraulic standing frame			

Communication	Independent with or without
	equipment
		Adaptive devices as indicated
		   (e.g., tendinosis splint; writing
		   splint for keyboard use, button
		   pushing, page turning, object
		   manipulation)			

Transportation	Independent driving from wheelchair	Modified van with lift Sensitized hand controls Tie-downs			
Homemaking	Some assist with light meal preparation; total assist for all other homemaking	Adaptive devices as indicated			
Assist required	Personal care: 6 hr/day Homecare: 4 hr/day		10[a]	17[a]	8–24[a]

Level C7–8

Functionally relevant muscles innervated: latissimus dorsi; sternal pectoralis; triceps; pronator quadratus; extensor carpi ulnaris; flexor carpi radialis; flexor digitorum profundus and superficialis; extensor communis; pronator/flexor/extensor/abductor pollicis; lumbricals (partially innervated)

Movement possible: elbow extension; ulnar/wrist extension; wrist flexion; finger flexions and extensions; thumb

Patterns of weakness: paralysis of trunk and lower extremities; limited grasp and dexterity secondary to partial intrinsic muscles of the hand

NSCISC sample size: FIM = 43/assist = 35

Respiratory	Low endurance and vital capacity secondary to paralysis of intercostals; may require assist to clear secretions				
Bowel	Some total assist	Padded tub bench with commode cutout or shower/commode chair Adaptive devices as indicated	1–4	1	1–4

(Continued)

TABLE 26.1   Expected Functional Outcomes—cont'd

Expected Functional Outcome		Equipment	FIM/ASSISTANCE DATA		
			Exp	Med	IR
Bladder	Independent to some assist	Adaptive devices as indicated	2–6	3	1–6
Bed mobility	Independent to some assist	Full electric hospital bed or full to king standard bed			
Bed/wheelchair transfers	Level: independent Uneven: independent to some assist	With or without transfer board	3–7	4	2–6
Pressure relief/ positioning	Independent	Wheelchair pressure-relief cushion Postural support devices Pressure-relief mattress or overlay may be indicated			
Eating	Independent	Adaptive devices as indicated	6–7	6	5–7
Dressing	Independent upper extremity; independent to some assist in lower extremities	Adaptive devices as indicated	4–7	6	4–7
Grooming	Independent	Adaptive devices as indicated	6–7	6	4–7
Bathing	Upper body: independent Lower body: some assist to independent	Padded tub transfer bench or shower/ commode chair Adaptive devices as needed Handheld shower	3–6	4	2–6
Wheelchair propulsion	Manual: independent on all indoor surfaces and level outdoor terrain; some assist with uneven terrain	Manual: rigid or folding lightweight or folding wheelchair with modified rims	6	6	6
Standing/ambulation	Standing: independent to some assist Ambulation: not indicated	Hydraulic or standard standing frame			
Communication	Independent	Adaptive devices as indicated			
Transportation	Independent in car if independent with transfer and wheelchair loading/ unloading; independent in driving modified van from captain's seat	Modified vehicle Transfer board			
Homemaking	Independent light meal preparation and homemaking; some to total assist for complex meal preparation and heavy housecleaning	Adaptive devices as indicated			
Assist required	Personal care: 6 hr/day Homecare: 2 hr/day		8[a]	12[a]	2–24[a]

Level T1–9

Functionally relevant muscles innervated: intrinsics of the hand, including thumbs; internal and external intercostals; erector spinae; lumbricals; flexor/ extensor/abductor pollicis

Movement possible: upper extremities fully intact; limited upper trunk stability; endurance increased secondary to innervation of intercostals

Patterns of weakness: lower trunk paralysis; total paralysis of lower extremities

NSCISC sample size: FIM = 144/assist = 122

Respiratory	Compromised vital capacity and endurance				
Bowel	Independent	Elevated padded toilet seat or padded tub bench with commode cutout	6–7	6	4–6
Bladder	Independent		6	6	5–6
Bed mobility	Independent	Full to king standard bed			
Bed/wheelchair transfers	Independent	May or may not require transfer board	6–7	6	6–7

(Continued)

TABLE 26.1 Expected Functional Outcomes—cont'd

Expected Functional Outcome		Equipment	FIM/ASSISTANCE DATA		
			Exp	Med	IR
Pressure relief/ positioning	Independent	Wheelchair pressure-relief cushion Postural support devices as indicated Pressure-relief mattress or overlay may be indicated			
Eating	Independent		7	7	7
Dressing	Independent		7	7	7
Grooming	Independent		7	7	7
Bathing	Independent	Padded tub transfer bench or shower/ commode chair Handheld shower	6–7	6	5–7
Wheelchair propulsion	Independent	Manual rigid or folding lightweight wheelchair	6	6	6
Standing/ambulation	Standing: independent Ambulation: typically not functional	Standing frame			
Communication	Independent				
Transportation	Independent in car; including loading and unloading wheelchair	Hand controls			
Homemaking	Independent with complex meal preparation and light housecleaning; total to some assist with heavy housecleaning				
Assist required	Homemaking: 3 hr/day		2[a]	3[a]	0–15[a]

Level T10-L1

Functionally relevant muscles innervated: fully intact intercostals; external obliques; rectus abdominis

Movement possible: fair to good trunk stability

Patterns of weakness: paralysis of lower extremities

NSCISC sample size: FIM = 71/assist = 57

Respiratory	Intact respiratory function				
Bowel	Independent	Padded standard or raised padded toilet seat	6–7	6	6
Bladder	Independent		6	6	6
Bed mobility	Independent	Full to king standard bed			
Bed/wheelchair transfers	Independent		7	7	6–7
Pressure relief/ positioning	Independent	Wheelchair pressure-relief cushion Postural support devices as indicated Pressure-relief mattress or overlay may be indicated			
Eating	Independent		7	7	7
Dressing	Independent		7	7	7
Grooming	Independent		7	7	7
Bathing	Independent	Padded tub transfer bench Handheld shower	6–7	6	6–7
Wheelchair propulsion	Independent all indoor and outdoor surfaces	Manual rigid or folding lightweight wheelchair	6	6	6
Standing/ambulation	Standing: independent Ambulation: functional, some assist to independent	Standing frame Forearm crutches or walker Knee-ankle-foot orthosis (KAFO)			
Communication	Independent				
Transportation	Independent in car, including loading and unloading wheelchair	Hand controls			

(Continued)

TABLE 26.1   Expected Functional Outcomes—cont'd

Expected Functional Outcome		Equipment	FIM/ASSISTANCE DATA		
			Exp	Med	IR
Homemaking	Independent with complex meal preparation and light housecleaning; some assist with heavy housecleaning				
Assist required	Homemaking: 2 hr/day		2[a]	2[a]	0–8[a]

Level L2-S5

Functionally relevant muscles innervated: fully intact abdominals and all other trunk muscles; depending on level, some degree of hip flexors, extensor, abductors; knee flexors, extensors; ankle dorsiflexors, plantar flexors

Movement possible: good trunk stability; partial to full control of lower extremities

Patterns of weakness: partial paralysis of lower extremities, hips, knees, ankle, foot

NSCISC sample size: FIM = 20/assist = 16

Respiratory	Intact function				
Bowel	Independent	Padded toilet seat	6–7	6	6–7
Bladder	Independent		6	6	6–7
Bed mobility	Independent	Full to king standard bed			
Bed/wheelchair transfers	Independent		7	7	7
Pressure relief/ positioning	Independent	Wheelchair pressure-relief cushion Postural support devices as indicated			
Eating	Independent		7	7	7
Dressing	Independent		7	7	7
Grooming	Independent		7	7	7
Bathing	Independent	Padded tub bench Handheld shower	7	7	6–7
Wheelchair propulsion	Independent all indoor and outdoor surfaces	Manual rigid or folding lightweight wheelchair	6	6	6
Standing/ambulation	Standing: independent	Standing frame			
	Ambulation: functional, some assist to independent	Forearm crutches or cane as indicated KAFO or ankle-foot orthosis (AFO)			
Communication	Independent				
Transportation	Independent in car, including loading and unloading wheelchair	Hand controls			
Homemaking	Independent with complex meal preparation and light housecleaning; some assist with heavy housecleaning				
Assist required	Homemaking: 0–1 hr/day		0–1[a]	0[a]	0[a]

Exp, Expected FIM score; IR, NSCISC interquartile range; Med, NSCISC median.
[a]Hours per day.
From Consortium for Spinal Cord Medicine, Paralyzed Veterans of America. *Outcomes Following Traumatic Spinal Cord Injury: Clinical Practice Guidelines for Health-Care Professionals.* Washington, DC: The Consortium; 1999.

status changes during the course of therapy. Many considerations must be weighed to make appropriate short-term and long-term decisions, and it is the responsibility of the team to be aware of how aging affects this population.

In individuals with SCI, aging is often accelerated by secondary effects of the disability such as muscle imbalance, infections (urinary and respiratory), deconditioning, pain, and joint degeneration secondary to overuse (Paulson, 1994). Urinary problems brought on by years of catheterization, bladder infections, and urinary retention are common. Other aging-related problems for SCI survivors include osteoporosis, arthritis and joint degeneration, constipation, weakening of already precarious skin, substance abuse, and the need for increased personal care over time.

Twenty years postinjury is the typical point at which aging problems begin to increase, as at least one of four SCI survivors in the United States has survived more than 20 years postinjury with a significant portion of those individuals prematurely experiencing aging problems (Pierce & Nickel, 1977). Individuals with SCI onset in their later years have different patterns of functional outcomes, program needs, and financial resources than do those with onset in their earlier

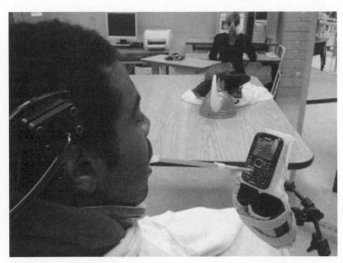

Fig. 26.9 C4 quadriplegic texting on cell phone with mouthstick and custom-adapted wheelchair mount.

years. A person who experienced SCI resulting in quadriplegia in their 20s (the age when the majority of SCIs occur) sees the degenerating conditions of premature aging become evident usually before the fourth decade (Freed, 1990). Therefore an individual in the fourth decade who was once independent in transfers at home and loading a wheelchair in and out of a vehicle may now require assistance due to degeneration of the shoulder muscles. This person may consider trading a car for an accessible van with additional modifications.

Likewise, someone at a level that usually permits functional independence (e.g., T10 paraplegia) may need personal care assistance and consider a power wheelchair with the onset of premature aging. Although use of a manual wheelchair provides the advantage of cardiopulmonary conditioning, the weight of the wheelchair combined with the distance from shoulder to push rim during propulsion can damage a weak or imbalanced shoulder complex.

Table 26.1 presents expectations of functional performance of SCI 1 year postinjury at each of the eight levels of injury (C1−3, C4, C5, C6, C7−8, T1−9, T10-L1, L2-S5) (Bashar & Hughes, 2018). The outcomes reflect a level of independence that can be expected of a person with motor-complete SCI, given optimal circumstances. The OTA should have a good understanding of aspects of each level to accurately communicate with other members of the interdisciplinary team regarding the client's clinical and treatment status.

The categories presented reflect expected functional outcomes in the areas of mobility, ADL, instrumental ADL (IADL), and communication skills. The guidelines are based on consensus of clinical experts, available literature on functional outcomes, and data compiled from Uniform Data Systems (UDS) and the National Spinal Cord Injury Statistical Center (NSCISC).

Within the functional outcomes for people with SCI listed in Table 26.1, a series of essential daily functions and activities have been identified along with the attendant care likely to be needed to support the predicted level of independence at 1 year postinjury. These outcome areas include the following:

- *Respiratory, bowel, and bladder function.* The neurologic effects of SCI may result in deficits in the ability of the individual to perform basic body functions. Respiratory function includes the ability to breathe with or without mechanical assistance and to adequately clear secretions. Bowel and bladder functions include the ability to manage elimination, maintain perineal hygiene, and manage clothing before and after elimination. Adapted or facilitated methods of managing these bodily functions may be required to attain expected functional outcomes (Bashar & Hughes, 2018).
- *Bed mobility, bed/wheelchair transfers, wheelchair propulsion, and positioning/pressure relief.* The neurologic effects of SCI may result in deficits of the skills required for the individual to perform activities for mobility, locomotion, and safety. Adapted or facilitated methods of managing these activities may be required to attain expected functional outcomes in standing and ambulation (Bashar & Hughes, 2018).
- *Standing and ambulation.* SCI may result in deficits in standing ability for exercise, psychological benefit, or ambulation for functional activities. Adapted or facilitated methods of management may be outcomes in standing and ambulation (Bashar & Hughes, 2018).
- *Eating, grooming, dressing, and bathing.* The neurologic effects of SCI may result in deficits in the individual's ability to perform these ADLs. Adapted or facilitated methods of managing ADL may be necessary to attain expected functional outcomes (Bashar & Hughes, 2018).
- *Communication (keyboard use, handwriting, and telephone use).* The neurologic effects of SCI may result in deficits of the individual's ability to communication. Adapted or facilitated methods of communication may be required to attain expected functional outcomes (Bashar & Hughes, 2018).
- *Transportation (driving, attendant-operated vehicle, and public transportation).* Transportation activities are critical for individuals with SCI to become maximally independent in their community. Adaptations may be required to help the individual meet the expected functional outcomes (Bashar & Hughes, 2018).
- *Homemaking (meal planning and preparations and home management).* Adapted or facilitated methods of managing homemaking tasks may be required to attain expected functional outcomes. Individuals with complete SCI at any level will require some level of assistance with some homemaking activities. The hours of assistance with homemaking activities are presented in Table 26.1 (Bashar & Hughes, 2018).
- *Assistance required.* Table 26.1 lists the number of hours that may be required from a caregiver to assist with personal care and homemaking activities in the home. Personal care includes hands-on delivery of all aspects of

self-care, mobility, and safety interventions (Bashar & Hughes, 2018).

- *Homemaking assistance* is also included in the recommendation for hours of assistance and includes activities previously presented. The number of hours presented in both the panel recommendations and the self-reported CHART data is representative of skilled and unskilled and paid and unpaid hours of assistance. The 24-hour-a-day requirement noted for the C1–3 and C4 levels includes the expected need for unpaid attendant care to provide safety monitoring (Bashar & Hughes, 2018). Adequate assistance is required to ensure that the individual with an SCI can achieve the outcomes set forth in Table 26.1. The hours of assistance recommended do not reflect changes in assistance required over time as reported by long-term survivors of SCI, nor do they take into account the wide range of individual variables mentioned throughout this chapter that may affect the number of required hours of assistance (Consortium for Spinal Cord Medicine, Paralyzed Veterans of America, 1999). Whether the representative individuals with SCI in the individual categories attained the expected functional outcomes for their specific level of injury is unclear. Also unclear is whether there were mitigating circumstances such as age, obesity, or concomitant injuries that would account for variability in assistance reported. An individualized assessment of needs is required in all cases.

- *Equipment requirements.* Minimum recommendations for DME and adaptive devices are identified in each of the functional categories. The most commonly used equipment is listed, with the understanding that variations exist among SCI rehabilitation programs and that use of such equipment may be necessary to achieve the identified functional outcomes. Additional equipment and devices that are not critical for most individuals at a specific level of injury may be required for some individuals. The equipment descriptions are generic to allow for varying program philosophies and financial resources. Rapid changes and advances in equipment and technology occur and must be considered. Health care professionals should remember that the recommendations set forth in Table 26.1 are not intended to be prescriptive but rather to serve as a guideline. The importance of individual functional assessment of people with SCI before making equipment recommendations cannot be overemphasized. All DME and adaptive devices must be thoroughly assessed and tested to determine medical necessity, to prevent medical complications (e.g., postural deviations, skin breakdown, pain), and to foster optimal functional performance. Environmental control units and telephone modifications may be necessary for safety and maximal independence, and each person must be individually evaluated for the need for this equipment. Recommendations for disposable medical products are not included in this table.

- *Functional Independence Measure (FIM).* Evidence for the specific levels of independence provided in Table 26.1 relies on both expert consensus and data from the previously utilized FIM in large-scale, prospective, and longitudinal research conducted by the NSCISC. The FIM was the most widely used disability measure in rehabilitation medicine, and although it may not incorporate all characteristics of disability in individuals recovering from SCI, it captures many basic disability areas. The FIM consists of 13 motor items and 5 cognitive items that are individually scored from 1 to 7. A score of 1 indicates complete dependence and a score of 7 indicates complete independence (see Table 26.1). The sum of the 13 FIM motor score items can range from 13, indicating complete dependence for all items, to 91, indicating complete independence for all items. The FIM was a measure completed by health care professionals in acute rehabilitation; other observers (including the client, family members, and caregivers) can contribute information to the ratings. Each of these observers may represent a different type of potential bias.

- Although the sample sizes of the FIM data for certain neurologic-level groups are quite small, the consistency of the data adds confidence to the interpretation. Other pertinent data regarding functional independence must be factored into outcome analyses, including medical information, client factors, social role participation, quality of life, and environmental factors and supports.

- In Table 26.1, the available FIM data are reported in three areas. Although the FIM is no longer widely used, it provides a uniform way to examine functional outcomes. The FIM data provide data 1-year postinjury of 405 survivors with complete SCI and a median age of 27 years. The NSCISC sample size for FIM and Assistance Data is provided for each level of injury. Different outcome expectations clearly should apply to different client subgroups and populations. Some populations are likely to be significantly older than those referenced, and functional abilities may be limited by advancing age (Penrod et al., 1990; Yarkony, Roth, Heinemann, & Lovell, 1988).

- *Home modifications.* To provide the optimal opportunity for individuals with SCI to achieve the identified functional outcomes, a safe and architecturally accessible environment is necessary. An accessible environment must take into consideration, but not be limited to, entrance and egress, mobility in the home, and adequate setup to perform personal care and homemaking tasks.

Research

Research in clinical settings and scientific laboratories around the world focuses on understanding the nature of SCI and defining the nervous system's response to this injury. The scientific community seems increasingly optimistic that it will be possible someday to restore function after SCI. This optimism is based on the combined research efforts of scientists in many different disciplines. It is important for all clinicians treating SCI to be aware of the scientific and technological advances so as to better educate clients while providing them with realistic and comprehensive rehabilitation interventions for their immediate and long-term needs (Bashar & Hughes, 2018).

SUMMARY

SCI can result in substantial paralysis of the limbs and trunk. The degree of residual motor and sensory dysfunction depends on the level of the lesion, whether the lesion was complete or incomplete, and the area of the spinal cord that was damaged.

After SCI, bony realignment and stabilization are established through surgical intervention, via an external immobilization device, or through a combination of both methods. The many possible complications of SCI include skin breakdown, rapid loss of bone density, and spasticity.

OTs and OTAs facilitate the client's achievement of optimal independence and functioning. Areas of focus are physical restoration of available musculature, self-care, independent living skills, short-term and long-term equipment needs, environmental accessibility, and educational, vocational, and leisure activities. The psychosocial adjustment of the client is important, and the OT and OTA offer support throughout every phase of the rehabilitation process.

REVIEW QUESTIONS

1. Describe the functional and prognostic differences between complete and incomplete lesions.
2. When reference is made to C5 in quadriplegia, what is meant in terms of level of injury and functioning muscle groups?
3. What are some medical complications common to clients with SCIs that can limit achievement of functional potential?
4. How does postural hypotension affect function, and how should a caregiver respond?
5. What are the signs of autonomic dysreflexia, and how should a caregiver respond?
6. What is the role of the OTA in the prevention of pressure sores?
7. What additional muscle power does the client with C6 quadriplegia have over the client with C5 quadriplegia? What is the major functional advantage of this additional muscle power?
8. What is the first spinal cord lesion level that has full innervation of the UE musculature?
9. List five goals of occupational therapy for the client with SCI.
10. What are some of the first self-care activities that the client with a C6 SCI should be expected to accomplish?
11. List four assistive devices commonly used by persons with quadriplegia and tell the purpose of each.
12. Why would a person with paraplegia require homemaking assistance if he or she is independent in all self-care and mobility?

REFERENCES

Amador, M. J., Lynne, C. M., & Brackett, N. L. (1998). Contemporary information regarding male infertility following spinal cord injury. *SCI Nursing.*, *15*(3), 61–65.

American Spinal Injury Association. (1992). *Standards for neurological and functional classification of spinal cord injury*. Chicago, IL: The Association.

Bashar, J., & Hughes, C. (2018). Spinal cord injury. In H. M. Pendleton, & W. Schultz-Krohn (Eds.), *Pedretti's occupational therapy: Practice skills for physical dysfunction* (8th ed., pp. 904–928). St Louis, MO: Elsevier.

Bromley, I. (1998). *Tetraplegia and paraplegia: A guide for physiotherapists*. 5th ed. New York, NY: Churchill Livingstone.

Consortium for Spinal Cord Medicine, Paralyzed Veterans of America. (1999). *Outcomes following traumatic spinal cord injury: Clinical practice guidelines for health-care professionals*. Washington, DC: The Consortium.

Freed, M. M. (1990). Traumatic and congenital lesions of the spinal cord. In F. J. Kottke & J. F. Lehmann (Eds.), *Krusen's handbook of physical medicine and rehabilitation*. Philadelphia, PA: WB Saunders.

Hanak, M., & Scott, A. (1983). *Spinal cord injury: An illustrated guide for health care professionals*. New York, NY: Springer-Verlag.

Heinemann, A. W., Magiera-Planey, R., Schiro-Geist, C., & Gimines, G. (1987). Mobility for persons with spinal cord injury: an evaluation of two systems. *Archives of Physical Medicine and Rehabilitation*, *68*(2), 90–93.

Hill, J. P. (Ed.), (1987). *Spinal cord injury: A guide to functional outcomes in occupational therapy*. Rockville, MD: Aspen.

Krantz, G., Tolan, V., Pontarelli, K., & Cahill, S. M. (2016). What do adolescents with developmental disabilities learn about sexuality and dating? A potential role for occupational therapy. *Open Journal of Occupational Therapy*, *4*(2), 5.

Malick, M. H., & Meyer, C. M. H. (1978). *Dynamic hand orthoses: Manual on the management of the quadriplegic upper extremity*. Pittsburgh, PA: Harmarville Rehabilitation Center.

Miękisiak, G., Łątka, D., Jarmużek, P., Zaøuski, R., Urbański, W., & Janusz, W. (2019). Steroids in acute spinal cord injury: all but gone within 5 years. *World Neurosurg.*, *122*, e467–e471. Available from doi:10.1016/j.wneu.2018.09.239.

National Institute of Neurological Disorders and Stroke (2019). Brown-Séquard syndrome information page. https://www.ninds.nih.gov/Disorders/All-Disorders/Brown-Sequard-Syndrome-Information-Page.

Paulson, S. (1994). *Santa Clara Valley Medical Center spinal cord injury home care manual*. (3rd ed.). San Jose, CA: Santa Clara Valley Medical Center.

Penrod, L. E., Hegde, S. K., & Ditunno, J. F., Jr. (1990). Age effect on prognosis for functional recovery in acute, traumatic central cord syndrome. *Archives of Physical Medicine and Rehabilitation*, *71*(12), 963–968.

Pierce, D. S., & Nickel, V. H. (1977). *The total care of spinal cord injuries*. Boston, MA: Little, Brown.

Soleyman-Jahi, S., Soleyman-Jahi, S., Yousefian, A., et al. (2018). Evidence based prevention and treatment of osteoporosis after spinal cord injury: a systematic review. *European Spine Journal*, *27*(8), 1798–1814.

Spencer, E. A. (1993). Functional restoration. In H. L. Hopkins & H. D. Smith (Eds.), *Willard and Spackman's occupational therapy* (8th ed.). Philadelphia, PA: JB Lippincott.

Whiteneck, G. G., & Charlifue, S. W. (Eds.), (1993). *Aging with spinal cord injury*. New York, NY: Demos Medical Publications.

Wilson, D. J., McKenzie, M. W, & Barber, L. M. (1984). *Spinal cord injury: A treatment guide for occupational therapists*. Thorofare, NJ: Slack.

Yarkony, G. M. (1994). *Spinal cord injury: Medical management and rehabilitation*. Gaithersburg, MD: Aspen.

Yarkony, G. M., Roth, E. J., Heinemann, A. W., & Lovell, L. L. (1988). Spinal cord injury rehabilitation outcome: the impact of age. *Journal of Clinical Epidemiology, 41*(2), 173—177.

SUGGESTED READING

Field-Fote, E. (2009). *Spinal cord injury rehabilitation (Contemporary Perspectives in Rehabilitation)*. Philadelphia, PA: FA Davis.

Klein, S. D., & Karp, G. (2004). *From there to here: Stories of adjustment to spinal cord injury*. Baltimore, MD: No Limits Communication.

Mayo Clinic. (2010). *Guide to living with a spinal cord injury: Moving ahead with your life*. New York: Demos Health.

Paralyzed Veterans of America. (2020). *Spinal cord injury and disease*. Washington, DC: Paralyzed Veterans of America. https://www.pva.org/research-resources/spinal-cord-injury-information/

Sisto, S. A., Druin, E., & Macht Sliwinski, M. (2008). In: *Spinal cord injuries, management and rehabilitation*. St Louis, MO: Mosby.

Somers, M. F. (2009). *Spinal cord injury: Functional rehabilitation* (3rd ed.). Upper Saddle River, NJ: Prentice Hall.

27

Neurogenic and Myopathic Dysfunction

Mary Beth Selby

OBJECTIVES

After reading this chapter, the student or the occupational therapy practitioner will be able to do the following:

1. Describe the causes of lesions that result in motor unit dysfunction.
2. Name the clinical conditions that are characterized as motor unit dysfunction.
3. Identify the clinical manifestations of motor unit dysfunction conditions.
4. Contrast the goals and methods of occupational therapy treatment programs for the various motor unit conditions.

KEY TERMS

Motor unit
Neurogenic
Myopathic
Lower motor neuron dysfunction
Poliomyelitis
Contractures
Postpolio syndrome

Guillain-Barré syndrome
Peripheral nerve injury
Atrophy
Regeneration
Myasthenia gravis
Muscular dystrophies

INTRODUCTION

The **motor unit** is the elementary functional unit in the motor system (Mattle & Mumenthaler, 2016). Its components are the motor neurons and the muscle fibers that it innervates (George, 2018; Hamby, 2017; Mattle & Mumenthaler, 2016). Diseases of the motor unit generally cause muscle weakness and atrophy of skeletal muscle and may be **neurogenic** (originating in the nerves) or **myopathic** (originating in the muscle). Neurogenic disorders affect the nerve cell bodies or the peripheral nerves. Myopathic diseases affect the neuromuscular junction or the muscle itself (Mattle & Mumenthaler, 2016). Since these conditions are commonly seen in clinical practice, it is beneficial for the occupational therapy assistant (OTA) to be familiar with the symptoms of each, the course of the disease, and occupational therapy interventions.

The neurons of the motor unit originate in the spinal cord and include the cell body and axons (George, 2018). These are part of the lower motor neuron system. A lesion to any of the neurologic structures of the lower motor neuron system will result in **lower motor neuron dysfunction** (deGroot, 1991; Manter, Gilman, Gatz, & Newman, 2003; Mattle & Mumenthaler, 2016). Lesions can result from (1) infections—poliomyelitis, Guillain-Barré syndrome; (2) nerve root compression (due to trauma—bone fractures and dislocations, lacerations, traction, penetrating wounds, and friction or poor positioning); (3) toxins—lead, phosphorus, alcohol, benzene,

and sulfonamides; (4) neoplasms—neuromas and multiple neurofibromatosis; (5) vascular disorders—arteriosclerosis, diabetes mellitus, and peripheral vascular anomalies; (6) degenerative diseases of the central nervous system—amyotrophic lateral sclerosis; and (7) congenital malformations (Douglas & Aminoff, 2019; Kiernan & Barr, 2009; Walter, 1992; Winhammar, Rowe, Henderson, & Kiernan, 2005). These are considered neurogenic disorders. This chapter will discuss in depth peripheral neuropathies (poliomyelitis and postpolio syndrome), peripheral nerve injuries (brachial plexus injuries, long thoracic nerve injuries, and axillary nerve injuries), and neuromuscular disorders (myasthenia gravis and muscular dystrophy).

NEUROGENIC DISORDERS

Poliomyelitis

The active immunization program (using the Salk and Sabin vaccines) in the United States since the mid-1950s has essentially eradicated poliomyelitis in the Western Hemisphere. New cases are rare. The last polio cases reported in the United States were in 1999. They were vaccine-associated paralytic polio cases caused by live oral polio vaccine. In 2009 only 1579 confirmed cases of polio were reported globally (Centers for Disease Control and Prevention, 2015). Adults who had poliomyelitis in early life in the United States and those from countries that lacked the benefits of immunization and rehabilitation are referred to occupational therapy for vocational evaluation or improvement of quality of life (Centers for Disease Control and Prevention, 2015; George, 2018; Schell & Gillen, 2019; Walter, 1992).

Poliomyelitis is a contagious viral disease that affects the anterior horn cells of the gray matter of the spinal cord and the motor nuclei of the brainstem. It results in a flaccid paralysis that may be local or widespread. The lower extremities, accessory muscles of respiration, and muscles that promote swallowing are primarily affected, but upper extremity (UE) involvement may also occur. Marked atrophy may be seen in the involved extremities, while deep tendon reflexes may be absent. Because poliomyelitis destroys the anterior horn cells, sensory roots are spared and sensation is intact. **Contractures** (permanent shortening of the muscles, tendons, and ligaments) can occur early in the course of the disease. In cases of local paralysis, the asymmetry of muscles pulling on various joints may promote deformities such as subluxation, scoliosis, and contractures. In severe cases osteoporosis (bone atrophy) may weaken the long weight-bearing bones (tibia and femur), and pathologic fractures can occur (Jester, 2014; Manter et al., 2003; Mattle & Mumenthaler, 2016).

The medical treatment for poliomyelitis during the acute phase includes bed rest, positioning, and applications of warm packs to reduce pain and promote relaxation. Because no known cure for poliomyelitis exists, the disease must run its course. The medical aspects of rehabilitation may include reconstructive surgery such as tendon transfer, arthrodesis, and surgical release of fascia, muscles, and tendons. Other rehabilitation measures may include therapeutic stretching, casts, muscle reeducation, orthoses, and bracing for standing or stability (Centers for Disease Control and Prevention, 2015; George, 2018).

Occupational Therapy Intervention Process. The OTA will most likely provide treatment to clients in the postacute phase who are in the rehabilitation stage. It is hypothesized that during the recovery process, in an effort to compensate for the loss of neurons, surviving motor neurons sprout new endings to restore function to muscles (Kiernan & Barr, 2009). Rehabilitation includes instruction in range of motion (ROM), muscle reeducation and graded strengthening, precautions against fatigue, psychological support, and retraining in activities of daily living (ADL).

Movement for the client who is recovering from acute poliomyelitis proceeds from passive ROM (PROM) to active ROM (AROM), depending on the client's level of voluntary control. Muscle reeducation should be preceded by gentle stretching exercises. All active motions should be performed under careful supervision of the therapist or assistant. Compensatory movement should be avoided. A limited but correct movement is preferred to a larger but incorrect movement. Completion of active movements in front of a mirror may enhance client observation and self-correction of

motions accordingly (Jester, 2014; Schell & Gillen, 2019; Winhammar et al., 2005).

Muscle reeducation is accomplished in a graded fashion. At first the client should learn muscle-setting exercises—alternating contraction and relaxation of muscles without moving the joints. Isometric exercises and electromyographic (EMG) biofeedback may be beneficial. As the client progresses, the clinician can apply light resistance manually before using resistance equipment. This allows the therapy practitioner to estimate directly the client's physical strengths and weaknesses. Weakened muscles must be protected at all times. Muscles that cannot resist the force of gravity are supported during exercise and rest periods. As a rule, resistive exercises are not attempted until the muscle can carry out a complete ROM against gravity. Weakened or flaccid muscles can be splinted at night to counteract the force of gravity or the pull of the stronger antagonist muscles. During resistive exercises the clinician should stress correct body positioning, joint alignment, and energy conservation. Periods of rest should be included in the exercise program. Activities that incorporate the same movements and musculature as the exercises are encouraged (George, 2018).

The goals for resistive exercises in the rehabilitation of a client with poliomyelitis are (1) to strengthen fully functioning muscles and (2) to strengthen weakened muscles by integrating them into a larger movement that permits the performance of a given activity. After 8 months, if the muscle cannot contract completely against gravity, it is unlikely that additional muscle strength will return. At this point the emphasis should be on maintaining existing muscles and functional ADL (George, 2018; Jester, 2014).

Psychological support for both client and family should be a part of the treatment program. The occupational therapy practitioner should anticipate and respect the client's fears and anxieties about the disabling effects of the disease. The client may need encouragement and positive experiences to develop an optimistic outlook during the rehabilitation process. The family may also need assistance in adjusting to the client's disability and new limitations. The occupational therapist (OT) or OTA should address these psychosocial issues with both the client and the family during treatment. Additional support may be secured through a referral to the psychology service in the rehabilitation facility (Conrad, Doering, Rief, & Exner, 2010; George, 2018; Lynch, Craig, & Peng, 2011; Ogawa et al., 2016).

As the rehabilitation process progresses, the precautions against physical and body fatigue continue. Assistive devices, splints, and mobile arm supports may be used to gain independence in ADL. After the acute medical problems have subsided, the recovery stage may last as long as 2 years (George, 2018; Schell & Gillen, 2019).

The OT or OTA should administer a self-care evaluation to determine a baseline of function. Dressing activities may include donning and doffing orthoses. Assistive devices should be tailored to the needs of the client (Robinault, 1973). It may also be advantageous to begin activities for prevocational and vocational exploration. Clients' quality of life can be improved if they are employed and productive. The prognosis for successful rehabilitation depends on the personality of the client and the perseverance of the clinician.

Postpolio Syndrome

Occupational therapy practitioners are seeing more clients with postpolio syndrome in rehabilitation centers. Clients who had polio earlier in life are experiencing additional weakness and other disabling symptoms years after the initial disease (Douglas & Aminoff, 2019; Theis, 2010). The numbers of such persons have increased, in part because of the influx of immigrants from Southeast Asia and Latin America who suffered the original infection in their native lands. It is estimated that more than 440,000 polio survivors are living in the United States. Of those, some 25% to 60% may be experiencing symptoms of postpolio syndrome (National Institute of Neurological Disorders & Stroke, 2019). Postpolio syndrome causes health and functional problems, and clients who are affected are likely to be referred for occupational therapy services (Schell & Gillen, 2019).

Postpolio syndrome is a combination of impairments occurring in individuals who have experienced poliomyelitis many years ago and have functioned quite satisfactorily in the interim. It is primarily characterized by increased weakness of muscles that were previously affected by the polio infection. This is considered to possibly be due to chronic strain of weakened musculature and ligaments or dysfunction in reinnervated motor units (George, 2018; Reed, 2014). Symptoms include fatigue, slowly progressing muscle weakness, and (at times) muscular atrophy. Joint pain and increasing skeletal deformities such as scoliosis are also common. The severity of the postpolio syndrome depends on the degree of residual weakness and disability after the original polio attack. Persons with only mild polio generally experience more mild postpolio symptoms. Those who experienced more severe polio with greater weakness may develop greater loss of function with postpolio syndrome (National Institute of Neurological Disorders & Stroke, 2019). One hypothesis about postpolio syndrome is that it occurs when motor neurons with excessive sprouting can no longer maintain the metabolic demands. Thus slow deterioration of individual terminals results (Manter et al., 2003; National Institute of Neurological Disorders & Stroke, 2019).

Fatigue is the most debilitating symptom because it limits activity yet is not apparent to others. The fatigue may be severe and out of proportion to the apparent physical demands of the activity and can be overwhelming (George, 2018; National Institute of Neurological Disorders & Stroke, 2019; Theis, 2010). An increase in difficulties with ADL accompanies the symptoms. Problems with functional mobility, transfers, home management, driving, dressing, eating and swallowing, and bladder and bowel control may occur (George, 2018; Theis, 2010).

Effective remedies aim to prevent muscle fatigue, improve body mechanics, and conserve energy. In general, it has been observed that clients who adjust their lifestyles experience improvement of symptoms and stabilization of function (National Institute of Neurological Disorders & Stroke, 2019; Schell & Gillen, 2019).

Occupational Therapy Intervention Process. When a diagnosis of postpolio syndrome has been made, the affected person may be referred for rehabilitation services. Occupational therapy practitioners evaluate client factors to assess how they affect ADL, occupational performance, and psychosocial status. Gait and orthotic needs should be evaluated as well (National Institute of Neurological Disorders & Stroke, 2019). The OTA may participate in this assessment process in specific areas where proficiency and competence have been demonstrated.

The first step in the occupational therapy intervention process is the development of an occupational profile. This can be completed by the OT or OTA through interviewing the client to ascertain valued occupational roles and obtain an activity profile of daily life. The client should be asked to report which activities cause pain or fatigue, which activities have been curtailed or eliminated because of symptoms, when symptoms are most likely to occur (time, circumstances), and what kinds of aids, equipment, and human assistance are presently used.

Assessment of client factors can be completed by the OT with input from the OTA. These assessments include manual muscle testing if indicated. It should be noted that, due to being easily fatigued, postpolio muscles may actually function at levels of strength lower than estimated from scores on the manual muscle test and that UE strength varies markedly throughout the ROM (George, 2018; Theis, 2010). Joint ROM measurements are important if contractures and muscle imbalances are present.

An assessment of psychosocial status is necessary to select the best approach for the client to facilitate rehabilitation efforts and to adjust to new limitations. Changes in physical capacities and curtailment of valued life skills confront the individual with psychological issues of coping, adjustment, and adaptation. These may be as traumatic as they were at the time of the original illness. Reactions such as denial, anger, frustration, and hopelessness must be recognized, addressed, and processed.

As a group, persons who originally had polio assumed that the disease was over, that disability was in the past, and that any residual weakness would not worsen. They worked hard to overcome the effects of the initial paralysis and often performed well, achieved high levels of personal fulfillment, became well integrated into society, and so disappeared as a disabled group. The onset of new symptoms disrupts the performance and lifestyle achieved through years of hard work. Old remedies are ineffective in ameliorating the new limitations. The person often struggles to accept the reality of the circumstances. As a result, the clinician should introduce change gradually. Small changes may be more easily accepted than major ones, even if the latter are obviously necessary (Centers for Disease Control and Prevention, 2015; George, 2018; National Institute of Neurological Disorders & Stroke, 2019; Schell & Gillen, 2019).

The client is confronted, for a second time, years after the disability was thought to be stabilized, with the notion of being disabled and with limited function and diminished participation in valued life activities. A supportive and realistic approach and client education are key to lifestyle modification (Centers for Disease Control and Prevention, 2015; National Institute of Neurological Disorders & Stroke, 2019; Schell & Gillen, 2019; Simon & Collins, 2017).

Exercise should be used cautiously because, if overdone, it could aggravate pain and damage muscles with fewer functioning motor units. Muscles weakened by disuse may benefit from gentle strengthening exercises that do not result in fatigue and that improve activity tolerance (Reed, 2014). Participation in ADL that provide gentle resistance may also help improve and maintain muscle strength. Exercises for muscles used for ADL should be used judiciously, and carefully supervised, so as not to be stressed further (George, 2018). Clients should be encouraged to be active within limits of their comfort and safety. A regular routine of activity or gentle exercise allows clients to positively impact their own health. Long-term strengthening or maintenance exercises are recommended only for muscles that show no EMG evidence of prior polio involvement. Further weakness, discomfort, pain, muscle spasm, or chronic fatigue resulting from exercise are signs of overuse caused by excessive activity (George, 2018; National Institute of Neurological Disorders & Stroke, 2019; Theis, 2010).

Pain can be managed or alleviated by improving body mechanics, supporting weakened muscles, and promoting lifestyle modification. The OTA can teach correct body mechanics in daily living tasks such as work and home management, functional mobility, and transfers. Orthoses may be used to support weakened muscles and prevent deformity with muscle imbalance. Activities and lifestyle should be modified to reduce fatigue, stress, and overuse of muscles. Weight reduction may be necessary for some clients (Newton-Triggs & Rogers, 2014; Williams, Fini, & Joyce, 2019).

OTAs can play an important role in the facilitation of positive lifestyle modifications. Clients must avoid overuse of muscles. Evaluation and retraining in ADL, along with activity modification, can be beneficial using assistive devices, energy conservation, and work simplification. The client and clinician should set priorities for occupational role performance. Energy conservation for the most valued activities may mean sacrificing less valued ones to be done by others or to be done with the assistance of equipment such as orthoses, assistive devices, or functional mobility aids (Reed, 2014; Theis, 2010). Adaptive devices are sometimes viewed by the person with postpolio syndrome as devices used by the disabled and are therefore rejected by the person or by the family. Often the device is more easily accepted when it is introduced as a tool to get a job done.

Guillain-Barré syndrome (GBS; also known as acute idiopathic neuropathy, infectious polyneuritis, and Landry syndrome) is an acute inflammatory condition involving the spinal nerve roots, peripheral nerves, and (in some cases) cranial nerves. GBS often follows a viral illness, immunization, or surgery and may affect both sexes at any age (Douglas & Aminoff, 2019; George, 2018; Hamby, 2017; Mattle & Mumenthaler, 2016; Reed, 2014; Utsugisawa, Nagane, & Akaishi, 2016; Walter, 1992; Zaretsky, Richter, & Eisenberg, 2005).

GBS has a rapid onset. Initially no fever presents, but pain and tenderness of muscles, weakness, and decreased deep tendon reflexes occur. As the disease progresses, it produces motor weakness or paralysis of the limbs, sensory loss, and muscle atrophy. Fatigue is also experienced, and in many cases it can be quite debilitating (Merkies & Kieseier, 2016; Ranjani et al., 2014). The prognosis in GBS is varied. In severe cases cranial nerves 7 (facial), 9 (glossopharyngeal), and 10 (vagus) may be involved, and the client may have difficulty speaking, swallowing, and breathing. If vital centers in the medulla are affected, the client may experience respiratory failure and require tracheostomy or assisted ventilation. In many of the cases, the client completely recovers within a few weeks to a few months with relatively few residual effects (Douglas & Aminoff, 2019; George, 2018).

Occupational Therapy Intervention Process. Rehabilitation can be initiated when the client is medically stabilized. Comprehensive rehabilitation goals should be coordinated with the physician, nurse, physical therapist, and other members of the team. The client may be referred to occupational therapy while still paralyzed. This initial phase of evaluation and treatment focuses on PROM, positioning, and splinting to protect weak muscles and prevent contracture and deformity. Restful activities (watching television and light social visits) are encouraged. As improvement occurs and more active motion is possible, occupational therapy interventions include gentle, nonresistive activities (light ADL), which can alleviate joint stiffness and prevent muscle atrophy and contractures (George, 2018; Hamby, 2017; Reed, 2014). The OT or OTA should grade the activity program to the client's physical tolerance level. Fatigue should be avoided, and psychological support should be provided (Ashley Nikita, 2014; Merkies & Kieseier, 2016; Schell & Gillen, 2019).

After the occupational profile is completed, the OT, with input from the OTA, can complete the assessment of occupational performance. This may include strength testing, ROM measurement, sensory testing, and ADL. The evaluation process may be fatiguing, so it may be helpful to spread it out over a few days (Reed, 2014).

PROM should begin with gentle movement of the proximal joints and should proceed only to the point of pain. As the client's tolerance increases, active assisted ROM (AAROM), AROM, and light exercises may be introduced. The program should stress joint protection, and the clinician should look for muscle imbalance and substitution patterns. Progressive resistive exercises should be used conservatively. Throughout the intervention process the clinician should avoid bringing the muscles to the point of fatigue and irritating inflamed nerves.

As the client's strength and tolerance increase, resistance can be gradually and moderately increased within daily tasks.

The clinician may introduce sedentary or tabletop activities during the early stages of recovery. As the client's strength increases, activities promoting more resistance such as leather work, textiles, and ceramics can be added. Grooming, self-care, and other ADL should be included as soon as the client's level of independence increases. Slings and mobile arm supports may be used to alleviate muscle fatigue and promote independence. Activities should be varied between gross and fine motor, as well as resistive and nonresistive to prevent undue fatigue. Participation in ADL should be continuously evaluated and modified to determine which activities the client can perform, where assistive or adaptive equipment is necessary, when energy conservation techniques are necessary, and where independence can be maximized (Ashley Nikita, 2014; Drory, Bronipolsky, Bluvshtein, Catz, & Korczyn, 2012; George, 2018; Hamby, 2017). Typically, as physical function improves, the OT or OTA can recommend discontinuing the use of adaptive equipment or techniques to enable a return to normalcy.

Psychological support is important throughout the treatment program. The clinician should try to facilitate a feeling of self-worth, convey a positive attitude, and provide encouragement throughout the therapeutic process. Because the prognosis for recovery is good, the activities should be mentally stimulating and purposeful to the client. The clinician should also respect the client's level of pain tolerance during stretching and ROM exercises (Ashley Nikita, 2014; George, 2018).

Peripheral Nerve Injuries

Peripheral nerve injury results in muscle weakness or flaccid paralysis. The loss of muscle innervation results in **atrophy** and hyporeactive or absent deep tendon reflexes.

Sensation along the cutaneous distribution of the nerve will also be lost. Trophic changes such as dry skin, hair loss, cyanosis, brittle fingernails, painless skin ulcerations, and slow wound healing in the area of involvement may also be present. Occasionally, minute muscle contractions called fasciculations may be seen on the surface of the skin overlying the denervated muscle belly. As a result of disturbances of sympathetic fibers of the autonomic nervous system, the ability to sweat above the denervated skin surfaces will be lost.

The client may experience paresthesia (i.e., sensations such as tingling, numbness, and burning or pain [causalgia]), particularly at night. Moreover, if the nerve damage was caused by trauma, edema will be a prominent clinical manifestation. EMG examinations may reveal extremely small muscle contractions called fibrillations (Côté, Amin, Tom, & Houle, 2011; deGroot, 1991; Kiernan & Barr, 2009; Manter et al., 2003; Mattle & Mumenthaler, 2016; Willmott, 2015).

Extensive peripheral nerve damage may produce deformity if contractures, joint stiffness, and poor positioning are allowed to occur. Disfigurement of the hands is particularly noticeable and may produce some psychological complications. Other complications may include osteoporosis of bone and epidermal fibrosis of the joints.

The medical-surgical management of peripheral nerve lesions depends on the type of injury that has occurred and may include microsurgery, nerve grafts or transplants, and injections of alcohol, vitamin B_{12}, and phenol.

Peripheral nerve **regeneration** begins about 1 month after the injury. The rate of regeneration depends on the nature of the nerve lesion. If the nerve root has been cleanly severed and surgically repaired, the rate of regeneration will vary from 0.5 inch (1.3 cm) to 1 inch (2.6 cm) per month. Peripheral nerve injuries caused by burns, sepsis, or crushing will present other complications to the healing process (National Spinal Cord Injury Statistical Center, 2013; Phelps & Walker, 1977). Age is another factor; children usually have a faster rate of regeneration than do adults (Morrison, Pathier, & Horr, 1978). In addition, proximal lesions regenerate faster than distal lesions, and injuries to mixed nerves are slower to recover than single nerves (Russell, 2015). Early medical treatment

CASE STUDY

Holly

Holly is a 36-year-old who developed lower extremity (LE) pain, weakness, and numbness in all four extremities, severe fatigue, and facial droop after experiencing a minor respiratory illness. Holly was hospitalized and diagnosed with Guillain-Barré syndrome. She quickly transitioned to the inpatient rehabilitation unit of the hospital. Holly was referred to physical therapy to address her LE weakness and mobility impairments, as well as to speech therapy for her facial droop and assessment of swallow function. During the occupational therapy evaluation Holly required moderate to maximal assist with all basic ADL and moderate assist with functional transfers. She was unable to ambulate. Holly had full AROM of her shoulders, elbows, wrists, and fingers. Her strength was 3 / 5 in all major muscle groups. She fatigued quickly. The occupational treatment plan included adaptive device training for lower body dressing (LBD), toileting, and showering. Functional transfer training included use of adaptive devices and techniques, as well as instruction in safety strategies. She was instructed in energy-conservation techniques during all functional tasks to prevent overfatigue and maximize her independence. Holly participated in low-resistance and aerobic exercises to gradually improve her functional strength and activity tolerance. Because Holly had never heard of her diagnosis, education regarding the course of the disease and appropriate precautions was also a part of her treatment. As her strength returned, her OT and OTA introduced standing tolerance during functional tasks and participation in instrumental ADL (IADL). After 4 weeks, Holly was independent in basic ADL, light meal prep, functional transfers, and functional mobility within household distances; thus she returned home with her husband. She required assist from her husband for grocery shopping and cleaning and was unable to yet return to work. She was referred to outpatient physical and occupational therapy to continue to address strength deficits as well as to improve job-related skills so that she could return to work as a soda distribution plant manager.

may require suturing the nerve and immobilizing the involved extremity to ensure good apposition of the severed nerves. In the past, full recovery of muscles was not probable because regenerated fibers lose about 20% of their original diameter and conduct impulses at a slower rate (deGroot, 1991; Kiernan & Barr, 2009; Manter et al., 2003; Mattle & Mumenthaler, 2016). Microsurgery has resulted in an improved regenerative process in recent years (Seddon, 1975).

Because peripheral nerves can regenerate, the course of recovery can be somewhat predictable. Although the clinical signs of regeneration do not always follow a specific sequence, the following clinical signs of nerve regeneration can be expected:

- *Skin appearance:* As the edema subsides and collateral blood vessels develop, the circulatory system should become more normalized. The skin should improve in its color and texture.
- *Primitive protective sensations:* The first signs of cutaneous sensation will usually be the gross recognition of crude pain, temperature, pressure, and touch.
- *Paresthesia:* Tingling or paresthesia ("pins and needles") distal to the presumed site of the lesion may indicate that regeneration is occurring.
- *Scattered points of sweating:* As the parasympathetic fibers of the autonomic nervous system regenerate, the sweat glands will recover their functions.
- *Discriminative sensations:* The more refined sensations such as the ability to identify and localize touch, joint position (proprioception), recognition of objects in the three-dimensional form (stereognosis), movement (kinesthesia), and two-point discrimination should be returning at this point.
- *Muscle tone:* Flaccidity will decrease, and muscle tone will increase. An important principle is that paralyzed muscles must first sense pressure before tone and movement can be realized.
- *Voluntary muscle function:* The client will be able to move the extremity first with gravity eliminated and then proceed to full ROM as strength increases. At this point graded exercises can begin.

Brachial Plexus Injury. The nerve roots that innervate the UE originate in the anterior rami between the C4 and T1 vertebrae. This network of lower anterior cervical and upper dorsal spinal nerves is collectively called the brachial plexus. This important nerve complex can be palpated just behind the posterior border of the sternocleidomastoid as the head and neck are tilted to the opposite side (Boltshauser, 2019; Mattle & Mumenthaler, 2016; Newton-Triggs & Rogers, 2014).

Lesions to the brachial plexus usually result from traumatic injuries. Birth trauma is the primary mechanism of injury in infants, which results in Erb palsy or Klumpke paralysis. Erb palsy is caused by a lesion to the C5–6 nerve roots, which give rise to the median nerve. Paralysis and atrophy occur in the deltoid, brachialis, biceps, and brachioradialis muscles. This manifests clinically by a hypotonic and medially rotated arm with limited functional movement.

Klumpke paralysis results from injury to the C8 and T1 nerve roots, which give rise to the ulnar nerve and effects the distal UE. Paralysis and atrophy occur to the wrist flexors and the intrinsic muscles of the hand (George, 2018; Mattle & Mumenthaler, 2016).

Long Thoracic Nerve Injury. The long thoracic nerve (C5–7) innervates the serratus anterior muscle, which anchors the apex of the scapula to the posterior of the rib cage. This injury is most often caused by carrying heavy weights on the shoulder, by trauma to the neck, and through axillary wounds. It results in winging of the scapula, difficulty flexing the outstretched arm above shoulder level, and difficulty protracting the shoulder or performing scapular abduction and adduction.

The treatment for long thoracic nerve injuries involves stabilizing the shoulder girdle to limit scapular motion. In severe cases, surgery may be indicated to relieve the excessive mobility of the scapula. Occupational therapy intervention focuses on facilitation of maximal functional independence through therapeutic activity, strengthening, and activity modification (such as using a reacher to compensate for decreased shoulder ROM).

Axillary Nerve Injury. The axillary nerve arises from the posterior cord of the C5–6 spinal nerves and innervates the deltoid and teres minor muscles. It is rarely damaged by itself, but it is often damaged along with traumatic injury to the brachial plexus. This lesion will cause weakness or paralysis of the deltoid muscle, resulting in limitations in horizontal abduction, lateral shoulder hyperesthesia (extreme sensitivity to pain or touch), and asymmetry of the shoulders. Muscle transplantation may be provided in cases of extensive and permanent nerve damage, to allow for arm abduction (Mattle & Mumenthaler, 2016; Seddon, 1975).

Treatment involves positioning to prevent deformity, maintain or improve ROM, and improve circulation. AROM and PROM should be completed daily for shoulder abduction. Adaptation to daily tasks should be done to protect the muscles from excessive stretch and to facilitate independence by compensating for movement deficits (e.g., through use of a long-handled assistive device). Postsurgical treatment should include EMG and biofeedback to facilitate muscle reeducation and prostheses (such as a foam rubber pad) to compensate for asymmetry. See Chapter 29 for more information regarding UE rehabilitation.

Occupational Therapy Intervention Process. The goal of occupational therapy intervention for peripheral nerve injuries is to assist the client in regaining the maximum level of motor function and independence in performance areas. Treatment is directed to the stage of recovery and focuses on remediation and compensation for sensory, motor, and performance deficits. The rate of return and the residual impairments depend largely on the severity of the lesion and the quality of care during the rehabilitation process. Table 27.1 offers a useful summary of the major nerve roots and clinical manifestations of their lesions.

TABLE 27.1 Clinical Manifestations of Peripheral Nerve Lesions

Spinal Nerves	Nerve Roots	Motor Distribution	Clinical Manifestations
Brachial Plexus			
C5–7	Long thoracic	Shoulder girdle, serratus anterior	Winged scapula
C5, C6	Dorsal scapular	Rhomboid major and minor, levator scapulae	Loss of scapular adduction and elevation
C7, C8	Thoracodorsal	Latissimus dorsi	Loss of arm adduction and extension
C5, C6	Suprascapular	Supraspinatus, infraspinatus	Weakened lateral rotation of humerus
C5, C6	Subscapular	Subscapularis, teres major	Weakened medial rotation of humerus
C6–8, T1	Radial	All extensors of forearm, triceps	Wrist drop, extensor paralysis
C5, C6	Axillary	Deltoid, teres minor	Loss of arm abduction, weakened lateral rotation of humerus
C5, C6	Musculocutaneous	Biceps brachii, brachialis, coracobrachialis	Loss of forearm flexion and supination
C6–8, T1	Median	Flexors of hand and digits, opponens pollicis	Ape-hand deformity, weakened grip, thenar atrophy, unopposed thumb
C8, T1	Ulnar	Flexor of hand and digits, opponens pollicis	Claw-hand deformity, interosseous atrophy, loss of thumb adduction
Lumbosacral Plexus			
L2–4	Femoral	Iliopsoas, quadriceps femoris	Loss of thigh flexion, leg extension
L2–4	Obturator	Adductors of thigh	Weakened or loss of thigh adduction
L4, L5, S1–3	Sciatic	Hamstrings, all musculature below the knee	Loss of leg flexion, paralysis of all muscles of leg and foot
L4, L5, S1, S2	Common peroneal	Dorsiflexors of foot	Foot drop, steppage gait, loss of eversion
L4, L5, S1–3	Tibial	Gastrocnemius, soleus, deep plantar flexors of foot	Loss of plantar flexion and inversion of foot

From H.J. Hislop, & Brown, A.D. (2013). *Danies and Worthington's muscle testing: Techniques of manual examination* (9th ed.), Philadelphia, W.B. Saunders.

The occupational therapy practitioner may be involved during the acute and rehabilitation phases of treatment. During the acute phase (immediately after surgery), treatment aims to reduce edema and prevent deformity. Immobilization splints are used to stabilize the extremity and protect the site of injury (Radomski & Latham, 2014; Schell & Gillen, 2019).

See Chapter 30 for more information on postoperative management of peripheral nerve repair.

Postoperative edema management can be achieved through positioning, manual therapy, and compression. Elevation of the extremity above the heart will facilitate edema drainage. Manual massage gently moves excess fluids into the lymphatic

CASE STUDY

Garrett

Garrett is a 45-year-old construction worker with a severe, traumatic brachial plexus injury to his right UE following a motorcycle accident. After surgical repair he was referred to outpatient occupational therapy to maximize functional use of his UE and to return to independence with all ADL. On initial evaluation Garrett presented with severe pain throughout his right UE and had no active movement. His PROM was limited to 70 degrees of shoulder flexion and 60 degrees of abduction. His elbow also had extremely limited PROM due to pain and stiffness. Garrett was developing moderate to severe tightness in his wrist and digit flexors. He required minimal assist upper body dressing (UBD), LBD, grooming, and showering. A treatment plan that consisted of physical agent modalities (such as hot packs before exercise to decrease joint stiffness and increase soft tissue elasticity and transcutaneous electrical nerve stimulation [TENS] to decrease pain) was established. It also included ADL training using one-handed techniques for basic ADL. Garrett also participated in

aggressive PROM and stretching to improve joint mobility and was given a home exercise program to supplement his therapy services. A resting hand splint was fabricated for support and stability of his wrist and hand, as well as to prevent contractures. Garrett progressed well with his functional independence and was able to independently perform BADL using one-handed techniques after two sessions of occupational therapy. With pain management, splinting, and exercise he was able to return to full PROM in his UE after 1 month. As his peripheral nerves regenerated, his occupational therapy treatment plan was upgraded to include AROM and neuromuscular facilitation techniques to obtain functional use of his UE. Due to his motivation and compliance with therapy techniques, including strict adherence to all recommendations and exercises, Garrett now has full AROM in his hand, wrist, and elbow and 120 degrees of shoulder flexion and abduction. He is able to independently use his right UE for all self-care tasks but continues to require bilateral assist for heavier household and work-related duties due to continued strength impairments.

system to improve edema drainage. External elastic supports provide compression, which can also be used to alleviate edema.

Assessment of ADL and muscle strength should be completed to identify difficulties with essential performance tasks. A graded functional activity and exercise program should be established as the client's muscle function returns. Resistive activities such as cooking, woodworking, ceramics, leather work, and copper tooling may be used in conjunction with isometric and isotonic exercises when muscle function is adequate. Care should be taken to avoid overwork and fatigue. Activity modification could include one-handed methods of ADL and use of assistive devices such as long-handled reaching aids and one-handed kitchen tools. If sensory dysfunction is present, sensory reeducation can be used to assist the client in establishing appropriate responses to sensory stimuli. Sensory reeducation for peripheral nerve injuries is discussed in Chapters 22 and 30.

DISEASES OF THE NEUROMUSCULAR JUNCTION

Some motor unit disorders originate in diseases of the junction between the motor nerve and the muscle it innervates.

Myasthenia gravis is a disease of chemical transmission at the nerve-muscle synapse or neuromuscular junction. It results in weakness of skeletal muscle (Carmichael, 2016; Mattle & Mumenthaler, 2016). It occurs at all ages but primarily affects younger women and older men (McDonald & Joyce, 2012; Utsugisawa et al., 2016). Medical management of these clients varies and may include removal of the thymus gland (thymectomy), treatment with pharmacologic agents, or plasmapheresis (blood filtering) (Carmichael, 2016; Douglas & Aminoff, 2019; Kornfeld, Ambinder, & Mittag, 1981; Mattle & Mumenthaler, 2016; Ruff & Fehr, 2014; Utsugisawa et al., 2016; Walter, 1992).

Myasthenia gravis is characterized by abnormal fatigue of voluntary muscle (Mattle & Mumenthaler, 2016). It can affect any of the striated skeletal muscles of the body but in particular targets the muscles of the eyelids and eyes and oropharyngeal muscles. Therefore the muscles most often affected are those that move the eyes, eyelids, tongue, jaw, and throat. The limb muscles may also be affected. The muscles that are used most often fatigue sooner (Carmichael, 2016; Mattle & Mumenthaler, 2016; Walter, 1992). Therefore the client may have double vision, drooping of the eyelids, and difficulty with speech or swallowing as muscles fatigue.

Clients with myasthenia gravis may experience life-threatening respiratory crises that require hospitalization and the use of a ventilator. The incidence of these crises has declined significantly in recent years probably because of increased use of thymectomy (Carmichael, 2016; Mattle & Mumenthaler, 2016; Walter, 1992). The intensity of the disease fluctuates, and its course is unpredictable (Walter, 1992). Spontaneous remissions occur frequently, but relapse is usual (Hamby, 2017; Mattle & Mumenthaler, 2016). Remissions

or decrease in symptoms and improvement in strength and function can last for years. However, there may be exacerbations of unpredictable severity induced by exertion, infection, or childbirth (Hamby, 2017). The prognosis for myasthenia gravis varies with each individual, but for most it is a progressively disabling disease; the client may ultimately become bedridden with severe permanent paralysis. Death usually results from respiratory complications (Douglas & Aminoff, 2019; Hamby, 2017; Mattle & Mumenthaler, 2016; Schell & Gillen, 2019).

Occupational Therapy Intervention Process

The primary role of the occupational therapy practitioner is to help the client regain muscle power and build activity tolerance without causing fatigue. The client's muscle strength should be monitored at regular intervals. Factors that contribute to fatigue and the effects of medications should be taken into account as well. Documentation should include significant changes in muscle strength and changes in the client's physical appearance (such as ptosis of the eyelids, drooping facial muscles, or alterations of breathing or swallowing). Reports to the physician should include this information.

Occupational therapy treatment should include gentle, nonresistive activities that are meaningful to the client. The activities should be graded so that they do not fatigue the client. Overexertion and respiratory dysfunction need to be prevented. Intervention strategies should include energy conservation, work simplification, and activity modification to reduce effort during daily activities (Ruff & Fehr, 2014). Client education should be provided about these strategies to prevent overexertion and exacerbation. Activity modifications may include adaptive equipment such as long-handled equipment, mobile arm supports, and orthotics (George, 2018; Reed, 2014; Zaretsky et al., 2005). Environmental modifications, such as removal of architectural barriers and bathroom adaptations, can be recommended. Assistive technology, such as electronic communication devices and environmental controls, can be installed in the client's home if needed.

MYOPATHIC DISORDERS

Muscular dystrophies (MD) are a group of motor unit disorders caused by disease of the muscles. They comprise nine genetic, degenerative diseases primarily affecting voluntary muscles (Muscular Dystrophy Association, 2019a; 2019b). The four major types of MD (Mattle & Mumenthaler, 2016; Walter, 1992) involve the progressive degeneration of muscle fibers with intact neuronal innervation and sensation. The progressive weakness occurs as the axon progressively innervates a fewer number of muscle fibers (McDonald & Joyce, 2012).

Duchenne and Becker MD

Duchenne MD is inherited as an X-linked recessive trait that only affects males. It is usually diagnosed between the ages of 18 and 36 months. Muscle weakness begins in the pelvic girdle and legs and then spreads to the shoulder girdle. The child has difficulty walking and demonstrates a waddling type of gait known as Trendelenburg gait. Most boys utilize a wheelchair for mobility by age 12. This disease progresses to the point of the client becoming bedridden, and death usually occurs by the age of 30 (Mattle & Mumenthaler, 2016; Muscular Dystrophy Association, 2019; Reed, 2014; Schell & Gillen, 2019; Walter, 1992). Becker MD presents with a later onset, slower course, and far less predictability. Though Duchenne and Becker MD affect boys almost exclusively, in rare cases Becker MD can affect girls (Muscular Dystrophy Association, 2019a; 2019b; 2019c; 2019d).

Other MD

Facioscapulohumeral MD has its onset in adolescence. It primarily affects muscles of the face and shoulder girdle. It progresses slowly and does not shorten life expectancy (Walter, 1992). It is inherited through an autosomal dominant gene and affects males and females equally (Mattle & Mumenthaler, 2016).

Myotonic MD causes weakness and myotonia (tonic spasm of muscles) that makes relaxation of muscle contraction difficult. It is inherited through an autosomal dominant gene and affects males and females. In addition to the myotonia, it involves the cranial muscles and shows a pattern of limb weakness that is distal rather than proximal (Mattle & Mumenthaler, 2016; Muscular Dystrophy Association, 2019; Walter, 1992). Other symptoms involve the gastrointestinal system, vision, heart, or respiration. Learning disabilities occur in some cases. The more severe congenital form begins at birth. The more common form may begin in teen or adult years (Muscular Dystrophy Association, 2019).

Limb-girdle dystrophies are a group of disorders that present with weakness and atrophy of the muscles around the shoulders and hips (limb girdles). These problems usually progress slowly. Cardiopulmonary complications sometimes occur in the later stages of the disease.

Occupational Therapy Intervention Process

This group of diseases is degenerative, and decline of muscle function cannot be prevented. The primary goal of occupational therapy is to support occupational performance by assisting the client in maintaining maximal independence in ADL and IADL for as long as possible. Self-care activities, assistive devices for independence, and leisure activities are key elements of the treatment program. Active exercises, especially low-impact aerobic exercise, may be helpful, but overexertion and fatigue should be avoided (Douglas & Aminoff, 2019). For clients with respiratory involvement, exercises for breathing control may be administered by the physical therapist (Hamby, 2017; Schell & Gillen, 2019; Simmonds & Wideman, 2011).

Rehabilitation measures are vital to delaying deformity and achieving maximal function within the limits of the disease and its debilitating effects. Medical management is largely palliative. In later stages caregiver education and positioning is important. Gentle passive stretch should be taught to the family with emphasis on maintaining good body alignment and joint integrity. Instruction in bed positioning is provided to prevent further trunk, hip, and extremity contractures. Wheelchair prescription and mobility training may be included, and power wheelchairs are necessary in some instances (George, 2018; McDonald & Joyce, 2012; Reed, 2014).

The wheelchair may require a special seating system or supports to minimize scoliosis and to prevent or reduce hip and knee flexion contractures and ankle plantar flexion deformity. A wheelchair lap board, suspension slings, or mobile arm supports are indicated to optimize self-feeding, writing, reading, use of a computer, and tabletop leisure activities when there is significant shoulder girdle and upper limb weakness. Built-up utensils may be helpful when grip strength declines. Home and workplace modification may be necessary for some clients (George, 2018; Schell & Gillen, 2019).

Psychosocial problems and educational and vocational requirements also need attention from the occupational therapy practitioner. Deficits in cognitive function and verbal intelligence have been reported in some types of MD. Depression and personality disorders may be concomitant problems (Kornfeld et al., 1981). Client and family education is an important part of the occupational therapy program. A supportive approach to the client and family is helpful as function changes and as new mobility aids, assistive devices, and community resources become necessary (Robinault, 1973; Schell & Gillen, 2019).

SUMMARY

The motor unit consists of the lower motor neuron, neuromuscular junction, and muscle. Some motor unit disease conditions are reversible, and others are degenerative. The OT and OTA both play vital roles in the management of clients with motor unit dysfunction. Provision of positioning, exercise, pain management techniques, and orthoses is necessary in the treatment of these clients. ADL skills, including self-care, home management, mobility, and work-related tasks, are central to recovery of function. Compensatory measures such as energy conservation, work simplification, and joint protection techniques are important elements of the occupational therapy intervention program. Assistive devices, communication aids, and mobility equipment, as well as training in their use, may be necessary. Psychosocial considerations and client and family education are important aspects of the occupational therapy program.

REVIEW QUESTIONS

1. Name three causes of lesions that will result in motor unit dysfunction.
2. Describe the differences in the occupational therapy treatment programs for clients with poliomyelitis and postpolio syndrome.
3. Describe the symptoms of postpolio syndrome.
4. What are the elements of the occupational therapy program for the client with postpolio syndrome?

5. Describe the occupational therapy intervention for Guillain-Barré syndrome.
6. List at least six clinical manifestations of peripheral nerve injury.
7. Describe the sequential signs of recovery after peripheral nerve injury.
8. Describe some treatment strategies for peripheral nerve injuries.
9. Describe four noninvasive methods for modulating pain perception.
10. Discuss the clinical signs of myasthenia gravis.
11. Describe the role of occupational therapy for clients who have myasthenia gravis.
12. What is the primary treatment precaution in myasthenia gravis?
13. Name and differentiate four types of MD. Which one primarily affects children?
14. What are the occupational therapy treatment goals for MD?

REFERENCES

Ashley Nikita, S. B. (2014). Inside Guillain-Barré syndrome: an occupational therapist's perspective. *SAJOT, 44*(3). Available from https://search.proquest.com/docview/1759941933?accountid=143111.

Boltshauser, E. (2019). Differential diagnosis in neurology and neurosurgery: a clinician's pocket guide. *Neuropediatrics, 50*(4), 271—272.

Carmichael, S. T. (2016). Emergent properties of neural repair: elemental biology to therapeutic concepts. *Annals of Neurology, 79*(6), 895—906.

Centers for Disease Control and Prevention. (2015). Poliomyelitis [PDF file]. Available from https://www.cdc.gov/vaccines/pubs/pinkbook/downloads/polio.pdf.

Conrad, N., Doering, B. K., Rief, W., & Exner, C. (2010). Looking beyond the importance of life goals. The personal goal model of subjective well-being in neuropsychological rehabilitation. *Clinical Rehabilitation, 24*(5), 431—443.

Côté, M., Amin, A. A., Tom, V. J., & Houle, J. D. (2011). Peripheral nerve grafts support regeneration after spinal cord injury. *Neurotherapeutics, 8*(2), 294—303.

deGroot, J. (1991). *Correlative neuroanatomy* (21st ed.). Norwalk, CT: Appleton & Lange.

Drory, V. E., Bronipolsky, T., Bluvshtein, V., Catz, A., & Korczyn, A. D. (2012). Occurrence of fatigue over 20 years after recovery from Guillain-Barré syndrome. *Journal of the Neurological Sciences, 316*(1-2), 72—75.

Douglas, V. C., & Aminoff, M. J. (2019). Nervous system disorders. In M. A. Papadakis, S. J. McPhee, & M. W. Rabow (Eds.), *Current medical diagnosis & treatment* New York, NY: McGraw-Hill.

George, A. H. (2018). Disorders of the motor unit. In H. M. Pendleton, & W. Schultz-Krohn (Eds.), *Pedretti's occupational therapy: Practice skills for physical dysfunction* (pp. 931—945). St Louis, MO: Elsevier.

Hamby, J. R. (2017). The nervous system. In H. Smith-Gabai, & S. E. Holm (Eds.), *Occupational therapy in acute care* (pp. 339—352). Bethesda, MD: American Occupational Therapy Association, Inc.

Jester, R. (2014). Rehabilitation and the orthopaedic and musculoskeletal trauma client. In S. Clarke, & J. Santy-Tomlinson (Eds.), *Orthopaedic and trauma nursing: An evidence-based approach to musculoskeletal care* (pp. 59—66). Oxford, UK: John Wiley & Sons, Ltd.

Kiernan, J. A., & Barr, M. L. (2009). *Barr's the human nervous system: An anatomical viewpoint* (9th ed.). Philadelphia, PA: Wolters Kluwer Health & Lippincott Williams & Wilkins.

Kornfeld, P., Ambinder, E. P., Mittag, T., et al. (1981). Plasmapheresis in refractory generalized myasthenia gravis. *Archives of Neurology, 38*, 478.

Lynch, M. E., Craig, K. D., & Peng, P. W. H. (2011). *Clinical pain management: a practical guide*. Hoboken, NJ: Blackwell Publishing, Ltd.

Manter, J. T., Gilman, S., Gatz, A. J., & Newman, S. W. (2003). *Manter and Gatz's essentials of clinical neuroanatomy and neurophysiology* (10th ed.). Philadelphia, PA: F. A. Davis.

Mattle, H., & Mumenthaler, M. (2016). *Fundamentals of neurology: An illustrated guide*. New York, NY: Thieme Publishers.

McDonald, C. M., & Joyce, N. C. (2012). Neuromuscular disease management and rehabilitation, part II: specialty care and therapeutics. *Physical Medicine and Rehabilitation Clinics of North America, 23*(4), xiii—xvii.

Merkies, I. S. J., & Kieseier, B. C. (2016). Fatigue, pain, anxiety and depression in Guillain-Barré syndrome and chronic inflammatory demyelinating polyradiculoneuropathy. *European Neurology, 75*(3-4), 199—206. Available from https://search.proquest.com/docview/1781542469/EAF87958CF0E4DA3PQ/7?accountid=143111.

Morrison, D., Pathier, P., & Horr, K. (1978). *Sensory motor dysfunction and therapy in infancy and early childhood*. Springfield, IL: Charles C Thomas Publisher.

Muscular Dystrophy Association. (2019a). Limb-girdle muscular dystrophy (LGMD). Available from https://www.mda.org/disease/limb-girdle-muscular-dystrophy.

Muscular Dystrophy Association. (2019b). What is myotonic dystrophy. Available from https://www.mda.org/sites/default/files/2019/06/MDA_DM_Fact_Sheet_June_2019.pdf.

Muscular Dystrophy Association. (2019c). Duchenne Muscular Dystrophy (DMD). Available from https://www.mda.org/disease/duchenne-muscular-dystrophy.

Muscular Dystrophy Association. (2019d). Becker muscular dystrophy (BMD). Available from https://www.mda.org/disease/becker-muscular-dystrophy.

National Institute of Neurological Disorders and Stroke. (2019). Postpolio syndrome fact sheet. Available from https://www.ninds.nih.gov/Disorders/Client-Caregiver-Education/Fact-Sheets/Postpolio-Syndrome-Fact-Sheet.

National Spinal Cord Injury Statistical Center. (2013). An update on spinal cord injury: epidemiology, diagnosis, and treatment for the emergency physician. *Trauma Report*. Available from https://search.proquest.com/docview/1266769814?accountid=143111.

Newton-Triggs, L., & Rogers, J. (2014). The musculoskeletal system and human movement. In S. Clarke, & J. Santy-Tomlinson (Eds.), *Orthopaedic and trauma nursing: An evidence-based approach to musculoskeletal care* (pp. 27—48). Oxford, UK: John Wiley & Sons, Ltd.

Ogawa, T., Omon, K., Yuda, T., Ishigaki, T., Imai, R., Ohmatsu, S., et al. (2016). Short-term effects of goal-setting focusing on the life goal concept n subjective well-being and treatment engagement in subacute inpatients: a quasi-randomized controlled trial. *Clinical Rehabilitation, 30*(9), 909—920.

Phelps, P. E., & Walker, E. (1977). Comparison of the finger wrinkling test results to establish sensory tests in peripheral nerve injury. *The American Journal of Occupational Therapy.*, *31*(9), 565–572.

Radomski, M. V., & Latham, C. A. T. (2014). *Occupational therapy for physical dysfunction* (7th ed.). Baltimore, MD: Lippincott Williams & Wilkins.

Ranjani, P., Khanna, M., Gupta, A., Nagappa, M., Taly, A. B., & Haldar, P. (2014). Prevalence of fatigue in Guillain-Barre syndrome in neurological rehabilitation setting. *Annals of Indian Academy of Neurology, 17*(3), 331–335.

Reed, K. L. (2014). *Quick reference to occupational therapy* (3rd ed.). Austin, TX: Pro-Ed.

Robinault, I. (1973). *Functional aids for the multiple handicapped.* New York, NY: Harper & Row.

Ruff, C. C., & Fehr, E. (2014). The neurobiology of rewards and values in social decision making. *Nature Reviews Neuroscience, 15*(8), 549–562.

Russell, S. (2015). *Examination of peripheral nerve injuries: An anatomical approach* (2nd ed.). New York, NY: Thieme Medical Publishers, Inc.

Schell, B. A. B., & Gillen, G. (2019). *Willard & Spackman's occupational therapy* (13th ed.). Philadelphia, PA: Wolters Kluwer.

Seddon, H. J. (1975). *Surgical disorders of the peripheral nerves* (2nd ed.). New York, NY: Churchill Livingstone.

Simmonds, M. J., & Wideman, T. (2011). Physical therapy and rehabilitation. In M. E. Lynch, K. D. Craig, & P. W. H. Peng (Eds.), *Clinical pain management: A practical guide* (pp. 183–190). Hoboken, NJ: Blackwell Publishing Ltd.

Simon, A. U., & Collins, C. E. R. (2017). Lifestyle redesign for chronic pain management: a retrospective clinical efficacy study. *The American Journal of Occupational Therapy, 71*(4), 1–7.

Theis AL. (2010). What is the best practice in occupational therapy for treating clients with postpolio syndrome? A systematic literature review [Graduate research project]. Available from https://search.proquest.com/docview/743816926?accountid=143111.

Utsugisawa, K., Nagane, Y., Akaishi, T., et al. (2016). Early fast-acting treatment strategy against generalized myasthenia gravis. *Muscle & Nerve, 55*(6), 794–801.

Walter, J. B. (1992). *An introduction to the principles of disease* (3rd ed.). Philadelphia, PA: WB Saunders.

Williams, L. M., Fini, H. M., & Joyce, N. C. (2019). Neuromuscular disease: motor neuron disorders. In R. Mitra (Ed.), *Principles of rehabilitation medicine*. New York, NY: McGraw-Hill.

Willmott, H. (2015). *Trauma and orthopaedics at a glance.* Chichester, UK: John Wiley & Sons, Ltd.

Winhammar, J. M. C., Rowe, D. B., Henderson, R. D., & Kiernan, M. C. (2005). Assessment of disease progression in motor neuron disease. *Lancet Neurology, 4*(4), 229–238.

Zaretsky, H. H., Richter, E. F., & Eisenberg, M. G. (2005). *Medical aspects of disability: A handbook for the rehabilitation professional* (3rd ed.). New York, NY: Springer Publishing.

28

Arthritis and Lower Extremity Joint Replacement

Mary Elizabeth Patnaude

ARTHRITIS

The word *arthritis* means "joint inflammation." The condition affects the joints and the tissue surrounding the joints. Arthritis causes pain and limited movement by damaging body tissue, either by wear and tear or inflammation. Inflammation can be localized or systemic, affecting multiple joints throughout the body. According to the Centers for Disease Control and Prevention (CDC), there are over 100 types of arthritis (USDHHS/CDC, 2015). Three of the most commonly occurring forms of arthritis are rheumatoid arthritis (RA), osteoarthritis (OA), and gout (Arthritis Foundation, 2019a).

Prevalence of Arthritis

Arthritis is one of the most prevalent health conditions diagnosed by doctors. It affects over 54 million Americans. More than 23 million Americans experience arthritis-attributed activity limitation (AAAL) (Arthritis Foundation, 2019a; USDHHS/CDC, 2015). The disease affects one in three adults in rural areas and over half of adults in urban areas (Arthritis Foundation, 2019a; USDHHS/CDC, 2015). For older adults the rate is even higher.

Types of Arthritis

Rheumatoid Arthritis. Rheumatoid arthritis is a **chronic**, **systemic**, **autoimmune** disorder. It is long lasting (chronic) and involves multiple body systems (systemic). In RA the immune system of the body attacks itself (autoimmune). RA most commonly damages joints, but in a small percentage of persons it may also damage the blood vessels, heart, lungs, or eyes (Arthritis Foundation, 2020b).

RA occurs most commonly between the ages of 30 and 40, and affects women three times more often than men (Arthritis Foundation, 2020b). The body's response to this attack leads to inflammation of the joint capsule or lining, known as **synovitis** (Deshaies, 2018). Synovitis causes an increased production of synovial fluid, which stretches the joint capsule, tendons, and ligaments. These structural changes weaken the joint and its structures (Deshaies, 2018).

The disease process for RA varies from person to person. Pain may be chronic or acute. Most commonly, individuals experience chronic **inflammation** of the joints throughout the lifespan. In some cases, the disease progresses continuously. In others, it progresses with exacerbations and periods of complete or incomplete remission. Some may have a single episode of joint inflammation and an extended remission. Remissions provide a period of pain relief but do not signify that the disease is cured. Joint damage occurring during exacerbations is not reversed. The progressive joint damage done by long-term inflammation leads to chronic pain (Deshaies, 2018). **Acute pain**, the body's physiologic reaction to tissue damage, has a defined beginning and end (Engel, 2018). The acute pain in RA is caused by the tissue damage during periods of exacerbation (Deshaies, 2018).

The systemic symptoms characteristic of RA include fatigue, loss of appetite, fever, diffuse achiness, morning stiffness, and weight loss. The long-term nature of the disease, as well as its uncertain course, may lead to decreased motivation to engage in meaningful occupations. Long-term occupational deprivation and chronic pain may also lead to depression.

Clinical features of RA. Joint swelling caused by RA results from an abundance of synovial fluid, enlargement of the synovium, and thickening of the joint capsule. These changes weaken the joint capsule, tendons, and ligaments. Inflamed joints are warm, swollen, tender, red, and difficult or painful to move. The inflammation and pain may cause decreased range of motion (ROM), strength, and endurance. Chronic inflammation invades cartilage, bone, and tendons. It secretes damaging enzymes. If left uncontrolled, this damage leads to scar tissue formation, which will fuse the joints, leaving them rigid and immovable (American Occupational Therapy Association, 2014; Andrade, Brandão, Pinto, & Lanna, 2016; Arthritis Health Professions Selection Task Force, 1980; Felson, 2017).

RA affects the joints bilaterally, but not always symmetrically (Andrade et al., 2016). One side, often the dominant hand, may be more severely impaired. RA most commonly affects the joints of the wrist, thumb, and hand (proximal interphalangeal [PIP] and metacarpophalangeal [MCP] joints). It may also affect the elbows, shoulders, neck, jaw, hips, knees, ankles, and feet (American Occupational Therapy Association, 2014; Andrade et al., 2016; Felson, 2017).

If not managed well, RA may lead to a variety of hand deformities. A common sign of RA is the fusiform (spindle-shaped) swelling in the PIP joints (Fig. 28.1). Finger deformities, resulting from a weakening of the joint structures, include swan-neck, boutonnière, and ulnar drift. The swan-neck deformity is characterized by fixed hyperextension of the PIP joint and flexion of the distal interphalangeal (DIP) joint, and often flexion of the MCP joint (Fig. 28.2). These finger postures cause difficulty forming both power and precision grasps. The boutonnière deformity, caused by detachment of the central slip of the extensor tendon, manifests as fixed PIP flexion and DIP hyperextension (Fig. 28.3). Boutonnière deformity of the thumb is commonly seen in RA. It leads to flexion of the thumb MCP joint and hyperextension of the IP joint. Ligamentous instability, resulting from stretching or lengthening of the collateral ligaments of the fingers, can lead to **joint laxity**. Joint laxity can cause loss of hand function by decreasing stability needed for pinch and finger dexterity

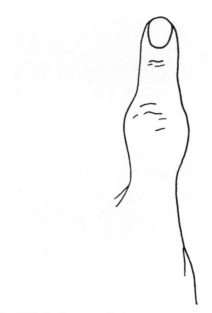

Fig. 28.1 Fusiform swelling.

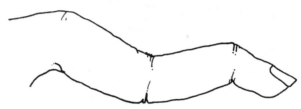

Fig. 28.2 Swan-neck deformity results in proximal interphalangeal (PIP) hyperextension and distal interphalangeal (DIP) flexion.

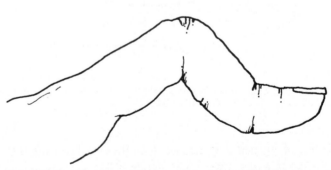

Fig. 28.3 Boutonnière deformity results in distal interphalangeal (DIP) hyperextension and proximal interphalangeal (PIP) flexion.

(Fig. 28.4). Weakened ligaments may also lead to joint subluxation or dislocation (Fig. 28.5). Ulnar drift, the extreme ulnar deviation of the MCP joint, is also a common symptom of RA (Fig. 28.6). Normal muscle action of the long finger flexors, which pull in an ulnar direction, causes this deformity when gripping forces act on the unstable joints.

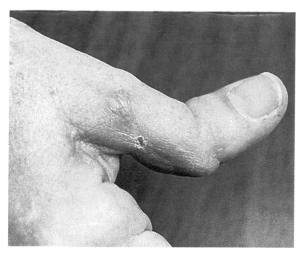

Fig. 28.4 Joint laxity (instability). (From ARHP Arthritis Teaching Slide Collection, American College of Rheumatology.)

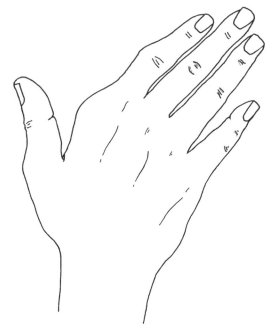

Fig. 28.6 Metacarpophalangeal (MCP or MP) joint ulnar drift.

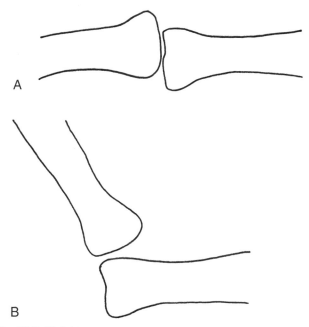

A

B

Fig. 28.5 (A) Subluxation. (B) Dislocation. (From Melvin JL. *Rheumatic Disease in the Adult and Child: Occupational Therapy and Rehabilitation.* 3rd ed. Philadelphia, PA: FA Davis; 1989.)

Osteoarthritis and Degenerative Joint Disease.

Osteoarthritis, also known as degenerative joint disease (DJD), occurs when the cushioning provided by cartilage in the joints breaks down (American Occupational Therapy Association, 2019; Arthritis Foundation, 2020a). This breakdown leads to joint pain and stiffness. Mechanical forces on the joint caused by too much weight, weak muscles, or misalignment are the primary cause of damage. However, localized inflammation, which is the body's primary response to tissue injury, can lead to increased damage (Felson, 2017). OA most commonly affects the knees, but can be seen in other joints such as the hip, shoulders, wrists, and hands. It is often referred to as the wear-and-tear disease because the involved joints wear down

with age, overuse, or injury. Risk factors for OA include history of joint injury, genetics, obesity, and female gender (especially after age 50) (American Occupational Therapy Association, 2019; Arthritis Foundation, 2020a).

Clinical features of OA. Degenerative joint damage, characterized by OA, begins when the smooth cartilage on the ends of the bone softens and loses its elasticity, leaving it vulnerable to damage. Over time, the damaged cartilage wears away, allowing the bones to rub together. When bones rub together with no lubrication, friction occurs. The bone friction causes pain, bone thickening (hypertrophy), and bone spurs. Bone spurs (bony growths or **osteophytes**) are formed where the ligaments and capsule attach to the bone. Damaged pieces of cartilage or bone may break off and become embedded in the joint fluid. The sediment in the joint, and/or the irregularity of the joint surfaces, may lead to an audible or palpable noise or grinding, known as **crepitus** (Felson, 2017). Fluid-filled cysts may form in the bone, near the joint or in the joint capsule. As a result of the damage, the joint may become stiff or unstable, leading to pain and restricted ROM.

The symptoms of OA may begin as acute pain, such following major orthopedic surgery, such as anterior cruciate ligament (ACL) surgery. It may also manifest as chronic pain that worsens over time. Initially, localized pain is felt in the affected joints following overuse or long periods of inactivity. Eventually, the decreased movement caused by pain will lead to weakening of the surrounding musculature, which leads to poor alignment. This poor alignment causes the joint damage mentioned earlier. Advanced OA leads to impaired coordination and posture (American Occupational Therapy Association, 2019; Andrade et al., 2016; Arthritis Foundation, 2020a).

Osteophytes that form in the fingers or at the carpometacarpal (CMC) joint of the thumb indicate cartilage damage, and can lead to finger deformities (American Occupational Therapy Association, 2019; Andrade et al., 2016; Felson, 2017). Bouchard nodes (Fig. 28.7A) form at the PIP joint, and Heberden nodes (see Fig. 28.7B) form at the DIP. Nodes at the thumb CMC joint, a common site of OA, can cause the joint to become subluxed, with a squared appearance (Fig. 28.8) (Arthritis Foundation, 2020a). These nodes feel hard to the touch, may be painful or tender, and lead to decreased ROM in the fingers. This can limit grasping and hand dexterity.

Gout. An excess of uric acid in the body causes **gout**, an inflammatory form of arthritis (Vannucchi, 2012). The cause is unknown, or **idiopathic**. The uric acid forms crystals, which deposit in and around joints causing inflammation and intense pain (Vannucchi, 2012). Gout affects over 8 million people (about 6 million men and 2 million women), representing about 3.9% of the US population (Zhu, Pandya, & Choi, 2011). Risk factors include genetic predisposition, advanced age, hypertension, high alcohol intake, and high body mass index (Vannucchi, 2012).

Gout can be characterized in four stages (Vannucchi, 2012). In asymptomatic gout, clients develop high blood levels of uric acid, which leads to crystal deposits in the joints but no pain. Some of these clients never develop symptoms. Symptomatic gout presents with a rapid onset of acute pain. The most common site of involvement is in the first metatarsal phalangeal (MTP) joint, also known as the big toe, but can progress to multiple joints. At its onset, the client will experience an inflamed joint that is hot, red, and extremely painful (Fig. 28.9). Although the initial symptoms often resolve without treatment, continued medical treatment helps to reduce the uric acid in the blood to prevent further flares (Vannucchi, 2012).

If medication fails to limit high uric acid in the blood, the patient reaches the final stage, known as chronic gout (Vannucchi, 2012). The accumulation of urate crystals in the joints can erode the cartilage, synovial membranes, tendons, and soft tissue, resulting in joint deformity.

INTERVENTIONS FOR ARTHRITIS

Management of arthritis focuses on the underlying causes of tissue damage. In RA, the body's immune response causes

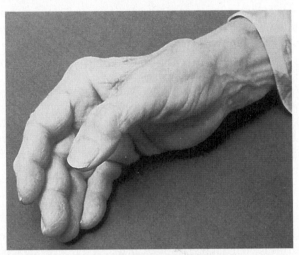

Fig. 28.8 Arthritic changes in the carpometacarpal joint of the thumb result in a squared appearance. (From the ARHP Arthritis Teaching Slide Collection, American College of Rheumatology.)

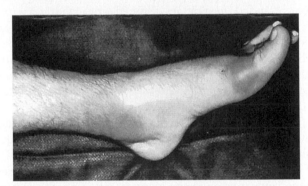

Fig. 28.9 Podagra—gout. (From the ARHP Arthritis Teaching Slide Collection, American College of Rheumatology.)

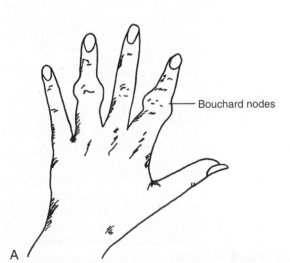

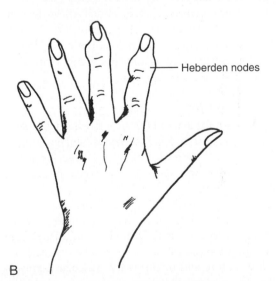

Fig. 28.7 Osteophyte formation in the (A) proximal interphalangeal joints (Bouchard nodes) and (B) distal interphalangeal joints (Heberden nodes) is characteristic of osteoarthritis.

systemic inflammation, which damages joints. OA is caused by mechanical stressors on tissue, which cause localized inflammation, wear, and tear. Gout results from an excess of uric acid in the body. Medical management includes targeted use of medication to prevent and reduce joint damage, and surgical intervention to correct painful and nonfunctional joints. Occupational therapy focuses on prevention, strengthening, and improving occupational engagement.

Medication Interventions

RA is an autoimmune disease. Therefore treatment focuses on medications that modify the disease process (England, 2018). Disease-modifying antirheumatic drugs (DMARDs) and biologic response modifiers (BRMs) are used alone or in combination to slow joint damage by suppressing the immune system (England, 2018). Examples of these drugs include methotrexate, gold salts, hydroxychloroquine, etanercept, and infliximab. The key to the effectiveness in these treatments relies on the ability for the physician to individually select the plan that works best for each individual client (Arthritis Foundation, 2019a). Current researchers are focusing on doing just that.

Medications for OA target the localized inflammation induced as the body's response to tissue damage. Recent developments include medications delivered early in the disease process, which target receptors in the joints to reduce or prevent the development of OA (Arthritis Foundation, 2020a). Steroids reduce inflammation but can have serious side effects, so limiting their use is important. Recent advances in these medications include longer-acting and delayed-release injection corticosteroids (Arthritis Foundation, 2019a).

The primary strategy for medical management of gout involves reducing the amount of uric acid in the blood. This often needs to be lifelong therapy (Vannucchi, 2012).

In acute flare-ups of gout, the medical focus is on decreasing inflammation and pain. Nonsteroidal anti-inflammatory drugs (NSAIDs) are used to reduce inflammation and pain in both OA and RA. Examples of NSAIDs include ibuprofen, naproxen, and aspirin. Analgesic medications relieve the pain associated with gout. Analgesics taken orally include acetaminophen and prescription pain medications. Topical analgesics include agents such as anti-inflammatory medications, camphor, salicylates, or capsaicin.

Surgical Intervention

Surgical intervention for RA and OA occurs when joint damage causes extreme pain and limits engagement in occupation. There are many surgical options available for severe arthritis. This chapter will focus on synovectomy, tendon repair, and arthroplasty.

In RA, synovectomy (removal of the diseased synovium) and tenosynovectomy (removal of diseased tendon sheath) are performed to prevent further complications. These surgeries relieve symptoms and slow the process of joint destruction or tendon rupture and help preserve vascular supply to the joint. Tendon surgery (including tendon relocation, tendon repair, tendon transfer, and tendon release) is considered

a corrective strategy for specific hand impairments. Tendon surgery is most often performed on the extensor tendons of the hand and wrist (Deshaies, 2018).

Surgeons perform joint fusion, or arthrodesis, by placing hardware, such as pins or rods, in the joints to cause bones to fuse (Arthritis Foundation, 2020b). They also replace severely damaged joints with prosthetic implants that provide the motion of the natural joint using arthroplasty. When the entire joint is replaced, the procedure is known as total arthroplasty. Surgeons complete this procedure on many joints. The most common are total hip arthroplasty (THA) and total knee arthroplasty (TKA).

THA involves replacement of the acetabulum of the hip and the femoral head. A high-density polyethylene socket is fitted into the acetabulum, and a metallic prosthesis replaces the femoral head and neck (Fig. 28.10). The surgeon either uses acrylic cement to affix the component to the bone or uses a prosthesis in which the bone can grow around it. Surgeons may use an anterior or a posterior approach. With an anterior or anterolateral approach, the patient will be unstable in external rotation, adduction, and extension of the operated hip and must observe precautions to prevent these movements for 6 to 12 weeks. With a posterior or posterolateral approach, the patient must be cautioned not to move the operated hip in specific ranges of flexion (usually 60–90 degrees) and not to internally rotate or adduct the leg. Failure to maintain **hip precautions** during muscle and soft tissue healing may result in hip dislocation (Fig. 28.11) (Michlovitz, 1990).

TKA involves cutting away the damaged portions of the distal femur and proximal tibia and attaching a prosthesis for the new joint. The type of prosthesis used depends on the severity of joint damage (Figs. 28.12 and 28.13). The prosthesis may be

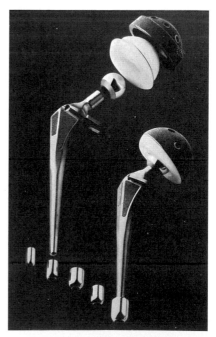

Fig. 28.10 Modular total hip prosthesis designed for bony ingrowth. (From Kottke FJ: *Krusen's Handbook of Physical Medicine Rehabilitation.* 4th ed. Philadelphia, PA: WB Saunders; 1990.)

Postoperative Precautions for Total Hip Arthroplasty: By Procedure

Approach	No Flexion Beyond 90 Degrees	No Internal Rotation	No Adduction Past Midline	No Extension	No External Rotation	No Abduction
Anterior	X	X	X	X	X	
Lateral	X	X	X	X	X	
Posterior	X	X	X			

Fig. 28.11 Postoperative hip precautions.

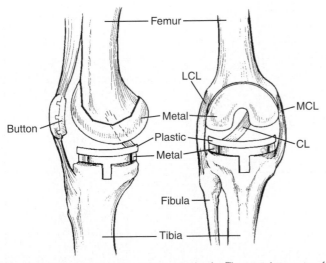

Fig. 28.12 Porous-coated total knee prosthesis. Note resurfacing features of components and beaded surfaces for biologic fixation. (From Kottke FJ: *Krusen's Handbook of Physical Medicine Rehabilitation.* 4th ed. Philadelphia, PA: WB Saunders; 1990.)

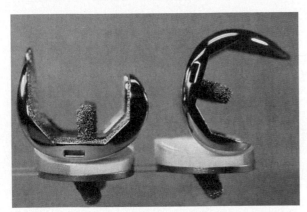

Fig. 28.13 Total knee replacement prosthesis. The metal aspects of the prosthesis cover the distal portion of the femur and the end of the tibia. There is a polyethylene plastic-bearing surface (plastic) between the metallic aspects of the two surfaces. The patella is replaced by a polyethylene button. The medial collateral ligament (MCL), lateral collateral ligament (LCL), and cruciate ligaments (CL) are retained.

cemented or not cemented to the bone. Clients given cemented prostheses can often bear weight as tolerated postoperatively. Clients given noncemented prostheses must usually observe nonweight-bearing (NWB) precautions

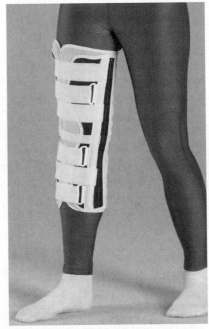

Fig. 28.14 A knee immobilizer is used to support and stabilize the knee joint during mobility. (Courtesy DeRoyal, Powell, TN.)

postoperatively. Patients may use a **knee immobilizer** (Fig. 28.14) to provide support to the knee when moving in and out of the bed and ambulating. Postsurgical knee pain should be addressed by the entire treatment team.

OCCUPATIONAL THERAPY

Occupational therapy practitioners, including occupational therapists (OTs) and occupational therapy assistants (OTAs), utilize a multimodal approach to treatment for their clients living with arthritis. The goal of intervention is to safely maximize independence in occupations and improve quality of life (American Occupational Therapy Association, 2019). Arthritis affects clients differently, so the first step in the occupational therapy intervention process must begin by the OT determining functional abilities and limitations, with input from the OTA, utilizing standardized and nonstandardized measures. OTs and OTAs formulate a dynamic intervention plan to address all the client's needs and improve occupational performance.

OCCUPATIONAL THERAPY TREATMENT PROCESS

Assessment of Occupational Performance

The initial step of the evaluation plan is the formulation of an occupational profile, which provided information on the client's occupational history, daily living routines, values, and needs (American Occupational Therapy Association, 2014). This type of interview may be conducted by the OT or the OTA, using an informal structure, or with a structured format such as the Arthritis Evaluation Checklist (Fig. 28.15).

ARTHRITIS EVALUATION CHECKLIST

Name: _____ Diagnosis: _____

Referral: _____

Initial Interview:

Which joints bother you the most? _____

Pain: (0–10 scale)   at rest _____   on movement _____   constant _____   Description _____

Do you experience morning stiffness? _____   Duration? _____

Which medications are you presently taking? _____

Since taking the medication, have you noticed any of the following? (circle)

                    headaches   nausea   itching   rash   ringing in ears   other _____

Surgeries? _____

Exercise program? _____

Splints? _____

What do you know about arthritis? _____

What are your goals? _____

UPPER EXTREMITY ROM:

		RIGHT		LEFT		COMMENTS
		Active	Passive	Active	Passive	
Shoulder	Extension/flexion					
	Adduction/abduction					
	Internal rotation					
	External rotation					
Elbow	Extension/flexion					
Forearm	Supination					
	Pronation					
Wrist	Flexion					
	Extension					
	Ulnar/radial deviation					

Limitations:

HAND PLACEMENT EVALUATION:

Key: 0—Easily   2—With moderate difficulty
       1—With minimal difficulty   3—Unable

	RIGHT	LEFT	COMMENTS
Reach overhead			
Touch top of head			
Touch mouth			
Touch back of neck			
Touch behind back			

Fig. 28.15 Arthritis evaluation checklist.

HAND	RIGHT	LEFT	COMMENTS
9 hole peg (seconds)			
Grip strength			
Pinch: lateral, 3-jaw			
Opposition			

Sensation:

Soft tissue and hand deformities noted: (including flexion contractures, swan neck, boutonnière, ulnar deviation, subluxation, edema, redness, warmth)

_____

_____

FUNCTIONAL ABILITIES: Key: 0—Easily   2—With moderate difficulty
                              1—With minimal difficulty   3—Unable
                                          COMMENTS

Grasp spoon or fork	
Carry to mouth	
Cut meat	
Drink from glass/cup	
Bilateral activities	
Button	
Manipulate coins	
Turn key in lock	
Write name	
Turn pages	
Use telephone	
Open doors	
Open jars	

Endurance: _____

Marital status: _____ Family members/supportive persons at home: _____

Household responsibilities: _____

Do you have difficulty in ADL? _____

Architecture: _____

Vocational responsibilities: _____

RECOMMENDATIONS: Adaptive equipment (circle):   key extension   feeding device   writing device   telephone device

       car door opener   dressing stick   buttonhook   other _____

Splints: _____

Joint protection: _____

Home program: _____

Evaluation completed by: _____ Date: _____

Fig. 28.15 (Continued)

Since pain is a major symptom of arthritis it must be assessed in the evaluation. A numeric pain rating on a scale of 0 (no pain) to 10 (greatest pain) can be used. In addition, the client can be asked to provide qualifiers, such as location of pain, time of day in which it occurs, and its effect on occupational performance. Assessment of signs of acute inflammation such as pain, heat, swelling, and/or redness should be noted (American Occupational Therapy Association, 2014; Felson, 2017).

The OT determines whether to use standardized or nonstandardized assessments to evaluate ROM, strength, coordination, sensation, and cognition (see Chapters 6, 7, 8, and 9).

These assessments may be done by the OT or the OTA (if competency in these areas has been demonstrated). Alternative methods of assessment may be utilized if necessary, to prevent stress on the joints. For example, grip and pinch strength may be tested with an adapted blood pressure cuff and measured in mm Hg (Andrade et al., 2016; Felson, 2017). Manual muscle testing must be done with caution to avoid pulling unstable joints out of alignment. Sensation testing, such as light touch, pain, temperature sense, and proprioception, may reveal impairments due to nerve compression or damage.

Evaluation of occupational performance in activities of daily living (ADL) and instrumental activities of daily living (IADL) should be done by selecting the appropriate assessments to identify the client's strengths, deficits, and contextual demands (American Occupational Therapy Association, 2014) (see Chapter 13). To get the most accurate assessment, it is important for this to be done as close to the actual time each activity is performed and in the environment that closely matches the natural context. Due to factors such as morning stiffness and fatigue, a client's abilities may vary throughout the day. Ideally, a home evaluation should be done in the patient's home. Onsite or simulated activities may be used to assess employment performance. Additional information to be documented include factors such as morning stiffness, medication regimen, and activity tolerance. The OT or OTA may also note whether the patient understands and utilizes energy conservation techniques to manage fatigue and joint protection techniques to ensure proper positioning (Andrade et al., 2016; Engel, 2018; Felson, 2017).

Pain and endurance often vary from day. Therefore the evaluation should include documentation about how the client's occupational performance differs from day to day.

Arthritis affects the entire person, so in the evaluation process, the occupational therapy practitioner should screen for cognitive and psychosocial deficits (Deshaies, 2018). The disease is painful and unpredictable, which may result in depression, denial, and anxiety. Psychological stressors may exacerbate the symptoms of the disease (Harris, 1981). Cognition testing may be necessary because depression may cause deficits in attention span, short-term memory, and problem-solving skills. Psychosocial factors to be considered during assessment include coping strategies and support structures.

Intervention Process
Occupational Therapy Intervention.
When designing an intervention plan, OTs and OTAs need to consider any surgical procedures performed. In postoperative clients, surgical precautions need to be followed. In both operative and nonoperative clients, OTs and OTAs utilize preparatory methods and tasks, occupations and activities, and education and training throughout the intervention process (American Occupational Therapy Association, 2014). Specific interventions include physical agent modalities (PAMS), rest, therapeutic exercise, therapeutic activity, postoperative positioning, positioning with orthotics, and client education (Deshaies,

2018). Researchers found positive outcomes associated with interventions focused on increasing physical activity and patient education to decrease pain and improve occupational engagement (Ekelman, Hooker, Davis, Klan, & Newburn, 2014; Poole et al., 2017).

Decreased strength, decreased dexterity, pain, and decreased activity tolerance have a strong correlation to activity limitations in clients with arthritis (Andrade et al., 2016). The goal of treatment is to decrease pain and inflammation, improve strength and dexterity, and improve endurance for occupational engagement (Andrade et al., 2016). Every intervention plan should be individually designed based on the client's severity of symptoms, general health status, lifestyle, and personal goals.

Physical agent modalities are considered preparatory methods. They should be used to prepare the client for engagement in occupation to reduce pain, manage inflammation, and increase ROM. PAMs utilized include thermal (heat, cold), mechanical (ultrasound), and electrical (transcutaneous electrical nerve stimulation [TENS] and biofeedback). Cold packs reduce inflammation and edema. Heat (paraffin wax and hot packs) reduces stiffness and increases mobility. Mechanical and electrical modalities relieve pain (Arthritis Health Professions Selection Task Force, 1980; Felson, 2017). In most states, the use of PAMs requires advanced certification. Clients may utilize modalities at home to improve mobility. This may include taking a warm bath or shower. The client should be educated on their use. For example, application of heat should be limited to 20 minutes to prevent increasing inflammation and edema (Arthritis Health Professions Selection Task Force, 1980; Felson, 2017; Fries, 1986). State licensure boards require varying levels of training and certification for application of PAMs. OTAs must be aware of their state licensure requirements, and acquire the required training if they use them as preparatory treatments for clients with arthritis.

Therapeutic Activities and Exercise.
Therapeutic activities and exercise promote joint function, muscle strength, and endurance (Fig. 28.16). OTAs should coordinate with other providers, such as physical therapy, to avoid overworking any group of muscles. See Table 28.1 for exercises to prevent deformity. OTAs must be aware of client factors, such as pain, mobility, and disease level, when providing interventions (Ekelman et al., 2014). Strong evidence exists to support the benefits of aerobic and resistive exercises, as long as they are performed at the appropriate level for the particular client (Ekelman et al., 2014). Intervention programs should begin slowly, then gradually increase in intensity, duration, and frequency of the various activities (Andrade et al., 2016). Splints, braces, and positioning devices may be used throughout the stages to provide joint rest and stability. The patient may perform self-care activities as tolerated while incorporating the principles of joint protection. During the acute stage, active assistive exercises and exercises with gravity eliminated may be performed within the limits of pain tolerance. As the patient's abilities improve, the activities will progress to

---

ARTHRITIS RANGE OF MOTION EXERCISES

The following exercises will help you to maintain your mobility. Do only those checked by the therapist.

INSTRUCTIONS

1. Start doing five of each exercise two times per day.
2. Progress to ten of each, two times per day.
3. Do all exercises *slowly* while sitting.
4. If having an active flare-up, cut down or eliminate exercises. After symptoms subside, start at the beginning to build up tolerance.

Shoulder

___ Hold your hands on your shoulders and make small to large circles with your elbows. Go clockwise and then counterclockwise.

___ With your hands on your shoulders, bring your elbows together in front of you and then spread your elbows apart to the side and as far back as you can reach.

Elbow

___ Hold your hands on your shoulders. Bring them out straight in front of you with your palms up.

___ With your elbows bent at your side, turn your palms up and down.

___ Roll up a newspaper and hold onto the ends of it with each hand facing down. Rest the paper on your knees. Bend your elbows to bring the paper to your right shoulder and back to your knees. Bend your elbows to your left shoulder and back to your knees.

Wrist

___ Hold your hand facing down. Make a fist as you bend your wrist up. Open your fingers as you bend your wrist down.

___ Hold your hands together in a praying position. Keeping your hands together and moving only your wrist, point your fingertips away from and toward you.

Hands

___ Touch your thumb to each finger.

___ Make a fist and stretch your fingers open and out.

Please call if you have any questions.

Fig. 28.16 Arthritis range of motion exercises.

include active and resistive exercises. The exercises should be done at the best time of the day for the patient—that is, when the patient feels more limber and has the least pain (such as after a warm shower or a short time after receiving pain medication) (Andrade et al., 2016; Felson, 2017).

In the acute stage, gentle passive and active ROM exercises to the point of pain (without stretch) should be done twice daily. As few as one to two repetitions of complete joint range are necessary to prevent loss of ROM (Engel, 2018; Felson, 2017). However, several attempts at movement may be necessary before full range is achieved. The patient may complete self-ranging exercises of the neck, elbows, and hands, but the therapy practitioner should passively range the shoulder to promote muscle relaxation (Felson, 2017). Isometric exercises without resistance may be completed to preserve strength. One to three contractions per muscle group per day is the recommended number (Engel, 2018; Felson, 2017). Resistive exercises and stretching at the end range should be avoided during the acute phase (Engel, 2018; Felson, 2017).

Rest. Rest is a form of activity modification. It is an important part of treatment that contributes to reduced inflammation

TABLE 28.1   Treatment for Specific Deformities

Deformity	Possible Medical Care	Treatment Methods	Splinting	Methods to Avoid
Swan-neck deformity	Synovectomy in the early stages	Daily ROM to each finger joint and gentle stretches for the PIP joints and intrinsics	Three-point finger splint for the PIP joint to prevent hyperextension	Isotonic, isometric, and resistive exercise
Boutonnière deformity	Synovectomy and tendon repair	Daily ROM to each finger joint, gentle assisted and active extension of the PIP joints, and active DIP flexion with the PIP extended	Extension mobilization or resting splints for the PIP joints	Isotonic, isometric, and resistive exercise
Trigger finger	Steroid injections	Tendon protection techniques—heat/ice for inflammation, avoidance of repetitive gripping activities	Trigger finger splint	Gripping exercises or activities
MP ulnar drift	Synovectomy Tendon realignment Joint replacement	Daily ROM to MP joints with emphasis on MP extension and radial deviation; joint protection techniques	Soft ulnar deviation splints during the day; immobilization splints with the MP joints in neutral deviation and 30 degrees of flexion at night	Isotonic, isometric, and resistive exercise Positions of deformity
MP volar palmar subluxation-dislocation	Joint replacement or repair	AROM of the MP joints emphasizing extension; joint protection techniques	Resting splints at night	Positions of deformity
Wrist subluxation	Arthroplasty or arthrodesis	—	Wrist support during the day and immobilization splint at night	—
Elbow synovitis	Steroid injections; synovectomy and resection of the radial head; arthroplasty	Rest for acute synovitis; use of cold; daily AROM and PROM exercise; isotonic or isometric exercise	Resting splint or splint for stabilization	Overuse
Shoulder synovitis	Steroid injections; applicable surgery	AROM and isotonic exercises preceded by hot packs	—	Slings

AROM, Active range of motion; DIP, distal interphalangeal; MP or MCP, metacarpophalangeal; PIP, proximal interphalangeal; PROM, passive range of motion; ROM, range of motion.

and increased energy levels. The need for rest varies from individual to individual and depends on disease activity. Greater amounts of bed rest may be required during severe exacerbation of disease symptoms, as experienced in RA. For many, short naps during the day, to balance work and rest, may be enough. Activity modification to provide rest to specific joints may be done with orthotics. For example, a hand-based orthotic to support the thumb may be beneficial during prolonged fine motor tasks. Psychological rest may be experienced with a short diversion from routine activities or a refocusing of attention on enjoyable instead of stressful events (Arthritis Health Professions Selection Task Force, 1980; Banwell, 1986; Ekelman et al., 2014).

Positioning. Proper positioning and joint alignment are beneficial ways to modify activity to rest joints, reduce joint stress, and prevent deformity. Sleeping in a nonweight-bearing position, such as on the opposite side of an involved hip, may help prevent joint stress. Positioning to prevent deformity and contractures is recommended. Sleeping without a pillow under the knees and with a small neck pillow will help avoid flexion contractures. Periods of lying prone may be helpful in maintaining full extension of the hips and knees. Maintenance of good postural alignment when standing and sitting also prevents deformities and undue stress to the muscles and joints. Adaptive equipment, such as chairs with elevated seats and armrests, will improve the client's ability to transfer from seated to standing, reduce stress on upper extremity joints, and help maintain postoperative precautions (Engel, 2018; Felson, 2017).

> **! ALERT**
>
> Patients with MCP ulnar drift should *not* exercise into composite fist (full fist) or use putty to do this because contraction of long finger flexors promotes ulnar drift. Instead, direct the patient to keep MPs (same as MCPs) extended while working on finger flexion.

> **CLINICAL PEARL**
>
> Exercises for RA tend to focus on antideformity positions:
> - To prevent MCP deformity, complete activities and exercises that position the hand in MP (MCP) extension and radial deviation. In RA, MP flexion and ulnar deviation lead to deformity.
> - To prevent the loss of PIP extension and the increase of DIP hyperextension seen in boutonnière deformity, complete activities and exercises that position the fingers in PIP extension and DIP flexion.
> - To prevent the excessive PIP hyperextension and DIP flexion seen in swan-neck deformity, complete activities and exercises that position the fingers in PIP flexion and DIP extension.

As the client begins to experience less acute flareups, activities and exercises that move the joints through the full ROM, with a gentle passive stretch at the end range, may be completed. Isotonic exercises and graded isometric exercises may be performed with caution to minimize stress to the joints (Engel, 2018; Felson, 2017). As the client continues to move from an acute to an inactive chronic phase of disease, more intense stretches at the end range of joint mobility, as well as carefully chosen resistive exercises, may be included during exercise and therapeutic activities, and daily living tasks (Andrade et al., 2016; Engel, 2018; Felson, 2017). Clients should listen to their body and respect pain during performance of exercise and activities. The assessment of pain should help guide the OTA in determining the correct type and amount to perform. The OT and the OTA remain mindful of the client's goals to determine whether their joints will benefit from a strengthening program. If pain resulting from exercise lasts longer than 1 hour, the vigor of the exercise should be reduced (Engel, 2018; Felson, 2017).

Education. Education in joint protection techniques should be a foundation of interventions with clients who have arthritis. These techniques may help prevent damage and increase participation in occupation. They are especially helpful in preventing hand deformities in clients with RA and/or OA (Arthritis Health Professions Selection Task Force, 1980; Banwell, 1986; Engel, 2018; Murphy & Lawson, 2018). Education in postoperative precautions for clients who received total joint replacements should also occur (see Fig. 28.11 for precautions following THA).

The following joint protection techniques and intervention strategies will be helpful to OTAs providing patient education to clients with arthritis.

1. *Respect pain.* Pain signals that possible tissue damage is occurring and indicates that there may be too much stress on the joint. Although clients with arthritis may feel that they can "tough it out," ignoring pain will often lead to more pain and joint damage. Pain that persists 1 to 2 hours after completing a task indicates that the activity may have caused too much stress on joints and that activity modification is warranted. Helpful modifications include breaking the task into smaller steps, with rest in between, modifying the joint position, or utilizing adaptive equipment to complete the task. Clients should avoid activities that put strain on painful joints (Arthritis Health Professions Selection Task Force, 1980; Banwell, 1986; Engel, 2018; Murphy & Lawson, 2018).

2. *Maintain muscle strength and joint ROM.* Therapeutic exercises and activities, which require that joints be used to the full available ROM, will result in maintenance of muscle strength and joint ROM. For example, when ironing, sweeping, or mopping, the client should use long, flowing strokes, straightening and bending the arms as much as possible (Fig. 28.17). To ensure the use of full shoulder ROM during reach, clients should store light items such as cereal or noodles in high cabinets (Arthritis Health Professions Selection Task Force, 1980; Banwell, 1986; Engel, 2018; Murphy & Lawson, 2018).

3. *Avoid positions that put stress on joints and lead to deformity.* Activity modification should be used to ensure

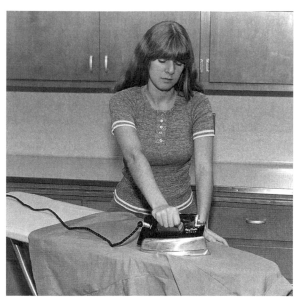

Fig. 28.17 During ironing, full extension at the elbow can be practiced.

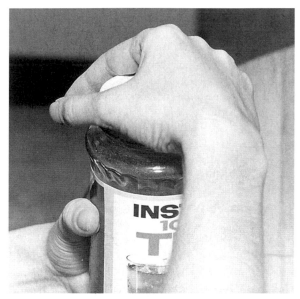

Fig. 28.18 Jar is twisted off with palm of right hand, or with left hand and opened with right hand, to prevent ulnar drift.

that joints are used in their most stable position. For example, using built-up handles on household items, such as pots, can assist the client in avoiding a tight grip while cooking (Arthritis Health Professions Selection Task Force, 1980; Banwell, 1986; Engel, 2018; Murphy & Lawson, 2018). Some other examples to avoid excess pressure on the finger include modifying the grip on a knife to mimic holding a dagger, using a pizza cutter instead of a knife, and holding a vegetable peeler parallel to the MP joints rather than diagonally across the palm (Arthritis Health Professions Selection Task Force, 1980; Banwell, 1986; Engel, 2018; Murphy & Lawson, 2018). In addition, clients should avoid hand positions requiring squeezing or twisting. For example, rather than squeezing a cleaning cloth between the fingers, it may be wrung out by spreading the hand flat over it or by squeezing it between the palms. Adaptive methods to avoid twisting while opening a jar include leaning on the jar with the palm of the hand and turning the lid with shoulder motion or holding the jar in a drawer as the cap is twisted (Arthritis Health Professions Selection Task Force, 1980; Banwell, 1986; Engel, 2018; Murphy & Lawson, 2018) (Fig. 28.18). There are also commercially available devices available for opening jars. To discourage the development of ulnar drift deformities, clients should utilize movements that turn their hands toward the thumb (radially). Some example of this include using the right hand to open a jar and the left hand to close it, stirring counterclockwise with the right hand and clockwise with the left hand, and avoiding using fingers to pick up a mug (Banwell, 1986; Engel, 2018; Murphy & Lawson, 2018).

4. *Avoid staying in one position for a long time.* Staying in one position leads to fatigue and stiffness. Activity

modifications to avoid this include using a book stand to hold a book rather than holding it with flexed fingers, using a nonskid surface to hold a bowl while stirring or placing the bowl in a partially open drawer, and never beginning an activity that cannot be stopped immediately if pain or fatigue sets in (Arthritis Health Professions Selection Task Force, 1980; Banwell, 1986; Engel, 2018; Murphy & Lawson, 2018).

5. *Use the strongest joints and muscles available.* Use of larger joints reduces stress on the smaller joints. For example, carrying a purse on the shoulder instead of in the hands makes use of the larger shoulder joint, rather than the fingers. Other examples include pushing doors open with the side of the arm or the whole body instead of the hand, adding cloth loops to drawer pulls so that they can be opened with the forearm, using palms with the fingers straight instead of bent fingers to pick up a coffee mug, and using the stronger leg first to go up the stairs and last to go down the stairs. Maintaining a healthy body weight will also help to avoid stress on the weight-bearing joints (Arthritis Health Professions Selection Task Force, 1980; Banwell, 1986; Engel, 2018; Murphy & Lawson, 2018).

6. *Distribute the workload over several joints.* Use oven mitts to carry hot dishes. Carry heavy loads close to the body using the arms rather than the hands. Slide objects along the counter instead of carrying them. If necessary, lift objects by scooping them up with forearms and both palms turned upward. Stress and pain may also be reduced by wearing a wrist splint during functional activities (Arthritis Health Professions Selection Task Force, 1980; Banwell, 1986; Engel, 2018; Murphy & Lawson, 2018).

Orthotic Intervention. Orthotics are used to support the joint in an optimal position for function and to provide rest and support (Engel, 2018; Felson, 2017). See Chapter 19 for detailed information regarding the principles of orthotic intervention. There is evidence to support the use of orthotics in clients with arthritis to prevent deformity, relieve pain, and increase grip strength (Ekelman et al., 2014). However, their use may increase stiffness and their efficacy may be decreased by inadequate client training and improper use (Ekelman et al., 2014). The most common orthotics fabricated for clients with arthritis are hand immobilization orthoses, a wrist immobilization orthosis (Fig. 28.19), an ulnar drift positioning orthotic (Fig. 28.20), and finger-based immobilization orthotics such as silver rings (Fig. 28.21).

Occupational Performance. Occupational therapy should maximize the ability of clients with arthritis to increase vitality, limit disease progression, and prevent activity limitation (Andrade et al., 2016). Activity tolerance can be increased by the grading of activities. For example, during an acute flareup, a client may complete bathing and hygiene at the sink rather than taking a full bath or shower. As the client gains strength and endurance, he or she will be able to resume a daily shower or bath and add resistance of using a loofah. Adaptive equipment and joint protection techniques can be used to effectively modify many tasks, such as bathing, dressing, home management, and leisure activities.

Energy Conservation. Energy conservation techniques are useful to clients with arthritis to maximize participation in occupation (Ekelman et al., 2014; Engel, 2018; Felson, 2017). OTAs can provide education about these techniques and assist clients in applying them to daily living. These techniques include balancing work and rest and work simplification.

Assistive Devices. See Chapter 13 for in-depth explanations of adaptive devices to increase participation in occupation. Table 28.2 provides a list of assistive devices.

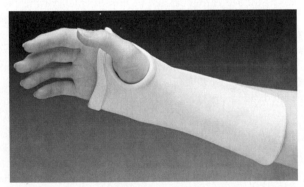

Fig. 28.19 Wrist immobilization splint. (From North Coast Medical, Inc., San Jose, CA.)

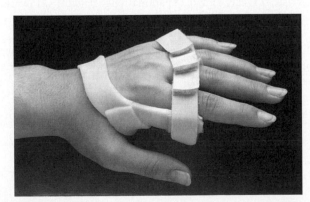

Fig. 28.20 Ulnar drift positioning splint. (From North Coast Medical, Inc., San Jose, CA.)

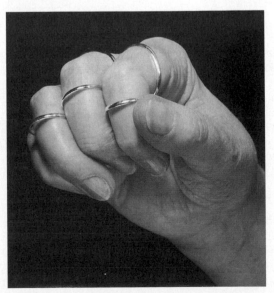

Fig. 28.21 Silver ring splint. (Courtesy Silver Ring Splint Company, Charlottesville, VA.)

TABLE 28.2   Assistive Devices

Problem	Principle	Examples
Decreased range of motion	Lengthen the handle on objects Organize objects within easy reach	Reachers, long-handled shoe horn, extended mop handle, long-handled bath sponge, revolving space saver, pegboards
Impaired grasp	Enlarge the circumference of handles	Built-up soft handles, large pens, universal cuffs
Instability	Stabilize objects and provide support for safety	Nonskid mats, suction brushes, handrails, grab bars
Decreased energy	Facilitate performance, energy-conservation techniques	Lightweight tools, electrical tools, Zim jar opener, sit with proper posture while working, pacing of activities, balancing of rest and activity
Potential for joint deformities	Increase leverage Prevent static or prolonged holding	Extended faucet handles, enlarged handles, adapted key holder, vegetable peeler held at MPs, lever-type doorknobs Book stand, bowl holder
Decreased strength	Modify work heights Raise the height of beds and chairs to make standing easier	Raised toilet seats, shower seats

MPs, Metacarpophalangeals.

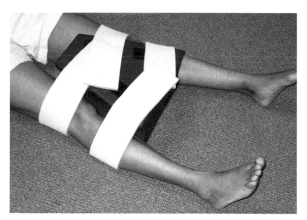

Fig. 28.22 Patient is positioned with an abduction wedge to maintain hip precautions.

CLINICAL PEARL

Proper body mechanics are imperative to effectively utilize assistive devices. The OTA should provide thorough training in all devices and observe the client during use to ensure this. Education on joint protection should be included in adaptive device training. Practice and therapist feedback will ensure safe use of devices, which will lead to better outcomes. Fig. 28.22 illustrates a positioning device for clients following total joint arthroplasty.

Discharge Planning. Discharge planning begins with the initial referral to occupational therapy. Active participation by the client throughout the intervention process will lead to better follow-through after discharge (Arthritis Health Professions Selection Task Force, 1980; Mann, Hurren, & Tomita, 1995). Education of clients and their families will help them access the resources available to them. When nearing discharge, clients may have more questions that need answering, and information repeated. This is okay because repetition and reinforcement are the keys to education. Examples that relate directly to the client are often most effective for teaching (Andrade et al., 2016). Home programs, developed by the OT and OTA, which include topics mentioned earlier, should be implemented for the client to continue after discharge. Verbal and written instructions geared to the patient's level of education and understanding may also reinforce carryover.

Fig. 28.23 provides a case study on Mrs. B, a client with RA. The case of Mrs. Johnson, who recently had a TKA, is presented in Fig. 28.24.

SUMMARY

RA, OA, and gout represent three commonly occurring forms of arthritis. They have different etiologies but cause similar impairments: pain, inflammation, joint damage, and decreased activity tolerance. These impairments can be reduced or eliminated with tailored medication regimens, exercise, surgery, and occupational engagement. OTAs can assist clients in achieving positive outcomes through therapeutic exercise and activity, preparatory activities, and patient education. The intervention process is dynamic, and the best outcomes will be achieved when they are individually tailored to each client.

REVIEW QUESTIONS

1. What clinical feature causes joint damage in RA?
2. What are the major differences between OA and RA?
3. When are occupational therapy services indicated for the treatment of clients with gout?
4. What are three systemic signs of RA?

Case Study: Mrs. B

Mrs. B. is a 36-year-old woman with RA. The onset was 3 years ago. She is married with an 8-year-old daughter. She lives in a three-bedroom, single-level home, with her husband and daughter. Her primary role is as a stay at home mom. She works a part-time job at a florist shop, designing and constructing wreaths, and arranging flowers. She enjoys this work and the money is a necessary part of the family budget.

Her RA is characterized by intermittent exacerbations affecting her bilaterally in the elbows, wrists, MP joints, and PIP joints. She demonstrates minimal limitations in ROM and strength in all these joints.

She demonstrates ulnar deviation, MP subluxation, boutonnière deformity and wrist subluxation. These deformities are not fixed, but still flexible. She has been on a course of anti-rheumatics and biologics to medically manage the disease process. She utilizes energy conservation and rest to prevent flares. She has been advised to avoid strenuous activity and resistance and to avoid fatigue.

Mrs. B. was referred to OT during the acute phase of a recent exacerbation. The intervention goals included maximizing participation, limiting loss of ROM and strength, preventing permanent deformity, and client education. She will be treated using both biomechanical and rehabilitation intervention approaches.

Strengths: Supportive and intact family unit; flexible employer allowing work modification, cognition WNL, motivated, bilateral LES WNL

Weaknesses: Muscle weakness, limited ROM, potential deformity, pain at rest and increased with activities, fluctuating vocational role, decreased independence in ADL, interruptions in valued roles (wife, mother, employee), psychosocial symptoms (social withdrawal during exacerbations), decreased endurance

Client Factors	Stage of Treatment	Intervention Objectives	Intervention Objectives	Gradation
Muscle weakness	Acute	Increase muscle strength to improve independence in ADL and maximize occupational performance	• Isometric exercise (no resistance) • Elbow and wrist flexion and extension, 1 set of 3, one time per day; active ROM exercises: elbow and wrist, flexion and extension, 1 set of 3, one time per day; self-care to tolerance	Increasing endurance, adaptive equipment training, grading of ADL tasks, functional mobility training.
Decreased ROM limiting participation in job tasks	Acute	Increase ROM of affected joints, to WFL, to enable independence in ADL and job tasks.	Active or active-assisted ROM exercises: flexion and extension of elbow, MP, PIP, wrist, radial and ulnar deviation; complete exercises in warm bath or shower or immediately after bathing, to increase flexibility.	As condition improves to subacute stages, complete gentle active and passive stretches at end range.
Potential deformity, moderate assistance needed for ADL, maximal assistance needed for IADL, increased pain with activity	Acute	Client will perform self-care with modified independence (utilizing adaptive equipment and joint protection techniques).	Patient education in joint protection techniques, activity modifications (built up handles on toothbrush, hairbrush, eating utensils, tools used at work, etc.), and adaptive equipment (button hook, washing mitt, etc.). Intervention activities: household and work tasks utilizing adaptive equipment and joint protection techniques.	As synovitis subsides, reduce the use of adaptive equipment and increase activity to tolerance.
Decreased muscle strength	Subacute	Increase in strength from fair to good, to increase independence in ADL and improve performance of job tasks.	Light IADLs (ironing, dust mopping, dish washing) to increase activity tolerance; isometric exercise with resistance; flexors and extensors of elbow, wrist, MPs and PIPs, 10 repetitions, 3 times per day.	Perform more aggressive stretches as tolerated. Engage in IADLs requiring more resistance, such as folding towels and loading the washing machine.
Decreased ROM	Subacute	Increase ROM in bilateral upper extremities to increase independence in ADL and improve performance of job tasks.	Active ROM exercises: flexion and extension of elbows, wrists, MPs and PIP joints; gentle passive stretching at end range; participation in IADLs requiring full ROM and light resistance such as: dust mopping, folding linens, and ironing.	

Fig. 28.23 Mrs. B. case study.

Case Study: Mrs. Johnson

Mrs. Johnson is a 50-year-old single parent of a 12-year-old daughter, who works as an administrative assistant at a local college. She ran long-distance in high school until a knee injury curtailed her running. Currently, she runs only 3–4 times per month. She participates in church activities and supervises her daughter's Girl Scout troop, and is active in outdoor activities. She has gained 100 pounds over the past three years. She experiences pain on both knees most days. She recently participated in a work-based weight loss program, resulting in a 50 pound weight loss. Despite the weight loss, she continued to experience knee pain. She consulted with an orthopedist, who diagnosed her with bilateral knee DJD.

Her increased knee pain limits her participation in many activities with her daughter and in her church. She is most upset at not being able to ride a bike or do more active kinds of things with her daughter. She wants to set a good example for health and exercise but is limited by her bilateral knee pain. Mrs. Johnson states, "Getting in and out of the car is excruciating!" She uses a cane for walking and feels really old. She recently underwent bilateral TKA (surgeries spaced 1 week apart). Her goals are to relieve pain, become more active, to be able to enjoy being a mom and church member, and to improve her self-esteem through exercise and weight loss.

Strengths: Family support (sister), pre-teen daughter able to manage self-care, supportive church friends, accessible home (ranch)

Weaknesses: BMI >30, limited recovery time (6 weeks PTO available from work), interruption in valued roles (especially mothering)

Client Factors	Stage of Treatment	Intervention Objectives	Intervention Objectives
Dependence in toileting	Acute	Increase independence in toilet hygiene and clothing management.	Increasing endurance, adaptive equipment training, grading of ADL tasks, functional mobility training.
Maximum assistance needed for transfers	Acute	Increase independence with bed mobility.	Transfer training, training in donning and doffing knee immobilizer, functional mobility training.

After 1 week, Mrs. Johnson was discharged to home with therapy. At this point she was able to complete all ADLs at the level of modified independent. The OT recommended a home evaluation for IADL training. She also recommended that Mrs. Johnson continue to employ joint protection techniques to prevent further diagnoses of DJD in other joints.

Fig. 28.24 Mrs. Johnson case study.

5. What are the clinical signs of joint inflammation?
6. When should resistive exercise be utilized in clients with RA?
7. What adaptive equipment helps maximize independence in ADL for clients with arthritis?
8. In what ways should the OTA take into account the medication regimen of each client?
9. Name three activity modifications that should be taught to patients with RA.
10. What areas of occupational performance should be evaluated in clients with arthritis?
11. Why is rest an important part of treatment for clients with arthritis?
12. Identify five principles of joint protection.
13. Describe how energy conservation techniques can be applied to daily activities.
14. Identify five assistive devices and describe why they are useful for patients with arthritis.

REFERENCES

American Occupational Therapy Association. (2014). OT practice framework: domain & process (3rd ed.). *The American Journal of Occupational Therapy, 68*(Suppl. 1), S1–S48.

American Occupational Therapy Association. (2019). Living with arthritis. https://www.aota.org/~/media/Corporate/Files/AboutOT/consumers/Adults/Arthritis/Arthritis%20tip%20sheet.pdf.

Andrade, J. A., Brandão, M. B., Pinto, M. R. C., & Lanna, C. C. (2016). Factors associated with activity limitations in people with rheumatoid arthritis. *The American Journal of Occupational Therapy, 70*, 7004290030. Available from http://doi.org/10.5014/ajot.2016.017467.

Arthritis Foundation. (2019a). American Academy of Orthopaedic Surgeons Fact Sheets. Atlanta, GA: The Arthritis Foundation. https://www.arthritis.org/getmedia/e1256607-fa87-4593-aa8a-8db4f291072a/2019-abtn-final-march-2019.pdf.

Arthritis Foundation. (2019b). What's the next big advance in arthritis treatment? Arthritis Today 2018/2019; 4.

Arthritis Foundation. (2020a). Osteoarthritis. https://www.arthritis.org/about-arthritis/types/osteoarthritis/.

Arthritis Foundation. (2020b). Rheumatoid arthritis: the basics about the disease that affects 1.3 million Americans. http://www.arthritis.org/rheumatoid-arthritis.php.

Arthritis Health Professions Selection Task Force. (1980). Arthritis teaching slide collection for teachers of allied health professionals. New York, NY: The Arthritis Foundation.

Banwell, B. (1986). Physical therapy in arthritis management. In: G. Ehrlich, (Ed.), *Rehabilitation management of rheumatic conditions.* (2nd ed.) Baltimore, MD: Williams & Wilkins.

Deshaies, L. (2018). Arthritis. In H. M. Pendleton, & W. Schultz-Krohn (Eds.), *Pedretti's occupational therapy: Practice skills for physical dysfunction* (8th ed.). St. Louis, MO: Mosby.

Ekelman, B. A., Hooker, L., Davis, A., Klan, J., Newburn, D., et al. (2014). Occupational therapy interventions for adults with rheumatoid arthritis: an appraisal of the evidence. *Occupational Therapy In Health Care*, 28(4), 347–361. Available from https://doi.org/10.3109/07380577.2014.919687.

Engel, J. (2018). Pain management. In H. M. Pendleton, & W. Schultz-Krohn (Eds.), *Pedretti's occupational therapy: Practice skills for physical dysfunction* (8th ed.). St. Louis, MO: Mosby.

England, B. R. (2018). What is most important in rheumatoid arthritis treatment—where are you, who are you, or where are you going? *The Journal of Rheumatology*, 45(10), 1341–1343. Available from https://doi.org/10.3899/jrheum.180395.

Felson, D. (2017). Arthritis. What works. What doesn't. *Nutr Action News*, 3–6. (October).

Fries, J. F. (1986). Arthritis: A comprehensive guide to understanding your arthritis. Reading, MA: Addison-Wesley.

Harris, E. (1981). Rheumatic arthritis: the clinical spectrum. In: W. H. Kelley (Ed.), *Textbook of rheumatology*. Philadelphia, PA: WB Saunders.

Mann, W. C., Hurren, D., & Tomita, M. (1995). Assistive devices used by home-based elderly persons with arthritis. *The American Journal of Occupational Therapy*, 49(8), 810.

Michlovitz, S. L. (1990). Thermal agents in rehabilitation. (2nd ed.). Philadelphia, PA: FA Davis.

Murphy, L. F., & Lawson, S. (2018). Orthopedic conditions: hip fractures and hip, knee and shoulder replacements. In H. M. Pendleton, & W. Schultz-Krohn (Eds.), Pedretti's occupational therapy: Practice skills for physical dysfunction (8th ed.). St. Louis, MO: Mosby.

Poole, J., Makena, B., Siegel, P., Velasco, E., Latham, A., & Quinlan, J. (2017). Effectiveness of occupational therapy interventions for adults with osteoarthritis: a systematic review. *American Journal of Occupational Therapy* (71, p. 63).

US Department of Health and Human Services/Centers for Disease Control and Prevention (USDHHS/CDC). (2015). Prevalence of arthritis and arthritis-attributable activity limitation by urban-rural county classification-United States. *MMWR*, 66, 527.

Vannucchi, P. (2012). Understanding, diagnosing, and treating gout. *Podiatr Manage*, 191–200. (April/May).

Zhu, Y., Pandya, B. J., & Choi, H. K. (2011). Prevalence of gout and hyperuricemia in the US general population. *Arthritis Rheumatism*, 63(10), 3136–3141. Available from 10.1002/art.30520.

29

Upper Extremity Rehabilitation

Shelby E. Hutchinson

OBJECTIVES

After reading this chapter, the student or the occupational therapy practitioner will be able to do the following:

1. Differentiate the roles of the occupational therapist and the occupational therapy assistant in the evaluation and treatment of the patient with an injured hand.
2. Explain the general principles for conducting assessments of range of motion, strength, sensibility, edema, soft tissue, and function.
3. Explain the treatment principles for selected acute hand injuries.
4. Practice specific assessments and treatment techniques under supervision.
5. Explain the impact of a hand injury on physical, cognitive, psychological, and contextual performance areas.

KEY TERMS

Observation
Range of motion (ROM)
Active ROM (AROM)
Passive ROM (PROM)
Edema
Manual muscle testing (MMT)
Grip strength
Pinch strength
Joint play
Joint mobilization
Extrinsic assessment
Intrinsic assessment
Sensibility
Sensory reeducation
Sympathetic function

Evaluation of hand function
Coban
Heat
Sensory desensitization
BTE Technologies
Weight well
Theraband
Hand grips
Functional activities
Immobilization approach
Early passive motion
Early active motion
Contracture
Complex regional pain syndrome (CRPS)
Cumulative trauma disorder (CTD)

INTRODUCTION

Upper extremity (UE) injuries account for approximately one third of all injuries (Kasch, 1988). Therefore it is important for occupational therapists (OTs) and occupational therapy assistants (OTAs) in the physical dysfunction practice area to be familiar with the occupational therapy process for these clients. UE dysfunction can occur from injury or disease. Work-related hand and finger injuries account for over 1 million visits to the emergency department (Rempel, 1992). Manufacturing, construction, and the retail trade produce the highest number of work-related hand injuries (Schier & Chan, 2007). Most of those injured are men between the ages of 25 and 44 years (Rempel, 1992). Hand injuries also commonly occur during household activities, while participating in sports, and from motor vehicle accidents. Diseases that cause

UE dysfunction include arthritis and congenital anomalies. UE dysfunction costs $19 billion in direct and indirect costs and often leads to long-term disability (Kasch, 1988). For example, only 15% of those with severe cerebrovascular accidents ever recover full hand function (Kasch, 1988).

The hand is vital to human function and appearance. The hand touches, gives comfort, and expresses emotions. Like the face, it is exposed for all to see and therefore has cosmetic importance. To facilitate engagement on meaningful occupation, it must flex, extend, oppose, and grasp thousands of times daily. A hand injury can interfere with the person's ability to participate fully in meaningful roles, occupations, and activities; jeopardize the family's livelihood; and compromise self-esteem. The loss of hand function through injury or disease affects more than the mechanical tasks that the hand performs. Hand injury has a psychological impact (Larson, 2006; Oerlemans et al., 2000).

Hand rehabilitation, or hand therapy, has grown as a specialty area in occupational and physical therapy. Hand therapy is defined, in part, as "the art and science of rehabilitation of the upper quarter of the human body. Hand therapy is the merging of occupational therapy and physical therapy theory and practice that combines comprehensive knowledge of the upper quarter, body function, and activity" (Oxford Grice et al., 2003). Treatment techniques have evolved from both professions.

This chapter provides a fundamental knowledge base for treating clients with UE dysfunction to the OTA who is interested in developing skills in this area. Hand rehabilitation requires advanced and specialized training for the OTA and close supervision by an OT. Assessment of client factors related to UE dysfunction should be completed by the OT with input from the OTA who has demonstrated service competency. Physical agent modalities (PAMs) may be used in preparation for or as an adjunct to purposeful activity (American Occupational Therapy Association, 1997). Each state has practice laws regarding the use of PAMs. Some states require specialty certification. OTs and OTAs should be aware of the laws within the state in which they practice.

UE rehabilitation is commonly referred to as hand therapy. It can be provided in treatment settings ranging from private therapy offices, to outpatient rehabilitation clinics, to hospitals. In all settings, knowledge of healing time and evidence-based treatment will lead to successful treatment. For example, it is important to keep in mind that after trauma or surgery, the body must repair the damaged tissue, such as bone. A series of complex overlapping cellular-level events occur. These events begin at the time of injury and may continue for many months. The healing process is divided into three phases: inflammatory, proliferative, and remodeling (Fess, 2002; Shacklock, 2005). Occupational therapy treatment guidelines differ depending on the phase of wound healing and mechanism of injury. The OT and OTA should consult with the referring physician regarding treatment modalities. Therapeutic use of self is important to gain client trust and cooperation, and to address the psychological effects of the injury. If the client does not feel that the treatment is meaningful and fully cooperates in the process, gains will be limited.

OCCUPATIONAL THERAPY INTERVENTION PROCESS

Occupational Profile

An occupational profile will provide the occupational therapy practitioner with the information about how the client's habits, routines, and roles have been affected by the hand injury. To plan an effective intervention, the OT and the OTA must understand the medical condition and the patient's concerns regarding present and future ability to participate in meaningful occupations. This can be done through an

informal interview or through a standardized assessment such as the Canadian Occupational Performance Measure (COPM) (Koman, Li, Smith, & Smith, 2011). During the interview, the OTA may be asked to gather demographic information about the patient, such as age, pain levels, hand dominance, medical history, vocation, avocational interests, and the patient's goals for therapy. Other pertinent information to be gathered includes documentation of surgical procedures and clarification of physician's orders. Review of imaging (x-rays or magnetic resonance imaging [MRI]) and other test results may provide more clarity on the client's condition. All of this information will assist the OT in setting goals and developing the intervention plan.

Assessment of Occupational Performance

Observation. The assessment begins with an **observation** of the client. This may begin when the client enters the clinic or office. Observe the patient's posture. Notice if the client is able to independently complete paperwork or needs assistance. Notice how the client is holding the injured extremity. Is it carefully guarded, or is it ignored? Are there any dressings or wrappings on the extremity? The position of the UE at rest, as well as the carrying posture, can yield valuable information about the dysfunction and the patient's response to it. The hand and arm must be carefully observed and inspected. The skin condition should be noted. Document lacerations, sutures, evidence of recent surgery, temperature, moistness of skin, edema, odor, contractures, and mobility of skin. If observed, trophic changes (dryness, thinning, and decreased sweating) in the skin should be documented. Occupational performance can be assessed by observing the client performing bilateral activities of daily living (ADL) tasks such as buttoning a button, donning a shirt, opening a jar, and threading a needle.

CLINICAL PEARL

In most cases the client's opposite extremity can provide the treating therapist with excellent information into what the injured hand's appearance, strength, range of motion, and overall function would be at baseline. Comparing the extremities will allow the therapist to generate realistic goals for treatment.

Assessment of Client Factors and Performance Skills. Movement is assessed by looking at active and passive mobility of joints, deformities, contractures, tendon integrity, and ligamentous laxity (Fig. 29.1). Peripheral nerves are evaluated indirectly via the sensibility and muscle strength assessments. A goniometer can be used to objectively measure joint **range of motion** (ROM), first **actively** (**Active Range of Motion, AROM**) and then **passively** (**Passive Range of Motion, PROM**) (Fig. 29.2).

Edema is the first stage of healing of an acute injury. It increases the size or volume of the hand, which can lead to further tissue damage. Hand volume is measured to assess the presence of edema and to determine the effect of treatment

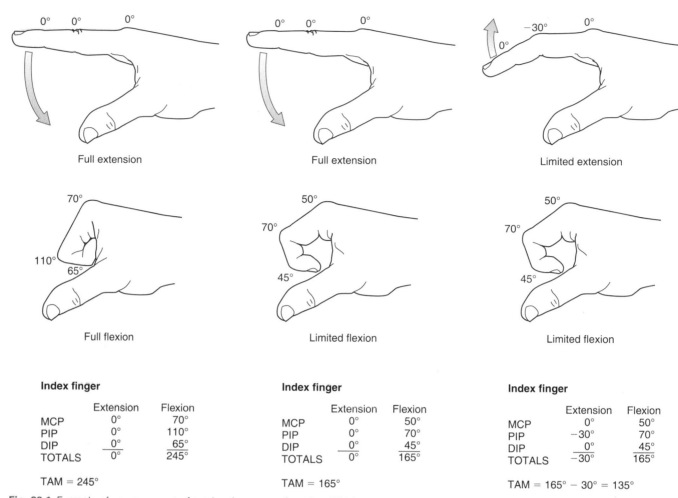

Fig. 29.1 Example of measurement of total active range of motion *(TAM)* in the hand. *DIP,* Distal interphalangeal; *MCP,* metacarpophalangeal; *PIP,* proximal interphalangeal.

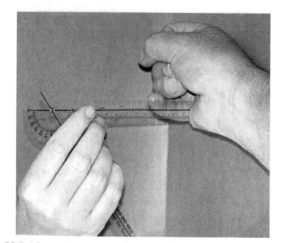

Fig. 29.2 Measuring distance between finger pulp and distal palmar crease.

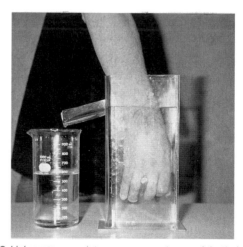

Fig. 29.3 Volumeter used to measure volume of both hands for comparison. Increased volume indicates edema.

and activities. By measuring the volume at different times of the day, the effects of rest versus activity and of splinting or treatment techniques designed to reduce edema may be determined. A volumeter (Coldham, Lewis, & Lee, 2006) may be used to assess hand edema (Fig. 29.3) because it has been shown to be accurate to 10 mL (Walsh, 2011) when used in the prescribed manner. The edema assessment is performed as described in Box 29.1.

BOX 29.1 Volumeter Assessment of Edema

1. Fill the plastic volumeter until the water reaches spout level. Allow excess water to drip out of the spout. Empty and dry the beaker thoroughly.
2. Instruct the patient to slowly immerse his or her hand into the plastic volumeter, being careful to keep the hand in the midposition, until the web space between the middle and ring fingers rests gently on the dowel rod. The hand must not press onto the rod.
3. Keep the hand still and in position until no more water drips into the beaker.
4. Pour the water from the beaker into a graduated cylinder.
5. Place the cylinder on a level surface, and read the amount of water displaced.

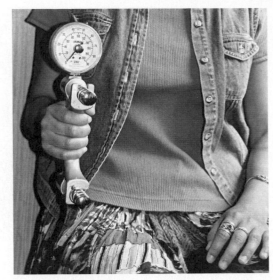

Fig. 29.4 Jamar dynamometer is used to measure grip strength.

Not all patients are candidates for the volumeter. Contraindication for use of a volumeter include open wounds, sutures, staples, or pins. In these instances, a tape measure or a jeweler's ring sizer can be used to measure parts of the hand or forearm. Measurements should be taken before and after treatment, especially after the application of thermal modalities or an orthotic.

Strength Assessment. UE strength assessment should be performed after the patient has been cleared for full-resistive activities, usually 8 to 12 weeks after injury or surgery. Strength is measured through **manual muscle testing (MMT)** (see Chapter 8), grip strength, and pinch strength.

Grip strength can be assessed with a dynamometer (Fig. 29.4). The recommended patient position (MacDermid, 2002) is seated with the shoulder adducted and neutrally rotated, the elbow flexed at 90 degrees, the forearm in the neutral position, and the wrist between 0 and 15 degrees of ulnar deviation. The patient is asked to squeeze using maximal effort. The dynamometer can be held lightly by the examiner so the patient will not drop the instrument. The uninvolved hand is measured for comparison. Normative data may be used to compare strength scores (Kamentz, 1985; Louis et al., 1984). Variables such as age will affect strength measurements.

Pinch strength is tested with either of the commercially available pinch gauges (Fig. 29.5). Two-point pinch (thumb tip to index fingertip), lateral or key pinch (thumb pulp to lateral aspect of the middle phalanx of the index finger), and three-point pinch (thumb tip to tips of index and long fingers) are measured. The patient position is the same as for grip testing, and the patient is asked to give maximal effort without pain, if possible (Fig. 29.6).

Assessment of Joints

ROM (see Chapter 7) measurements should be taken to assess AROM and PROM because joints may develop dysfunction after trauma, immobilization, or disuse. Limited ROM is often caused by tightness in the ligaments and other soft tissues that surround a joint. **Joint play** (Mathiowetz, Remmells, & Donoghue, 1985; Waylett-Rendell & Seibly, 1991) involves the small, passive, involuntary movements

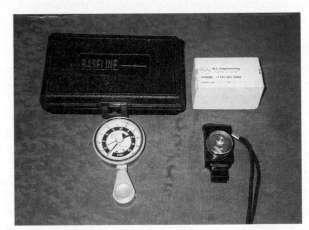

Fig. 29.5 Baseline and B&L Engineering pinch gauges.

that must occur inside the joint at the joint surfaces. These movements must be present for a joint to express normal ROM (Mathiowetz et al., 1985). Because these motions are passive and not under voluntary control, they cannot be produced at will and can be facilitated only by someone other than the patient (Kelsey & McEwing, 1997). The technique to assess or help to restore these motions is called **joint mobilization** (Moscony, 2007). An example of this is joint distraction, in which the OT firmly but gently applies a traction (pulling) force at the joint, thereby stretching the ligaments surrounding that joint. Guidelines must be followed for applying joint mobilization techniques and require additional training for OTAs.

Extrinsic assessment and **intrinsic assessment** identify whether decreased ROM is being caused by tightness of the extrinsic muscles/tendons (origins outside of the hand proper) or intrinsic muscles/tendons (origins and insertions inside the hand proper). This is determined by passively placing joints —metacarpophalangeals (MCPs), proximal interphalangeals

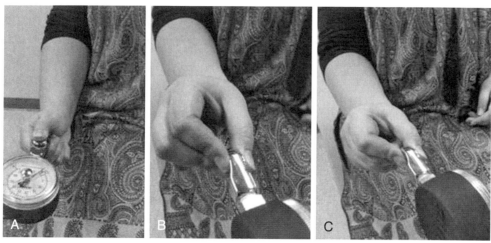

Fig. 29.6 Pinch gauge is used to measure pinch strength in a variety of prehension patterns. (A) Lateral pinch. (B) Three-jaw chuck. (C) Two-point pinch.

(PIPs), and distal interphalangeals (DIPs)—in a series of recommended positions (American Society for Surgery of the Hand, 1990).

Sensory Testing

Any patient who has sustained a direct injury to a peripheral nerve or who is suspected of having a condition that may compress a peripheral nerve needs to be fully assessed in the area of **sensibility**. The ability of the hand to function, explore, and interact with the environment depends on sensibility (Anthony, 1993). Sensibility testing is done to (1) assess the recovery of a nerve after laceration and repair, (2) determine the presence of a nerve compression syndrome and the return of nerve function after surgical decompression, and (3) determine the efficacy of conservative treatment to reduce compression. Sensibility testing can begin with sensory mapping of the entire volar surface of the hand (Callahan, 2002). The areas are carefully marked and transferred to a permanent record, usually a diagram of the hand. Mapping should be repeated at monthly intervals during nerve regeneration.

A variety of tests may be required to adequately assess sensibility. These tests can be divided into four categories: (1) threshold tests for pain, vibration, temperature, and touch pressure; (2) functional tests to assess the quality of sensibility or what Moberg described as "tactile gnosis," such as stationary and moving two-point discrimination and the Moberg Pick-up Test; (3) objective tests that do not require active participation by the patient, including the O'Riain wrinkle test, the triketohydrindene hydrate (Ninhydrin) sweat test, and nerve conduction studies (Coldham et al., 2006); and (4) provocative or stress tests that either attempt to reproduce the patient's complaints of pain or determine if a peripheral nerve is regenerating at the appropriate rate.

Threshold Tests

Vibration. Tuning forks of 30 and 256 cycles per second (cps) are used for assessing the return of vibratory sensation after nerve repair as regeneration occurs and as a guideline for

initiating a **sensory reeducation** program (Cyriax, 1985; Dellon, 1984). Commercially available vibrometers may also be used to detect abnormal sensation. Vibration and the Semmes-Weinstein monofilament tests (Bell-Krotoski, 2002) are more sensitive in picking up a gradual decrease in nerve function in the presence of nerve compression where the nerve circuitry is intact. Therefore vibration, Semmes-Weinstein, and electrical testing are reliable and sensitive tests for early detection of carpal tunnel syndrome and other nerve compression syndromes. Vibration and Semmes-Weinstein tests can be performed in the clinic with no discomfort to the patient and are excellent screening tools when nerve compression is suspected (Bell-Krotoski, 2002; Fishman, 1995–2010). The Semmes-Weinstein monofilament test provides the most accurate instrument for assessing cutaneous pressure thresholds (Bell-Krotoski, 2002). The test uses 20 nylon monofilaments, of increasing thickness, housed in plastic handheld rods. Markings on the probes range from 1.65 to 6.65. Normal fingertip sensibility has been found to correspond to the 2.44 and 2.83 probes.

The monofilaments must be applied perpendicular to the skin and are applied until the monofilament just begins to bend. Results can be graded from normal light touch (probes ≥ 2.83) to loss of protective sensation (probes ≤ 4.56). There are commercially available pocket-size monofilament touch tests containing five monofilaments that are easy to use and are in protective cases (Fig. 29.7A).

Touch Pressure. Moving touch is tested with the eraser end of a pencil. The eraser is placed in an area of normal sensibility and, with light pressure, is moved to the distal fingertip. The patient notes when the perception of the stimulus changes. Light and heavy stimuli may be applied and noted (Cyriax, 1985). Constant touch is tested by pressing with the eraser end of the pencil, first in an area with normal sensibility and then moving distally. The patient responds when the stimulus is altered; again, light and heavy stimuli may be applied (Cyriax, 1985).

Functional Tests

Static Two-Point and Moving Two-Point Discrimination.
Discrimination requires the patient to distinguish between two direct stimuli. These tests elicit information about the patient's potential for function. To assess static two-point discrimination, a variety of commercially available devices, such as the Disk-Criminator (Lister, 1993) or Touch-Test Two-Point Discriminator (see Fig. 29.7B), are used. The Disk-Criminator is a small tool with parallel prongs of variable distances apart. It has blunted ends that will not hurt the patient and should produce replicable results. The patient is touched with the device and asked to indicate whether he or she perceives one or two points (Box 29.2).

Moving two-point discrimination is slightly more sensitive than stationary two-point discrimination (Law, Baptiste, & Carswell, 1998), and it provides information about the patient's potential to manipulate objects in the hand. Two-point values increase with age in both sexes (as the skin becomes less discriminating), with the smallest values occurring between the ages of 10 and 30. Women tend to have smaller values than men, and no significant differences exist between dominant and nondominant hands (Law et al., 1998).

Modified Moberg Pick-Up Test.
Recognition of common objects is the final level of sensory function. Moberg used the phrase "tactile gnosis" to describe the ability of the hand to perform complex function by feel. Moberg described the Pick-Up Test in 1958 (Coldham et al., 2006), which Dellon (1984) later modified. This test is used with either a median nerve injury or a combined injury of median and ulnar nerves. Clinically, it takes twice as long to perform the tests with vision occluded than with vision not occluded. The therapist performs the test as described in Box 29.3.

Objective Tests

Sympathetic Function.
The wrinkle test and the Ninhydrin test are objective tests of **sympathetic function**. Recovery of the sympathetic function (sweating, pain, and temperature

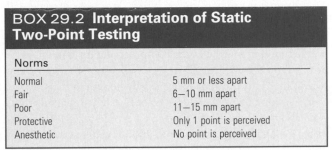

BOX 29.2 Interpretation of Static Two-Point Testing

Norms	
Normal	5 mm or less apart
Fair	6–10 mm apart
Poor	11–15 mm apart
Protective	Only 1 point is perceived
Anesthetic	No point is perceived

From American Society for Surgery of the Hand. The Hand, Examination and Diagnosis. 3rd ed. New York, NY: Churchill Livingstone; 1990.

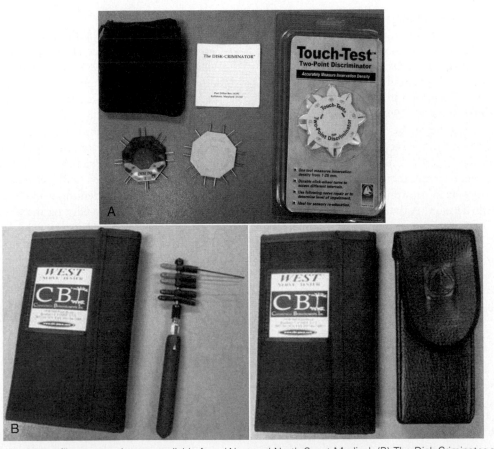

Fig. 29.7 (A) Pocket-sized monofilament touch tests available from West and North Coast Medical. (B) The Disk-Criminator and the Touch Test Two-Point Discriminator can be used to assess static or moving two-point discrimination.

BOX 29.3 Modified Moberg Pick-Up Test

1. Place 9 or 10 small objects (coins, paper clips, etc.) on a table.
2. Ask the patient to place them one at a time in a small container as quickly as possible while looking at them. Time the patient.
3. Repeat the test for the opposite hand with vision.
4. Repeat the test for each hand with the vision occluded.
5. Ask the patient to identify each object, one at a time, with and then without vision.
6. Observe substitution patterns that may be used when the patient cannot see the objects.

---

discrimination) may occur early but does not correlate with functional recovery (Cyriax, 1985). O'Riain (Moscony, 2007) observed that denervated skin does not wrinkle. Therefore nerve function may be tested by immersing the hand in water for 5 minutes and noting the presence or absence of skin wrinkling. This test may be especially helpful in diagnosing a nerve lesion in young children or cognitively impaired adults. The ability to sweat is also lost in a nerve lesion. A Ninhydrin test (Callahan, 2002; Moscony, 2007) evaluates sweating of the finger. Other signs of sympathetic dysfunction are smooth, shiny skin; nail changes; and "pencil pointing," or tapering of the fingers (Von Der Heyde, 2007).

Provocative Tests

Tinel sign and Phalen test are considered "provocative" tests in nerve compression syndromes because they are used to elicit a pathologic response of the nerve. During the first 2 to 4 months after nerve repair, axons regenerate and travel through the hand at a rate of about 1 mm per day or 1 inch (2.54 cm) per month. Tinel sign may be used to follow this regeneration (Laseter & Carter, 1996). The test is performed by tapping gently along the course of the nerve, starting distally and moving toward the nerve repair site to elicit a tingling sensation in the fingertip. The point at which tapping begins to elicit a tingling sensation is noted and indicates the extent of sensory axon growth. As regeneration occurs, hyperesthesias will develop. Although this hypersensitivity may be uncomfortable to the patient, it is a positive sign of nerve growth. A treatment program for desensitization of hypersensitive areas can be initiated as soon as the skin is healed and can tolerate gentle rubbing and immersion in textures. Desensitization is discussed further in the treatment section of this chapter. The examiner may attempt to elicit a Tinel sign in nerve compression disorders such as carpal tunnel syndrome. The therapist taps the median nerve at the level of the wrist (Callahan, 2002; Mathiowetz et al., 1985). The Tinel sign is considered positive if the patient reports tingling along the course of the nerve distally when tapped. The Phalen test will also produce the nerve paresthesias present in compression of the median nerve. The patient is asked to hold the wrist in a fully flexed position for 60 seconds. The test is considered positive if tingling occurs within this time (Callahan, 2002; Mathiowetz et al., 1985).

Functional Testing

Evaluation of hand function or performance is important because the physical evaluation does not measure the patient's ingenuity and ability to compensate for the loss of strength, ROM, and sensation or for the presence of deformities. The results of the physical evaluation will, however, increase the therapist's understanding of functional impairment and of why patients function the way they do (Mathiowetz et al., 1985).

The OT and/or OTA should observe the effect of dysfunction on use of the hand during ADL. In addition, a standardized performance evaluation such as the Jebsen Hand Function Test (Hung, Chan, Chang, Tsang, & Leung, 1990) can be administered. With service competency, delegated administration of some of these tests may be within the scope of the OTA.

Jebsen Hand Function Test. This test provides objective measurements of standardized tasks with norms for patient comparison. It is a short, inexpensive test that is easily assembled by the administrator. The test consists of seven subtests: (1) writing a short sentence, (2) turning over 5-inch cards three times, (3) picking up small objects and placing them in a container, (4) stacking checkers, (5) eating (simulated), (6) moving large empty cans, and (7) moving large weighted cans. Norms are provided for dominant and nondominant hands for each subtest and are also divided by sex and age. The authors provide instructions for assembling the test and specific instructions for administering it (Hung et al., 1990).

Dexterity Tests. Dexterity is the ability to manipulate small objects with the fingers with speed and accuracy (Apfel & Carronza, 1992). The Nine-Hole Peg Test (Gelberman, Szabor, Williamson, & Dimick, 1983) is one of the most commonly used dexterity tests. It is quick and easy to administer and is norm tested. Other tests of hand dexterity are the Crawford Small Parts Dexterity Test (Crawford & Crawford, 1981), the Bennett Hand Tool Dexterity Test (Bennett, 1981), the Purdue Pegboard Test (Stewart Pettengill & vanStrein, 2011), and the Minnesota Manual Dexterity Test (Evans & Burkhalter, 1986). The Valpar Corporation has developed norm-referenced tests that measure an individual's ability to perform work-related tasks. This information can be used in predicting the likelihood of successful return to a specific job. These tests are especially useful when administering a work capacity evaluation. Tests may be purchased and come with standardized norms and instructions for administration and scoring (Mathiowetz et al., 1985).

CLINICAL PEARL

Do not use the tools of any assessment (such as Nine-Hole Peg Test or any other test for dexterity) for treatment activities. The retest would not be valid because there would be a learning effect for the patient.

Patient-Reported Measures

Outcome measure tools are primarily by self-report (i.e., the patient determines the answers to specific questions). Initial

BOX 29.4 Categories of Functional Outcome Measures

Generic Measures:
    Canadian Occupational Performance Measure (COPM)
    Short Form 36 (SF36)
    Short Musculoskeletal Functional Assessment (SMFA)
Regional Measures:
    Disabilities of the Arm, Shoulder, and Hand (DASH)
    Michigan Hand Questionnaire (MHQ)
    Patient-Rated Wrist/Hand Evaluation (PRWHE)
Disease-Specific Measures:
    Arthritis Impact Measurement Scales (AIMS2-SF)
    Australian/Canadian Osteoarthritis Hand Index (AUSCAN)
    Rotator Cuff Quality of Life (RC-QOL)

From Von Der Heyde R. Assessment of functional outcomes. In: Cooper C, ed. Fundamentals of Hand Therapy. St Louis, MO: Mosby Elsevier; 2007:98–111.

hand evaluations are beginning to include outcome measures to determine a patient's health status, functional status, and overall satisfaction level. A therapist does not observe function or behavior. There are three categories (Thomas, Moutet, & Guinard, 1996) of outcome measures: generic measures, which compare overall health conditions; regional measures, which look at specific body systems or areas; and disease-specific measures (Box 29.4 provides a partial list of outcome measures by category). The DASH (Disability, Arm, Shoulder, and Hand) and the Michigan Hand Questionnaire are often selected for use in a hand therapy clinic because these tools direct their questions to the outcomes related to the UE (Bear-Lehman & Poole, 2011). The Barthel ADL Index is widely used to assess lifestyle task performance; a newer tool, the MAM (Manual Ability Measure), is being developed to look at hand function across diagnostic categories (Chen, Granger, Peimer, Moy, & Wald, 2005).

INTERVENTION TECHNIQUES

Edema Management

Edema is a normal consequence of trauma but must be quickly and aggressively treated to prevent permanent stiffness and disability. Within hours of trauma, vasodilation and local edema occur. Early control of edema is ideally achieved through elevation, massage, compression, and AROM. The patient is instructed at the time of injury to keep the hand elevated, and a compressive dressing is applied to reduce early swelling. Pitting edema is present early and can be recognized as a bloated swelling that "pits" when pressed by the examiner's finger. This may be more pronounced on the dorsal surface where the skin is looser and where venous and lymphatic systems provide return of fluid to the heart. Active motion is especially important to produce retrograde venous and lymphatic flow; AROM moves this fluid back into the general circulatory system.

If swelling continues, a serofibrinous exudate (a fluid that contains both serum and fibrin) invades the area. Fibrin is

deposited in the spaces surrounding the joints, tendons, and ligaments, resulting in reduced mobility, flattening of the arches of the hand, tissue atrophy, and further disuse (Taleisnik, 1985). Normal gliding of the tissues is reduced, and stiffness and pain in the hand often result. Scar adhesions are likely to form and further limit tissue mobility. If untreated, these losses may become permanent. Early recognition of persistent edema through volume and circumference measurement is important. Several of the suggested edema control techniques may be necessary.

Elevation. Early elevation with the hand above the heart is essential. Slings should be avoided if possible because they tend to reduce blood flow because of the flexed elbow posture and may lead to shoulder stiffness, such as adhesive capsulitis or locking of the elbow due to heterotopic ossification, as well. Resting the hand on pillows while seated or lying down is effective. Resting the hand on top of the head or using devices that elevate the hand with the elbow in extension have been suggested. Suspension slings may be purchased or fabricated.

The patient should use the injured hand for ADL within the limitations of resistance prescribed by the physician. Light ADL that can be accomplished while the hand is in the dressing are permitted because these facilitate gentle active ROM.

Contrast Baths. Contrast baths, immersing the hand alternately in warm water and then cold water, have traditionally been used by many therapists to help reduce edema and facilitate ROM in hand-injured patients. The alternating of warm and cool water will cause vasodilation and vasoconstriction, resulting in a pumping action on the edema. Many patients report that they like contrast baths. Although the technique is described in textbooks, little research has been done on its effectiveness. Practitioners are urged to study the literature and make an informed decision before using this treatment strategy; the OTA should consult with the supervising OT.

Retrograde Massage. The practitioner, client, or family member may perform retrograde massage frequently throughout the day. The massage assists in blood flow and lymph drainage. Start the massage distally and stroke smoothly and lightly in a proximal direction with the extremity in elevation (Cyriax, 1985). Active motion should follow the massage if possible, but avoid muscle fatigue.

Manual Edema Mobilization. Artzberger (2002) described a massage technique she developed based on manual lymphatic treatment (MLT), a treatment technique used for people with lymphedema. She modified MLT and coined the term "Manual Edema Mobilization (MEM)" for this new technique and began to use it on subacute hand patients with some success. MEM is used in cases where the impairment of the lymph system is temporary (edema) rather than caused by damage to the lymphatic system (lymphedema). This technique is grounded in a thorough understanding of the anatomy and physiology of the lymphatic system, as well as research data (Artzberger, 2002). OTs and OTAs are encouraged to study and take hands-on continuing education courses to develop service competency in this massage technique (Artzberger, 2002).

Pressure Wraps. Light compression may be applied throughout the day with a light **Coban** wrap, an Isotoner glove, or a custom-made garment by Bioconcepts or Jobst (Fig. 29.8). Wrapping with Coban elastic (Dommerholt, 2004) may be used to reduce edema (Fig. 29.9). Starting distally, the finger is wrapped snugly with Coban. Care must be taken not to pull the Coban too tightly because it can restrict circulation. Each involved finger should be wrapped distal to proximal until the wrap is proximal to the edema. The wrap remains in place for 5 minutes and then is removed. Active exercise may be done while the finger is wrapped or immediately after. Measurements should be taken before and after treatment to

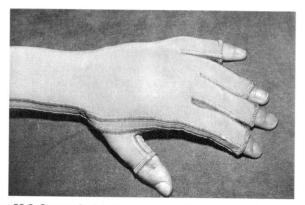

Fig. 29.8 Custom-fit Jobst garment may be used to reduce edema and to reduce or prevent hypertrophic scar formation after burns or trauma.

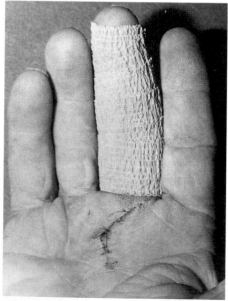

Fig. 29.9 One-inch Coban is wrapped with minimal pressure from distal to proximal.

document an increase in ROM and a decrease in edema. The wrapping may be repeated three times a day. Any method of compression should not be constricting and must be discontinued if ischemia results. Elastic Ace bandages may be used for larger areas. An elastic bandage of 3 or 4 inches in width may be used when the entire hand and forearm require a gentle pressure wrap. A variety of pressure wraps are used by hand centers. Tubular gauze and Digisleeves (American Society for Surgery of the Hand, 1990) provide compression to a specific finger. No single method is superior to the other. A combination of techniques used at different stages of healing and according to patient comfort may be most effective.

Physical Agent Modalities. Two modalities are particularly helpful in the reduction of edema: neuromuscular electrical stimulation (NMES) and high-voltage pulsed-current (HVPC) stimulation. Both modalities are applied in such a way as to facilitate a muscle contraction, thereby improving the muscle's ability to pump. Improved pumping action will boost lymphatic return, which will reduce edema (Kietrys, Barr, & Barbe, 2011). These modalities must be used in conjunction with purposeful activity. OTs and OTAs need documented competency to utilize them.

Active ROM. Normal blood flow depends on muscle activity. Active motion does not mean wiggling the fingers, but rather maximum available ROM done firmly and with purpose. Casts and splints must allow mobility of uninjured parts while protecting newly injured structures. The shoulder and elbow should be moved several times a day. The importance of AROM for edema control, tendon gliding, and tissue nutrition cannot be overemphasized.

Treatment for Decreased ROM

ROM. To improve ROM, the practitioner must answer the following questions:
- What is the available PROM?
- Is muscle strength available?
- Can the tendons glide?

PROM gives information about noncontractile structures such as ligaments surrounding the joint. PROM is assessed by the therapist moving the joint throughout its available range. AROM gives information about the contractile units moving the joint. When PROM is greater than AROM, there is a problem with the contracting unit (i.e., muscle weakness or tendon adherence). If PROM is limited, the therapist must address the specific cause of the limitation and choose treatment strategies to improve AROM.

To improve PROM, the OT may use a combination of the following: modalities to improve tissue elasticity, joint mobilization techniques to restore joint play, PROM to the involved joint, and dynamic or static progressive splinting. The OTA may supplement these PROM treatment strategies with specific exercises or activities that target the involved structures. The clinician must be sensitive to the patient's age and interest when selecting activities. As with any rehabilitation program, the patient should be provided with a specific home exercise program that will supplement and reinforce therapy.

Soft Tissue Mobilization. Many hand therapy patients present with wounds caused by trauma or surgical intervention. Scar tissue formation, necessary for healing, forms on all wounds. The OT and OTA use techniques to modify and remodel the scar to help preserve soft tissue mobility. Tissues that have restored gliding have different scar architecture from those that do not develop the ability to glide. With gliding, the scar resembles the state of the tissues before injury, whereas the nongliding scar remains fixed on or adherent to the surrounding structures. Controlled tension on a scar has been shown to facilitate remodeling. Scar formation is also influenced by the patient's age and the quantity of scar deposited (Taleisnik, 1985).

Pressure. A hypertrophic scar, or a scar that is randomly laid down and thickened, cannot glide properly and therefore may restrict AROM, contribute to deformity, or be cosmetically unacceptable. The principal technique used to modify a scar is the application of pressure. Several types of commercially available products, when used in combination, enable the clinician to manage scars effectively. For example, the following products can be used as the contact medium with the skin: Otoform, Silastic Elastomer, and Prosthetic Foam. These products are generally held in place with pressure devices such as Coban wrap, Isotoner gloves, Ace bandages, or pressure elastic garments. Pressure should be applied for most of the 24-hour period and removed for bathing and exercise. As the scar changes in response to pressure, the contact medium needs to be replaced. For patients with burns, a custom-measured pressure garment is worn 23 hours per day and may need to be worn for 6 to 18 months, depending on the severity of the burn.

Massage. Gentle to firm massage of the scarred area with a thick ointment such as lanolin, Deep Prep, or Aliprep Deep Tissue massage cream will rapidly soften scar tissue. Massage should be followed with active hand use so that tendons will glide against the softened scar (Cyriax, 1985). Vibration to the area with a small, low-intensity vibrator will have a similar effect (Jebsen, Taylor, Trieschmann, Trotter, & Howard, 1969). Active exercise with facilitation techniques, exercise against resistance, or functional activity should follow vibration. Massage and vibration may be started 4 weeks after the injury.

Heat in the form of a paraffin bath, hot packs, or fluidotherapy immediately followed by stretching while the tissue cools will provide stretch to scar tissue. Gently wrapping the scarred or stiff digit into flexion with Coban during the application of heat will often increase mobility in the area. Heat should not be used with insensate areas or if swelling persists (Kaltenborn & Evjenth, 1989). Scar reduction techniques can be carried out by the OTA under close supervision of an OT.

AROM and Physical Agent Modalities. AROM provides an internal stretch against a resistant scar. NMES, high-voltage direct-current ultrasound, and a continuous passive motion machine may be used to assist a motion when the patient cannot achieve active range because of scar adhesions or weakness (Harden & Bruehl, 2006; Kietrys et al., 2011). These modalities help increase motor activity and help remodel the scar.

Normalization of Sensation. As an injury to the hand resolves, the hand or a portion of it may be either hypersensitive or hyposensitive, having either too much or too little sensation. To facilitate the return of function to the peripheral or digital nerve, a program of sensory reeducation may be used. Alternatively, a patient may have a hypersensitive area, one that is excessively sensitive to even the lightest touch, making it almost impossible for that person to manipulate ordinary items. In this case, a program of **sensory desensitization** is indicated.

The goal of sensory reeducation is to maximize the functional level of sensation. All programs emphasize a variety of stimuli used in a repetitive manner to bombard the sensory receptors. A sequence of eyes-closed, eyes-open, eyes-closed is used to provide feedback during the training process. Sessions are limited in length to avoid fatigue and frustration. To avoid further trauma, objects must not be potentially harmful to insensate areas. A home program should be provided to reinforce learning that occurs in the clinical setting. Several authors (Callahan, 2002; Cyriax, 1985; Von Der Heyde, 2007) have found that sensory reeducation can result in improved functional sensibility in motivated patients. Objective measurement of sensation after reeducation must be performed and then compared with initial testing to accurately assess the success of the program. A program of sensory reeducation does not begin until the patient has at least protective sensibility.

Sensory desensitization techniques are based on the theory that nerve fibers that carry pain sensation can be positively influenced through the use of pressure, rubbing, vibration, transcutaneous electrical nerve stimulation (TENS), percussion, and active motion. Hypersensitivity is sometimes the result of a lacerated nerve, but a too tight cast or splint may also cause nerve irritation requiring a program of sensory desensitization (Melvin, 1989).

Yerxa et. al (1983) have described a desensitization program that "employs short periods of contact with three sensory modalities: dowel textures, immersion or contact particles, and vibration." This program allows the patient to rank 10 dowel textures and 10 immersion textures on the degree of irritation produced by the stimulus. Treatment begins with a stimulus that is irritating but tolerable. The stimulus is applied for 10 minutes three or four times a day. The vibration hierarchy is predetermined and is based on cycles per second of vibration, the placement of the vibrator, and the duration of the treatment. The Downey Hand Center hand sensitivity test can be used to establish a desensitization treatment program and to measure progress in decreasing hypersensitivity (Waylett Rendal, 1988; Yerxa et al., 1983).

Strength Training

Acute care is followed by a gradual return of motion, sensibility, and preparation to return to normal ADL. Strengthening of the injured and neglected extremity usually begins in the clinic but will be much more effective if carried over with a written home program. The following are some examples of strength training programs.

Computerized Evaluation and Exercise Equipment. Cedaron Medical, Inc. manufactures Dexter ImpairmentCare, which is a computerized evaluation system (www.cedaron.com). The system allows therapists to complete a UE evaluation using some of the tools previously discussed in this chapter. A printed report is then generated with the evaluation data. The system can also calculate the patient's Permanent Impairment Level as established by the American Medical Association. The Dexter Evaluation and Therapy System can be used to evaluate the patient, record and report the results of evaluation, establish an exercise program, record the results of each therapy session, and compare changes in the individual's strength or ROM. Any clinician using the Dexter system is encouraged to get sufficient training and to review the published validity studies (Bellace, Healy, Besser, Byron, & Hohman, 2000; Brown et al., 2000).

BTE Technologies (formerly Baltimore Therapeutic Co.) manufactures several large computer-assisted systems to meet the evaluation and rehabilitation needs of occupational and physical therapists (BTE Technologies, 2011). The Simulator II (Fig. 29.10) system is primarily used for UE rehabilitation. A variety of handles and tools can be attached to the system to serve three functions: (1) provide UE strengthening exercise such as shoulder flexion and extension, (2) simulate UE industrial tasks such as climbing a ladder or auto repair, and (3) simulate ADL tasks such as ironing or putting on shoes. When using the Simulator II for strength training, set the resistance low and gradually increase the resistance with concurrent increases in the length of exercise.

Resistive Pulley Weights. The **weight well** (Barber, 1978) (Fig. 29.11) is one type of resistive pulley system that is commercially available. A variety of handle shapes are attached to rods with suspended weights. The rods are turned against resistance throughout the ROM to encourage wrist flexion and wrist extension, pinch, pronation and supination patterns, and full grasp and release of the injured hand. The weight well can be graded for resistance and repetitions and is an excellent tool for progressive resistive exercise. Pulley systems can have single or double handles and can be mounted on walls and/or ceilings for shoulder and general UE resistive exercise. Not all systems will include an attachment for the hand and wrist.

Theraband is a 6-inch-wide (15.2-cm-wide) rubber sheet available by the yard and color-coded by degrees of resistance. It can be cut into any length and is used for resistive exercise for the UE. Use of the Theraband is limited only by the therapist's imagination; it can be adapted to diagonal patterns of motion, wrist exercises, or follow-up treatment of tennis elbow,

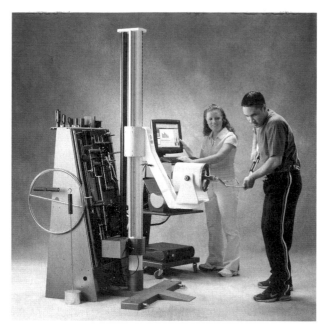

Fig. 29.10 Simulator II from BTE Technologies for upper extremity rehabilitation.

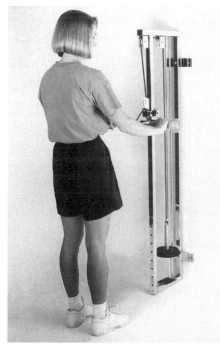

Fig. 29.11 Weight well used for upper extremity and pinch and grip strengthening. (Courtesy Karen Schultz Johnson.)

among other uses. The Theraband can be combined with dowel rods and other equipment to provide resistance throughout the ROM. It is inexpensive and easy to incorporate into a home treatment program.

Hand grips of graded resistance are available from rehabilitation supply companies and sporting goods stores. They can be purchased with various resistance levels and used for progressive resistive hand exercises. The practitioner is cautioned against using overly resistive spring-loaded grippers such as those sold in sporting goods stores. These devices may be beneficial to the seasoned athlete but are usually too resistive for the recently injured. Therapy putty can be purchased in bulk and in grades of resistance. It is color-coded to allow an easy progression as the client's strength improves. It can be adapted to most finger motions and is easily used as part of a home program; the amount given to the patient is adjusted to hand size and strength.

Household items such as spring-type clothespins have been used to increase strength of grasp and pinch. Imaginative use of common objects may originate with the clinician or the patient and is highly beneficial and motivating.

Functional activities are an integral part of rehabilitation of the hand. By engaging in occupation-based activities early, the patient will, in most cases, be able to achieve long-term goals in desired performance areas (Amini, 2004). Functional activities may include crafts, games, dexterity activities, ADL, and work samples. Many of the treatment techniques described to this point are used to condition and prepare the hand for normal use.

Activities should be started as soon as possible at whatever level the patient can perform them, with adaptations to compensate for limited ROM and strength. Activities should be used in conjunction with other treatments. The OT must continually assess the patient's functional capacities and initiate changes in the treatment program to introduce a graded program of activities as soon as possible in the restorative phase of healing.

Vocational and avocational interests and goals should be noted at the time of initial evaluation and taken into account when planning treatment so that the patient can eventually resume meaningful life roles. Incorporating these types of activities into treatment will improve patient carryover and facilitate faster healing times secondary to the concept of muscle memory. Activities should be graded from light to heavy resistance and from gross to fine dexterity. For example, crafts have been found to work extremely well with hand injuries. Therapeutic activities in this category may include macramé, weaving, clay, leather, and woodworking. When integrated into a program of total hand rehabilitation, they provide another milestone of achievement rather than a diversion to fill up empty hours.

Activities that do not have an end product but provide practice in dexterity and ADL skills also fit into the category of functional activities. Developmental games and activities that require pinch or grasp and release may be graded and timed to increase difficulty. ADL boards that have a variety of opening and closing devices provide practice for use of the hand at home and increase self-confidence. Often a hobby can be adapted for use in the clinic. Fly-tying (making lures for trout from string and feathers) is a difficult dexterity activity but one that will be enjoyed by avid fishermen. Golf clubs and fishing poles can be adapted in the clinic to allow an early return to a favorite form of relaxation. Humor and interaction with the therapists and other patients provide vital but intangible benefits.

Clinical Application for Select Hand Injuries

Amputation. A traumatically amputated fingertip or partial finger amputation may occur with the use of machinery such as saws and snow blowers (see Chapter 31).

The goal of surgery is to ensure good skin coverage of the amputated part. The occupational therapy goals are wound care, edema reduction, scar management, desensitization, and restoration of ROM (of digit and surrounding structures) and function. Edema reduction must be addressed to avoid damage to the replanted digit. See previous discussion for specific techniques to address goals. If hypersensitivity occurs in the residual limb, see earlier strategies for sensory reeducation.

In addition, evaluation for a prosthesis may be required. Prosthetics can lead to improved functional use of the digit and rebuild patient self-confidence (Fig. 29.12). With appropriate rehabilitation, a single partial finger or fingertip amputation should have limited impact on a person's ability to return to full employment and meaningful activity.

> ### CLINICAL PEARL
>
> Suggest that patients with fingertip amputations purchase a Dr. Scholl's toe guard, which is lined with silicone to help reduce scar, shape tip, and help cushion against vibration.

Interventions for Acute Tendon Injuries

Tendon injuries are difficult to treat and make it difficult to restore normal function to injured hands and fingers (Kessler & Hertling, 1983). The hand is divided into anatomic tendon zones for both the flexor (palmar) and extensor (dorsal) surfaces (Kessler & Hertling, 1983) (Fig. 29.13). The purpose of the zone designation was to help the surgeon—and subsequently the therapist—better understand the treatment of a specific tendon injury. Surgical and rehabilitation protocols are often determined by the level, or zone, of injury.

When a tendon moves, it is said to "glide." When a person makes a fist, for example, the flexor digitorum superficialis and flexor digitorum profundus muscle bellies contract and the tendon portion of the muscle slides or glides proximally. At the same time, the extensor digitorum communis muscle

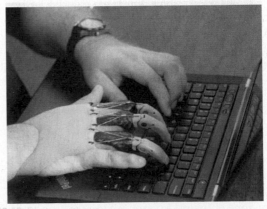

Fig. 29.12 Digit prostheses.

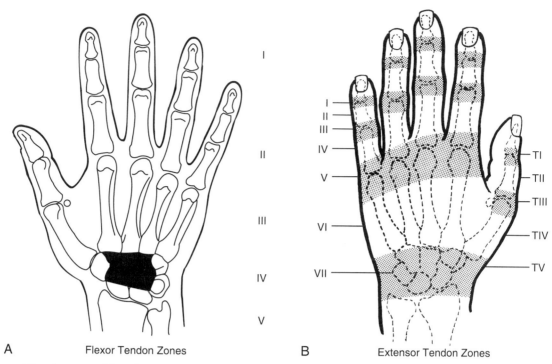

Fig. 29.13 Flexor (A) and extensor (B) tendon zones as determined by the First Congress of the International Federation of Societies for Surgery of the Hand, 1980. (From Kleinert HE, Sibrand S, Gill T. Flexor tendon injuries. *Surg Clin N Am.* 1981;61(2):268–269.)

must relax, allowing its tendon to glide distally and releasing to allow the fingers to fully flex in a fist position. An injury to a tendon that involves excessive scarring may cause a tendon to become adherent or stuck to other tissues or bone, preventing this necessary gliding. Tendon healing has three primary stages: (1) inflammatory (48–72 hours after surgery), which is the time that the tendon is most vulnerable and subject to rupture; (2) proliferative (approximately 5 days postsurgery until week 4), when tendon repair strength is slowly improving due to new collagen being laid; and (3) remodeling (week 4 until approximately 4–5 months after surgery), when full repair strength should be achieved but will not be that of the patient's preinjury strength (Voleti, Buckley, & Soslowsky, 2012).

Sometimes the tendon alone is injured, but more typically other structures are injured as well. The treatment protocols discussed in this chapter must be modified when other structures are injured in conjunction with the tendon. An understanding of tendon and hand anatomy and of the type of surgical repair is critical to rehabilitation of a patient with any tendon injury, as is good communication with the surgeon.

Flexor Tendon Injuries

The goal of flexor tendon surgery and rehabilitation is a strong repair that allows the tendon to glide freely (Sorock, Lombardi, Courtney, Cotnam, & Mittleman, 2001). Because of the complicated anatomy and mechanical considerations, treatment protocols have been developed for almost every level or zone of injury. A flexor tendon that has been injured

between the distal palmar crease and the insertion of the flexor digitorum superficialis (Zone II) is considered the most difficult to treat because the tendons lie in their sheaths in this area beneath the fibrous pulley system, and any scarring will cause adhesions. This area is often called "no man's land." The treatment strategies discussed in this chapter are primarily for tendons injured in Zones II and III.

Primary repair of the flexor tendons within these zones is attempted most often after a clean laceration. Several methods of postoperative management have been proposed with the common goal of promoting tendon glide and minimizing the formation of scar adhesions. Three methods of postoperative flexor tendon management are (1) immobilization, (2) controlled passive mobilization, and (3) early active mobilization (Table 29.1). Note: In each of the three rehabilitation methods, the patient is placed in a dorsal blocking splint to prevent wrist and finger extension. The wrist is positioned in 10 to 30 degrees of flexion with the MCP joints at 40 to 60 degrees of flexion and the PIPs and DIPs in full extension.

Immobilization Technique. This treatment strategy completely immobilizes the tendon for 3.5 weeks after tendon repair. Immobilization may not result in consistently good results because it often leads to scar adherence and may lead to a greater incidence of tendon rupture. However, in the presence of other injuries (e.g., a fractured phalanx that cannot be moved), this technique may be necessary. Also, if a patient appears unable to participate fully in treatment (as might be the case for a child or an individual with cognitive impairments), this method may be selected.

TABLE 29.1   Flexor Tendon Rehabilitation Protocol[a]

Treatment Protocol	Indications/ Discussion	Early Treatment Phase	Middle Treatment Phase	Late Treatment Phase
Immobilization	Patient under 10 years old Cognitively impaired When movement would adversely affect other healing structures Usually leads to adherent scar	0 to 3 weeks *Positioning Splint* Postoperative cast or dorsal blocking splint Wrist 10–30° flexion MCP 40–60° flexion IP full extension *Exercise:* AROM uninvolved shoulder, elbow	3 to 6 weeks *Positioning Splint* Change wrist to neutral *Exercise:* Passive finger flexion with wrist in 10° extension Tendon glide exercise (see Fig. 29.13)	4 to 6 weeks *Positioning Splint* Discontinue splint May need nighttime static extension splint *Exercise:* Blocking Light resistance Light ADL
Early passive mobilization protocols 1. Kleinert 2. Duran and Houser 3. Modified Duran	Early passive motion Facilitates tendon glide and decreases adherent scar formation	0 to 4.5 weeks (Duran & Houser) *Positioning Splint* Wrist 20° flexion MCP relaxed flexion IP extension *Exercise:* Passive PIP and DIP flexion/extension in protected position Modified Duran *Positioning Splint* Wrist varies from 20° flexion to 20° extension MCP 40–50° flexion Strap finger in extension at night and when not exercising *Exercise:* PROM as above Active extension of PIPs and DIPs with MCPs held in maximum flexion In OT clinic only: protected tenodesis	4.5 to 8 weeks (Duran & Houser) *Positioning Splint* Replace splint with wrist band with rubber band traction applied to finger *Exercise:* Active extension Blocking FDS glide Fisting	8 weeks (Duran & Houser) *Positioning Splint* Discontinued *Exercise:* Begin gentle graded resistance
Early active motion protocols 1. Washington 2. Indiana Protocol 3. Minimal Active Muscle Tendon Tension (MAMTT)	Generally favored protocols Places gentle active tension on the repaired tendon Therapist and MD must agree on protocol Patient must be able to comply fully with treatment regimen	0 to 4 weeks (Washington) *Positioning Splint* Wrist 30–45° flexion MCP 40–70° flexion IP full extension Rubber band traction with palmar bar pulley *Exercise:* Active IP extension to splint Passive flexion MCP, PIP, and DIP Composite passive flexion to distal palmar crease	4 to 6 weeks (Washington) *Positioning Splint* Week 5 begin nighttime splinting only, wrist changed to 15° flexion May apply wrist cuff with rubber band traction *Exercise:* Active tendon glides or "place & hold" exercise, cleared by MD Blocking flexion of PIP and DIP, cleared by MD Composite extension to neutral	6 to 8 weeks (Washington) *Positioning Splint* Discontinue protective splint but may begin dynamic PIP extension if indicated *Exercise:* Blocking to PIP and DIP Passive wrist, finger extension Light putty with MD approval Light ADL At 8 weeks can begin graded resistance

DIP, Distal interphalangeal; *FDS*, flexor digitorum superficialis; *IP*, interphalangeal; *MCP*, metacarpophalangeal; *PIP*, proximal interphalangeal. Data from Cifaldi CD, Schwarze L. Early progressive resistance following immobilization of flexor tendon repairs. *J Hand Ther.* 1991;4:111; Duran RJ, et al. Management of flexor tendon lacerations in zone 2 using controlled passive motion postoperatively. In: Hunter JM, Mackin E, Callahan A, et al, eds. *Rehabilitation of the Hand.* 3rd ed. St Louis, MO: Mosby; 1990; Evans RB, Thompson DE. The application of force to the healing tendon. *J Hand Ther.* 1993;6(4):266–284; Halikis MN, Manske PR, Kubota H, et al. Effect of immobilization, immediate mobilization, and delayed mobilization on the resistance to digital flexion using a tendon injury model. *J Hand Surg.* 1997;22(3):464–472; Schenck RR, Lenhart DE. Results of zone II flexor tendon laceration in civilians treated by the Washington regime. *J Hand Surg.* 1996;21 (6):984–987; Stewart Pettengill KM, van Strein G. Postoperative management of flexor tendon injuries. In: Mackin EJ, Callahan AD, Osterman AL, et al, eds. *Rehabilitation of the Hand and Upper Extremity.* 5th ed. Vol. I. St Louis, MO: Mosby; 2002.
[a]This table is meant only as a basic outline of the variety of rehabilitation protocols for a flexor tendon injury. Not all protocols have been listed or described under each category. It is the responsibility of the therapist to consult the appropriate and complete sources. It is expected that the OT will study the original complete protocols and be in contact with the surgeon before beginning tendon rehabilitation. The OTA must also have knowledge of tendon anatomy and the protocols to assist the OT in treatment.

Controlled Passive Motion. Duran and Houser (Duff & Estilow, 2011) suggested the use of controlled passive motion, which allows 3 to 5 mm of tendon excursion, to achieve optimal results after primary tendon repair. They found this practice sufficient to prevent adherence of the repaired tendons. On the third postoperative day, the patient begins a twice-daily exercise regimen of passive flexion and extension of six to eight motions for each tendon. Care is taken to keep the wrist flexed and the MCPs in 70 degrees of flexion during passive exercise. After 4.5 weeks the protective dorsal splint is removed, and the rubber band traction is attached to a wristband (Fig. 29.14). Active extension and passive flexion are done for 1 additional week and gradually increased over the next several weeks.

Early Active Motion. Dr. Harold Kleinert, a pioneer of flexor tendon surgery, was an early advocate of rubber band traction after repair of flexor tendons. This technique is often called the Kleinert technique. After surgical repair, rubber bands are attached to the nails of the involved fingers with a suture through the nail or with a hook held in place with cyanoacrylate glue. A dorsal blocking splint is fabricated from low-temperature thermoplastic material with the MCP joints held in about 60 degrees of flexion and the PIPs in gentle flexion. The patient must be able to fully extend the interphalangeal (IP) joints actively within the splint; otherwise, joint contractures will develop (see Fig. 29.14). Kleinert's original protocol has been modified but remains the basis for most of the early active motion protocols described in the literature and described briefly in Table 29.1. His protocol and the Washington approach use early active extension but passive flexion. The Indiana and MAMTT (minimal active muscle-tendon tension) protocols allow for early gentle supervised active flexion of the injured tendon. There is some evidence (Stralka, 1996) that early active motion such as "place-and-hold" exercises do result in greater finger motion after a Zone II tendon injury.

In the Kleinert and Washington protocols the patient wears the splint 24 hours a day for 3 weeks and is instructed to actively extend the fingers several times a day in the splint, allowing the rubber bands to pull the fingers into flexion. The movement of the tendon through the tendon sheath and pulley system minimizes scar adhesions while enhancing tendon nutrition and blood flow. The dorsal blocking splint is removed at 3 weeks, and the rubber band is attached to a wristband, which is worn 1 to 5 additional weeks, depending on the surgeon's judgment.

It is important to note that new protocols are currently being proposed, and the treatment of tendon repair is ever changing. The Saint John protocol, being one of the more recent approaches to flexor tendon rehabilitation, involves the patient remaining awake during surgery so that he or she can actively make a fist to ensure that there is no gapping of the tendon once repaired (Bell-Krotoski, 2011). During rehabilitation the patient partakes in a combination of PROM followed by partial AROM exercises through completing half fists instead of the more commonly used place-and-hold exercises postrepair. At 2 to 4 weeks the patient is progressed out of the traditional dorsal blocking orthotic to a short Manchester orthotic to improve mobility and decrease adhesions from forming to the newly repaired tendon. Though this technique for surgery and postrehabilitative treatment is not widely used yet, it does hold much promise and is an excellent example of both how surgery and treatment of flexor tendon repairs are progressing.

To be successful, all the early mobilization techniques require a motivated patient who thoroughly understands the program. Some early active mobilization protocols currently allow early active extension and flexion of the repaired tendons, as well as other changes (Cannon, 1993; Sorock et al., 2001). Only the most experienced OT who has good communication with the surgeon should attempt these treatment approaches.

Postacute Flexor Tendon Rehabilitation

Although each protocol has a specific and sometimes slightly different time line, when active flexion is begun out of the splint after any of the postoperative management techniques described previously, the patient should be instructed in exercises to facilitate differential tendon gliding (Ware & Sherbourne, 1992; Watson & Carlson, 1987). Wehbe (1987) recommends three positions—hook fist, straight fist, and composite fist—to maximize isolated gliding of the flexor digitorum superficialis and the flexor digitorum profundus tendons, as well as stretching of the intrinsic musculature and gliding of the extensor mechanism. These tendon glide exercises (Fig. 29.15) should be repeated 10 times in each position, two to three times daily. Isolated exercises to assist tendon gliding may also be performed with a blocking splint (Edmond, 1993) (Fig. 29.16) or by using the opposite hand (Fig. 29.17). The MCP joint is held in extension during blocking, so the intrinsic muscles that act on it cannot overcome the power of the repaired flexor tendons. Care should be taken not to hyperextend the PIP joint because this would overstretch the repaired tendons.

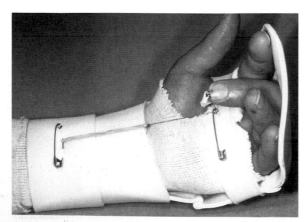

Fig. 29.14 The dorsal blocking splint allows for passive flexion of the digit(s) and full active extension at the proximal interphalangeal (PIP) and distal interphalangeal (DIP) joints.

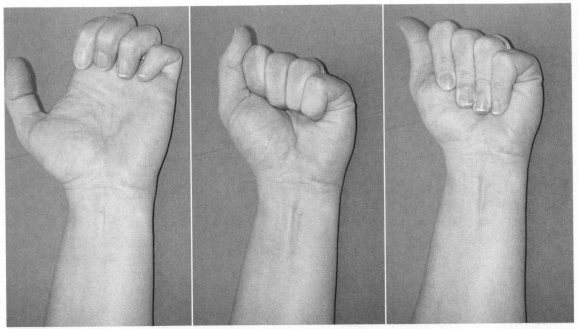

Fig. 29.15 Tendon gliding exercises. Patient starts with fingers in full extension and then makes each of these fist positions.

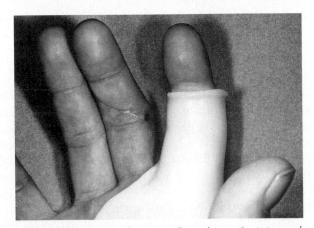

Fig. 29.16 A blocking splint can allow the patient to perform isolated tendon motion at a specified joint.

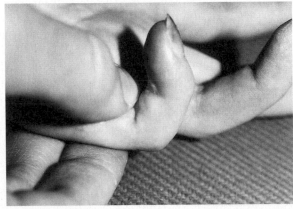

Fig. 29.17 Manual blocking of the metacarpophalangeal (MCP) during active flexion of the proximal interphalangeal (PIP) joint.

After 6 to 8 weeks, passive extension may be started and a volar finger splint may be necessary to correct a flexion contracture at a PIP joint. Alternately, the therapist may fabricate a cylindrical plaster splint to apply constant static pressure on the contracture (Bell-Krotoski, 2011) (Fig. 29.18).

After approximately 8 weeks, the patient may begin light resistive exercises, light ADL, and other activities. The patient must avoid lifting with or applying excessive resistance to the affected hand. Sports activities should be discouraged. However, activities such as working with soft clay, woodworking, and macramé are excellent. Full resistance and normal work activities may resume at 3 months postsurgery.

Although performance of ADL is generally not a problem, therapy providers should ask patients about any problems they may have or anticipate. Disuse and neglect of a finger,

especially the index finger, are common and should be prevented. Gains in finger flexion and extension may continue to be recorded for 6 months postoperatively. A functional to excellent result is obtained when there is minimal extension lag at the PIP and DIP joints and the finger(s) can flex to the palm.

Extensor Tendon Injuries. Extensor tendons are broad, thin, and structurally flat, which makes them more likely to become adherent to the tissue above (skin) and below (fascia, bone) after injury. They can rupture more easily than flexor tendons. Scar adherence limits extensor tendon gliding and can impair not only extension of the digits but also flexion. Incomplete extension is known as extensor lag. Three current treatment approaches to extensor tendon rehabilitation are

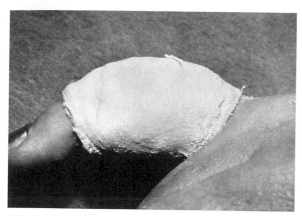

Fig. 29.18 Plaster cylindric cast used to apply gentle static stretch to proximal interphalangeal (PIP) joint.

(1) immobilization, (2) early controlled passive mobilization, and (3) early active motion. Extensor tendons are divided into zones (see Fig. 29.13), and rehabilitation depends on the zone of injury regardless of which of the three treatment methods is used.

The **immobilization approach** keeps the tendons in a shortened position through splinting or casting. Tendons are immobilized for 3 weeks; in week 4, gentle active motion of the repaired tendons is introduced. Extensor tendons injured proximal to the MCP joints often become adherent to the structures above and below them. This problem will require the OT to begin a splinting program. A removable volar splint is used between exercise periods to protect the tendon for 2 additional weeks. Dynamic flexion splinting may be started 6 weeks after surgery to regain flexion if needed.

Extensor tendons injured proximal to the MCP joint may be immobilized for 3 weeks. After this, the finger may be placed in a removable volar splint that is worn between exercise periods for an additional 2 weeks. Progressive ROM is begun after 3 weeks, and if full flexion is not regained rapidly, dynamic flexion may be started after 6 weeks.

Extensor tendon injuries that occur distal to the MCP joint require a longer period of immobilization (usually 6 weeks). A progressive exercise program is then initiated with dynamic splinting during the day and static splinting at night to maintain extension.

The **early passive motion** approach reverses what was done for the flexor tendons. The extensor tendons are held in extension by dynamic, gentle rubber band traction, and the patient is allowed to actively flex the fingers, thereby passively moving the repaired extensor tendons. These splints must have a dorsal component to provide a block to flexion so as not to move the tendons too much, which could lead to overstretching or rupture of the extensor tendon (English, Rehm, & Petzoldt, 1982; Evans, 1995). This method facilitates tendon strength and can prevent the scarring that ultimately limits motion and function.

The early active short arc program, developed by Evans (English et al., 1982; Evans, 1986), allows the tendon (except a Zone I injury) to actively move 3 days after surgery. The

therapist must take care to ensure that the stress applied by **early active motion** does not overpower the strength of the surgical repair. The splinting program is quite complex and specific, and it requires a skilled OT (English et al., 1982; Evans, 1986; Hardy & Freeland, 2011; Stanton-Hicks et al., 1995).

Peripheral Nerve Injuries

The peripheral nerve can be injured by one of the following mechanisms: (1) compression from within by a tumor or fracture; (2) external compression such as a hand or finger crushed in a machine or car door; (3) laceration by a fractured bone, knife, or lid of a can; (4) stretching, which deranges the internal structure of the nerve beyond its ability to function, as may occur in a motor vehicle accident when the arm and therefore brachial plexus may be stretched by a direct force; (5) inadvertent injection into a peripheral nerve; (6) radiation such as may be administered to the axillary lymph node area because of breast cancer; and (7) electricity. Peripheral nerves have both motor and sensory functions. Symptoms of peripheral nerve injuries include muscle weakness or paralysis and sensory loss in the area innervated by the injured peripheral nerve. The therapist who assesses the patient for nerve loss must be familiar with the muscles and areas that are innervated by the three major forearm nerves. A summary of UE peripheral neuropathies can be found in Table 29.2.

Peripheral Neuropathy

OTs may administer several quick clinical tests of the motor function of the individual peripheral nerves to detect impairment. The ulnar nerve may be tested by asking the patient to pinch a piece of paper between the thumb and index finger while the therapist tries to pull the paper way. This is called the Froment sign (Fig. 29.19). The therapist may also palpate the first dorsal interosseous muscle. The radial nerve may be tested by asking the patient to extend the wrist and fingers together (Fig. 29.20). Median nerve function is tested by asking the patient to oppose the thumb to the fingers (Chusid, 1985) (Fig. 29.21). Early signs of median nerve compression are commonly sensory in nature and may be tested by performing provocative tests such as the Phalen test and percussing over the median nerve at the wrist to elicit a Tinel sign, as described earlier in this chapter. Patients may also develop compression syndromes of the ulnar and radial nerves that will be indicated by paresthesias along the course of those nerves.

Radial Nerve. The radial nerve innervates the extensor and supinator group of muscles of the forearm. The sensory distribution of the radial nerve is a strip of the posterior upper arm and the forearm, the dorsum of the thumb, and the index and middle fingers and radial half of the ring finger to the PIP joints. Sensory loss of the radial nerve does not usually result in dysfunction or have serious functional ramifications. A dorsal splint that provides wrist extension, MCP extension, and thumb extension is provided to protect the extensor

TABLE 29.2 Nerve Injuries of the Upper Extremity

Nerve	Location	Affected	Test
Radial nerve (posterior cord; fibers from C5, C6, C7, C8)	Upper arm	Triceps and all distal motors; sensory to SRN	MMT, sensory test
Radial nerve	Above elbow	Brachioradialis and all distal motors; sensory to SRN	MMT, sensory
Radial nerve	At elbow	Supinator, ECRL, ECRB, and all distal motors; sensory to SRN	MMT, sensory
Posterior interosseous nerve	Forearm	ECU, ED, EDM, APL, EPL, EPB, EIP; no sensory loss	Wrist extension—if present indicates PIN rather than high radial nerve
Radial nerve at ECRB, radial artery, arcade of Frohse, origin of supinator	Radial tunnel syndrome	Weakness of muscles innervated by PIN; no sensory loss	Palpation for pain over extensor mass; pain with wrist flexion and pronation; pain with wrist extension and supination; pain with resisted middle finger extension
Median nerve (lateral cord from C5, C6, C7; medial cord from C8, T1)	High lesions (elbow and above)	Paralysis/weakness of FCR, PL, all FDS, FDP, I and II; FPL, pronator teres, and quadratus, opponens pollicis, APB, FPB (radial head), lumbricals I and II; sensory cutaneous branch of median nerve	MMT, sensory
Median nerve	Low (at wrist)	Weakness of thenars only	Inability to flex thumb tip and index fingertip to palm; inability to oppose thumb, poor dexterity
Median nerve under fibrous band in PT, beneath heads of pronator, arch of FDS, origin of FCR	Pronator syndrome	Weakness in thenars but *not* muscles innervated by AIN; sensory in median nerve distribution in hand	Provocative tests to isolate compression site
Median nerve under origin of PT, FDS to middle	Anterior interosseous nerve syndrome	Pure motor, no sensory; forearm pain preceding paralysis; weakness of FPL, FDP I and II, PQ	Inability to flex IP joint of thumb and DIP of index; increased pain with resisted pronation; pain with forearm pressure
Median nerve at wrist	Carpal tunnel syndrome	Weakness of median innervated intrinsics; sensory	Provocative tests, Tinel, sensory
Ulnar nerve at elbow (branch of medial cord from C7, C8, T1)	Cubital tunnel syndrome	Weakness/paralysis of FCU, FDP III and IV, ulnar intrinsics; numbness in palmar cutaneous and dorsal cutaneous distribution; loss of grip and pinch strength	Pain with elbow flexion/extension
Ulnar nerve at wrist	Compression at Guyon's canal	Weakness and pain in ulnar intrinsics	Reproduced by pressure at site

SRN, Superficial radial nerve; *MMT*, manual muscle test; *ECRL*, extensor carpi radialis longus; *ECRB*, extensor carpi radialis brevis; *ECU*, extensor carpi ulnaris; *ED*, extensor digitorum; *EDM*, extensor digiti minimi; *APL*, abductor pollicis longus; *EPL*, extensor pollicis longus; *EPB*, extensor pollicis brevis; *EIP*, extensor indicis proprius; *PIN*, posterior interosseous nerve; *FCR*, flexor carpi radialis; *PL*, palmaris longus; *FDS*, flexor digitorum superficialis; *FDP*, flexor digitorum profundus; *FPL*, flexor pollicis longus; *APB*, abductor pollicis brevis; *FPB*, flexor pollicis brevis; *AIN*, anterior interosseous nerve; *PT*, pronator teres; *FCR*, flexor carpi radialis; *PQ*, pronator quadratus; *IP*, interphalangeal; *DIP*, distal interphalangeal; *FCU*, flexor carpi ulnaris.

tendons from overstretching during the healing phase and to position the hand for functional use (Fig. 29.22).

Median Nerve. The median nerve innervates the flexors of the forearm and hand and is often called the "eyes" of the hands because of its importance in sensory innervation of the volar surface of the hands. Median nerve loss may result from lacerations, as well as from compression syndromes of the wrist such as carpal tunnel syndrome. Motor distribution of the median nerve is listed in Table 29.2. Sensory distribution of the median nerve includes the volar surface of the thumb, index, and middle fingers; the radial half of the ring finger and dorsal surface of the index and middle fingers; and the radial half of the ring finger distal to the PIP joints. The sensory loss associated with median nerve injury is particularly disabling because sensory innervation is lacking in the fingers that perform all pinch patterns. The patient is unable to judge the amount of pressure or force needed to accomplish a pinch task and so the task becomes almost impossible to do. When vision is occluded, the patient will

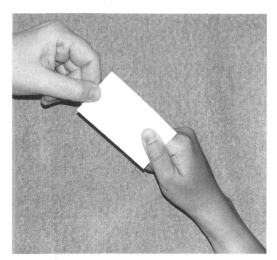

Fig. 29.19 Quick ulnar nerve function test.

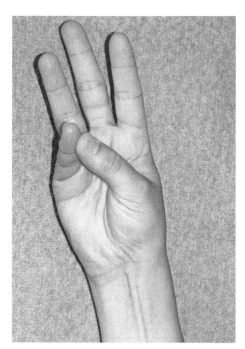

Fig. 29.21 Quick median nerve function test.

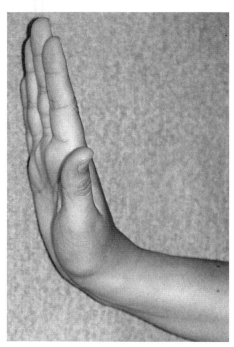

Fig. 29.20 Quick radial nerve function test.

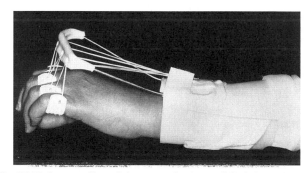

Fig. 29.22 Low-profile radial nerve splint is carefully balanced to pull metacarpophalangeal (MCP) joints into extension when wrist is flexed and allows the MCP joints to fall into slight flexion when wrist is extended, preserving normal balance between two joints and preventing joint contracture. (Courtesy Judy C. Colditz.)

substitute pinch to the ring and small fingers to compensate for this loss.

Splints that position the thumb in palmar abduction and slight opposition will increase functional use of the hand (Fig. 29.23). If clawing of the index and long fingers is present, a splint should be fabricated to prevent hyperextension of the MCP joints. Patients report that they avoid use of the hand with a median nerve injury because of lack of sensation rather than because of muscle paralysis. Despite this, the weakened or paralyzed muscles should be protected.

Ulnar Nerve. The ulnar nerve in the forearm innervates only the flexor carpi ulnaris, the median half of the flexor digitorum profundus, and the intrinsic muscles of the hand (see

Table 29.2). The sensory distribution of the ulnar nerve includes the dorsal and volar surfaces of the little finger and the ulnar half of the dorsal and volar surface of the ring finger. An ulnar nerve injury results in hyperextension of the MCP joints of the ring and small fingers (clawing) caused by action of the extensor digitorum communis that is not held in check by the third and fourth lumbricals (Moberg, 1958).

Splints should block hyperextension of the MCP joints (Fig. 29.24). The IP joints of the ring and small fingers will not demonstrate a great flexion deformity because of the paralysis of the flexor digitorum profundus. The hypothenar muscles and interossei will be absent. The wrist will assume a position of radial extension caused by the loss of the flexor carpi ulnaris.

Sensory loss of the ulnar nerve results in frequent injury (especially burns) to the ulnar side of the hand and small finger. Patients must be instructed in visual protection of the anesthetic area.

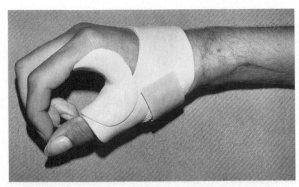

Fig. 29.23 A hand-based thumb-positioning splint may be used with median nerve injury to preserve the web space and to position thumb for function.

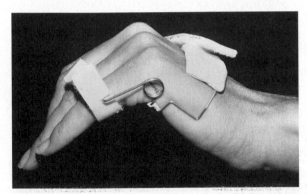

Fig. 29.24 A dynamic ulnar nerve splint blocks hyperextension of the metacarpophalangeal (MCP) joints, thus allowing extension of the proximal interphalangeal (PIP) joints. (Splint courtesy Mary Dimick, University of California—San Diego Hand Rehabilitation Center.)

Postoperative Management After Nerve Repair

After surgical nerve repair the hand is placed in a position that will minimize tension on the nerve. For example, after the repair of the median nerve the wrist will be immobilized in a flexed position. Immobilization usually lasts 2 to 3 weeks, after which protective gentle motion of the joints may begin. The clinician must exercise great care not to put excessive traction on the newly repaired nerve.

Correction of a **contracture** (soft tissue shortening around a joint) may take 4 to 6 weeks. Active exercise is the preferred method of gaining full wrist extension, although a light dynamic splint may be applied with the surgeon's supervision. Splinting to assist or substitute for weakened musculature may be necessary for an extended period during nerve regeneration. Splints should be removed as soon as possible to allow for active exercise of the weakened muscles. However, instructing the patient in correct patterns of motion is important so that substitution is minimized.

Initially, treatment is directed toward the prevention of deformity and correction of poor positioning during the acute and regenerative stages. PROM is an essential component of the clinic and the home exercise programs, so that as the muscle begins to work it does not have to move a tight or contracted joint. Patients must be instructed in visual protection of the anesthetic area. The patient's ADL status should be evaluated in case alternative methods or devices are needed for functional independence. Use of the hand in the patient's work should be evaluated, and the patient should be returned to employment with any necessary job modifications or adaptations of equipment as soon as possible.

Careful muscle, sensory, and functional testing is performed frequently (Fig. 29.25). As the nerve regenerates, splints may be changed or eliminated. Exercises and activities are revised to reflect the patient's new gains, and adaptive equipment should be discarded as soon as possible.

As motor function begins to return to the paralyzed muscles, a careful program of specific active and active-assistive exercises is devised to facilitate the return. The OT may use NMES (Donatelli & Owens-Burkhart, 1981) to provide an external stimulus to help strengthen the newly innervated muscle. When the muscle grade receives a good rating, functional activities are used to complete the return to normal strength.

An intact peripheral nerve gives sensory feedback and stimulates a motor response. As previously mentioned, the sensory dysfunction may be due to insufficient sensation of hypersensitivity.

Sensory reeducation attempts to help the patient learn to recognize and interpret normal sensory impulses. Sensory reeducation is not begun until the patient has protective sensibility. In both treatment strategies, the patient must understand the treatment objectives, be willing and able to carry out the prescribed program at home, and consciously incorporate his or her hand into daily tasks (Kleinert, Schepel, & Gill, 1981).

> **CLINICAL PEARL**
>
> Patients with UE peripheral nerve injury often experience intolerance to cold. The clinician may suggest a mitten or glove lined with Thinsulate to guard against pain experienced in a cold environment.

Upper Extremity Fractures

Fractures may occur in any bone. The realignment of a fractured bone is known as reduction. Reduction is achieved operatively (open) or nonoperatively (closed). Closed reductions are immobilized with a cast or an immobilization orthosis. Open reductions are immobilized with internal fixation devices such as Kirschner wires, metallic plates, and screws so that the desired position is maintained. External fixation may be used alone or in combination with internal fixation. The preferred position of immobilization of a hand fracture is wrist extension, MCP flexion, and PIP and DIP extension (Harden & Bruehl, 2006). This position is called the safe position (Fess, 2003) or intrinsic plus position (Harden & Bruehl, 2006) because it maintains the length of the collateral ligaments of the MCP, PIP, and DIP joints, thereby preserving the eventual mobility of the hand. Trauma to bone may also

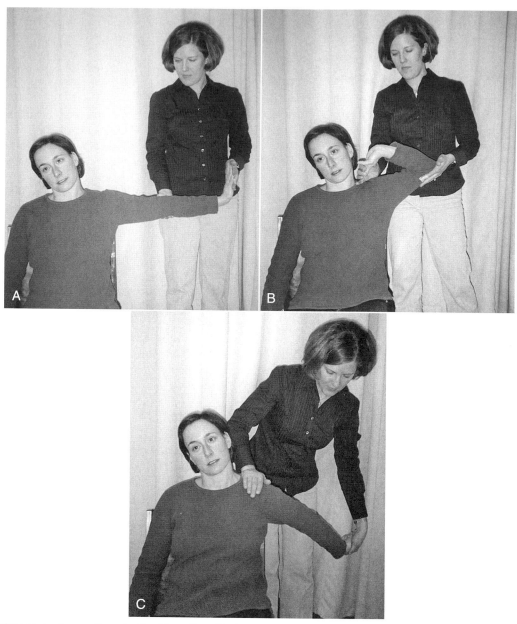

Fig. 29.25 Neurodynamic testing positions for the (A) median, (B) ulnar, and (C) radial nerves.

involve trauma to tendons and nerves in the adjacent area. Treatment must be geared toward the recovery of all injured structures. Joint contractures and tendon adherence can complicate postfracture hand rehabilitation (Harden & Bruehl, 2006).

In the first 3 to 5 weeks of treatment (immobilization), occupational therapy intervention focuses on edema reduction, skin or wound care, light functional use of the extremity, and AROM of the noninvolved joints proximal and distal to the fracture.

Once remodeling of the bone occurs, the surgeon will remove the immobilization apparatus (internal plates, screws, and pins are not usually removed) to allow movement and the specified amount of resistance. Early motion will prevent the adherence of tendons and reduce edema through stimulation

of the lymphatic and blood vessels. Assessment of the extremity occurs once the brace or cast is removed, and treatment for deficits should be addressed. A splint may be used to correct a deformity or to protect the hand or finger from additional trauma to the fracture site. An example of this type of splinting is the Velcro "buddy" splint (Fig. 29.26).

Wrist Fractures. The Colles fracture of the distal radius is the most common injury to the wrist (Breger Stanton, Lazaro, & MacDermid, 2009). It often results in limitations in wrist flexion and extension, and forearm pronation and supination. Use of splints, active motion that emphasizes wrist movement, and joint mobilization may be beneficial. The weight well (see Fig. 29.11) may be used to provide resistance to wrist motions.

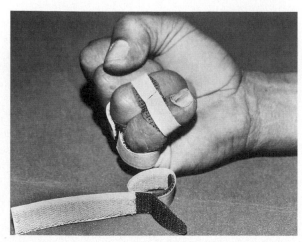

Fig. 29.26 Velcro "buddy" splint/strap may be used to protect a finger after a fracture or to encourage movement of a stiff finger.

The scaphoid is the second most commonly injured bone in the wrist (Breger Stanton et al., 2009) and is often fractured when the hand is extended at the time of injury. Fractures to the proximal portion of the scaphoid may result in nonunion because of its poor blood supply. Scaphoid fractures will require a prolonged period of immobilization, sometimes up to several months in a cast, with resulting stiffness and pain.

CLINICAL PEARL

For all distal fractures: Both passive and active ROM of the noninvolved joints are critical for preventing stiffness of shoulder and elbow. When the patient cannot use the hand and is not reaching overhead, around, and so forth, the proximal joints can easily become stiff.

Complex Regional Pain Syndrome

Complex regional pain syndrome (CRPS) is a painful disorder that can occur in the UE or lower extremity (LE) after injury or immobilization; it is characterized by pain, irregular blood flow, edema, changes in skin temperature and color, and often limitations of movement (de Mos et al., 2007). There are two subsets of CRPS: CRPS type I, which refers to the classic reflex sympathetic dystrophy (RSD), and CRPS type II, which presents with similar signs and symptoms but can be attributed to a diagnosed nerve injury (Box 29.5 lists diagnostic criteria). The degree of trauma in both types may not correlate with the severity of the pain and may occur after any injury, even a seemingly minor one. The syndrome appears to be triggered by a cycle of vasospasm and vasodilation after an injury. Abnormal edema and constrictive dressings or casts may be a factor in initiating the vasospasm. A vasospasm can decrease the blood supply to tissue; edema and pain result and contribute to the abnormal cycle of pain (Oatis, 2004). When circulation is decreased, the extremity becomes cool and pale. Fibrosis after tissue anoxia and

BOX 29.5 Diagnostic Criteria for Complex Regional Pain Syndrome

1. Pain that is out of proportion to initial event or injury
2. One symptom in each of the four categories:
   a. Sensory: acutely sensitive to touch
   b. Vasomotor:
      1. Changes in skin temperature, limb may be cooler or warmer than noninvolved side
      2. Changes in skin color—may be red, blue, pale, blotchy
   c. Sudomotor/edema: limb may be swollen, sweaty, or dry
   d. Motor/trophic:
      1. Decreased ROM
      2. Changes in nails, hair, and skin
3. One sign in two of the categories
   a. Sensory: aversion to pinprick or light touch
   b. Vasomotor: asymmetric skin color or temperature
   c. Sudomotor/edema: edema, sweating irregularities
   d. Motor/trophic: decreased ROM, weakness, tremors, changes in nails, hair or skin
4. Another diagnosis cannot explain signs and symptoms

From Harden RN, Bruehl SP. Diagnosis of complex regional pain syndrome: signs, symptoms, and new empirically derived diagnostic criteria. *Clin J Pain* 2006;22:415–419.

the production of protein-rich exudates results in joint stiffness. The patient may cradle the hand and prefer to keep it wrapped. There may be an exaggerated reaction to touch, especially light touch. Osteoporosis may be apparent on x-ray films by 8 weeks after trauma. Burning pain associated with CRPS type II is a symptom that may be alleviated by surgical interruption of the sympathetic nerve pathways. Millions of people in the United States may be affected with CRPS; (Stanton-Hicks et al., 1995) women are affected more frequently than men, the UE is more often involved than the LE, and fractures are the most common initiating event (de Moss et al., 2007). CRPS types I and II can present a real challenge to the treating physician and therapist. CRPS can be extremely disabling and is potentially a long-term condition that can prevent the patient from fully participating in valued life activities.

The goals of occupational therapy intervention for clients with CRPS are to control the symptoms of pain and edema, help normalize sensation, improve joint ROM, and facilitate independence in ADL. These may be achieved with compensatory strategies and/or assistive devices if necessary (Miller, Jerosch-Herold, & Shepstone, 2017). Treatment should begin as early as possible to prevent long-term consequences, such as complete dysfunction of the limb. Interventions must avoid aggravating pain or increasing inflammation. See earlier discussion for ways to control pain, increase ROM, decrease edema, and normalize sensation.

CRPS may trigger shoulder pain and stiffness, resulting in adhesive capsulitis or a frozen shoulder. Therefore early in the treatment program, AROM and functional activities should include the entire upper quadrant. Skateboard or pulley exercises are helpful in the early stages for active-assistive exercise of the shoulder. Splints that reduce joint stiffness should be used as tolerated. A tendency to develop CRPS should be suspected in any patient who seems to complain excessively about pain, appears anxious, and may report profuse sweating and temperature changes in the hand. Patients will tend to overprotect the hand. Early intervention with a structured therapy program of functional activities, group interaction, psychological support, and exercises that include all joints from the hand to the shoulder may prevent the occurrence of a fully developed pain syndrome. This problem is best recognized early and treated with tempered aggressiveness and empathy. The OTA who suspects a patient may be developing CPRS must report this immediately to the supervising OT.

Cumulative Trauma Disorder

Several terms have described the conditions that occur when the musculoskeletal system is subjected to repeated stress: *overuse syndromes, cervicobrachial disorders, repetitive stress or strain injuries (RSIs), repetitive motion injuries,* and ***cumulative trauma disorders (CTDs)***. In the United States the term CTD is most used. Cumulative disorders are thought to be work related and are often referred to as work-related musculoskeletal disorders (MSDs). MSDs are defined as "injuries or disorders of muscles, nerves, tendons, joints, cartilage, or spinal disks associated with risk factors at the workplace" (Kendall, McCreary, & Provance, 2005).

For example, a worker who is required to stand on an assembly line doing the same task repeatedly or type on a computer all day is at risk for MSD. Work-related high-risk factors for CTD are repetition, high force, awkward joint posture, direct pressure, vibration, and prolonged static positioning (Armstrong, 1992). The human body was not made to work this way, even though today's technology and productivity may encourage this behavior. CTD may take many weeks, months, or years to develop and may take just as long to resolve.

Cumulative trauma occurs when force is repeatedly applied to the same muscle or muscle group, causing an inflammatory response in the tendon, muscle, or nerve (Oatis, 2004). Muscle fatigue is an important aspect of cumulative trauma and can be relieved by rest. However, chronic fatigue, the usual condition of these patients, cannot be relieved by rest alone. In these circumstances, it is important to examine the patient's job requirements, as well as home and leisure activities.

Diagnoses associated with cumulative trauma usually fall within the following three categories: tendonitis, nerve compression or entrapment syndromes, and myofascial pain. Common examples of CTD involving the tendons are lateral epicondylitis (tennis elbow), medial epicondylitis (golfers' elbow), and de Quervain disease. Patients can also demonstrate nerve pain associated with CTDs. See previous discussion of treatment for peripheral nerve injury.

Myofascial pain may be caused by poor posture and positioning of the body out of normal alignment. This diagnosis is difficult to make because the pain is often referred to a distal area. An accurate diagnosis of any of these conditions is difficult and should be done by a skilled physician, often with input from an experienced OT.

In the acute phase, when muscle or tendon involvement exists, the goal of treatment is to reduce inflammation through rest. Immobilization orthoses (for rest) may be used in combination with anti-inflammatory medication. The therapy program consists of modalities to reduce pain and stretching to prevent joint stiffness. The patient should be instructed to avoid pain.

The exercise phase of treatment begins as the acute symptoms decrease. Gentle resistance exercises can be added on a warmed and stretched muscle. It should be increased slowly and should not result in increased pain. Patients are instructed to stretch at home, especially before activity, three times daily for an indefinite time.

In addition to abovementioned techniques, education related to postural awareness and ergonomic problem solving with the patient are critical to complete recovery. To control symptoms in the long term, patients must become aware of what triggers their symptoms and learn early intervention strategies if symptoms reappear. Modalities to reduce pain—splints, stretching, and modified activities—combined with proper body mechanics are usually effective. The key is that patients learn self-management techniques and take an active role in their treatment. When the patient's job demands have caused the CTD, an evaluation of the job site, tools used, and body mechanics during work activities may be indicated (see Chapter 16).

 CLINICAL PEARL

Begin your occupational therapy program with postural training exercises such as "chin tuck" exercises and "scapular pinching" that will lengthen anterior body muscles.

CLINICAL PEARL

Teach diaphragmatic breathing to take the stress off the intercostals and upper trapezius, which are accessory breathing muscles.

SUMMARY

The OT usually assesses the hand-injured patient with assistance from the OTA. The OT establishes the intervention strategy for each patient. The OTA may assist in certain defined areas and in some areas may carry out the treatment independently. OTAs who work in UE rehabilitation must be familiar with assessment and intervention concepts. OTAs who elect to work in this specialty area are encouraged to further develop service competency by participating in continuing education and onsite supervision.

CASE STUDY

JC is a 65-year-old retired police officer who injured his left, nondominant, hand in a home accident with a circular saw. He sustained a subtotal amputation of the tips of the index and middle fingers, which were successfully replanted. The ring finger, which could not be replanted, was amputated at the level of the DIP joint. The accident and surgery occurred on December 3; he is seen for the first time in occupational therapy on January 10. Pictured is the patient's hand at rest in comparison with the noninjured side (Fig. 29.27) and the patient attempting to make a fist (Fig. 29.28).

For results of JC's initial evaluation in occupational therapy, refer to Fig. 29.29. Consider the following questions:

1. Determine a problem list for JC and list problems in priority order. What rationale guides this order?

2. For each problem that you have described, discuss the intervention strategy you would use. What is your rationale for the strategy?
3. For each treatment strategy, describe exactly what the therapy practitioner would do, including patient position and therapist action.
4. Discuss the ADL areas in which the patient may have difficulty. What are the best recommendations for these possible limitations?

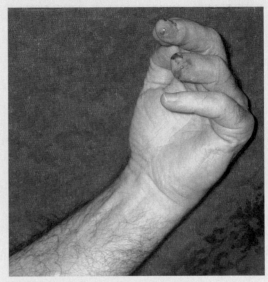

Fig. 29.28 Patient attempting to make a fist.

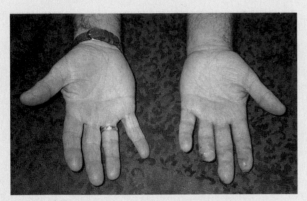

Fig. 29.27 Palmar surface, injured and noninjured hands.

REVIEW QUESTIONS

1. Describe the various sensory tests and their appropriate uses.
2. What are two tools used to measure edema? Discuss the rationale for each.
3. Name two objective tests of sympathetic function.
4. What is the only technique that is always appropriate for acute hand injury?
5. Name the components of a hand evaluation.
6. What are the benefits of using the Jebsen Hand Function Test?
7. If no goniometer is available, describe another method of evaluating gross finger flexion.
8. What are the goals of occupational therapy with a patient who has had a fingertip amputation?
9. Name the three types of pinch that are routinely assessed for strength. Name two functional activities for each of these pinch types.
10. Name the three levels of peripheral nerve injury.
11. Why is the median nerve sometimes referred to as the "eyes" of the hand?

12. Why does clawing occur in the small and ring fingers after ulnar nerve injury?
13. What splint position is indicated after a low-level median nerve injury that has resulted in paralysis?
14. Once a patient has been cleared for strengthening, name two clinic activities and two craft activities that will achieve this goal.
15. Describe two treatment strategies to reduce fingertip hypersensitivity.
16. Describe the appropriate splint immediately after flexor tendon repair. What is the rationale of the Kleinert protocol?
17. What is complex regional pain syndrome? What is the difference between CRPS type I and CRPS type II? What is a key caution when working with patients with CRPS?
18. Discuss the risk factors for work-related musculoskeletal or cumulative trauma at the workplace. What body tissues are affected by work-related musculoskeletal disorders? What is the goal of occupational therapy during the acute rehabilitation phase when working with a patient with this disorder?

OCCUPATIONAL THERAPY INITIAL EVALUATION RESULTS

Patient:	JC	
History:	Left carpal tunnel release 1991, no other relevant PMH	
Wound appearance:	Well-healed scars volar surface of index and middle fingers; amputation of ring finger at DIP joint	
Edema:	Moderate	

Circumference	Right	Left
Wrist	6.75 inches	6.75 inches
Midpalmar (DPC)	8.50 inches	8.25 inches
PIP joint ring fingers	2.50 inches	2.75 inches

Pain: 4 out of 10 (intermittent, not constant, patient bothered by numbness more than pain)

Hand active ROM — Right noninjured

Finger	MCP joint	PIP joint	DIP joint	TAM
Index	0/85	0/100	0/60	245
Middle	0/90	0/100	0/65	255
Ring	0/80	0/90	0/55	225
Small	0/80	0/85	0/60	225
Thumb	0/40	−/60		100

Hand active ROM — Left injured

Finger	MCP joint	PIP joint	DIP joint	TAM
Index	0/70	0/45	0/30	145
Middle	0/70	0/45	0/10	125
Ring	0/60	0/30	Amp	0/40
Small	0/70	0/50	0/10	130
Thumb	0/40	0/60		100

Finger tip to distal palmar crease

Finger	Right	Left injured
Index	0 cm	6 cm
Middle	0 cm	7 cm
Ring	0 cm	6 cm
Small	0 cm	5.5 cm

Strength (recorded in pounds)

Test	Right	Left injured
Gross grasp	105	20
2 point pinch	18	4
3 jaw chuck	22	8
Lateral	26	10

Dexterity

9-hole peg test	Right = 15 seconds	Left = 27 seconds

Sensibility

Semmes-Weinstein monofilament test

Finger tip	Radial side	Ulnar side
Thumb	3.61	3.61
Index	3.61	3.61
Middle	3.61	4.31
Ring (amp at DIP)	3.61	3.61
Small	3.61	3.61

Fig. 29.29 Case study: occupational therapy initial evaluation results.

REFERENCES

American Occupational Therapy Association. (1997). Physical agent modalities position paper. *The American Journal of Occupational Therapy*, 51(10), 870–871.

American Society for Surgery of the Hand. (1990). In: *The hand, examination and diagnosis.* (3rd ed.). New York: Churchill Livingstone.

Amini, D. A. (2004). Renaissance in occupational therapy and occupation-based hand therapy. *OT Practice*, 9(3), 11–15.

Anthony, M. S. (1993). Sensory evaluation. In: G. Clark, E. F. Shaw-Wilgis, & B. Aiello, et al. (Eds.), *Hand rehabilitation: A practical guide.* New York: Churchill Livingstone.

Apfel, E. R., & Carronza, J. (1992). In dexterity. In: *American society of hand therapists, clinical assessment recommendations.* 2nd ed. Chicago, IL: AHST.

Armstrong, T. J. (1992). Cumulative trauma disorders of the upper limb and identification of work-related factors. In: L. H. Millender, D. S. Louis, & B. P. Simmons (Eds.), *Occupational disorders of the upper extremity.* New York, NY: Churchill Livingstone.

Artzberger, S. M. (2002). Manual edema mobilization: treatment for edema in the subacute hand. In: E. J. Mackin, A. D. Callahan, & A. L. Osterman, et al. (Eds.), *Rehabilitation of the hand and upper extremity.* (5th ed.). Vol. I. St Louis, MO: Mosby.

Barber, L. M. (1978). Occupational therapy for the treatment of reflex sympathetic dystrophy and post-traumatic hypersensitivity of the injured hand. In: S. Fredericks, & G. S. Brody (Eds.), *Symposium on the neurologic aspects of plastic surgery*. St Louis, MO: Mosby.

Bear-Lehman, J., & Poole, S. E. (2011). The presence and impact of stress reactions on disability among patients with hand injury. *Journal of Hand Therapy, 24*, 89–93.

Bellace, J. V., Healy, D., Besser, M. P., Byron, T., & Hohman, L. (2000). Validity of the Dexter evaluation system's Jamar dynamometer attachment for assessment of hand grip strength in a normal population. *Journal of Hand Therapy, 13*(1), 46–51.

Bell-Krotoski, J. A. (2002). Sensibility testing with the Semmes-Weinstein monofilaments. In: E. J. Mackin, A. D. Callahan, & A. L. Osterman, et al. (Eds.), *Rehabilitation of the hand and upper extremity.* (5th ed.). Vol. I. St Louis, MO: Mosby.

Bell-Krotoski, J. A. (2011). Tissue remodeling and contracture correction using serial plaster casting and orthotic positioning. In: T. M. Skirven, A. L. Osterman, J. Fedorczyk, & P. Amadio (Eds.), *Rehabilitation of the hand and upper extremity.* (6th ed.). Vol. 2. Philadelphia, PA: Elsevier.

Bennett GK. (1981). *Hand-tool dexterity test.* New York, NY: Harcourt, Brace, Jovanovich.

Breger Stanton, D. E., Lazaro, R., & MacDermid, J. C. (2009). A systematic review of the effectiveness of contrast baths. *Journal of Hand Therapy, 22*(1), 57–69.

Brown, A., Cramer, L. D., Eckhaus, D., Schmidt, J., Ware, L., & MacKenzie, E. (2000). Validity and reliability of the Dexter hand evaluation and therapy system in hand-injured patients. *Journal of Hand Therapy, 13*(1), 37–45.

BTE Technologies. (2011). Smart physical therapy and physiotherapy equipment, occupational therapy equipment, & athletic training equipment. https://www.btetechnologies.com.

Callahan, A. D. (2002). Sensibility assessment for nerve lesions-in-continuity and nerve lacerations. In: E. J. Mackin, A. D. Callahan, & A. L Osterman, et al. (Eds.), *Rehabilitation of the hand and upper extremity.* (5th ed.). Vol. I. St Louis, MO: Mosby.

Cannon, N. M. (1993). Post flexor tendon repair motion protocol. *Indiana Hand Center News, 1*, 13–17.

Chen, C., Granger, C. V., Peimer, C. A., Moy, O. J., & Wald, S. (2005). Manual ability measure (MAM-16): a preliminary report on a new patient-centered and task-oriented outcome measure on hand function. *The Journal of Hand Surgery, 30*(2), 207–216.

Chusid, J. G. (1985). In: *Correlative neuroanatomy and functional neurology.* (19th ed.). Los Altos, CA: Lange.

Coldham, F., Lewis, J., & Lee, H. (2006). The reliability of one vs. three grip trials in symptomatic and asymptomatic subjects. *Journal of Hand Therapy, 19*(3), 318–327. Available from doi:10.1197/j.jht.2006.04.002.

Crawford, J. E, & Crawford, D. M. (1981). *Crawford small parts dexterity test manual.* New York, NY: Harcourt.

Cyriax, J. H. (1985). Clinical application of message. In: J. V. Basmajian (Ed.), *Manipulation, traction, and massage.* (3rd ed.). Baltimore, MD: Williams & Wilkins.

de Mos, M., de Bruijn, A. G. J., Huygen, F. J., Dieleman, J. P., Stricker, B. H., & Sturkenboom, M. C. (2007). The incidence of complex regional pain syndrome: a population based study. *Pain, 129*(1), 12–20.

Dellon, A. L. (1984). Evaluation of sensibility and reeducation of sensation in the hand. Baltimore, MD: Williams & Wilkins.

Dellon, A. L. (1983). The vibrometer. *Plastic and Reconstructive Surgery, 71*(3), 427–431.

Dommerholt, J. (2004). Complex regional pain syndrome—1: history, diagnostic criteria and etiology. *Journal of Bodywork and Movement Therapies, 8*, 167–177.

Donatelli, R., & Owens-Burkhart, H. (1981). Effects of immobilization on the extensibility of periarticular connective tissue. *The Journal of Orthopaedic and Sports Physical Therapy, 3*, 67–72.

Duff, S. V., & Estilow, T. (2011). Therapist's management of peripheral nerve injury. In: T. M. Skirven, & A. L. Osterman, et al. (Eds.), *Rehabilitation of the hand and upper extremity.* (6th ed.). Vol. I. Philadelphia, PA: Elsevier.

Edmond, S. L. (1993). *Manipulation mobilization extremity & spinal techniques.* St Louis, MO: Mosby.

English, C. B., Rehm, R. A., & Petzoldt, R. L. (1982). Blocking splints to assist finger exercise. *The American Journal of Occupational Therapy, 36*(4), 259–262.

Evans, R. B., & Burkhalter, W. E. (1986). A study of dynamic anatomy of extensor tendons and implications for treatment. *The Journal of Hand Surgery, 11*(5), 774–779.

Evans, R. B. (1986). Clinical management of extensor tendon injuries: the therapist's perspective. In: T. M. Skirven, & A. L. Osterman, J. Fedorczyk, & P. Amadio (Eds.), *Rehabilitation of the hand and upper extremity.* (6th ed.). Vol. 2. Philadelphia, PA: Elsevier.

Evans, R. B. (1995). Immediate active short arc motion following extensor tendon repair. *Hand Clinics, 11*(3), 483–512.

Fess, E. E. (2002). Documentation: essential elements of an upper extremity assessment battery. In: E. J. Mackin, A. D. Callahan, & A. L. Osterman, et al. (Eds.), *Rehabilitation of the hand and upper extremity.* (5th ed.). Vol. 1. St Louis, MO: Mosby.

Fess, E. E., Gettle, K., Phillips, C., & Jansen, J. R. (2004). *Hand and upper extremity splinting principles & methods.* (3rd ed.). St Louis, MO: Mosby.

Fishman, T. D. (1995-2010). Phases of wound healing. 1995-2010. http://medicaledu.com/phases.htm.

Gelberman, R. H., Szabor, M., Williamson, R. V., & Dimick, M. P. (1983). Sensibility testing in peripheral nerve compression syndromes: an experimental study in humans. *The Journal of Bone and Joint Surgery, 65*(5), 632–638.

Harden, R. N., & Bruehl, S. P. (2006). Diagnosis of complex regional pain syndrome: signs, symptoms, and new empirically derived diagnostic criteria. *The Clinical Journal of Pain, 22*(5), 415–419.

Hardy, M. A., & Freeland, A. E. (2011). Hand fracture fixation and healing: skeletal stability and digital mobility. In: T. M. Skirven, & A. L. Osterman AL, et al. (Eds.), *Rehabilitation of the hand and upper extremity.* (6th ed.). Vol. 1. Philadelphia, PA: Elsevier.

Hung, L. K., Chan, A., Chang, J., Tsang, A., & Leung, P. C. (1990). Early controlled active mobilization with dynamic splintage for treatment of extensor tendon injuries. *The Journal of Hand Surgery, 15*(2), 251–257.

Jebsen, R. H., Taylor, N., Trieschmann, R. B., Trotter, M. J., & Howard, L. A. (1969). An objective and standardized test of hand function. *The Archives of Physical Medicine and Rehabilitation, 50*(6), 311–319.

Kaltenborn, F. M, & Evjenth, O. (1989). In: *Manual mobilization of the extremity joints.* (4th ed.). Oslo, Norway: Olaf Norlis Bokhandel.

Kamentz, H. L. (1985). Mechanical devices of massage. In: J. V. Basmajian (Ed.), *Manipulation, traction and massage.* (3rd ed.). Baltimore, MD: Williams & Wilkins.

Kasch, M. C. (1988). Clinical management of scar tissue. *OT Health Care, 4*(3), 37–52.

Kelsey, J. L., & McEwing, G. (1997). Upper extremity disorders: frequency, impact, and cost in the united states. New York, NY: Churchill Livingstone.

Kendall, F. P, McCreary, E. K, & Provance, P. G., et al. (2005). *Muscles: Testing and function.* (5th ed.). Baltimore, MD: Williams & Wilkins.

Kessler, R. M, & Hertling, D. (1983). Joint mobilization techniques. In: R. M. Kessler, & D. Hertling (Eds.), *Management of common musculoskeletal disorders.* New York, NY: Harper & Row.

Kietrys, D. M., Barr, A. E., & Barbe, M. (2011). Pathophysiology of work-related musculoskeletal disorders. In: T. M. Skirven, & A. L. Osterman, et al. (Eds.), *Rehabilitation of the hand and upper extremity.* (6th ed.). Vol. 2. Philadelphia, PA: Elsevier:1769.

Kleinert, H. E., Schepel, S., & Gill, T. (1981). Flexor tendon injuries. *Surgical Clinics of North America, 61*(2), 267–286.

Koman, L. A., Li, Z., Smith, B. P., & Smith, T. L. (2011). Complex regional pain syndrome: types I and II. In T. M. Skirven, A. L. Osterman, J. Fedorczyk, & P. Amadio (Eds.), *Rehabilitation of the hand and upper extremity.* (6th ed.). Vol. 1. Philadelphia, PA: Elsevier.

Larson, R. N. (2006). Desensitization and reeducation. In: S. L. Burke, J. R. Higgins, & M. A. McClinton et al. (Eds.), *Hand and upper extremity rehabilitation.* St Louis, MO: Elsevier; 151–165.

Laseter, G. F., & Carter, P. R. (1996). Management of distal radius fractures. *Journal of Hand Therapy, 9*(2), 114–128.

Law, M., Baptiste, S., & Carswell, A., et al. (1998). In: *Canadian occupational performance measure.* (3rd ed.). Ottawa, Canada: CAOT Publications ACE.

Lister, G. L. (1993). In: *The hand: Diagnosis and indications.* (3rd ed.). New York, NY: Churchill Livingstone.

Louis, D. S., Greene, T. L., Jacobson, K. E., Rasmussen, C., Kolowich, P., & Goldstein, S. A. (1984). Evaluation of normal values for stationary and moving two-point discrimination in the hand. *The Journal of Hand Surgery, 9*(4), 552–555.

MacDermid, JC. (2002). Outcome measurement in the upper extremity. In: E. J. Mackin, A. D. Callahan, K. L. Osterman, & Amadio, P. (Eds.), *Rehabilitation of the hand and upper extremity.* (5th ed.). Vol. 1. St Louis, MO: Mosby.

Mathiowetz, V., Kashman, N., Vollard, G., Weber, K., Dowe, M., & Rogers, S. (1985). Grip and pinch strength: normative data for adults. *The Archives of Physical Medicine and Rehabilitation, 66* (2), 69–74.

Mathiowetz, V., Remmells, C., & Donoghue, L. (1985). Effects of elbow position on grip and key pinch strengths. *The Journal of Hand Surgery, 10*(5), 694–697.

Melvin, J. L. (1989). In: *Rheumatic disease occupational therapy and rehabilitation.* (3rd ed.). Philadelphia, PA: FA Davis.

Miller, L. K., Jerosch-Herold, C., & Shepstone, L. (2017). Effectiveness of edema management techniques for subacute hand edema: a systematic review. *Journal of Hand Therapy, 30*(4), 432–446. Available from doi:10.1016/j.jht.2017.05.011.

Moberg, E. (1958). Objective methods for determining the functional value of sensibility in the hand. *The Journal of Bone and Joint Surgery (Britain), 40-B*(3), 454–476.

Moscony, A. M. B. (2007). Common nerve problems. In: C. Cooper (Ed.), *Fundamentals of hand therapy.* St Louis, MO: Mosby Elsevier; 201–250.

Oatis C. A. (2004). *Kinesiology: The mechanics and pathomechanics of human movement.* Philadelphia, PA: Lippincott Williams & Wilkins.

Oerlemans, H. M., Oostendorp, R. A. B., deBoo, T., van der Laan, L., Severens, J. L., & Goris, J. A. (2000). Adjunctive physical therapy versus occupational therapy in patients with reflex sympathetic dystrophy/complex regional pain syndrome type I. *The Archives of Physical Medicine and Rehabilitation, 81,* 49–56.

Oxford Grice, K., Vogel, K. A., Le, V., Mitchell, A., Muniz, S., & Vollmer, M. A. (2003). A brief report—adult norms for a commercially available nine hole peg test for finger dexterity. *The American Journal of Occupational Therapy, 57*(5), 570–573.

Rempel, D. M. (1992). Work-related cumulative trauma disorders of the upper extremity. *JAMA, 267*(6), 838–842.

Schier, J. S., & Chan, J. (2007). Changes in life roles after hand injury. *Journal of Hand Therapy, 2-*(1), 57–68.

Shacklock, M. (2005). *Clinical neurodynamics: A new system of musculoskeletal treatment.* Sydney, Australia: Butterworth Heinemann.

Sorock, G. S., Lombardi, D. S., Courtney, T. K., Cotnam, J. P., & Mittleman, M. A. (2001). Epidemiology of occupational acute traumatic hand injuries: a literature review. *Safety Science, 38,* 241–256.

Stanton-Hicks, M., Jänig, W., Hassenbusch, S., Haddox, J. D., Boas, R., & Wilson, P. (1995). Reflex sympathetic dystrophy: changing concepts and taxonomy. *Pain, 63,* 127–133.

Stewart Pettengill, K. M., & vanStrein, G. (2011). Postoperative management of flexor tendon injuries. In: T. M. Skirven, & A. L. Osterman, J. Fedorczyk, & P. Amadio (Eds.), *Rehabilitation of the hand and upper extremity.* (6th ed.). Vol. 1. Philadelphia, PA: Elsevier.

Stralka, S. W. (1996). Reflex sympathetic dystrophy. In: S. B. Brotzman (Ed.), *Clinical orthopaedic rehabilitation.* St Louis, MO: Mosby.

Taleisnik, J. (1985). *The wrist.* New York, NY: Churchill Livingstone.

Thomas, D., Moutet, F., & Guinard, D. (1996). Postoperative management of extensor tendon repairs in zones V, VI, VII. *Journal of Hand Therapy, 9*(4), 309–314.

Voleti, P. B., Buckley, M. R., & Soslowsky, L. J. (2012). Tendon healing: repair and regeneration. *Annual Review of Biomedical Engineering, 14,* 47–71.

Von Der Heyde, R. (2007). Assessment of functional outcomes. In: C. Cooper (Ed.), *Fundamentals of hand therapy.* St Louis, MO: Mosby Elsevier: 98–111.

Walsh, M. T., (2011). Therapist's management of complex regional pain syndrome. In: T. M. Skirven, A. L. Osterman, J. Fedorczyk, & P. Amadio (Eds.), *Rehabilitation of the hand and upper extremity.* (6th ed.). Vol. 2. Philadelphia, PA: Elsevier.

Ware, J. J., & Sherbourne, C. D. (1992). The MOS 36-item short-form health survey (SF-36), part I: conceptual framework and item selection. *Medical Care, 30,* 473–483.

Watson, H. K., & Carlson, L. (1987). Treatment of reflex sympathetic dystrophy of the hand with an active "stress loading" program. *The Journal of Hand Surgery, 12*(5), 779–785.

Waylett-Rendell, J., & Seibly, D. (1991). A study of the accuracy of a commercially available volumeter. *The Journal of Hand Surgery, 4*(1), 10–13.

Waylett-Rendall, J. (1988). Sensibility evaluation and rehabilitation. *Orthopedic Clinics of North America, 19*(1), 43–56.

Yerxa, E. J., Barber, L. M., Diaz, O., Black, W., & Azen, S. P. (1983). Development of hand sensitivity test for the hypersensitive hand. *The American Journal of Occupational Therapy, 37* (3), 176–181.

30

Burns

Jessica Balland

OBJECTIVES

After reading this chapter, the student or the occupational therapy practitioner will be able to do the following:

1. List the functions of skin and identify changes caused by a burn injury.
2. List the treatment goals for the three phases of burn wound healing.
3. Discuss the value of elevated, antigravity positioning for the burn client and give one example.
4. Discuss scar management and give one example of a technique used to prevent or minimize scarring.
5. Prioritize rehabilitation goals to achieve maximum recovery with the least cost to the client.
6. List two ways the occupational therapy practitioner prevents infection transfer.
7. Prioritize adaptations for function and list two reasons why such adaptations are discontinued early for burned survivors.
8. Discuss the benefits and challenges of using videogames and Wii to improve motivation for rehabilitation.
9. List two additional diagnoses that benefit from burn-style rehabilitation.

KEY TERMS

Skin
Epidermis
Dermis
Burn
Eschar
Extent of the burn
Percentage of the total body surface area (%TBSA)
Edema

Autograft
Split-thickness skin graft (STSG)
Full-thickness skin graft
Hypertrophic scar
Contracture
Wound maturation stage
Skin conditioning (moisturizing)
External vascular supports/compression garments

INTRODUCTION

The annual incidence of burn-related injuries in the United States is decreasing. Current estimates suggest that 500,000 burn clients are treated annually in the United States. Of these, more than 45,000 require hospitalization. Thirty-five hundred (3500) deaths occur from residential fires, and 500 result from other causes such as motor vehicle and aircraft crashes, contact with electricity, chemicals or hot liquids and substances, and other sources of burn or freezing injury (American Burn Association, 2007). Improvements in comprehensive burn rehabilitation continue (American Occupational Therapy Association, 2014; Atiyeh, Gunn, & Hayek, 2005; Ehde, Patterson, Wiechman, & Wilson, 2000). Recovery after a burn is a long and arduous process (Celis, Suman, Huang, Yen, & Herndon, 2004; Helm, 1993; Hoffman, Doctor, Patterson, Carrougher, & Ferness, 2000). Severely burned survivors experience a myriad of continuing medical, functional, and psychosocial problems. Nonetheless, those who want to return to the level of function they had before their injuries can anticipate recovery near that capacity (Lund & Browder, 1944; Sungur et al., 2006).

Beyond ensuring their clients' survival, burn care professionals use advanced medical and surgical techniques and focus on minimizing pain and maximizing motion, functional recovery, and quality of life after a burn.

Although this chapter is concerned mainly with thermal burns, the reader is advised that burn-style rehabilitation is also being applied to conditions such as toxic epidermal necrolysis (in which the skin dies after exposure to a toxin such as spider bite or infection) and necrotizing fasciitis (in which the deep fascia and connective tissue die after toxic exposure).

SKIN

The **skin** (Fakhry, Alexander, Smith, Meyer, & Peterson, 1995; Glass & Bruns, 2000; Holavanahalli et al., 2000) is the largest organ of the body and serves primarily as an environmental barrier. Skin is waterproof, protects from infection,

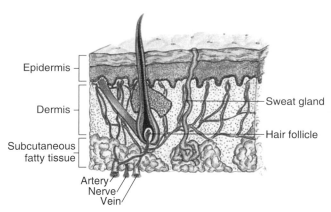

Fig. 30.1 Cross section of the skin. (From Potter PA, et al.: *Fundamentals of Nursing*, ed 10, 2021, Elsevier, St Louis.)

helps control body temperature, prevents fluid loss, provides vast sensory information, and contributes to identity.

Skin has two basic layers: the epidermis and the dermis (Fakhry et al., 1995; Glass & Bruns, 2000; Holavanahalli et al., 2000) (Fig. 30.1). The skin growth cells (germinal keratinocytes) are in the **epidermis**. The melanocytes (pigment or color-producing cells) are found at the dermoepidermal junction.

The **dermis** (Glass & Bruns, 2000) is composed of highly structured and organized collagen, wandering cells (white blood cells, macrophages, fibroblasts, endothelial cells), blood vessels, elastic fibers, and a gluelike substance of glycosaminoglycans (GAG) that is also known as ground substance. The dermis does not regenerate and heals by scar formation.

A **burn** is a permanent destruction of tissue caused by release of energy from an external agent. **Eschar**, pronounced "es-kar," is the dead epidermis and necrotic dermis that remain attached to the wound bed. Most thermal burns are of varying depths (Table 30.1).

When the skin is damaged, innumerable systemic, physiologic, and functional problems begin (Holavanahalli et al., 2000; Laubenthal et al., 1996; Neugebauer et al., 2008; Richard et al., 1996; Simons et al., 2003). The basis for safe burn treatment is detailed knowledge and understanding of normal skin anatomy, physiology, wound healing, and infection control; this expertise requires continuing study and research by all team members. With increasingly high levels of training in staff, hospital stay is reduced and outcomes improve in burn centers (Serghiou et al., 2007; Sheridan et al., 2000; Sungur et al., 2006). In the acute stage of a burn injury, the focus of all team members, including occupational therapists (OTs) and certified occupational therapy assistant (COTAs), is on assisting in the stabilization and survival of the client.

OBJECTIVE MEASURES OF BURN INJURY SEVERITY

Percentage of Total Body Surface Area Involved

The **extent of the burn** is classified as a **percentage of the total body surface area (%TBSA)** burned. Two methods used to estimate burn size are the rule of nines and the Lund and Browder chart (Leung et al., 1984). The rule of nines, developed in the 1940s by Pulaski and Tennison and communicated by word of mouth, divides the body surface into areas of 9%, with the perineum making up 1%. Although simple, the rule of nines is relatively inaccurate, especially for children (Fig. 30.2). The Lund and Browder chart (Leung et al., 1984) provides a more accurate estimate of %TBSA involved and is used in most burn centers.

Burn Depth

An accurate depth of burn is difficult to estimate. Assessment is based on experienced clinical observation of the appearance, sensitivity, and pliability of the wound (Esselman, Thombs, Magyar-Russell, & Fauerbach, 2006; Fakhry et al., 1995; Fricke, Omnell, Dutcher, Hollender, & Engrav, 1999). The burn is described as a superficial-, partial-, or full-thickness injury (see Table 30.1). For treatment planning, the team should remember that the wound is constantly changing and must be reassessed frequently (Iles, 1988; Parry et al., 2003).

Mechanism of Injury

Thermal injuries are caused by exposure to flames, steam, hot liquids, hot metals, electricity, radiation, toxic chemicals, or extreme cold. Heat injury accounts for most burns (American Burn Association, 2007; Sungur et al., 2006); about 75% of these accidents are preventable.

MEDICAL MANAGEMENT OF ACUTE BURN INJURIES

Acute Care

Burn injury causes extensive shifts of body fluids (Kowalske et al., 2003; Kurtz, 1999; Tredget et al., 2002; Yohannan et al., 2009). Fluids and electrolytes are replaced intravenously to prevent shock and death. This may result in severe **edema** (swelling). OTs and COTAs play a key role in edema management (see Chapter 29).

In circumferential full-thickness burns, the leathery eschar is inelastic, thus impairing normal circulation. Surgical intervention to improve circulation is an escharotomy (incision through destroyed skin) (American Occupational Therapy Association, 2014; Ehde et al., 2000). The procedure is usually painless because the nerve endings are destroyed in a full-thickness burn (Fig. 30.3).

Wound Care/Infection Control

A shower, shower cart hydrotherapy (SCH), submersion cleansing, or local cleansing of the wound and uninvolved areas is done on admission and, depending on dressings used, weekly or biweekly. Various topical agents are applied to reduce bacterial counts in the wounds. Since infection is a leading cause of burn-related complications, it is imperative that all staff observe universal infection control precautions according to the hospital's rules (see Chapter 3). All

TABLE 30.1 Depth of Injury Correlated With Anticipated Healing Time and Treatment Interventions

Injury Depth	Healing Time	Wound Outcome	Therapy Treatment Modalities
Superficial epidermis (first-degree burn)	1–5 days for spontaneous healing	No problems after healing	Elevation decreases limb pain. Wash wound to prevent infection. On healed wound, aloe or other moisturizer reduces dry skin and itching. Therapist rarely consulted.
Superficial dermis (superficial partial-thickness burn or second-degree burn)	14 days for spontaneous healing	Possible pigment (color) changes	Above, plus more careful wound care. Active elevated exercise to preserve joint function and improve wound circulation, especially venous return. Protective garments. Sunscreen. Acknowledge client's pain and inconvenience. Coordinate treatments with adequate analgesia.
Deep reticular dermis (deep partial-thickness burn or second-degree)	21 days[a] for spontaneous healing. (If grafted, see below.)	Probable pigment changes. Reduced skin durability. Severe scarring. Sensory changes. Sweating changes. Edema in dependent limbs, usually temporary	Above, plus: Therapists consulted by burn team. More frequent active elevated exercise. Elevated positioning or splints or both. Vascular support garments.[b] Healed areas may need inserts or silicone tapes to manage hypertrophic scars. Moisturization and lubrication to healed skin. Prolonged stretch to involved joints twice daily until contractures resolve. Daily living skills practice. Psychological therapy. Team collaboration to prevent stress disorder.
Subcutaneous tissue (full-thickness burn or third-degree burn)	Variable healing time. Graft needed or if small area, approximated wound edges with primary closure. Very large burn, cultured epithelial autograft (CEA)[c]	Same as above. Additional sweating loss. Possible loss of involved finger or toe nails. Possible additional sensory loss. No hair over grafts	Same as above plus: Postoperative positioning or immobilization. Initiate exercise despite pain, very slow weaning from analgesics and medications for stress. Vibration for itching. Additional education for skin precautions. Wear support/pressure garments and inserts and overlays to manage concave areas. Participate in peer support group. Early return to recreation and work, school, family, and community responsibilities.
Muscle, tendon, bone (fourth-degree burn, historic term, rarely used)	Healing time variable. Amputation or reconstructive surgery such as flaps needed[d]	Variable	Same as above plus: Deep tendon massage to prevent tethered skin. Adapted equipment. Prosthetic fitting and training if indicated. Additional counseling for stress. Watsu (water shiatsu) therapy for posttraumatic stress. Memory retraining. Participate in peer support group. Work retraining if unable to return safely to preburn employment.

[a]If surgeon grafts burn by 14 days, scar formation is reduced with improved functional outcome, less pain, and shortened length of hospital stay.
[b]Gradient pressure progressively decreases the rate of pressure applied by an elastic bandage or cylindrical pressure sleeve, keeping the most pressure on the distal limb and the least pressure around the proximal area of the extremity.
[c]Areas of cultured epithelial autograft (CEA) show permanent fragility; loss of temperature control; dry, blister-prone skin with permanently changed sensation.
[d]Early amputation with closure using noninjured tissue shortens length of hospital stay, decreases pain and wound breakdown, improves prosthesis fit, and simplifies prosthesis use. However, wounds are rarely of single depth, through skin and muscle.

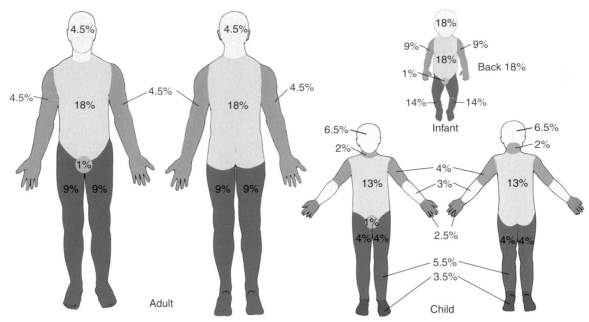

Fig. 30.2 Rule of nines. (From Elsevier Inc.: *ICD-10-CM/PCS Coding: Theory and Practice, 2019/2020 Edition*, 2019, Elsevier, St Louis.)

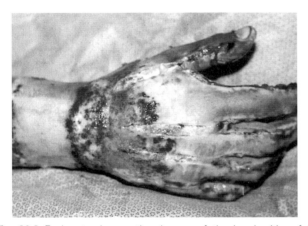

Fig. 30.3 Escharotomies on the dorsum of the hand with a full-thickness burn injury.

equipment, materials, and surfaces must be disinfected between client contacts. All family, staff, and visitors wash hands frequently and consistently.

Skin Grafting

Surgery decreases hospital length of stay, pain, and scar or contracture complications when the depth and extent of the wound will require 3 or more weeks for healing (Sheridan et al., 2000). With the client anesthetized, the surgeon excises (removes) the eschar, controls bleeding in the recipient area, and places an autograft. An **autograft** is a surgical transplantation of the person's own skin from an unburned area (donor site). The sheet or meshed (perforated evenly by machine) **split-thickness skin graft** (**STSG**) is applied to the clean excised wound (graft recipient site). As the size of a survivable burn increases, available donor sites for autograft decrease. For this reason, alternatives to autografts such as the cultured epidermal autograft (CEA), other cultured skin substitutes,

biologic dressings/temporary graft, or synthetic coverings are being explored (American Burn Association, 2007; American Occupational Therapy Association, 2014; Ehde et al., 2000). When the wound is limited in size but the defect is so deep that tendon survival or graft adherence is extremely doubtful, a plastic surgeon covers the area with a microvascular skin flap autograft. Because a **full-thickness skin graft** requires donor wound closure by an STSG or by edge-to-edge closure, it is usually reserved for reconstruction.

Pain

Pain (de Lateur, Magyar-Russell, Bresnick, Bernier, & Ober, 2007; Ferguson, Franco, Pollack, Rumbolo, & Smock, 2010; Neugebauer et al., 2008) is defined as an unpleasant sensory and emotional response to a stimulus associated with actual or potential tissue damage (Neugebauer et al., 2008). The amount of pain experienced by each client is unpredictable and varied; it is influenced by burn depth and location, client age, gender, ethnicity, education, occupation, history of drug or alcohol abuse, and psychiatric illness. A burn medication protocol includes long-acting narcotics for background pain, short-acting drugs for procedural pain, and medications to decrease anxiety. Procedural pain occurs during activities such as wound cleansing, dressing changes, or therapy (Baker, Russell, Meyer, & Blakeney, 2007; Falkel, 1994; Parry et al., 2003). Occupational therapy treatment will be more effective and better tolerated by the client if scheduled when pain medications are at peak effectiveness. As the wound heals, a client gradually decreases the dosage and frequency of drugs and usually requires minimal pain medications after wound closure.

Scar Formation

A **hypertrophic scar** is a hard, red, collagenous bundle of connective tissue raised above the surface of the burn wound (Atiyeh et al., 2005; Fricke et al., 1999; Kurtz, 1999;

TABLE 30.2 Antideformity Positioning, Equipment, and Techniques

Body Area	Antideformity Position	Equipment/Technique
Mouth	Varied	Regular food (i.e., not cut into small pieces), straw for thick liquids, exercise, microstomia splint
Ears/face	Positions that prevent pressure	No pillows, ear protection headgear, cutout cushions in airbed, head of bed elevated to decrease edema and risk of aspiration
Neck	Neutral/slight extension	No pillow (or neck extended by foam wedge), elevation and head cutout airflow or bead bed, foam neck splint conformer, multiple rings of plastic tubing collar (sometimes called *watsu*, or water shiatsu), triple component neck splint
Chest/abdomen	Trunk extension, shoulder retraction	Head of bed lowered, towel roll beneath spine, clavicle straps
Axilla	Shoulder abduction 90–100 degrees	Arm boards, foam wedges, overhead traction slings, axillary total contact splint, clavicle straps, overhead wheeled walker
Elbow/forearm	10 degrees short of full elbow extension, forearm neutral	Foam wedge pillows, arm boards, conformer splints, dynamic splints
Wrist/hand	Wrist extension 30 degrees, thumb abducted and extended, MCP flexion 50–70 degrees, IP extension	Elevation above heart with pillows or foam wedges when lying down or sitting; suspension slings, deltoid aid, overhead bar on wheeled walker with overhead bar for walking
Hip/thigh	Neutral extension, hips abducted 10–15 degrees	Bed elevation changed for prone/side-lying positions, trochanter rolls, pillow between knees, wedges to abduct hips
Knee/lower leg	Knee extension for circumferential burn, slight flexion for anterior burn	Foot of bed positioned to elevate feet when sitting in bed, knee conformer, casts, dynamic splints, knee extension with feet elevated when sitting, normal gait when walking
Ankle/foot	Neutral or 0–5 degrees dorsiflexion	Cutout heel cushions, airflow bed with foot cushion, custom splint, cast, AFO, pillow under calf to prevent pressure on heels, footstool elevation when sitting, heel-to-toe motion when walking, slow normal to large step gait during ambulation

Note: All positioning must be varied throughout 24 hours. Any position held for many days can result in contractures. *AFO*, Ankle-foot orthosis; *IP*, interphalangeal; *MCP*, metacarpophalangeal.

Leslie et al., 1996). Initially, healed burn wounds usually appear red and flat. Hypertrophic scars commonly become visible 6 to 8 weeks after wound closure. The functional or cosmetic significance of hypertrophic scars varies with the anatomic location of the wound. Race, age, and the location and depth of the burn wound have been reported to influence hypertrophic scarring (Kurtz, 1999; Leslie et al., 1996; Schneider et al., 2008; Supple, 2010).

Contracture Development

Normal wound healing occurs by contraction of the edges of the wound into one another to close it (American Occupational Therapy Association, 2014; Schneider et al., 2008). This mechanism of healing is compounded by the fact that the position of comfort for someone recovering from a severe burn is one that reinforces contractures. Clients who have been severely burned feel more comfortable when positioned with both the lower and upper extremities flexed and adducted. Without active stretching of the healing wound, the new collagen fibers in the wound will shorten, leading to **contracture** (Atiyeh et al., 2005; Blakeney, Moore, Meyer, Bishop, & Murphy, 1995; Fricke et al., 1999; Helm, 1993). A contracture is the limitation in joint range of motion (ROM) caused by shortened soft tissue, tendons, ligaments, blood vessels, and nerves or by calcium deposits surrounding the involved joint. See Table 30.2 for strategies to manage contractures and joint deformities.

Psychosocial Factors

During hospitalization, the client may experience fear, isolation, dependency, and pain. Potential psychological reactions include posttraumatic stress disorder (de Lateur et al., 2007), depression, withdrawal, reactions to disfigurement, regression, and anxiety and uncertainty about the ability to resume work, family, community, and leisure roles (Atiyeh et al., 2005; Bailes, Reder, & Burch, 2008; de Lateur et al., 2007; Helm, 1993). COTAs and OTs provide client education to facilitate the adjustment, coping, and self-direction needed for the client to resume participation in meaningful occupation.

Burn Rehabilitation

Team. The multidisciplinary burn care team consists of the client and family, physicians, nurses, physical therapists (Sheridan et al., 1999) and physical therapy assistants (Reeves, 2004), OTs (Sheridan et al., 1999), COTAs (Parry et al., 2003), dietitians, social workers, respiratory therapists, art and play therapists, massage therapists, recreational therapists (Helm, Herndon, & deLateur, 2007), personal clergy, case managers, visiting caregivers, chaplains, and vocational counselors. Nationally, team members available to the burn client vary widely (Bailes et al., 2008; Baker et al., 2007; Fricke et al., 1999; Reeves, 2004; Richard et al., 1996; Schneider et al., 2006). Specific role delineation varies with state licensure or certification regulations and with hospital or facility policies (Bailes et al., 2008; Baker et al., 2007; Esselman et al., 2006).

Phases of Recovery

Burn management can be divided into three overlapping phases: (1) acute care, (2) surgical and postoperative care, and (3) rehabilitation (inpatient and outpatient) (Reeves, 2004).

The acute care phase occurs in the first 72 hours after a major burn injury. If the wound is superficial, a person experiences only this phase.

The surgical and postoperative phase follows the acute phase. The risk of wound infection, sepsis, and septic shock are increased in this phase. Infection control is paramount.

The final phase is the postgrafting or wound maturation period when the client is medically stable. This phase may occur on an inpatient or an outpatient basis. Factors that affect outcomes of healing are the original depth and %TBSA of the burn, the quality of wound healing, type of scar formation, and effective team collaboration. The final phase is the longest, most rigorous, and most challenging for the clients, family, and staff. The COTA intervention will assist the client to increase independence in activities of daily living (ADL), increase engagement in meaningful occupations such as hobbies, manage adaptive equipment (such as compression garments), and increase endurance and ROM (through therapeutic exercise).

OCCUPATIONAL THERAPY PROCESS IN BURN REHABILITATION

OTs and COTAs collaborate with the interdisciplinary team to coordinate services so that clients with burns can benefit from the skills and viewpoints of all disciplines. In this setting, occupational therapy practitioners utilize knowledge of the complex interaction of the context and environment (such as hospital setting and infection control) with client factors (such as skin and medical status) and performance skills (such as ability to move) to facilitate independence in performance of meaningful occupations, such as ADL and instrumental activities of daily living (IADL) (American Occupational Therapy Association, 2014). The therapeutic approaches, energy, and creativity utilized during the process of occupational therapy service delivery provides valuable resources to the burned client and the family. Table 30.3 lists examples of intervention strategies for each stage of recovery.

The COTA plays a role on the team at a burn center where recovering clients with burns, who may have received skin grafts, receive rehabilitation. The goal of treatment is to have them return home to resume work, school, and community roles. The COTA, in collaboration with the OT, may provide inpatient and outpatient services focusing on ADL, IADL, and therapeutic exercise and activities.

ASSESSMENT OF OCCUPATIONAL PERFORMANCE

Occupational Profile

The assessment process should be initiated within 24 to 48 hours of admission to the facility (Kurakazu & Hirai, 2018). As always, it begins with the gathering of the occupational profile, which can be completed through an informal interview or a standardized assessment (American Occupational Therapy Association, 2014). In addition, a chart review

TABLE 30.3	Interventions at Each Stage of Burn Rehabilitation		
Burn Intervention	**Phase of Treatment**	**Goal of Intervention**	**Methods**
Therapeutic Exercise	Acute Care Postoperative Phase	Edema management Increase in AROM Prevention of contracture Endurance	PROM AROM Graded progressive exercise BTE Technologies Biodex (Figs. 30.7, 30.8, 30.9) Work simulator
Positioning	Acute Care Postoperative	Edema management Immobilization in antideformity position	Elevation (Fig. 30.4) Maintenance of grafts
Orthotics	Acute Care	Prevention of contracture	Volar wrist immobilization (Fig. 30.5) • 30 degrees wrist extension • 50–70 degrees of MCP flexion • Full extension of IP, PIP, DIP joints
ADL and IADL	Postacute	Increasing independence in self-care Activity tolerance	Bathing Dressing Light housekeeping Play (Fig. 30.10)

ADL, Activities of daily living; *AROM,* active range of motion; *DIP,* distal interphalangeal; *IADL,* independent activities of daily living; *IP,* interphalangeal; *MCP,* metacarpophalangeal; *PIP,* proximal interphalangeal; *PROM,* passive range of motion.

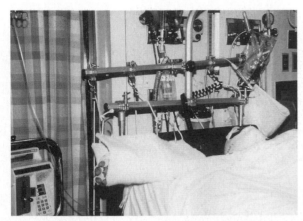

Fig. 30.4 Supine shoulder positioning using overhead traction and felt slings.

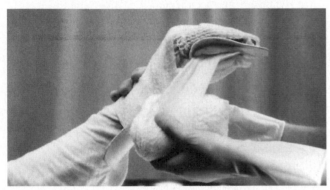

Fig. 30.5 Postburn hand splint. Note wrapping approach for the thumb.

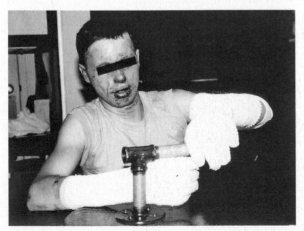

Fig. 30.6 A commonly used pipe tree is a good activity for hand exercise after a burn injury.

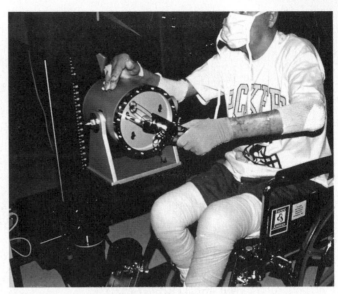

Fig. 30.7 A presized intermediate glove is worn all the time, including during exercise and activity, to condition the skin and control edema. BTE Technologies (www.btetech.com) provides work simulation. Note elastic wraps to legs, toe to groin, bilaterally.

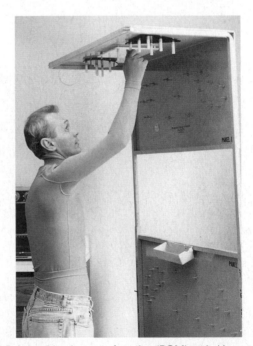

Fig. 30.8 A combined range of motion (ROM) and skin-conditioning activity. Use of the Valpar whole body ROM for upper extremity exercise while wearing compression garments.

nication, or family interviews, may be necessary to gather the most comprehensive interview possible.

Assessment of Client Factors

This portion of the evaluation can be done by the OT with input from the COTA. The burn wounds should be examined to determine the extent and depth of injury and critical

should be completed to gain information on burn etiology, medical history, secondary diagnoses, and precautions. If the client has injuries resulting in dependency on a ventilator or alterations on consciousness, alternative methods of commu-

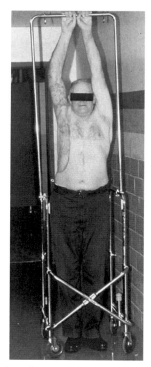

Fig. 30.9 Wheeled walker equipped with an overhead bar helps client stretch axillary contracture during ambulation.

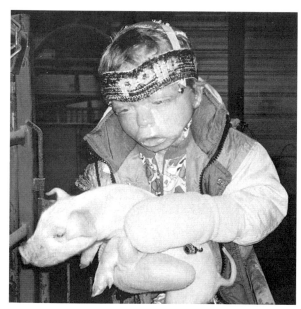

Fig. 30.10 Mittens, layered clothing, and scarves protect child doing winter chores from frostbite.

areas involved. In addition, factors such as edema, sensation, ROM, coordination, hand dominance, and cognition should be assessed (Kurakazu & Hirai, 2018). Client factors such as spiritual and cultural values and psychological factors should be considered with the goal of facilitating resumption of meaningful occupation to the maximal extent possible (Kurakazu & Hirai, 2018). See Table 30.1 for summary of outcomes expected for burn survivors.

Intervention Process

As previously mentioned, the focus of rehabilitation in the acute care phase is to support the medical management and survival of the client, while preventing or limiting client factors that will lead to poor outcomes, such as infection or contracture. OTs and COTAs provide positioning, therapeutic exercise and occupations to manage edema, promote healing, and facilitate activity tolerance, all within the limits set by physician orders. For example, the COTA may adapt self-care activities, such as grooming, to be done at bed level to

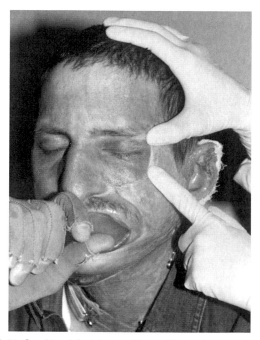

Fig. 30.11 Combined facial stretching with hand strengthening. A client wearing an Isotoner glove for hand edema uses a syringe case to stretch the left cheek pouch while an OTA stretches the facial contracture band. Note the neck splint.

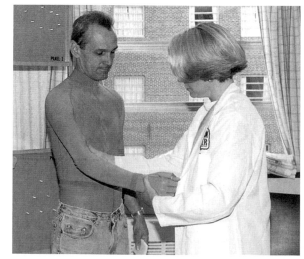

Fig. 30.12 Assess the fit of custom-made compression garments frequently to ensure adequate compression for scar management.

facilitate tolerance of upright sitting posture and encourage the client to move out of positions of deformity and comfort.

In the surgical and postoperative phases, OTs and COTAs provide interventions to facilitate independence in ADL and IADL that promote adherence to postoperative precautions. For example, if a skin graft was completed, ADL must be completed in a way that does not endanger the graft. This may involve adapting the task or utilizing adaptive equipment, such as a dressing stick. This would avoid movement that may stretch skin beyond tolerance of wound boundaries because the graft area is often immobilized after surgery. The preferred position and length of immobilization vary by physician preference and burn center protocol; however, the area is usually immobilized in extension for 1 to 7 days (Richard et al., 1996; Richard et al., 2009).

In the **wound maturation stage** (postgrafting), wound closure begins and continues to full healing. A mature wound is soft, flat, durable, and supple. The color will closely match the client's healthy skin. Time from grafting to maturation varies, but can occur between a few months and 2 years

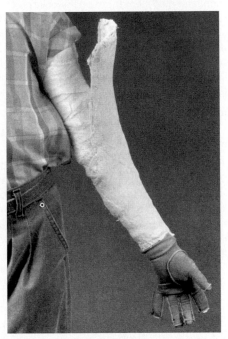

Fig. 30.15 Treatment of elbow scar contracture with a serial fall-out elbow cast applied at maximum elbow extension at night blocks flexion and allows full, painless extension by morning when the cast is removed. After several weeks, contracture does not reform and the cast is discontinued.

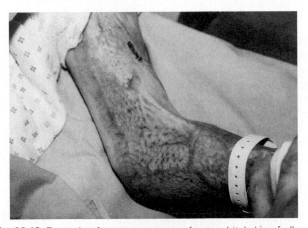

Fig. 30.13 Example of scar contracture of antecubital skin of elbow. Note taut, shortened skin when elbow is extended.

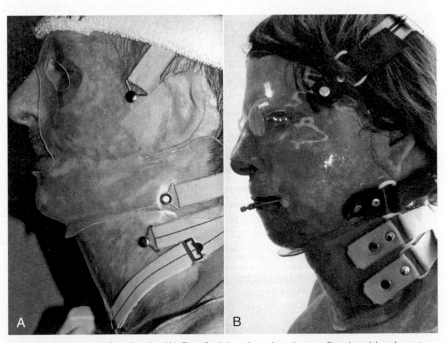

Fig. 30.14 Transparent facial orthosis and neck orthosis. (A) Day facial and neck orthoses fitted to blanch or turn raised scar tissue white. (B) Night face and neck orthoses with humidity domes for eyes and microstomia prevention appliance for mouth stretch.

CASE STUDY

Jacy is a 36-year-old, right hand–dominant, college-educated man of Native American heritage. He is recently married to Halona, his wife. Jacy believes in the use of healing stones as an alternative or adjunct to Western medicine. He is employed full time at an airline. Jacy and Halona both receive insurance coverage from his job. His job duties include drafting, computer design, and management of onsite building construction. Halona is employed full time as a laboratory technician at a local hospital. His family's financial well-being is dependent on him returning to work. Both Jacy's and Halona's incomes are needed to meet financial obligations, such as mortgage payments and new home remodeling. Jacy enjoys watching sports, riding his motorcycle, and completing home repairs and renovations.

Jacy sustained partial- and full-thickness burns on his right face, neck, chest, axillary folds, arm, and hand. The burns cover 20% of his total body surface area (TBSA). The injury occurred when a carburetor he was examining backfired causing his clothes to catch fire. Jacy was hospitalized for 21 days. During that time, he received STSG meshed skin grafts to his right hand and STSG sheet grafts to his face.

Occupational Therapy Process

Acute Care Phase	Current Status	Short-Term (1-Week) Goals (Including Education)
Upper extremity (UE), lower extremity (LE), face, trunk function Range of motion (ROM) Strength Sensation Mobility	ROM—eyelids do not close when asleep Mouth has increased from small to medium size microstomia prevention appliance (MPA) Shoulder flexion and abduction limited to 0–150 degrees; elbow flexion limited to 10–90 degrees Right wrist extension decreased—unable to extend wrist actively past neutral, approximately 20-degree wrist extension after 20 minutes of prolonged stretch Supination limited to 20 degrees actively and 60 degrees passively bilaterally Hand function—active ROM: metacarpophalangeals (MCPs) 0–45 degrees, proximal interphalangeals (PIPs) 15–30 degrees, distal interphalangeal (DIP) 0 degrees Unwilling to do prolonged stretch independently because of pain and medication sleepiness When cued, does relaxation breathing before exercise Increased sensitivity to touch and cocontraction from pain in past week Distraction from pain, irritation from nasogastric feeding tube, coughing up secretions Needs cueing for each exercise Since off ventilator, ambulates to chair independently and forgets tall walker Good functional strength	Close eyelids tightly three to five times each hour from 6 AM to 11 PM to elongate contracting upper and lower lids, so he avoids corneal scratches or edema, keeps the ability to see, read, and do vocational and avocational activities. Increase mouth stretches to 6 cc tube by next week so that he can eat normal foods and safely be intubated for general anesthesia. Improve wound healing by keeping right UE flexible and participating more vigorously in active ROM in all joints burned within limits of pain, endotracheal tube, and intravenous lines to improve wound healing and assist return to work activities. Four times daily, reach for bed traction bar above head with both hands, hold stretch, count to 15, exaggerate extension to prepare for self-feeding. As soon as vent discontinued, use Baltimore Therapeutic Equipment in rehabilitation clinic and soft foam gripper increasing to rubber band exerciser when IPs closed so that he can use hands for driving. Remember to use overhead walker for ambulating. Learn quad sets and ankle pumps to use when grafted. Discuss pain and distraction with surgeon and psychologist, use recommendations, and share information with therapist.
Positioning and edema management Foam wedge Traction	Positioning—no head pillow because of face and neck burns, elevated head off bed; shoulders at 90 degrees forward flexion in chair, at 90-degree abduction in bed (using bedside table to support end of wedge); elbow extension; forearm in neutral; hands slightly elevated Pillow behind neck when in chair to allow neck extension when sitting	Keep injured areas elevated. Use wedges or airplane bed attachment at all times. Change position every 2 hours when awake by elevating head of bed, flexing knees, turning, and when off vent dangling; sitting, standing, or walking. Be able to state importance of using tall walker for edema control when ambulating. Beginning middle of week, when off vent, independently direct elevation and move furniture to achieve elevated positioning for arms and, if needed, legs. Review positioning with OTA each afternoon.
Orthotics	Wears large or extra-large MPA	Keep MPA in mouth all night and loosen (not remove) to avoid discomfort of insertion and removal. Change to wearing 5–30 minutes of each waking hour as soon as tolerated.

(Continued)

Occupational Therapy Process—cont'd

Acute Care Phase	Current Status	Short-Term (1-Week) Goals (Including Education)
Splints	Uses Exu-Dry pad or equivalent neck dressing to improve neck contours	
Casts		
Support garments	Wears wrist-hand-finger orthosis in IP extension, MP flexion, wrist 30-degree extension, thumb abduction/flexion secured with Kerlix coarse mesh gauze wrap at bedtime Wears elastic wraps on legs during day	Remember to ask for wrist-hand-finger orthosis at bedtime. Remove leg elastic wraps at bedtime as soon as tolerated.
Daily living skills (evaluation done by OTA and OT)	Unable to pick up anything because of open fingertips Uses elastic wrap or tape on comb, toothbrush, fiber pen, spoon and fork for eating because of hand edema Needs assistance bathing Cannot apply lotion to dry lips before eating or moisturize healed areas yet Can remove elastic wraps with help Cannot don own clothing because of too much wound drainage, tube feeding supplements, and gas pains causing clothing to be temporarily too tight around waist	Operate nurse call button with foot or arm by middle of week. Independently eat, brush teeth, comb hair, sign forms, and clean glasses by end of week using gross grasp. Family will bring large jogging shorts and shirt. Slip-on shoes after grafting.
Client and family involvement with therapy	Given outpatient instruction book for education in anticipated course of wound, graft, and donor healing Home therapy program and education reviewed with wife and parents on several occasions Written exercise program being followed by client—still needs maximum help from therapist at this point, facial and hand edema interfere, groggy from medications, and does not remember exercises from one session to the other Works with vigor and is cooperative during therapy sessions when analgesia effective Wears healing stones	Family will begin to learn active ROM exercise program for face, neck, UEs and follow through in the evening with client. Work on memory, negotiation, and teamwork during therapy. Take responsibility to inform others of desires and wishes. Family will follow through with client's independent exercises and therapy program. Change Velcro healing stone pocket as needed.
Equipment		Use foam wedge, overhead walker, foam tape, and large handles temporarily for utensils.

Follow-Up Intervention

In the outpatient phase, the treatment plan is updated and the face orthotic is refitted. These appointments occur every 2 weeks for a minimum of 2 months. At that point, the scar formation is well managed, and visits are scheduled one time per month. Jacy is discharged from all therapy once scar maturation occurs.

(in children it can take up to 5 years) (Richard & Ward, 2005; Ricks & Meager, 1992). At this point, external life support and monitoring tubes have likely been discontinued since the client is now medically stable.

Throughout all stages of rehabilitation, the focus of occupational therapy intervention is on maximizing independence and minimizing deformity and contractures (Harris & Harris, 1999). For example, a plastic face mask or neck splint may be used to stretch facial and neck muscles, minimize neck flexion contractures, and soften scars. Intervention may also focus on client and family education, to empower the maintenance of precautions and implementation of healthy habits that facilitate healing (Field, Peck, Hernandez-Reif, Krugman, & Burman, 2000; Johnson, 1994; Leslie et al., 1996; Manning, 2002; Richard et al., 2009; Ricks & Meager, 1992; Suman & Herndon, 2007). The intervention plan is continuously updated as the client gains skills and prepares for discharge to the next level of care, likely to home.

The focus of intervention in outpatient rehabilitation is restoration of motivating habits and routines that will boost self-confidence, encourage social interaction, and assist in resumption of roles and routines (such as a parent, student, or employee). In addition, this stage includes follow-up visits to the physician and fittings for orthotics and compressive garments (if applicable). After discharge from an inpatient setting, the client resumes function in a way that will preserve grafts and not damage delicately healed wounds. The client will be able to independently don and remove vascular supports and complete self-care, including bathing, **skin conditioning (moisturizing)**, and wound care, with minimal assistance.

At this stage, clients have likely recovered at least 80% of their previous active range of motion (AROM) and strength. They are likely able to tolerate prolonged stretching, to prevent further contractures and joint deterioration. This allows functional use of the upper and lower extremities to facilitate full participation in home and community occupations.

They have likely developed enough endurance to perform at least 2 hours of work-equivalent activity and 8 hours of IADL, such as light housekeeping or meal preparation. The goal of intervention will be for them to recover sufficient coordination, ROM, and endurance to be independent in all ADL and IADL without the need for activity modification (such as use of adaptive equipment) (Figs. 30.6 to 30.8.).

Clients should be able to independently complete long-term management and care of postburn body structures, such as grafted skin and damaged vascular structures. This may include edema management, infection control (to prevent cellulitis), prosthetic and orthotic use (overlays and compression garments for scar management), sun protection (sunscreen clothing), and prevention of hypothermia.

If needed, clients will participate in coordinated planning for discharge from burn care and explore resources for resumption of vocational or educational roles (vocational rehabilitation or school counselor). They will become comfortable participating in valued occupations while wearing orthotics, **external vascular supports**, prosthetics, and/or **compression garments**. They will participate in hiring any needed personal care or homemaking assistants to resume occupational roles (Figs. 30.11, 30.12, 30.13, 30.14, and 30.15).

All of this takes place within the context of them learning to cope constructively with stress symptoms, changed body appearance, intimacy issues, and adjustment to disability. This may occur by them seeking assistance from supports, such as a psychologist, counselor, or family members. Finally, the OT and COTA will complete a home assessment to provide recommendations for any adaptive equipment, mobility aids, or home modifications needed to facilitate safety and independence.

SUMMARY

Advances in burn care continue to improve burn injury outcomes. Today, most clients recovering from a burn injury can expect to return to a life closely resembling that of before the burn. This will include early return to school or work. The American Burn Association (American Burn Association, 2007) (ABA) Guidelines for the Operation of Burn Centers do not specify a particular client-to-therapist ratio, only that there must be one full-time equivalent burn therapist (either an occupational or physical therapist) assigned to the burn center. The guidelines further specify that staffing must be based on client activity but do not specify ratios or acuity

considerations. Some burn centers have developed their own frequency of therapy guidelines (Baker et al., 2007).

The OT and COTA provide exercise, ADL, IADL, skin-conditioning activities, positioning techniques, splints, casts (American Burn Association, 2007), client education, vascular support, and compression garments. Reassessment of client needs and function throughout recovery promotes effective and economical treatment progression.

REVIEW QUESTIONS

1. What are the two layers of the skin?
2. Why may a client need temporary adaptations for self-care during the acute care phase?
3. What is the primary objective for positioning during acute care?
4. Why are clients immobilized postoperatively?
5. How soon after grafting can gentle, active ROM be resumed?
6. How soon after grafting should an intermediate garment or support dressing be applied?
7. Why are skin-conditioning activities used in burn rehabilitation? Name two examples of skin-conditioning techniques.
8. When a splint is ordered in the acute phase, what is the preferred wearing schedule? Why?
9. What is the primary cause of dysfunction after a burn injury?
10. Which points should be covered in a home program?
11. What are possible causes of limitations in ADL during the rehabilitation phase?
12. How does a client recover work skills?
13. Are splints always used during the rehabilitation care phase?
14. Name three interventions to prevent sunburn.
15. When should client education about burn injury and rehabilitation begin?

REFERENCES

American Burn Association. Burn care resources in North America; 2007. https://ameriburn.org/who-we-are/media/burn-incidence-fact-sheet/.

American Occupational Therapy Association. (2014). OT practice framework: domain & process (3rd ed.). *Am J Occup Ther*, 68(1) (Suppl. 1), S1–S48.

Atiyeh, B. S., Gunn, S. W., & Hayek, S. N. (2005). State of the art in burn treatment. *World Journal of Surgery*, 29, 131–148.

Bailes, A. F., Reder, R., & Burch, C. (2008). Development of guidelines for determining frequency of therapy services in a pediatric medical setting. *Pediatric Physical Therapy*, 20, 194–198.

Baker, C. P., Russell, W. J., Meyer, W., III, & Blakeney, P. (2007). Physical and psychologic rehabilitation outcomes for young adults burned as children. *Archives of Physical Medicine and Rehabilitation*, 88, S57–S64.

Blakeney, P., Moore, P., Meyer, W., III, Bishop, B., Murphy, L., et al. (1995). Efficacy of school reentry programs. *The Journal of Burn Care & Rehabilitation, 16*, 469–472.

Celis, M. M., Suman, O. E., Huang, T. T., Yen, P., & Herndon, D. N. (2004). Effect of a supervised exercise and physiotherapy program on surgical interventions in children with thermal injury. *The Journal of Burn Care & Rehabilitation, 24*, 57–61.

de Lateur, B. J., Magyar-Russell, G., Bresnick, M. G., Bernier, F. A., Ober, M. S., et al. (2007). Augmented exercise in the treatment of deconditioning from major burn injury. *Archives of Physical Medicine and Rehabilitation, 88*, S18–S23.

Ehde, D. M., Patterson, D. R., Wiechman, S. A., & Wilson, L. G. (2000). Post-traumatic stress symptoms and distress 1 year after burn injury. *The Journal of Burn Care & Rehabilitation, 21*(2), 105–111.

Esselman, P. C., Thombs, B. D., Magyar-Russell, G., & Fauerbach, J. A. (2006). Burn rehabilitation: state of the science. *American Journal of Physical Medicine & Rehabilitation, 85*, 383–413.

Fakhry, S. M., Alexander, J., Smith, D., Meyer, A. A., & Peterson, H. D. (1995). Regional and institutional variation in burn care. *The Journal of Burn Care & Rehabilitation, 16*, 86–90.

Falkel, J. E. (1994). Anatomy and physiology of the skin. In R. L. Richard, & M. J. Staley (Eds.), *Burn care and rehabilitation principles and practice*. Philadelphia, PA: FA Davis.

Ferguson, J. S., Franco, J., Pollack, J., Rumbolo, P., & Smock, M. (2010). Compression neuropathy: a late finding in the postburn population: a four-year institutional review. *Journal of Burn Care & Research, 31*(3), 458–461.

Field, T., Peck, M., II, Hernandez-Reif, M., Krugman, S., Burman, I., et al. (2000). Postburn itching, pain, and psychological symptoms are reduced with massage therapy. *The Journal of Burn Care & Rehabilitation, 21*(3), 189–193.

Fricke, N. B., Omnell, M. L., Dutcher, K. A., Hollender, L. G., & Engrav, L. H. (1999). Skeletal and dental disturbances in children after facial burns and pressure garment use: a 4-year follow-up. *The Journal of Burn Care & Rehabilitation, 20*(3), 239–249.

Glass, T. M., & Bruns, M. M. (2000). Exercises for pediatric burn therapy. San Antonio, TX: Therapy Skill Builders.

Harris, S., & Harris, J. (1999). *Permachart Quick Reference Guide. The skin.* Concord, Ontario: Papertech, Inc.

Helm, P., Herndon, D. N., & deLateur, B. (2007). Restoration of function. *Journal of Burn Care & Research: Official Publication of the American Burn Association, 28*, 611–614.

Helm, P. A. (1993). The status of burn rehabilitation services in the United States: results of a national survey. *The Journal of Burn Care & Rehabilitation, 13*(6), 656–662.

Hoffman, H. G., Doctor, J. N., Patterson, D. R., Carrougher, G. J., & Ferness, T. A., III (2000). Virtual reality as an adjunctive pain control during burn wound care in adolescent clients. *Pain, 85*(1-2), 305–309.

Holavanahalli, R., Cromes, G., Kowalske, K., & Helm, P. (2000). Factors predicting satisfaction with life over time in clients following a major burn injury. The Journal of Burn Care & Rehabilitation, 21, s139.

Iles, R. L. (1988). *Wound care: The skin.* Kansas City, MO: Marion Laboratories.

Johnson, C. (1994). Pathologic manifestations of burn injury. In R. L. Richard, & M. J. Staley (Eds.), *Burn care and rehabilitation principles and practice*. Philadelphia, PA: FA Davis.

Kowalske, K., Holavanahalli, R., Serghiou, M., Esselman, P., Ware, L., Delateur, B., & Helm, P. (2003). Contractures following burn injuries in children and adults—a multicenter report. *The Journal of Burn Care & Rehabilitation, 24*, S85.

Kurakazu, D., & Hirai, A. H. (2018). Burns and burn rehabilitation. In H. M. Pendelton, & W. Schultz-Krohn (Eds.), *Pedretti's occupational therapy: Practice skills for physical dysfunction* (8th ed.). St Louis, MO: Mosby.

Kurtz, L. (1999). Creating productivity standards. *OT Practice*, 26–30.

Laubenthal, K. N., Lewis, R. W., et al. (1996). Prospective randomized study of the effect of pressure garment therapy on pain and pruritus in the maturing burn wound. *American Burn Association, 28*, 161.

Leslie, G., et al. (1996). Native Americans: a challenge for the pediatric burn team (poster). *American Burn Association, 28*, 147.

Leung, K. S., Cheng, J. C., Ma, G. F., Clark, J. A., & Leung, P. C. (1984). Complications of pressure therapy for post-burn hypertrophic scars: biochemical analysis based on 5 clients. *Burns, 10*(6), 434–438.

Lund, C., & Browder, N. (1944). The estimation of area of burns. *Surg Gynecol Obstetr, 79*, 352–355.

Manning, G. (2002). *Love, Greg & Lauren.* New York, NY: Bantam Books.

Neugebauer, C. T., Serghiou, M., Herndon, D., & Suman, O. E. (2008). Effects of a 12-week rehabilitation program with music and exercise groups on range of motion in young children with severe burns. *Journal of Burn Care & Research, 29*(6), 939–948.

Parry, I. S., Doyle, B., Mollineaux, C., Palmieri, T. L., & Greenhalgh, D. G. (2003). Foot drop in children with burn injury. *The Journal of Burn Care & Rehabilitation, 24*, S100.

Reeves, S. U. (2004). Adaptive strategies after severe burns. In C. H. Christiansen, & K. M. Matuska (Eds.), *Ways of living: Adaptive strategies for special needs* (3rd ed.). Bethesda, MD: AOTA Press.

Richard, R., Baryza, M. J., Carr, J. A., Dewey, W. S., Dougherty, M. E., et al. (2009). Burn rehabilitation and research: proceedings of a consensus summit. *Journal of Burn Care & Research, 30*(4), 543–573.

Richard, R., et al. (1996). Algorithm to guide burn client treatment by physical therapist assistants (PTAs). *American Burn Association, 28*, 160.

Richard, R., & Ward, R. S. (2005). Splinting strategies and controversies. *The Journal of Burn Care & Rehabilitation, 26*, 392–396.

Ricks, N., & Meager, D. (1992). The benefits of plaster casting for lower extremity burns after grafting in children. *The Journal of Burn Care & Rehabilitation, 13*(4), 465–468.

Schneider, J. C., Holavanahalli, R., Helm, P., Goldstein, R., & Kowalske, K. (2006). Contractures in burn injury: defining the problem. *Journal of Burn Care & Research, 27*(4), 508–514.

Schneider, J. C., Holavanahalli, R., Helm, P., O'Neil, C., Goldstein, R., et al. (2008). Contractures in burn injury part II: investigating joints of the hand. *Journal of Burn Care & Research, 29*(4), 606–613.

Serghiou, M., Ott, S., Farmer, S., Morgan, D., Gibson, P., & Suman, O. (2007). *Comprehensive rehabilitation of the burned client.* In: D. Herndon (Ed.) *Total burn care* (3rd ed., pp. 620–651). Philadelphia, PA: Elsevier.

Sheridan, R., Hinson, M. I., Liang, M. H., Nackel, A. F., Schoenfeld, D. A., et al. (2000). Long-term outcome of children surviving massive burns. *JAMA: the Journal of the American Medical Association, 283*(1), 69–73.

Sheridan, R., Weber, J., Prelack, K., Petras, L., Lydon, M., et al. (1999). Early burn center transfer shortens the length of hospitalization and reduces complications in children with serious burn injuries. *The Journal of Burn Care & Rehabilitation, 20* (5), 347–350.

Simons, M., King, S., & Edgar, D. (2003). Occupational therapy and physiotherapy for the client with burns: principles and management guidelines. *The Journal of Burn Care & Rehabilitation, 24*(5), 323–335.

Suman, O. E., & Herndon, D. N. (2007). Effects of cessation of a structured and supervised exercise conditioning program on lean mass and muscle strength in severely burned children. *Archives of Physical Medicine and Rehabilitation, 88*(12 Suppl. 2), S24–S29.

Sungur, N., Ulusoy, M. G., Boyacgi, S., Ortaparmak, H., Akyuz, M., et al. (2006). Kirschner-wire fixation for postburn flexion contracture deformity and consequences on articular surface. *Annals of Plastic Surgery, 56*(2), 128–132.

Supple, K. G. (2010). Handle with care. *Advance Physical Therapy Rehabilitation Medicine, 16*(23), 60–63.

Tredget, E., Anzarut, A., Shankowsky, H., & Logsetty, S. (2002). Outcome and quality of life of massive burn injury: the impact of modern burn care. *The Journal of Burn Care & Rehabilitation, 23*, S95.

Yohannan, S. K., & Schwabe, E., Sauro, G., & Kwon, R. (2009). The Wii gaming system for rehabilitation of an adult with lower extremity burns: a case report. Proceedings from the 2009 American Burn Association. *The Journal of Burn Care & Rehabilitation, 43*:S65.

RESOURCES FOR CUSTOM-MADE GARMENTS

Barton Carey

P.O. Box 421

Perrysburg, OH 43552

(800) 421-0444

Bio-Concepts

2424 E. University Dr.

Phoenix, AZ 85034

(800) 421-5647

RESOURCES FOR OVERLAY AND INSERT MATERIALS

Liquid Silicone

Any splint supply catalog

Silon Woundcare Products

Bio Med Sciences

7584 Morris Court, Suite 218

Allentown, PA 18106

(800) 257-4566

INTERNET WEBSITES AND BLOGS

http://www.burntherapist.com/QuarterlySplints.htm

www.healthgamesresearch.org (Robert Wood Johnson Foundation, Pioneer Portfolio)

www.humanagames.com

www.games4rehab.com

http://www.wiihabilitation.org/

www.wiihabilitation.co.uk/resources.shtml

31

Amputation and Prosthetics

Kyle Borges

OBJECTIVES

After reading this chapter, the student or the occupational therapy practitioner will be able to do the following:

1. Appreciate the role of occupational therapy within the context of the rehabilitation team.
2. Understand the relationship between levels of amputation and the function of the client.
3. Appreciate the importance of maximizing the client's skill with prosthetics.
4. Understand why recovery can be slow and physically draining for the patient and family.
5. Teach new methods for basic and advanced activities of daily living with prosthetics.

KEY TERMS

Transhumeral amputation
Transradial amputation
Cosmesis
Socket
Phantom pain
Body-powered prosthesis
External-powered (myoelectric) prosthesis
Terminal device (TD)
Early postoperative prosthesis

Transfemoral amputation
Transtibial amputation
Syme amputation
Rigid removal dressing
SACH foot
Pylon
C-leg
Ischial weight-bearing prosthesis

INTRODUCTION

The vast majority of people who undergo amputations do not know what to expect when they come to the medical center. This traumatic crisis will affect both the family and the patient. A successful rehabilitation program requires the coordinated efforts of the rehabilitation team. These efforts include teamwork, surgical management, preprosthetic training, pain management, psychological support, and training in the use of both body-powered and myoelectric prostheses. Throughout the occupational therapy treatment process, an ongoing collaboration between the occupational therapist (OT) and occupational therapy assistant (OTA) occurs.

Amputation or loss of limb occurs congenitally or as a result of trauma or disease (Larson & Gould, 2020). Congenital amputation is the absence of a limb or part at birth (O'Sullivan, Cullen, & Schmitz, 2020). Acquired amputation is the loss of part or all of an extremity resulting from trauma or surgery (Larson & Gould, 2020). The focus of this chapter will be on upper extremity (UE) and lower extremity (LE) amputations sustained in adulthood. Acquired amputations result from surgery and trauma (Stoner, 2020). Surgical amputations of both UEs and LEs are performed in cases of severe infections or gangrene, to remove cancerous tumors, and in cases of severe injury in which extremities are not salvageable.

The rehabilitation of the individual with limb loss requires a team approach. The skills of many health care professionals contribute to a successful team. These include a general or vascular surgeon, orthopedic surgeon, plastic surgeon, physiatrist, prosthetist, OT, OTA, physical therapist, social worker, psychologist, pastoral counselor (spiritual guidance), and vocational counselor. Occupational therapy intervention before surgery emphasizes psychological support, education on prosthetic options available, training for the postoperative exercise program, and introduction to one-handed survival techniques for activities of daily living (ADL).

UPPER LIMB AMPUTATIONS

Causes and Incidences of Amputations

In 2005, 1.6 million persons were living with the loss of a limb in the United States. It is estimated that by 2050, 3.6 million people will have undergone limb amputation. Annual hospital costs for those who undergo amputations are $4 billion (Pedretti & Pasquinelli, 2020). Thirty-eight percent of all amputations are due to diabetes-related disease of the vascular system. Lower limb amputations are most commonly due to vascular disease. Eighty-two percent are related to diabetes or peripheral vascular disease, especially in those over age 60 (DiDomenico, 2020; Dillingham, Pezzin, & MacKenzie, 2002). African American men experience the highest rates of amputation due to vascular disease (Dillingham et al., 2002). Prevention of diabetes-related vascular disease could reduce the number of amputations by 10% (225,000 individuals) (Wright, 2020).

Upper limb amputations most often result from trauma following motor vehicle accidents (MVAs), work-related injuries, recreational injuries, tumors, burns, electrical injuries, and war injuries. Rates for trauma-related and cancer-related amputation declined by approximately 50% in the 20 years from 1984 to 2004 (National Limb Loss Information Center, 2005).

UPPER LIMB AMPUTATIONS

Classification of Upper Amputation Levels

Levels of amputations of the UE are illustrated in Fig. 31.1. Although some individuals may still refer to limb loss as "above elbow" and "below elbow," the current terms utilized are **transhumeral** and **transradial**. These terms more accurately indicate the bone transected by the surgery.

Amputation level significantly affects function. The higher (more proximal) the level of amputation, the greater the functional loss and the more the client must depend on the prosthesis for function and **cosmesis** (appearance). Higher-level amputations require more complex and extensive prostheses and prosthetic training.

Shoulder forequarter and shoulder disarticulation (SD) amputations result in the loss of all arm and hand functions.

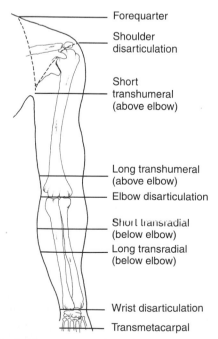

Forequarter

Shoulder disarticulation

Short transhumeral (above elbow)

Long transhumeral (above elbow)

Elbow disarticulation

Short transradial (below elbow)

Long transradial (below elbow)

Wrist disarticulation

Transmetacarpal

Fig. 31.1 Levels of upper extremity amputation.

Short transhumeral amputation will result in the loss of all hand, wrist, and elbow functions, as well as the loss of shoulder rotation. Long transhumeral and elbow disarticulation amputations will result in the loss of hand, wrist, and elbow functions while preserving shoulder function.

Short transradial amputations result in loss of hand and wrist function, forearm pronation and supination, and reduction in the force of elbow flexion. Shoulder function remains in most. Long transradial amputations result in the loss of hand and wrist function and most forearm pronation and supination. Elbow function and force of elbow flexion will be good. The wrist disarticulation will result in complete loss of hand and wrist function; pronation and supination remain unaffected.

Transmetacarpal or partial hand amputations occur across the metacarpal bones. Functions of all the unaffected joints remain intact. The level of hand function available depends on whether the thumb was amputated or left (Bucchieri, Poole, & Schmidt, 2020). A variety of custom made prostheses are available for each level of amputation.

Surgical Management

The primary goal of surgical amputation is to preserve the length of the residual limb to improve prosthetic suspension and force transmission from the residual limb to the **socket**. Surgical procedures include the beveling distal bones, transaction of the nerves (which are allowed to retract into proximal soft tissues to prevent adherence to the scar or prosthetic trauma), appropriate myofascial closure of muscle, myodesis (suturing appropriate underlying muscle to bone), and appropriate placement of skin incision line(s). This avoids skin breakdown over bony prominences and skin adherence to the underlying bone (Friedman, 2020b). Effective surgical management results in a well-shaped residual limb that can be fitted with a prosthesis allowing for maximal prosthetic function. During and after medical and surgical interventions, team members try to facilitate the psychosocial adjustment of the patient and family members.

Postoperative Management

A surgical amputation without complications usually results in an acute care stay of 3 to 4 days. Within these several days, therapists make initial contact and begin preprosthetic training. This includes preparing the residual limb to utilize a prosthesis and offering emotional and psychological support, all to achieve maximal independence in ADL.

Postoperative Complications

Complications following amputation surgery can occur in multiple body systems. These include neuromas (nervous system), contractures (musculoskeletal system), and skin breakdown (integumentary system). In addition, pain management is important for clients experiencing hypersensitivity and phantom limb phenomena.

Neuromas may occur in upper and lower limbs after amputation. A neuroma is a bulbous benign tumor that may develop at the proximal end of a severed nerve. It is generally made up of nerve fibers and Schwann cells. Treatment may include surgical excision and/or modification of the prosthetic sock (Pedretti & Pasquinelli, 2020).

Contractures of ligaments and muscles, which would otherwise allow for good motion of a joint, is another risk factor following amputation. They most often occur in the joint above the amputation if full range of motion (ROM) is not initiated postoperatively and if the client rests the extremity in a flexed position for comfort. Contractures interfere with prosthetic fitting and training due to significant joint stiffness and loss of ROM.

Prolonged muscle inactivity leads to weakness. Therefore postoperative treatment includes early out of bed mobility. Prolonged immobility and bed rest following an amputation will lead to longer recovery time and an increase risk of complications.

Skin breakdown is most often caused by uneven pressure on the residual limb. Other causes include poor blood supply to and decreased sensation in the residual limb. Skin inspection can help avoid this breakdown and should be taught to postoperative clients.

Pain Management

Hypersensitivity of the residual limb often occurs postoperatively. In these cases, a program to normalize sensation will ease discomfort caused by tactile stimulation. For a full explanation of desensitization, see Chapter 29. Postoperative rehabilitation for clients with amputations should include a desensitization program leading to a level of sensation that allows for maximal functioning.

Most clients experience phantom pain in the residual limb. **Phantom pain** is a burning and shooting pain and a squeezing sensation in the residual limb. This is likely due to abnormal sensory processing within the nervous system. Fortunately, phantom limb pain tends to improve with time (Esquenazi, 2004; US Department of Health and Human Services 1993).

Phantom sensation refers to the sensations felt in the residual limb. Most individuals who experience a traumatic amputation feel it. These sensations include numbness, tingling, temperature changes, pressure, itching, and muscle cramps. In addition, some individuals feel as if they can still move or control the residual limb, leading to some attempting to walk following lower limb loss. The length of time in which individuals experience phantom sensation varies. Some experience it for a few months while for others it may linger for many years, despite decreasing in intensity (Esquenazi, 2004; US Department of Health and Human Services, 1993).

PREPROSTHETIC TRAINING

An interview with the client and family provides the OT and OTA with information regarding life before the amputation. This includes roles and habits, home environment, and client factors. The OT, with input from the OTA, completes a preprosthetic evaluation to assess client factors and to introduce a self-care training program. This information is used to establish an intervention plan. The goals of this preprosthetic stage are to promote fitting of a prosthesis through residual limb shrinkage and desensitization. Other goals include maintaining functional ROM of the proximal joints, building prosthetic skill, facilitating adjustment to the loss, and maximizing independence in self-care (Lyons, 1983).

Several areas need to be addressed during this stage to ensure that the residual limb heals well and can tolerate a prosthesis. This includes good skin integrity, residual limb shape, and adequate joint ROM and muscle strength. Therefore the following areas should be addressed during the preprosthetic stage of intervention.

Skin hygiene will help preserve skin integrity following amputation and is an important part of the training program. The tight socket and the prosthetic sock can cause a lot of perspiration. Keeping the skin clean and dry, as well as inspecting it for redness and breakdown, is important in the healing process. Other things included in a program of skin hygiene include using antiperspirants, socks, or liners with the prosthesis to reduce perspiration and avoiding compromising the fit or function of the prosthetic (Orr, Glover, & Cook, 2018).

Movement will help keep the skin mobile and prevent decreased circulation. Therefore the client is encouraged to move and use the residual limb as much as possible during the healing period. In addition to assisting in healing, movement will help give normal proprioceptive input to the brain and prevent muscle atrophy and contractures that may result.

Shrinking and shaping the residual limb is necessary to form a tapered-shaped limb that will tolerate a prosthesis. Compression aids in the shrinking and shaping process. This can be done with an elastic Ace bandage, a tubular bandage, or a shrinker sock applied to the residual limb. A figure-8 method is used when an elastic bandage is applied to the limb. Care must be taken to apply the bandage smoothly, evenly, and not too tightly from the distal to the proximal end of the residual limb. Circular wrapping, which may cause loss of circulation and further tissue loss, should not be used. The elastic bandage should be rewrapped several times a day to keep the correct tension. The patient is instructed to wrap the residual limb when not wearing the postoperative prosthesis.

Full joint ROM and muscle strength can be maintained through participation in occupation and through a therapeutic exercise program tailored for the client. These exercises may be initiated once the client receives clearance from the physician. Therapeutic exercise should encourage the use of the residual limb, maintain ROM of joints proximal to the amputation site, and strengthen muscles of the arm and shoulder. Adequate muscle strength and endurance is needed to operate the prosthesis (American Occupational Therapy Association, 2020). See Chapter 29 for an in-depth explanation of therapeutic exercises to improve ROM and strength.

It is common for new clients to experience depression and anxiety for up to 2 years postamputation. Other psychosocial challenges experienced by clients are social discomfort (adjusting to the fact they appear different from other people) and body-image anxiety (adapting to a changed body image) resulting from activity restriction, depression, and anxiety (Horgan & MacLachlan, 2004).

Therefore psychological support is an important part of this phase of treatment. Responses to amputations have often been compared with the grieving process. Clients experience identifiable stages of denial, anger, depression, coping, and acceptance (Friedman, 2020a). Some individuals will progress through these stages and ultimately adapt to the loss. The cause of the amputation may contribute significantly to individual responses. Psychosocial factors associated with positive psychosocial adjustment to the amputation include an individual's disposition toward optimism, an individual's active coping mechanisms, and the quality of the social support systems available. Other positive factors include controlled pain, a good prosthetic fit, and the comprehensive care provided by the team.

PROSTHETIC TRAINING

Choosing the Prosthesis

The team educates the client on the types of prostheses and helps the client make the decision as to which one to choose. Many factors are taken into account, such as the client's age, cognitive status, and type of amputation. The OT and OTA may help the client understand the options and the functional implications of each type.

There are two main types of prostheses, **body-powered** and **external-powered** (**myoelectric**). Body-powered prostheses (mechanical), such as one with a hook as a **terminal device** (**TD**), are controlled by cables and muscle power. This type requires limb movement and strength and is less cosmetically pleasing, but it is the most durable. External-powered (myoelectric) prostheses rely on an external motor or battery for power. Although these may provide more proximal function, greater grip strength, and a more pleasing appearance, they are heavy and expensive (Box 31.1).

BOX 31.1 Advantages and Disadvantages of Myoelectric Prostheses

Advantages
Improved cosmesis
Increased grip force (approximately 25 lb in an adult myoelectric hand)
Minimal or no harnessing
Ability to use overhead
Minimal effort needed to control device
Closely corresponds to human physiologic control

Disadvantages
Cost of prosthesis
Frequency of maintenance and repair
Fragile nature of glove and need for frequent replacements
Absence of sensory feedback (some sense of proprioceptive feedback provided in a body-powered prosthesis)
Slow response of electric hand
Increased weight

Body-Powered Components

Prosthetic Sock. A prosthetic sock is worn over the residual limb. It absorbs perspiration and protects from discomfort or irritation that results from direct contact of the skin with the socket of the prosthesis. It accommodates volume change in the residual limb and aids with fit and comfort of the residual limb in the socket (Scott et al., 1985; Wellerson 2020).

Harness. The harness is used to suspend the prosthesis and to anchor the control cables. The figure-8 harness is a common design, but others are available. Extra straps may be added to the figure-8 design as needed. The higher the level of amputation, the more complex the harnessing system must be. Variations in available muscle power and ROM may necessitate variations in the harness design. A properly fitted harness is important for both comfort and function.

Cable and Components. The cable is made of stainless steel and is contained in a flexible stainless-steel housing. It is fastened to the prosthesis by a retainer unit made of a base plate and a retainer butterfly or by a housing crossbar and a leather loop. A ball or ball swivel fitting at one end of the cable attaches it to the TD while a T-bar or hanger fittings at the other end attach it to the harness (Weeks, Anderson-Barnes, & Tsao, 2010).

Socket. The forearm **socket** for the transradial below-elbow (BE) client may be made of plastic resins or carbon graphite. The latter is lightweight, comfortable, and durable. The socket may have a single or double wall. The socket must be stable on the residual limb to allow the wearer full power and control of the prosthesis. The transradial socket may be constructed to allow remaining pronation and supination to be used. The single wall socket is used when the outside diameter of the distal end of the residual limb is sufficient to permit tapering to the wrist unit. The double wall socket is used when the residual limb is too short or slender to achieve the desired contour or tapering. The inner wall conforms to the residual limb, and the outer wall gives the required length and contour for the forearm replacement. The socket must fit snugly and firmly but allow full ROM at the first available joint.

Osseointegration is a procedure in which a suspension system connects the prosthesis directly to the bone via a partially external titanium implant. There is no need for a socket. This procedure is useful for those who suffer complication related to using a prosthesis, such as skin breakdown and residual limb edema (Esquenazi, 2004).

Elbow Unit. The elbow unit on the transhumeral above-elbow (AE) prosthesis allows the maximal ROM possible. It also allows locking of the elbow in various degrees of motion and positioning of the prosthesis for arm rotation. This is done with a manual control friction turntable unit.

Wrist Unit. The wrist unit is usually selected for its ability to meet the needs of the client in daily living and vocational activities (Scott et al., 1985). It orients the terminal device in the forearm socket and serves as a disconnecting unit so that TDs may be interchanged. Once positioned, the wrist unit is held in place by one of a number of lock options: friction lock, quick disconnect, locking unit, or flexion unit.

- The friction lock slips on and is easy to position; however, this lock can easily slip off when heavy objects are carried.
- The quick disconnect allows for easy changing of TDs that have specialized functions.
- A locking unit option is chosen when there is a need to prevent rotation during grasping and lifting.
- A wrist flexion unit allows for improved self-care functions in midline, such as shaving, buttoning, and perineal care. It is especially helpful for a bilateral UE client.

Terminal Devices

Current prosthetic devices cannot completely substitute for every hand function, which together are anatomically and physiologically complex. All prostheses lack sensory feedback and provide only limited mobility and dexterity. Prosthetic hands provide three-jaw chuck pinch, and hooks provide lateral pinch. Slip control is a recently introduced technology that can improve prehension to prevent accidental dropping of objects (Esquenazi, 2004).

Passive and active TDs are available. Passive TDs are designed for cosmesis. They do not have movable parts and can only function as a gross assist. The passive hand and mitt-shaped prostheses are examples of passive TDs. The passive hand is a cosmetically pleasing and socially acceptable hand that is positioned in a static grasp position. The mitt shape is similar to a cupped hand and is recommended for infants. This TD may be used as a shock absorber in sports for younger children.

Active TDs are designed for function and not for cosmesis. The hook and the mechanical hand (Fig. 31.2) are examples of active TDs. The hook TD may be made of aluminum or stainless steel alone or in combination with titanium. The hook may have canted or lyre-shaped fingers and usually has a neoprene or polyethylene gripping surface to protect grasped objects and prevent slippage. The hook is the most functional, durable, and commonly prescribed and used TD. Several types of hooks are available to meet individual needs. The farmer's and carpenter's hooks make handling tools easier, and narrow-opening hooks may be used for handling fine objects.

On the hook TD, the number of rubber bands controls the amount of grasp pressure. Training usually begins with one rubber band, and the number increases to three to four rubber bands as training progresses. The mechanical hand is a functional hand that may be attached to the wrist unit and is activated by the same control cable that operates the hook. The fingers are controlled at the metacarpophalangeal (MCP) joints by the prosthesis control cable. The hand TD sacrifices grip force (2 lb maximum) for improved cosmesis. A natural-looking plastic glove fits over the mechanical hand (Scott et al., 1985).

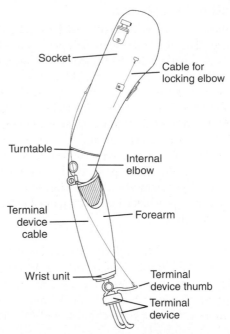

Fig. 31.2 Component parts of standard above-elbow prosthesis. (Modified from Santschi W, ed. *Manual for Upper Extremity Prosthetics*. 2nd ed. Los Angeles, CA: University of California Press; 1958.)

Terminal devices are used to attempt to replicate five types of grip/prehension.

- Precision grip, which includes the pads of the thumb and index finger in opposition, providing the ability to pick up or pinch small objects
- Tripod grip/three-jaw chuck pinch, in which the pad of the thumb is opposed to the index and middle finger
- Lateral grip/key pinch, in which the pad of the thumb is lateral to the index finger, which is employed in turning a key in a lock
- Hook power grip, where the distal and proximal interphalangeal joints are flexed, and the metacarpals are straight such as in holding a briefcase
- Spherical grip, in which the tips of all fingers are flexed, such as in opening a round doorknob (Esquenazi, 2004).

Materials and construction used in prosthetic components continue to improve. These include lightweight socket fabrication materials (carbon graphite or high-temperature flexible thermoplastics), custom-fitting techniques, suspension systems (such as osseointegration), slip controls, power sources, and electric controls (Esquenazi, 2004).

The advantages of body-powered prosthesis include their durability and their ability to be exposed to environmental conditions (e.g., water and dirt). They provide proprioceptive feedback. They require lower maintenance costs than myoelectric prostheses.

The disadvantages include the restriction caused by the harness and the high amount of force exerted on the residual limb. They also provide a decreased grip force compared to myoelectric options and are difficult to control for individuals with higher level amputations.

Myoelectric Components

A myoelectric prosthesis is controlled by electrical signals from muscles. The first practical myoelectric-controlled prosthesis was demonstrated in 1948 (Jacobsen, Knutti, Johnson, & Sears, 1982). In the next several decades a considerable research effort followed; as a result, myoelectric prostheses have been improved so much that their clinical value is well established (Jacobsen et al., 1982). The concept of myoelectric control is simple: An electric signal from a muscle is used to control the flow of energy from a battery to a motor. The muscles in the residual limb produce the control signal by contracting through voluntary control. The motor is activated by the signal, and a prosthetic hand, wrist, or elbow is directed to move into action.

Socket/Suspension. Socket design is very important to the functional use of the myoelectric prosthesis. When the prosthetist is designing the socket for the client, the following areas must be considered: (1) residual limb comfort, (2) overall cosmesis, (3) electrode contact, and (4) suspension style.

Residual limb comfort within the socket will often determine the wear and use pattern of the prosthesis. The socket must not compromise skin integrity by causing pressure points or pressing on sensitive areas of the residual limb. The client will not wear or use the device if it is not comfortable.

The same principle applies to the overall appearance of the prosthesis. To encourage the patient's acceptance, the prosthetic socket should be pleasing in skin tone, size, length, and muscle bulk. It is most essential that the socket design provide constant contact between the skin and the electrodes with very little movement of the arm within the socket. Without careful design and fit of electrode to muscle site contact, the operation of the prosthesis will be difficult (if not impossible), thus setting the patient up for failure.

Finally, the socket design determines the type of suspension to be used. For clients with transradial (BE) amputations, self-suspension is always an option. This means the total elimination of a harness and its restriction of movement. In most cases the client with a transhumeral (AE) amputation still requires a harness in addition to self-suspension to distribute the weight of the prosthesis. The type of suspension used should be determined by the length of the residual limb, the client's preference based on comfort and ease of prosthetic application and removal, and the prosthetic use pattern. The three types of suspension are sleeve, supracondylar, and suprastyloid suspension (Brenner, 2020).

The prosthetist is the expert on the various socket suspensions available. However, the therapy practitioner must know the suspension options to assist the patient and the prosthetist in choosing one that will best meet the functional demands of the patient.

Battery. The battery (Fig. 31.3) provides the energy to run the motor that operates the component parts of the prosthesis. A removable rechargeable 6-volt lithium ion battery is used. The battery operates the prosthesis during the day and

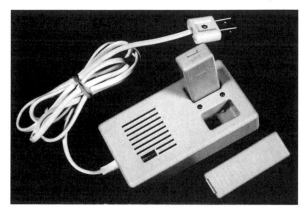

Fig. 31.3 Battery of a myoelectric arm is inserted in a battery charger and charged overnight.

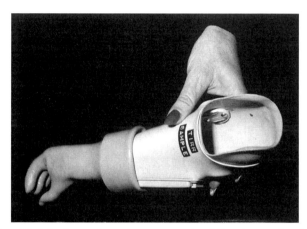

Fig. 31.4 Surface electrodes recessed within the wall of a myoelectric socket detect muscle contractions.

is recharged at night. The client may have several batteries to interchange as needed. The charge time of a battery varies from 6 to 24 hours of use, depending on the capacity and age of the battery. The capacity of these batteries to hold a charge will decrease in time, eventually requiring complete replacement of the battery. The battery is positioned at the surface of the prosthesis to allow for easy removal for charging. On the transradial prosthesis, the battery is located on the forearm; on the transhumeral prosthesis, the battery is fitted at the elbow joint or is internal. The prosthetist positions the battery for easy removal and a pleasing appearance.

Electrodes. Surface electrodes (Fig. 31.4) are mounted inside the socket at predetermined muscle sites that display strong myoelectric signals. Good electrical contact is the key to achieving a usable myoelectric prosthesis. The **electrode** reads the muscle activity and sends a message to the controller that moves the motor at the terminal device. For instance, in the case of a transradial amputation, electrodes are placed on the wrist extensors and finger flexors. The electrodes read a signal from the finger flexors, send a message to the motor to bend the fingers, and the prosthetic hand responds by closing. In the case of transhumeral amputation, the electrodes are placed on the triceps to open the hand and the biceps to close the hand. These sites are also used to send the signal to the elbow device, triggering elbow flexion from the biceps and elbow extension from the triceps.

Shoulder Unit. When a patient has a shoulder disarticulation or a forequarter amputation, a shoulder unit is used. It provides cosmesis for a symmetric body appearance. Passive and friction components permit manual positioning of the shoulder but no active function.

Elbow Unit. Myoelectric-controlled elbow units are available for clients with transhumeral amputations. The client with a high-level amputation requires an electric elbow because the force required to pull the mechanical prosthetic cable to operate a TD or mechanical elbow is too great for a short residual limb. Previously, prosthetic choices for these individuals were greatly limited. The development of the electric elbow has made it possible to restore UE function to clients with amputations as high as a shoulder disarticulation. The motions of elbow flexion and extension are controlled by electrical signals from the muscle surface. When a muscle contracts, the muscle membrane generates an electric potential. The control unit senses, amplifies, and processes this potential. The same muscle sites used for hand control are used for elbow movement. Therefore no retraining of new muscle sites is needed. No large shoulder movements are required, only the natural contraction of the triceps and biceps, which allows for more natural, smooth body movements. Through myoelectric control, the elbow unit has 21 available stopping positions within the range of 15 to 150 degrees of elbow flexion (Jacobsen et al., 1982) and can perform flexion and extension movement patterns. A passive humeral rotation joint provides side-to-side positioning of the forearm. The elbow unit can sustain a maximum load of 50 lb when locked and 2 lb when not locked (Jacobsen et al., 1982). Elbow units weigh 2 lb, and the electric hand weighs 1 lb. This extra 3 to 4 lb of weight is worth it to clients who develop enough competence to use it, since they greatly increase the functional use of the prosthesis.

Wrist Unit. There are several available wrist unit options: (1) passive friction wrist, (2) quick-disconnect wrist, (3) flexion wrist, and (4) electric wrist rotator. The quick-disconnect wrist is the most commonly used wrist component in a myoelectric prosthesis because it allows for faster manual positioning of the wrist than a myoelectric signal, it eliminates additional movements otherwise needed for prosthetic movement, and it allows for easy exchange of TDs.

Terminal Devices. Myoelectric prostheses most frequently utilize an electric hand as a terminal device (Fig. 31.5). They are available in sizes to fit everyone from small children to adults. The mechanism is covered with a latex glove made to match the remaining hand utilizing many skin tones and

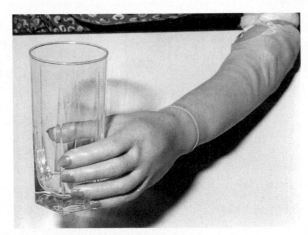

Fig. 31.5 Myoelectric hand.

features. The hand opens and closes at varying widths, but finger movement cannot be isolated and grip force cannot be graded. The grip is strong (25-lb force). The Greiffer TD provides quick handling and precise manipulation of small objects. It features a 38-lb grasp, parallel gripping surfaces, and a flexion joint for dorsal and volar wrist flexion (Roeschlein & Domholdt, 1989). It can be fitted with accessories for specific activities, such as sports, unusual work tasks, and leisure activities. It is useful for active adults needing to perform heavy upper-body activities, such as heavy work in industry or farming. The prosthetist is a good resource for these specialized TDs.

Progression of the Prosthesis

Assuming an client enters the prosthetic rehabilitation process at the time of surgery and has no complications, has good funding sources, has an optimal length of the residual limb, and is motivated for treatment, the progression would proceed as follows: (1) immediate/**early postoperative prosthesis**, (2) preparatory mechanical prosthesis, (3) preparatory myoelectric prosthesis, (4) definitive mechanical prosthesis, and (5) definitive myoelectric prosthesis. In many cases this progression is not practical or realistic. Many factors interfere with the preferred prosthetic progression. The progression differs from patient to patient, depending on variables such as residual limb length, funding sources, patient motivation, and time of entry into the rehabilitation process. A patient can start or stop at various points in the progression as a result of these factors.

Immediate/Early Postoperative Prosthesis. An immediate prosthesis and an **early postoperative prosthesis** are identical in fabrication. The name given varies with the time of fabrication. The immediate prosthesis is applied in surgery at the time of final closure. The early postoperative prosthesis is applied sometime after surgery but before suture removal. In both cases the socket is made from fiberglass casting tape wrapped around the residual limb. A thermoplastic frame is attached to the socket, and the terminal device and elbow unit are stabilized onto this frame (Brenner, 2020). If an elbow unit is required, a lightweight manual hinge elbow is placed on this prosthesis with eight set-locking points to position the elbow. A figure-8 harness with a simple cable to control the TD is used. Only one rubber band is provided for grip force at this stage. The prosthesis is used mainly as a gross stabilizer. The immediate/postoperative prosthesis introduces the patient to prosthetic use and wear and provides a rigid dressing for edema control and proprioceptive input (Brenner, 2020).

PREPARING FOR THE PROSTHESIS

Preparatory Mechanical Prosthesis

The preparatory mechanical prosthesis is applied when full healing is complete and the sutures are removed, usually 10 to 14 days after surgery. The socket is fabricated from a plaster mold of the residual limb for a customized fit. The socket is made of clear plastic to allow for monitoring of residual limb changes in volume and socket fit. The preparatory prosthesis is made from more durable materials than the postoperative prosthesis and can be used like a definitive (final) prosthesis. Its construction permits easy interchangeability of parts and components to evaluate which works best for this patient. The purpose of the preparatory mechanical prosthesis is to manage edema, condition tissues to accept the prosthetic socket, determine optimal functioning of parts, demonstrate the client's motivation and compliance, and give the client a chance to try out the mechanical prosthesis (Brenner, 2020).

The preparatory prosthesis allows the patient to develop skill and strength while determining which specifications work best. It is more cost effective to make changes to this (temporary) prosthesis. Thus patients are free to evaluate their prosthetic needs.

Preparatory Myoelectric Prosthesis

A preparatory myoelectric prosthesis is a cost-effective way to analyze the patient's ability to use the prosthesis and to evaluate the components best suited to the patient's needs. The preparatory myoelectric prosthesis is fitted similarly to the final prosthesis, except that it has a transparent test socket to monitor electrode contact and evaluate socket stability. A fitting frame is attached to the socket to provide a surface for the electronic components to be attached. A standard protective outer glove is placed over the electronic hand for cosmesis and protection of the inner shell of the hand. Suspension, socket design, and electrode placement are all easily changeable to allow the patient to explore options. The purpose of the preparatory myoelectric prosthesis is to determine the client's motivation and commitment to the prosthesis, to evaluate appropriate components and suspension systems, to condition the tissues in a self-contained socket, and to determine the patient's use, skill, and wear patterns with myoelectric control (Pedretti & Pasquinelli, 2018).

Definitive Mechanical Prosthesis. Once the patient has determined the components needed, has established a full wear pattern with good prosthetic skill, and has reached full residual limb maturation, a definitive mechanical prosthesis is considered. The definitive prosthesis is designed around choices made by the patient in the preparatory stage. The definitive prosthesis is fabricated with durable parts and provides a good cosmetic appearance.

Definitive Myoelectric Prosthesis. Myoelectric prostheses cost between $20,000 and $45,000. Therefore the preparatory myoelectric prosthesis is an essential step to determine if the cost to the client will result in a useful device. The design of the final product incorporates the components that were determined to best suit the client during the preparatory myoelectric prosthesis stage.

Prosthesis Training Program

Wear and Use Schedule. The wear and use schedule begins with the client wearing it for 15 minutes, three times a day, with 5 minutes of active use. By the third day, the wear schedule is increased to 30 minutes of wear, three times a day, with 10 minutes of active use. Wear and active use progressively increase on an individual basis. After each period of wear, the client needs to check the residual limb to identify pressure spots and problems with healing. An activity list provides suggestions to build skills. Examples of skill-building activities include picking up small objects such as paper clips, wrapping presents, and playing cards. Most prosthetic skill training occurs on an outpatient basis. Instructions are graded from simple to complex, to avoid overwhelming the patient and to encourage use of the prosthetic device.

Components of Mechanical Prosthetic Training. A preparatory mechanical prosthesis is fabricated immediately after the sutures are removed. Once the patient has this device, training can begin full force with emphasis on prosthetic wear, skill, use, acceptance, grip-strength tolerance, a two-handed pattern, and a return to independence in ADL, work, and leisure activities. Other goals include retraining dominance if necessary, normalizing sensation in the residual limb, and strengthening the residual limb.

- *Introduction to prosthetic parts:* The client should learn the names and functions of the parts of the prosthesis to facilitate communication with team. This helps clients to convey information about having difficulties with the prosthesis or if the prosthesis needs repairs.
- *Donning and removing the prosthesis:* The client dons the residual limb sock with the remaining arm. To apply the prosthesis, the client places it on a table or bed and pushes the residual limb between the control cable and Y-strap from the medial side into the socket (Fig. 31.6A). The remaining arm is then slipped into the axilla loop. The client grasps the harness and lifts it over the head so that it is positioned properly in back (see Fig. 31.6B). The shoulders are shrugged to shift the harness forward and into the correct position. To remove the prosthesis, the client slips the axilla shoulder strap off on the sound side with the TD and then slips the shoulder strap off on the amputated side. The harness is slipped off like a coat.

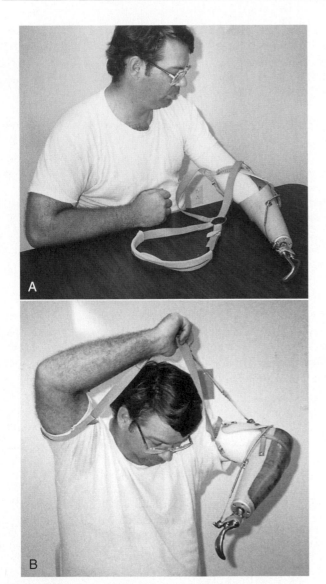

Fig. 31.6 Donning a mechanical prosthesis.

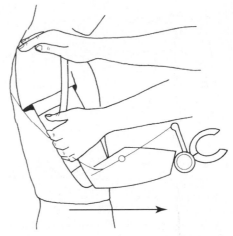

Fig. 31.7 Therapist moves residual limb forward to attain cable tension and terminal device opening.

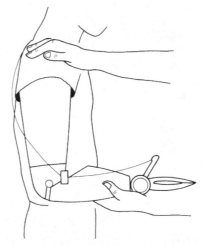

Fig. 31.8 Therapist passively flexes elbow to cause slackening of control cable.

Controls Training

- *TD control training:* All amputations proximal to the wrist require a TD. Biscapular abduction and humeral flexion on the amputated side are the motions necessary to operate the TD. The clinician passively moves the patient through the motions (Fig. 31.7). During this procedure the client watches the TD operate and gains a sense of the tension on the prosthesis control cable. The client then repeats the motions without assistance and verbalizes the actions that occurred during operation. The clinician instructs the client to repeat all of the motions in one continuous sequence in both sitting and standing positions until they are smooth and natural (Weeks et al., 2010). The client will then be instructed to open and close the TD in a variety of ranges of elbow and shoulder motion. TD opening and closing should be accomplished easily with the elbow extended, at 30 degrees, 45 degrees, 90 degrees, and with full elbow

flexion, as well as with the arm overhead, down at the side, out to the side, and leaning over to floor level (Wellerson, 2020).
- *Elbow control training:* Transhumeral amputations require that the client learn to flex the mechanical elbow. Once again, humeral flexion and scapular abduction are the control motions. The clinician passively flexes the prosthesis into full elbow flexion, noting that the control is slackened by this maneuver (Fig. 31.8). The clinician then flexes the client's shoulder forward and asks the client to hold this position while the clinician lets go (Fig. 31.9). The client gains a sense of the control cable tension across the scapula from this maneuver. The client is asked to relax the residual limb to the side of the body once again, slowly allowing the forearm to extend (Fig. 31.10). The client is then asked to again flex the humerus and abduct the scapula to accomplish elbow flexion and relax the residual limb back slowly into shoulder extension to achieve elbow extension. This is

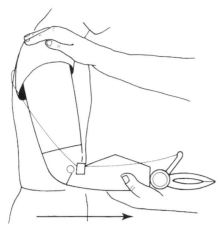

Fig. 31.9 Forearm is moved forward to maintain elbow flexion, thus creating tension on control cable.

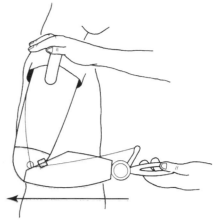

Fig. 31.11 Therapist pushes humerus into hyperextension to lock elbow.

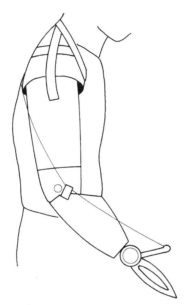

Fig. 31.10 Client relaxes residual limb to allow controlled extension of forearm.

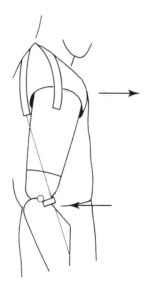

Fig. 31.12 Shoulder is rolled forward, scapula abducted, and humerus hyperextended to lock or unlock elbow at various points in range of motion.

repeated until the client gains enough control of cable tension to accomplish elbow flexion and extension smoothly and with ease (Wellerson, 2020). The clinician then teaches elbow locking by passively pushing the humerus into hyperextension with the elbow flexed, thus locking the elbow (Fig. 31.11). The clinician brings the arm back to the neutral position and then releases, demonstrating that the elbow mechanism is locked. The clinician repeats this maneuver, demonstrating that the elbow is now unlocked. The client is then asked to lock the elbow by moving the humerus into hyperextension and rolling the shoulder forward, using scapular depression and abduction at the same time to lock the elbow. The client is then asked to practice locking and unlocking the elbow in various ranges of elbow flexion and extension until full flexion and extension are obtained (Fig. 31.12) (Wellerson, 2020).

Use Training

Once the controls are mastered, use training begins. The first stage is prepositioning the TD. Prepositioning involves rotating the TD to the best position to grasp an object or perform a given activity. The goal of prepositioning the TD should be to allow clients to approach an object or activity as they would with a normal hand and to avoid overreaching and similar awkward body movements that might be used to compensate for poor prepositioning. Along with prepositioning, prehension training should begin with large, hard objects such as blocks, cans, and jars and progress to soft and then crushable objects such as rubber balls, sponges, paper boxes, cones, and paper cups. These objects should be placed at various heights and positions that demand prepositioning and TD opening and closing, elbow flexion, and locking and unlocking, at various heights.

The client should be encouraged to use a problem-solving approach to these and other tasks to determine the best position for the TD, as well as appropriate use of the sound arm and the prosthesis in activities. Use training should progress to performance of necessary ADL. The client is encouraged to analyze and perform activities of personal hygiene and grooming, dressing, feeding, home management, communication and environmental hardware use, avocation, and vocation as independently as possible. The OTA may help the client achieve success by training with a special method or gadget or repetitious practice (Weeks et al., 2010).

Components of Myoelectric Prosthetic Training. Myoelectric prosthetic training takes place simultaneously with mechanical prosthetic training. Once the patient has developed good skill and use with the mechanical prosthesis and can tolerate learning another skill, muscle site testing and weight training are introduced. A typical treatment session at this point might focus on mechanical prosthetic functional use training for 15 minutes, muscle site training for 15 minutes, and weight training for the remaining 30 minutes. The therapist must thoroughly understand the myoelectric prosthesis and be able to differentiate patient errors from possible equipment malfunctions. The ability to pinpoint the source of the problem (whether it be equipment or operator error) is the key to successfully teaching and training the client about myoelectric control.

The goals of the myoelectric training program are as follows:
- To operate the prosthesis automatically with minimal effort
- To care for the prosthesis
- To use the prosthesis smoothly and efficiently for commonly encountered tasks
- To analyze the best methods for unusual or new tasks (Schuch & Pritham, 1994)

Signal training. Signal training is the process of learning to produce the muscle signals necessary to operate the myoelectric prosthesis (Schuch & Pritham, 1994). Electrodes placed on the residual limb are connected to a feedback system that lets the patient know when the control muscles are contracting and at what level of intensity. Signal training helps the patient develop the ability to produce clear, strong contractions without wasting energy and to relax the control muscles even when the rest of the arm is actively moving (Orr et al., 2018). Once the muscle sites are located by the OT, the OTA uses the same biofeedback device for training. Individuals with an amputation must receive adequate training and practice in initiating the desired muscle contractions before receiving the myoelectric prosthesis. The patient's success and effectiveness in using the prosthesis are closely related to the quality of the muscle site training process.

Weight training. The OT designs a shoulder strengthening home exercise program to improve management of the added weight of the myoelectric prosthesis. The OTA may implement the weight-training program while providing instruction to ensure follow-through. Theraband, free weights, and weight-training equipment all work equally well to accomplish this goal. The prosthetist can provide a socket, equaling the weight of the myoelectric prosthesis, several weeks before receiving the prosthesis to accustom the client to wearing the additional weight.

Care and donning of prosthesis. Care of the prosthesis includes charging the batteries, cleaning it, and caring for the glove. The method of donning it is determined by the type of suspension and socket design that the patient uses. Multiple methods can be used. It is always donned with the electronics in the off position.

Use training. Use training combines skill-building activities to learn prosthetic control and functional activities to encourage carryover of skills in daily tasks, culminating in an occupational task important to the patient (American Occupational Therapy Association, 2014; American Occupational Therapy Association 2020). Training must begin with learning to use the myoelectric hand in simple approach, grasp, and release activities. Classic therapeutic activities for hand control can be used, such as the pegboard or hook-and-loop fastening (Velcro) checkers. The patient should be able to judge the amount of hand opening or closing required to pick up an item. For instance, if the patient is trying to pick up a cotton swab, full hand opening would not be necessary and would demonstrate a lack of control. The clinician emphasizes good problem-solving skills for the patient to first position the TD in the optimum position for the specific activity. It is a common error for the client to adjust the body with compensatory large-body motions rather than adjusting or prepositioning the hand first.

Training must also include the mastery of the gripping force of the terminal device. This involves close visual attention to grade the muscle contraction to get a specific result in the calibration of the myoelectric hand. Too strong a grasp will result in crushing an object that is being held (Fig. 31.13). Training with foam cups, sponges, and cotton balls will help develop the control needed to grasp and lift and move paper

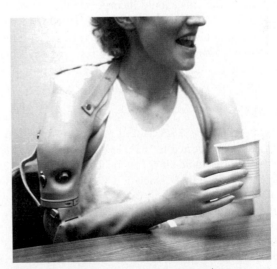

Fig. 31.13 Above-elbow client demonstrates how too strong a grasp will crush the object being held.

cups, eggs, potato chips, and sandwiches; ultimately, the patient can learn sufficient sensitivity to hold someone's hand. Eventually the movements will take less cognitive effort and become automatic. Each session should focus on both functional training and skill-building activities. Occupationally based two-handed tasks should include those the patient finds difficult and those that fit the patient's interests. The therapist should observe the patient closely when he or she is performing a functional task and ask the following questions: (1) Is the patient using the prosthesis spontaneously in the activity? (2) Is it being used as a gross stabilizer or in a nonactive pattern of use? (3) Does the patient use large compensatory body movements instead of prepositioning the components to the optimal position? (4) Is the patient overshooting the target? and (5) Is the patient using the proper grip force? Appropriate activities to focus on deficit areas can be selected on the basis of these answers.

Vocational and leisure activities. As training proceeds and the patient develops a sense of self-acceptance and comfort with the amputation, the clinician should broach the subject of return to work. If possible, job requirements can be discussed and then practiced in a simulated step-by-step process. Ideally, the clinician could make an onsite visit, and several requirements of the job could be practiced. If changes and adjustments to the work environment are necessary, the clinician could advise on these modifications (see Chapter 16, Work).

Leisure and social participation contribute to significant physical and psychological well-being and are critically important. The terminal devices for recreational activities are not myoelectric but can be placed on the socket of a myoelectric prosthesis. Therapeutic Recreation Systems (TRS) has some excellent adaptation components (American Occupational Therapy Association, 2020).

Expected Outcomes

At the completion of a training program, patients should be proficient in the use and care of both the mechanical and myoelectric prostheses and should demonstrate a full-day wear pattern. Patients should incorporate the use of a prosthesis into all occupational tasks, and they should demonstrate good spontaneous prosthetic use with skilled precision of movement. They should also have resolved psychological issues related to limb loss and have a realistic outlook on the usefulness of the prosthesis as a replacement arm.

Role of the OTA

UE client training is a specialized area of treatment. A program is usually directed by a skilled and experienced senior clinician. Under guidelines established by the American Occupational Therapy Association (AOTA), the OT would complete the evaluation and prosthetic checkout and establish the goals and treatment plan. Under close supervision the OTA may implement a program for the patient with an amputation. Close supervision is essential because of the complex problems and degree of change commonly seen, which may require a modified treatment approach or reevaluation by the OT. The OTA is responsible for keeping the supervising OT informed of all changes in patient performance and any other pertinent facts. As treatment progresses and changes are noted, the OTA may contribute suggestions for program modifications or additions that will help the patient reach the established goals. Communication and feedback between the OT and the OTA are keys to a successful program.

LOWER LIMB AMPUTATIONS

Levels of Amputation

Levels of lower limb amputation, described with current terminology, are shown in Fig. 31.14. The higher the level of amputation is, the greater the functional loss of the part and the more the client will depend on the prosthesis for function and cosmesis. The higher level amputation requires more complex and extensive prostheses and prosthetic training. Hemipelvectomy and hip disarticulation amputation results in loss of the entire LE; thus hip, knee, ankle, and foot functions are lost (O'Sullivan et al., 2020; Orr et al., 2018). **Transfemoral** (above-knee) **amputations** (AKAs) and knee disarticulation amputations result in loss of knee, ankle, and foot motion. The residual limb of the transfemoral amputated limb can vary in length from 10 to 12 inches (5.4–30.5 cm) below the greater trochanter (O'Sullivan et al., 2020; Orr et al., 2018).

Transtibial (below-knee) **amputations** (BKAs) result in a residual limb that is approximately 4 to 6 inches (10.1–15.2 cm) in length from the tibial plateau (O'Sullivan et al., 2020; Orr et al., 2018). Other classification systems further delineate

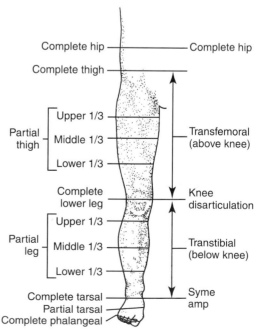

Fig. 31.14 Levels of amputation and functional losses in lower extremity. (From O'Sullivan SB, Cullen K, Schmitz T. *Physical Rehabilitation: Evaluation and Treatment Procedures*. Philadelphia, PA: FA Davis; 1981.)

the amputations into thirds: Upper, middle, and lower third indicate the distance below the ischium for transfemorals. For the transtibials, these divisions indicate the distance below the tibial plateau (O'Sullivan et al., 2020). The **Syme amputation** is equivalent to an ankle disarticulation and results in loss of ankle and foot function (Banerjee, 2020). In a transmetatarsal amputation, the foot is severed through the metatarsal bones and the ankle function remains intact (Banerjee, 2020). Loss of the small toes does not result in functional impairment. Loss of the great toe, however, prevents toe-off during ambulation (Spencer, 2020).

Occupational Therapy Intervention

The focus of intervention is on positioning, transfer training, strengthening of UE, ADL and instrumental activities of daily living (IADL), dynamic balance (with and without a prosthesis), strengthening the LE for the client to perform IADL (with and without a prosthesis), driving, prevocational and vocational activities, leisure education, and facilitating reintegration into the community. Critical to these aims are the provision of family education, a home visit, a home program, and provision of appropriate durable medical equipment (DME) for the home such as tub seats, tub benches, raised toilet seats, and grab bars. The OTA may assist the OT or assume responsibility for many of these areas once service competency with this population is achieved.

Preoperative care includes psychological support tailored to the backgrounds and lifestyles of each client, which will influence the client's abilities to cope with the loss of a limb. Support groups can help clients express feelings. Group members are generally sensitive to others' needs and encourage constructive and creative thinking, which helps to motivate initiative and self-assurance. Visits by other clients who have adjusted to the loss of a limb can also offer support.

CASE STUDY

Cathy is an 18-year-old, right-hand-dominant Chinese American girl who, at age 17, sustained a right transradial amputation in an automobile accident. She was fitted with a cable-driven harness with a hook TD. She now desires a cosmetic hand and training with a myoelectric prosthesis.

Occupational History and Profile
Cathy is a high school senior. She has lived in the United States for the past 3 years, since her family (both parents, one other sibling) emigrated from Guangdong province in China. She plans to attend college next year and has been awarded a full scholarship. She spends her time studying and helping her parents with household chores. She occasionally works as a receptionist in her family's restaurant. She enjoys downloading music, taking photographs, and hanging out with her girlfriends.

Client Factors and Performance Skills
The OT assessed passive and active ROM, muscle strength, sensory function, and coordination of both UEs. The left UE was within normal limits on all measures; the amputated right UE showed some distal sensory loss but good coordination, ROM, and strength across existing joints. Cathy performed all basic ADL, including makeup application skillfully.

Cathy stated that she wanted the myoelectric hand for cosmetic reasons because she felt self-conscious going away to college wearing a hook. She also said she was afraid no one would want to go out with her.

Interventions
Outpatient occupational therapy was provided at a rehabilitation hospital three times a week for 45 to 60 minutes. The OT and the prosthetist worked with Cathy to place the controls. The OTA trained Cathy in using the myoelectric device for basic ADL (BADL) and IADL. Cathy was very motivated and had strong family support. Therefore she progressed rapidly in wearing time and skill in calibration and positioning of the device. She completed training in time for the fall semester.

Preprosthetic Training

OTs and OTAs can incorporate the preprosthetic training as part of the ADL routine, beginning with residual limb care (residual limb wrapping, skin inspection, and donning and doffing stockings and prosthesis). Physical therapists manage wound care and application of physical agent modalities for pain control and promotion of wound healing. The level of the amputation influences the occupational therapy process.

Rigid Removal Dressing. The **rigid removal dressing** (i.e., cast or a stiff solid dressing of plaster of Paris or other material) is applied postoperatively to ensure control of swelling, to apply firm pressure, and to contour the residual limb in preparation for the permanent prosthesis. The cast is changed approximately every 10 days or earlier if the cast becomes loose until the residual limb is healed and ready for a permanent artificial leg (Fig. 31.15). The cast is held in position with a canvas band and secured with a Velcro strap. Alternatively, suspension straps can be used to overcome the weight of the cast.

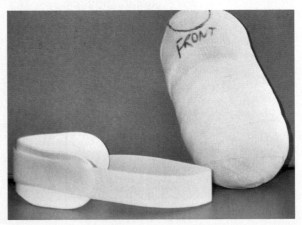

Fig. 31.15 Rigid removal dressing with Velcro strap.

Suspension Straps. The suspension straps can go to the waist or shoulder belt to keep the cast in position. The end of the cast can be made to take a simple training prosthesis (usually called a *pylon*) so that training in standing and walking can be started immediately. A typical pylon is shown in Fig. 31.16.

The casts are normally designed to take only 30 to 45 lb of body weight. Too much weight on the cast may result in slow healing or even cause the wound to open. An adjustment quadrilateral socket attached to the upright of a bail suspension and a solid ankle cushion heel (**SACH foot**) are used for

the foot (Orr et al., 2018). An immediate postoperative prosthesis for the LE client allows greater independence early on in the rehabilitation program.

Types of Prostheses

The **pylon** is a temporary artificial leg. The pylon will serve as a working prosthesis to allow the client to use the residual limb and proximal musculature, maintain joint ROM, and provide a sense of pressure, motion, and weight that may be similar to that of the actual prosthesis (Spencer, 2020).

The computerized **C-leg** system from Otto Bock features a microprocessor-controlled knee-shin system. It is customizable and allows for increased comfort while ambulating a variety of surfaces and inclines. The client can safely and easily climb stairs and uneven terrain. Although it is expensive (approximately $60,000), this device provides state-of-the-art function and versatility and is consistently used for wounded military personnel with transfemoral amputations (Fig. 31.17) (Howard, 2005).

The Canadian-type disarticulation prosthesis meets the needs of the hemipelvectomy and hip disarticulation client (Fig. 31.18). This prosthesis is suspended from the pelvis and equipped with hip and knee joints and a SACH foot. Pelvic movements provide energy for use of the limb (Spencer, 2020).

The Syme client uses the Canadian-type Syme prosthesis or a plastic Syme (Fig. 31.19). This prosthesis consists of a total contact plastic socket and SACH foot; there is no ankle joint (Spencer, 2020).

Transmetatarsal and toe amputations do not require prostheses. These clients need a shoe-toe filler (Spencer, 2020). In the complete tarsal, the amputation is the same as in the Syme. In the partial tarsal the instep is intact. In the complete phalangeal, all the toes are amputated.

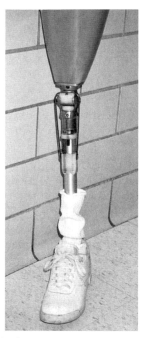

Fig. 31.16 A typical pylon.

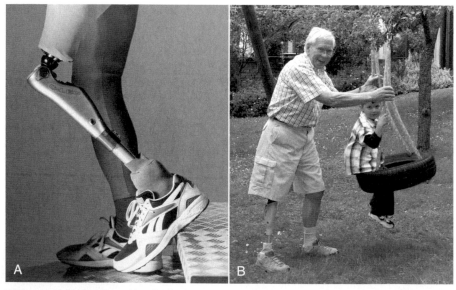

Fig. 31.17 (A) Otto Bock C-leg system. (B) Man with a C-leg playing with his grandson. (Courtesy Otto Bock HealthCare, Minneapolis, MN.)

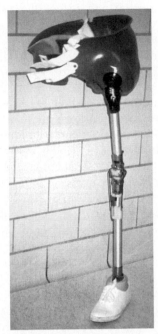

Fig. 31.18 The Canadian prosthesis meets the needs of the hemipelvectomy and hip disarticulation client.

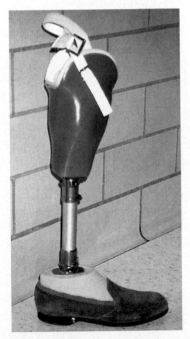

Fig. 31.19 Plastic Syme prosthesis.

Postoperative management includes edema management, exercise, balance, and pain management. For transfemoral (AK) and transtibial (BK) with swelling (edema) at the residual limb site, the practitioner instructs the client on how to apply the elastic wrap(s) in a figure-8 pattern to prevent a tourniquet effect. The elastic wrap(s) should be placed around the residual limb site with firm pressure distally that decreases as the wrapping continues proximally. Bandages are reapplied three or four times a day (Pezzin, Dillingham, MacKenzie, Ephraim, & Rossbach, 2004). If the client cannot wrap properly, a residual limb shrinker (an elastic stocking to control edema) is worn when the prosthesis is not being worn. Maintaining postoperative ROM in the involved extremity is necessary to maintain joint integrity and prevent contractures. Because balance can be affected by the loss of the LE, additional training will be required for ADL. Pain management is important. The aim is to decrease pain whenever possible.

Occupational Therapy Evaluation

The OT and OTA work in close partnership with all the rehabilitation team members to obtain information on the new client in the rehabilitation unit. The OT and OTA have important and distinct roles in the practice setting. The OTA's responsibilities in the initial evaluation process may include data collection from chart review, interviews with patient and family members, general observations, behavioral checklists, and administering standardized tests once competency is demonstrated (in accordance with the OTA's experience and the facility's regulations). The OTA and OT should both have the following knowledge of the patient's medical condition: (1) date and level of amputation (including complications during hospitalization), (2) reason for amputation, (3) exact site and level of amputation, (4) periods of dependent positioning allowed by physician, (5) wear schedule for the prosthesis, and (6) other medical conditions that might influence treatment (e.g., fractures, vascular involvement, medication, edema, infection, lab values, pertinent comorbidities) (Lyons, 1983). The occupational therapy evaluation should cover the following areas: physical functions and skills, ADL, assessment of vocational interests/pursuits, home safety and accessibility, and architectural barriers within the community.

The occupational therapy plan of care requires assessment, reassessment, and ongoing communication between the OT and OTA to provide a truly individualized course of treatment to a person with an amputation. The assessment of the ROM, muscle strength, sensation, coordination, balance, vision, pain, and activity tolerance of the person with an amputation will be performed by the OT. A comprehensive and ongoing assessment of the person's prior level of function and occupational profile will provide guidance in determining discharge disposition. The OT prepares the intervention plan for any complex problem involving physical, emotional, or cognitive factors that arise throughout the course of treatment. The OTA implements the plan under the guidance and supervision of the OT. The OTA observes for any changes from the initial assessment and reports these to the OT; in collaboration with the OTA, the OT can change the plan of care as needed to ensure individualized treatment is provided on the basis of information gathered and reported by the OTA. The OTA provides training for the routine/structured techniques for ADL, bed mobility, wheelchair mobility, seating and positioning, transfers, toileting, hygiene, and dressing, with supervision from the OT as directed by the established plan of care.

An OTA can gather data regarding IADL, leisure, and social interests and pursuits and report such findings to the OT; however, it is the responsibility of the OT to integrate these findings into the plan of care in order for the OTA to provide intervention. The OTA can also provide training for IADL such as homemaking, meal preparation, laundry, shopping, and cleaning. The OTA can lead groups on home safety and accessibility, exercise, pacing and energy conservation, home modifications, discharge planning, work simplification, and joint protection and may document the individual's participation. OTs or experienced, service-competent OTAs can complete a home assessment to identify architectural barriers within the individual's home and community. The OT and OTA will formulate the occupational therapy discharge and follow-up plan.

Basic Activities of Daily Living

Positioning. Prevention of muscle and joint contracture is an important postoperative goal because these are common problems seen in clients with lower limb loss (Lyons, 1983; Orr et al., 2018). Clients with transfemoral amputations are at risk of developing a flexion, external rotation, and abduction contracture of the affected hip. Clients with transtibial amputations are at risk for an external rotation deformity of the hip and flexion of the knee (Orr et al., 2018). Daily ROM exercise can help prevent this. Placing pillows under the residual limb should be avoided. Proper positioning reduces excessive edema in a limb when seated in a wheelchair (Fig. 31.20) (Orr et al., 2018). The OTA needs to consider the seating and positioning of the person with an amputation. Proper cushion selection can assist with obtaining neutral hip alignment and prevent pelvic obliquity, thereby reducing the risk of developing contractures. Appropriate cushions also address comfort

and pain management and reduce the risk of decubitus ulcers.

Residual limb hygiene. Once the wound is healed and sutures are removed, the residual limb should be washed with warm water and dried with a towel. Lotion or alcohol is not recommended. As part of the ADL routine, the OTA should instruct the client on residual limb inspection with a long-handled mirror to ensure the skin is intact.

Dressing training. Most clients with lower limb loss can independently dress their upper body but require assistance for LE dressing. LE dressing should be graded with increasing difficulty, from performing in bed, to sitting [bedside to sink-side], to standing (Orr et al., 2018). Socks and shoes should be donned while sitting. A sock aid, long-handled shoe horn, long-handled reacher, and elastic shoelaces may ease donning and doffing for the individual with loss of flexibility, poor sitting balance, or impaired vision. A footstool may also be useful.

Bed mobility. Bed mobility activities can promote independence without rails or an overhead trapeze bar. Clients with lower limb loss are encouraged to roll from side to side, perform bridging activities with knee and hip flexion, and push the foot of the existing limb so that they can push up in bed and don LE clothing over the hips (Fig. 31.21) (Orr et al., 2018). Bed mobility is an important aspect to master in preparation for bedside ADL and transfers.

Wheelchair mobility and parts management.
The wheelchair will be the main source of postoperative mobility for some persons with LE amputations and should be assessed by the OT (see Chapter 15, Moving in the Environment for information on wheelchair training).

Transfer training. The unilateral LE client generally uses a standing pivot transfer (90-degree pivot), transferring toward the existing limb when possible. Having the individual practice transfers toward the amputated side or 180-degree pivots increases independence when he or she is transferring in more restrictive environments (e.g., a bathroom or bedroom) (Orr et al. 2018). The use of a pivot disc with crutches and/or a standard walker can assist with stand pivot transfers. Sliding board transfers may be taught to clients with bilateral

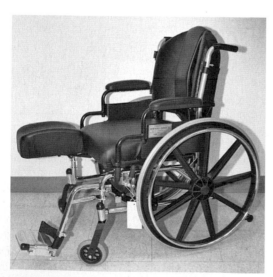

Fig. 31.20 Proper positioning reduces excessive edema in a limb when individual is in a wheelchair.

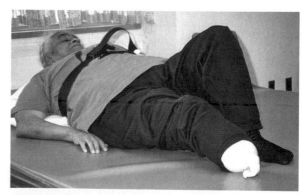

Fig. 31.21 Bridging, a bed mobility skill called for pushing up in bed to don lower extremity.

lower limb loss and to those with a weak existing limb; however, UE and core strength should be assessed before attempting slide board transfers. Clients with bilateral lower limb loss may consider purchasing a wheelchair with a zippered or removable back to allow transfer by sliding backward to a surface and by sliding forward to return to the wheelchair (anterior/posterior) (Lyons, 1983). Transfer training for a person with an amputation should be practiced for various surfaces and situations such as toilet transfers, tub/shower stall transfers with and without a seat or bench, bed transfers to and from a chair or wheelchair, and transfers from wheelchair to and from a chair.

Bathing. Bathing is a self-care activity that includes dressing and undressing, transferring to and from shower chair or tub transfer bench, and balancing while managing the water controls (faucets) and body parts. Adaptive devices (i.e., long-handled bath brush, flexible shower hose, grab bars, and a tub-transfer bench/chair) can promote independence and safety (Orr et al. 2018).

Balance activities. The prerequisite to performing ADL and IADL is balance. The person with an amputation must have good dynamic sitting and standing balance while performing LE dressing activities and while bathing, transferring, reaching for objects in cupboards overhead, and retrieving objects from the floor. These tasks may be done from the wheelchair and while wearing an immediate postoperative prosthesis. The occupational therapy practitioner must provide graded functional activities to facilitate postural adjustment in all planes (Orr et al., 2018). The occupational therapy practitioner must also address core strengthening and UE strengthening to assist with balance.

Pain management. No specific protocol for the treatment of phantom sensation and pain exists. Medication, biofeedback, and other compensatory techniques can decrease the pain and sensation. The OT can instruct the person with an amputation on techniques such as applying pressure (to tolerance), rubbing, tapping, and other modalities such as heat or cold applications on the residual limb for relief (Lyons, 1983). An experienced OTA will observe the client's performance and collaborate with the OT when problems arise. Alternative treatment ideas to address pain management that can be addressed by the OTA include deep breathing, yoga, tai chi, visualization, and progressive muscular relaxation.

Energy conservation and work simplification. The person with an amputation will expend more energy during ADL than a person of the same sex, age, and stature who has no amputations (Banerjee, 2020). Energy expenditure increases with age and obesity (Orr et al., 2018). The OTA should incorporate pacing in all activities to prevent fatigue and injury. The OTA should determine the person's activity tolerance through vital signs, rate of perceived exertion, and use of the BORG scale (see Chapter 34).

Home management. Living alone will require independence and safety during homemaking tasks. Home management should be addressed near discharge but should be considered day 1 on initial evaluation and may involve a combination of individual and group sessions. Areas discussed and practiced are preparing simple and full meals, purchasing food, cooking, serving, cleaning, doing laundry (light and heavy), cleaning house, stripping and making beds (a hospital bed and double bed), and working at various levels (e.g., with a wheelchair, walker [standard or wheeled], cane, and crutches [axillary or loftstrand] with or without prosthesis) (Orr et al., 2018).

Driving. State laws regarding driving after LE amputation vary. The occupational therapy practitioner should know the law before recommending that the individual resume driving. When appropriate, the individual should be referred to a driver safety specialist for a driving assessment (see Chapter 15, Moving in the Environment).

Prevocational and vocational activities. The evaluation will determine whether the person with an amputation can return to his or her previous job. The basic elements are psychological testing, including interest and achievement; establishment of an initial vocational plan; vocational counseling; work evaluation, including definition of functional skills and assessment of architectural barriers in the work environment; driver education and vehicle modification as needed; communication with state vocational rehabilitation agencies, insurance companies, and other sponsors; job analysis and modifications; and follow-up (see also Chapter 16, Work).

Leisure and social participation. Recreation and the constructive use of leisure time enhance quality of life. Many individuals may view mobility limitations as obstacles to returning to premorbid leisure activities. Thus the overall program should include using community recreational resources, learning new leisure skills, making adaptations for previous leisure skills and interests, and refining of functional abilities related to specific leisure activities. Community skills groups feature both discussion and reentry trips to develop the skills necessary to take an active role in recreational opportunities (Kegel, Webster, & Burgess, 1980). Recreational LE prostheses are available for golf, swimming, and skiing (Orr et al., 2018) (see also Chapter 17).

Community reintegration. Ultimately, the individual must gain independence in and accessibility to the community. Here, the person with an amputation attempts to manage curbs, inclines, steps, uneven surfaces, and elevators. The individual should be encouraged to problem-solve specific architectural barriers.

Discharge planning. Discharge planning includes educating the family, providing home exercise programs, and securing necessary DME. A home visit may be completed in anticipation of discharge (Roeschlein & Domholdt, 1989).

During family education, the OT or OTA demonstrates skills taught and encourages the patient and family to practice with the recommended DME. The therapist observes for safety, corrects any unsafe practices, and decides if further education is warranted. It is important to determine if the discharge situation will provide appropriate social support. The OT and OTA work collaboratively, as the following case study illustrates.

CASE STUDY

Marna: Lower Extremity Amputation

Marna is a 76-year-old African American woman. She had a surgical right transtibial amputation due to poor circulation. The residual limb is well healed, and there is good residual limb shrinkage. No significant medical issues are present, and there were no complications during hospitalization.

Referral

A referral was sent to occupational therapy to increase function in basic ADL, mobility, transfers, and IADL with a prosthesis and walker. The estimated length of stay is 14 days.

Marna was assigned to the client unit. The OT reviewed Marna's medical chart in conjunction with the OTA to obtain data sent from the acute care facility.

Occupational History and Profile

Marna is a retired postal worker. She reported having completed 1 year of college. She enjoys the following leisure activities: playing cards, visiting friends, bowling, and traveling with her husband (Louie) to Georgia to visit family members.

Marna lives with Louie in a single-family home. There are three steps to enter the front of the home with bilateral hand rails, as well as a ramp leading up to the side door. Her bedroom and a full bathroom are located on the first floor with a tub. Louie is in poor health and is in a wheelchair. He cannot assist her physically; however, accommodations have been made to the home already: There is a handheld shower with grab bars and a tub bench, as well as a raised toilet seat and grab bars near the toilet. Marna will need to be independent with adaptive equipment and devices for self-care skills and transfers with the **ischial weight-bearing prosthesis** and a standard walker. She will also need to be able to complete light meal preparation for both Louie and herself. Marna is also responsible for medication management for both Louie and herself, as well as financial management. Marna's niece, Stella, will perform the heavier home management activities such as laundry and housekeeping and other personal business in the community such as grocery shopping, driving, and obtaining medication from the pharmacy.

Client Factors and Performance Skills

The OTA's admissions interview included an introduction to the occupational therapy program. Marna was aware of her deficits and appeared motivated. The assessment began with UE passive ROM and active ROM, manual muscle test, and tests of sensory, coordination, pain, edema, skin, visual, and cognition performance by the OT. ADL performance, transfer status positioning, and activity tolerance were assessed collaboratively by the OT and OTA. A treatment plan was developed after completion of all the assessments. Areas of deficits were identified. Short-term and long-term goals were identified with Marna, who played an active part in setting goals.

Interventions

Marna was treated by the OTA in daily sessions of 45 to 60 minute. The OTA consulted daily with the OT. Adaptive devices (i.e., long-handled bath brush, dressing stick, stocking aid, reacher) were issued to improve Marna's self-care skills at bed or wheelchair levels. Transfers were initially performed with a sliding board to compensate for Marna's decreased activity tolerance. At discharge, Marna's mobility and transfers were independent at walker with walker basket level with prosthesis. She was able to complete light meal preparation in the kitchen such as obtaining a beverage from the refrigerator and making soup and sandwiches, as well as transporting items to the table. Marna was educated on energy-conservation techniques and was able to demonstrate 100% understanding and integration of these techniques during her occupational therapy sessions. Dressing the LE posed some problems initially, but Marna was independent with adaptive equipment at discharge. Marna was reassessed daily for areas that required more improvement. Family instruction was completed with Louie and Stella present. A home evaluation was also completed by the OT and OTA to determine Marna's ability to use current DME already in the home. Marna made significant progress in the rehabilitation program. She returned home with good family support and a UE home exercise program. Home therapy was recommended at discharge to ensure a safe transition into the home.

Three weeks after discharge, Louie informed the staff that Marna had died. Marna will be remembered for her determination to regain her skills and return to the community.

SUMMARY

Rehabilitation and prosthetic training of the client following upper limb loss is a complex specialty practice area and is managed by an experienced OT in collaboration with the prosthetist and other rehabilitation team members. The OTA may assist, particularly in use training, donning and removing, and transfer of skills to ADL and work and leisure activities.

The rehabilitation of an individual with lower limb loss requires the skills of many health care specialists, including OTs and OTAs. Occupational therapy intervention should focus on positioning, ADL training, and maintaining and improving ROM and strength in the residual limb to accept a prosthesis and to increase engagement in meaningful occupations. The OT and OTA also assess the feasibility of the client's returning to work and resuming or exploring leisure skills.

Facilitating psychological adjustment is another major role of the clinician working with the UE and LE clients and their family members. The OT and OTA must collaborate to maximize the client's skills for reentry into the workforce and community.

REVIEW QUESTIONS

1. Define the following abbreviations: AE, TD, BE.
2. Which arm functions are lost—and which functions are retained—in a long transradial amputation?
3. List the advantages and disadvantages of a myoelectric prosthesis.
4. Which motions accomplish TD opening with a mechanical prosthesis?

5. Which five questions should be asked when one is observing a client in an activity?

6. What is the recommended initial wearing period for the postoperative prosthesis?

7. What does "prepositioning the TD" mean?

8. Why is it important to wrap the residual limb?

9. What are the responsibilities of the OTA in initial evaluation of the client with lower limb loss?

10. Which method can be used postoperatively to ensure control of residual limb swelling and to contour the residual limb for the permanent prosthesis?

11. Why is the client with lower limb loss instructed *not* to place pillows under the hip and knee?

12. Clients sometimes feel as if their missing limb is moving. What is this phenomenon called?

13. Which adaptive devices can ease donning of an LE prosthesis for an individual with loss of flexibility?

14. Which method can be used to teach the LE client to don pants in bed?

15. Which transfer approach is generally used by the LE client?

16. For which activities must the LE client have good dynamic balance?

17. For the LE client, which areas are assessed, discussed, and practiced in home management?

18. What will be reviewed by the OT or OTA during family education?

19. Describe what is included in discharge planning for the LE client.

REFERENCES

American Occupational Therapy Association. (2014). *Occupational therapy practice framework: Domain and process*. (3rd ed.). *The American Journal of Occupational Therapy*, 68 (s1), s1–s48.

American Occupational Therapy Association. (2020). *Project to delineate the roles and functions of occupational therapy personnel*. Rockville, MD: The Association.

Banerjee, S. J. (2020). *Rehabilitation management of clients*. Baltimore, MD: Williams & Wilkins.

Brenner, C. D. (2020). In: *Atlas of limb prosthetics*. (2nd ed.). St Louis, MO: Mosby.

Bucchieri, J., Poole, B. T., & Schmidt, C. C., et al. (2020). Restoration of thumb function after partial or total amputation. In: E. J. Mackin, A. D. Callahan, & T. M. Skirven et al., (Eds.), *Rehabilitation of the hand and upper extremity*. (5th ed.). St Louis, MO: Mosby.

DiDomenico, R. (2020). Lower limb amputation in the elderly: meeting the rehabilitation challenge. *Focus Geriatrics Care Rehabilitation 4*, 1–8.

Dillingham, T. R., Pezzin, L. E., & MacKenzie, E. J. (2002). Limb amputations and limb deficiency: epidemiology and recent trends in the United States. *Southern Medical Journal*, 95, 875–883. http://www.client-coalition.org/fact_sheets/amp_-stats_cause.html.

Esquenazi, A. (2004). Amputation rehabilitation and prosthetic restoration. From surgery to community reintegration. *Disability and Rehabilitation*, 26(14/15), 831–836.

Friedman, L. W. (2020a). *The psychological rehabilitation of the client*. Springfield, IL: Charles C Thomas.

Friedman, L. W. (2020b). *The surgical rehabilitation of the client*. Springfield, IL: Charles C Thomas.

Horgan, O., & MacLachlan, M. (2004). Psychosocial adjustment to lower-limb amputation: a review. *Disability and Rehabilitation*, 26(14/15), 837–850.

Howard, WJ Chief, Occupational Therapy Service, Walter Reed Army Medical Center, Washington DC. Personal communication, July 25, 2005.

Jacobsen, S., Knutti, D. F., Johnson, R. T., & Sears, H. H. (1982). Development of Utah artificial arm. *IEEE Transactions on Bio-Medical Engineering*, 29(4), 5.

Kegel, B., Webster, J., & Burgess, E. M. (1980). Recreational activities of lower extremity clients: survey. *Archives of Physical Medicine and Rehabilitation*, 61, 258.

Larson, C. B., & Gould, M. (2020). In: *Orthopedic nursing*. (8th ed.). St Louis, MO: Mosby.

Lyons, B. G. (1983). The issue is: purposeful versus human activity. *The American Journal of Occupational Therapy*, 37, 493.

National Limb Loss Information Center. (2005). Amputation statistics by cause: limb loss in the United States. https://www.amputee-coalition.org/resources/limb-loss-statistics/.

Orr, A. E., Glover, J. S., & Cook, C. L. (2018). Amputations and prosthetics. In H. M. Pendleton, & W. Schultz-Krohn (Eds.), *Pedretti's occupational therapy: Practice skills for physical dysfunction* (8th ed., pp. 1083–1116). St Louis, MO: Mosby.

O'Sullivan, S., Cullen, K., & Schmitz, T. (2020). *Physical rehabilitation: Evaluation and treatment procedures*. Philadelphia, PA: FA Davis.

Pedretti, L., & Pasquinelli, S. (2018). Amputations and prosthetics. In: L. Pedretti, & B. Zoltan (Eds.), *Occupational therapy: Practice skills for physical dysfunction*. (3rd ed.). St Louis, MO: Mosby.

Pezzin, L. E., Dillingham, T. R., MacKenzie, E. J., Ephraim, P., & Rossbach, P. (2004). Use and satisfaction with prosthetic limb devices and related services. *Archives of Physical Medicine and Rehabilitation*, 85, 723–729.

Roeschlein, R. A., & Domholdt, E. (1989). Factors related to successful upper extremity prosthetic use. *Prosthetics and Orthotics International*, 13, 14–18.

Schuch, C. M., & Pritham, C. H. (1994). International organization terminology: application to prosthetics and orthotics. *Journal of Prosthetics and Orthotics*, 6(1), 29–33.

Scott, R., Caldwell, R. R., Sanderson, E. R., & Wedderburn, Z. (1985). Understanding and using your myoelectric prosthesis. *UNB Monogr Myoelectric Prostheses*, New Brunswick: Bioengineering Institute.

Spencer, E. (2020). Amputations. In: H. L. Hopkins & H. D. Smith (Eds.), *Willard and Spackman's occupational therapy*. (5th ed.). New York, NY: JB Lippincott.

Stoner, E. K. (2020). Management of the lower extremity client. In: F. J. Kottke, G. K. Stillwell & J. F. Lehmann (Eds.), *Krusen's handbook of physical medicine and rehabilitation*. (3rd ed.). Philadelphia, PA: WB Saunders.

US Department of Health and Human Services. (1993). Vital and health statistics: prevalence of selected impairments, 1977. *Series*, 10, 155–129.

Weeks, S. R., Anderson-Barnes, V. C., & Tsao, J. W. (2010). Phantom limb pain. *Neurologist*, 16(5), 277–286.

Wellerson, T. L. (2020). *A manual for occupational therapists on the rehabilitation of upper extremity clients*. Dubuque, IA: Brown.

Wright G. (2020). *Controls training for the upper extremity client* [film]. San Jose, CA: Instructional Resource Center, San Jose State University.

RECOMMENDED READING

Atkins, D. J., & Alley, R. D. (2003). Upper-extremity prosthetics: an emerging specialization in a technologically advanced field. *OT Practice*, 8(3), CE1–CE8.

Atkins, D. J., & Meier, R. H., (Eds.) (2020). *Comprehensive management of the upper-limb client*. New York, NY: Springer-Verlag.

Christian, A. (2020). *Lower limb amputation: A guide to living a quality life*. New York, NY: Demos Medical Publishing.

Klute, G. K., Kantor, C., Darrouzet, C., Wild, H., Wilkinson, S., Iveljic, S., et al. (2009). Lower limb client needs assessment using multistakeholder focus group approach. *Journal of Rehabilitation Research & Development*, 46(3), 293–304.

Pedretti, L. W., & Early, M. B. (2020). *Occupational therapy: Practice skills for physical dysfunction*. (5th ed.). St Louis, MO: Mosby.

Reed, K. L. (2020). *Quick reference to occupational therapy*. (2nd ed.). Gaithersburg, MD: Aspen.

Van der Linde, H., Hofstad, C. J., Geertzen, J. H. B., Postema, K., & Van Limbeek, J. (2007). From satisfaction to expectation: the patient's perspective in lower limb prosthetic care. *Disability and Rehabilitation*, 29(3), 1049–1055.

Watt, J. (2005). On the road to recovery at Brooke Army Medical Center. *OT Practice*, 10(14), 16–18.

Yeager, A. (2004). Low-tech adaptive devices for upper-extremity amputations. *OT Practice*, 9(8), 12–16.

RESOURCES

American Academy of Orthotics and Prosthetics. http://oandp.org/.
Client Coalition of America. http://www.client-coalition.org/aca_about.html.
Client Information Network. www.amp-info.net.
Hosmer-Dorrance, manufacturer of components. http://hosmer.com/.
Otto Bock, supplier of prosthetics. http://www.ottobockus.com/.
Therapeutic Recreation Systems (TRS), Inc.
2450 Central Ave #D
Boulder, CO 80301-2844
(800) 279–1865
(303) 444–4720.

Cardiac Dysfunction and Chronic Obstructive Pulmonary Disease

E. Joy Crawford

OBJECTIVES

After reading this chapter, the student or the occupational therapy practitioner will be able to do the following:

1. Describe the cardiovascular and respiratory systems and their functions.
2. Identify cardiovascular and pulmonary conditions that are typically addressed in occupational therapy practice.
3. Describe the medical management of cardiac and pulmonary disease.
4. Identify signs and symptoms of cardiac and respiratory distress.
5. Explain how to assess and monitor patient's responses to activities during therapeutic interventions.
6. Discuss psychosocial considerations for persons with cardiovascular or pulmonary disease.
7. Describe methods recommended by occupational therapy practitioners to enhance independence, simplify tasks, conserve energy, and manage stress.

KEY TERMS

Myocardium
Ischemia
Myocardial infarction (MI)
Cardiac rehabilitation
Congestive heart failure (CHF)
Cardiac risk factors
Percutaneous transluminal coronary angioplasty (PTCA)
Coronary artery bypass graft (CABG)
Median sternotomy
Endoscopic atraumatic coronary bypass
Signs of cardiac distress

Heart rate
Blood pressure
Rate pressure product (RPP)
Chronic obstructive pulmonary disease (COPD)
Pulmonary rehabilitation
Dyspnea control postures
Pursed-lip breathing (PLB)
Diaphragmatic breathing
Cardiovascular responses to activity
Basal metabolic equivalent (MET)
Energy conservation

INTRODUCTION

The Centers for Disease Control and Prevention (CDC) reported that heart disease is the leading cause of death in the United States, accounting for more than 630,000 deaths each year (Carrieri-Kohlman, Douglas, & Gormley, 1995); comparatively, chronic lower respiratory disease was the third leading cause of death in 2014 (Centers for Disease Control & Prevention, 2017). The number of individuals reporting having a diagnosis of chronic obstructive pulmonary disease (COPD) has reached almost 15.7 million, with the actual number unknown as not all adults with the disease may be aware that their pulmonary issues are related to COPD (Centers for Disease Control & Prevention, 2017). Considering these facts, and the medical and functional implications associated with these diseases, the role of occupational therapy with this patient population is vital.

Individuals with disorders of the cardiovascular or pulmonary system can be severely limited in endurance and performance of activities of daily living (ADL). Occupational therapy services can benefit such individuals. An understanding of the normal function of the cardiopulmonary system, the pathology of cardiopulmonary disease, common risk factors, clinical terminology, medical interventions, precautions, and standard treatment techniques will guide the certified occupational therapy assistant (COTA) in providing effective care and promoting recovery of function in persons with a compromised cardiovascular or pulmonary system.

Every cell of the body has three major requirements for life: (1) a constant supply of nutrients and oxygen, (2) continual removal of carbon dioxide and other waste products, and (3) a relatively constant temperature. The cardiovascular and pulmonary systems play key roles in these processes.

CARDIOVASCULAR SYSTEM

Anatomy and Circulation

The heart and blood vessels work together to maintain a constant flow of blood throughout the body. The heart, located between the lungs, is pear shaped and about the size of a fist. It functions as a two-sided pump. The right side pumps blood from the body to the lungs; simultaneously, the left side pumps blood from the lungs to the body. Each side of the heart has two chambers, an upper atrium and a lower ventricle.

Blood flows to the heart from the venous system. It enters the right atrium, which contracts and squeezes the blood into the right ventricle. Next, the right ventricle contracts and ejects the blood into the lungs, where carbon dioxide is exchanged for oxygen. Oxygen-rich blood flows from the lungs to the left atrium. As the left atrium contracts, it forces blood into the left ventricle, which then contracts and ejects its contents into the aorta for systemic circulation (Fig. 32.1). Blood travels from the aorta to the arteries and through progressively smaller blood vessels to networks of tiny capillaries. In the capillaries, blood cells exchange their oxygen for carbon dioxide.

Each of the ventricles has two valves: an input valve and an output valve. The valves open and close as the heart muscle (**myocardium**) contracts and relaxes. These valves control the direction and flow of blood.

The heart is living tissue and requires a blood supply (arterial and venous system) of its own or it will die. Coronary arteries cross over the heart muscle to supply the myocardium with oxygen-rich blood. The coronary arteries are named for their location on the myocardium (Fig. 32.2). Cardiologists

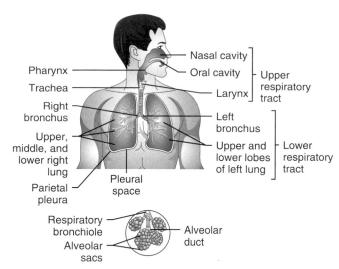

Fig. 32.2 Coronary circulation. (From Goodman CC, Fuller KS. *Goodman and Fuller's Pathology: Implications for the Physical Therapist.* 5th ed. St Louis: Elsevier; 2021.)

refer to these arteries by abbreviations, such as *LAD* for left anterior descending. A blockage of the LAD will interrupt the blood supply to the left ventricle. Because the left ventricle supplies the body and brain with blood, a heart attack caused by LAD blockage can have serious consequences (Andreoli, Fowkes, & Zipes, 1983; Elliot, Anbe, & Armstrong, 2004; Mythos for SoftKey, 1993–1995). Review Fig. 32.2 and locate the LAD. This is the general area of Frederick's heart attack in the accompanying case study.

Mechanism of Heart Contraction

The heart has an electrical conduction system that regulates contraction and relaxation of the myocardium (Fig. 32.3). Electrical impulses usually originate in the right atrium at the sinoatrial (SA) node and travel along internodal pathways to the atrioventricular (AV) node, through the bundle of His, to the left and right bundle branches, and finally to the Purkinje fibers. Nerve impulses normally travel this pathway 60 to 100 times every minute, causing both atria to contract and then both ventricles. The SA node responds to vagal and sympathetic nervous system input (Andreoli et al., 1983). Heart rate increases in response to exercise and anxiety and decreases in response to relaxation behaviors such as deep breathing and meditation.

Electrical impulses generated below the SA node cause the heart to contract abnormally. Some conduction irregularities can be life threatening. Impulses generated by the heart's conduction system can be studied by electrocardiography (ECG). ECG is used to assist in diagnosing cardiac disease (Andreoli et al., 1983; Dubin, 2000).

PATHOLOGY OF CARDIAC DISEASE

Ischemic Heart Disease

Cardiovascular disease (CVD) refers to diseases of the heart or blood vessels. Atherosclerosis is a CVD process that develops over

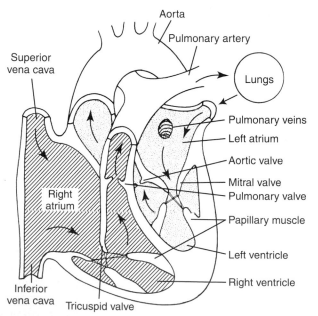

Fig. 32.1 Anatomy of the heart. (Modified from Guyton AC. *Textbook of Medical Physiology.* 8th ed. Philadelphia, PA: Saunders; 1991.)

CASE STUDY

Frederick

An occupational therapist (OT) has evaluated Frederick, a 48-year-old realtor, who experienced 10/10 substernal chest pain, nausea, and shortness of breath during closing of a large commercial transaction. In preparing for the closing, he had continued to work despite extreme fatigue, occasional chest pain, and shortness of breath. He was diagnosed with an acute anterolateral myocardial infarction (MI) complicated by acute congestive heart failure (CHF). After being stabilized in an acute hospital, he was discharged to a skilled nursing facility (SNF) for further therapy.

Frederick wants to return to his family and his real estate work. He is a married father of three children, ages 13, 11, and 7. His wife works full time and cannot manage his care at home until he is self-sufficient. He was referred to occupational therapy for ADL evaluation and progression of activity.

Evaluation Summary

Medical history: unremarkable. Risk factors: age, sex, family history, and a sedentary lifestyle. Current clinical status: Normal sinus rhythm, enlarged left ventricle, and diffuse coronary artery disease. He performed a 2 basal metabolic equivalent (MET) seated sponge bath with minimal assistance. Vital signs were appropriate during the evaluation, except systolic blood pressure fell 20 mmHg in recovery (3 minutes after completion of bathing), and patient became symptomatic (nausea and shortness of breath). Symptoms and vital signs stabilized after 5 minutes of rest. Frederick reports smoking one pack of cigarettes a day for the past 30 years. He states that he drinks socially, a few beers on weekends.

Frederick is anxious. He eats his meals in bed. He transfers independently and per physical therapy can safely walk to the bathroom. He expressed concern that he will die "before age 50, just like Dad." Before his MI, Frederick enjoyed playing catch with the kids and taking occasional walks with his wife. He describes himself as a "weekend warrior."

Problem List

1. Decreased functional capacity and endurance for self-care
2. Lack of ability to pace activity and monitor own signs and symptoms
3. Lack of knowledge of the benefits of energy conservation strategies
4. Potential for alteration in sexual function
5. Positive risk factors of sedentary lifestyle and cigarette smoking
6. Anxiety amplified by family history of cardiac death

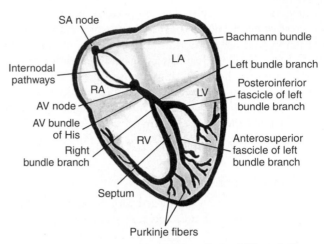

Fig. 32.3 Cardiac conduction. (Modified from Andreoli KG, et al. *Comprehensive Cardiac Care: A Text for Nurses, Physicians, and Other Health Practitioners.* St. Louis, MO: Mosby; 1983.)

affects arteries supplying the brain, heart, kidneys, or legs (American Heart Association, 2019). The leading cause of death for men and women in the United States is atherosclerotic CVD (Collins, Langbein, & Fehr, 2001). Coronary artery disease (CAD) refers to atherosclerosis of the arteries supplying the heart muscle.

If a coronary artery is partially or completely blocked, the heart may not get enough oxygen (a condition called **ischemia**). Persons with CAD may be free of symptoms at rest but develop angina, a type of chest pain, while eating or during exercise, exertion, or exposure to cold. Angina varies from individual to individual. Rest, medication, or both may relieve angina, usually without permanent heart damage. However, angina is a warning sign and should not be ignored.

Chest pain that is not relieved by rest or medication is indicative of a **myocardial infarction** (**MI**), or heart attack. A physician should evaluate the patient promptly. During an MI, part of the heart muscle dies. If a substantial part of the heart is damaged, the heart will stop (cardiac arrest) and the person may die. Once hospitalized, heart attack survivors are managed in a coronary care unit, where they are closely observed for complications. Ninety percent of all persons who have had an MI will develop arrhythmia (Borg, 1982). Close medical management is imperative.

For about 6 weeks after an MI, tissue damage can spread if the heart works too hard. A delicate balance of rest and activity must be maintained for **cardiac rehabilitation** so that the heart can heal without the patient becoming deconditioned. In about 6 weeks, scar tissue forms and the risk of extending the MI decreases. Scar tissue does not contract with each heartbeat, so the heart will not pump as well. Graded exercise can strengthen the healthy part of the myocardium and improve cardiac output.

Frederick has CAD and had ignored his symptoms (shortness of breath, fatigue, and chest pain). The CAD became significant enough to cause an MI. His heart muscle was damaged by loss of its blood supply. During his rehabilitation, Frederick must learn to listen to and respect the signs and symptoms that he previously disregarded.

a period of many years (Goldman, Hashimoto, & Cook, 1981). The walls of arteries can become injured by years of cigarette smoking or high blood pressure. Once the wall is damaged, it becomes irregular in shape and prone to collecting plaque (fatty deposits, like cholesterol). Platelets also gather along the arterial wall and clog the artery (which is called a lesion). The artery narrows and allows less blood to pass through it. Atherosclerosis may occur in any part of the body but is most dangerous when it

Frederick's recovery is also complicated by heart failure. **Congestive heart failure (CHF)** results when the heart cannot pump effectively, and thus fluid backs up into the lungs or the body. Fluid overload is serious because it puts a greater workload on the heart. Straining causes further congestion. Usually, CHF can be controlled with diet, medications, and rest. Patients who experience difficulty resuming their former level of activity after acute CHF may limit their own recovery. Persons with acute CHF can attain optimal function through graded activity.

Valvular Disease

Heart valves may become damaged with disease or infection, resulting in CHF, ischemia, volume overload, or pressure overload. If the aortic valve fails to close properly (aortic insufficiency), CHF or ischemia may result. In another disorder of the aortic valve, aortic stenosis (calcification), pressure overload occurs. The left ventricle, which is working harder to open the sticky valve, enlarges, and cardiac output decreases. Ventricular arrhythmia, cerebral insufficiency, confusion, syncope (fainting), and sudden death may result. Surgery to correct valve problems may be recommended. Volume overload results when fluid accumulates in the lungs and causes shortness of breath. The overload increases the potential for irregular and ineffective contractions in both atria (atrial fibrillation). Consequently, blood flow through the heart slows, and blood clots (emboli) may develop in the ventricles. Many cerebrovascular accidents are caused by emboli ejected from the heart into the circulatory system of the brain.

Cardiac Risk Factors

The Framingham study (Covino, Stern, & Stern, 2011) identified many factors that put people at risk for developing atherosclerosis. **Cardiac risk factors** fall into the following three major categories: (1) unchangeable factors—heredity, male gender, and age; (2) changeable factors—cholesterol levels, cigarette smoking, high blood pressure, and an inactive lifestyle; and (3) contributing factors—diabetes, stress, and obesity. The more risk factors a person has, the greater the risk of developing CAD. Four risk factors—smoking, diabetes, hypertension, and excessive weight—have been associated with left ventricular enlargement, which is a major cause of CHF (American Heart Association, 2018).

Reduction of risk factors is an important goal for the patient and requires support from the rehabilitation team. Prevention of cardiac disease is ultimately in the hands of the individual. Health care professionals, aware of the changes that persons with heart disease must make to reduce risk factors, can facilitate these changes via education, dialogue, and affirmation of the individual's responsibility. It takes years for most CVD to develop. Early prevention can avert or delay the onset. Which risk factors did Frederick have, and into what category might each be classified?

Medical Management

Emergency personnel will administer aspirin to persons who experience a heart attack if they have not taken any before the onset of symptoms. In the emergency department the patient is evaluated to determine whether reperfusion (opening blood flow) of the coronary blood vessels would be helpful. The patient may be given intravenous fibrinolytic therapy (clot-busting medication) or surgery to restore the blood flow. These emergency measures improve chance of survival and limit cardiac damage (Antman et al., 2004).

Various surgical options can correct circulatory problems associated with CAD. Balloon angioplasty (or **percutaneous transluminal coronary angioplasty [PTCA]**) and **coronary artery bypass grafts (CABGs)** are most common. In PTCA, a balloon catheter is guided through the circulatory system into the coronary arteries. The site of the lesion is pinpointed, and the balloon inflated, pushing plaque against the arterial wall. When the balloon is deflated, improved circulation to the myocardium usually results. During a PTCA a wire mesh tube, called a stent, may be implanted into the coronary artery to keep the artery open.

In CABG, the surgeon opens the patient's chest by cutting through the sternum (**median sternotomy**) and spreading the ribs to expose the heart. Diseased sections of the coronary arteries are bypassed with healthy blood vessels from the saphenous veins, internal thoracic artery, or radial artery, with the goal of improving circulation. Following a sternotomy, a patient may be required to follow sternal precautions for 4 to 6 weeks. These precautions, and the length of time that they must be adhered to, may vary from surgeon to surgeon. Recent literature reviews suggest that prolonged precautions may delay the return to daily life activities (Adams, Lotshaw, & Exum, 2016). The OT and COTA should follow policy guidelines set by their facility. General precautions following a sternotomy include:

- Avoiding shoulder flexion beyond 90 degrees
- No asynchronous movements of the upper extremity
- Avoiding reaching behind the back
- No pushing or pulling
- No lifting more than 5 to 10 lb
- Avoidance of activities that cause sternal noises, such as popping or clicking

The less invasive **endoscopic atraumatic coronary bypass** procedure (endo-ACAB) does not require a sternotomy as the heart is accessed via the ribs. This approach does not require sternal precautions, and the recovery time is much faster (Vassiliades, Reddy, & Puskas, 2007).

Other cardiac surgical interventions the OT and COTA should be aware of are heart valve replacements. Since surgical procedures may vary, precautions will be dependent on the procedure. The COTA should clarify any precautions prior to providing occupational therapy interventions.

When the heart's pumping ability is severely reduced, a heart or heart/lung transplantation may be performed. If the operation is successful, the patient may be rehabilitated to a level of function that is significantly higher than in the months before surgery.

Cardiac Medications

Knowledge of the purpose and side effects of cardiac medication provides a framework for understanding the patient's response to activity. Table 32.1 lists common cardiac medications. Cardiac medications are adjusted at frequent intervals until an optimal therapeutic response has been attained. Adverse signs and symptoms should be reported to the physician or nurse promptly. In most settings the nurse is responsible for contacting the physician.

Psychosocial Considerations

Following the diagnosis of a cardiac condition, or having experienced a cardiac event, it is not uncommon for individuals to report sadness, anxiety, or deceased quality of life (Pozuelo, 2019). The length of time in which these symptoms and feelings last may vary from person to person (Pozuelo, 2019). Of

TABLE 32.1 Common Cardiac Medications—Modified from Cardiac Medications at a Glance: American Heart Association, 2008

Category	Common Names	Purpose	Uses
Anticoagulants	Coumadin (warfarin) Enoxaparin (Lovenox) Heparin	Prevents blood clots	Helps to prevent harmful clots from forming. May prevent clots from becoming larger and causing more serious problems. Often prescribed to prevent stroke.
Antiplatelet agents	Aspirin Ticlopidine Clopidogrel Dipyridamole	Prevents blood clots by preventing platelets from sticking together	Helps prevent clotting in patients who have had a heart attack, unstable angina, and other forms of CVD. Usually prescribed preventively, when plaque buildup is present.
Angiotensin-converting enzyme (ACE) inhibitors	Benazepril (Lotensin) Captopril (Capoten) Enalapril (Vasotec) Fosinopril (Monopril)	Expands blood vessels and decreases resistance. Allows blood to flow more easily and makes the heart's work easier	Used to treat CVD including HTN and CHF.
Angiotensin II receptor blockers (or inhibitors) (ARBs)	Candesartan (Atacand) Eprosartan (Teveten) Irbesartan (Avapro)	ARBs prevent this chemical from having any effects on the heart and blood vessels. Dampens BP.	Used to treat or improve symptoms of cardiovascular conditions including HTN and CHF.
β-blockers	Nadolol (Corgard) Propranolol (Inderal) Atenolol (Tenormin) Other drugs ending in "olol"	Decreases the heart rate and cardiac output, which lowers BP and makes the heart beat more slowly and with less force.	Used to lower BP. Used with therapy for cardiac arrhythmias and in treating angina. Used to prevent repeated heart attacks.
Calcium channel blockers	Diltiazem (Cardizem) Verapamil (Isoptin, Calan)	Interrupts the movement of calcium into the cells of the heart and blood vessels.	Used to treat HTN, angina, and some arrhythmias.
Diuretics	Lasix (furosemide) Dyazide Hydrochlorothiazide (HCTZ)	Lowers BP, decreases edema through increased urination	Used to help decrease BP and excessive fluid buildup in tissues of the body.
Vasodilators	Isosorbide dinitrate (Isordil) Nesiritide (Natrecor) Hydralazine (Apresoline) Nitrates (NTG) Minoxidil	Relaxes blood vessels and increases the supply of blood and oxygen to the heart while reducing its workload.	Used to decrease angina.
Cardiac glycosides (digitalis preparations)	Digoxin Lanoxin	Increases the force of the heart's contractions, which can be beneficial in heart failure and for irregular heart beats.	Used to relieve heart failure symptoms
Statins	Atorvastatin (Lipitor) Simvastatin (Zocor)	Can lower blood cholesterol levels	Used to lower LDL ("bad") cholesterol, raise HDL ("good") cholesterol and lower triglyceride levels.

BP, Blood pressure; *CHF*, congestive heart failure; *CVD*, cardiovascular disease; *HTN*, hypertension.

the individuals who receive a CABG, 30% to 40% may experience some degree of depression (Scalzi and Burke, 1992), while 15% of those with the diagnosis of cardiac disease may experience depression (Pozuelo, 2019). In some cases, patients may experience denial of their condition, which may have a significant negative impact on their overall health and wellbeing (Covino et al., 2011). In some instances the help of a mental health professional is indicated.

Individuals entering cardiac rehabilitation programs may suffer from psychological distress that is related both to physical compromise and to psychological factors (Jette and Downing, 1996). Individualized assessments that focus on social, psychological, and occupational status of patients can be helpful in tailoring therapeutic intervention for optimal functional outcomes (McKenna, Mass, & Tooth, 1998). Education and supportive communication may reduce anxiety and alleviate frustration (Gentry and Haney, 1975). As patients begin to resume more normal activities, feelings of helplessness may begin to subside. New habits and routines may be explored and developed as the patient begins to engage in valued occupations.

Consider Frederick and his psychosocial response. Did he express any anxiety during his evaluation? What healthy coping mechanisms to decrease anxiety are available to Frederick? What aspects of his history would be of concern?

Cardiac Rehabilitation

Cardiac rehabilitation is a program aimed at educating persons with CVD to improve their cardiac condition, improve physical conditioning, reduce symptoms of cardiac distress, improve overall health, and prevent cardiac problems. Working with the health care team, individuals recovering from acute MI, CABG, and other cardiac procedures are instructed in guided exercise to improve their recovery. Through active engagement in the rehabilitation process, individuals learn to manage and improve their health.

During the first 1 to 3 days after an MI, stabilization of the cardiac patient's medical condition is usually attained. This acute phase is followed by a period of early mobilization. Phase 1 of treatment (inpatient cardiac rehabilitation) focuses on monitored low-level physical activity, including self-care; reinforcement of cardiac and postsurgical precautions; instruction in energy conservation and graded activity; and establishment of guidelines for appropriate activity levels at discharge. Via monitored activity, the ill effects of prolonged inactivity can be averted, and medical problems, poor responses to medications, and atypical chest pain can be addressed.

Phase 2 of treatment, outpatient cardiac rehabilitation, usually begins at discharge. During this phase exercise can be advanced while the patient is closely monitored on an outpatient basis.

Community-based exercise programs follow in phase 3. Some individuals require treatment in their place of residence because they are not strong enough to tolerate outpatient therapy.

When patients engage in a comprehensive cardiac rehabilitation program, health care costs can be significantly reduced and positive health effects can result (Levin, Perk, & Hedback, 1991). Patients who acquire skills in relaxation and breathing control after an MI have been found to need fewer hospitalizations and

have less expensive medical management even 5 years post MI (Oldridge, Guyatt, & Fischer, 1988). Increased functional independence, prevention of disability, and a decreased need for custodial care have been attained in elderly cardiac rehabilitation patients (Ferrara, Corbi, & Bosimini, 2006). Acute inpatient rehabilitation consists of monitored ADL and instruction in cardiac and postsurgical precautions, energy conservation, graded activity, and risk factor management. The patient is also instructed in guidelines for discharge activities. The ill effects of prolonged inactivity can be averted by means of monitored activity while medical problems, poor responses to medications, and atypical chest pain can be rooted out. Cardiac rehabilitation may continue in the home, community, or outpatient setting.

Prompt, accurate identification of the signs and symptoms of cardiac distress and immediate modification of treatment are imperative. If any **signs of cardiac distress** (Table 32.2) are observed during treatment, the proper response is to stop the activity, have the patient rest, seek emergency medical help if the symptoms do not resolve, report the symptoms to the team, and modify future activity to decrease the workload on the heart. Part of the occupational therapy intervention for Frederick should include identification of adverse response to activity. What signs and symptoms did Frederick ignore before his heart attack? Frederick would be unlikely to stop an activity when signs of cardiac distress occur if he could not recognize them in himself. During his evaluation, Frederick's blood pressure dropped after assisted seated sponge bathing. He also experienced nausea and shortness of breath. What precautions should the OT or COTA review with Frederick before his next treatment session?

The Borg Rate of Perceived Exertion (RPE) scale measures perception of workload (Antman et al., 2004). Patients are shown the scale (which ranges from 6–20) and instructed that a rating of 6 means no exertion at all and a 20 equals the most strenuous activity they have ever performed. After the activity, they are asked to appraise their feelings of exertion and rate the task.

Tools for Measuring the Patient's Response to Activity

Heart rate, blood pressure, rate pressure product, and ECG readings are other measures for evaluating the cardiovascular system's response to work.

Heart Rate. **Heart rate** (beats per minute) can be monitored by palpating the radial, brachial, or carotid pulse. The radial pulse is located on the volar surface of the wrist, just lateral to the radial head. The brachial pulse is slightly medial to the antecubital fossa. The carotid pulse, located lateral to the Adam's apple, should be palpated gently because overstimulation can cause the heart rate to fall. The COTA must establish service competency in palpating the carotid pulse before attempting palpation independently.

Heart rates can be regular (even) or irregular. Although an irregular heart rate is abnormal, many persons function quite well with one. To determine the heart rate, one applies the

TABLE 32.2	**Signs and Symptoms of Cardiac Distress**
Sign/Symptom	**What to Observe**
Angina	Look for chest pain that may be squeezing, tight, aching, burning, or choking in nature. Pain is generally substernal and may radiate to the arms, jaw, neck, or back. More intense or longer-lasting pain forewarns of greater ischemia.
Dyspnea	Look for shortness of breath with activity or at rest. Note the activity that brought on the dyspnea and the amount of time that it takes to resolve. Dyspnea at rest, and with resting respiratory rate over 30 breaths per minute, is a sign of acute CHF. The patient may need emergency medical help.
Orthopnea	Look for dyspnea brought on by lying supine. Count the number of pillows the patient sleeps on to breathe comfortably (1, 2, 3, or 4 pillows of orthopnea).
Nausea/emesis	Look for vomiting or signs that the patient feels sick to the stomach.
Diaphoresis	Look for a cold, clammy sweat.
Fatigue	Look for a generalized feeling of exhaustion. The Borg Rate of Perceived Exertion (RPE) scale is a tool used to grade fatigue.
Cerebral signs	Ataxia, dizziness, confusion, and fainting (syncope) are all signs that the brain is not getting enough oxygen.
Orthostatic hypotension	Look for a drop in systolic blood pressure of greater than 10 mm Hg with change of position from supine to sitting or from sitting to standing.

second and third fingers flat (not tips) to the pulse site. If the pulse is even (regular), count the beats for 10 seconds and multiply the finding by 6. When the heart rate is irregular, the number of beats should be counted for a full minute.

A sudden change in heart rate from regular to irregular should be reported to the physician. In addition, patients can be taught to take their own pulses and monitor their heart rates' responses to activity. As a general rule of thumb, the heart rate should rise in response to activity.

Blood Pressure. **Blood pressure** is the pressure that the blood exerts against the artery walls as the heart beats. A stethoscope and blood pressure cuff (sphygmomanometer) are used to determine blood pressure indirectly. Place the cuff snugly around the patient's upper arm just above the elbow, centering the bladder of the cuff above the brachial artery. Inflate the cuff while palpating the brachial artery to 30 mmHg above the point at which a pulse is last felt. With the earpieces of the stethoscope angled forward in the ears, the practitioner places the dome of the stethoscope over the patient's brachial artery. The practitioner supports the patient's arm in extension with the brachial artery and the stethoscope gauge at the patient's heart level. The practitioner deflates the cuff at a rate of approximately 2 mmHg per second. Listening carefully, the practitioner first hears two sounds that correspond to the systolic blood pressure. The practitioner listens for when pulse fades (diastolic blood pressure). This procedure should be practiced under immediate supervision until competency is established.

Rate Pressure Product. Heart rate and blood pressure will fluctuate in response to activity. Cardiac output is affected by both. **Rate pressure product (RPP)** measurement gives a more accurate indication of how well the heart is pumping. RPP is the product of heart rate and systolic blood pressure ($RPP = HR \times SBP$). It is usually a five-digit number but is reported in three digits by dropping the last two digits (e.g., HR $100 \times SBP\ 120 = 12000 = RPP\ 120$). During any activity RPP should rise at peak and return to baseline in recovery.

ECG provides another objective measure of heart activity. It takes hours of instruction, study, and practice to become proficient in ECG reading and interpretation. The COTA can become qualified to read an ECG after receiving advanced training by a qualified clinical instructor and demonstrating service competency. See Dubin's *Rapid Interpretation of ECG* (Dubin, 2000) as a resource on the subject.

Many similarities exist between the evaluation and treatment of persons with cardiac disease and those with pulmonary dysfunction. A review of the pulmonary system and chronic obstructive pulmonary disease follows.

ANATOMY AND PHYSIOLOGY OF RESPIRATION

While the heart provides oxygen-rich blood to the body and transports carbon dioxide and other waste products to the lungs, the respiratory system exchanges oxygen for carbon dioxide. The cardiac and pulmonary systems are interdependent. If no oxygen were delivered to the bloodstream, the heart would soon stop functioning for lack of oxygen; conversely, if the heart were to stop pumping, the lungs would cease functioning for lack of a blood supply.

The respiratory system supplies oxygen to the blood and removes waste products, primarily carbon dioxide, from the blood. Air enters the body through the nose and mouth and travels through the larynx or voice box to the pharynx. From there it continues downward into the lungs by way of the trachea or windpipe. If the trachea or pharynx becomes blocked, a small incision may be made into the trachea to allow air to freely pass into the lungs. This procedure is called a tracheotomy.

Two main bronchi branch off from the trachea, carrying air into the left and right lungs. The bronchi continue to branch off into smaller tubes called bronchioles. Bronchioles segment into smaller passages called the alveolar ducts. Each alveolar duct divides and leads into three or more alveolar sacs. The entire respiratory passageway from bronchi to alveolar ducts is often called the pulmonary tree.

CASE STUDY

Petua

Petua is a 64-year-old woman with a 3-year history of chronic obstructive pulmonary disease. She was released from the acute care hospital 3 days ago, having been stabilized after an acute exacerbation of COPD. She is widowed and lives alone in a small, one-bedroom apartment. She has one daughter who is married, works full time, and has one child. Petua was referred to occupational therapy for pulmonary rehabilitation. An OT evaluated her and established a treatment plan for the COTA to follow.

Evaluation Summary

Petua has been smoking cigarettes since age 20 and currently smokes one pack per day. She has had three prior exacerbations of COPD. She states that she cannot quit smoking because all of her friends smoke. Her apartment is on the first

floor and is across the street from a grocery store. There is a first-floor laundry room in her building. Petua's daughter lives three blocks away and checks on her daily. She empties the bedside commode that Petua uses at night and provides groceries and dinner. Petua wants to empty the commode herself. She is extremely anxious and demonstrates only minimal understanding of pursed lipped and diaphragmatic breathing. The home health aide provides maximum assistance with sink-side seated bathing. Petua experiences dyspnea on exertion and does not apply breathing techniques to activity. She gets herself a light breakfast and snack with a complaint of severe dyspnea on exertion. Petua does not use her prescribed oxygen during activity because it is too heavy to carry around. According to physical therapy, she was a limited community ambulator before her recent hospitalization.

Each alveolar sac contains more than 10 alveoli. A fine, semipermeable membrane separates the alveolus from the capillary network. Across this membrane, oxygen is transported and exchanged for carbon dioxide. Exhaled carbon dioxide travels upward through the pulmonary tree and out through the mouth and nose.

The muscle power for breathing air into the lungs, or inspiration, is provided primarily by the diaphragm. Originating from the sternum, the ribs and lumbar vertebrae, and the lumbocostal arches, the diaphragm forms the inferior border of the thorax. The muscle fibers of the diaphragm insert into a central tendon. Innervated by the left and right phrenic nerves, the diaphragm comes downward as it contracts, enlarging the volume of the thorax and causing a drop in pressure in the lungs. Air then enters the lungs, equalizing lung and outside air pressures. Accessory muscles—the intercostals and scalene—are also active during inspiration. They maintain the alignment of the ribs and help elevate the rib cage, respectively.

At rest, expiration is primarily a passive relaxation of the inspiratory musculature. Forced expiration requires active contraction of the abdominal muscles to compress the viscera and squeeze the diaphragm upward in the thorax. Expiration can be further forced by flexing the torso forward and pressing with the arms on the chest or abdomen. As the volume of the thorax decreases, air is forced out of the lungs. Fig. 32.4 shows the structure of the respiratory system (Brannon, Foley, & Starr, 1997; Mythos for SoftKey, 1993–1995).

Innervation of the Respiratory System

Breathing is mostly involuntary. A person does not have to think to take a breath. The autonomic nervous system controls breathing. With anxiety and increased activity, the sympathetic nervous system will automatically increase the depth and rate of inspiration. Parts of the brain provide the central control for breathing; they adjust their response to input from receptors in the lungs, the aorta, and the carotid body.

Although the act of breathing is primarily involuntary, there is also a volitional component that allows for measured and deliberate mediation of the outflow of breath during activities requiring

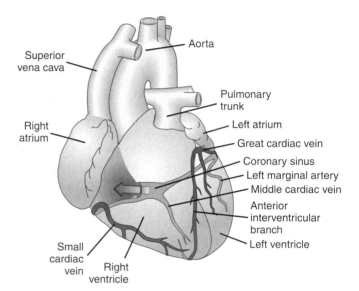

Fig. 32.4 Major structures of the respiratory system. (From McCannce SE, McCance KL. *Understanding Pathophysiology*, St Louis: Elsevier; 2017.)

controlled breathing such as swimming or playing the harmonica (Brannon et al., 1997; Mythos for SoftKey, 1993–1995).

CHRONIC OBSTRUCTIVE PULMONARY DISEASE

Common chronic disorders of the lungs for which pulmonary rehabilitation is ordered include **chronic obstructive pulmonary disease (COPD)** and asthma (Brannon et al., 1997). COPD (actually a group of diseases) is characterized by "damage to the alveolar wall and inflammation of the conducting airways" (American Thoracic Society, 1962) and includes emphysema, peripheral airway disease, and chronic bronchitis. More than 15.7 million Americans have been diagnosed with COPD (Centers for Disease Control and Prevention, 2019). The CDC speculates that the number is actually higher, as 50% of adults with impaired pulmonary function are believed to have COPD but are undiagnosed (Centers for Disease Control and Prevention, 2019).

The most common signs of COPD are daily coughing, shortness of breath, and increasing fatigue with exercise (Santa Clara Valley Medical Center, 2007). In COPD the onset of physical disability is typically gradual, with dyspnea on exertion representing the initial phase of disability. The disease evolves toward shortness of breath at rest. Uncoordinated, ineffective breathing patterns contribute to shortness of breath (Collins et al., 2001).

Asthma is characterized by irritability of the bronchotracheal tree and is typically episodic in its onset. Individuals with asthma may be free of symptoms for periods of time between the episodes of wheezing and dyspnea (Farzan, Phillips, & Farzan, 1985). A genetic predisposition seems to influence development of asthma in some individuals. Allergic causes of asthma may include pollens and respiratory irritants such as perfume, dust, pollen, and cleaning agents. If left untreated, a severe asthmatic episode may result in death (American Thoracic Society, 1962; Brannon et al., 1997).

Pulmonary Risk Factors

Smoking is the primary cause of COPD. The best method for preventing COPD or for controlling it is to not smoke (Santa Clara Valley Medical Center, 2007). Because cigarette smoke is a pulmonary irritant, it may also be a causative agent in asthmatic episodes. Other environmental irritants such as air pollution and chemical exposure are contributory risk factors in the development of COPD and asthma (American Thoracic Society, 1962; Brannon et al., 1997).

Medical Management

COPD is a progressive, chronic disease process. The onset of the disease process is gradual. Medications prescribed for pulmonary disease include anti-inflammatory agents (e.g., steroids, cromolyn sodium), bronchodilators (e.g., albuterol, theophylline) that help to open the airways, and expectorants (e.g., iodides, guaifenesin) that help loosen and clear mucus. Oxygen therapy, at a specific liter flow, may also be prescribed. Some persons on oxygen therapy may be tempted to increase the liter-per-minute flow, erroneously thinking that more is better. This practice can result in CO_2 retention and lead to right heart failure.

Persons with acute respiratory distress initially may be managed on a ventilator before being weaned to oxygen. Ventilators provide a mechanical assist to the process of inspiration. Ventilators will not slow the end-stage disease process of COPD.

When a patient's endurance decreases enough to impair ADL performance, the physician may refer the patient to occupational therapy (American Thoracic Society, 1962; Brannon et al., 1997).

Signs and Symptoms of Respiratory Distress

Dyspnea is the most obvious sign that an individual is having difficulty breathing. In its most severe form, the patient is short of breath at rest. Persons with this level of dyspnea will be unable to utter a short phrase without gasping for air. When reporting that a patient has dyspnea, the practitioner should note the precipitating factors (e.g., "Mr. S. becomes short of breath when washing his face while seated in front of the sink").

Other signs that the body is not getting enough oxygen include extreme fatigue, a nonproductive cough, confusion, impaired judgment, and cyanosis (a blue tinge to the skin) (American Heart Association, 2018; Bragg, 1975).

Psychosocial Considerations

COPD is a progressive and debilitating physical illness, and the psychosocial effects of the disease are considerable. Depression and anxiety are not uncommon and occur more frequently among those with COPD than those with other chronic illnesses or those in the general population (Yohannes, Kaplan, & Hanania, 2018). In fact, patients with COPD are 85% more likely to develop anxiety (Yohannes et al., 2018). Dyspnea-related anxiety (fear related to shortness of breath and inability to manage symptoms) leads to avoidance of physical exertion (Carrieri-Kohlman et al., 1995). A spiral of functional decline can follow in which the individual stops participating in activities that cause symptoms, lowering one's physical capacity for activity. This leads to deconditioning in which the individual experiences shortness of breath in activities that are progressively less physically demanding. Controlling and reducing dyspnea-related anxiety is important; patients can be taught breathing techniques using guided mastery and can be made more aware of symptoms and their management (Carrieri-Kohlman et al., 1995). Progressive muscle relaxation has been shown to be successful for controlling dyspnea and anxiety and for lowering heart rate (Renfroe, 1988).

PULMONARY REHABILITATION

The goals of **pulmonary rehabilitation** are to stabilize or reverse the disease process and return the patient's function to its highest capacity. A multidisciplinary rehabilitation team working with the patient can design an individualized treatment program to meet this end. An accurate diagnosis, medical management, therapy, education, and emotional support are components of a pulmonary rehabilitation program. OTs and COTAs are often part of the team that also includes the physician, nurse, and patient. Respiratory therapists, dietitians, physical therapists, social workers, and psychologists may also be team members. When occupational therapy is part of the pulmonary rehabilitation team, the outcome for severely disabled COPD patients is improved (Lorenzi, Cilione, & Rizzardo, 2004). Knowledge of specialized pulmonary treatment techniques is imperative to treating persons with pulmonary disease.

Treatment Techniques

Dyspnea Control Postures. Breathlessness can be reduced in patients with COPD by having them adopt **dyspnea**

control postures. When sitting, the patient bends forward slightly at the waist while supporting the upper body by leaning the forearms on the table or thighs. When standing, leaning forward and propping the body on a counter or shopping cart may relieve the problem.

Pursed-Lip Breathing. **Pursed-lip breathing** (**PLB**) is thought to prevent tightness in the airway by providing resistance to expiration. This technique increases use of the diaphragm and decreases accessory muscle recruitment (Breslin, 1992). PLB is sometimes instinctively adapted by persons with COPD, whereas others may need to be instructed in the technique. Instructions for PLB are the following: (1) Purse your lips as if you are going to whistle; (2) slowly exhale through pursed lips—you should feel some resistance; (3) inhale deeply through your nose; and (4) it should take you twice as long to exhale as it does to inhale.

Diaphragmatic Breathing. Another breathing pattern that calls for increased use of the diaphragm to improve chest volume is **diaphragmatic breathing**. Many persons learn this technique by placing a small paperback novel on the abdomen just below the thorax. The person lies supine and is instructed to inhale slowly and make the book rise. Exhalation through pursed lips should cause the book to fall.

Desensitization. As individuals with COPD experience dyspnea during activity, manage their anxiety, and monitor and adjust their breathing in a controlled therapeutic environment, they begin to become desensitized to dyspnea-related anxiety. The therapist reinforces dyspnea control postures, paced activity, and breathing techniques while ensuring safe performance of activity. Oxygen saturation monitors, when available, provide another measure of safety. When oxygen saturation drops below 90%, activity should be stopped (Migliore, 2004).

Relaxation. Progressive muscle relaxation in conjunction with breathing exercises can be effective in decreasing anxiety and in controlling shortness of breath. One technique involves tensing muscle groups while slowly inhaling and then following with relaxation of the muscle groups when exhaling twice as slowly through pursed lips. It is helpful to teach the patient a sequence of muscle groups to tense and relax. One common sequence involves tensing and relaxing the face; then the face and the neck; then the face, neck, and shoulders; and so on down the body to the toes. A calm, quiet, and comfortable environment is important for the novice in learning any relaxation technique. Biofeedback in conjunction with relaxation therapy promotes a more rapid mastery of relaxation skills (Green, Walters, & Green, 1969).

Management of Dyspnea Guidelines for Practice (McKenna et al., 1998). Migliore (2004) developed guidelines for the treatment of individuals with COPD. Treatment focuses initially on control of respiration at rest. Initial patient competency is attained in PLB and diaphragmatic breathing with dyspnea control postures. Biofeedback (paced breathing, metronomes, and recording

of the patient's breathing pattern) reinforces learning. Clients are then progressed to controlled breathing with activity. Management of dyspnea-related anxiety is attained by therapeutic discussions to improve the patient's understanding of how poor breathing patterns create false danger signals and signs or symptoms of true hypoxia. Using both individual and group treatment, Migliore's guidelines provide the clinician with an organized and meaningful approach to treatment.

Other Treatments and Considerations. Physical therapists may teach chest expansion exercises, a series of exercises intended to increase the flexibility of the chest. Percussion, postural drainage, and vibration are other techniques used to loosen secretions and assist with draining them from the lungs. Other team members usually teach these techniques.

Humidity, pollution, extremes of temperature, and lack of air movement have been reported to have a deleterious effect on persons with respiratory ailments. These factors should be taken into consideration when one is planning activities.

EVALUATION AND TREATMENT OF PERSONS WITH CARDIOPULMONARY DYSFUNCTION

Occupational therapy intervention can promote improvements in performance of ADL for persons with limitations caused by chronic respiratory or cardiovascular limitations. The following information is to be used for both cardiac and pulmonary conditions, occurring separately or together.

Evaluation Process
Review of the Medical Record. A review of the medical record will identify the patient's medical history (diagnosis, severity, associated conditions, and secondary diagnoses), social history, test results, and precautions. Although the COTA may not perform the initial evaluation of the patient, familiarizing oneself with changes in the patient's condition as documented in the medical record should be standard practice.

Patient Interview. It is common courtesy and good medical practice to begin every patient encounter with an introduction and an explanation of the purpose of treatment. Good interview skills include asking the right questions, listening to the patient's response, and observing patients as they respond. Look for signs of anxiety, shortness of breath, confusion, difficulty comprehending, fatigue, posture, endurance, ability to move, and family dynamics. Interview questions should not only seek clarification of information that was not clear in the medical record but also clarify the patient's understanding of his or her condition and treatment.

Not uncommonly, patients may have cardiac *and* pulmonary conditions. Patients with a history of angina should be asked to describe their angina. If they also had an MI, patients should be asked if they can differentiate between angina and MI chest pain and pulmonary symptoms. Clarification of symptoms before treatment can prove invaluable should symptoms arise.

Asking patients to describe a typical day, identify activities that bring on shortness of breath or angina, and tell how their physical limitations interfere with the things they enjoy doing most in life will reveal problems that are relevant to the patient.

Clinical Assessment of Performance Skills. The purpose of the clinical assessment is to establish the patient's present functional ability and limitations. The content of an OT's clinical assessment will vary from patient to patient and setting to setting. Persons with impairments of the cardiovascular system will be monitored for heart rate, blood pressure, and signs and symptoms of cardiac distress during an evaluation of tolerance to postural changes and a functional task. Table 32.3 summarizes appropriate and inappropriate **cardiovascular responses to activity**. Individuals with disorders of the respiratory system must be monitored for signs and symptoms of respiratory distress. Range of motion, strength, and sensation may be grossly assessed within the context of the ADL evaluation. The patient's cognitive and psychosocial status will become apparent to the skilled clinician through interview and observation.

After the evaluation, the OT has sufficient information to formulate a treatment plan. In consulting the patient about the treatment plan, the clinician informs the patient of the expected outcome of treatment and verifies that goals will be meaningful and relevant to the patient.

Intervention

Both Frederick and Petua have a decreased functional capacity for self-care. They share a similar goal of wanting to take a standing shower (3.5 **basal metabolic equivalents [MET]**) and tolerate being out of bed for most of the day. The clinical techniques and cueing provided by the OT or COTA will be unique to the condition of each of them. In reading this treatment section and comparing Frederick's cardiac condition to Petua's compromised respiratory status, consider which interventions would be most appropriate for each individual.

Progression of treatment for persons with cardiovascular impairment or respiratory impairment is guided by present clinical status, recent functional history, response to current activity, and prognosis. Persons with significant cardiac or pulmonary impairment, limited recent functional ability, inappropriate orthostats (cardiovascular responses to changes in position [e.g., sit to stand]) or poor reaction to activity, and a poor prognosis

will progress slowly in comparison with individuals with little impairment of the heart or lungs, a recent history of normal functional ability, appropriate responses to orthostats and activity, and a good prognosis. The COTA should keep these factors in mind when treating persons with cardiopulmonary deficits.

In both case studies in this chapter, the patients might benefit from working on seated bathing during the next therapy session, but the focus of treatment will be different for each. Frederick's session might focus on early recognition of symptoms, pacing his self-care, and exhaling on exertion. Petua's treatment would include coordination of PLB and diaphragmatic breathing with activity and use of dyspnea control postures at rest. If tolerated, dyspnea control postures could be extended to a simple light hygiene task such as seated oral hygiene.

Energy costs of an activity and the factors that influence them can further guide the COTA in the safe progression of activity. Oxygen consumption suggests how hard the heart and lungs are working, providing an indication of the amount of energy required to complete a task. Resting quietly in bed requires the least amount of oxygen per kilogram of body weight, 1 MET, roughly 3.5 mL O_2 per kilogram of body weight. As activity increases, more oxygen is required to meet the demands of the task. For instance, dressing requires 2 MET, or roughly twice the amount of energy that lying in bed takes. Guided by a MET table (Table 32.4) and the patient's response to activity, the COTA can determine a logical treatment progression tailored to the patient's prognosis and goals. As a general rule, once patients tolerate an activity (i.e., seated sponge bathing) with appropriate responses, they can progress to the next higher MET level activity (i.e., standing sponge bath).

At all times during interactions with patients, therapy personnel focus on attaining the safest and highest level of function. With a cardiac rehabilitation patient in denial, the COTA might best focus on paced activity and teaching the patient to recognize and identify symptom exacerbation as a time to stop and rest. In pulmonary rehabilitation the focus shifts to performing compensatory breathing strategies and dyspnea control postures. Here patients are learning to push their limits safely; education focuses on improving patient understanding that increased work requires increased respiratory effort. By focusing on helping the patient learn appropriate activity responses, the COTA guides the patient toward improving independent function in a safe and sustainable manner.

TABLE 32.3 **Cardiovascular Response to Activity**		
	Appropriate	**Inappropriate**
HR	Increases with activity, to no more than 20 beats/min above resting heart rate	HR more than 20 beats/min above RHR with activity, RHR ≥ 120, HR drops or does not rise with activity
BP	SBP rises with activity	SBP ≥ 220 mm Hg, postural hypotension (≥10–20 mm Hg drop in SBP), decrease in SBP with activity
Signs and symptoms	Absence of adverse symptoms	Excessive shortness of breath, angina, nausea and vomiting, excessive sweating, extreme fatigue (RPE ≥ 15), cerebral symptoms

BP, Blood pressure; *HR*, heart rate; *RPE*, rate of perceived exertion; *RHR*, resting heart rate; *SBP*, systolic blood pressure.

TABLE 32.4 Basal Metabolic Equivalent Table of Areas of Occupation

MET Level	Activities of Daily Living	Instrumental Activities of Daily Living, Work, Play, and Leisure
1–2	Eating, seated (Lorenzi et al., 2004); transfers, bed to chair; washing face and hands; brushing hair (Lorenzi et al., 2004); walking 1 mph	Hand sewing (Centers for Disease Control and Prevention, 2017), machine sewing, sweeping floors (Centers for Disease Control and Prevention, 2017), driving automatic car, drawing, knitting (Pozuelo, 2019)
2–3	Seated sponge bath (Pozuelo, 2019), standing sponge bath (Pozuelo, 2019), dressing and undressing (Jette and Downing, 1996), seated warm shower (Pozuelo, 2019), walking 2–3 mph, wheelchair propulsion 1–2 mph	Dusting (Lorenzi et al., 2004); kneading dough (Centers for Disease Control and Prevention, 2017); hand washing small items (Centers for Disease Control and Prevention, 2017); vacuuming, electric (Lorenzi et al., 2004); preparing a meal (Jette and Downing, 1996); washing dishes (Pozuelo, 2019); golf (Pozuelo, 2019)
3–4	Standing shower, warm (Jette and Downing, 1996); bowel movement on toilet (Centers for Disease Control and Prevention, 2017); climbing stairs at 24 ft/min (Pozuelo, 2019)	Making a bed (Jette and Downing, 1996), sweeping, mopping, gardening (Pozuelo, 2019)
4–5	Hot shower (Jette and Downing, 1996), bowel movement on bedpan (Jette and Downing, 1996), sexual intercourse (Pozuelo, 2019)	Changing bed linens (Lorenzi et al., 2004), gardening, raking, weeding, rollerskating (Green et al., 1969), swimming 20 yards/min (Pozuelo, 2019)
5–6	Sexual intercourse (Pozuelo, 2019), walking up stairs at 30 feet/min (Pozuelo, 2019)	Biking 10 mph level ground (Pozuelo, 2019)
6–7	Walking with braces and crutches	Swimming breaststroke (Pozuelo, 2019), skiing, playing basketball, walking 5 mph, shoveling snow, spading soil (Pozuelo, 2019)

The duration of any physical activity must also be taken into account when determining activity guidelines. Obviously, persons who have difficulty performing a 2 MET activity must still use a commode (3.5 MET) or bedpan (5 MET) for their bowel management. A person can perform at a higher than usual MET level for brief periods without adverse effects.

Sexual activity at 5 MET is often a grave concern to persons with impaired cardiovascular function and their partners. Sexual intercourse is intermittent in its peak demands for energy. Patients often can return to sexual intercourse once they can climb two flights of steps in 1 minute with appropriate cardiovascular responses (Scalzi and Burke, 1992). Providing the patient with information as to when it is safe to resume sexual activity can reduce anxiety surrounding the resumption of sexual intercourse. Discussing sexual activity guidelines with the patient and partner may further decrease anxiety. The patient should be instructed to monitor heart rate and symptoms of cardiac distress before and after intercourse. In addition, the patient and partner should be informed that cardiac medications can affect the patient's libido. The patient should be encouraged to inform the physician of problems related to sexual activity. Medications can often be adjusted to alleviate these problems.

Energy Conservation

When patients learn to conserve their energy resources, they can perform at a higher functional level without expending more energy. The basic principles of **energy conservation** and work simplification, covered in Chapter 28 and other chapters, should prove useful in teaching persons with cardiovascular or pulmonary compromise how to decrease energy demands on the body while promoting function. The role of the COTA is to assist the patient with identifying relevant roles and tasks and determining how those tasks and roles may be modified to maximize independence and enhance quality of life. Environments may be modified, tasks simplified, roles revisited, and routines tweaked to promote participation.

Exhaling with exertion is an energy conservation strategy particularly helpful for persons with compromised cardiac or pulmonary function. This technique helps control the rate of increase of systolic blood pressure with activity. It is important for the patient to practice energy conservation skills during treatment. Therapeutic support is critical in learning. Both Frederick and Petua would benefit from this technique.

Patient and Family Education

OTs and OTAs, as members of the health care team, share the responsibility for patient and family education. Cardiac and/or pulmonary anatomy, disease process, symptom management, risk factors, diet, exercise, and energy conservation must be taught and reinforced to patient and family members by the team. Including family members in an education program provides support indirectly to the patient through the family unit. Such support is critical when a patient depends on the help of a family member to accomplish everyday tasks.

In progressing treatment for Frederick and Petua, their individual goals will evolve into the areas of instrumental ADL. For Frederick, sexual activity guidelines, guidelines for resuming sporting activities with his youngsters, and return to work are all possible venues for further therapeutic intervention. Petua has expressed an interest in basic homemaking tasks (emptying her commode). Given the proximity of laundry facilities to her apartment, independence in personal laundry may be of interest to her. Smoking cessation is essential for optimal outcomes for Petua.

SUMMARY

Healthy individuals can meet the varying demands of their bodies for oxygen because their heart and respiratory rates adjust to meet oxygen demand. When the cardiovascular and/or pulmonary system is compromised, the ability to perform normal activity declines. This chapter is designed to guide the OT and COTA in the treatment of persons with impairments of the heart or lungs.

REVIEW QUESTIONS

1. Describe the heart's size and explain the function of its right and left sides.
2. What do the heart valves control?
3. Explain the significance of the coronary arteries in heart disease and heart attacks.
4. Identify the symptoms of cardiac distress. Explain why modifying activity in response to them is important.
5. Explain the significance of left ventricular dysfunction.
6. Using the MET chart, identify a safe self-care task for a person who can function at 2.5 MET.
7. If the patient could perform a seated sponge bath but could not stand because of a secondary disability, which activity would you choose to promote progress in rehabilitation? Explain.
8. Describe the appropriate therapeutic response when a patient develops chest pain during activity.
9. What is COPD?
10. Name the breathing techniques used in pulmonary rehabilitation and their purposes.
11. Describe dyspnea control postures.
12. Explain how treatment concerns for activity tolerance vary and are similar for persons with cardiac compromise and those with respiratory conditions.
13. Using the cardiac medications chart, explain how cardiac medications might affect heart rate or blood pressure.
14. What are cerebral signs? What do they signify, and why is this important? What action would you take if a patient were to suddenly develop cerebral signs?

EXERCISES

1. Demonstrate dyspnea control postures in sitting and standing.
2. Teach your partner pursed-lip and diaphragmatic breathing.
3. Choose a cooking task. Explain how to modify the activity by using three energy conservation principles.
4. Determine your partner's heart rate and respiratory rate.
5. Have your partner run in place for 3 minutes. Immediately take your partner's blood pressure and heart rate. Calculate the RPP for before and immediately after activity. Was your partner's response appropriate?
6. Pretend that your partner is Frederick (see case study) and that he is asking about when it will be safe for him and his wife to resume sexual activity. How will you respond?
7. Pretend your partner is Petua (see case study). She has a resting respiratory rate of 33. While panting, she tells you to "Leave" (pant) "me" (pant) "alone" (pant). Demonstrate an appropriate response.

REFERENCES

Adams, J., Lotshaw, A., Exum, E., et al. (2016). An alternative approach to prescribing sternal precautions after median sternotomy, "keep your move in the tube." *Proceedings (Baylor University Medical Center), 29*(1), 97–100. Available from: https://doi.org/10.1080/08998280.2016.11929379.

American Heart Association. (2018). Understand your risks to prevent a heart attack. http://www.heart.org/HEARTORG/Conditions/HeartAttack/UnderstandYourRiskstoPreventaHeartAttack/Understand-Your-Risks-toPrevent-a-Heart-Attack_UCM_002040_Article.jsp#.XX5npShKhPY.

American Heart Association. (2019). Atherosclerosis. What role does cholesterol play? http://www.heart.org/HEARTORG/Conditions/.../Atherosclerosis_UCM_305564_Article.jsp#.XX5c-ChKhPY.

American Thoracic Society. (1962). Definitions and classifications of chronic bronchitis, asthma, and pulmonary emphysema. *The American Review of Respiratory Disease, 85*(8), 762–768.

Andreoli, K. G., Fowkes, V. K., Zipes, D. P., et al. (1983). *Comprehensive cardiac care: A text for nurses. physicians and other health practitioners* (5th ed.). St. Louis, MO: Mosby.

Antman, E. M., Anbe, D. T., Armstrong, P. W., et al. (2004). ACC/AHA guidelines for the management of patients with ST-elevation myocardial infarction: a report of the American College of Cardiology/American Heart Association Task Force on Practice Guidelines (Writing Committee to Revise the 1999 Guidelines for the Management of Patients With Acute Myocardial Infarction). *Journal of the American College of Cardiology, 4*(3), 671–719.

Borg, G. A. (1982). Psychosocial bases of perceived exertion. *Medicine & Science in Sports & Exercise, 14*(5), 377–381.

Bragg, T. L. (1975). Psychological response to myocardial infarction. *Nursing Forum, 14*(4), 383–395.

Brannon, F. J., Foley, M. W., Starr, J. A., et al. (1997). *Cardiopulmonary rehabilitation: Basic theory and application* (3rd ed.). Philadelphia, PA: FA Davis Company.

Breslin, E. H. (1992). The pattern of respiratory muscle recruitment during pursed-lip breathing. *Chest, 101*(1), 75–78.

Carrieri-Kohlman, V., Douglas, M. D., Gormley, J. M., et al. (1995). Desensitization and guided mastery: treatment approaches for the management of dyspnea. *Heart & Lung, 22*, 226–234.

Centers for Disease Control and Prevention. (2017). Heart disease fact sheet. https://www.cdc.gov/dhdsp/data_statistics/fact_sheets/fs_heart_disease.htm.

Centers for Disease Control and Prevention. (2019). Basics about COPD. https://www.cdc.gov/copd/basics-about.html.

Collins, E. G., Langbein, W. E., Fehr, L., et al. (2001). Breathing pattern retraining and exercise in persons with chronic obstructive pulmonary disease. *AACN Clinical Issue, 12*, 202–209.

Covino, J. M., Stern, T. W., & Stern, T. A. (2011). Denial of cardiac illness: consequences and management. *The Primary Care Companion for CNS Disorders, 13*(5). Available from: https://doi.org/10.4088/PCC.11f01166.

Dubin, D. (2000). *Rapid interpretation of EKGs* (6th ed.). Tampa, FL: Cover Publishing.

Elliot, M. A., Anbe, D. T., Armstrong, P. W., et al. (2004). ACC/AHA guidelines for the management of patients with ST-elevation myocardial infarction, executive summary: a report of the American College of Cardiology/American Heart Association Task Force on Practice Guidelines (Writing Committee to Revise the 1999 Guidelines for the Management of Patients With Acute Myocardial Infarction). *Circulation, 110*(5), 588−636.

Farzan, S., Phillips, M. L., & Farzan, D. (1985). *A concise handbook of respiratory diseases* (2nd ed.). Reston, VA: Pearson.

Ferrara, N., Corbi, G., Bosimini, E., et al. (2006). Cardiac rehabilitation in the elderly: patient selection and outcomes. *The American Journal of Geriatric Cardiology, 15*(1), 22−27.

Gentry, W. D., & Haney, T. (1975). Emotional and behavioral reaction to acute myocardial infarction. *Heart & Lung, 4*(6), 738−745.

Goldman, L., Hashimoto, B., Cook, E. F., et al. (1981). Comparative reproducibility and validity of systems for assessing cardiovascular functional class: advantages of a new specific activity scale. *Circulation, 64*(6), 1227−1234.

Green, E., Walters, E. D., Green, A. M., et al. (1969). Feedback technique for deep relaxation. *Psychophysiology, 6*(3), 371−377.

Jette, D. U., & Downing, J. (1996). The relationship of cardiovascular and psychological impairments to the health status of patients enrolled in cardiac rehabilitation programs. *Physical Therapy, 76*(2), 130−139.

Levin, L. A., Perk, J., & Hedback, B. (1991). Cardiac rehabilitation: a cost analysis. *The Journal of Internal Medicine, 230*(5), 427−434.

Lorenzi, C. M., Cilione, C., Rizzardo, R., et al. (2004). Occupational therapy and pulmonary rehabilitation of disabled COPD patients. *Respiration, 71*, 246−251.

McKenna, K., Mass, F., & Tooth, L. (1998). Predictions of quality of life after angioplasty. *Scandinavian Journal of Occupational Therapy, 5*, 173−179.

Migliore, A. (2004). Management of dyspnea guidelines for practice for adults with chronic obstructive pulmonary disease. *Occupational Therapy in Health Care, 18*(3), 1−20.

Mythos for SoftKey. (1993−1995). *Bodyworks 4.0: Human anatomy leaps to life.* Cambridge, MA: SoftKey International.

Oldridge, N. B., Guyatt, G. H., Fischer, M. E., et al. (1988). Cardiac rehabilitation after myocardial infarction. Combined experience of randomized clinical trials. *JAMA, 260*(7), 945−950.

Pozuelo, L. (2019). Depression and heart disease. Cleveland Clinic. https://my.clevelandclinic.org/health/diseases/16917-depression--heart-disease.

Renfroe, K. L. (1988). Effect of progressive relaxation on dyspnea and state anxiety in patients with chronic obstructive pulmonary disease. *Heart & Lung, 17*(4), 408−413.

Santa Clara Valley Medical Center. (2007). *Chronic Obstructive Pulmonary Disease (COPD).* San Jose, CA.

Scalzi, C., & Burke, L. (1992). Myocardial infarction: behavioral responses of patient and spouses. In S. L. Underhill, E. S. Woods, & E. S. Sivarajan Froelicher (Eds.), *Cardiac nursing.* Philadelphia, PA: JB Lippincott.

Vassiliades, J. T. A., Reddy, V. S., Puskas, J. D., et al. (2007). Long-term results of the endoscopic atraumatic coronary artery bypass. *The Annals of Thoracic Surgery, 83*(3), 979−985. Available from: https://doi.org/10.1016/j.athoracsur.2006.10.031.

Yohannes, A. M., Kaplan, A., & Hanania, N. A. (2018). COPD in primary care: key considerations for optimized management: anxiety and depression in chronic obstructive pulmonary disease: recognition and management. *The Journal of Family Practice, 67*, S11−S18. Available from: https://doi.org/10.3949/ccjm.85.s1.03.

Oncology

Ann Burkhardt

OBJECTIVES

After reading this chapter, the student or the occupational therapy practitioner will be able to do the following:
1. Describe cancer and its diagnosis and medical-surgical treatments.
2. Identify strategies for helping clients cope with side effects of chemotherapy and radiation.
3. Describe the role of occupational therapy in the treatment of cancer clients.
4. Identify techniques to be used in addressing a variety of occupational therapy goals with cancer clients.

KEY TERMS

Neoplasm
Cancer
Carcinoma
Sarcoma
Lymphoma
Leukemia
Paraneoplastic syndrome
Chemotherapy
Blood levels
Radiation therapy

Immunologic approaches
Nanotechnology
Mastectomy
Life review therapy
Radical neck dissection
Stomas
Colostomy
Urostomy
Palliative care

INTRODUCTION

Cancer is a broad category of conditions found when a tumor, or **neoplasm** (new abnormal growth of cells), is present in the body. A **cancer** is an abnormal tissue that grows and spreads or that may metastasize (move and start in new sites) throughout the body. Cancers may be low grade, with a natural history of slow development and spread, or may be high grade, with a tendency to grow quickly and spread rapidly. The cancer type is diagnosed by the tissue from which it first develops. For example, if a person has breast cancer that metastasizes to the lung, the biopsy of the lung lesion will contain breast cancer cells, not lung cancer cells. This condition would be labeled "breast cancer metastatic to the lung."

The cancer is further defined by the tissue in which it arises. For example, a **carcinoma** arises from epithelial tissue, a **sarcoma** from connective tissue, a **lymphoma** from the cellular components of lymph nodes, and **leukemia** from blood-forming organs such as the bone marrow. Many cancers are solid tumors or masses in the tissue of origin. Cancers arising in the bone marrow are often characterized by abnormal blood cell counts such as those associated with anemia. When cancers arise in endocrine tissues (glands), the cancer may produce a pseudohormone that mimics a hormone normally present in the bloodstream. In these instances, the free-circulating hormone level will be abnormally elevated. People occasionally show neurologic signs (e.g., seizures, cognitive changes) caused by the free circulation of the pseudohormones. This is an example of **paraneoplastic syndrome**, a group of symptoms indirectly caused by the presence of cancer elsewhere in the body. Because no solid tumor is present, the paraneoplastic syndrome is sometimes the first clinical sign of a cancer that is difficult to diagnose.

Medical Background Information

Some cancers have observable, palpable masses and people can self-detect them as they check out their own bodies on a regular basis. Individuals can participate in preventative health measures. For example, breast self-examinations are something health care professionals teach women to do, feeling their breasts while showering or bathing at least on a monthly basis. For example, a woman could detect a mass the size of a pea in her breast. Once detected, she should see her physician for further assistance with diagnosis. A great number of palpable masses (breast lumps) are nonmalignant; however, the lump must be assessed histologically (cells viewed under a microscope) to determine the composition of the lump.

From a public health perspective (Cancer Treatment Centers of America, 2018), a person should arrange screening at regular intervals for several cancer diagnoses as a part of preventative health. Individuals can be encouraged to be proactive in following through with these screening tests as recommended by their local department of health, their insurer, and/or their health care providers. The recommendations may vary, so it is important to choose a source for advice and follow-through. For example, women who are at average risk for breast cancer have yearly mammograms from ages 40 to 49. Earlier mammography screening is advised for women who have genetic predisposition, for example. Other cancers that can be preventatively screened include colon cancer (colonoscopy), skin cancers (visual assessment, full body scan), prostate cancer (manual palpation, prostate-specific antigen [PSA] blood testing), and genitourinary cancers in women (uterus, cervix, vaginal, Pap smear).

A variety of x-rays and scans are used to assist in the diagnosis of cancer. A lung cancer, for instance, may be detected initially by chest x-ray. The x-ray is the initial screening test. It is crude and not clear in its definition but still sensitive enough to be used for cancer screening. Moreover, it is much less expensive than a computed tomography (CT) scan or magnetic resonance imaging (MRI) procedure. Mammograms—x-rays of the breast tissue—are used to detect breast tumors.

CT scans may be done with or without the use of contrast dye. Contrast dye is radioactive and circulates in the bloodstream, outlining all vascular (blood vessel) structures. To receive the nutrients they need to grow, tumors usually develop vascular networks that are highlighted by dye during this test. CT with contrast dye is a fairly good tool to diagnose the presence of a solid tumor.

MRI is helpful in the diagnosis of soft tissue lesions. No radiation is used in an MRI, a scan that uses magnetic properties of biologic tissues to form the basis of an image. Abnormal tissues respond to magnetic radiofrequencies differently than do normal tissues and produce a different image in an MRI. The scan cannot differentiate, however, among blood clots, cancers, or demyelinating plaques (like those found in clients with multiple sclerosis). Gadolinium is a magnetically active material used with the MRI as a contrast dye. It enhances the image of the vascular system with magnetic properties of the dye. MRI is particularly helpful for diagnosing spinal disorders.

Bone scans are tomographic scans (serial x-rays that, when viewed in composite, produce a three-dimensional representation of the segment of the body scanned) of the skeletal system. Contrast dye is injected 2 hours before the scan is taken. Bone scans are helpful in diagnosing metastatic lesions to bone and some primary bone tumors. They are used to stage cancers that metastasize to bone such as breast cancer and prostate cancer. They are also used for regular, routine follow-up for persons with an initial diagnosis of these cancers to check for recurrence of the cancer.

A positron emission tomography (PET) scan is used to look at the structure and function of body tissues and is effective at spotting tumors in the body (Brazier, 2017).

Biopsies are surgical procedures in which a section or segment of tumor is removed so that a pathologist may examine it to determine a diagnosis. Biopsies can be done in several ways (e.g., scrape, smear, needle biopsy).

Regional lymph nodes may be suspected of involvement, either from a primary cancer, such as lymphoma, or as a sign of regional spread of disease, as in breast cancer. Lymph nodes are dissected at the time of a surgery to detect regional spread of the cancer and to stage the cancer. Imaging with ultrasound is sometimes used instead of biopsy of lymph nodes for staging a cancer.

Staging of Cancer

A few systems are in use for staging cancers, but most are based on the same underlying principles. At diagnosis, the cancer may be localized to one region. At this point, the cancer is usually an early stage and may be classified as stage I disease. Cancer that has spread to an adjacent local region of the body such as from the right breast to the right axilla is classified as stage II disease (a tumor and one metastasis). If the disease spreads to another organ such as from the breast to the lung, then stage III disease is evident. When multiple systems/organs are involved and the disease is widespread, stage IV is present (National Cancer Institute, 2015).

Another staging system commonly used is the tumor, node, and metastasis (TNM) system. Tumor (T) represents the number of actual tumor sites, primary and metastatic. Node (N) refers to the number of positive or involved lymph nodes that have cancer present in a surgical pathology sample. Metastasis (M) may be regional or widespread (National Cancer Institute, 2015).

Staging of the disease is helpful, along with other information concerning the specific cancer, in determining a treatment course and prognosis for the client. The past few years have seen an improvement in the treatment of several forms of advanced stage (IV) cancer, thus resulting in higher rates of survival with improved quality of life. For example, hormone-mediated cancers such as breast cancer and prostate cancer are being managed by combining a drug that blocks formation of bony metastases with hormone site blockers or chemotherapy regimens.

Treatment

After a diagnosis and staging of cancer, choices are made concerning treatment. Most solid tumors are removed surgically. Removal of the mass plus a margin of normal tissue taken from the surrounding area lessens the risk of local spread to normal tissues. When a tumor is encapsulated, tightly localized in its own capsule, sometimes a limited resection or lumpectomy is sufficient. If a tumor has invaded some of the local region or structures, a resection removes the tumor and the involved structures as a whole mass. If the surgery removes bone, sometimes reconstructive or joint replacement surgeries may be necessary to improve cosmetic appearance or function. When a tumor is aggressive but interferes with a normal body function, a surgical bypass procedure may prolong function or alleviate pain. If a tumor has invaded surrounding tissues and structures and the neurovascular bundle (nerves and their blood supply), sometimes an amputation is the surgery of choice.

In recent years, many cancer diagnoses have been viewed as chronic illnesses. People who have been in remission for up to decades after their initial diagnosis and treatment may have exacerbations, or recurrence of disease. The demand for rehabilitation and improvement in quality of life has increased because longevity has improved, and people are learning to take charge of their own continuing care during intervals when they are not under direct treatment.

Medical Oncology and Chemotherapy. Tumors are composed of different types of tissue, so the same treatment will not work for all tumors. Some tumor cells are sensitive to chemotherapy agents. **Chemotherapy** is a means of affecting change with chemicals. Most chemotherapeutic agents are toxic to normal tissues, as well as cancer cells, so side effects are inevitable.

Chemotherapy works in several ways (CancerNet, 2019). It can be used as a neoadjuvant (pretreatment), before surgery or radiation therapy, to shrink tumors. Chemotherapy can also be used as an adjuvant (adjunct treatment), after surgery or radiation therapy, to destroy any remaining cancer cells. Additionally, chemotherapy can be used as the sole treatment for some cancers (e.g., to treat cancer of the blood or lymphatic system, such as leukemia or lymphoma). Further, chemotherapy can be used to treat recurrent cancer, for cancers that come back after treatment. Finally, chemotherapy can be used as a palliative treatment, to suppress (but not cure) metastatic cancer that has returned or spread. Moderate evidence indicates that rehabilitation can be beneficial both before and after chemotherapy treatment (Hunter et al., 2017a).

Chemotherapy drugs can interfere with the tumor cells' genetic material, so the tumor cells stop dividing, multiplying, and surviving (CancerNet, 2019). Tumor cells often have a higher metabolic rate than normal cells, so they take up the chemicals and die first before the normal tissue shows signs of destruction.

Other chemotherapies work by bonding with the surface of the cancer cells and blocking their interaction with other cells (CancerNet, 2019). Because many cells rely on interactions with other cells to travel through membranes and become biologically active, this mechanical blocking mechanism stops their ability to act. Monoclonal antibodies, hormones, and some antitumor antibiotics act in this manner (CancerNet, 2019).

Clients who accept the concept of chemotherapy typically dread the side effects. The drugs are poisonous to normal tissues and can affect almost any body organ. For instance, many chemotherapies deplete the bloodstream of platelets, cells that help to clot blood. A person whose platelet count is low bleeds easily (CancerNet, 2019). Simple activities such as brushing teeth may provoke abnormal bleeding. Overuse of a joint can trigger bleeding into a joint space or a muscle compartment, which can abnormally raise the pressure in the enclosed area and cause the normal tissues to die. In extreme cases, a compartment syndrome may result. If this goes undetected and the tissues become necrotic, an amputation may be necessary to save the person's life. Occupational therapists (OTs) and occupational therapy assistants (OTAs) play a role in rehabilitation by staying informed about blood cell counts, monitoring sensory and motor function, and informing the doctor of any changes involving a limb.

OTs and OTAs should be informed about **blood levels** (Braveman et al., 2017), such as white blood cell and platelet counts and hematocrit, when making treatment choices in rehabilitation (Table 33.1). The crisis with platelets may last only a few days, when the chemotherapy is at the maximum level in the bloodstream. Once the platelets begin to recover, more normal and increasingly stressful activities may be graded to adjust to the change and restore normal function, and to increase occupational engagement.

Neutropenia is a severe impairment of the immune response with decreased resistance to infection. A cold can cause severe illness in someone who is immunosuppressed. Neutropenic clients may be kept on protective isolation to limit the risk of cross infection.

Anemia reduces an individual's tolerance for treatment. The oxygen level in the system is depleted because of reduced hemoglobin. OTs and OTAs play a role in instructing clients about managing fatigue. This can be done through energy conservation techniques, such as pacing. Recent research shows there is strong evidence that exercise is safe and beneficial for most cancer types at all stages, including end of life, regardless of age (Hunter et al., 2017b). Exercise, particularly aerobic exercise, reduced cancer-related fatigue (Garrity et al., 2018). With overactivity, the person may require oxygen to recover from shortness of breath. All types of occupational participation, including self-care and exercise, should be prioritized to encourage a sense of self-direction and to maximize functional ability.

Neurotoxic (toxic to nerves) chemotherapeutic agents may cause peripheral neuropathy (see Chapter 27). The person may have both motor and sensory involvement of the peripheral nerves, experiencing diminished (hypoesthesia) or heightened (hyperesthesia) sensory awareness, particularly in the hands and feet. The loss of protective sensation caused by decreased sensory awareness may place clients at risk for cutting, burning, or entrapping a limb. In clients with heightened sensory awareness, intense pain and burning sensations

TABLE 33.1	Blood Values Reference Chart	
Complication	**Normal Range**	**Precaution**
Neutropenia (white blood cell count)	47.6–76.8%	Avoid exposure to infection
Platelets (thrombocytopenia)	<130,000	Avoid resistive activities Avoid skin breakage
Hematocrit (anemia)	Men: 40–54% Women: 37–47%	Monitor vitals and respiratory rate

TABLE 33.2 Peripheral Neuropathy and Precautions in Activities of Daily Living

Clinical Sign	Functional Problem	Solution
Numbness	Loss of sharp and dull perception, at risk for cutting and burning limb	Use vision, cueing, and adapted equipment
Burning pain	Cannot tolerate anything touching hand or foot	Wear toning gloves, cloth gloves, soft padding, and socks. Use relaxation techniques
Proprioceptive loss	Unaware of where arm and leg are in space	Teach cueing and position for safety

may decrease activity tolerance for activities of daily living (ADL) and instrumental activities of daily living (IADL). OTs and certified OTAs (COTAs) may utilize sensory reeducation with clients experiencing peripheral neuropathy (see Chapter 29). For example, sensory stimulation may decrease pain (massage and exposure to graded textures). In addition, compression garments (toning gloves or tubular support bandages) may regulate the painful sensation and provide comfort and protection of the limb. Table 33.2 provides a summary of precautions regarding treatment of peripheral neuropathy.

Some chemotherapies cause alopecia (hair loss), one of the most obvious outward signs that identify a person who has a serious illness and may invoke the social stigma of cancer. It can affect eyebrows, pubic hair, and extremity hair. Since hair is a significant element of individual identification, this can be an especially troubling side effect. Hair usually grows back after completion of chemotherapy treatment, but the person may experience premature graying, other color shifts, and changes in texture and distribution of hair. Some people respond well to the suggestion to use wigs or hairpieces; others prefer to wear hats, scarves, or turbans; some prefer to go bald. It is a personal choice. OTs and OTAs may be helpful in identifying the choices and providing community resources, names of stores, and access to catalogs for clients with cancer.

Some chemotherapies and radiation can damage reproductive organs. Clients should be informed of the effects of the cancer treatment on the ability to reproduce (have children by natural means). Men can have sperm frozen in a sperm bank for future use. Embryos can also be frozen for later use. Even adolescents who do not currently have a sexual partner may choose this option to keep future choices open.

Radiation Therapy. **Radiation therapy** uses radioactive materials to kill or control the growth of cancer cells. Some (but not all) cancers are sensitive to radiation; therefore it is not always the treatment of choice. However, when a tumor is sensitive to its beams, radiation can be curative on its own or in combination with a chemotherapeutic agent.

The radioactive isotope may be placed in a machine that pinpoints the location of the tumor. A lead plate protects tissues from exposure until the person is correctly positioned and ready for treatment. External beam radiation directs the radiation over a set field, exposing the tumor and surrounding tissues to treatment. The beam can also be directed to a specific spot by placing a cone over the lens of the linear accelerator (radiation machine), thus concentrating the beam in one specific region. Exposure is given over a period of days, weeks, or months to deliver a total dose of radiation that could not be tolerated in one dose (because the radiation burns the tissues). Near the completion of treatment, the person may experience radiation burning. The radiologist will ask the client to avoid using lotions, creams, perfumes, and soaps on the treatment zone because these products could increase the probability of a burn by changing the surface composition of the skin (National Cancer Institute, 2015).

Radiation can also be administered through implantation of radioactive seeds into the tumor bed or affected gland (brachytherapy). The seeds are removed when treatment is completed. The treatment course for brachytherapy is usually a few days to a week. The radioactive seed is either implanted directly into the tissues or inserted through a flexible straw. Brachytherapy is used in the treatment of thyroid cancer, prostate cancer, some cancers of the genitourinary tract in women, and soft tissue carcinomas. While a client is radioactive with the seed implanted, personnel must take special precautions. Lead aprons are often available for short-term direct contact with the client. The chart usually states the maximum time allowed for exposure to health care providers, thus limiting the rads delivered to the caregiver. Lead chariots (shields) are often provided at the doorway of the client's room. The caregiver is protected behind the chariot, but can speak with the client inside the room.

In addition to its curative effect, radiation can also be used to treat cancer pain. Radiation may reduce pain in two ways: (1) by decreasing the size of a mass that is pressing on structures or nerves, or (2) by deadening the perception of the nerve. Radiation is particularly helpful with spinal tumors and bony metastases (Cancer Treatment Centers of America, 2018).

The side effects of radiation may be seen immediately (as in the case of radiation burns), over time, or in conjunction with the healing process. Fibrosis is a form of scarring that may result from radiation. Some of the modalities used to treat burns have been found helpful in treating radiation fibrosis in its early stages (see Chapter 30). For example, silicone gel pads may keep the tissues soft, hydrated, and pliable.

Participation in daily occupations during the scar management phase may help to reverse the soft tissue contracture effect (National Cancer Institute, 2015). Soft tissues are soft in part because of their elastic properties and their relationship to fascia, the tissue layer beneath the skin. Fascia covers the muscle compartments and reduces the effect of friction that occurs with normal movement and work. When the soft tissues are irradiated, they are burned. On healing, the tissues stiffen and harden. Beneath the skin, the fascia may also lose its elasticity and resilience. The person who receives radiation therapy may report pulling, tightening, or stiffness associated with the fibrotic change. The client may describe the body as feeling hard, even like wood.

Radiation to the region of the head and neck may contribute to the development of dysphagia, or swallowing disorders. Initially, the irradiated tissues are inflamed and swollen. Open sores can form in the oral cavity and oropharyngeal cavity, thus slowing the swallowing reflex and diminishing the function of the musculature supporting the swallowing mechanism. Food can spill into the airway and be aspirated (breathed into the lungs) (Little et al., 1998).

Head and neck irradiation can also cause stiffening of the muscles of the jaw, mouth, neck, and shoulder. Scar management, range of motion (ROM), and movement activities are helpful in restoring normal function and preventing pain and discomfort.

Radiation may also cause neutropenia. Therefore care should be taken to protect from cross infection. This can be done through infection control measures such as handwashing and personal protective equipment such as masks (Chapter 3) and avoiding proximity with anyone who is ill.

Radiation can also cause myelopathy (pathologic loss of the myelin surrounding a nerve) and neuropathy (weakness or sensory loss). This can be temporary or permanent. Permanent nerve damage may result in functional impairment. An example of a type of nerve damage caused by radiation is brachial plexopathy (see Chapters 27 and 29). Occupational therapy treatment includes positioning (for comfort and prevention of deformity) and activity modification with the use of adapted equipment (to compensate for decreased strength and ROM). In addition, modalities, stress reduction techniques, and relaxation may be used for both acute and chronic pain management (see Chapter 29).

Cancer treatment and survival with a diagnosis of cancer typically interrupt and alter normal activities. The client may experience change in expectations concerning future roles and may need to define new roles. OTs and OTAs can help by facilitating participation in the occupations that are most meaningful to each client.

Clients who receive radiation may experience alopecia. The response and management are the same in this instance as in the management of alopecia after chemotherapy.

Recent Advances in Cancer Treatment. Immunologic approaches, such as vaccines, have become more common in use for some cancers. These include monoclonal antibodies and tumor-agnostic therapies. Monoclonal antibodies can bond with proteins on the surface of cancer cells and flag those cells for detection by the immune system for destruction. Tumor agnostic treatment is another form of immune therapy that treats any kind of cancer if the cancer has the specific molecular alteration targeted by a drug that works by slowing down the immune system. These drugs treat adults and children with solid metastatic tumors or with unresectable tumors that cannot be treated with surgery. The tumors must also have a molecular alteration called

microsatellite instability—high (MSI-H) or deoxyribonucleic acid (DNA) mismatch repair deficiency (dMMR). Tumors that have MSI-H or dMMR have difficulty repairing damage to their DNA. As a result, they often develop large numbers of mutations in their DNA. The mutations produce abnormal proteins on the tumor cells that make it easier for immune cells to find and attack the tumor.

Hormonal therapy treatments change the levels of hormones in the body. Hormones are chemicals the body makes to control the activity of specific types of cells or organs. Hormone levels control several types of cancers such as some breast and prostate cancers.

Targeted therapy treatments target and disable genes or proteins found in cancer cells that the cancer cells need to grow. **Nanotechnology** is being advanced for use in the treatment of cancers. Nanoparticles are being used both to target specific malignant cells as direct transporters of chemotherapy to the malignancy and in diagnostic scanning procedures to transport contrast materials directly to a malignancy so that spread of disease can be directly visualized and pinpointed. It is anticipated that nanotechnology will dramatically lessen side effects of chemotherapy and make targeting of malignant cells more exact and direct.

PERSONAL MEANING AND A DIAGNOSIS OF CANCER

A diagnosis of cancer may cause the individual to reflect more deeply on the personal meaning of life, death, health, and illness. Creswell (2012) described the psychological context for personal meaning as the following:

1. The meaning of an experience to a person
2. The description the person gives about, and the interpretation derived from, the experience
3. The examination of the essence of the structures of the experience

Liminality, the sense that one personally recognizes the finality of one's life, has been described by Little and colleagues (1998). The experience of liminality initially produces a feeling of loss of control and the need to seek sources of rational straightforward answers. Over time, awareness of one's liminality persists, but living with the reality becomes bearable.

Royeen and Duncan (2001) have described meta-emotion as the cognitive awareness of one's emotion and how one uses emotion to experience life moment to moment. The process is an intertwining of emotion and meaning. According to Royeen and Duncan, emotion is a constituent part of occupation. Over time emotion cannot exist without occupation as a constituent part.

Padilla (2003) described occupational meaning as the insider's perspective. Meaning is experienced as it is being lived. Features or items that a person perceives to be meaningful can be analyzed with respect to their role as structural units of meaning. When a person is living with a diagnosis of cancer, his or her sense of personal meaning will be influenced by the severity and context of problems or challenges that emerge, in particular with regard to how these changes influence personal values and broaden or narrow participation in the process of living. Occupational therapy treatment planning and intervention is based on the information gathered in an occupational profile. This can provide a basis for problem solving that will enable clients with cancer to participate in the occupations, life roles, activities, and tasks that are meaningful and important to them. This will provide a sense of self-control and sustainability leading to an active presence in their own continued process of living. OTs and OTAs provide clients, who are living with chronic, potentially life-threatening illness, the tools to do what they want and need to do every day (Box 33.1).

Moderate evidence supports the idea that a variety of psychosocial interventions are beneficial in treatment of people who have cancer. A systematic review found that psychosocial interventions increased quality of life for people with advanced-stage cancer. Short-term life review increased spiritual well-being for people with terminal cancer, and stress management groups increased psychosocial adjustment among breast cancer survivors (Hunter et al., 2017a).

Breast Cancer

During the early postoperative phase after breast cancer surgery, the arm on the side of surgery is at risk for loss of ROM because the surgical incision may extend under the arm and thus limit chest wall and myofascial (soft tissue) gliding. Within the first 2 to 3 weeks after surgery, the client should move gently to protect the incision and promote healing. In the next phase, the client should stretch to regain normal movement in the arm. Because inpatient hospitalization is short (2 days for a **mastectomy** [removal of a breast]; 1 day for lumpectomy), outpatient and community group programs to encourage movement are appropriate and needed. In addition, education about sensory changes perceived as discomfort or pain, which occur normally after breast surgery, is necessary. Education helps to encourage movement and allay fear as to the meaning of the pain. Strong evidence exists that providing client education reduces anxiety (Hunter et al., 2017a).

Education concerning lymphedema (swelling of the arm on the side of surgery that can occur because lymph nodes

were removed or damaged) is also crucial. Clients with lymphedema should take special care to avoid trauma (cuts, insect bites, burns, and repetitive strain injuries) to the arm on the surgical side. Community agencies may provide support groups and exercise programs. Putting clients in touch with these programs can be beneficial. Examples of programs include the Reach To Recovery® program or Look Good Feel Better® program of the American Cancer Society, SHARE, or ENCORE. Clients appreciate information about resources available for breast prostheses (e.g., corsetieres), wigs, salons, and other camouflage (hats or turbans). Occupational therapy practitioners may initiate, coordinate, and lead groups for a Look Good Feel Better® program.

During chemotherapy and radiation therapy treatment, clients can benefit from movement programs to restore normal motion to the arm on the side of treatment. Radiation therapy can cause adhesive capsulitis (a stiffening and hardening of the glenohumeral joint capsule resulting in a loss of rotation and mobility of the shoulder joint) that leads to frozen shoulder in the irradiated shoulder as radiation fibrosis develops. Continuation of stretching exercises, especially overhead and shoulder rotation movements (scaption), is important for prevention of reflex muscle spasm and pain syndromes. Due to chemotherapy, breast cancer survivors may also experience peripheral neuropathy. Table 33.3 (also Table 33.2) summarizes side effects, precautions, and techniques.

Research has shown that women with breast cancer who attend support groups tend to have a better quality of life and extended longevity even if they are in the advanced stage of disease. From a research perspective, little is known about the healing power of prayer and spiritual development. Moderate evidence now exists that short-term life review (Hunter et al., 2017a) increased spiritual well-being for people with terminal cancer. **Life review therapy** involves adults referring to their past to achieve a sense of peace or empowerment about their lives.

Improved perception of the value of complementary medicine is promoting research in several allopathic medical centers regarding techniques such as stress reduction, massage, and energy therapies (e.g., therapeutic touch, reiki). This potential area of development and participation is useful for occupational therapy practitioners who use groups in treatment settings. Functionally based standardized tests can be used to demonstrate improved functional outcomes with the use of complementary techniques. Moderate evidence exists that yoga, regardless of type, benefits mental health, quality of life, sleep, and sense of well-being and decreases stress. Qi gong improved quality of life, mood, fatigue, and immune response and reduced inflammation (Hunter et al., 2017b).

Moreover, some clients may have defined psychiatric diagnoses and may require occupational therapy intervention based on that diagnosis. For instance, adjustment disorder may occur in some clients as a result of their diagnosis or a change in their condition. It is not uncommon for clients with acute lymphedema to experience anxiety, which results in a tendency to overfocus on details. These clients may require counseling and drug therapy to moderate their anxiety.

TABLE 33.3 Functional Impact and Management of Side Effects from Cancer Treatment

Treatment	Side Effect	Functional Impact	Rehabilitation Management
Radiation stretching	Burn (acute)	Avoid touch	Active ROM
	Burn (subacute)	Soft tissue contracture	Scar management, stretching
	Myelopathy	Plexopathy	Positioning, ADL compensatory strategies
Chemotherapy	Neutropenia	Immunocompromise, fatigue	Protective isolation, paced activity
	Thrombocytopenia (low platelet count)	Decreased activity tolerance	Avoidance of skin breaks, paced activity
	Anemia	Shortness of breath, decreased activity tolerance	Frequent rest periods
	Peripheral neuropathy	Decreased sensation	Safety education and activity modification
Surgery	Incision	Movement limitation	Time for incision to heal (~10 days), stretching after healing
	Referred pain	Reluctance to move	Coordination of pain medications with treatment, education regarding actual risk
	Phantom pain	Sleep disturbance, decreased activity tolerance	Application of light pressure to the area, education regarding meaning and actual risk

ADL, Activities of daily living; *ROM*, range of motion.

Depression may also be associated with a cancer diagnosis. Depression may be reactional and appropriate to the situation or based on neurochemical changes. Meaningful activities graded to assure success may be helpful to foster the development of self-esteem and improve the symptoms of depression. In addition, structured activity can limit distractions and redirect the focus of the individual from a feeling of being overwhelmed to one of tolerating and coping with life in the present. Successful completion of a structured activity may also provide hope because concrete evidence of a positive change results. Moderate evidence supports the use of traditional psychosocial strategies, yoga, and exercise to reduce anxiety and depression.

Lung Cancer

In the early postoperative phase, clients who have undergone surgery to remove a portion of the lung may depend on oxygen because of shortness of breath. Occupational therapy intervention should focus on the implementation of energy conservation and work simplification techniques to facilitate independence in ADL. It is advisable to monitor the client's vital signs, including respiratory rate (the number of breaths per minute), pulse, and blood pressure. In inpatient rehabilitation settings, it may be possible to monitor activity tolerance with a pulse oximeter (a digital machine with a finger electrode that measures the percentage of oxygen consumed). The goal is for the client to do as much activity as physical tolerance allows. Moderate evidence exists that deep breathing exercise can help to reduce anxiety and panic associated with the emotional distress of feeling short of breath (Hunter et al., 2017a). It also supports the use of nonpharmacologic interventions, such as problem solving, energy conservation, and education, to reduce the symptom of breathlessness (Hunter et al., 2017b).

The surgery for lung cancer, thoracotomy, involves a wide excision from the center of the chest to under the arm, terminating laterally at the spine. After the initial healing of the incision, the client may benefit from scar management and sensory reeducation for paresthesia (see Chapter 29).

Gentle general conditioning exercises (GCEs) may assist the client with increasing activity and respiratory tolerance. A program of GCEs may be taught to the client or caregiver for a self-treatment regimen to support the occupational therapy program. The caregiver and client can also be instructed in a ROM and positioning program for the shoulder on the side of surgery.

Head and Neck Cancer

Cancers of the head and neck region require surgical resection, usually augmented by radiation therapy and in some cases chemotherapy. The procedures most commonly done with oropharyngeal cancer clients require removal of cervical and submaxillary lymph nodes. The procedures for which occupational therapy is consulted most often are neck dissections (radical or modified radical) and resections involving the oropharynx and tongue.

Radical neck dissection involves removing the lymph nodes and vessels from the border of the jaw, the strap muscles of the neck, and the trapezius muscle. The spinal accessory nerve (cranial nerve XI) may be impaired by a radical dissection. This nerve gives rise to the long thoracic nerve, which innervates the serratus anterior and sternocleidomastoid (SCM). Therefore damage to this nerve may cause scapular winging due to decreased innervation of serratus anterior, which may cause a painful shoulder with decreased ROM (see Chapter 27). It may also cause decreased neck strength and ROM due to damage to the SCM. After surgery, some scar tissue must be allowed to develop in the neck to substitute for the lost function of the SCM, which aligns the head at midline. Some neck stiffness tends to result and is necessary. However, what is not necessary is scarring of the tissues that are radiated. Scar management (see Chapter 29), gentle active ROM, and positioning with cervical support pillows will be helpful in restoring more normal skin quality and preventing pain and deformity of the neck.

Head and neck cancer clients also are at risk for developing oral-motor dysphagia. Strong evidence supports the use of neuromuscular electrical stimulation in conjunction with traditional swallowing training to facilitate greater recovery than swallowing training alone for adults after head and neck cancer treatment (Hunter et al., 2017b). However, the swallowing team may find the client can eat only if the diet is limited in consistency, or food will be aspirated. Some of these clients will be unable to eat orally and may need to be tube-fed for some time. If the client's diet is limited, liquids may have to be thickened with an agent to guarantee the consistency of the bolus. In addition, clients may require special positioning or timed sitting after eating so that they do not aspirate after meals.

The swallowing specialist, usually the speech therapist or OT, provides the instructions. The OTA may be responsible for following through on the feeding program, using guidelines from a supervisor. See Chapter 11 to review interventions for mealtime occupations.

Again, training of the caregiver and client is important for follow-through on exercise and activity programs. It is essential with dysphagia because the ability to swallow and protect one's airway is a vital (life-supporting) function.

Bone Tumors and Soft Tissue Sarcomas

Bone tumors and soft tissue sarcomas are usually first seen in the extremities. The surgical management depends on numerous factors, including the type of tumor, the aggressiveness of the tumor, the status of the circulatory supply to the limb, the age and general health of the client, and the functional prognosis. Some of the bone tumors are primary in bone, but most are metastases from other cancers. Soft tissue tumors are usually primary in nature. Some develop from prenatal influences and are called "embryonic in origin." Some of these tumors are highly malignant and difficult to treat effectively.

If a tumor is aggressive and the blood or nerve supply to the limb is impaired, the client may require an amputation (see Chapter 31). If the tumor is present but the blood and nerve supply are intact, it may be possible to salvage the limb. In this instance, the distal portion of the limb is preserved, the portion of bone is removed with some healthy tissue (a margin), and a prosthesis is implanted and cemented into place. Amputees from cancer are rehabilitated similarly to amputees from other causes. However, some cancer amputations remove the total hindquarter or forequarter.

Occupational therapy focuses on positioning and ADL. The client will require training in positioning with the fracture brace and the sling, as well as self-ROM (with precautions as prescribed by the surgeon) and activities to restore hand strength and function. Cosmetic shoulder pads are also helpful in restoring the illusion of bulk to the arm because there will be loss of muscle and soft tissue with surgery.

Because many of these clients are children or adolescents, parental training is important. Compliance with the use of the fracture brace and sling is crucial to prevent fracture of the limb and dislocation of the indwelling prosthesis.

Colon and Bladder Cancers

Clients with colon or bladder cancer have **stomas**—openings from the surgically resected site to the outside of the body—after surgery. **Colostomy** stomas (which have an opening between the colon and body surface) and **urostomy** stomas (which have an opening between the body surface and the organs that produce and collect urine) are common. Clients may also undergo chemotherapy as part of their treatment. They may develop peripheral neuropathy and lose fine motor sensibility and function—the very type of feeling and movement they must rely on to independently remove and clean their colostomy and urostomy bags and sites.

The occupational therapy practitioner may be asked to work collaboratively with the enterostomal nurse and the client to develop strategies to restore independent function in stoma care and hygiene. Changing a clamp or using a built-up tool and practicing this adapted technique is often the single skill needed for discharge of these clients to the community.

This group can also benefit from peer support group activities because the presence of the stomas and the side effects of the disease and treatment affect body image, self-perception, sexual functioning, and life roles. Table 33.4 summarizes cancer conditions commonly seen in occupational therapy settings.

ISSUES CONCERNING DEATH AND DYING

People who confront life-threatening illnesses are forced to face their own mortality. Grief is a common reaction and a necessary part of the adjustment process and is preceded by a dynamic interplay of behaviors or stages described by Kübler-Ross as denial, bargaining, anger, depression, hope, and acceptance (Kübler-Ross, 2014). At any given point the client may exhibit one or several of these behaviors. Usually one stage prevails at a given time over the others. Denial is characterized by thoughts such as, "A mistake has been made. This cannot be happening to me." Bargaining is manifested by thoughts such as, "If I do this one thing, then it will be all right." Anger may be volatile at times and may also be outwardly directed at a number of objects, including (at times) the therapist. When people are predominantly angry, they may not tolerate therapy.

Depression is manifested by feelings of helplessness and hopelessness. When people are depressed, motivation generally wanes. Hope implies that some change for the good is possible. This restores motivation and participation in therapeutic goals. Acceptance is rarely achieved. Great faith or self-actualization must be possessed for a person to accept the inevitable. Once acceptance is reached, therapy may no longer be a goal, unless the person has personal goals or requires the intervention of the therapist for comfort measures (Padilla, 2003; Royeen & Duncan, 2001).

It may be hard for the therapy staff to react normally around the dying client. It is difficult for most people to feel comfortable around death because it forces each of us to face our own individual issues, beliefs, and fears. Knowing the right thing to do or say is part of the art of **palliative care**. For some

TABLE 33.4 Cancer Conditions Commonly Treated in Rehabilitation Settings

Type of Cancer	Side Effect Causing Physical Disability[a]	Possible Rehabilitation Diagnoses
Brain	Mass effect of the tumor displacing brain tissue Postradiation necrosis	Hemiparesis, quadriparesis, cognitive impairment Visual impairment, sensory impairment, ADL impairment, dysphagia
Head and neck	Facial disfigurement, sensory and motor loss (surgery) Oropharyngeal loss	Decreased movement of face or neck, shoulder pain and instability Facial/regional disfigurement, dysphagia, ADL impairment
Spinal	Sensory and motor loss below the level of the tumor	Paraparesis, quadriparesis, bowel and bladder dysfunction, pain, ADL impairment
Leukemia and lymphoma	Blood cell count changes, neurologic signs	Weakness, fatigue, deconditioning, neuropathy, dysphagia, ADL impairment
Bone	Amputation, limb-sparing postsurgical complications	Mobility impairment, ADL impairment, wounds and scars, pain
Soft tissue	Amputation, scar adhesions, radiation fibrosis	Mobility impairment, ADL impairment, wounds and scars, pain
Colon and bladder	Colostomy, urostomy	Peripheral neuropathy, impaired mobility, ADL changes—toileting, bathing, and dressing
Lung	Postsurgical oxygen dependence and thoracic surgical movement limitations	Shortness of breath, ADL impairment, decreased mobility
Breast	Myofascial and joint changes in chest wall and shoulder Sensorimotor compromise in arm (brachial plexopathy) Uncontrolled lymphedema in arm, ADL impairment	Decreased mobility in arm, pain, myofascial scarring Muscle imbalance, sensory changes
Metastatic	Multiple organ and system involvement	Pain, fatigue, deconditioning, pain, impaired mobility, sensorimotor changes Cognitive changes

ADL, Activities of daily living.

[a]There may be accompanying psychological sequelae: depression (situationally or organically based), anxiety (including adjustment disorders), and hallucinations (related to medications or organic/disease processes). In addition, people with diagnoses of cancer often face issues concerning role adjustment and adaptation.

people, it is enough for a caregiver to be accountable and present; the physical act of following up indicates caring and support.

Some clients may seek existential (religious and spiritual) meaning (Padilla, 2003; Royeen & Duncan, 2001). The response of the caregiver is individualized and depends on the individual caregiver's comfort and willingness to engage in the therapeutic use of self. If the caregiver is uncomfortable, the client could be assisted in contacting a spiritual or religious advisor. In this case, the clinician should just say, "I am not comfortable discussing this with you" or "I don't feel comfortable speaking about this topic."

Providing or facilitating activities that help the person deal with issues concerning death can be helpful. Some examples are creating memory books for significant others who will be left behind and writing personal diaries with humorous or special events—the stories that define the dying individual's life roles and experiences. Clients may also wish to write letters to family members or friends to resolve issues or say goodbye.

Palliative care also has its physical aspects. Techniques of comfort care that could be used are positioning, massage, complementary medicine (e.g., guided imagery, stress management,

aromatherapy, therapeutic touch), adaptive devices, and rearrangement of the physical environment to allow maximum access for the client with limited mobility. The practitioner can help maintain the client's dignity by helping with toileting activities and strategies.

SUMMARY

Cancer is a cluster of diseases with unique and identifiable problems for the occupational therapy practitioner to evaluate and treat. Although at one time many people did not survive cancer, with advances in medical care diagnoses are being made earlier and clients are being successfully treated for many cancer conditions. Many cancers are now viewed as chronic illnesses.

The role of the occupational therapy practitioner for the person with cancer is always changing. The practitioner must be a good detective to search out the clues in each instance that may guide treatment. Skillful intervention interweaves the principles of physical disability practice and of mental health practice. Evidence is supporting the value of occupational therapy intervention for persons who have diagnoses of cancer (Hunter et al., 2017a, 2017b).

The partnership of the OT and OTA is imperative in cancer treatment, perhaps even more than in other areas of practice because case management for these conditions is highly technical. The OTA may perform many of the same evaluations and treatments used with the general physically disabled and mental health populations.

REFERENCES

Braveman, B., Hunter, E. G., Nicholson, J., Arbesman, M., & Lieberman, D. (2017). Occupational therapy interventions for adults with cancer. *The American Journal of Occupational Therapy*, 71(5), 7105395010p1-7105395010p5. Available from doi:10.5014/ajot.2017.715003.

Brazier, Y. (2017). What is a PET scan, and are there risks? *MNT*. Available from https://www.medicalnewstoday.com/articles/154877.

CancerNet. (2019). Understanding chemotherapy. <https://www.cancer.net/navigating-cancer-care/how-cancer-treated/chemotherapy/understanding-chemotherapy>.

Cancer Treatment Centers of America. (2018). Cancer screenings: who should be screened and what cancers can be detected? <https://www.cancercenter.com/community/blog/2018/03/cancer-screenings-who-should-be-screened-and-what-cancers-can-be-detected>.

Creswell, J. W. (2012). *Qualitative inquiry and research design: Choosing among five traditions*. Thousand Oaks, CA: Sage.

Garrity, K., Fink, T., & Arrigo, M. (2018). Fatigue and functional outcomes in cancer rehabilitation. *The American Journal of Occupational Therapy*, 72(4 Suppl. 1), 7211505101. Available from doi:10.5014/ajot.2018.72S1-RP201B.

Hunter, E. G., Gibson, R. W., Arbesman, M., & D'Amico, M. (2017a). Centennial topics—systematic review of occupational therapy and adult cancer rehabilitation: part 2. Impact of multidisciplinary rehabilitation and psychosocial, sexuality, and return-to-work interventions. *The American Journal of Occupational Therapy*, 71, 7102100040. Available from do:10.5014/ajot.2017.023572.

Hunter, E. G., Gibson, R. W., Arbesman, M., & D'Amico, M. (2017b). Systematic review of occupational therapy and adult cancer rehabilitation: part 1. Impact of physical activity and symptom management interventions. *The American Journal of Occupational Therapy*, 71(2), 7102100030p1-7102100030p11. Available from doi:10.5014/ajot.2017.023564.

Kübler Ross, E. (2014). *On death and dying: What the dying have to teach doctors, nurses, clergy and their own families*. New York, NY: Simon & Schuster.

Little, M., Jordens, C. F., Paul, K., Montgomery, K., & Philipson, B. (1998). Liminality: a major category of the experience of cancer illness. *Social Science and Medicine*, 47, 1485—1494.

National Cancer Institute. (2015). Cancer staging.<https://www.cancer.gov/about-cancer/diagnosis-staging/staging>.

Padilla, R. (2003). Clara: a phenomenology of disability. *The American Journal of Occupational Therapy*, 57(4), 413—423.

Royeen, C. B., & Duncan, M. (2001). Meta-emotion of occupation: a new twist for mental health. Paper presented at the American Occupational Therapy Association Annual Conference, Philadelphia.

RECOMMENDED READING

Baltisberger, J., & Howel, D. (2016). A mixed-methods study of mothering during chemotherapy for breast cancer. *The American Journal of Occupational Therapy*, 70(4 Suppl. 1), 7011505158p1. Available from doi:10.5014/ajot.2016.70S1-PO5088.

Braveman, B., & Hunter, E. G. (2017). *Occupational therapy practice guidelines for cancer rehabilitation with adults (AOTA Practice Guidelines Series)* (1st ed). Bethesda, MD: American Occupational Therapy Association.

Braveman, B., Hunter, E. G., Nicholson, J., Arbesman, M., & Lieberman, D. (2017). Occupational therapy interventions for adults with cancer. *The American Journal of Occupational Therapy*, 71(5), 7105395010p1—7105395010p5. Available from doi:10.5014/ajot.2017.715003.

Burkhardt, A., & Weitz, J. (1991). Oncologic applications for silicone gel sheets in soft-tissue contractures. *The American Journal of Occupational Therapy*, 45(5), 460—462. Available from doi:10.5014/ajot.45.5.460.

Darragh, A., Vicary, K., Hock, K., Gaerke, L., & Flinn, S. (2017). Home-based intervention for chemotherapy-induced peripheral neuropathy. *American Journal of Occupational Therapy*, 71(4 Suppl. 1), 7111515238p1. Available from doi:10.5014/ajot.2017.71S1-PO3156.

Doyle Lyons, K., Newman, R. M., Kaufman, P. A., et al. (2018). Goal attainment and goal adjustment of older adults during person-directed cancer rehabilitation. *American Journal of Occupational Therapy*, 72(2), 7202205110p1—7202205110p8. Available from doi:10.5014/ajot.2018.023648.

Garrity, K., Fink, T., & Arrigo, M. (2018). Fatigue and functional outcomes in cancer rehabilitation. *American Journal of Occupational Therapy*, 72(4 Suppl. 1), 7211505101p1. Available from doi:10.5014/ajot.2018.72S1-RP201B.

Hopkins, S., Radomski, M. V., Finkelstein, M., et al. (2017). Focus forward: outcomes of a brief occupational therapy intervention for cancer-related cognitive dysfunction. *American Journal of Occupational Therapy*, 71(4 Suppl. 1), 7111520274p1. Available from doi:10.5014/ajot.2017.71S1-PO1053.

Hunter, E. G., Gibson, R. W., Arbesman, M., & D'Amico, M. (2017). Systematic review of occupational therapy and adult cancer rehabilitation: part 1. Impact of physical activity and symptom management interventions. *American Journal of Occupational Therapy*, 71(2), 7102100030p1-7102100030p11. Available from doi:10.5014/ajot.2017.023564.

Hunter, E. G., Gibson, R. W., Arbesman, M., & D'Amico, M. (2017). Systematic review of occupational therapy and adult cancer rehabilitation: part 2. Impact of multidisciplinary rehabilitation and psychosocial, sexuality, and return-to-work interventions. *American Journal of Occupational Therapy*, 71(2), 7102100040p1-7102100040p8. Available from doi:10.5014/ajot.2017.023572.

Sleight, A. G. (2017). Occupational engagement in low-income Latina breast cancer survivors. *American Journal of Occupational Therapy*, 71(4 Suppl. 1), 7111505075p1. Available from doi:10.5014/ajot.2017.71S1-RP304D.

Sleight, A. G., & Stein Duker, L. I. (2016). Toward a broader role for occupational therapy in supportive oncology care. *American Journal of Occupational Therapy*, 70(4), 7004360030p1-7004360030p8. Available from doi:10.5014/ajot.2016.018101.

34

HIV Infection and AIDS

Katlyn Kingsbury

OBJECTIVES

After reading this chapter, the student or the occupational therapy practitioner will be able to do the following:

1. Discuss the physical, mental health, and environmental factors associated with HIV disease that impede and enable engagement in occupation.
2. Understand the impact of HIV on body structures and functions, life activity, and social participation.
3. Understand the occupational therapy process for adults with HIV disease.
4. Understand the stages of HIV disease and its impact on occupational performance and participation.
5. Develop wellness strategies (in collaboration with the occupational therapy practitioner) for adults with HIV disease.

KEY TERMS

Human immunodeficiency virus (HIV)
Acquired immunodeficiency syndrome (AIDS)
Context
Adaptations
Cultural competence

Cultural effectiveness
Occupational role
Wellness
Control
Occupational choices

INTRODUCTION

Human immunodeficiency virus (HIV) attacks a person's immune system, the system that fights against infections calling specialized cells (T cells/B cells) to assist when a foreign substance is recognized in the body. It was discovered in 1982 when researchers were investigating an unusual diagnosis of a rare form of cancer and pneumocystis pneumonia (PCP) in five men from New York and California (US Department of Health & Human Services, 2001). In the months following, the condition was identified in others, including those who utilized intravenous (IV) drugs and individuals receiving frequent blood transfusions (i.e., individuals with hemophilia). Unfortunately, HIV claimed the lives of hundreds before its mechanism of transmission (contact with certain bodily fluids: blood, semen, breast milk, etc.) was discovered.

An individual infected with the virus may be asymptomatic for many years. According to the Centers for Disease Control and Prevention (CDC) (Centers for Disease Control and Prevention, 2019a), there are more than 1 million people living with HIV in the United States with 1 of 7 (approximately 14%) having no awareness of the infection (Mayo Clinic, 2018). Therefore the virus may severely damage the immune system before diagnosis, putting people at increased risk for developing other dangerous conditions/illnesses.

Advances in treatment transformed this terminal illness to a chronic illness. Occupational therapists (OTs) and certified occupational therapy assistants (COTAs) utilize occupations to assist clients with chronic diseases to lead productive, active, participatory, and meaningful lives. Therefore occupational therapy can play an important role in the lives of individuals living with the chronic disease known as HIV.

According to the CDC, sexual contact remains the most common form of transmission of HIV (Centers for Disease Control and Prevention, 2019a). Sixty-six percent of newly diagnosed individuals are male and 215 of those are between the ages of 13 and 24 (Centers for Disease Control and Prevention, 2019a). The CDC identified the following behaviors as those that may increase the risk of infection: unprotected sex, IV drug use, and substance use/abuse (Centers for Disease Control and Prevention, 2019a). Occupational therapy may play a role in assisting at-risk individuals to enact healthy behavioral and lifestyle changes and by providing client education on health and sexual activity (Centers for Disease Control and Prevention, 2019c). OTs and COTAs provide holistic care, improving the likelihood of improved overall health and well-being.

HIV is a complex infection that manifests in several stages that can progress at varying speeds, durations, and presentations (Box 34.1). It culminates in a condition known as **acquired immunodeficiency syndrome (AIDS)**; as the end stage of the infection, individuals in earlier stages of HIV do not have AIDS. In the initial stage of infection (acute HIV), which occurs within 2 to 4 weeks of transmission, the

---

BOX 34.1 World Health Organization Clinical Staging of HIV/AIDS for Adults and Adolescents With Confirmed HIV Infection

Clinical Stage 1

Asymptomatic
Persistent generalized lymphadenopathy

Clinical Stage 2

Moderate unexplained weight loss (<10% of presumed or measured body weight)[a]
Recurrent respiratory tract infections (sinusitis, tonsillitis, otitis media, and pharyngitis)
Herpes zoster
Angular cheilitis
Recurrent oral ulceration
Papular pruritic eruptions
Seborrhoeic dermatitis
Fungal nail infections

Clinical Stage 3

Unexplained[b] severe weight loss (>10% of presumed or measured body weight)
Unexplained chronic diarrhea for longer than 1 month
Unexplained persistent fever (>37.6° C intermittent or constant, for >1 month)
Persistent oral candidiasis
Oral hairy leukoplakia
Pulmonary tuberculosis (current)
Severe bacterial infections (such as pneumonia, empyema, pyomyositis, bone or joint infection, meningitis, or bacteremia)
Acute necrotizing ulcerative stomatitis, gingivitis, or periodontitis

Unexplained anemia (<8 g/dL), neutropenia (<0.5 × 109/L) or chronic thrombocytopenia (<50 × 109/L)

Clinical Stage 4[c]

HIV wasting syndrome
Pneumocystis pneumonia
Recurrent severe bacterial pneumonia
Chronic herpes simplex infection (orolabial, genital, or anorectal of >1-month duration or visceral at any site)
Esophageal candidiasis (or candidiasis of trachea, bronchi, or lungs)
Extrapulmonary tuberculosis
Kaposi sarcoma
Cytomegalovirus infection (retinitis or infection of other organs)
Central nervous system toxoplasmosis
HIV encephalopathy
Extrapulmonary cryptococcosis, including meningitis
Disseminated nontuberculous mycobacterial infection
Progressive multifocal leukoencephalopathy
Chronic cryptosporidiosis (with diarrhea)
Chronic isosporiasis
Disseminated mycosis (coccidioidomycosis or histoplasmosis)
Recurrent nontyphoidal *Salmonella bacteremia*
Lymphoma (cerebral or B-cell non-Hodgkin) or other solid HIV-associated tumors
Invasive cervical carcinoma
Atypical disseminated leishmaniasis
Symptomatic HIV-associated nephropathy or symptomatic HIV-associated cardiomyopathy

[a] Assessment of body weight in pregnant woman needs to consider the expected weight gain of pregnancy. Retrieved from http://www.who.int/hiv/pub/guidelines/HIVstaging150307.pdf, September 17, 2010.
[b] Unexplained refers to where the condition is not explained by other causes.
[c] Some additional specific conditions can also be included in regional classifications (such as reactivation of American trypanosomiasis [meningoencephalitis and/or myocarditis] in the WHO region of the Americas and disseminated penicilliosis in Asia).

---

individual is highly contagious and may present with flulike symptoms (headache, achiness in muscles and joints, sore throat, etc.). In the next stage (clinical latent infection/chronic HIV), which may last many years, the individual is often asymptomatic except for persistent generalized lymphadenopathy (PGL). In the final stage (AIDS), the individual experiences severe symptoms (night sweats, recurring fevers, chronic diarrhea, fatigue, weight loss, etc.). At this stage, individuals are at high risk for opportunistic infections that typically do not affect individuals with properly functioning immune systems, leading to further decline in health. However, advances in HIV treatment in the United States prevent many individuals with HIV from developing AIDS (Centers for Disease Control and Prevention, 2019a; Mayo Clinic, 2018). The World Health Organization (WHO) has categorized the stages of infection as well as the symptoms present within each stage. This categorization can be utilized to further understand the body structures and functions impacted throughout the HIV/AIDS disease process (Weinberg and Kovarik, 2010).

The COTA may provide services to individuals in any stage of infection to facilitate the maximal level of occupational performance possible. This can be done through an

emphasis on holism and mind-body-spirit. Goals related to mastery and independence celebrate wellness, life, and living —not illness, death, and dying. To provide client-centered and holistic care, OTs and COTAs must evaluate the occupational performance of clients within the **context** of their environment and culture.

Client Factors

COTAs address client factors related to physical and mental health when working with individuals living with HIV/AIDS. Persons with HIV will likely experience a variety of impairments to body structures and functions over time, influencing their occupational participation. The disease effects individuals differently, but the following factors are likely to be seen with this population:

- Fatigue
- Peripheral and central nervous system disorders
- Visual impairments
- Cardiac problems
- Pain
- Weakness (neuromuscular)
- Changes in posture, gait, range of motion (ROM), strength, coordination, balance

- Changes in cognition (particularly affecting safety in carrying out tasks)

These physical client factors can and often do lead to changes in all areas of occupation (American Occupational Therapy Association, 2014). These include activities of daily living (ADL), instrumental activities of daily living (IADL), rest and sleep, education, work, play and leisure, and social participation. Additionally, these factors often lead to altered performance patterns within and a person's habits and routines (e.g., increased time needed to complete basic IADL [BIADL] and IADL).

As a result of the reciprocal nature of mind and body, physical changes often impact the psychosocial status and mental health of individuals living with HIV and AIDS (e.g., depressed mood as a result of decreased physical ability to participate in meaningful leisure activities). Individuals may experience dysfunction in mental health such as difficulty coping with the diagnosis and increased stress relating to current and future effects of the disease, even if they are not experiencing the aforementioned physical impairments. The complexity of the infection, and its varied course for each person, results in uncertainty regarding what comes next (e.g., next diagnosis, results of a new blood test, new symptoms). The stress this causes may severely limit the individual's performance patterns (occupational habits, roles, routines, or activities). The person's identity may become consumed by the aspects of the disease, rather than being based on how he or she can function on a day-to-day basis. COTAs can assist people with managing their daily lives and help them cope with the many new challenges that come with living with HIV or AIDS, no matter the stage or severity of illness. Other psychosocial and mental health considerations include but are not limited to:

- Anxiety (often manifested in physical symptoms)
- Depression
- Guilt over being infected or the possibility of having infected others
- Preoccupation with illness or death
- Lack of interventions, limited access to health care, lack of insurance
- Anger (at the disease, lack of interventions, lack of social support, etc.)
- Neuropsychiatric problems (forgetfulness, apathy, withdrawal, memory loss)
- Altered self-image because of cancer or severe weight loss
- Lack of control over environment
- Hopelessness and helplessness
- Lack of meaning in daily activity and sense that life is meaningless
- Altered goals, plans, dreams for the future
- Grief and bereavement issues
- Societal stigma

It is important to understand that individuals cope with illness in a variety of ways—some effectively and some ineffectively. COTAs can help individuals identify and implement the most effective coping strategies for them and increase their understanding of **adaptations** that can be made to foster their ability to engage in meaningful and necessary occupations within a variety of contexts.

Environmental Factors

The context and environment of persons living with HIV/AIDS include not just the physical setting in which they live, but also the social, personal, cultural, temporal, and virtual contexts and environments in which they experience transactional relationships with occupation and participation (American Occupational Therapy Association, 2014). Occupational performance and functioning improve when the COTA incorporates contextual observations and awareness into interventions and understands the constant interaction between a person, his or her environment, and occupational performance.

Physical Environment. People with symptomatic HIV (and associated physical impairments) might have, for example, difficulty negotiating steps (at their home, places of worship, school, etc.) or visual-motor impairments affecting driving, shopping, and community mobility. A complex external physical environment (e.g., setup of one's home or place of work) may make access and occupational participation within that environment difficult for an individual with HIV or AIDS who is experiencing increased fatigue, decreased strength/ROM, or pain. Other physical challenges may include sensory problems that can alter balance and increase pain that can result in reduced safety in a variety of physical environments. It is also important to consider the physical contexts that were present prior to one's diagnosis of HIV/AIDS (e.g., a person born with only one upper extremity).

Social Environment. Over the history of the disease, individuals with it have experienced stigmatization and discrimination, which sometimes led to them being seen as social pariahs or outcasts. COTAs should take these social factors into account when designing interventions to maximize their understanding of these clients and their experience as an occupational being. As with any chronic illness, relationships with significant others, family members, and work associates may change because of an HIV diagnosis. The discrimination experienced by some with HIV/AIDS may make going to the hospital or other health care facility frightening, rather than a relief. Since the COTA may be one of the first people to physically touch a person with HIV following diagnosis, through ADL, ROM, strengthening, or a creative intervention, it is essential for the contact to be accepting, caring, and therapeutic in nature. Therapeutic touch that embodies acceptance and compassion can be as important to the person with HIV as any medication. Most importantly, the clinician who is skilled in therapeutic use of self and who has the goal of developing a healthy and nondiscriminatory therapeutic relationship can enable a person with HIV/AIDS to carry on despite the diagnosis and its impact on daily occupations.

Personal Context. An individual's personal context is defined as "demographic features of the individual, such as age, gender, socioeconomic status, and educational level, that are not part of a health condition" (p. S8) (American Occupational Therapy Association, 2014). This context must be considered by the OT and COTA to provide interventions that are relevant and meaningful to the individual (age-appropriate activities, information provided at level consistent with the individual's education level, etc.). Doing so will enable the person to engage in interventions more effectively, increasing his or her therapeutic potential.

Cultural Context. As with other diagnoses, the person with HIV may come from any population or group of people. Occupational therapy interventions that are culturally specific and uniquely defined enhance patient health and promote well-being. Such interventions can demonstrate that the COTA cares about and is attentive to the particular needs of that one individual, helping to establish rapport and a trusting therapeutic relationship. **Cultural competence** and **cultural effectiveness** are vital aspects of providing occupational interventions that effectively consider an individual's cultural context. OTs and COTAs who strive for increased cultural competence and effectiveness are better suited to provide interventions that embody respect and acceptance for their clients, resulting in an improved therapeutic relationship and outcomes (Black, 2017).

CASE STUDY[a]

Mr. J

Mr. J., a 38-year-old white male, was admitted to the hospital 6 months after an initial diagnosis of AIDS and after his first incident of pneumocystis pneumonia. He was referred to occupational therapy in the morning of the day of his hospital discharge for neuropathy in both feet. Mr. J. is a well-educated and well-traveled bank executive of French descent who speaks five languages. He rarely communicates with members of his nuclear family, who live outside the United States, and he lives with his supportive partner of 5 years. Due to the nature of the acute care (i.e., referred to occupational therapy in the morning and discharged that afternoon) situation, assessment consisted only of interview and role, ADL, and biomedical assessments.

Assessment revealed Mr. J. to be independent in all self-care, home maintenance, and mobility activities except for minor standing balance deficits. No cognitive or sensory deficits were noted other than mild lower extremity neuropathy. Strength, active ROM (AROM), and coordination were all functional for task performance. Mr. J. complained of diminished endurance, affecting his occupational habits and pursuits of interests, including exercise, history, collecting, photography, movies, concerts, classical music, and swimming. He had narrowed his leisure activities to include listening to classical music when he "felt up to it." He felt out of control and believed that HIV had taken over. He openly discussed his prognosis and his religious beliefs, examining his unresolved relationship with God and the possibilities of an afterlife. The OT referred him to Dignity (a gay Catholic organization), the unit social workers, and the hospital chaplain.

Critical Thinking Questions

1. What goals can you identify that Mr. J. might desire?
2. What interventions (in addition to those discussed earlier) would be appropriate?
3. What aspects of each environment/context are at play here?

[a]Adapted and reprinted with permission from Pizzi M. The model of human occupation and adults with HIV infection and AIDS. *Am J Occup Ther.* 1990;44(3):42–49.

Occupational Therapy Intervention Process

Participation in meaningful occupation can help people make better use of time, prevent dysfunction, and influence an individual's health (Meyer, 1977). Analyzing occupational performance, through an occupational profile, can assist clients with HIV/AIDS to maintain a balance between work, rest, and sleep, which will lead to optimal health. An occupational profile provides the first step in the intervention process. It should be used to analyze the interaction of these factors in client wellness.

Environment Factors. Due to the interplay between person, environment, and occupation, people are continuously influencing and being influenced by environment. The physical, social, temporal, attitudinal, and cultural environments are key to understanding occupational performance and creating adaptations to promote health and well-being. Occupations provide the most meaning when they are developed within the context of a familiar environment. For example, facilitating a chef or a homemaker in a wheelchair to make a home-cooked meal for a family gathering can include all aspects of the environment, and the task is meaningful for the individual.

Occupational Roles. Role functioning (mastery and progress toward developing an **occupational role**) should be incorporated in intervention goals and activities to promote and strengthen an individual's occupational well-being. For example, if a patient is employed and identifies as a worker, interventions designed to restore work habits, routines, and task performance would be appropriate. If a patient has no occupational role, role development might be important if that patient has no habits, routines, or meaningful activity during the day.

Wellness. Wellness and health promotion have been emphasized both as interventions and as outcomes (Pizzi, Reitz, & Scaffa, 2006). According to the CDC, prevention programming has had a colossal impact on the reduction and overall stabilization of new case rates of HIV in the United States since the 1980s (Centers for Disease Control and Prevention, 2019c). Research indicates that prevention programming designed to address the specific contexts and factors that place particular groups at risk are increasingly effective. The client-centered and holistic nature of the profession uniquely qualifies OTs and COTAs to design and implement prevention programs.

Meaningful occupations in which a person can successfully engage promote **wellness**. Wellness programming, facilitated and led by the COTA, can be implemented with individuals, populations, and communities. Engagement in productive occupations and purposeful, occupation-based activities adapted by the COTA and OT can support immune system health, which is important for those with HIV/AIDS. An example of this may be a strengthening program (in collaboration with the physical therapist) done through engagement in favorite occupations (such as yoga), balanced with

Demographics
Name: Age: Sex:
Lives with (relationship)
Identified caregiver:
Race: Culture: Religion: —practicing:
Primary occupational roles:
Primary diagnosis:
Secondary diagnosis:
Stage of HIV:
Past medical history:
Medications:

Activities of Daily Living (using ADL performance assessment)
Are you doing these now?
Do you perform homemaking tasks?
For areas of difficulty: Would you like to be able to do these again like you did before? Which ones?

Work
Job: When last worked:
Type of activity at job:
Work environment:
If not working, would you like to be able to?
Do you miss being productive?

Play/Leisure
Types of leisure activities engaged in:

Are you doing these now?
If not, would you like to?   Which ones?
Would you like to try other things as well?

Is it important to be independent in daily living activities?

Physical Function
Active and passive range of motion:
Strength:
Sensation:
Coordination (gross and fine motor/dexterity):
Visual/perceptual:
Hearing:
Balance (sit and stand):
Ambulation/transfers/mobility:
Activity tolerance and endurance:
Physical pain:
Location:
Does pain interfere with doing important activities?
Sexual function:

Cognition (attention span, problem solving, memory, orientation, judgment, reasoning, decision-making, safety awareness)

Time Organization
Former daily routine (prior to diagnosis):
Has this changed since diagnosis?   If so, how?

Are there certain times of day that are better for you to carry out daily living tasks?

Do you consider yourself regimented in organizing time and activity or pretty flexible?

What would you change if anything in how your day is set up?

Fig. 34.1 Pizzi Assessment of Productive Living (PAPL) for adults with HIV infection and AIDS. (Courtesy Michael Pizzi.)

rest, leisure, and good nutrition. This balance may be achieved through the COTA assisting a client to organize routines and prioritize goals to make the best use of time. Techniques to do this may be utilizing a time log or activity log that corresponds to how the person uses time.

A person with HIV might perceive that life is short and that time cannot be wasted. This exploration can provide the person with HIV insight into how he or she is able to utilize time in an effective and meaningful way to perform all necessary and desired occupations on a daily basis. Offering practical, functional, and meaningful occupation-based care throughout the therapy process is as essential in helping those with HIV/AIDS reach their goals as it is when working with individuals with any diagnosis.

Body Image and Self-Image
In the last six months, has there been a recent change in your physical body and how it looks? How do you feel about this?

Social Environment (Describe support available and utilized by patient)

Physical Environment (Describe environments in which patient performs daily tasks and level of support or impediment for function)

Stressors
What are some things, people, and situations that are or were stressful?
What are some current ways you manage stress?

Situational Coping
How do you feel you are dealing with:
    a. Your diagnosis
    b. Changes in the ability to do things important to you
    c. Other psychosocial observations

Occupational Questions
What do you consider to be important to you right now?

Do you feel you can do things important to you now? In the future?

Do you deal well with change?

What are some of your hopes, dreams, aspirations? What are some of your goals?

Have these changed since you were diagnosed?   How?

Do you feel in control of your life at this time?

What do you wish to accomplish with the rest of your life?

Plan:

Short-term goals:

Long-term goals:

Frequency:

Duration:

Therapist:

Fig. 34.1, cont'd.

ASSESSMENT OF OCCUPATIONAL PERFORMANCE

The OT, with input from the COTA, utilizes a variety of tools to assess occupational performance. These can include the physical assessment of ROM, strength, balance, and participation in ADL. These can also include psychosocial assessments such as depression scales and coping assessments. The Pizzi Assessment of Productive Living (PAPL) for adults with HIV disease (Fig. 34.1) provides an overview of areas that could be assessed in clients with HIV and suggests interventions to address them. The COTA contributes to the assessment process by completing parts of the occupational profile and ADL evaluation.

Intervention Process

The OT and COTA use the information gathered in the evaluation process to develop a client-centered plan of care. This plan includes goals developed in collaboration with the client.

The client-centered nature of the occupational therapy process can serve to empower clients with HIV and AIDS.

Proper infection control procedures must be maintained throughout the intervention process with all clients, including those with HIV/AIDS. Gloves should be worn whenever there is a possibility of contact with blood or body fluids. Masks should be worn when either the client or practitioner has symptoms of an airborne illness, such as a cold or flu. Gowns should be worn in the case of certain infections. Each facility has procedures and policies. See Chapter 3 for more specifics relating to infection control and safety in the clinic.

Restoring and maintaining function and preventing dysfunction in self-chosen occupations related to the person's life and lifestyle are the focus of clinical interventions. In addition to traditional clinical interventions, it is important to consider nutrition as it relates to supporting emotional and physical health, as well as a healthy immune system. Nutritional education can be incorporated into adaptive homemaking skills and ADL.

Alternative therapies may be used to complement traditional care and reduce stress. These include visualization, imagery, massage, meditation, therapeutic touch, and manual therapies. Some individuals also use herbal remedies. These should be used with caution and discussed with the physician, as they may have an effect on medical interventions. Some of the techniques utilized, such as manual therapy and massage, may require additional training. COTAs should refer to the practice guidelines in their state to assess requirements and competencies needed to administer them.

The extensiveness of the HIV disease process, as well as the multitude of ways in which individuals are affected by it, may cause some clients to feel a loss of **control** in the process. The complexity of care in a hospital setting, which requires coordination of many care providers, may also cause individuals to feel a loss of control over how their time is spent. The feelings of loss of control may be ameliorated through the provision of **occupational choices** within all interventions/sessions. For example, the COTA could devise a list of 5 to 10 activities to increase physical or mental health and well-being. The COTA can allow the client to choose three for the session. This will contribute to improvement in client-centered care and provide an experience of control and choice to clients. Clients are their own expert on who they are and how best they "do" their lives; COTAs are the facilitators of health through their care, compassion, and knowledge of the power of occupation in people's lives.

Providing control and choices at each session conveys a healthy respect for the person with HIV and helps to establish rapport. It also symbolizes caring at its best. Helping the person to adapt a routine or habit of daily living can promote healthier living. Illness of any kind disrupts a routine of activity. A progressive and chronic disease constantly interrupts routine. The COTA should work with the person with HIV to determine the best and worst times of day for activity and energy output. Is the person a morning or evening person? What is the normal routine of the person's day? How can the health care provider help to adapt the routine to make it as comfortable as possible? This is an often overlooked but vital part of interventions and overall caring that the OTA can implement.

Generalized weakness and fatigue disrupt routines and activity performance. Incorporating energy conservation, work simplification, and other strategies and adaptive devices can help maintain task performance. Positioning for the bedbound or frail patient can prevent pressure ulcers and promote healthier sleep and rest patterns.

Ergonomic and appropriate positioning for tasks will optimize comfort and engagement in favored occupations. Learning the use of adaptive equipment is vital for any person with functional limitations. A reacher could be useful for a person with decreased ROM; lap trays, feeding equipment, and writing implements for people with hand neuropathies; and dressing sticks and sock aids for lower extremity dressing are just some examples of commonly used equipment. The COTA must ensure that the person wants to use the equipment and knows how to use it.

Factors contributing to psychosocial stress must also be considered. These can include (1) absence of a cure for the

CASE STUDY

Mr. J., Part 2

Occupational therapy recommendations for Mr. J. included adaptive equipment for safety during bathing. Physical activity was tailored to his interests, values, and occupational choices. A new routine of daily living emphasized energy-conservation techniques such as balancing activity and rest to maintain productivity. Additionally, adaptations to Mr. J.'s worker role (transition from office to home) were recommended to maintain his participation in his highly valued work role.

Mr. J. was admitted to the hospital 1 year later with his third episode of PCP and severe neuropathy in both feet. This caused considerable pain even at rest, and other physical limitations resulted in increased dependence in his daily occupations.

This time the occupational therapy assessment was performed with the primary nurse and Mr. J.'s partner, Mr. F., in attendance. Their participation gave a more comprehensive perspective and helped meet the needs and goals of both Mr. J. and his caregiver.

Assessment

Mr. J. had poor endurance and severe pain in both feet, which limited standing tolerance to less than 2 minutes. His AROM, strength, coordination, vision, and cognition were within functional limits. No neuropathy was noted in his hands, but he had a flexion contracture as a result of a painful tubercular nodule that caused difficulties with writing and holding utensils.

Mr. J.'s daily living routine was severely altered, and his occupational roles of worker, homemaker, and hobbyist were affected. His partner reported that Mr. J. spent increased time in bed, watching television or listening to music. Mr. J. less frequently came to the dining room for meals and increasingly requested that his meals be served to him in bed. This caused his partner distress. Although he wanted to help Mr. J., Mr. F. wanted guidance in how much assistance to give and how much encouragement he should give for him to do things more independently.

Mr. F. reported that Mr. J. demonstrated anger and depression related to helplessness and hopelessness, but he refused mental health care. He participated in no leisure activity, was apathetic, and felt hopeless regarding current and future occupational performance. He preferred for caregivers to support his dependency rather than facilitate independence. His occupational performance varied considerably at different times of the day, and with different caregivers. For example, he would often perform tasks for the OT but not for the nurses. This created differing opinions among staff regarding his level of occupational performance.

Critical Thinking Questions

1. What questions are raised by Mr. J.'s behavior?
2. What questions are raised about his physical decline?
3. What interventions are most appropriate for him?

CASE STUDY

Mr. J., Part 3

Discussion among team members led to development of a structured and consistent approach that focused on sharing control of timing and choice of activities with Mr. J. The program of care was adapted to his preferences and promoted wellness by making interventions more meaningful to him.

The physical environment of the hospital was adapted, and items from Mr. J.'s home were brought in to create a more familiar physical space. Throughout the rehabilitation process, the OT worked with Mr. J.'s partner in his caretaker role. Attention was given to restructuring Mr. F.'s other roles, routines, time management, and activities to diminish his stress level, validate his own caregiving abilities, and work through impending loss of a partner. Mr. F. found these interventions helpful. He also stated that he felt like withdrawing from Mr. J. because of guilty feelings and impending loss. The OT helped him focus on positive aspects of life and living.

Despite Mr. J.'s ability and choice to eat independently, his mother was observed feeding him. In acknowledging her overwhelming need to resume the role of caregiver, a role soon to be relinquished, the interventions team continued to learn the lesson of asking, "Whose need is it? Whose need is greater?"

Mr. J.'s interventions focused on occupational and physical therapy, including a balance among self-care, mobility, work, and leisure tasks. The program incorporated rest and his medical regimen, including vital signs and IV medications. As much as possible, he was given the opportunity to organize his schedule, which helped him to normalize his routine and incorporate new activities. Mr. J. chose to follow a program of holistic activities that included massage and back rubs, imagery and visualization, therapeutic touch, exercise, balance and gait training, and personal and instrumental ADL. Important leisure and social activities such as listening to classical music, attending plays at the hospital, praying and meditating, reading, working, spending time with loved ones, resting, and sleeping were included. The intervention team included occupational and physical therapy, a nurse, a chaplain, a physician, a social worker, a recreation therapist, and Mr. J.'s significant others.

In addition, the occupational therapy program included the following:

- Provision of and teaching in use of adaptive equipment (tub bench, handheld shower, built-up handles for utensils, writing adaptations)
- Joint self-ranging, exercise, and upper extremity—strengthening occupations
- Energy conservation

- Development of new leisure tasks and engagement in those formerly enjoyed
- Discussion and activities centered around role changes and adaptation of favored roles (e.g., setting up tasks at bedside to continue his work in banking)
- Family and partner education to develop competence and confidence and to reduce fear in caring for Mr. J.

At the beginning of Mr. J.'s second hospitalization, a home program was designed to give direction, focus, and purpose and to establish goals for his hospitalization. (This is realistic and does not provide false hope to people with HIV because HIV is a process with great variability.)

Although Mr. J. hoped he would be discharged home, he came to accept that it was not possible as his medical condition rapidly worsened. His occupational therapy program was adapted accordingly. One month before Mr. J.'s death, his mother, father, and sister visited him. The OT discussed the rehabilitation program with them; interventions were expanded to meet their needs to assist Mr. J. with his personal care, passive ROM, and work and leisure tasks and to incorporate their support for Mr. J.

At his highest level of function during his 6 weeks of hospitalization, Mr. J. participated in daily exercise, walked to and from therapy, engaged in work-related tasks, and was independent in personal care. At his lowest level of functioning, Mr. J. was positioned for comfort, had classical music at his bedside, and participated in as much personal care as he chose, which occasionally consisted of finger feeding while in bed.

As the nuclear family slowly became involved in Mr. J.'s care, the benefits of an occupation-centered approach were evident. The family restored their own forsaken occupational roles (particularly that of caregiver) and participation in occupations once enjoyed by the entire family assisted in healing old wounds. Open communication and self-expression were facilitated by the restoration of these roles and occupations. Mutual love, forgiveness, and support were shared among all family members, which assisted Mr. J. in envisioning his life as complete. The nuclear family first met Mr. J.'s partner at the bedside, and they immediately supported each other, which eased the loss felt by everyone when Mr. J. died.

Critical Thinking Question

1. When a patient's functional abilities vary from day to day and decline, the occupational therapy practitioner must modify interventions to match the person's abilities. Identify several instances of such modifications in the case of Mr. J.

---

disease, (2) disruption of routines by interventions and regimens that may include 30 pills three times a day, (3) constant doctor and clinical appointments, (4) real and perceived discrimination, and (5) work roles and relationships that are lost because of the diagnosis. These factors experienced by people living with HIV/AIDS may not be seen as commonly with other diagnoses. Another consideration is that the individual may have lost friends, family members, or significant others to the disease. Unresolved grief and bereavement issues and

anger may exacerbate anxiety and other psychosocial factors related to HIV. The COTA must always note this possibility during interventions.

Health promotion and wellness programming are essential. HIV has become a chronic illness managed well by medications and improved health care strategies. OTAs have an opportunity to establish positive, healthy community-based programming that helps people with HIV remain active, resilient, and strong.

SUMMARY

Through carefully developed interventions, COTAs can play an important role in developing activities to promote health and well-being for people with HIV/AIDS. This should be done in conjunction with the OT, by frequently checking back with the client to ensure the process meets his or her needs. This occupation and client-centered approach to care will enhance health and well-being for clients living with HIV/AIDS. Therefore occupational therapy services can provide clients with HIV/AIDS tools to improve their quality of life, transition more easily to and live productively in the community, enable active occupational participation, and live longer and successful lives.

REVIEW QUESTIONS

1. Describe the stages of HIV disease relative to their impact on occupational performance.
2. Describe the physical, psychosocial, and environmental factors to consider when working with adults with HIV.
3. Discuss the contextual considerations when implementing interventions.
4. Describe and discuss several themes related to occupational therapy intervention when working with people with HIV.
5. Describe and explain various interventions used in occupational therapy when working with adults with HIV, using the occupational therapy practice framework to guide you.
6. Discuss and explain how wellness approaches in occupational therapy guide clinical interventions for adults with HIV. How might you develop a wellness and prevention program for this population?

REFERENCES

American Occupational Therapy Association. (2014). Occupational therapy practice framework: domain and process (3rd ed.). *The American Journal of Occupational Therapy, 68*(Suppl. 1), S1–S48. Available from doi:10.5014/ajot.2014.682006.

Black, R. M. (2017). Cultural impact on occupation. In K. Jacobs, & N. MacRae (Eds.), *Occupational Therapy Essentials for Clinical Competence* (pp. 13–28). Thorofare, NJ: SLACK Incorporated.

Centers for Disease Control and Prevention. (2019a). Basic statistics. https://www.cdc.gov/hiv/basics/statistics.html.

Centers for Disease Control and Prevention. (2019b). HIV and youth. https://www.cdc.gov/hiv/group/age/youth/index.html.

Centers for Disease Control and Prevention. (2019c). HIV prevention works. https://www.cdc.gov/hiv/policies/hip/works.html.

Mayo Clinic. (2018). HIV/AIDS. https://www.mayoclinic.org/diseases-conditions/hiv-aids/symptoms-causes/syc-20373524.

Meyer, A. (1977). The philosophy of occupational therapy. *The American Journal of Occupational Therapy, 31*(10), 639–642.

Pizzi, M., Reitz, S. M., & Scaffa, M. E. (2006). Wellness and health promotion for people with physical disabilities. In H. Pendleton, & W. Schultz-Krohn (Eds.), *Pedretti's occupational therapy for physical dysfunction.* St Louis, MO: Elsevier.

US Department of Health & Human Services. (2001). Centers for Disease Control and Prevention. First report of AIDS. *MMWR, 50*(21). Available from https://www.cdc.gov/mmwr/PDF/wk/mm5021.pdf.

Weinberg, J. L., & Kovarik, C. L. (2010). The WHO clinical staging system for HIV/AIDS. *American Medical Association Journal Ethics, 12*(3), 202–206.

RECOMMENDED READING

Bedell, G. (2000). Daily life for eight urban gay men with HIV/AIDS. *The American Journal of Occupational Therapy, 54,* 197–206.

Braveman, B. H. (2001). Development of a community-based return to work program for people with AIDS. *Occupational Therapy in Health Care, 13*(3/4), 113–131.

Galantino, M. L., & Pizzi, M. (1991). Occupational and physical therapy for persons with HIV disease and their caregivers. *Journal of Home Health Care Practice, 3*(3), 46–57.

Kielhofner, G., Braveman, B., Finlayson, M., Paul-Ward, A., Goldbaum, L., & Goldstein, K. (2004). Outcomes of a vocational program for persons with AIDS. *The American Journal of Occupational Therapy, 58*(1), 64–72.

Phillips, I. (2002). Occupational therapy students explore an area for future practice in HIV/AIDS community wellness. *AIDS Patient Care and STDS, 16,* 147–149.

Pizzi, M. (1989). Occupational therapy: creating possibilities for adults with HIV infection, ARC, and AIDS. *AIDS Patient Care, 3,* 18–23.

Pizzi, M. (1992). Women and AIDS. *The American Journal of Occupational Therapy, 46*(11), 1021–1026.

Pizzi, M. (1991). Adaptive human performance and HIV infection: considerations for therapists. In: M. L. Galantino, (Ed.), *Clinical assessment and interventions in HIV: Rehabilitation of a chronic illness.* Thorofare, NJ: Slack.

Pizzi, M. (1996). *HIV infection and AIDS: A professional's guide to wellness, health and productive living.* Silver Spring, MD: Positive Images and Wellness.

Pizzi, M. (Ed.), (1990). HIV/AIDS. *The American Journal of Occupational Therapy (Special Issue)*; 44(3).

Pizzi, M., et al. (1991). HIV infection and occupational therapy. In: J. Mukand (Ed.), *rehabilitation for patients with HIV disease.* New York, NY: McGraw-Hill.

Pizzi, M., & Hinds-Harris, M. (1990). Infants and children with HIV infection: Perspectives in occupational and physical therapy. In: M. Pizzi, & J. Johnson, (Eds.), *Productive living strategies for people with AIDS.* New York, NY: Haworth Press.

Schindler, V. (1988). Psychosocial occupational therapy intervention with AIDS patients. *The American Journal of Occupational Therapy, 42,* 507–512.

Solomon, G. F., Temoshok, L., O'Leary, A., & Zich, J. (1987). An intensive psychoimmunologic study of long surviving persons with AIDS. *Annals of the New York Academy of Sciences, 496,* 647–655.

Spence, D. W., Galantino, M. L., Mossberg, K. A., & Zimmerman, S. O. (1990). Progressive resistance exercise: effect on muscle function and anthropometry of a select AIDS population. *The Archives of Physical Medicine and Rehabilitation, 71,* 644–648.

RESOURCES

AIDS Education and Training Centers National Resource Center. http://www.aidsetc.org/aidsetc?page = home-00-00. Resources including PowerPoint slides, CDs, and educational handouts.

Centers for Disease Control and Prevention. http://www.cdc.gov/ hiv/default.htm. Provides most updated information about HIV/AIDS and programming for the disease, including prevention guides, brochures, and slides.

World Health Organization (WHO). http://www.who.int/hiv/en/. Provides updated information on HIV from an international perspective.

INDEX

Page numbers followed by *f* indicate figures; *b,* boxes; *t,* tables.